AF673374

Clinical Pharmacy and Pharmacotherapeutics

Second Edition

Clinical Pharmacy and Pharmacotherapeutics

Second Edition

Ravishankar. K.
M.Pharm, Ph.D.
Principal and Professor, Department of Pharmacology,
Aditya College of Pharmacy, Surampalem.

Kiranmayi. G. V. N
M.Pharm (Ph.D)
Associate Professor, Department of Pharmacology,
Aditya College of Pharmacy, Surampalem.

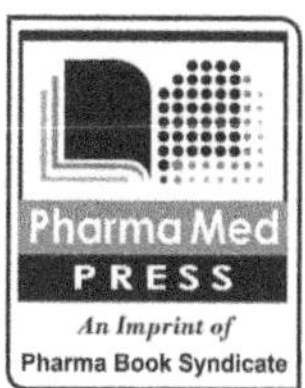

PharmaMed Press
An imprint of Pharma Book Syndicate

A unit of BSP Books Pvt. Ltd.

4-4-309/316, Giriraj Lane,
Sultan Bazar, Hyderabad - 500 095.

Clinical Pharmacy and Pharmacotherapeutics, ***Second Edition***
by Ravishankar K. and Kiranmayi G.V.N

Second Edition 2018
First Edition 2013

Published by

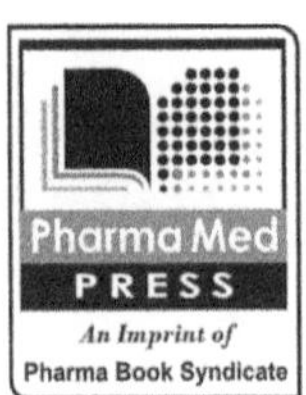

PharmaMed Press
An imprint of Pharma Book Syndicate

A unit of BSP Books Pvt. Ltd.

4-4-309/316, Giriraj Lane, Sultan Bazar, Hyderabad - 500 095.
Phone: 040-23445605, 23445688; Fax: 91+40-23445611
E-mail: info@pharmamedpress.com
www.pharmamedpress.com/pharmamedpress.net

ISBN: 978-93-86819-63-5 (Hardback)

Dedication

To our mentors, who inspired the journey of discovery, championed the passions, and exposed the frontiers.

To our colleagues, who enriched the path, multiplying the dimensions beyond imagination.

To our institutions, which nurtured the nascent trajectory and fostered the ultimate destination.

Preface

We have been gratified by the popularity of the first edition of **Clinical Pharmacy and Pharmacotherapeutics.** In the last four years, since the first edition of this book was published we have received suggestions from readers commenting on the book and suggesting how it could be improved. We have also built up a large file of ideas based on our own experiences in reading, writing, and editing and in examining and supervising theses. With the aid of all this information we have completely revised the book. The most obvious changes in this second edition are the new chapters.

In preparing this edition, we have incorporated hundreds of clarifications suggested by our own teaching experience and encouraging comments of colleagues. The second Edition of **Clinical Pharmacy and Pharmacotherapeutics** is a new book which covers many general and important topics. The colour style has increased the clarity of presentation and total information content.

This edition emphasizes several new themes which includes communication skills for clinical pharmacist, Medication History Interview, Evidence Based Medicine, Pharmaceutical Care Plan, Polypharmacy and Medication Errors, The Role of the Pharmacist in Disease Management, Case Presentation, Patient Counseling, Gastro Esophageal Reflux Disorder, Ascites, Dysphagia, Alcoholic Hepatitis, Hepatitis, Drug Induced Hepatotoxicity, Pancreatitis, Benign Prostate Hyperplasia, Diabetic Nephropathy, Urinary Stone Disease, Ischemic Heart Disease, Atrial Flutter, Hypertrophic Cardiomyopathy, Pulmonary Hypertension, Cystic Fibrosis, Hemoptysis, Alzheimer's Disease, Anxiety Disorders, Major Depressive Disease, Headache, Stroke, Obsessive Compulsive Disorder, GI Infections, Sexually Transmitted Diseases, Sepsis and Septic Shock, Cushing's Disease, Addisons Disease, Pheochromocytoma, Breast Cancer, Prostate Cancer, Colorectal Cancer, Diabetic Retinopathy, Acne Vulgaris, Drug Dependence and Drug Abuse and many new case studies pertaining to wide variety of diseases are discussed.

This sequence of new chapters builds new information on a foundation of information already assimilated. However, these new chapters can be used equally well in courses and curricula that present these topics in a different sequence. Within each chapter, emphasis is placed on discussion of drug groups and prototypes rather than offering repetitive detail about individual drugs.

Major features that make this book particularly useful in integrated curricula include different sections comprises of new important topics that specifically address the clinical choice and use of drugs in patients and the monitoring of their effects.

Significance of this book includes:

- Different Case Studies pertaining to wide variety of diseases are discussed; explicit answers and discussions are provided in the text of Part IV.
- Many important new chapters were added.
- A Drug Summary Table is placed in most of the chapters; these provide a concise recapitulation of the most important drugs.
- New illustrations with full color were provided with significant information which would help and clarify important concepts.
- Expanded coverage of new topics in Part I, II & III were highlighted.

We strongly believe that this book would satisfy the need of many students of B.Pharmacy, Pharm D and M. Pharmacy to the maximum extent. Many new and interesting topics are covered and the readers don't have to search for an alternative. We authors in confidence claim that the best we are providing for the benefit of all students.

- Authors

Acknowledgement

We are grateful to GOD for guiding us to conceptualise, develop and complete the book. Indeed, without His help and will, nothing is accomplished.

At the outsight we express our sincere pranams to the lotus feet of our esteemed Professor and Pharmacologist **Prof. Dr. D. Visweswaram** for giving us valuable education and what we are today is because of him.

We would like to extend our heartiest gratitude to **Mrs. R. K. Durga** , Jr. Assistant for extending her help in preparing this book.

We express our sincere thanks to our beloved Chairman, **Sri N. Sesha Reddy Garu**, Ex MLA, Anaparthy and Vice Chairman, **Sri. N. Satish Reddy Garu,** Aditya Group of Institutions, Surampalem for their encouragement.

We would like to convey our special thanks to our publishers - BSP Books Pvt. Ltd., for accepting and publishing our book and extending their whole hearted cooperation.

Our sincere thanks to all our well wishers who supported us.

- Authors

Contents

Preface (vii)

Acknowledgement (ix)

PART - I

GENERAL

CHAPTER 1

Introduction to Clinical Pharmacy 3

CHAPTER 2

Communication Skills for Clinical Pharmacists 13

CHAPTER 3

Medication History Interview 27

CHAPTER 4

Evidence-Based Medicine 33

CHAPTER 5

Pharmaceutical Care Plan 68

CHAPTER 6

Rational Drug Use 77

CHAPTER 7

Polypharmacy and Medication Errors 82

CHAPTER 8

Drug Interactions 91

CHAPTER 9

Adverse Drug Reactions (ADR) 118

CHAPTER 10

The Role of the Pharmacist in Disease Management 126

CHAPTER 11

Case Presentation 137

CHAPTER 12

Patient Counseling 144

CHAPTER 13

Parenteral Nutrition 162

CHAPTER 14

Pharmacovigilance 170

CHAPTER 15

Essential Drugs 184

CHAPTER 16

Therapeutic Drug Monitoring 190

PART - II

LIFE STAGES

CHAPTER 17

Posology 201

CHAPTER 18

Drug therapy in Neonates and Paediatrics 206

CHAPTER 19

Drug Therapy in Geriatric Patients 213

CHAPTER 20

Dose and Dosage Schedule of Digoxin 216

CHAPTER 21

Drug Dosing Adjustments in Patients with Renal Failure 221

PART - III

PHARMACOTHERAPEUTICS

GASTRO INTESTINAL DISORDERS

CHAPTER 22

Peptic Ulcer Disease 229

CHAPTER 23

Inflammatory Bowel Disease 240

CHAPTER 24

Diarrhea 251

CHAPTER 25

Constipation 259

CHAPTER 26

Nausea and Vomiting 266

CHAPTER 27

Gastro Esophageal Reflux Disorder 272

CHAPTER 28

Ascites 281

CHAPTER 29

Dysphagia 289

HEPATIC DISORDERS

CHAPTER 30

Liver Disease 294

CHAPTER 31

Alcoholic Hepatitis 302

CHAPTER 32

Hepatitis 310

CHAPTER 33

Drug Induced Hepatotoxicity 318

CHAPTER 34

Pancreatitis 348

RENAL DISORDERS

CHAPTER 35

Acute Renal Failure 356

CHAPTER 36

Chronic Kidney Disease 361

CHAPTER 37

Benign Prostatic Hyperplasia (BPH) 366

CHAPTER 38
Diabetic Nephropathy 371

CHAPTER 39
Urinary Stone Disease 383

CARDIOVASCULAR DISORDERS

CHAPTER 40
Hypertension 389

CHAPTER 41
Heart Failure 399

CHAPTER 42
Arrhythmia 409

CHAPTER 43
Dyslipidemia 417

CHAPTER 44
Coronary Artery Disease 425

CHAPTER 45
Ischaemic Heart Disease 430

CHAPTER 46
Atrial Flutter 436

CHAPTER 47
Hypertrophic Cardiomyopathy 443

RESPIRATORY DISORDERS

CHAPTER 48
Asthma 447

CHAPTER 49
Chronic Obstructive Pulmonary Disease 458

CHAPTER 50
Pulmonary Hypertension 466

CHAPTER 51
Cystic Fibrosis 475

CHAPTER 52
Hemoptysis 482

NEUROLOGICAL AND PSYCHOLOGICAL DISORDERS

CHAPTER 53
Insomnia and Anxiety 487

CHAPTER 54
Schizophrenia 497

CHAPTER 55
Epilepsy 503

CHAPTER 56
Parkinson's Disease 514

CHAPTER 57
Pain 520

CHAPTER 58
Alzheimer's Disease (AD) 528

CHAPTER 59
Anxiety Disorders 536

CHAPTER 60

Major Depressive Disease 551

CHAPTER 61

Headache 567

CHAPTER 62

Stroke 588

CHAPTER 63

Obsessive Compulsive Disorder 596

INFECTIONS

CHAPTER 64

Respiratory Tract Infections 606

CHAPTER 65

Urinary Tract Infections 622

CHAPTER 66

Infective Meningitis 631

CHAPTER 67

Tuberculosis 634

CHAPTER 68

HIV Infection 643

CHAPTER 69

GI Infection 651

CHAPTER 70

Sexually Transmitted Diseases 660

CHAPTER 71

Sepsis and Septic Shock 674

PROTOZOAL INFECTIONS

CHAPTER 72

Malaria 684

CHAPTER 73

Filaria 693

ENDOCRINE DISORDERS

CHAPTER 74

Thyroid Disorders 699

CHAPTER 75

Parathyroid Disorders 710

CHAPTER 76

Diabetes Mellitus 715

CHAPTER 77

Cushing's Syndrome 733

CHAPTER 78

Addisons Disease 747

CHAPTER 79

Pheochromocytoma 774

OBSTETRICS AND GYNECOLOGICAL DISORDERS

CHAPTER 80

Menstrual Cycle Disorders 790

CHAPTER 81
Menopause 808

CHAPTER 82
Drug Therapy in Pregnancy 812

CHAPTER 83
Drug Therapy in Lactation 824

MALIGNANT DISORDERS

CHAPTER 84
Leukemia 829

CHAPTER 85
Lymphoma 836

CHAPTER 86
Breast Cancer 842

CHAPTER 87
Prostate Cancer 852

CHAPTER 88
Colorectal Cancer 862

RHEUMATIC DISORDERS

CHAPTER 89
Rheumatoid Arthritis 888

CHAPTER 90
Osteoarthritis 898

CHAPTER 91
Gout and Hyperuricemia 906

EYE DISORDERS

CHAPTER 92
Glaucoma 912

CHAPTER 93
Diabetic Retinopathy 918

SKIN DISORDERS

CHAPTER 94
Psoriasis 934

CHAPTER 95
Skin Disorders and Cutaneous Drug Reactions 944

CHAPTER 96
Acne Vulgaris 949

MISCELLANEOUS

CHAPTER 97
Male Sexual Dysfunction 957

CHAPTER 98
Drug Dependence and Drug Abuse 961

CHAPTER 99
Nutraceuticals 978

CHAPTER 100
Pharmacoeconomics 985

CHAPTER 101
Pharmacogenomics 991

PART - IV
CASE STUDIES

CHAPTER 102

Cardiovascular Case Studies 1001

CHAPTER 103

Respiratory Case Studies 1008

CHAPTER 104

Central Nervous System Case Studies 1011

CHAPTER 105

Gastro Intestinal Case Studies 1014

CHAPTER 106

Infection Case Studies 1017

CHAPTER 107

Endocrine Case Studies 1021

CHAPTER 108

Malignant Case Studies 1023

CHAPTER 109

Skin Case Studies 1025

CHAPTER 110

Liver Case Studies 1029

CHAPTER 111

Miscellaneous Case Studies 1031

PART - V
PROBLEMS

CHAPTER 112

Problems based on Paediatric Dose Calculations 1037

CHAPTER 113

Problems based on Clearance 1043

CHAPTER 114

Problems based on Absorption Half Life 1045

CHAPTER 115

Problems based on Elimination Half life 1049

CHAPTER 116

Problems based on Area Under Curve (AUC) 1053

CHAPTER 117

Problems based on Wagner Nelson Method 1055

CHAPTER 118

Problems based on One Compartment Oral Absorption 1059

CHAPTER 119

Problems based on Two Compartment Model IV Bolus 1062

CHAPTER 120

Problems based on Non Compartmental Analysis 1066

APPENDIX - I

General Medical Abbreviations 1067

APPENDIX - II

Glossary of Medical Terms 1084

APPENDIX - III

Drug Induced Disorders 1098

COLOUR PLATES 1103

INDEX 1119

PART - I GENERAL

1 Introduction to Clinical Pharmacy
2 Communication Skills for Clinical Pharmacists
3 Medication History Interview
4 Evidence Based Medicine
5 Pharmaceutical Care Plan
6 Rational Drug Use
7 Polypharmacy and Medication Errors
8 Drug Interactions
9 Adverse Drug Reactions (ADR)
10 The Role of the Pharmacist in Disease Management
11 Case Presentation
12 Patient Counseling
13 Parenteral Nutrition
14 Pharmacovigilance
15 Essential Drugs
16 Therapeutic Drug Monitoring

CHAPTER 1

Introduction to Clinical Pharmacy

Clinical pharmacy is the branch of Pharmacy where pharmacists provide patient care that optimizes the use of medication and promotes health, wellness, and disease prevention. Clinical pharmacists care for patients in all health care settings but the clinical pharmacy movement initially began inside hospitals and clinics. Fig. 1.1 indicates the role of clinical pharmacy in patient care.

CLINICAL PHARMACIST

Clinical pharmacist is the expert in therapeutic use of medication therapy, evaluation and recommendation of drugs to the patient and other health care professionals. The term clinical pharmacy is being used to describe the new growth of pharmacists. It comprises of functions necessary to discharge a particular set of social responsibilities related to therapeutic drug use in the following major categories.

1. Dispensing and administering drugs
2. Documenting professional services
3. Direct patient involvement
4. Reviewing drug use
5. Education
6. Consolation

AIM OF CLINICAL PHARMACY

The aim of clinical pharmacy is to ensure the patient's maximum well being and to play a meaningful role in the safe and rational use of drugs.

The main roles of clinical pharmacy are:

1. To assist the physician in doing a better job of prescribing and monitoring drug therapy for the patient.
2. To assist medical and paramedical staff and documenting medication indications correctly.
3. To maximize the patients' compliance in drug use process.

SCOPE OF CLINICAL PHARMACY

Clinical pharmacy services are of considerable importance in all the hospitals because; Clinical Pharmacy can serve as a guide to the physician for the safe and rational use of drugs. A clinical pharmacist can help to achieve economic hospital by planning safe drug policies, for suggesting means of reductions of waste, by preventing misuse of drugs and in the preparation of budget by forecasting future means of hospital based upon their drug utilization process.

The scope of clinical pharmacy is of utmost appreciation in the following areas:

1. Drug information
2. Drug utilization
3. Drug distribution
4. Drug selection

5. Drug evaluation
6. Pharmacy education and teaching
7. Rationalization and Optimization of drug therapy
8. Monitoring of drug therapy
9. Evaluation of desired outcomes
10. Assessment of therapeutic endpoints
11. Reduction of Medication Related Problems through Pharmaceutical Interventions
12. Monitoring plans.

QUALITIES OF CLINICAL PHARMACIST

The clinical pharmacist should have the following qualities.

1. Good communication skills
2. Clinical skills
3. Professional relationship
4. Empathy
5. Monitoring drug therapy

ROLE OF CLINICAL PHARMACIST IN HEALTH CARE TEAM

The Clinical Pharmacist has the following roles.

1. Taking medication history of the patient
2. Drug interactions
3. Selection of drug therapy
4. Drug monitoring
5. Adverse drug reactions
6. Management of drug policies
7. Research and development programme
8. Drug information

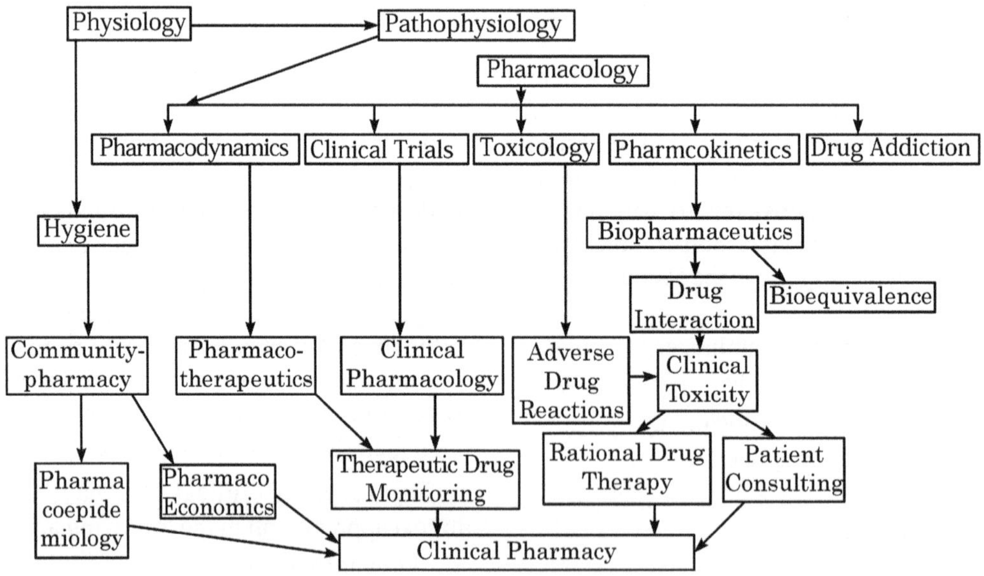

FIGURE 1.1

Role of clinical pharmacy in patient care.

DUTIES OF CLINICAL PHARMACIST

The daily routine duties of Clinical Pharmacist are,

1. Assisting pharmacokinetic consultations with necessary follow up.
2. Monitoring drug therapy schedule.
3. Taking rounds with health care team
4. Teaching pharmacy students
5. Patient counseling
6. Review of hospital forbid art
7. Preparation of drug monograph to be reviewed by pharmacy and the therapeutic community of hospital.
8. To serve as a systemic guideline for the documentation of clinical pharmacy activities (PWDT)

In this manner, clinical pharmacy is totally patient oriented and deals with rationale of drug therapy.

CLINICAL PHARMACOKINETICS

Clinical Pharmacokinetics is the science of the rate of movement of drugs within biological systems, as affected by the absorption, distribution, metabolism, and elimination of medications.

It involves,

- Study of the time course of a drug's movement through the body.
- Understanding of what the body does to (or with) the drug.
- Application of Therapeutic Drug Monitoring (TDM) and individualization of drug therapy

Pharmacokinetics (PK) - What the body does to the drug

- Absorption; distribution, metabolism, excretion (ADME)

  Pharmacodynamics (PD) - What the drug does to the body
- Drug concentration at the site of action or in the plasma is related to a magnitude of effect

Pharmacokinetic processes depend on two fundamental kinetic processes-zero order kinetics and first order kinetics.

Zero order kinetics: Zero order kinetics is where the plasma concentration of a drug decreases at a constant rate. A graph of this will show a linear relationship between time from peak concentration and plasma concentration (Fig. 1.2).

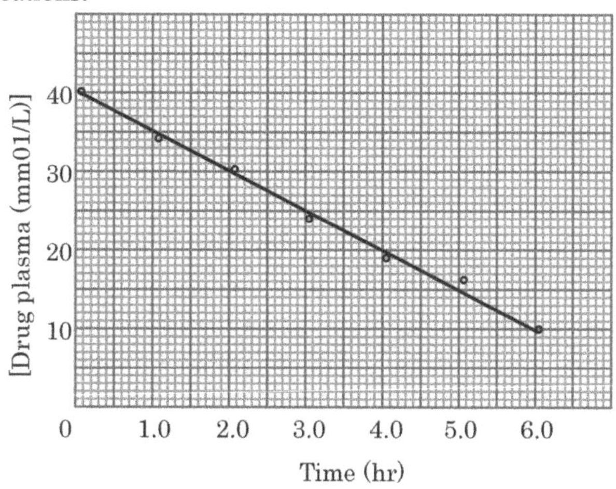

FIGURE 1.2

Zero order kinetics.

Examples of zero-order processes

1. The entry of drug into the circulation during intravenous infusion.
2. The absorption of many depot forms of administration e.g., Fluphenazine decanoate in oil (used in schizophrenia).

First-Order Reaction

A first-order reaction depends on the concentration of only one reactant (a unimolecular reaction). Other reactants can be present, but each will be zero-order (Fig. 1.3).

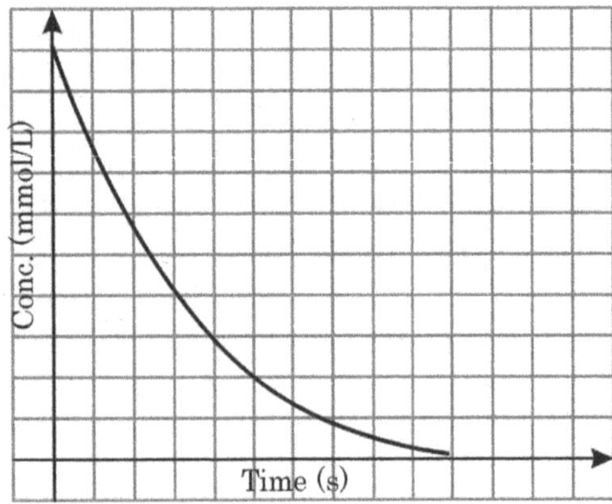

FIGURE 1.3

First order kinetics.

PHARMACOKINETIC PROCESSES

ABSORPTION

- Must be able to get medications into the patient's body
- Drug characteristics that affect absorption:
  - Molecular weight, ionization, solubility, and formulation
- Factors affecting drug absorption related to patients:
  - Route of administration, gastric pH, contents of GI tract

ABSORPTION IN THE PEDIATRIC PATIENT

- Gastrointestinal pH changes
- Gastric emptying
- Gastric enzymes
- Bile acids and biliary function
- Gastrointestinal flora
- Formula/food interaction

DISTRIBUTION

- Membrane permeability
  - cross membranes to site of action
- Plasma protein binding
  - bound drugs do not cross membranes
  - malnutrition = ↓ albumin = ↑ free drug
- Lipophilicity of drug
  - lipophilic drugs accumulate in adipose tissue
- Volume of distribution

PEDIATRIC DISTRIBUTION

- Body Composition
  - ↑ total body water and extracellular fluid
  - ↓ adipose tissue and skeletal muscle
- Protein Binding
  - albumin, bilirubin, α_1-acid glycoprotein
- Tissue Binding
  - compositional changes

METABOLISM

- Drugs and toxins are seen as foreign to patients bodies
- Drugs can undergo metabolism in the lungs, blood, and liver
- Body works to convert drugs to less active forms and increase water solubility to enhance elimination

- Liver - primary route of drug metabolism
- Liver may be used to convert pro-drugs (inactive) to an active state

TYPES OF REACTIONS

- Phase I (Cytochrome P450 system)
- Phase II

PHASE I REACTIONS

- Cytochrome P450 system
- Located within the endoplasmic reticulum of hepatocytes
- Through electron transport chain, a drug bound to the CYP450 system undergoes oxidation or reduction
- Enzyme induction
- Drug interactions

PHASE I REACTIONS TYPES

- Hydrolysis
- Oxidation
- Reduction
- Demethylation
- Methylation
- Alcohol dehydrogenase metabolism

PHASE II REACTIONS

- Polar group is conjugated to the drug
- Results in increased polarity of the drug
- Types of reactions
  - Glycine conjugation
  - Glucuronide conjugation
  - Sulphate conjugation

ELIMINATION

- Pulmonary: expired in the air
- Bile: excreted in feces
  - enterohepatic circulation
- Renal
  - glomerular filtration
  - tubular reabsorption
  - tubular secretion

PEDIATRIC ELIMINATION

- Glomerular filtration matures in relation to age, adult values reached by 3 years of age
- **Neonate:** decreased renal blood flow, glomerular filtration, and tubular function yields prolonged elimination of medications
- Aminoglycosides, Cephalosporins, penicillin's : longer dosing interval

BASIC CLINICAL PHARMACOKINETIC PARAMETERS

The three basic pharmacokinetic parameters of first order elimination are:

(i) Volume of Distribution (V_d)
(ii) Clearance (Cl)
(iii) Half Life ($t_{1/2}$)

Above parameters have specific well defined utility.

(i) ***Volume of Distribution (V_d):*** Apparent volume of distribution is the volume of serum plasma or blood that is occupied by the drug in the body

V_d is a proportionality constant that equates the serum drug concentration (SDC) to the total amount of drug in the body. V_d has no physiological basis and thus it does not relate to volume of serum, blood or total body water.

$$V_d = \frac{\text{Dose}}{\text{Serum Drug Concentration}}$$

Since elimination of drug occurs from the moment of drug input the equation more commonly used is;

$$V_d = \frac{\text{Clearance}}{\text{Elimination rate constant}}$$

It helps to:

(i) Determine a loading dose of a drug.

(ii) Determine amount of drug in the body.

(iii) Make qualitative assessment of distribution of drug in the body.

(ii) *Clearance (Cl):* Cl is a descriptive term used to evaluate the efficiency of drug removal from body. Drugs are cleared primarily by kidneys (Clr) and liver (Clh). Clearance can be expressed as an estimate of efficiency flow, a sum or a ratio.

Cl = Clh + Clr + Clearance of other eliminating organs.

Clearance is a proportionality constant that relates the rate of drug elimination to the SDC. It is a flow rate measured in units of volume per time (i.e. milliliters per minute. Cl helps to determine the steady state concentration that will be achieved from a specific maintenance dosage.

Elimination of drug from body follows two patterns:

(i) *First order elimination* (Linear or concentration independent): Here the rate of elimination is directly proportional to the concentration of drug in serum i.e. as serum drug concentration rises the drug is eliminated at a faster rate.

(ii) *Michaelis – Menten elimina-tion* (non-linear or concentration dependent): Here the rate of elimination does not change in proportion to changes in serum concentration i.e., as serum drug concentration rises, rate of elimination increases less than proportionately e.g. phenytoin. For such drugs careful monitoring of drug levels is essential.

If the Cl of a drug is known, then the rate of drug elimination can be calculated by multiplying the Cl by the SDC (assuming first order drug elimination).

(iii) ***Half Life ($t_{1/2}$):*** Half life is the time required for the serum drug concentration to get decreased to one half, irrespective of the starting concentration. This is illustrated in Fig.1.4. Each down stroke represents a halving of the plasma concentration and each across stroke is the time taken for that halving to occur i.e., the half – life.

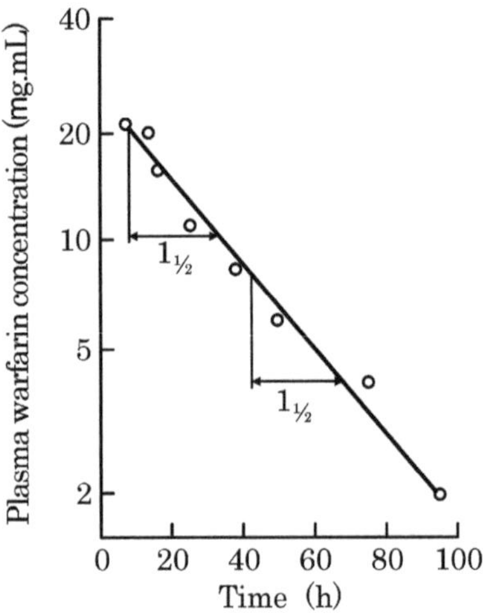

FIGURE 1.4

The principle of half-life ($t_{1/2}$). When plasma concentration versus time data are linear in a semi-logarithmic plot, the time it takes for the plasma concentration to fall from any value to half that value is a constant, the half-life.

The following are the uses of half-life:

(i) *As a guide to the time it takes for a drug to be eliminated from the body:* For most drugs, the half-life measured in plasma or serum, is directly related to the half life of the drug in the tissues. However, some drugs have short half-lifes in the plasma but are stored in the tissue, from which they are released slowly; this is true of the vitamin A analogues.

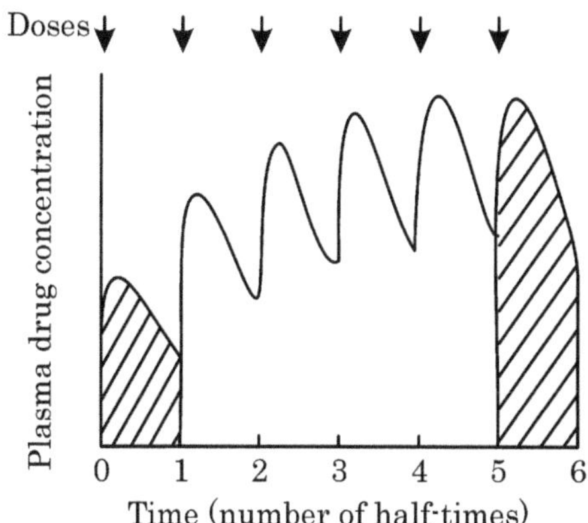

FIGURE 1.5

The theoretical plasma concentrations of a drug over a period of time during its repeated oral administration.

(ii) *As a guide to the rate of accumulation of drug in the body during multiple dosing (Fig 1.5):* It is only variable that determines the rate of which drug accumulates in the body during regular multiple dosing. For example, if we consider the regular oral administration of a drug that is rapidly absorbed. After the first dose, the concentration of drug in plasma rises sharply as the drug is absorbed, it reaches a peak and then starts to fall, as the drug is distributed around the body and eliminated. After the second dose, the rise in concentration to the next peak is the same as after the first dose, but because the new peak is higher than the first, the rate of fall is faster (first-order kinetics). After each successive dose, the increase in the plasma concentration is same but, because the peak is always higher, the size of the fall after peak becomes progressively larger with successive doses. Eventually the size of the fall in plasma concentration after the peak is as great as the size of the preceding rise and a steady state is reached. At steady state, the amount of drug eliminated from the body in a single dose interval is the same as the amount that enters it.

Strictly speaking this is not a true steady for two reasons:

(i) Because plasma concentrations are fluctuating all the time.
(ii) Even the mean of those concentrations does not reach a true steady value until infinite time.

However, for practical purpose, a steady state is said to have occurred after four to five half-lifes, when 94-97% the eventual steady state value will have been reached.

No. of half-life	B % accumulated	Total
1	50	50%
2	50 + 25	75%
3	50 + 25 + 12.5	87.5%
4	50 + 25 + 12.5 + 6.25	93.75%
5	50 + 25 + 12.5 + 6.25 + 3.125	96.9%

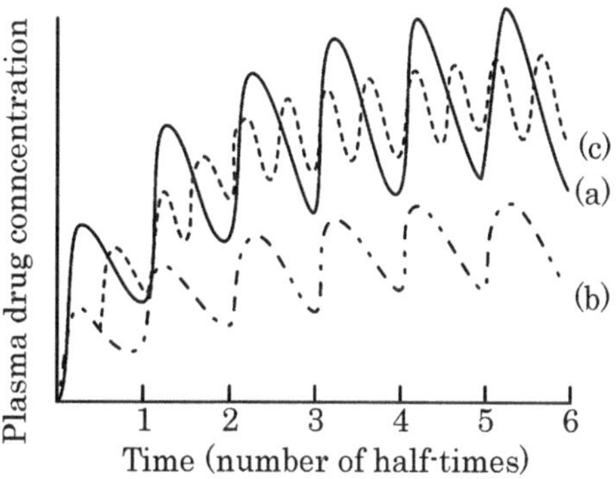

FIGURE 1.6

The effects of varying the dose and frequency of administration on the time taken to reach steady state and the eventual steady-state plasma concentration.

This means that the time taken to reach steady state depends only on half-life of the drug, and neither on the size of the dose nor frequency of administration (Fig. 1.6)

(iii) *As a guide to the relationship between the loading dose and maintenance dose:* When a drug has a longer half life than 24 hours (e.g. digoxin 40 hours; Digitoxin 7 days) it takes several days or weeks (4 – 5 half lifes) of regular administration of the same daily dose before the steady state plasma concentration are reached. Such a delay may be unacceptable. So if a loading dose can be given followed by administration of a regular maintenance dose to maintain the steady state (Fig. 1.7).

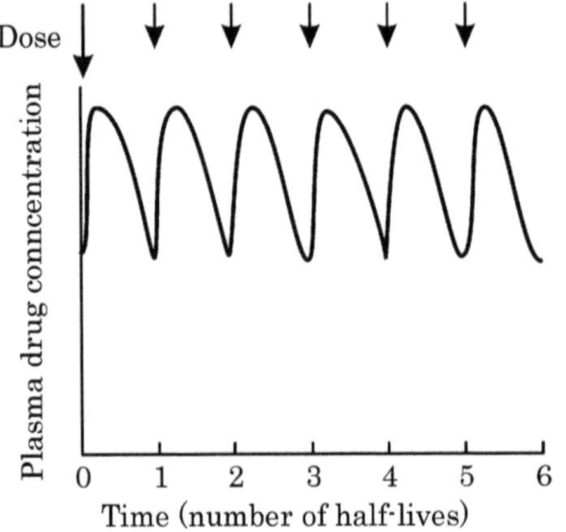

Figure 1.7

The effect of an initial loading dose. If the correct loading dose is given, a steady state can be achieved rapidly and then maintained by giving a smaller maintenance dose.

Even when the half life of a drug is short, it is sometimes desirable to give a loading dose if a very rapid effect is required e.g. Lidocaine in the treatment of cardiac arrhythmias.

Relationship between half-life ($t_{½}$), Clearance (Cl), volume (V) and Steady State Concentration (C_{ss})

1. Cl and V are independent pharmacokinetic parameters not influencing each other and whose values determine the elimination rate constant (or half life) of drug from the serum and the C_{ss} achieved after maintenance dosing.
2. Half life is a dependent function whose value depends on Cl (inversely proportional) and V (directly proportional).
3. Cl can be considered as representing the sum of all drug elimination process in the body and V represents the distribution of drug and is influenced by the pharmacodynamic characteristics of the clearing agent.
4. The C_{ss} achieved after constant Iv infusion (e.g. Lidocaine theo-phylline) or mean C_{ss} achieved after multiple oral dosage depends on Cl only, it is not influenced by V.

METHODOLOGY FOR CLINICAL PHARMACOKINETIC STUDY

1. Scheme of Administration: Both single dose and multiple dose studies should be performed within the recommended dose range and dose intervals.

Multiple dose studies should be whenever possible continued long enough to establish steady state concentrations of the drug and for such steady state levels, their dose-dependence and variability should be determined. Accumulation kinetics of drug predicted from the kinetic constants obtained from single dose studies should be verified experimentally; different dosage should be included in one study to determine dose dependence and to decide whether changes from linearity to non linearity occur at dosage levels which are normally used. After discontinuation of a prolonged treatment, the possibility of very slow terminal decrease in plasma concentrations, which can reflect the existence of a deep compartment, should be investi-gated. This might explain the discrepancy between the long action of the substance and the apparent short elimination half life as measured after a single dose administration.

2. Subject Selection

(a) *Initial studies*: Initial studies are generally performed in a restricted number of fasting healthy adult volunteers in well defined controlled conditions. When the substance carries too serious a risk to healthy volunteers (e.g. anti-cancer drugs, they are conducted in patients suffering from diseases for which the drug is considered to be indicated.

(b) *Further studies:* Further studies should be conducted in patients suffering from diseases for which the drug is claimed to be indicated. The relation between dose, plasma concen-tration and therapeutic effects, where this is feasible should be studied. Particularly, it should be established that the pharma-cokinetic behavior of the drug in patients corresponds to that in healthy subjects. The full range of kinetic studies need only be repeated in patients if studies indicate that the pharmacokinetics in this group differ from those in healthy volunteers.

(c) *Influence of various patho-physiological states:* It is very useful to know the kinetics of drugs in a very large number of pathophysiological situations; however, it is clear that this knowledge requires multiple, long and expensive studies which cannot all be performed before licensing.

Therefore, the only studies which should be reasonably submitted before marketing are those which seem to be necessary in regard to the properties, indications, contra-indications, routes of elimination, scheme of administration of the drug and those which are required to define the necessary dosage changes which cannot be calculated from the pharma-cokinetic parameters available from volunteers under standar-dized conditions and in patients without functional disturbances of the systems of absorption, distribution or elimination.

In so far as the indications render this relevant, kinetics should be studied in patients at extreme of age 9 infants, children and elderly). For drugs intended to be orally administered, it is important to study the effects of food on absorption. Other factors like body weight, time of day, environment factors, genetic differences, alcohol, smoking habits, concomitant medication, sex, may influence the results and the interpretation of later clinical studies. Then the kinetic studies should be extended accordingly.

3. Sampling and Analysis of Drug Concentration: The number of blood samples should be large enough and the timing appropriate to allow a adequate determination of the absorption and/or distribution and elimination phases. Plasma concentrations in the post absorption phase should possibly, be determined at above two or three half lifes to avoid confusion between distribution and elimination half lifes. If there is an evidence for a very long terminal half life, plasma concentration should be followed for a much longer time. If urinary data are obtained, the urine should be collected until there is no further detectable excretion of parent drug or metabolites within the limits of the method used. The stability of the substance during sampling and storage requires careful attention.

The samples are then analyzed by various methods like spectro-photometry, HPLC etc.

Specificity, accuracy (as regards recovery) and precision (sensitivity and reproducibility) of the methods should be mentioned. Both for technical reasons and safety cold analytical methods are often to be preferred to tracer radioactive techniques. If radioactive isotopes are used, the tracer dose should always be combined with a quantity of non labeled drug within the therapeutic dose range. However, in most cases it is necessary to develop suitable cold analytical methods to separate and assay quantitatively the metabolites and / or the parent compound. The mathematical methods are then used (graphical representation, computer analysis, pharmacokinetic formulas) to get various pharmacokinetic parameters. Proper statistical analysis of the data obtained should be made and the inter and intra individual variations estimated in at least some of the studies whether the number of subjects is large enough.

REFERENCES

1. Holford NHG, Sheiner LB. Understanding the dose–effect relationship: clinical application of pharmacokinetic–pharmacodynamic models. Clin Pharmacokinet 1981: 6: 429-453.
2. Duffull SB, Robinson BA. Clinical pharmacokinetics and dose optimisation of carboplatin. Clin Pharmacokinet 1997: 33: 161-183.
3. Winter ME. Aminoglycosides. In Basic Clinical Pharmacokinetics, Applied Therapeutics Inc, Vancouver,1994: 128.
4. Holford NHG. A size standard for pharmacokinetics. Clin Pharmacokinet 1996: 30: 329-332.
5. Lin JH, Lu AYH. Inhibition and induction of cytochrome P450 and the clinical implications. Clin Pharma-cokinet 1998: 35: 361-390.
6. Clinical Pharmacy Defined (Pharmacotherapy 2008; 28(6): 816-817).

CHAPTER 2

Communication Skills for Clinical Pharmacists

INTRODUCTION

Communication in the context of pharmacy practice is concerned primarily with health and illness. The concept of *'health'* can be viewed in six different dimensions (Table 2.1).

Table 2.1

Six dimensions of health

1. *Physical health:* concerned solely with the mechanistic function of the body.
2. *Mental health:* the individual's ability to think clearly and rationally.
3. *Emotional health:* the ability to understand, express and deal with emotions and respond appropriately to the emotional state of others.
4. *Social health:* the ability to successfully develop, maintain and terminate relationships.
5. *Spiritual health:* religious, moral and ethical beliefs, which may lead to peace of mind.
6. *Societal health:* the wider community, including such issues as inequality, poverty, prejudice, crime and un-employment.

The relational dimension of care has grown in importance in recent years, with a remarkable change in the nature of practitioner-patient relationships. From a professional practice standpoint, it has instilled a greater consciousness of service quality, whilst from a consumer perspective, it articulated standards whereby services could be judged for overall quality and satisfaction. One effect of this has been to raise the expectations of patients about what they are entitled to as consumers of health care services. The production and display of a practice leaflet in each community pharmacy, detailing the pharmaceutical services available, is but one example of this consumer-oriented approach.

THE NEED FOR GOOD COMMUNICATION

Interpersonal communication is a two-way, transactional, process. The interactive style is to a large extent shaped, and even determined, by the other person. For instance, a pharmacist who is dealing with a happy, young mother showing off her newborn infant will behave very differently compared to when dealing with a recently bereaved 80 year old widow. Pharmacists must be cognisant of the goals, nature and expectations of each individual patient. In their study of information-giving in community pharmacies there were two groups of patients active and passive. Active patients received almost twice as much information as passive ones, although in a follow-up one day after their visit, it was found that both groups had forgotten two-thirds of the information they had been given. Interestingly, those patients who complain most about the amount of information or explanation they have been given may paradoxically be better informed than those who do not complain. The results of this research at the practitioner-patient interface under the headings are summarised in Table 2.2 and discussed below.

Table 2.2

Key issues of practitioner-patient interaction
1. Patients often do not clearly understand, or forget the information they are given
2. Patients are not satisfied with the advice and information they are given
3. Lack of patient-practitioner concordance
4. Patient satisfaction and concordance are related
5. Inattentiveness to the patient's psychosocial needs

The main findings here are:

- The more information given the more is forgotten. In general patients forget approximately half the information they are given by practitioners
- Patients remember best what they hear first, as well as what they consider to be most important
- Patients often have minimal biological knowledge, such as the location of vital organs
- Patients with a higher level of medical knowledge recall more of what they are told
- A patient's age is not necessarily an indicator of retentive ability
- Patients who are highly anxious at one extreme, or not at all anxious at the other, remember less than those with a moderate level of anxiety
- Many patients, even if they do not understand, do not like to ask questions
- Complicated oral or written instructions compromise understanding

Patients are often dissatisfied with the advice and information they are given

Dissatisfaction with advice is usually linked to the following factors:

- Poor practitioner rapport-building skills, e.g. poor level of eye contact, little empathy, and lack of encouragement
- Patients not receiving the amount of information they require
- Limited time available for the consultation
- Lack of specificity and precision in the information given
- The way in which information is provided
- Being unable to access the right person to deal with their problem

LACK OF PATIENT-PRACTITIONER CONCORDANCE

In all practitioner-patient exchanges there is an imbalance, or asymmetry in the perspectives and roles of the individuals concerned. For example, the practitioner has the knowledge base and the status that the patient does not usually have, while the latter has the condition that the former does not have. This can lead to discordance in the relationship. The concept of concordance has been advocated to empower patients to meet their specific needs. Concordance is based on the notion that the consultation is a negotiation between practitioner and patient acting as equals, with the aim of achieving a therapeutic alliance. The importance of achieving this alliance is underscored by the research literature, which abounds with evidence of therapeutic failure.

PATIENT SATISFACTION AND CONCORDANCE ARE RELATED

Lack of adherence with clinical advice has been shown to be directly related to the following factors:

Inattentiveness to patients' psychosocial needs

Research demonstrates reluctance by practitioners to discuss the psychosocial dimensions of a patient's wellbeing. Patients react negatively to this, particularly as they deem their emotional needs to be as important, if not more important, than their physical needs. Dissatisfaction is, therefore, often attributed to: empathy, and lack of encouragement

- Patients not receiving the amount of information they require
- Limited time available for the consultation
- Lack of specificity and precision in the information given
- The way in which information is provided
- Being unable to access the right person to deal with their problem
- Level of satisfaction with the consultation
- The persuasiveness and credibility of the practitioner and of the information provided
- Patients' perceptions of the severity of their condition and their vulnerability to it
- The duration and complexity of the treatment regime
- Treatment effectiveness
- Patients' expectations, outlook and attitude
- Influence of family and friends
- The level of supervision provided

Inattentiveness to patients' psychosocial needs

- Overly directive practitioners.
- Practitioner insensitivity to the patient's feelings, concerns and opinions.
- A concentration purely on the patient's medical condition to the exclusion of accompanying worries—listening only to facts and ignoring feelings.
- Failure to tune in to the patient's nonverbal cues which signal other needs.
- Lack of support to manage a condition where coping rather than a cure is the only realistic option.

Given all of the above issues, the necessity for the pharmacist to become a skilled communicator is apparent. The key benefits which will ensue are shown in Table 2.3.

Table 2.3

Consequences of the pharmacist as a skilled communicator
• Patient outcomes get improved. • Patient satisfaction with services gets improved. • More patient-friendly pharmacy practice. • Reduction in patient anxiety. • Increased pharmacist status. • Enhanced pharmacist satisfaction and self-esteem. • Decrease in complaints and litigation.

By contrast when pharmacists' communication is ineffective the consequences are equal and opposite of the above. The likely outcomes are shown in Table 2.4.

Table 2.4

Consequences of the pharmacist as an unskilled communicator
• Reduced adherence to therapeutic regimes. • Decreased satisfaction with the content and process of the communication. • Insensitivity to the needs of customers. • Increased worry and concern amongst patients. • Decreased pharmacist status. • Job dissatisfaction. • Loss of business and reduced client base. • Increases in formal complaints and legal action.

KEY COMMUNICATION SKILLS

A study of communication among pharmacists identified eleven key skill areas, together with relevant sub-skills, through analysis of video recordings of actual practice. These are presented in Table 2.5 in rank order of perceived importance. Knowledge and application of these skills are fundamental to effective practice and they are summarized below.

Table 2.5

Rank order of effective communication skills and sub-skills

1. Building rapport
   - i. Preserving confidentiality
   - ii. Being helpful
   - iii. Being available/accessible
   - iv. Showing genuine concern
   - v. Offering reassurance
   - vi. Politeness in manner
   - vii. Showing interest in the patient
   - viii. Showing warmth
   - ix. Engaging
   - x. Showing pleasure
   - xi. Accommodating patient's needs
   - xii. Use of humor
   - xiii. Greeting by name
2. Explaining
   - i. Reasoned instructions
   - ii. Explaining for reassurance
   - iii. Informing
   - iv. Repetition
   - v. Reinforcing/emphasizing
   - vi. Directing
3. Questioning
   - i. Other medication taken
   - ii. Symptoms-related
   - iii. Exploring situation
   - iv. Patient details
   - v. Showing interest
4. Listening
   - i. Showing sympathy/empathy
   - ii. Encouraging patient to provide information
   - iii. Showing interest (beyond the problem)
5. Nonverbal communication
   - i. Eye contact
   - ii. Tone of voice
   - iii. Examining patient
   - iv. Proximity
   - v. Positioning
   - vi. Using hand gestures
   - vii. Smiling and nodding
   - viii. Standing still
   - ix. Touch
   - x. Illustration/demonstration
6. Suggesting/Advising
7. Opening
   - i. Identifying patient by name (prescription check)
   - ii. Greeting, general
   - iii. Greeting by name
8. Closing
   - i. Polite closing
   - ii. Thanking patient
   - iii. Initiating ending of interaction
9. Assertiveness
   - i. Pharmacist politely standing ground
   - ii. Enhancing credibility by referring to view of other health professionals
10. Disclosing personal information
11. Persuading
12. Communication and Disability

Table 2.5 *Contd...*

BUILDING RAPPORT

There are two motivations for pharmacists to maintain rapport with patients. Firstly, to present themselves as health care practitioners and secondly, the development and preservation of patient loyalty, necessary to sustain business success. Building rapport was the skill most frequently employed by community pharmacists, indicating that the relationship element of practice was particularly important. In addition, patients were more influenced by, and followed the advice of, practitioners with whom they formed a good relationship. Indeed, there is clear evidence that we require fewer reasons for accepting recommendations from friends than from strangers. The existence of a good relationship also allows for the expression of negative emotions by the practitioner (e.g. anger, anxiety, frustration), and this is related to greater patient adherence to the advice and direction offered. Genuine concern communicated by the pharmacist is reciprocated by a desire in the patient to please the practitioner by following treatment directives. Many strategies contribute to the initiation, maintenance and enhancement of relationships. Among the most important are demonstrating friendliness and warmth, using the patient's name, expressing genuine interest and concern for patients and their needs, discussing shared interests, demonstrating appropriate sympathy and empathy, referring to previous encounters, being readily available, employing appropriate humor and preserving confidentiality. Another crucial dimension of rapport building is that of offering reassurance. Negative media publicity about medicines has increased patients' need for reassurance concerning their therapy. In anticipation of questions such as 'is it safe to continue taking this?' pharmacists need firstly to deal with the factual aspect of the fear. Table 2.6 represents a four-step model of reassurance. In parallel, pharmacists should use a range of reassurance strategies in order to address related emotional concerns (Table 2.7).

Table 2.6

A four step model of reassurance
1. Provision of general background information
2. Review of scientific/clinical evidence
3. A summary of the balance of risk: benefits
4. Recommended action

Table 2.7

Reassurance strategies
• Showing a willingness to listen to patient concerns
• Conveying a competent professional approach
• Using reassuring nonverbal communication (e.g. eye contact, close interpersonal distance, appropriate touch)

EXPLAINING

Client satisfaction occurs across three domains:

- Affective satisfaction is a product of factors such as empathy, friendliness and trust.
- Behavioral satisfaction is determined by factors such as how the client's needs/problems are ascertained, length of waiting time and the pace of the interaction. The establishment of good rapport contributes to both of these dimensions.

- Cognitive satisfaction relates to the explanations given by the pharmacist to the patient. Here the emphasis is on providing advice, information and instruction in sufficient detail and using language which can be readily understood. The understanding, retention and utilization of advice and information can be effected by pharmacists using the techniques shown in Table 2.8.

Table 2.8

Strategies used by pharmacists to ensure patients understand, retain and use advice and information
• Place the most important points at the beginning and at the end of any interaction • Emphasize key points • Give specific instructions • Provide only essential information in order to prevent overload • Simplify complicated messages • Use examples and analogies relevant to the patient's experience • Have a logical structure that patients can follow • Present the oral message fluently • Converse at the patient's pace • Repeat instructions • Accompany the oral message with a written or visual aid • Address the needs of special patient groups (e.g. braille labels for the visually impaired; instruction leaflets in ethnic minority languages) • Provide a demonstration • Encourage the patient to repeat the demonstration • Monitor the extent of patient understanding • End the consultation with a summary of key points

QUESTIONING

The traditional medical model of health care has been that while patients might know what they want, health professionals, through their superior knowledge, believe they know what patients actually need. More recently, this imbalance between patient and practitioner goals has been strongly questioned. The predominant view now is that patients should be empowered to negotiate their own needs and be involved in the decisions involving all aspects of their care. This means that pharmacists in partnership with patients must agree the needs to be met. The acronym FUN (First Uncover Needs) is useful, in that it is only when the needs of patients have been fully established that the interaction can progress satisfactorily and messages be specifically tailored to address them. While there are recurring patient questions (Table 2.9), it is important to respect the individuality of each patient and find out exactly what their specific needs and circumstances are. This means that pharmacists must pay careful attention to their questioning style.

The research evidence consistently points to a predominantly closed style of questioning by pharmacists and an interviewing style in which the pharmacist controls and directs the consultation. Closed and leading questions restrict the scope of responses, often requiring only a 'Yes' or 'No' answer, and assume prior knowledge on the part of the questioner, such that the information gathered maybe incomplete or inaccurate potentially resulting in compromised action. For this reason pharmacists need to develop effective interviewing techniques which will be objective in the collection of data and open to the needs of patients. A distinction can be

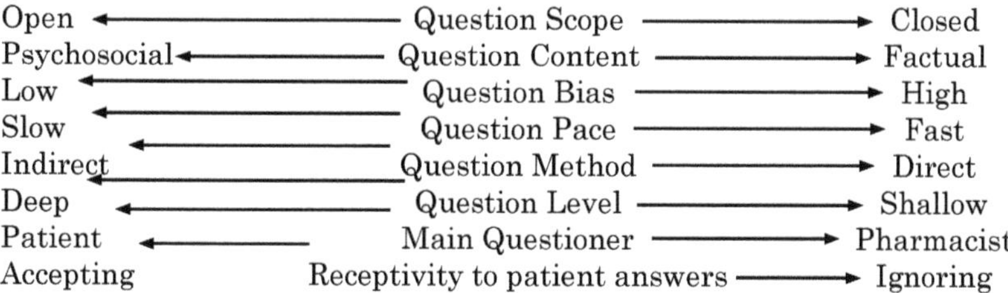

FIGURE 2.1

Facilitative and restrictive questioning.

made between facilitative and restrictive questioning styles. As shown in fig 2.1, the facilitative style allows patients to be centrally involved in the consultation. The style of the questions tends to be open, their content includes psychosocial dimensions, there is a low level of bias in terms of fewer leading questions, the pace is appropriate to the patient, and the health professional encourages patient questions and is accepting of responses.

Table 2.9

Questions commonly asked by patients

- 'Why me?'
- 'Why now?'
- 'Why this particular illness?'
- 'What is this medicine for?'
- 'How do I take it?'
- 'Are there any side-effects?'
- 'How long do I need to take it for?'
- 'What will happen if I don't take it?'
- 'What is going to happen to me?'

In order to use questions effectively pharmacists should employ the strategies outlined in Table 2.10.

Table 2.10

Effective questioning

- Reduce the number of closed questions and use more open questions

Table 2.10 *Contd...*

- Ask only one question at a time
- Structure the sequence of questions to follow a logical pattern
- Use probing questions to follow up on patients' responses
- Increase participation by pausing both after asking a question and after the patient's initial response
- Encourage patients to ask questions
- Avoid questions that will bias responses
- Show concerted attention in delivering the question

LISTENING

As well as asking appropriate questions, pharmacists should listen carefully to what the patient has to say. Evidence from public surveys consistently demonstrates a very strong desire for community pharmacists to spend more time listening fully to patient concerns. Good listening behavior demands concentrated effort and is indicated both verbally and nonverbally. 'Active listening is very hard work initially and demands considerable attention and practice but the advantages in terms of eliciting information and developing a good therapeutic relationship with a patient is worth the investment of time'.

To optimize effective listening, the points in Table 2.11 should be borne in mind:

Table 2.11

Optimizing effective listening
• Do not stereotype the patient • Be objective • Show nonverbal indicators of interest and attention (eye contact head nods, etc) • Arrange a conducive environment, avoiding distractions • Be prepared to listen • Keep an open, analytical mind, searching for the central thrust of the message • Identify supporting arguments and facts • Do not dwell on one or two aspects at the expense of others • Delay judgment or refutation, until you have heard the entire message • Verbally follow up on what the patient has said (questions, reference to previous statements, summaries, etc.)

NONVERBAL COMMUNICATION

There are two core purposes of nonverbal behaviour. First, *message comprehension and recall* is facilitated by the use of nonverbal behaviours, such as communicative gestures (e.g. raising three fingers to signal 'three' of something). Second, *relational communication,* such as the expression of liking and friendship, is conveyed by a range of behaviours including: direct body and facial orientation, a close conversational distance, consistent eye contact, head nods, a forward leaning and open posture, smiles and pleasant facial expressions, frequent gestures, and appropriate touch. Nonverbal communication is especially important in pharmacy for the four main reasons shown in Table 2.12.

Table 2.12

Four reasons for the particular importance of nonverbal communication in pharmacy
1. The role of patients as consumers of health care gives them the time and opportunity to monitor closely the nonverbal behavior of the pharmacist

Table 2.12 *Contd...*

2. Fear and uncertainty about their illness increases the attention they pay to the pharmacist's often subtle nonverbal cues that indicate how and what they should be feeling
3. Patients often do not fully understand the verbal message, or believe it not to be wholly truthful, and so they analyse nonverbal cues for information on which to base their judgements about their condition
4. The patient's treatment or condition may interfere with their ability to communicate verbally. Nonverbal signals then become the prime channel for communication

While the pharmacist must be skilled in the use of nonverbal behaviour, the interpretation and assessment of the patient's nonverbal messages is also very important. For example, a patient showing nonverbal signs of embarrassment should be taken to a more private area of the pharmacy for the consultation. In addition, pharmacists also need to make important decisions about the truthfulness of what the patient is saying, especially if drug abuse or misuse is suspected. A range of research studies on deception indicators have revealed commonly recurring verbal and nonverbal behaviours (Table 2.13).

Table 2.13

Indicators of deception
Nonverbal deceptive indicators • Increased pupil dilation and blinking • More self-manipulations and gestures unrelated to the speech content • Speaking at a higher pitch • Greater number of speech errors and hesitations
Verbal deceptive indicators • Shorter response length • More generalities (fewer specific references about people, places and temporal ordering of events)

Table 2.13 *Contd...*

- More irrelevant information unrelated to the central theme
- Greater equivocation
- Considerable 'levelling', which is tendency to use terms such as *'all', 'every', 'none'*, or *'nobody'*

SUGGESTING/ADVISING

A comparison of consultations revealed one skill that was commonly employed when dealing with over the counter (OTC) items but not used by pharmacists when handling prescription-related encounters. This skill, termed suggesting/ advising, was defined as the offer of a personal/professional opinion about a particular course of action, while simultaneously allowing the final decision to lie with the patient. Examples of this skill included: *'Have you tried an inhalation at all? Sometimes it can help...'. 'I think you'd be better taking the adult cough mixture because it just thins the phlegm and* then you cough it up yourself...' It may be that in the OTC context, patients have to fully negotiate their own needs (and pay directly for the service), and this in turn demands a more comprehensive response from the pharmacist. This is in contrast to the situation where the *'written order'* from the doctor (the prescription) following a medical consultation may already have dealt with many of the patient's needs, and the pharmacist does not wish to appear to *'intervene'*. At the same time, there are degrees of suggestion by the pharmacist, with some more forcefully expressed than others, to emphasise their importance. These were prefaced by expressions such as: *'I would strongly recommend you...'. ' You would be well advised to...'.*

OPENING

As the saying goes, *'You don't get a second chance to make a first impression', and* indeed the manner in which the pharmacist meets and greets the patient will influence how the former is perceived. The main steps involved in effective openings are shown in Table 2-14.

CLOSING

It is important to terminate the consultation smoothly and satisfactorily, so that it comes to a natural end with both parties having achieved their goals. To achieve an effective closure, the checklist in table 2-15 should be borne in mind.

Table 2.14

Main steps in effective openings

- Greet the patient using their name if possible *('Good morning, Mrs Iverson. How are you today?')*
- Use appropriate nonverbals (move towards the patient, smile, engage in eye contact, etc.)
- Carefully observe the patient's nonverbal communication to determine the degree of privacy required
- Take up a suitable location for the consultation and give the patient undivided attention
- Use an approach which underlines to the patient that their involvement is both expected and desired
- Establish fully what the patient's needs and concerns are and convey to the patient your acceptance of these
- Check out *'what has gone before'*, as appropriate
- Reward the patient for seeking advice *('It's wise to ask about this)*

Table 2.15

Achieving effective closure of communication
• Summarise and remind the patient of the main points covered • Obtain feedback to check the patient understands what has been explained • Make future links *(e.g. 'Take these tablets for a week and then come back and see me')* • Motivate and encourage the patient about the benefits of the treatment regime (e.g. *'These will ease the pain immediately and the itch will* • Refer the patient elsewhere if appropriate *('You need to go and see your doctor...')* • Praise the patient *(e.g.'You were right to come and see me')* • Use closure indicators to show that the consultation will soon be ending (orienting away from the patient—pointing your feet towards the dispensary is a subtle yet gentle indicator of imminent termination; and saying something like: *'Well we've covered just about everything...'*) • Employ final closure markers, use the patient's name, and try to include a non-task comments (e.g. *'OK. Bye, Mrs Karpoov. Take care of that slippery footpath.'*).

ASSERTIVENESS

The ability to assert oneself confidently is essential for effective social functioning. This involves standing up for personal rights and expressing personal thoughts and feelings openly, while at the same time respecting the rights of others. An assertive approach is particularly important when:

- Making reasonable requests of others
- Refusing to comply with unreasonable requests
- Handling unreasonable refusals

However, within the health setting it would seem that certain groups, including pharmacists, find this skill quite difficult to implement, especially when dealing with other professionals and with ancillary health care workers. At the same time, it is now well established that *'assertion is a learned skill, not a "trait" that a person "has" or "lacks"*. His means that pharmacists who have difficulty in being assertive can learn to overcome such inhibition. In fact there are three main behavioral styles of relevance here:

1. *Nonassertive style.* This style involves being subservient, self effacing and apologetic, using hesitant speech with low voice volume, avoiding eye contact, fidgeting frequently, not expressing opinions, and forgoing personal rights rather than becoming involved in any possibility of *'unpleasantness'*.
2. *Assertive style.* This involves the person seeking equality with others, readily expressing opinions and feelings, addressing contentious issues, speaking in a firm yet conversational tone, engaging in eye contact, and protecting the rights of themselves and others.
3. *Aggressive style.* This style involves vehemently expressing opinions, being selfopinionated and overbearing, reveling in contentious issues, speaking loudly and abusively, interrupting others and glaring at them, and taking no cognizance of their rights.

Of these styles, assertiveness has been clearly shown to be the most effective. Submissive people are not well respected, while aggressive individuals are actively disliked. When assertion is used skilfully, with due recognition given to the rights of others, then the most positive outcomes are obtained. The use of assertiveness often involves three elements, which may be illustrated in a situation where the pharmacist is confronted with a dubious prescription.

- Description of the situation—*'This prescription has been altered'*
- Description, plus indication of noncompliance—*'This prescription has been altered and therefore I can't dispense it'*
- Description, noncompliance, plus request for the situation to be changed—*'This prescription has been altered and therefore I can't dispense it. Can you get your doctor to confirm this alteration?'*

DISCLOSING PERSONAL INFORMATION

Self-disclosure is the act of verbally and/or nonverbally communicating to others personal information . It can be nonverbal, in that we can either hide feelings such as worry, happiness etc., or openly express them in our facial expressions, posture, and so on. However, most research on self-disclosure focuses upon the verbal component, and here the key defining feature is the use of a personal selfreference pronoun such as *'I', 'me', 'mine'* etc. Thus, the difference between the statements *'diabetes is very worrying'* and *'I am very worried about diabetes'* is that the former may or may not be a self-disclosure, whereas the latter definitely is.

A knowledge and skilled use of self-disclosure is important in pharmacy for two main reasons. First, to effect an accurate diagnosis, patients must openly and honestly disclose personal details about their condition. Pharmacists therefore must use tactics that encourage patients to fully explain their situation. They can increase the level of self-disclosure from patients by:

- Establishing a relationship of trust, confidence, acceptance and empathy
- Having a professional personal appearance
- Providing a private environment in which personal matters can be discussed freely
- Dealing with patients in a receptive, caring, and unhurried style

Second, pharmacists have to decide what, and when, it is appropriate to self-disclose to patients. Here, self-disclosure can be divided into two main types—the pharmacist's own personal experiences, and the pharmacist's personal reactions to the patient's disclosures. Both are appropriate, but must be used judiciously. The first type can help to reassure patients that what they are experiencing is not unusual (a technique known as 'normalising'), and also help to develop rapport by demonstrating shared experiences (e.g. 'I know what you're going through. When we had our first child, she kept us awake…'). However, patients do not expect a great deal of disclosure from pharmacists, and so the second type is more common. Here, the focus of attention stays firmly upon the patient, and the pharmacist shows a willingness to become involved in their 'world' ('I really am determined to help you stop smoking…').

PERSUADING

Given the wealth of evidence indicating that patients often fail to follow advice about treatment regimes, knowledge of the influencing tactics that can serve to increase patient compliance is important. A range of effective persuading strategies has been identified. To influence patients the pharmacist should: Capitalize on their professional relationship with patients: we are more likely to be influenced by people we like, and for whom we have high regard. A positive pharmacist-patient relationship is the key to successful persuasion. In fact, the forceful delivery of negative messages within a positive relationship often leads to increased acceptance by a patient of the health threatening nature of their condition.

Engage feelings of threat and fear: this is an important influencing tactic in encouraging people to change their behavior. In the health context, the success of this approach depends upon four factors:

1. The magnitude and severity of the negative outcome
2. Its probability of occurring if nothing is done to avoid it
3. The effectiveness of the recommended response to remove the threat
4. The patient's belief in being able to adhere to the recommended treatment

Invoke moral appeals to promote positive health behavior: this is an effective tactic since breaches the moral code usually produce feelings of guilt. For example, a pregnant woman could be encouraged to give up smoking by telling her: *'You have a duty to your unborn child to give it the healthiest possible start in life, so you really must stop smoking.*

Include logical arguments delivered with few hesitations or expressed doubts: a 'powerful' authoritative speech style (few hesitations or expressed doubts, coupled with the use of intensifies such as *'definitely', 'absolutely* etc.) increase the influencing power of an argument.

Underline the power of the message: This is enhanced when the pharmacist projects a professional image in terms of personal appearance and bearing, and when the pharmacy, in its design, layout, product range and display, portrays a professional image.

These, then are the key communication skills central to effective pharmacy practice. There are no hard and fast rules about when, with which patients, or under what conditions, they should be used. Rather, the pharmacist must decide which combination of skills best meets the needs and requirements of each individual patient. However, for some patients, special communication efforts need to be made, owing to the nature of their conditions.

COMMUNICATION AND DISABILITY

Overcoming patients' communication difficulties is a major hurdle to effective patient

Counseling. This is especially the case when counseling patients who:

- Are confused about their medication
- Have age-related medication problems
- Are anxious about treatment

The groups of patients who may have particular communication difficulties are shown in Table 2.16.

Table 2.16

Patients who may have communication difficulties
• Disabled patients using wheelchairs • The visually impaired • The deaf or hard of hearing • Those who do not speak English • The elderly who are mentally ill • Those with learning disabilities

The area of learning disabilities was explored in the Report on Mental Health Foundation Committee of Inquiry (1996) which provided a salutary insight into the range of communication problems faced by this group of people. The following quotation is indicative of the type of problem such individuals experience.

The doctor gave me some tablets, but I had no idea what they were. He explained to me. but I didn't understand. It was Latin. People with learning disabilities find it hard to take tablets. They don't know what they are. They're afraid they will take the wrong kind of tablets and die.'

More recently, in an evaluation of 611 patients admitted to a University Hospital general medical service, 15.9% were found to have one or more disabilities affecting communication . Nine percent had altered mental states, 4.7% vision impairments, 2.8% speech impairments and 0.5% hearing impairments. Disability was more apparent in older age groups.

Clearly where communication difficulties exist and where they are not effectively managed, patient care is compromised and levels of patient dissatisfaction rise. There is, therefore, a crucial need for practitioners to be sensitive to the communication needs of such patients and to have developed strategies to facilitate effective dialogue between both parties.

The approach must operate at two levels, at the strategic or institutional level and at the personal level. At the strategic level clients' needs should be identified and defined, services should then be planned on the basis of need, implemented on a managed basis and monitored for effectiveness and quality. At the personal level, it will be concerned with the particular 'accommodations' that need to be in place to facilitate communication. Some examples are given in Table 2.17 .

A particular case in point is the inability of some patients to speak the language of the country in which they are resident. This is especially the case among ethnic minorities. Much has been done in respect of information produced in the ethnic minority languages and the importance of producing medicines-related information in such formats cannot be overemphasised.

Table 2.17

Facilitating effective communication in disability

Disability	Accomodation
Visually impaired	Large print Braille
Hearing impaired	Audiotape materials Assistive listening devices Sign language and interpretation
Speech impairment	Tracheotomy speech adapters Communication boards
Impaired mental states	Compliance aids Surrogate sources of information e.g. carers

REFERENCES

1. Allen, M. and Preiss, R. (Eds.) (1998) *Persuasion: Advances Through Meta-Analyses,* Hampton Press, New Jersey.
2. Armstrong, D. (1991) What do patients want? Someone who will answer their questions. *British Medical Journal,* **303**, 261–262.
3. Audit Commission (1993) *What Seems to be the Matter: Communication Between Hospitals and Patients,* HMSO, London.
4. Blenkinsopp, A., Robinson, E. and Panton, R. (1994) Do pharmacy customers remember the information given to them by the community pharmacist? In: G.Harding, S.Nettleton

and K.Taylor (Eds.), *Social Pharmacy: Innovation and Change,* Pharmaceutical Press, London, pp. 84–94.

5. Buller, D. and Burgoon, J. (1996) Interpersonal deception theory. *Communication Theory,* **6**, 203–242.
6. Cipolle R.J., Strand L.M. and Morley P.C. (1998) *Pharmaceutical Care Practice,* McGraw-Hill, New York.
7. Davis, H. and Fallowfield, L. (1991) *Counselling and Communication in Health Care,* John Wiley, Chichester.
8. Department of Health (1992) *The Patient's Charter,* HMSO, London.
9. Dickson, D., Hargie, O. and Morrow, N. (1997) *Communication Skills Training for Health Professionals* (2nd Edn.) Chapman and Hall, London.
10. Ebert, D.A. (1998) Communication disabilities among medical inpatients. *New England Journal of Medicine,* **339**, 272–273.
11. Ewles, L. and Simnett, I. (1992) *Promoting Health: A Practical Guide* (2nd Edn.) Scutari Press, London.
12. Hargie, O. and Morrow, N. (1988) Interpersonal communication 3. Assertiveness skills. *Pharmacy Update,* **4**, 243–247.
13. Hargie, O. and Morrow, N. (1991) The skill of self disclosure, parts 1 and 2. *Chemist and Druggist,* **235**, 343–344 and 769–770.
14. Hargie, O., Morrow, N. and Woodman, C. (2000) Pharmacists' evaluation of key communication skills in practice. *Patient Education and Counselling,* **39**, 61–70.
15. Hargie, O., Saunders, C. and Dickson, D. (1994) *Social Skills in Interpersonal Communication.* Routledge, London.

CHAPTER 3

Medication History Interview

A medication history is an accurate, complete and detailed account of all prescribed and non-prescribed medications that had taken by a patient or is currently taking prior to a newly initiated institutionalized or ambulatory care.

It provides valuable insights into patients' adherence, allergic tendencies to social drug use pharmacological and non-pharmacological treatments and probable self-medication with alternative and complementary medicines.

Medication history interview mainly related with patient Interviewing in collecting the data medical history.

GOALS

The medication history interview's main goal is to obtain information on aspects of drug use that may assist in patient over all care. The information gathered can be utilized to:

- Compare medication profiles with the medication administration investigate and record the discrepancies.
- Verify medication history taken by other staffs and provide additional information where appropriate.
- Allergies and adverse reactions have to be documented.
- Screen for drug interactions.
- Patient medication compliance should be monitored.
- The rationale for drug prescribed should be assessed.
- Assess the evidence of drug abuse.
- Appraise the drug administration techniques.
- The requirements for medication aids should be identified.
- Document patient initiated medication administration.

What is to be Documented?

To review and identify suitable additional treatments, current medical treatment, medical professionals will require reliable and complete medication history. Research has established that the pharmacist provide the most accurate medication history when compared to all other health professionals. Pharmacists are well prepared to fulfill and plays an very important role.

A well structured, prepared approach helps to obtain relevant complete information. The below information is commonly recorded:

- Currently or recently prescribed medicines.
- OTC medication.

- Vaccinations.
- Alternative or traditional remedies.
- Description of reaction and allergies to medicines.
- Medicines found to be ineffective.
- Past treatment courses Adherence and the use of the adherence aids.

Interviewing the Person

- Self introduction
- Informing the person for what reason you are there
- The client should be made aware of the importance of maintaining an medication list in the chart.

Information Sources

- Patient
- Guardian or family
- Vials of the Medication / Bubble packs
- List of Medications
- Community Pharmacy
- Medication history
- DPIN (Drug Programs Information Network)

Questions to Ask

- Is there development of any allergies or adverse reactions to medications that are used previously and if so what were the reactions.
- Which medications are you currently taking?

  The medication name

  The type of dosage form

  The dosage used

  The routes of drug administration

  Number of times a drug is used

  Are there any specific period of time for usage of the drug

  The reason behind the usage of the medication

Table 3.1

Alcohol Use Categories (Adults)

Category	Men	Women
Lifetime abstainer	<12 drinks in lifetime	<12 drinks in lifetime
Former infrequent drinker	≥12 drinks in lifetime but <12 drinks in any single year and no drinks in the past year	≥12 drinks in lifetime but <12 drinks in any single year and no drinks in the past year
Current drinker	≥12 drinks in lifetime and ≥1 drink in the past year	≥12 drinks in lifetime and ≥1 drink in the past year
Infrequent drinker	1-11 drinks in past year	1-11 drinks in past year
Light drinker	≤3 drinks per week	≤3 drinks per week
Moderate drinker	>3 and up to 14 drinks per week	>3 and up to 7 drinks per week
Heavier drinker	>14 drinks per week (>2 drinks per day on average)	>7 drinks per week (>1 drink per day on average)
Binge drinker	≥5 drinks in about 2hours	≥4 drinks in about 2 hours

Adapted from Schoenborn CA, Adams PF, Barnes PM, et al: Health behaviors of adults: United States, 1999-2001. National Center for Health Statistics. *Vital Health Stat* 10(219):1-79, 2004; National Institute of Alcohol Abuse and Alcoholism: NIAA council approves defnition of binge drinking. *NIAAA Newsletter* (3):3, 2004.

- What medications are taken by the person either regularly or as needed basis?
- What are the over-the-counter (non-prescription) medications taken by the person either regularly or as needed basis?
- Which herbal or natural medicines taken by the person either regularly or as needed basis?
- Vitamins or other supplements that are taken by the person?

MEDICATION HISTORY TAKING TIPS

- Open-ended questions (what, how, why, when) with yes/no questions

  Balance should be balanced.
- pose only non-biased questions .
- leading questions should be avoided
- vague responses (non-compliance) should be explored
- judgmental comments should be avoided
- 24 hours survey (morning, lunch, supper, bedtime) approaches should be used

  Systematic review (head to toe review)

  Prescribers link should be monitored (family physician, specialists)
- Review each medication vials if they are available with the patients

  content of bottle should be Confirmed

  Instructions on prescription vials are to be Confirmed
- Review each medication available with patient and confirm that it is current

Other Questions

- Did the patient started recently any new medication
- Is there any change in the dose or stop any of the medications recently by the physician?
- whether there is any change in the dose or stopped any of the medications recently

Other Questions to Determine the Effectiveness/Compliance

- Is the medications causing side effects that are used currently?
- Whether is there any change in dose or stopped any medications due to the side effects.
- whether the medicine usage is stopped whenever the person feels better?
- is administration of the medicine is stopped if it makes feel worse?

Client Education

- Ownership should be encouraged
- Advise the client to bring the medications at each visit to the hospital
- client was informed to carry the list of current medications (prescription and OTC)
- family members/ caregivers are encouraged to get involved
- one pharmacy only should be encouraged

Reconciliation and Documentation

Upon discovering a problem

The list should be updated if minor (eg : OTC taken as needed)

Other physicians prescribed medications should be included (eg : specialist)

If the person is not taking the medication as prescribed it should be informed to the physician

Document in the Client's Chart

The date of the Medical Record completed and initial on the medication reconciliation status record. Important information in the progress notes should be indicated.

MEDICATION HISTORY INTERVIEW DOCUMENTATION FORM

Patient name:	I.P. No:	Date of Admission:	
Age:	Height:	Weight:	BMI:
Qualification:		Occupation:	
Recent Hospitalization:		Duration of Hospitalization:	
Reasons for Previous Hospitalization (If applicable):			
Reasons for Current Hospitalization:			

Past Prescription Medications (Drug name) (Start Date) (Dose prescribed) (Schedule) (Indication)				

Past Non-Prescription Medications (Drug name) (Start Date) (Dose prescribed) (Schedule) (Indication)				

Complementary and Alternate Medicines (Start Date) (Dose prescribed) (Schedule) (Indication)				

Current Non-Prescription Medications (Start Date) (Dose prescribed) (Schedule) (Indication)				

Current Prescription Drugs (Drug name) (Start Date) (Dose prescribed) (Schedule) (Indication)				

<table>
<tr><td colspan="4">Immunizations (Vaccine and date given)</td></tr>
<tr><td colspan="4">Allergies (Date, description of event, Treatment)</td></tr>
<tr><td colspan="4">Adverse Drug Reactions (Attach PvPI form if applicable)</td></tr>
<tr><td colspan="2">Social History : Marital Status</td><td colspan="2">Occupation</td></tr>
<tr><td colspan="4">Tobacco: 1ppd (pack per day) x 1year = 1 pack year history</td></tr>
<tr><td colspan="4">Alcohol: Life time abstainer ☐ Former infrequent drinker ☐ Current drinker ☐
Infrequent drinker ☐ Light drinker ☐ Moderate drinker ☐
Heavier drinker ☐ Binge drinker ☐</td></tr>
<tr><td colspan="4">Dietary Information</td></tr>
<tr><td>(Diet restrictions)</td><td>(Diet supplements)</td><td>(Stimulants)</td><td>(Suppressants)</td></tr>
<tr><td colspan="2">Family Chart</td><td colspan="2">Assessment of Patient Compliance</td></tr>
</table>

MEDICATION HISTORY CHECKLIST FOR THE PRECEPTOR

Format:

- [ ] The date and time of the interview is noted.
- [ ] The history is signed (and co-signed).

Details:

- [ ] All medications are referred as per the guidelines
- [ ] The start date is noted for all drugs
- [ ] Stop date is noted for past drugs
- [ ] Dose and interval are noted for all drugs
- [ ] Indication is noted for all drugs
- [ ] Actual use of each medication is noted
- [ ] Details of all adverse reactions are noted
- [ ] Details of medication allergies are noted

Components:

- [ ] Patient demographics
- [ ] Current Prescription medications
- [ ] Current Non-prescription medications
- [ ] Current CAM medications
- [ ] Past prescription medications
- [ ] Past Non-prescription medications
- [ ] Past CAM medications
- [ ] Immunizations
- [ ] Dietary information
- [ ] Assessment of adherence

CHAPTER 4

Evidence-Based Medicine

It concentrates on the scientific method as the key source of knowledge in making clinical decisions. It is defined as "The Precise, Diligent, and Rational use of best evidence in decision making about the individual patient care, while interlinking clinical experience with the best available evidence from a systematic search."

SOURCES OF KNOWLEDGE

It utilizes the scientific method as a key source of knowledge for clinical decision making. However, in addition to the scientific method, there are also various other sources of knowledge.

1. Reference to tradition – accepting certain truths. **Problem:** many traditions are not evaluated for validity nor tested against potentially superior alternatives.
2. Reference to authority – placing trust in those who are authorities or experts on an issue. **Problem:** this method reduces the necessity for critical analysis and confirmation of validity and does not encourage testing of potentially superior alternatives.
3. Trial and error – applying multiple attempts to find a solution by chance. Used when no other basis for making a decision exists. **Problem:** this method results in a haphazard and not correct one to attain the knowledge.
4. Logical reasoning – involving deductive reasoning—a systematic method for drawing conclusions.
5. Scientific method – applying a logical sequential process to develop a conclusion. This process involves identifying the problem, organizing collection of data, objectively analyzing the data, and interpreting the findings.

THE SOLUTION

The 5-Step Evidence-Based Medicine process exhibits the following characteristics:

- Offer less complexity
- Offers time-sensitive decision making support by alleviating time-intensive methods
- Maintains rigor
- Categorizes evidence quality in a simple and logical manner
- Provide a process designed specifically for pharmacy practitioners making drug therapy decisions

This process involves five steps defining the clinical question. **Step one** defining the clinical question is essential in providing direction to the remaining four steps of this

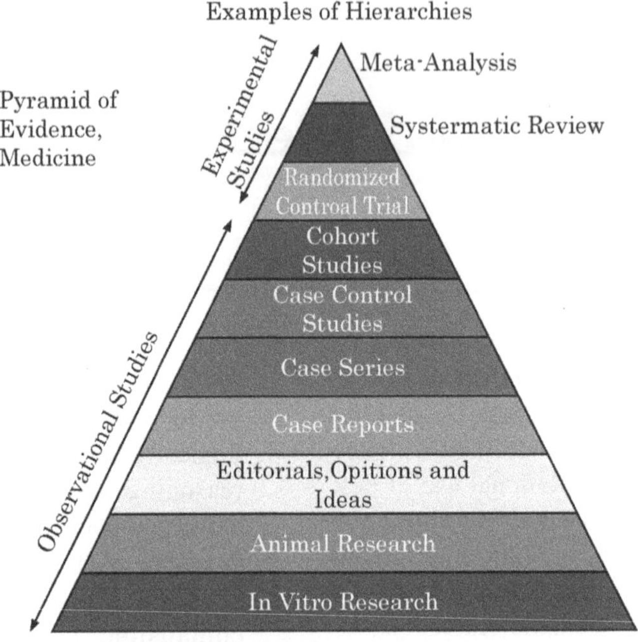

FIGURE 4.1

System of hierarchy of Evidence Based Medicine.
(Source: http://libraryguides.nau.edu/pbc/pa)

evidence-based medicine process. This step may be the tough one in the process because it involves the conversion of a clinical problem into an answerable clinical question.

Step two involves searching the literature for articles associated with this clinical question.

Many of the practitioners will not conduct extensive and sophisticated database searches to ensure a comprehensive review of the pertinent literature.

Step three is evaluating literature found. Again, the assumption is that the reader has completed at least a basic critical evaluation course with some exposure to biostatistics.

Step four is determining the quality of identified and critically evaluated evidence. Several different hierarchies of evidence are available to accomplish this step.

Step five is drawing a conclusion with proper evidence, which involves the creation of a specific statement supported by the data and other special considerations/special populations provided by the evidence.

DEFINE THE CLINICAL QUESTION

Step 1 – Define the Clinical Question

The first step of the 5-Step Evidence-Based Medicine Process, Define the Clinical Question, may be the most difficult one because it involves the translation of a clinical problem into an answerable clinical question. Defining and structuring an appropriate clinical question are both critical. According to a survey conducted by the Drug Information Service at the Medical College of Virginia Hospitals, the original clinical question asked was significantly different from the actual question that needed to be answered 85% of the time. This problem suggests the need for applying some type of systematic process to ensure the most accurate definition of the clinical question. One approach using a logical and systematic manner to define the problem and clarify the clinical question has been proposed by drug information specialists. The goal of this approach is to understand the context and scope of the problem.

Framing the Clinical Question Using PICO: (Patient Intervention Comparison Outcome)

Accurately defining the clinical question is essential to providing direction for the remaining four steps of the evidence-based medicine process outlined in this book. Those steps include retrieving the pertinent literature, critically evaluating the literature, categorizing the quality of the evidence, and developing a recommendation that can be justified. A generic, minimally defined clinical question does not provide the required direction for these steps.

EXAMPLE 1

Using Minimal Detail to Define the Clinical Questions

An example of a generic, minimally detailed clinical question is taking a newly marketed non injectable insulin product and asking if this product should be added to a preferred drug list within an institution. The following can be determined from this minimal information:

1. context – a preferred drug list formulary management activity for an institution
2. scope – a population-based decision for a specific institution that may have a particular patient population such as indigent and/or Medicaid

With this example, only the context and scope of the question are provided. The details necessary to define the true clinical question are missing. Using the PICO approach, the definitive details of the clinical question can be determined.

An accepted approach for framing the clinical question is provided by Sackett and colleagues using an acronym approach referred to as PICO. This approach includes the following components:

Patients – What individual patient or patient population is associated with the clinical question? Are there any patient subgroups that require special attention?

Interventions – What interventions can be used in this clinical situation?

Comparison – What additional interventions can be considered and compared to the chosen intervention?

Outcome – What is the end result most desired for the individual patient, patient population, and/or patient subgroup?

EXAMPLE 2

PICO Approach Defined

The Patient population includes both type 1 and 2 diabetics either just initiating therapy or having been on insulin for a period of time. A special subgroup of patients to consider might include those with a "needle phobia" or those who want a more practical way to administer insulin when out in public.

The Intervention is the non- injectable insulin. Related questions would further define how the intervention is administered and provide a description of the device needed for administration, frequency of administration, and dosing equivalency to inject table insulin.

The Comparison includes inject table in sulins and other interventions such as competitor non inject table insulins, insulin stimulators, and insulin enhancers.

The Outcome is adequate glycemic control as measured by fasting blood glucose levels and HbA1C without the problems and inconveniences associated with injectable insulin

Using this PICO approach now allows development of a well defined clinical question as illustrated in Example 3.

EXAMPLE 3

The Well-Defined Clinical Question

"Are there safety and/or convenience benefits associated with this noninjectable insulin compared to inject table insulin, other non injectable insulins, insulin stimulators, or insulin enhancers to provide normal blood glucose and glycemic control in type 1 and 2 diabetic patients? Is there a difference in patient motivation to use the non-injectable insulin between patients just initiating versus maintaining insulin therapy and/ or those patients with 'needle phobia'?"

EFFECTS ON OTHER EVIDENCE-BASED MEDICINE ACTIVITIES

Once the clinical question has been accurately defined, the following activities associated with the evidence-based medicine process can be initiated.

- Identify specific search terms for use in retrieving pertinent information (Example 4).

EXAMPLE 4

Specific Search Terms

- The specific intervention's trade name
- Names of other competing non-injec table insulins
- Names of insulin stimulators
- Names of insulin enhancers
- Names of injectable insulins
- Type 1 diabetes
- Type 2 diabetes
- Fasting blood glucose
- HbA1C
- "Needle phobia"

- Determine the relevance of the search results now that the details of the patient population, intervention, comparisons, and desired outcomes are known.
- Focus information retrieval and critical evaluation efforts toward the pertinent evidence as the specific patient population, intervention, comparison, and desired outcomes have been identified by the defined clinical question.
- Develop a recommendation more efficiently and effectively based on observations made possible by a well-defined clinical question during the critical evaluation of the evidence (see Example 5).

EXAMPLE 5

Specific Observations

- Determine if there are safety and/or convenience benefits associated with using non-injectable insulin versus identified alternative therapies.

- Determine if there is a difference in patient motivation to use non-injectable insulin between type 1 and type 2 diabetic patients
- Determine if there is a difference in patient motivation to use non-injectable insulin in patients initiating injectable insulin therapy for the first time versus patients already maintained on injectable insulin.
- Consider if a subgroup of patients with "needle phobia" is more likely to utilize the non-injectable insulin compared to those without this problem.

TIPS FOR DEFINING THE CLINICAL QUESTION

Important points to consider when defining the clinical question include the following:

- Describe a group of patients with similar characteristics as those in the problem or situation you are trying to define with the clinical question.
- Identify the primary intervention.
- Identify the primary desired outcome and how that outcome is measured in the clinical setting.

PROBLEMS TO BE AVOIDED

Finally, some common problems are associated with defining the clinical question that should be avoided:

- Complex clinical situations resulting in numerous questions identified can be handled by dissecting the situation into smaller, less complex, and more manageable problems requiring fewer questions.
- Too little or complete lack of adequate background information can be handled by further questioning key people associated with the clinical situation.
- Lack of time to complete an evidence-based medicine analysis can be due to an overabundance of clinical problems associated with the situation. Judicious prioritization identifying those clinical problems having the greatest impact on a patient or institution is one way to deal with this issue.

RETRIEVE PERTINENT INFORMATION

Step 2 – Retrieve Pertinent Information

The second step of this 5-Step Evidence-Based Medicine process, Retrieving Pertinent Information, involves creating a comprehensive search strategy to identify all of the pertinent evidence available relative to the clinical question. This information can be retrieved from a variety of databases and compendia. To complete this step, the pharmacy practitioner needs a basic understanding of common databases and standard search strategies. An incomplete search strategy may cause the omission of key information and may result in an inappropriate recommendation affecting the treatment and/or safety of the patient. Once this strategy is defined and completed, the next step is to refine the search results. Search strategies and the techniques used to organize search results will be discussed in this chapter. Retrieving Pertinent Information is an extremely important step in the 5-Step Evidence-Based Medicine Process because it builds the foundation for this process.

DECIDING WHERE TO START

To ensure that recommendations are supported by the best available evidence, it is important for a clinical practitioner to understand the steps used to provide a successful search. An effective search strategy begins broad with the use of tertiary resources and narrows to primary resources. Tertiary resources include textbooks and compendia (e.g., Micromedex, LexiComp, Clinical Pharmacology, Facts and Comparisons). These resources are used for gathering general background information pertaining to the clinical question. Secondary resources are indexing and abstracting services that simplify the search and identify primary literature. Some examples include PubMed (or Medline), International Pharmaceutical Abstracts, Iowa Drug Information Services, and EMBASE. Primary resources refer to journals containing original research, including randomized controlled trials, review articles, case studies, and meta analyses. The resources discussed above are crucial in carrying out the 5-Step Evidence-Based Medicine Process.

CREATING THE SEARCH STRATEGY

Broad to narrow search

A precise search strategy is critical to ensure all pertinent evidence is identified. Too much or too little detail in the search strategy can result in limited usable evidence. For instance, specific search terms can limit the results while the use of more general search terms often provides excessive amounts of non-relevant information.

EXAMPLE 6

Using General and Specific Search Terms

The defined clinical question is whether Drug A is as effective as Drug B regarding improvement of bone density in the treatment of osteoporosis.

Specific Search Terms:
Drug A brand name
Drug B brand name
General Search Terms:
Drug A generic name
Drug B generic name
Osteoporosis
Bone Density
Drug A—all approved indications besides osteoporosis
Drug B—all approved indications besides osteoporosis

1. Use of specific search terms listed above can limit the search to those articles where only the brand name appears. More possible "hits" may appear if the search is made somewhat more general by searching both the brand and generic names of Drug A and Drug B.
2. Searching by brand and generic names of Drug B could result in too general of a search if Drug B has been on the market long enough to lose patent exclusivity. In this case, not all the generic products identified with this search are going to be pertinent to the situation. For instance, if the brand name product is the only oral form and this is the route pertinent to the clinical question, then only the brand name drug would be of interest.

BIBLIOGRAPHIC SEARCHING

Once the original search is complete, a technique referred to as bibliographic searching can aid in optimizing results of the search. The technique involves reviewing citations of previously identified pertinent information in the original search. This technique can help identify additional literature as well as help in discovering additional search terms that may be useful to broaden the original search. Bibliographic searching helps create a network or "spider web" of information relating to the subject and helps ensure search results are thorough and complete, thus leading to a strong and confident recommendation.

ORGANIZING SEARCH RESULTS—SEARCH AND SIFT TECHNIQUE

Applying the skills in Step 4 – Categorize the Quality of Evidence to the retrieval process can maximize efficiency of the literature search and make an overwhelming list of search results manageable. A technique referred to as "Search and Sift" helps the clinician prioritize and organize search results by the quality of evidence and allows evidence to be eliminated that is not pertinent to the clinical question.

The technique involves "sifting" through the abstracts of search results using key words identified from the Ten Major Considerations to quickly determine the quality of evidence. This technique also helps eliminate lower quality, less reliable evidence.

EXAMPLE 7

Using the "Search and Sift" Technique

As a practitioner, you have been asked to provide guidance on the prophylaxis of stress ulcers. After identifying and reviewing the available therapeutic guidelines on stress ulcers, you determine the need to update the original evidence-based guidelines published in 1998. You will need to first retrieve the pertinent information that has become available since this guideline was published.

USING THE INTERNET AS A RESOURCE

Search results available from various Internet search engines, such as Google, should be used with caution. Because the Internet is so widely available, the source of information is not always clear. A good example is Wikipedia, an online "dictionary" which allows any individual to contribute regardless of the source or validity of information. Additionally, not all medical literature is indexed on the Internet, further limiting the results of the search. In remote cases, a general Internet search may be useful; however, caution is advised. Results from the Internet should be reserved as the last resort only after an exhaustive search of appropriate databases has been completed.

Several factors should be considered before using information obtained from the Internet in an evidence-based medicine analysis:

1. Documented medical evidence is present with citations, not just opinions
2. Website credibility
3. Author's credibility
4. Date of publication
5. Unbiased tone used
6. Peer reviewed

EVALUATE LITERATURE

Step 3 – Evaluate Literature

After the clinical question has been defined and all pertinent information in answering it has been retrieved, the practitioner will perform a critical literature evaluation on all primary material collected. This third step in the 5-Step Evidence-Based Medicine Process is vital to determine any major limitations in a study and the impact they may have on the results and/or primary outcomes of the study.

Most practitioners have experience in critical literature evaluation. Multiple item checklists are used to identify and evaluate important aspects of a study. While these multiple item lists can be helpful to the evaluator due to the great detail and number of specific points given to address within a study, they can also be time consuming and daunting for the practitioner. Health care professionals have a limited amount of time when deciding what articles to read and critically evaluate.

MULTIPLE ITEM CHECKLISTS

Often multiple item checklists are used as a teaching aid for students who are evaluating literature. An example of a multiple item checklist is provided at the end of this chapter. While these lengthy lists serve a purpose when orienting students to the critical literature evaluation process, they can be a barrier to the busy practitioner trying to assess studies in time-sensitive situations. Many items on multiple item checklists do not have a major impact on the study's overall validity nor do they shed much light on the reliability of the evidence provided by a study. In narrowing down these extensive checklists to the Ten Major Considerations, practitioners will find critical literature evaluation much more functional. The amount of time needed to thoroughly evaluate the integrity of an article is greatly reduced by using the Ten Major Considerations.

TEN MAJOR CONSIDERATIONS

Once the Ten Major Considerations have been integrated into the practitioner's thought process, reading articles and determining their relevance become different. Major limitations that could have a significant impact on the study's integrity are taken into account, thus allowing the practitioner to recognize potential problems with the overall outcome of the study. By evaluating articles from this perspective, the practitioner is able to quickly identify the overall quality of evidence as well as which articles are worth reading.

The Ten Major Considerations provide the practitioner with a concise and quick method to critically evaluate literature, a method that is much less daunting and time consuming compared to using a multiple item checklist. The Ten Major Considerations are presented in the table above and in detail below.

1. Is power set and/or met?

Power is the ability of a study to detect statistically significant differences between treatment groups, when such a difference truly does exist. Once a study is verified as a randomized controlled trial, the practitioner can establish whether or not power was met. To determine this, the description for power should be found in the statistical section of most studies. When deciding whether or not a particular study met power, the practitioner should ask the following questions:

- What is power set at?
- How many patients are needed to meet power?
- What type of analysis is performed on the primary outcome measurements—per protocol or intent-to-treat?
- Does the number of patients used in the analysis meet the sample size required to meet power? If so, one should feel confident that enough patients are included to show a difference if one exists.

EXAMPLE 8

Power is Met

In a study conducted sample size was based on estimated differences in average asthma exacerbation rate between two different therapies. "To identify difference of 20% in the relative risk of exacerbations between salmeterol/ fluticasone propionate (SFC) and formoterol/ budesonide (FBC) combinations, at a two-sided á=0.05 significance level with 90% power using the Normal approximation to the Poisson regression techniques, 525 patients per group were required." Intent-to-treat analyses were used for both primary and secondary outcome measures, with the primary outcome being rate of asthma exacerbations over a 6-month period. The final intent-totreat analysis included 694 patients from the SFC group and 697 patients from the FBC group.

This example clearly states that 525 patients are needed in each treatment group to meet power for the primary outcome. This study undoubtedly met this requirement with both the SFC and BC treatment groups, including well over 525 patients in their final analyses (n=694 and n=697, respectively). It is also important to determine whether or not as per protocol or intent-to-treat analysis was completed when determining power. A per protocol analysis requires knowing the number of patients that completed the study. An intent-to-treat analysis requires knowing the number of patients randomized into the study groups. Note that a modified intent-to treat analysis includes specific criteria that must be met once a patient is randomized into the study (e.g., must have received at least one dose of the study drug or had at least one follow-up visit).

Understanding the importance of power in a study can be of great benefit for the practitioner trying to decipher what literature is worth reading in his or her limited time. In situations where power is not met or not calculated, the next question asked is: "Does a difference exist between treatment groups?" If a statistically significant difference is noted between treatment groups, the fact that the study did not meet power becomes less of a concern. If no statistically significant difference is found between treatment groups, a possibility exists that there were not enough people enrolled in the trial to detect a significant difference. This is a concern. Therefore, a clinician makes best use of time by reading trials that either did meet power or did not meet power but showed a statistically significant difference (potential type II error).

EXAMPLE 9

Power Is Not Met

In a trial performed by Gonzales et al., all study participants were randomized and all efficacy data was compared via intent-to-treat analysis. "A sample size of 335 participants per group was estimated as providing 90% power for a 2-tailed x2 test with ?=0.05 for the comparison between varenicline and bupropion SR for the 4-week continuous abstinence rate based on an odds ratio (OR) of 1.72 vs a bupropion SR response rate of 28.6%." Four-week continuous rates of abstinence between trial weeks 9 through 12 were confirmed via exhaled carbon monoxide. Varenicline (n=352) proved superior to placebo (n=344) (95% CI, 2.70–5.50; P<.001) and buproprion SR (n=329) (95% CI, 1.40–2.68; P<.001).

Are dosages and treatment regimens appropriate? It is important to look at the dosage and/or treatment regimen used for each treatment group in a study. A potential major limitation can exist if a dosage and/or treatment regimen being used is not typically what is seen for the specific indication being addressed. This can help the practitioner recognize if sub- or supra-therapeutic dosing may have an effect on study results. It is also important to consider whether or not equivalent doses of study drugs are being compared. For instance, in a comparative trial evaluating cholesterol-lowering agents, one would not want simvastatin 80 mg to be compared to atorvastatin 10 mg. This comparison could potentially provide an advantage for one drug over the other and confound the results.

EXAMPLE 10

Doses and Regimens are Appropriate

In a study very low birth- weight infants received fluconazole for prevention of fungal infections. For 2 weeks, infants were given 3 or 6 mg of fluconazole every third day; after the 2-week period, this became every other day. Normal saline was given on this same timetable to the placebo group. The study drug was administered intravenously through a catheter, if in use, or an orogastric tube.

In this example, a determination needed to be made in regards to appropriate dosing in the pediatric population. The main concern is safety of the dosage given in this study. Once safety is established, it is then appropriate to determine whether the dose of fluconazole used is similar to doses previously used for this indication.

It is not always clear whether a dosage and/or regimen is appropriate when looking at a study that is investigating a non-FDA approved indication. The safety of the dosage and/or treatment regimen is the primary concern. This can often be determined by reviewing other approved indications for the treatment in question to determine if dosages being used in the trial fall within these approved dosage ranges. In addition, some literature may address dosing for the particular non- FDA approved indication being studied.

EXAMPLE 11

Doses and Regimens for a Non-FDA Approved Indication

A trial examining clomiphene and metformin's efficacy in infertility associated with polycystic ovarian syndrome (PCOS). Metformin and clomiphene were begun concurrently upon study initiation. Patients received met for min 500 mg and clomiphene 50 mg, metformin 500 mg and matching clomiphene placebo matching metformin placebo and clomiphene 50 mg, or just placebo. Subjects receiving metformin 500 mg increased their dosage to two tablets twice daily (maximum dose of four tablets) depending on their tolerability of the drug. Subjects randomized to clomiphene were given one 50-mg clomiphene tablet to be taken for 5 days beginning on the third day of menses. Documentation of adequate ovulation determined whether clomiphene dosage should be maintained. A dosage increase of one additional 50- mg tablet per day was made in patients with no response or minimal response to clomiphene.

In cases where a study is evaluating a non- FDA approved indication like the above example for metformin and polycystic ovarian syndrome (PCOS), the first concern should be for the safety of the particular dosage regimen in patients. Lexi- Comp and Clinical Pharmacology are resources that may include recommended dosing for non-FDA approved indications. If unable to confirm appropriate dosing using these resources, the practitioner's next step is to ensure dosing is within appropriate ranges seen in indications in which the medication has been approved. In this case, the non-FDA approved dose for met for min in PCOS is listed in Clinical Pharmacology as 500 mg three times daily. While the above study uses a higher dosage for PCOS than reported in Clinical Pharmacology (two 500-mg tablets twice daily), it is still considered appropriate because it is not out of range when looking at an FDA-approved indication for metformin such as diabetes.

2. Is the length of the study appropriate to show effect?

A study conducted for an inadequate length of time can result in no treatment effect seen when there really is potential for an effect. In most situations, the concern will be whether or not the trial was conducted for a long enough period of time. For instance, some anti-depressant medications requires 4–6 weeks to see any effect or improvement in patients. A study involving these agents only lasting 3 weeks may not be an adequate amount of time to show any significant differences in efficacy.

3. Are inclusion criteria adequate?

Inclusion criteria are developed primarily to ensure the correct patient population is used to determine efficacy. To participate in any well-designed study, subjects must meet certain criteria before being approved for inclusion in a trial. Investigators identify specific parameters such as age, disease state and/or stage of disease state, sex, treatment history, and other medical conditions that may influence trial results. When inclusion criteria are not properly defined, the possibility exists that a study may be using patients not representative of the population that the investigators intended to treat. Correctly selecting the inclusion criteria for a trial can have a large impact on whether or not the study is clinically relevant to the question being asked. Choosing to include patients outside the target disease state or whose demographics are not appropriate for the desired population may have an impact on the results of the study. In these cases, clinical judgment must be used to determine the extent of the effect.

EXAMPLE 12

Inclusion Criteria

Patients who met proper criteria for migraine with or without aura as determined by the International Headache Society (IHS) were enrolled in the trial. Subjects were required to be in good health and to have had at least a 6-month history of migraines, experiencing between one and eight attacks per month. Enrolled subjects were both male and female aged 18–65 years.

When determining whether or not inclusion criteria are appropriate, it is important to keep in mind why criteria are developed in the first place. Trial investigators must ensure that the correct patient population is used to determine efficacy, otherwise a study may be evaluating a population that is not representative of the one they set out to treat. In the example shown above, it was the investigator's intent to compare two migraine medications within the same class and the effect they had on patients with acute migraine. The inclusion criteria developed in this example resulted in a patient population appropriate for the study. Practitioners who are evaluating inclusion criteria should always ask whether the patient population enrolled is representative of the population they intend to treat.

When evaluating a study for adequate inclusion criteria, the practitioner should also identify any inclusion criteria not mentioned that would be important to the specific trial. If certain inclusion criteria are identified as absent, the practitioner must assess whether or not there is a potential effect on the results due to this deficit.

4. Are exclusion criteria adequate?

Patient safety is the primary focus when establishing exclusion criteria. This is the investigator's opportunity to exclude any patients who may be at risk for increased adverse events and other safety issues by participating in the trial. Just as investigators determine specific parameters or guidelines to establish those patients to be included in a trial, parameters are also established for patients who will be excluded because of safety reasons. Factors such as co-morbid conditions and concurrent medications that have the possibility of increasing the risk of adverse events are taken into consideration.

Exclusion criteria not only ensure safety in a study but guard against inclusion of patients who could potentially decrease one's ability to determine if results are due to the study treatment or another factor. Below are a few examples of these potential factors:

- Previous exposure to the study treatment/similar treatment within 6 months of the study
- Any current medication use that could bias the results
- Certain co-morbid conditions and/or disease states
- Previous procedures affecting the study drug or disease state in question

It is also important to identify instances when exclusion criteria are too restrictive, thus creating a study less relevant to the specific patient population requiring treatment.

EXAMPLE 13

Exclusion Criteria

A multi-center trial to assess low-dose Orlistat effects on body weight of mild to moderately overweight individuals was conducted by Anderson et al. Subjects were excluded if they had any of the following: prior weight loss surgery, prior weight loss of 3 kg or more in the past 3 months, use of any medications that have an effect on weight loss within the past 6 months, bulimia and/or laxative abuse, untreated thyroid disease, history within the past 6 months of CABG or angioplasty procedure with cardiovascular disease, diabetes currently controlled by medication, recent smoking cessation within last 6 months, and use of any medications that interact with orlistat. Pregnant or breastfeeding women were not included.

When determining whether a study has selected appropriate exclusion criteria, emphasis is placed on patient safety. It is the investigator's job to make sure all patients who potentially could be safety risks are excluded from the trial. Many times this means learning more about the medication being studied and its adverse effects. The above exclusion criteria in the orlistat trial adequately addressed safety concerns such as drug interactions, pregnancy, and cardiovascular considerations.

The above trial also accounted for concurrent medications and/or underlying disease states that could have impacted the results. For instance, investigators excluded patients with untreated thyroid disease such as hypothyroidism or any use of pharmacological agents within the last 6 months affecting body weight. With the exclusion of these factors, the investigators decreased the possibility that results of the trial would show anything but the effect orlistat had on weight loss of patients enrolled in the study.

EXAMPLE 14

Exclusion Criteria are Not Adequate

In a study conducted ,treatments for acute migraine were compared. The antimigraine medications were allowed except for the use of NSAIDs, daily analgesics, or propranolol. Pregnant or lactating women were not eligible for inclusion into the study.

The above study defined many exclusion criteria that were appropriate for ensuring the safety of trial participants when using the triptan medications. Unfortunately, the authors neglected one major safety issue with the triptan medications: cardiovascular concerns. Serotonin receptor agonists, such as the triptans, may increase the potential for cardiovascular side effects; this should be addressed within the exclusion criteria. When evaluating the adequacy of exclusion criteria, the practitioner should be familiar with all safety concerns of the particular medication or treatment being studied.

5. Is the study blinded?

An adequately blinded study guards against investigator and subject bias. Typically, one would like to see double-blinded studies because they attempt to prevent the largest degree of investigator or patient bias in a trial. In single-blinded studies (where either the investigator or patient is not blinded to the intervention), there is a greater chance for bias to confound the results.

The exact method of blinding is seldom explained in the article. Rather, a statement that the study was blinded is usually seen. The practitioner should question whether there were any potential barriers . for example a peculiar smell or taste characteristic of the study drug should also be reproduced for the control(s) to maintain blinding. That smell or taste in some cases can be masked for the study drug. In either situation, an explanation of how this was handled should be provided. If there is no explanation, the practitioner must assume the issue was not addressed. Blinding is considered a major limitation when this occurs; however, the practitioner still needs to assess whether that major limitation had any effect on the overall results/conclusions.

EXAMPLE 15

Blinding

A double-blind, placebo-controlled trial in patients with pulmonary hypertension performed used a stratified central-randomization scheme to allocate patients to their four respective treatment groups (sildenafil 20, 40, or 80 mg or placebo). Dose escalation took place for the first 7 days of the study for those patients assigned to the 80-mg treatment group. They received 40 mg three times daily for 7 days and then moved up to 80 mg three times daily. Dummy dose escalation was also performed for the other three treatment groups during the first 7 days.

Although the trial described above was double blinded and took measures to conceal dose escalation in the sildenafil 80-mg treatment group, there is still potential for blinding to be flawed. Sildenafil's side effect profile includes incidence of penile erection in male patients, which could potentially cause patients to become unblinded to their respective treatment groups. The authors do not address thispotential weakness in the blinding of the study.

6. Did randomization result in similar groups?

When randomization is successful, each patient has an equal chance of being assigned to one treatment group versus the other(s). Even more critical is that the trial ends up with very similar groups demo-graphically following randomization. If a significant disparity is found between treatment groups, there is concern about whether the results observed are due to the study drug or a difference that was present between groups from the start. For instance, in a clinical trial evaluating the efficacy of an asthma medication, it is important that a similar number of smokers are randomized to each treatment group. If groups are dissimilar, the results seen may not accurately depict the medication's efficacy and may potentially be due to a lower or higher number of smokers being randomized to a particular group.

The demographics table in a study is useful for confirming similar treatment groups. When dissimilarities are found, it is important to question what impact or clinical relevance the dissimilarity could have had on the results. For instance, disease states often have many levels of severity. If one treatment group has more severe patients than the other after randomization, the drug's efficacy may be falsely reported as reduced in that group compared to the group with less severe patients. The practitioner must also be aware of any additional demographic information that should have been collected or discussed but was not. If this occurs, it is important to question what impact this discrepancy may have had on the results.

EXAMPLE 16

Similar Groups after Randomization and Statistics

A modified table below illustrates baseline characteristics seen in a trial evaluating the effects on fracture rate of continuing or stopping alendronate after 5 years of treatment .

The above example demonstrates how some trials display demographic data. Statistics were run on the demographic data above, helping the practitioner to detect any significant differences seen in baseline characteristics after randomization. When studies provide statistical information on baseline data, it makes identifying significant differences much easier. For instance, if p-values were not provided, one might question whether or not a significant difference was seen. No significant differences were seen in the above example. If a significant difference had been seen, the practitioner should question what impact the difference would have had on the results of the trial.

EXAMPLE 17

Similar Groups after Randomization and No Demographic Table

In a study conducted "the baseline demographics of the placebo and orlistat groups were similar. Of the 378 subjects, 94.4% were female (n=357), 89.2% were white (n=337), average (+SD) age was 46.2 + 11.41 years, baseline weight was 72.8 + 6.97 kg, and BMI was 26.8 + 0.96 kg/m2."

Not all studies will address the similarity of demographics among treatment groups after randomization in the same way. For instance, the above example is from a trial that just briefly mentioned groups were similar in the text of the article. No chart or statistics were given. In these cases, the practitioner must decide whether this major consideration was adequately addressed and what impact may be seen on the results.

Although a chart was provided in this study to illustrate baseline characteristics, the table was not analyzed for statistically significant differences seen. In these instances, the practitioner must use clinical judgment to determine if any demographic information appears to be significantly different. If something is identified, the next step is questioning what effect that difference will have on results.

When analyzing data using a per protocol analysis, one should ensure that groups are similar at the end of the study. A per protocol analysis utilizes the results seen in each of the treatment groups at the completion of a study. Patients withdraw from studies for various reasons, which can result in different groups at the end of the trial. When evaluating a study using a per protocol analysis, the evaluator should attempt to determine if the groups are similar at completion of the trial. When a difference between groups occurs at the end of a study, it is important to question what impact or clinical relevance the dissimilarity may have on results.

Finally, it is important to remember that even a well planned and adequately conducted randomization can fail and result in dissimilar groups. In this instance, the practitioner evaluating the study must determine if these differences have any significant impact on the results.

7. Are appropriate statistical tests used for type(s) of data analyzed?

The reader must determine if the appropriate statistical test was used for the type of data analyzed. This particular consideration tends to create the most difficulty for the practitioner. Using the incorrect statistical test for the type of data analyzed can have serious negative impact on the results, making them impossible to interpret accurately. When the incorrect statistical test is used for the type of data analyzed, the results should not be trusted unless the authors have provided an adequate explanation why the tests in question were used. Luckily for the practitioner, this determination does not have to be such a tedious and puzzling process. When one is equipped with the right tools, identifying the correct statistical test in a trial can be straightforward. A good understanding of the different types of data (nominal, ordinal, interval, and ratio) used in trials and access to an appropriate statistical test reference is all that is necessary. A chart detailing when certain statistical tests should or should not be used is found in

8. Are evaluation measurements standard, validated, or accepted practice?

When choosing how to accurately measure the primary outcome of a study, the investigators should select evaluation measurements that are validated or accepted in practice. In addition, it is important to verify that the outcome measure being used is relevant to the disease state in question. For instance, weight loss should not be used as a primary outcome measure in a trial investigating the efficacy of an oral diabetic agent in lowering blood glucose levels.

EXAMPLE 18

Appropriate Evaluation Tool

In a trial performed the efficacy of sildenafil versus placebo for primary pulmonary hypertension was studied. The Naughton protocol was used to help evaluate the primary endpoint of the study, which was "change in exercise time on treadmill."

It is important to establish the appropriateness of both the primary outcome of a study as well as the evaluation tool used to measure that primary outcome. Determining whether an outcome measure and/or evaluation tool is validated or accepted in practice can be done in a variety of different ways. For instance, the above example uses "change in exercise time on treadmill" as the primary outcome measure and the Naughton protocol as the evaluation tool. A quick literature search confirms that both this outcome measure and evaluation tool is frequently used when looking at the disease state of primary pulmonary hypertension. Also, the Naughton protocol is described in many clinical exercise physiology textbooks as being an approved method for treadmill tests. Therefore, both the outcome measure and tool are validated and accepted methods in practice.

Even if the results of a study are statistically significant, they are questionable and potentially not applicable if an inappropriate evaluation method is used to measure the primary outcome.

If you are unfamiliar with an outcome measure or test being used in a particular study, further investigation is warranted. When the measurement or test in question is referenced, the practitioner can go to the reference cited to determine if the measurement or test has been validated and/or is an accepted practice. In cases where the evaluation tool in question has not been referenced, the following questions may be asked when determining the appropriateness of the outcome measure or test.

- Do studies looking at this same outcome use this particular evaluation tool?
- Is this method or test validated?
- Does the evaluation method being used measure something that is clinically relevant to the disease state or medication being studied?
- Is this a new trend being used to evaluate this specific outcome?

CATEGORIZE QUALITY OF EVIDENCE

Step 4 – Categorize Quality of Evidence

After completing the critical evaluation of a specific trial, the practitioner needs to categorize the quality of evidence.

For instance, a randomization scheme, comparison group, and adequate sample size are specific study design characteristics. In addition, key attributes that strengthen or weaken the basic study design are considered.

These key attributes are represented by the Ten Major Considerations that were previously used to critically evaluate articles. Both components of the quality of evidence equation (specific study design characteristics and key study attributes) are required for an accurate categorization of the quality of evidence.

Levels of Evidence—Specific Study Design Characteristics

A ranking system referred to as levels of evidence is utilized to categorize studies based on quality of design.

Several methods exist to categorize a study's level of evidence.1–8 The method used in this chapter provides a simple, straightforward, and logical approach. The process is based on four specific study design characteristics that assist in categorizing studies by their respective levels of evidence. These specific study design characteristics are

1. Interventional or observational study design
2. Controlled or non-controlled study design
3. Randomized or non-randomized study design
4. Power set/met or not set/met for the study design

EXAMPLE 19

Relationship Between Study Design Characteristics and Levels of Evidence

A randomized, controlled trial comparing two different drugs for use in irritable bowel syndrome could be

- Level I if powered to show a difference if one really existed.
- Level II if power is not met or not initially set to show a difference if one existed. Studies used to observe changes such as incidence of constipation versus diarrhea associated with irritable bowel syndrome without intervention in a population of patients over time could be
- Level III if a prospective observational study design is used.
- Level IV if a retrospective observational study design is used.

  A testimonial of how well stress reduction exercises reduce irritable bowel symptoms in a single patient or series of patients would be considered
- Level V since no randomization scheme, control group, or set power exists.

The progression from Level I to Level V represents a decrease in quality of study design and, therefore, reliability of results provided by that particular trial. As the evidence used to develop a recommendation decreases in quality (Level I going to Level V), the overall strength of that recommendation also decreases. In other words, Level I evidence represents the highest possible level of study design quality; Level V evidence represents the lowest level of study design quality. Recommendations are developed from the highest level of evidence available. When no evidence exists, recommendations are made based on experience which can overestimate efficacy and underestimate safety risks.

FIVE QUESTIONS TO ASK

Five questions are asked to determine existence of these specific study design characteristics within a particular trial.

Diagrams are provided to help illustrate the differences between the five levels of evidence.

Question #1: Does the study have an intervention or is it strictly observational?

In other words, are patients being assigned a specific therapy or intervention?

Level I and Level II evidence are represented by trials with an interventional study design .The investigators are assigning a specific intervention to each subject. For instance, a trial to identify the effects of an anti-diabetic agent would require a group of subjects to be given the intervention (drug).

Levels III and IV evidence is represented by trials with an observational study design. In observational trials, investigators are merely observing the subjects and no intervention is being assigned. Subjects are chosen based on presence or absence of specific characteristics. A trial observing what complications occur to diabetic patients with lack of long-term glycemic control versus diabetic patients with long-term glycemic control is considered an observational trial.

Level V evidence is represented by trials with either an interventional or observational study design.

Note that trials utilizing an interventional study design represent the higher levels of evidence (Levels I, II). Those trials utilizing an observational study design represent a lower level of evidence (Level III, IV), and the trial design representing the lowest level of evidence is Level V. The progression from Level I to Level V evidence represents a decrease in quality of trial design and, therefore, reliability of results provided by that particular trial. A decrease in quality and reliability of evidence corresponds to a decrease in overall strength of the recommendation being developed.

Question #2: Does the study have a control group?

Level I and Level II evidence are represented by trials with a control group . Control groups provide a comparison to ensure that changes seen in the intervention group are due to something other than chance.

Level III and Level IV evidence are also represented by trials with a control group. This control group can be either prospective or retrospective in nature. As with interventional trials, the control group serves as a way to ensure that changes seen in the study group are due to something other than chance.

Level V evidence is represented by trials without a control group. Without a control group, there is no way to confirm that changes seen in a subject or group of subjects are due to something other than chance. Essentially, Level V trials are equivalent to personal testimonials. Level V trials typically consist of a single-case study, case series, and/or case report.

Note that trials containing a control group represent the higher levels of evidence (Levels I through IV). Those trials containing no control group represent the lowest level of evidence (Level V). The progression from Level I to Level V evidence represents a decrease in the quality of the trial design and, therefore, reliability of the results provided by that particular trial. Without high quality and reliable evidence, the strength of the recommendation is compromised.

Question #3: Does the observational study look forward or backward in time (prospective or retrospective)?

Level III evidence is represented by observational trials that look forward in time using prospective cohort groups of subjects. In prospective observational trials, the investigators define the disease and the predicted variables prior to the onset of disease. Subjects are chosen based on specific characteristics (e.g., smoking) and followed forward in time to observe the development of a specific outcome (e.g., lung cancer).

EXAMPLE 20

Level III Prospective Observational Trial

Level III evidence is represented by a trial such as the Harvard Nurse's Health Study II that is considered one of the most significant studies conducted on the health of women. This study has been following nurses and the progression of their health since 1989. An example of the results includes the long-term effect of moderate alcohol consumption on the nurse's cognitive function.

In this analysis, cognitive function was monitored over time in nurses consuming moderate quantities of alcohol. A similar group of nurses who were not consuming alcohol were followed simultaneously over the same time period and represent the prospective cohort comparison group.

Level IV evidence is represented by observational trials that look back in time using retrospective cohort or case control groups. For instance, investigators will examine the data for a group of subjects with a diagnosis of lung cancer and examine smoking history of the group to determine if an association exists between smoking and development of lung cancer.

EXAMPLE 21

Level IV Retrospective Observational Trial

An observational study is designed to examine the differences in lifestyle between patients that have developed esophageal cancer versus those who have not developed this disease. The investigators randomly select charts from an institution's medical records of patients who developed esophageal cancer. Various characteristics such as lifestyle are identified that may have led to the development of the esophageal cancer such as a consistent diet of extremely spicy foods.

Note that observational trials using a prospective design represent a higher level of evidence (Level III) than trials containing a retrospective design, which represent a lower level of evidence (Level IV). Trials using a prospective design have less potential for bias interfering with the results than those with a retrospective design. The progression from Level III to Level IV evidence represents a decrease in quality of the trial design and, therefore, reliability of results provided by that particular trial. Only high quality and reliable evidence can provide a strong recommendation.

Question #4: Is the study randomized?

Level I and Level II trials utilize a randomization scheme to assign patients to study groups (see Figure 6.6). Randomization, when done correctly, ensures each subject has an equal chance of being assigned to either of the study groups. The result of a trial with a successful randomization scheme has study groups with similar demographic characteristics following the randomization process; differences in an outcome measure between groups at the end of the study are more likely attributable to the intervention.

Level III, Level IV, and Level V trials do not utilize a randomization scheme to assign patients into various groups. Rather, subjects to be entered into the trial can be chosen at random. For instance, out of a potential subject pool of 500, the investigators randomly select 300 subjects for the study.

EXAMPLE 22

Random Selection of Subjects for Observational Trials

A prospective observational trial (Level III) examining the long-term effects of smoking would include subjects randomly selected from a pool of subjects with a history of smoking. These patients are followed forward in time to observe the development of specific outcomes (e.g., lung cancer).

Note that trials utilizing a randomization scheme to assign patients to study groups represent the higher level of evidence (Level I and Level II). Those trials utilizing no randomization scheme represent the lower levels of evidence (Levels III, IV, and V). A successful randomization scheme assures that each patient has an equal opportunity of being assigned to one group versus another, and this should result in demographically similar groups. Changes noted in the study results can then be attributed to something other than starting out with dissimilar groups. The progression from Level I to Level V evidence represents a decrease in quality of the trial design and, therefore, reliability of results provided by that particular trial. The strength of the recommendation is decreased when the quality and reliability of the evidence is low.

Question #5: If the study is an interventional randomized and controlled trial, is power met?

Level I evidence is represented by trials where power is set and met. In these trials, the sample size is adequate to show a difference between study groups, if a difference really exists.

Level II evidence is represented by trials where power is set and not met or power is not set or not mentioned at all. Power especially becomes important when no statistically significant difference is found between the treatment groups. In this situation, a difference between treatment groups may have been observed if additional patients were enrolled to meet power. For this reason, no definitive conclusion can be made that the groups are similar.

Note that trials where power is set and met represent the higher level of evidence (Level I). Those trials where power is set and not met or not mentioned represent the lower level of evidence (Level II). Basics for Interpretation power is used to determine an adequate sample size that will show a difference between treatment groups, if a difference really exists. The progression from Level I to Level II evidence represents a decrease in quality of the trial design and, therefore, reliability of results provided by that particular trial. Higher quality and reliability of evidence is associated with an overall increase in strength of the recommendation.

Ten Major Considerations—Key Study Attributes

As discussed earlier, the second part of the quality of evidence equation is the consideration of key study attributes that strengthen or weaken the basic study design. These key study attributes are represented by the Ten Major Considerations used to critically evaluate an article.

If one of the Ten Major Considerations (key studies attribute) is present in the study, that attribute is considered a major strength. However, if that same major consideration or key study attribute is absent or lacking, a major limitation is determined to exist for that study.

The next question to ask when a major limitation is identified is whether this limitation appears to have an effect on the overall study results. If the answer is yes to that question, then the overall quality of that trial is lessened, even though the level of evidence remains the same.

EXAMPLE 23

Major Limitation: Impact versus No Impact on Study Results

A Level I trial has a major limitation of randomization not resulting in similar groups. Upon further inspection, this appeared to have an effect on the results making them questionable. That Level I trial would have a lesser overall quality of evidence than a Level I trial with randomization identified as a major limitation and no effect on the results noted.

DEVELOP A CONCLUSION AND RECOMMENDATION

Step 5 – Develop a Conclusion and Recommendation

The fifth step of the 5-Step Evidence-Based Medicine Process, Develop a Conclusion and Recommendation may be the most important task and yet can be the most challenging for the practitioner. This is the step that provides a solid and defendable recommendation. The degree of confidence in the recommendation and the justifications supporting that recommendation are based on the quality of evidence available. Essentially, the recommendation is as strong as the supporting evidence. A recommendation developed following the 5-Step Evidence-Based Medicine Process is easy to support and defend because the highest quality of evidence has been utilized.

ORGANIZING THE PERTINENT INFORMATION

Once the evidence has been retrieved, analyzed, and categorized by quality, sorting the pertinent information by level of evidence is extremely helpful to begin developing a conclusion. By organizing the evidence from the highest to lowest in confidence (levels of evidence and major limitations), the practitioner can begin to identify the most reliable information to develop a conclusion.

DEVELOPING A CONCLUSION FROM THE SUMMARY

The conclusion becomes more apparent as results from the highest level of evidence are compared and contrasted in the Summary Table of Evidence Evaluated. By reviewing these findings in more detail, the practitioner will be able to identify the differences between the highest quality trials. These differences are important in fine-tuning the conclusion and one's degree of confidence in that conclusion.

For example, a conclusion that Drug A has equivalent efficacy compared to Drug B can be made from the single Level I trial with no major limitations. The major limitation of power not being met puts the first Level II trial in question. When power has not been met and there is no difference between treatment groups, the concern is that a difference may have been shown if enough patients had been entered to meet power.

After careful review, it is determined that there is no way to assess whether this major limitation had an effect on the overall study results; however, one should assume that it did affect the overall results. The second Level II trial has this same major limitation in addition to a question about whether the higher dose used for Drug A may have given that drug an unfair advantage. If a normal therapeutic dose of Drug A would have been used, Drug A may have been less effective than Drug B. There is no way to determine if this major limitation had an effect on the overall study results. To be on the conservative side, one should assume that this major limitation did have an effect on the overall results.

This example illustrates the necessity for including the major limitations to help determine overall confidence in a study's results. If major limitations are not taken into consideration, an inappropriate conclusion may be reached. Even with a high level of evidence, overall reliability of the trial could be reduced by one major limitation such as dissimilar groups after randomization.

It is crucial to determine whether the results appear to be affected by an identified major limitation. After this determination, a decision can be made to either include the trial results as reliable or discredit findings and exclude the trial.

DEVELOPING A RECOMMENDATION FROM THE CONCLUSION

From Conclusion to Recommendation

Even the simplest decision involves a process that must occur between forming a conclusion and developing a recommendation. Three components are involved in this.

The first component (quality of the evidence) is a result of Step 3: Evaluate Literature and Step 4: Categorize the Quality of Evidence of the 5-Step Evidence-Based Medicine Process outlined in this book. The quality of the available evidence is considered in addition to major strengths and limitations of studies that make up this available evidence. When developing a recommendation, the practitioner should know that the overall reliability of the evidence is important.

Logical reasoning, the second component, requires both deductive and inductive reasoning. This component provides practicality in forming the recommendation. For instance, when no head-to-head comparative trials exist or two drugs, other trials with identical control groups for each drug in similar patient populations may be used along with logical reasoning to draw conclusions that go into the recommendation.

The third component, clinical judgment, comes from experience as a clinical practitioner. Clinical judgment fills in gaps where evidence does not exist or is weak. For instance, a practitioner's clinical experience reveals that with a specific patient, drugs from the same pharmacological class have different degrees of efficacy. Based on this clinical judgment, the practitioner may suggest changing to a different drug in the same pharmacological class to assist in identifying the optimal agent.

For extremely complex decisions leading to recommendations, formal decision analysis processes are used. The primary tool utilized is the decision tree.

Type of Decision

An individual patient decision is represented by a typical treatment plan developed for a single patient. Both decisions are important and will affect health care for patients.

The population-based decision is typically made in a more conservative manner since many patients will be affected and little is known about the specifics of each patient in this population.

When details about a single patient's disease and medication history are known, the practitioner can customize the decision to fit that individual patient. Knowing these specifics allows the practitioner to use clinical judgment associated with that individual. With an understanding of the type of clinical decision being made (individual patient versus population-based), the practitioner can modify the final recommendation to fit the type of decision.

EXAMPLE 24

Developing a Recommendation Based on Type of Decision

Clinical Question – Is Drug A as efficacious and safe as Drug B, currently on the formulary?

Here is what we know from the evidence:

1. Conclusion from evidence – Drug A and Drug B have equivalent efficacy and safety with no specific advantage of one over the other. Drug A is considerably more expensive than Drug B.
2. This is supported by a Level I trial with no major limitations.
3. The two Level II trials are not considered since they were not powered to show a difference, if one existed and no difference between treatment groups was noted.
4. This is a population-based decision; therefore, a conservative stance needs to be taken with the clinical decision to be made here. If this were an individual patient decision, the practitioner would want to assess any subgroup analyses that may pertain to the specific patient. With this in mind, a completely different recommendation could be required.

   Recommendation Statement: I do not recommend adding Drug A to the formulary. (Note: The degree of confidence one has in this recommendation still need to be fully determined to adjust the overall tone of the statement. This will be explained in the next section.)

Confidence of the Recommendation

The confidence of a recommendation depends on the quality of evidence supporting that recommendation statement. The degree of confidence one has in the evidence is important when determining how strongly to state the recommendation. To assist in determining strength of the recommendation statement, the Grade of Recommendation

Tool is used. The highest level of evidence (Level I) is also the evidence that carries the greatest confidence.

EXAMPLE 25

Strength of Recommendation Statement Based on Confidence in Evidence

Taking the previous example where the conclusion was that Drug A and Drug B have equivalent efficacy based on a Level 1 study with no major limitations, it is clear that this Level of Evidence provides a Grade A Recommendation. This is the highest Level of Evidence available to support the recommendation and, therefore, a strong and firm tone should be used in the recommendation statement if no major limitations exist.

Format for the Recommendation

Recommendations should include a statement with justification points that support the recommendation. Although various formats can be used to present a recommendation, a clear and concise statement is important to ensure effective communication. This template can be modified to fit various styles, but two primary components should be present—a clear and concise recommendation statement followed by supportive justification points.

EXAMPLE 26

The Recommendation Statement

I strongly recommend that Drug A not replace Dug B on the formulary, but be reserved as second- line therapy for allergic conjunctivitis only after Drug B has been tried and failed.

Support for the Recommendation

Justification points provide clear and concise support, similar to "pillars," for the recommendation statement. Each justification point includes the efficacy, safety, special considerations/ special populations, and cost associated with a specific situation. Information obtained from the evidence should be addressed under each of these considerations:

Efficacy

- Summary of the highest level of evidence trial(s) beingused to develop the recommendation statement.
- Specifically what that evidence confirms. Any major limitations identified along with the determined impact that those limitations may have on the results, especially the primary outcome measure(s).
- Any outcomes that are of interest to the clinical question.

Safety

- Description of adverse drug reactions noted especially those different from the comparison group(s).
- A statement of overall safety profile and any safety concern(s). This should be obtained from information that includes the greatest number of patients exposed (usually, the Package Insert/Prescribing Information) to attempt to identify rare adverse drug reactions.

Special considerations/special populations

- This is a very broad scope category, and the content is highly dependent upon the defined clinical question. Some types of special considerations that would be appropriate to include are differences in dosing convenience and route of administration between the drugs in question.

- Any knowledge gained that addresses the advantages and/ or disadvantages of the study drug over existing therapy.
- Specific populations that need to be highlighted due to the drug's benefit or disadvantages on those populations should be addressed.
- Any knowledge gained from the study that provides an understanding of how and where this drug fits in overall therapeutic strategies and standard practice guidelines should be included.

Cost

- Differences in cost between the treatments studied including nursing/ pharmacy and other related costs, if possible.
- Differences in cost compared to current standard of care treatment.
- Any impact associated with these differences in cost (both savings and/or expenditures).

The following example illustrates effective use of justification points to support/ defend the previously developed recommendation statement.

APPLICATIONS

Incorporating Evidence-Based Clinical Decision Making into Clinical Practice

How do practitioners incorporate evidence-based decision making into clinical practice? By following the five-step process outlined throughout this book, pharmacy practitioners can assess the evidence available and make either **1.** firm recommendations and decisions based on results of rigorously controlled investigations or **2.** cautious recommendations and decisions when results of uncontrolled clinical observations exist. Evidence-based medicine, when used in pharmacy, is applied in various situations. This chapter will examine several examples of how pharmacy practitioners can use evidence-based medicine in clinical practice when making both individual patient decisions as well as population-based decisions.

Individual patient decisions are made frequently in pharmacy and often require a less conservative approach due to the fact that more information is available regarding an individual versus an entire population. Practitioners must look at the patient as a whole and consider many factors when making a recommendation or decision regarding an individual's health. As discussed previously, it is imperative to consider efficacy, safety, special considerations/ special populations, and cost when making a clinical decision or recommendation. This also applies to individual patients.

The clinician should apply the 5-Step Evidence-Based Medicine Process to determine if the treatment option is efficacious. Various sources of evidence should be reviewed such as interventional or observational clinical trials, case control studies, case series, or individual case studies. By assessing risk versus benefit, the practitioner can determine if the efficacy of the therapy outweighs the harm if any it may cause to the patient.

Other important aspects to consider when looking at the safety justification of a patient-specific decision are allergies, concomitant medications and potential drug interactions, current disease states and interactions that may be associated with them, and compliance/adherence concerns.

Special populations that should be considered include dosing convenience, route of administration, specific situations that may affect the patient positively or negatively, and advantages or disadvantages over lack of treatment or existing treatment. Specifically, "Is there a population that may especially benefit from the recommendation?" An angiotensin-converting enzyme inhibitor, for instance, would benefit a kidney failure patient who also has hypertension.

Finally, cost should be considered. "Can the patient afford the treatment?" "Are there patient assistance programs available to help with affordability of the therapy?" "Is there a significant cost associated with the treatment such as travel expenses or medical devices used for administration?" "Would any additional cost be outweighed by preventing future complications or morbidity or mortality?"

By factoring efficacy, safety, special considerations/special populations, and cost into forming a decision as well as assessing risk versus benefit, practitioners can be assured that an appropriate individual patient decision is made.

Population-based clinical decisions differ from individual ones in that a more conservative approach is required because fewer specifics are known. When formulating a recommendation for a population such as a medication class review, comparative analyses, or a formulary request, the clinician's decision is affecting a large number of people who have many different disease states, different medication regimens, and different compliance issues. These decisions, similar to individual patient decisions, also require the practitioner to consider efficacy, safety, special considerations/ special populations, and cost when making a recommendation.

The efficacy justification to support population-based decisions often is derived from evidence such as interventional or observational clinical trials, case control studies, or well designed meta-analyses or systematic reviews. The safety considerations of a population-based decision should be assessed by reviewing the evidence as well as the most current prescribing information.

As with individual clinical decisions, it is imperative that the following special considerations/special populations are taken into account for population-based recommendations: dosing convenience, route of administration, specific situations that may affect the population positively or negatively, and advantages or disadvantages of the treatment.

When formulating a recommendation for a population, practitioners have fewer known specifics regarding prescription coverage, patient income, and other variables; therefore, cost is typically one of the final components to consider. Sometimes the question is asked, "How much better should one drug be in terms of efficacy, safety, or special considerations/special populations to justify the additional expense?" If efficacy, safety, and special considerations/special populations are the same between comparative drugs, one can consider cost to be the primary determinant.

Examples

The following examples are provided to illustrate application of the evidence-based process described in this book to both individual patient and population-based decisions.

EXAMPLE 27

Individual Patient Clinical Decision/ Recommendation

This example illustrates how to use the 5-Step Evidence-Based Medicine Process to assist in making a clinical decision/ recommendation for an individual patient.

A physician wants to give BP, a male patient, Drug A for treatment of his osteoporosis instead of Drug B because Drug A can be given once per month whereas Drug B requires weekly administration. Somewhere the pharmacist read or heard that Drug A was not as effective in male osteoporosis as Drug B. Before the pharmacist calls the physician to discuss this issue, he or she should conduct an evidence-based medicine analysis to confirm that Drug A is not as effective as Drug B in male osteoporosis.

Patient Background:

63-year-old Male

No known drug allergies

Past medical history:

Hypertension—controlled on lisinopril

Type 2 diabetes—controlled on metformin and insulin glargine

Hypercholesterolemia—uncontrolled on simvastatin; ezetimibe added at most recent visit with physician

Prescription coverage that discounts all medications

Step 1: Define the Clinical Question

- Determine the actual question being asked so that an appropriate response is formed. For this example, the question would be "Is Drug A as effective as Drug B in the treatment of male osteoporosis for BP?"

Step 2: Retrieve Pertinent Information

A literature search was performed using two databases and the following search terms: Drug A (brand and generic names), Drug B (brand and generic names), osteoporosis, male. After reviewing the search results from both databases using appropriate limits and the search and sift technique, the clinician found two key articles. The clinician performed a bibliographic search by reviewing the references of the two articles found. This technique led to a case series. Overall, the literature search revealed the following articles:

- Article #1 – A randomized, double-blind, parallel group study in male patients with osteoporosis compared Drugs A and B. Power was set and met; that is, sample size was adequate to show a difference between study groups, if a difference really exists. One major limitation was noted; the groups were not similar after randomization. No other limitations were identified from the ten major considerations list. The results of the study showed that Drug B was superior to Drug A for the treatment of male osteoporosis, and this difference was statistically significant (p=0.001). There was no difference in the incidence or severity of adverse drug reactions between the two drugs. No special considerations/special populations were noted.

- Article #2 – A randomized, double-blind, crossover study in male patients with osteoporosis compared Drugs A and B for treatment. Power was set and met, thus indicating an adequate sample size has been used t show a difference between Drugs A and B, if a difference really exists. No other major limitations were noted. The results of this study showed that Drugs A and B are equivalent in efficacy for the treatment of male osteoporosis (p=0.26). In addition, no difference in the incidence or severity of adverse drug reactions between the two drugs was noted. No special considerations/special populations were identified. The two drugs were similar in price.
- Article #3 – A case series of male patients with osteoporosis was studied. These patients were observed over a 1-year period after being placed on Drug A by the primary physician. There was an improvement noted in bone density tests after 1 year of receiving Drug A. Some adverse drug reactions were noted, but they were anticipated based on the package insert information and were not severe. No special considerations/ special populations were noted.
- The two drugs are similar in price; however, Drug A is covered by prescription insurance.

Step 3: Evaluate Literature

Efficacy

- Critically evaluate each trial and determine if the article supports or refutes the use of Drug A over Drug B
  - Article #1 – The results of the study showed that Drug B was superior to Drug A for the treatment of male osteoporosis, and this difference was statistically significant (p=0.001).
  - Article #2 – The results of this study showed that Drugs A and B are equivalent in efficacy for the treatment of male osteoporosis (p=0.26).
  - Article #3 – There was an improvement noted in bone density tests after 1 year of receiving Drug A; however, statistics were not performed since there was no comparison group.
- Establish if each trial has major or minor limitations.
  - Article #1 – The groups were not similar in baseline bone mineral density scores after randomization, and this appeared to have potentially affected the results. No other major limitation was identified.
  - Article #2 – No major limitations from the ten major considerations list were noted
  - Article #3 – This study was a case series and, therefore, did not have a comparative group. Due to this study design, several of the ten major considerations were considered to be major limitations.

Safety

- Assess risk versus benefit of Drug A versus Drug B versus no treatment.
  - Article #1 – No difference was noted in the incidence or severity of adverse drug reactions between the two drugs.

- Article #2 – No difference was noted in the incidence or severity of adverse drug reactions between the two drugs.
- Article #3 – Some adverse drug reactions were noted, but they were anticipated based on the package insert information for Drug A and were not severe. Note there was no comparison group.

• Special considerations/special populations
• Establish if Drug A is dosed more or less conveniently than Drug B.

- Drug A is dosed once monthly compared to Drug B, which is weekly.

• Does the route of administration vary between drugs?
• Determine any potential advantages or disadvantages of Drug A versus Drug B.

Step 4: Categorize the Quality of Evidence

✓ Determine the level of evidence for each trial, including the major and minor limitations identified.

• Article #1 is a Level I trial with the major limitation that the two groups are not similar after randomization, which appears to have affected the results.
• Article #2 is a Level I trial with minor limitations.
• Article #3 is a Level V trial with major limitations

Step 5: Develop a Conclusion and Recommendation

✓ Develop a conclusion regarding the overall efficacy based on the evidence.

• Drug A is equivalent to Drug B in overall efficacy.

✓ Develop a conclusion regarding the overall safety based on the evidence.

• Drugs A and B have similar safety profiles.

✓ Review patient's allergies and potential drug-drug or drug–disease interactions to limit adverse events.

• No drug–drug interactions were identified with current therapy.

✓ Develop a conclusion regarding any special considerations/special populations.

• Drug A is administered significantly less frequently than Drug B.

✓ Develop a conclusion regarding the overall cost of medication specific to this individual patient based on the following:

• Can the patient afford this medication? - Insurance coverage BP's insurance covers Drug A.

- Patient assistance programs available

• Are there other cost concerns associated with the treatment?
• Are there long-term cost-saving benefits of Drug A or Drug B?

✓ Assign the appropriate grade of recommendation based on the quality of evidence available

✓ Develop a recommendation based on conclusions made and applied to this individual patient.

✓ Example:
I strongly recommend using Drug A for the treatment of osteoporosis in BP for the following reasons: (Grade A Recommendation)

• Efficacy – A Level I trial showed that Drugs A and B were equivalent in efficacy for treating male osteoporosis. A second Level I trial showed that Drug B was superior to Drug A in the treatment of male osteoporosis; however, this trial had a major limitation that discredited the results. As additional support, a case series noted an improvement in the bone density test after 1 year of receiving Drug A.

- Safety – There appeared to be no difference in adverse drug reactions between Drugs A and B. No drug–drug interactions were noted with BP's current medication regimen. BP has no known drug allergies; therefore, it's not an issue.
- Special considerations/special populations – Drug A would allow the patient once monthly dosing, thus possibly increasing compliance.
- Cost – Drugs A and B are similar in price. Drug A will be a less expensive choice for BP since his prescription insurance coverage includes Drug A.

EXAMPLE 28

Population-Based Decision/ Recommendation

This example illustrates how to compile a class review or comparative review to assist in the formulary management decision making process.

Step 1: Define the Clinical Question

✓ Determine the actual question being asked so that an appropriate response is formed. For this example, the question would be "Is there a specific drug(s) that is superior to the others within the class?"

Step 2: Retrieve Pertinent Information

✓ Become familiar with class by reading tertiary textbook resources, compendia class summaries, recent review articles, or class reviews.

✓ Identify medications to be compared and identify FDA-approved indications.

✓ Complete a literature search for Level I or II comparative trials by searching various databases. Using the "search and sift" technique, narrow the search to randomized, controlled trials with or without power met in human subjects. In order to ensure a thorough search is accomplished, be sure to complete a bibliographic search of all relevant articles.

- The search should compare drugs in the same class, not drugs compared to other classes or the drug compared to placebo, if possible.
- If head-to-head comparison trials do not exist, then consider using placebo-controlled trials or trials comparing the class to the same drug that maybe is outside of the class.

Step 3: Evaluate Literature

✓ Efficacy

- Review each trial and determine if the article supports or refutes the use of one drug over another.
- Establish if each trial has major or minor limitations.

✓ Safety

- Assess safety of the drugs within the class when compared in the literature.
- Obtain the most recent package inserts to help determine possible safety concerns; safety information should always be derived from package inserts rather than individual trials. Larger patient population exposure and possibly longer patient exposure are found in package inserts.

✓ Special considerations/special populations

- Establish if one drug is dosed more or less conveniently than the other(s).
- Does the route of administration vary between drugs?

- Determine if there are other potential advantages or disadvantages of the drugs within the class.

✓ Cost

- Is the cost significantly lower for one drug?
- Are there long-term cost-saving benefits?
- When formulating a recommendation for a population, fewer specifics are known regarding prescription coverage, patient income, and other variables; therefore, cost is typically one of the final components to consider when forming the recommendation.
- Identify differentiating characteristics for medications within the class by indication and use to aid in formulating evidence based conclusion.

Step 4: Categorize the Quality of Evidence

✓ Determine the level of evidence for each trial, including the major or minor limitations identified.

Step 5: Develop a Conclusion and Recommendation

✓ Develop a conclusion regarding the overall efficacy based on the evidence.

✓ Develop a conclusion regarding the overall safety based on the evidence.

✓ Develop a conclusion regarding any special considerations/special populations.

✓ Develop a conclusion regarding the overall cost of medication specific to this population on the following:

- Cost of Drug X versus Drug Y
- Long-term cost benefits of either drug

✓ Assign the appropriate grade of recommendation.

✓ Develop a recommendation statement based on conclusions and grade of recommendation to be applied to this population.

✓ Formulate evidence-based recommendation statement with appropriate justification:

- Efficacy
- Safety
- Special considerations/special populations
- Cost

EXAMPLE 29

Population-Based Decision/ Recommendation

This example illustrates how to compile a comparative review to assist in the formulary management decision making process.

A physician has requested the addition of Drug X to an institution's formulary to replace Drug Y for treatment of chronic obstructive pulmonary disease (COPD). The pharmacist has been asked to complete a comparative review of the two agents. In addition, an evidence-based medicine recommendation needs to be developed that the pharmacist can present and defend at the next P&T meeting for the institution.

Step 1: Define the Clinical Question

✓ Determine the actual question being asked so that an appropriate response is formed. For this example, the question would be "Should Drug X replaces Drug Y for COPD on the formulary?"

Step 2: Retrieve Pertinent Information

A search of the literature revealed the following evidence:

✓ Article #1 – A randomized, placebo-controlled trial was conducted using Drug X in patients with COPD. Power was not met, thus indicating that an adequate sample size was not used to show a difference between study groups, if a difference really exists. None of the other ten major considerations were discussed. Patients receiving Drug X showed greater improvement in trough FEV1 over placebo ($p<0.01$). These same patients also showed significant improvements in other outcome measures such as peak expiratory flow rate, decreased exacerbations, and health status scores. The only adverse effect that was noted to occur more frequently in the Drug X group was dry mouth. Patients receiving Drug X who also had impaired renal function were required to have dose frequency adjustments.

✓ Article #2 – A randomized, placebo-controlled trial was conducted using Drug X in patients with COPD. Power was set but not met, thus indicating that an adequate sample size was not used to show a difference between study groups, if a difference really exists. No other major limitations were noted. The patients receiving Drug X showed greater improvement from baseline than Drug Y in both trough FEV1 ($p<0.001$) and FVC ($p<0.05$) and maintained these effects throughout the study period. Patients receiving Drug X also experienced significantly greater improvement over Drug Y in peak expiratory flow rate ($p<0.01$). More patients in the Drug X group experienced dry mouth effects than those in the Drug Y group.

Due to the strict inclusion/exclusion criteria, no special considerations/special populations were identified. Drug X is more expensive than Drug Y. Patients had more difficulty using the drug dispensing device for Drug X versus Drug Y.

✓ Article #3 – A case report described 12 patients receiving Drug X who also experienced dry mouth. These patients were observed by their family physician who prescribed the drug to treat their COPD symptoms. No details were given.

Step 3: Evaluate Literature

✓ Efficacy

- Review each trial and determine if the article supports or refutes the use of Drug X over Drug Y.

- Article #1 – The results of the study showed that Drug X was superior to placebo, improving pulmonary function in COPD patients. Specifically, patients receiving Drug X showed greater improvement in trough FEV1 over placebo ($p<0.01$). These same patients also showed significant improvements in other outcome measures such as peak expiratory flow rate, decreased exacerbations, and health status scores.
- Article #2 – The results of the study showed that Drug X was superior to Drug Y, improving pulmonary function in COPD patients. Specifically, patients receiving Drug X showed greater improvement from baseline than Drug Y in both trough FEV1 ($p<0.001$) and FVC ($p<0.05$) and maintained these effects throughout the study period. Patients receiving Drug X also experienced significantly greater improvement over Drug Y in peak expiratory flow rate ($p<0.01$).
- Article #3 – No details were given regarding efficacy in this case report discussing the safety of Drug X in 12 patients.

- Establish if each trial has major or minor limitations.
  - Article #1 – Power was set, but not met. That is, an adequate sample size was not used to show a difference between study groups, if a difference really exists. However, because there was a statistically significant difference noted with the primary endpoint for Drug X compared to placebo, this is less of a concern. None of the other ten major considerations were discussed.
  - Article #2 – Power was set, but not met. That is, an adequate sample size was not used to show a difference between study groups, if a difference really exists. However, because there was a statistically significant difference noted with the primary endpoint for Drug X compared to placebo, this is less of a concern. None of the other ten major limitations were identified.
  - Article #3 – This was a case report, and, therefore did not have a comparative group. Due to this, there were several major limitations.

✓ Safety

- Assess safety of Drug X versus Drug Y when compared in the literature.
  - Article #1 – The only adverse effect that was noted to occur more frequently in the Drug X group was dry mouth. There was no difference in the incidence or severity of adverse drug reactions between the two drugs.
  - Article #2 – Dry mouth was the only adverse effect noted to occur more frequently in the Drug X group compared to Drug Y.
  - Article #3 – This was a case report describing 12 patients receiving Drug X that also experienced dry mouth.
- Retrieve the most current prescribing information to determine possible safety concerns.
  - Dry mouth is the most frequent adverse effect associated with Drug X.

✓ Special considerations/special populations

- Establish if Drug X dosed more or less conveniently than Drug Y.
  - Same dosing frequency
- Does the route of administration vary between drugs?
  - Patients had more difficulty using the drug dispensing device for Drug X versus Drug Y.
- Determine if there are other potential advantages or disadvantages of Drug X versus Drug Y.
- Are there any other specific situations that may affect the population positively or negatively?
  - Patients receiving Drug X who also had impaired renal function were required to have dose frequency adjustments.

✓ Cost

- Is the cost of Drug X significantly higher than Drug Y?
  - Drug X is more expensive than Drug Y.
- Are there long-term cost-saving benefits of Drug X or Drug Y?
- When formulating a recommendation for a population, practitioners have fewer known specifies regarding prescription coverage, patient income, and other variables; therefore, cost does not weigh as heavily and is typically one of the final components taken into consideration when forming the recommendation.

Step 4: Categorize the Quality of Evidence

✓ Determine the level of evidence for each trial:

- Article #1 is a Level II trial with major limitation of power.
- Article #2 is a Level II trial with major limitation of power.
- Article #3 is a Level V trial with major limitations.

Step 5: Develop a Conclusion and Recommendation

✓ Develop a conclusion regarding the overall efficacy based on the evidence.

- Drug X is superior in efficacy to Drug Y.

✓ Develop a conclusion regarding the overall safety based on the evidence.

- The frequency of dry mouth occurring was greater with Drug X than Drug Y.

✓ Develop a conclusion regarding any special considerations/special populations.

- The dispensing device was more difficult to use for Drug X than Drug Y.
- Patients with impaired renal function require dose frequency adjustments with Drug X.

✓ Develop a conclusion regarding the overall cost of medication specific to this population based on the following:

- Cost of Drug X versus Drug Y
  - Drug X is more expensive.
- Long-term cost benefits of either drug

✓ Assign the appropriate grade of recommendation

✓ Develop a recommendation statement based on conclusions made and applied to this population.

✓ Example:

Recommend replacing Drug Y with Drug X on the institution's formulary for treatment of COPD for the following reasons: (Grade B Recommendation)

- Efficacy – A Level II trial shows that Drug X is superior to placebo for improving pulmonary function in COPD patients. In addition, a Level II trial shows Drug X is superior to Drug Y in improving pulmonary function in COPD patients.
- Safety – With the exception of dry mouth, there appears to be no difference in adverse drug reactions between Drug X and Drug Y.
- Special considerations/special populations – In renal impaired patients, dosing frequency adjustment is necessary with Drug X in patients with COPD. Patients who may have difficulty handling the drug dispensing device for Drug X should consider treatment with Drug Y to ensure treatment is being administered properly.
- Cost – Drug X is more expensive than Drug Y; however, there is superior improvement in pulmonary function with Drug X that justifies the additional cost. This improvement in pulmonary function may lead to fewer emergency department visits and fewer hospitalizations, therefore, lowering overall cost.

REFERENCES

1. Kirkwood CF, Kier KL. Modified Systematic Approach to Answering Questions. In: Malone PM, Kier KL, Stanovich JE, eds. Drug Information: A Guide for Pharmacists. 3rd ed. New York, NY: McGraw-Hill Companies, Inc; 2006.
2. Calis KA, Sheehan AH. Formulating Effective Responses and Recommen-

dations: A Structured Approach. In: Malone PM, Kier KL, Stanovich JE, eds. Drug Information: A Guide for Pharmacists. 3rd ed. New York, NY: McGraw- Hill Companies, Inc; 2006.

3. Dahl R, Chuchalin A, Gor D, et al. EXCEL: A randomized trial comparing salmeterol/ fluticasone propionate and formoterol/ budesonide combinations in adults with persistent asthma. Respiratory Medicine. 2006; 100:1152– 1162.
4. Gonzales D, Rennard SI, Nides M, et al. Varenicline, an ?4?2 nicotinic acetylcholine receptor partial agonist, vs sustained-release bupropion and placebo for smoking cessation, a randomized controlled trial. JAMA. 2006; 296:47–55.
5. Manzoni P, Stolfi I, Pugni L, et al. A multicenter, randomized trial of prophylactic fluconazole in preterm neonates. N Engl J Med. 2007; 356:2483–2495.
6. Legro RS, Barnhart HX, Schlaff WD, et al. Clomiphene, metformin, or both for infertility in the polycystic ovary syndrome. N Engl J Med. 2007; 356:551–566.
7. Tfelt-Hansen P, Teall J, Rodriguez F, et al. Oral rizatriptan versus oral sumatriptan: A direct comparative study in the acute treatment of migraine. Headache. 1998; 38:748-755.

CHAPTER 5

Pharmaceutical Care Plan

Patient care planning involves systematically assessing a patient's health problems and needs, setting objectives, performing interventions, and evaluating results. Not all patients require a written PCP. Pharmacists must assess their own patients and identify specific areas on which to focus. For example, the pharmacist may want to identify patients with specific diseases (e.g., asthma, hypertension, diabetes mellitus, or hypercholesterolemia).

In order times, dispensing of drug was the main function assigned to pharmacist. With emergence of clinical pharmacist the pharmacist's contribution neither begins nor ends when drugs are dispensed. He must have a knowledge and understanding of the patient and able to consider present or future drug therapy in terms of patient's current status, his behavior, the objectives of the therapy and his prognosis. He should also be able to communicate on the appropriateness of drug therapy, benefits risk ratio and be able to suggest regimes. A complex relation bridges the patient, his disease and the treatment. The sequence of making drug treatment decisions and ultimately providing the patient with drugs is complex (Fig 5-1).

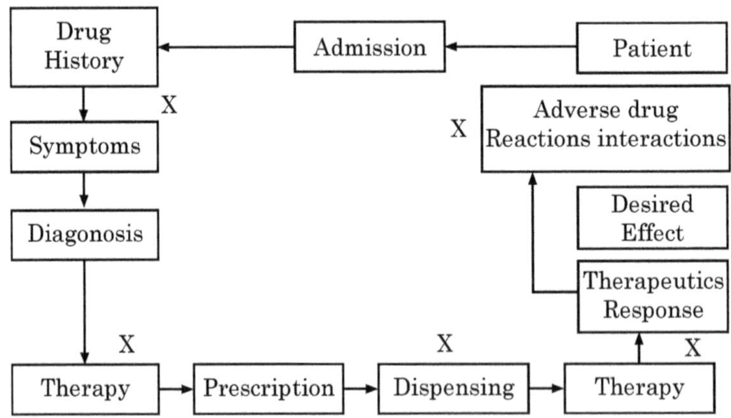

FIGURE 5.1

The Process of making drug therapy decisions.

(X) Indicate areas of involvement of the clinical or ward pharmacist

Pharmaceutical care plan (PCP) is a patient –concentrated systematic approach. The pharmacist designs a format to ensure proper usage of the drugs, achieve a definite result and improves the patient care by assuring the safety, effectiveness and cost-effectiveness.

It can be expressed diagrammatically, outlining each stage sequentially and identifying the likely cause failure of the treatment as well as focusing on the possible areas of involvement by the Clinical pharmacist.

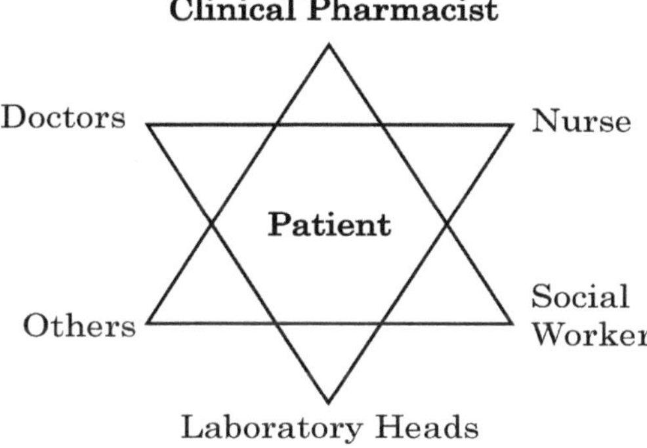

FIGURE 5.2

The health care team.

Drug often induces illness. They may also complicate disease. Medical and drug histories are usually recorded for each patient shortly after admission to a hospital. A patient is being looked after by several persons including clinical pharmacist who work together.

Along with dispensing a clinical pharmacist is expected to perform the following functions.

(A) History taking (B) Ward rounds (C) Checking the prescription and dispensing of drugs. (D) Patient Counseling (E) Therapeutic Drug Monitoring (F) Patient Compliance Monitoring (G) Adverse drug Reaction Monitoring (H) Pharmacoeconomics (I) Miscellaneous

A. History taking:

Doctors often take history of illness. The specific job of pharmacist is to take Medication history "it can be defined as systematic reporting of the drugs used earlier or currently by the patient. The prior use of certain drugs may even predispose a patient to ill-effects during either present or future therapy. Because of pharmacist's specialized knowledge, drug histories taken by them can be more informative than those obtained by medically trained personnel, especially where self medication with 'over the counter' medicines is concerned. Pharmacists also frequently find it easier to clarity confusion regarding the strength or brand of particular dosage forms than their medical colleagues. Hospital pharmacist has traditionally advised medical staff on drugs for general use within a hospital. He usually decides upon the source of supply and frequently works with medical and nursing colleagues to eliminate the use of duplicate or highly toxic drugs and rationalizes the range of drug kept and supplied by his department.

The pharmacist on the ward, however, is in a good position to advise on drug therapy before or at the time when prescription is written. In doing so he should have some idea of the efficacy and safety of treatment considered in terms of the incidence of side effects and possible adverse reactions.

In a study conducted over a 4-month period on a gynecological ward in a district general hospital, it was observed that significantly more items were reported by a pharmacist than by a doctor when medication histories were taken from the same patients in admission by both parties. It was noted that the doctor frequently failed to report self medication even where it was being taken in fairly large quantities. The pharmacists report also contained more information about adverse effects of therapy such as nausea, vomiting, dizziness, diarrhea and constipation.

Recognition and possible avoidance of such effects in future could significantly improve patient compliance with subsequently prescribed medication.

Components of History Taking: History taking a care medical process that provides central databases for all. It should include the following:

(a) Patient Details:
   1. Age 2. Gender 3. Ethnicity
   4. Occupation 5. Height 6. Weight

(b) Family History: Information about familial diseases (Grand parents, brother and sisters.)

(c) Social History: Include socio-economic status, dietary habits, life style (exercise, vocation, habits like smoking, drinking or illicit drug usage.

(d) Medical History: Includes childhood, past, recent or current diseases, chronic illnesses, current medication including 'over the counter drugs', allergy or any past adverse drug reactions noticed.

B. Ward rounds:

Ward round is a visit by health care professional (doctor with or without nurse, pharmacists or any paramedical staff like

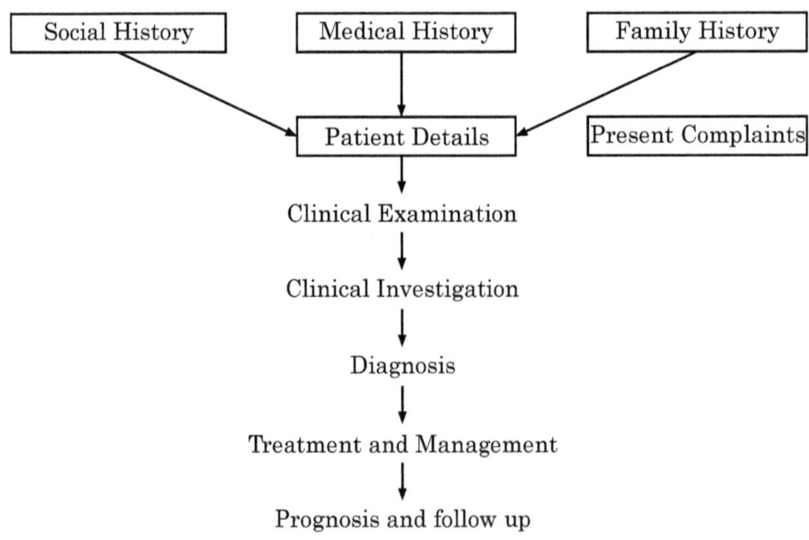

FIGURE 5.3

History Taking by Clinical Pharmacist.

technician or physiotherapist) to an indoor patient in a hospital. It is customary in India that only a doctor with nurse does the ward rounds. However, over passage of time, it has been realized that clinical pharmacist should accompany the doctor and nurse during ward round.

The times and frequency of visits to award by the pharmacist are also decided jointly by the doctor, pharmacist and the ward sister. The frequency depends upon the average length of stay per patient as well as the 'type' of patient and disease state dealt with on the ward in question. An Acute medical, surgical or admission ward requires a daily or even twice daily visit while long stay units where changes in drugs treatment occur infrequently could be adequately covered by a weekly or even monthly visit depending upon geographical location and the staff available. The time at which the pharmacist visits should ideally always be the same each day and should enable adequate contact with medical and nursing staff. The most convenient time to all concerned is just after or even during the main prescribing round.

Goals and Objectives of ward rounds

- To understand the patient's clinical status and progress.
- To get relevant information on drugs consumed, their effectiveness and adverse effects if any.
- To get information about medical compliance.
- Therapeutic drug monitoring.
- To get information on co-morbidity
- Planning for patient discharge or prolongation of stay.

Types of Ward Rounds:

Ward Rounds are conducted at secondary or tertiary health care center.

There are four types of ward rounds:

(a) Pre-Rounds: Visit to the patient ward by the post-graduate students of the medical college and / or the intern to perform the daily review of patient's health status is called pre-rounds. Such type of ward round is a part of training of the student. A clinical pharmacist can accompany the health care professional during such ward rounds, but will have limited learning opportunities since during such visits; less decisions of the disease management are made.

(b) Registrar / Resident Rounds: The visit to the patient ward, daily at a fixed time by the registrars or the resident doctors of the hospital are labeled as registrar / resident rounds. Further, such type of ward round in the intensive care units may be conducted multiple times a day depending on the seriousness of the patient's disease. Such kind of ward rounds can be very useful for the clinical pharmacists since they are extensive, exhausting and involve the teaching of clinical aspects to post-graduate students.

(c) Professor / Chief Rounds: A ward round participation involving interns, post-graduate students, registrars, residents and the experienced doctor (may or may not be a consultant) together is known as professor/chief rounds. It may be conducted daily, weekly, biweekly or bimonthly depending upon the availability of time. Such type of ward rounds involve, sorting out the problems encountered by the registrars or resident doctors in diagnosis, treatment and / or management of certain specific illnesses. Thus, the rounds become extensive and specialized for discussing complex and complicated problems. These types of ward rounds are therefore more challenging for clinical pharmacists.

(d) **Teaching Rounds:** The extensive, detailed ward rounds conducted at regular basis by the medical academicians and medical staff for the undergraduate medical students is called teaching rounds. A clinical pharmacist can join during such rounds but will have limited exposure since this type of ward rounds do not involve any kind of decision making.

C. Checking the Prescription and Dispensing of Drugs:

A traditional task of a pharmacist has been to perform a safety check on prescription and whilst on wards he is also able to monitor drug administration. This may give the appearance of evaluating the performance of medical and nursing colleagues. The motives and interests of clinical pharmacists must therefore, be made clears.

Hospital pharmacist's aim is to reduce drug errors, to encourage rational drug therapy and consequently to benefit the patient. They must not operate as doctor himself but as professionals, trained to complement the drug related services already provided by doctors, who are expert in their own field. The maintain credibility, pharmacists must not play on the mistakes and bad prescribing of some physician but develop a more constructive approach in which they can monitor drug therapy for the benefit of the patient and offer advice, not just information to the prescriber.

In hospitals which operate a stock of drug distribution to the wards without a comprehensive ward pharmacy service; prescriptions are frequently interpreted by nurses who may only consult the prescriber or perhaps other nursing colleague when the dose appears unusual or when there is a problem with its prescribing. There is very little attempt to detect inappropriate concurrent prescribing or potential drug interactions to both medical and nursing staff on the optimum dosage, dosing frequency, dosage forms, as well as the times and routes of administration. Drugs are sometimes used inappropriately due to lack of knowledge of formulation on the part of the prescriber. Having all the relevant information to hand on the ward, the clinical pharmacist is able to advice on the best formulation to suit a particular patient's needs. Likewise unnecessary or excessive drug use can be discouraged more effectively whilst on the ward than from a distance, where the relevant background information is not usually available.

Expected outcomes:

- Prevention or cure of a specific disease
- Relieving of or decrease in the patient's symptoms
- Halting or slowing the progression of the disease
- Counter the disease or symptoms

Goals of PCP:

- Diagnosis of the potential and actual drug related problems
- Determining the actual drug-related problems
- Reducing the drug-related problems

Various Steps in Pharmaceutical Care Plan:

- Development of a comprehensive database of the patient
- Illustrating the absolute and potential drug-related problems
- Developing the therapeutic goals
- Monitoring the important parameters with end points and frequency
- Reassessment and Evaluation

Setting up of a Data-Base of the Patient

- Enumeration of the Demographics of the patient (age, sex, height, weight,.....)
- History of past medical history and present disease
- Present usage of medicines and medication history of the patient
- Drug related allergy and intolerance to the drugs
- caffeine ,Smoking, alcohol, and drug abuse history
- Compliance history of the patient.
- Physical examination of the patient and abnormal laboratory results including renal and hepatic function

Assess the Actual Problem using SOAP Format Data:

S: Subjective: patient's chief complain or why came to hospital

O: Objective: traceable facts as vital signs, lab results, blood pressure

A: Assessment: the medical diagnosis on the given date

P: Plan: treatment plan including drugs, lab orders, referrals...

Drug Related Problems

After the creation of a patient database, the pharmacist should evaluate the patient's drug treatment:

1. Determine the patient for the problems related to the drugs.
2. Evaluate whether drug-related problems are being treated or not.
3. Assess whether the current drug therapy is applicable or not.
4. Estimate whether additional drug therapy is needed.
5. Determine if any of the drug-related problems may have been caused by medication.

Understanding of the types of drug-related problems that may occur facilitates the evaluation process. Most of the drug-related problems are the result of:

1. Not administering the appropriate drug
2. Receiving the wrong drug
3. Receiving too little of the drug
4. Receiving too much of the drug
5. Experiencing an adverse drug reaction
6. Experiencing a drug interaction
7. Not receiving the prescribed drug
8. Receiving a drug for which there is no valid medical indication

Development of Therapeutic Goals

Next, therapeutic goals must be established for each drug-related problem so that the pharmaceutical care planning process can be effective. Therapeutic goals should be definite, realistic and, if possible, measurable. Most therapeutic goals relate to:

1. Approach normal physiology (i.e., normalize blood pressure).

2. Slow progression of disease (i.e., slow progression of cancer).
3. Alleviate symptoms (i.e., optimize pain control).
4. Prevent adverse effects.
5. Control medication costs.
6. Educate the patient about his or her medication.

The development of a Pharmaceutical care plan can be compiled as a five step process involving the SOAP format (Subjective data, Objective data, Assessment, and Plan of care). Taking the example for an asthma patient, the process can be described as follows.

Step 1: Collection of Information

The pharmacist should collect an accurate medication history of the patient, including both prescription and nonprescription based drugs and the reasons for which those medications were prescribed. The pharmacist has to obtain information from the physician, which includes laboratory test results and hospitalizations. Then the pharmacist should get the permission from the concerned patient before soliciting this information. Once the obtained information is compiled, the preparation of a pharmaceutical care plan can be initiated.

Step 2: Identifying Problems

Based on the patient's medication profile in Figure 5-4, one problem evident is asthma. If applicable, other problem should be listed. In Figure 5-4, subjective and objective findings that are correlated to the problem were listed. Subjective findings are those that the patient feels(e.g., 'I feel tired all the time, "I woke up coughing").. the other findings are those that can be observed by the pharmacist (e.g., patient appears tired, high blood pressure , edema in ankles).

Step 3: Problem Assessment

The pharmacist plays an important role analyzing and integrating the information that is obtained in steps 1 and 2 and draws conclusions in developing a patient-specific PCP. For example, in the case of a person suffering with asthma case (Figure 5-4), the pharmacist may first identify the factors that increases the asthma. The pharmacist does not has to be involved in testing of the skin, nor does the pharmacist have to conduct a extensive history of all the factors that may have precipitated in the asthma. Also, the pharmacist has to determine if drugs (eg., aspirin, NSAIDS, or beta-blockers) caused or exacerbated the asthma .

Later on, the pharmacist has to assesses the severity of the condition of the asthma. This could be done (as shown in the plan) by determining the PEFR, examining the patient's daily symptoms and peak flow diary, or determining whether the patient had been hospitalized and placed on steroids or a mechanical ventilator.

Step 4: Plan Development

In step 4, the pharmacist establishes goals related the patient's problems and specifies an action which is aimed at reaching each goal. Each goal (i.e., required improvement) should be stated in terms of outcomes that indicate the extent of the solution to the problem. Often, the patient may has several problems, and the plan must be very good enough to have a positive effect on the patient health.

Patient Profile and PCP for an Ambulatory Patient with Asthma

Last name:	Poplar	*First name*: Hedda	*initial*. M.	
Address.	201 E. Wabash			
City, State Zip:	Anytown, State 12345			
Telephone.	556-1234			
Birth date:	*11-9-41* *Ht- 64'*	Wt. 185 lb	Sex.- F	Race: White
Allergies:	Aspirin (bronchospasm)			
Diagnosis(es):	Asthma			
Other information:	Smoker (cigarettes), obese			

Drug	**Strength**	**Regimen**	**Quantity**
TheoDur	300 mg	1 tablet orally	twice a day 100.
Albuterol	MDI 200 puffs/month	2 puffs every 4 hours	2 as needed

Asthma Problem(s)* Subjective and Objective Information Evaluation/Outcome(s)	**Assessment**	**Plan(s)/Goal(s)**
Coughs at night, SOB Follow up with patient on exertion, MDI weekly, low HRQOL	Poor asthma control frequent perhaps aggravated by cough, SOB exacerbations requiring and number undercompliance with medication regimen	Refer to smoking cessation program to evaluate smoking, obesity, and on exertion, Refer to dietitian of exacerbations
Check medication calendar and call physiologic well-being	Review at next refill: pill count MDI usage, amount, technique	Leads to decreased physical, social, and to remind about refills
PEFRs between 60% and Check to see if prescribed 80% of personal best corticosteroid be added	Inadequate anti-inflammatory medication Review use with patient	Suggest to physician that inhaled

Determine if PEFR Is more than 80% of personal best with PEFM

*Hedda Poplar is a 55-year-old white woman who presents at the pharmacy with new prescriptions for TheoDur and albuterol MDI. The pharmacist, take a medication and symptom history, measure a PEFR. and complete the patient profile in Figure 1. On the basis of the information, it was concluded that her main problem is asthma, but she is also overweight and smokes cigarettes. As the pharmacist develop the PCP for the patient, the pharmacist note her problem of asthma in column I and use the SOAP format (Subjective and Objective information, Assessment, and Plan) to document the problem. Document the patient's Subjective and Objective information. the pharmacist Assessment (column 2) Include general ideas about why she has the problem of asthma. In column 3, you develop a general plan to resolve the identified problem. Finally, In column 4, you list general and specific outcomes measures to ensure that your plan Is being met

HRQOL - health-related quality of life; MDI = metered-dose Inhaler; PCP = pharmaceutical care plan; PEFM = peak expiratory flow meter; PEFR =peak expiratory flow rate; SOB = shortness of breath.

FIGURE 5.4

Patient Profile and PCP for an Ambulatory Patient with Asthma.

Step 5: Evaluating the Outcomes

Outcomes are mainly used to evaluate the success of the Pharmaceutical care plan. The treatment plan must be manageable, measurable and meaningful. Outcomes are highly specific, measurable indicators for the goals of treatment. The outcomes must be identified in the planning process.

The therapeutic outcomes that are listed for asthma would include, but not be limited to, lower frequency and severity of acute exacerbations, fewer physician office visits, side effects elimination, PEFRs that never fall below 80% of previous personal-best predicted rates, fewer emergency department visits, and maintenance of activities that enhance the patient's quality of life and may have been limited by the disease.

The following components are to be included in the Documentation.

1. Patient data such as name, medical record number, location, date of hospital admission (if applicable). age, sex, height, weight, known medication or other allergies, and medication history.
2. Name of pharmacist(s) responsible for development and implementation of the PCP.
3. Patient problem(s) listed Individually in order of potential pharmacotherapeutic impact (highest to lowest priority). Subjective and objective data that lead to identification of a specific problem and potential drug-related problems should also be included.
4. Date on which problem of the patient was identified. Many diseases are chronic throughout the patient's entire life like urinary tract infection or upper respiratory tract infection usually resolve in 10 to 14 days.

REFERENCES

1. Strand LM, Cipolle RJ, Morley PC. Pharmaceutical care: an introduction. 1992. Upjohn Co. pp 14-29.
2. Strand LM, Cipolle RJ, Morley PC. Drug-related problems; their structure and function. Ann Pharmacother 1990; 24: 1093-7.
3. Canady BR, Yarborough PC. Documenting pharmaceutical care: creating a standard. Ann Pharmacother 1994; 28: 1292-6.
4. Gold ML, Fedder DO. Developing a pharmaceutical care plan. US Pharmacist 1992; 17(10):53-60.
5. Chase PA, Bainbridge J. Care plan for documenting pharmacist actvities. Am J Hosp Pharm 1993; 50:1885-8.
6. Rich DS. Pharmaceutical care plans. Hosp Pharm 1994; 29(2); 176-8.
7. Brown S. Clinical monitoring of home care patients. US Pharmacist 1996; 21(Suppl); 3-8.
8. Cameron KA. Preventing medication-related problems among older Americans. Man Care Int 1998; 11(10); 74-85.
9. Egging P. Implementing pharmaceutical care in the home setting. Pharmaguide 1995; 8(4); 1-9.

CHAPTER 6

Rational Drug Use

INTRODUCTION

A MAJOR GLOBAL PROBLEM

Irrational use of medicines is a major problem worldwide. WHO estimates that more than half of all medicines are prescribed, dispensed or sold inappropriately, and that half of all patients fail to take them correctly. The overuse, underuse or misuse of medicines results in wastage of scarce resources and widespread health hazards. Examples of irrational use of medicines include: use of too many medicines per patient ("poly-pharmacy"); inappropriate use of antimicrobials, often in inadequate dosage, for non-bacterial infections; over-use of injections when oral formulations would be more appropriate; failure to prescribe in accordance with clinical guidelines; inappropriate self-medication, often of prescription-only medicines; non-adherence to dosing regimes.

OUR GOAL

Ensure therapeutically sound and cost-effective use of medicines by health professionals and consumers improving the use of medicines by health workers and the general public is crucial both to reducing morbidity and mortality from communicable and non-communicable diseases, and to containing drug expenditure.

Ideally, therapeutically sound and cost-effective use of medicines by health professionals and consumers is achieved at all levels of the health system, and in both the public and the private sectors. A sound rational drug use programme in any country has three elements:

- **Rational use of medicines strategy and monitoring:** Advocating rational medicines use, identifying and promoting successful strategies, and securing responsible medicines promotion.
- **Rational use of medicines by health professionals:** Working with countries to develop and update their treatment guidelines, national essential medicines lists and formularies, and supporting training programmes on rational use of medicines.
- **Rational use of medicines by consumers:** Supporting the creation of effective systems of medicines information, and empowering consumers to take responsible decisions regarding their treatment.

The above elements were developed in close collaboration with the regional and country offices. They are formulated in such a way as to reflect the main responsibilities of a national essential medicines programme.

WHO ADVOCATES 12 KEY INTERVENTIONS TO PROMOTE MORE RATIONAL USE

1. Establishment of a multidisciplinary national body to coordinate policies on medicine use
2. Use of clinical guidelines
3. Development and use of national essential medicines list
4. Establishment of drug and therapeutics committees in districts and hospitals
5. Inclusion of problem-based pharmacotherapy training in under graduate curricula
6. Continuing in-service medical education as a licensure requirement
7. Supervision, audit and feedback
8. Use of independent information on medicines
9. Public education about medicines
10. Avoidance of perverse financial incentives
11. Use of appropriate and enforced regulation
12. Sufficient government expenditure to ensure availability of medicines and staff.

DEFINITION

Rational use means "prescribing right drug, in adequate dose for the sufficient duration and appropriate to the clinical needs of the patient at lowest cost." The concept of rational drug use is age old, as evident by the statement made by the Alexandrian physician Herophilus 300 B.C that is

"Medicines are nothing in themselves but are the very hands of god if employed with reason and prudence."

Rational drug use attained more significance nowadays in terms of medical, socio economical and legal aspect. Factors that have led sudden realization for rational drug use are.

1. **Drug explosion:** Increase in the number of drugs available has incredibly complicated the choice of appropriate drug for particular indication.
2. **Efforts to prevent the development of resistance:** Irrational use of drugs may lead to the premature demise of highly efficacious and life saving new antimicrobial drug due to development of resistance.
3. **Growing awareness:** Today, the information about drug development, its uses and adverse effects travel from one end of the planet to the other end with amazing speed through various media.
4. **Increased cost of the treatment:** Increase in cost of the drug increases economic burden on the public as well as on the government. This can be reduced by rational drug use.
5. **Consumer protection Act (CPA):** Extension of CPA in medical profession may restrict the irrational use of drugs.

REASONS FOR IRRATIONAL USE OF DRUGS

1. Lack of information: Unlike many developed countries we don't have regular facility which provides us up to date unbiased information on the currently used drugs. Majority of our practitioners rely on medical representatives. There are differences between pharmaceutical concern and the drug regulatory authorities in the interpretation of the data related to indications and safety of drugs.

2. Faulty and inadequate training and education of medical graduates: Lack of proper clinical training regarding writing a prescription during training period, dependency on diagnostic aid, rather than clinical diagnosis, is increasing day by day in doctors.

3. Poor communication between health professional and patient: Medical practitioners and other health professional giving less time to the patient and not explaining some basic information about the use of drugs.

4. Lack of diagnostic facilities/Uncertainty of diagnosis: Correct diagnosis is an important step toward rational drug therapy. Doctors posted in remote areas have to face a lot of difficulty in reaching to a precise diagnosis due to non availability of diagnostic facilities. This promotes poly-pharmacy.

5. Demand from the patient: To satisfy the patient expectations and demand of quick relief, clinician prescribe drug for every single complaint. Also, there is a belief that "every ill has a pill" All these increase the tendency of polypharmacy.

6. Defective drug supply system and ineffective drug regulation: Absence of well organized drug regulatory authority and presence of large number of drugs in the market leads to irrational use of drugs.

7. Promotional activities of pharmaceutical industries: The lucrative promotional programmes of the various pharmaceutical industries influence the drug prescribing.

HAZARDS OF IRRATIONAL USE OF DRUGS

Irrational use of drugs may lead to:

1. Ineffective and unsafe treatment
2. Exacerbation or prolongation of illness.
3. Distress and harm to patient
4. Increase the cost of treatment

MEASURES TO PROMOTE RATIONAL DRUG Use

Medicines (drugs) cannot be used rationally unless everyone involved in the pharmaceutical supply chain has access to objective information about the drug they buy and use. Knowledge and ideas about drugs are constantly changing and a clinician is expected to know about the new development in drug therapy.

The pre-requisites of rational drug use are

- Critical assessment and evaluation of benefits and risk of drug used.
- Compare the advantages, disadvantages, safety and cost of the drug with existing drug for some indication.

OBSTACLES EXIST IN RATIONAL DRUG USE

Various obstacles in rational drug use are:-

1. Lack of objective information and of continuing education and training in pharmacology.
2. Lack of well organized drug regulatory authority and supply of drugs.
3. Presence of large number of drugs in the market and the lucrative methods of promotion of drugs employed by pharmaceutical industries.
4. The prevalent belief that "every ill has a pill."

STEPS TO IMPROVE RATIONAL DRUG PRESCRIBING

Step 1: Identify the patient's problem based on symptoms and recognize the need for action.

Step 2: Diagnosis of the disease. Identify underlying cause and motivating factors. This may be specific as in infectious disease or non specific.

Step 3: List possible intervention or treatment. This may be non drug treatment or drug treatment. Drug must be chosen from different alternatives based on efficacy, convenience and safety of drugs including, drug inter-actions and high risk group of patients.

Step 4: Start the treatment by writing an accurate and complete prescription e.g., name of drugs with dosage forms, dosage schedule and total duration of the treatment.

Step 5: Given proper information instruction and warning regarding the treatment given e.g., Side effects (ADR), dosage schedule and dangers/risk of stopping the therapy suddenly.

Step 6: Monitor the treatment to check, if the particular treatment has solved the patient's problem. It may be:

(a) Passive monitoring – done by the patient himself. Explain him what to do if the treatment is not effective or if too many side effect occurs

(b) Active monitoring done by physician and he make an appointment to check the response of the treatment.

CONCLUSION

Indiscriminate use of drugs not only wastes scarce resources that could otherwise be spent on other essential services, but also leads to drug induced disease. The drug control authority, the teaching institutes, drug industries, N.G.O and the patient himself may be helpful for rational drug use. Drug authority must circulate the list of essential drugs which could be updated from time to time. It must monitor the safe and proper use of these drugs and enforce a uniform regulation for promotional literature. Teaching institute must conduct regular research work and proper training of undergraduates and post graduates. Motivation of NGO to organize various programmes for public awareness lastly, the patient himself should observe strict compliance to the physician' prescription and never indulge in self medication.

To conclude, the demands of rational drug use are:

1. Availability of essential and life saving drugs and unbiased drug information with generic name.
2. Adequate quality control and drug control.
3. Withdrawal of hazardous and irrational drugs.
4. Drug legislation reform.

REFERENCES

1. Irrational drug combinations; Need to sensitize undergraduates. Gautam, C.S. Aditya S. Ind. J. Pharmacol; Vol. 38, 3, June 06, 169-170.
2. Essential drugs and Rational Therapeutics Text book of Pharmacology S.D. Seth 1 s t Ed.1997, 783-791.
3. Essential drugs and Rational Therapeutics Text book of Pharmacology S.D. Seth 2ndEd.2004, 907-916
4. Organization behaviour and community health promoting rational drug use among health professionals UmaTekur and Isha Gupta Publication from state institute of health and family welfare; Rajasthan 2nd ed. 1998, 273-276
5. Rational drug use Organization behaviour and community health promoting rational

drug use among health professionals Adesh Mathur. Published by state institute of health and family welfare, Jaipur, 3 rd ed. 2001, 95-103

6. The rational use of drugs, Report on the conference of experts Nairobi, 25-29 Nov.1985 sponsored by W.H.O. Geneva.

7. Improving drug use Editorial, Action programme on essential drug No. 23 1997

8. Rational use of drugs Gurbani N K., Sharma Rameshwar and Dandiya P.C., Pharma Times, May 2000, 18-33

CHAPTER 7

Polypharmacy and Medication Errors

POLYPHARMACY

Polypharmacy is the simultaneous administration of multiple medications at a time. It is mainly related to the h the prescriptions and usage of too many or unnecessary drugs at dosages greater than therapeutically essential. However, usage of multiple medications may be needed sometimes for treating various diseases and can provides best care for patients (Table 7.1).

Table 7.1

Proportion of higher users of medications (as a percentage of those taking at least one medication*)

Number of medications	Total	under 65 years	65-74 years	75-84 years	over 85 years
4 or more	14.5	10.1	33.2	40.7	38.2
4 or more	4.6	2.6	13.1	17	16.2

*Excludes complementary medicines (vitamins, herbal preparations, etc).

ELDERLY PATIENTS AT INCREASED RISK

In general older people have higher rates of chronic illness and are more likely to be taking multiple medications. The usage of more medications at a time causes the risk of various side effects like collapse, confusion and functional decline. Improper vision, loss of hearing and memory capacity and there will be alteration of metabolic rates, which includes declining renal function will be experienced in older people.

The development of adverse reactions may go undetected because symptoms may be similar to those problems associated with older age like forgetfulness, weakness or tremor. These adverse reactions may also be misinterpreted as like a medical condition and lead to the prescription of more additional drugs.

Steps for managing Polypharmacy

1. Prevention: Avoid prescribing drugs for minor, non-specific or self-limiting complaints. Only prescribe when there is good evidence of likely efficacy as well as a strong need for the medication.

2. Regular medication review: An accurate medication history is necessary for patients who are using multiple medicines. This can be best achieved when the medication review is done in the home of the patient. The patient should be informed to get all the medications at each time of appointment which includes both prescribed and non-prescribed.

3. Non-pharmacological approaches: Instead of usage of medications for longer time life style modification should be implemented

4. Communication: Communicate with the patient about their expectations, problems, concern in using the medications and their conditions to follow the medication regimen. The changes in the medication regimen with the patient's other health care providers should be discussed and implemented.

5. Simplify: Reduce the medication regimen to the essential drugs. Consider only few dosage intervals and dose reduction when appropriate. Usage of optional, trivial and placebo medications should be reduced.

Table 7.2

Common examples

Medication	Original indication	Reason for reassessment	Possible action
Digoxin	Heart failure; in sinus rhythm	Heart failure well controlled with ACE inhibitor and diuretic	Consider ceasing digoxin
Nonsteroidal antiinflammatory Drugs (NSAIDs)	Osteoarthritis	Potential to exacerbate co-existing diseases; potential to cause gastrointestinal side effects	Prescribe regular paracetamol and cease or reduce use of the NSAID; intermittent use may be adequate
Low dose tricyclic Antidepressants	Insomnia and/ or anxiety	Potential to cause adverse effects such as hypotension which may predispose to falls	Withdraw slowly replacing with nonpharmacological measures

Table 7.3

Factors Associated With Geriatric Patient Polypharmacy

- Availability of nonprescription drugs
- High cost of prescription medications (leads to use of up to several other "alternatives" to reach same effect)
- Hoarding of old medications
- Inadequate patient knowledge of medications and medical conditions
- Increasing number of chronic health conditions
- Patients being treated by multiple prescribing physicians
- Patients using different sources of medication, often with little or no co-ordination between these sources
- Taking at least one medication for every diagnosis
- Tendency toward self-treatment/self medication

Table 7.4

Suggested polypharmacy screening questions

Polypharmacy: Useful Screening Questions for the Practitioner
• Does the patient take any dietary supplements, herbal medications, vitamins, or over-the-counter drugs?
• What pharmacies (both traditional and internet-based stores) did the patient use to fill prescriptions during the last two years?
• How many practitioners does the patient currently go to? What medications does each respective practitioner prescribe?
• Is the patient able to clearly read and understand labels on prescription medications that he/she is taking? Is the patient able to easily open the medication vial and appropriately take prescribed doses?
• When does the patient take his/her medications? Of those times, when are they more likely to forget to take medications? How often does he/she forget to take medications?
• Does the patient have any concerns or questions about his or her medication regimen?

Table 7.5

List of potential adverse outcomes associated with polypharmacy

Adverse drug reactions
• Arrhythmia
• Balance/gait disturbances (resulting in falls/injuries)
• Cognitive changes/confusion
• Constipation
• Cutaneous reaction/rash
• Gastric ulcers/bleeding
• Hypotension or hypertension
• Neurologic dysfunction (i.e., pseudoparkinsonism)
• Psychiatric side effects (depression, suicidal ideation, etc)
• Unexpected treatment failure
Drug-drug interactions (often very complex)
Increased costs of medication and/or treatment
Increased risk of hospitalization
Patient non-adherence (increased with complex regimens)
Various medication errors

Table 7.6

Proposed patient-centered strategies for reducing complications associated with polypharmacy

- Assist patients with making a comprehensive list of their prescription and over-the-counter medications. This should include the dose, frequency, strength, and duration of therapy
- Educate patients that medication nonadherence may lead to unnecessary medication changes
- Encourage patients to carry the list of their medications to every physician appointment and update this list whenever changes are made to their medication regimen
- Encourage patients to read all labels carefully and to use only one pharmacy (or as few pharmacies as possible)

MEDICATION ERRORS AND THEIR PREVENTION

Factors that are responsible for medication errors are as follows :

1. Misinterpretation of the prescription due to
   (a) Bad handwriting
   (b) Incomplete or insufficiently clear instructions
   (c) Alterations on the prescription sheet.
2. Failure to review treatment or to cancel a prescription.
3. Failure to adopt a uniform system of prescription.
4. Duplication of drug administration.
5. Failure to identify the individual patient correctly.
6. Absence of the prescription from the ward when required.
7. The required drugs not being available
8. Transfer of drugs from one container to another on the ward.
9. Setting out the doses in advance of the medicine round.
10. Variation in timing of medicine rounds.
11. Errors in prescribing including incompatibilities and failure to take account of previous drug treatment.
12. The large variety of drug used.
13. The increased mobility of patient within the award and within the hospital.
14. Patients taking their own drugs into the hospital.
15. The number of nurses involved in the administration of drugs to the patients due to shorter span of duty, part times and shift working.
16. The number of doctors who may prescribe for any patient.
17. Alteration to or inadequate labeling of drug.

Error Types:

(i) Omission error: It is defined as failure to administer an ordered dose. If the patient refuses to take the medicine it is not considered as medication error. Also in view of the recognized contraindication if the dose is not administered, no error in considered to have occurred.

(ii)Unauthorized drug error: This error means administration to the patient of a medication not authorized for the patient. This category includes a dose given dose given outside a stated set of clinical variable (e.g. medication ordered to administer only if the patient's blood pressure falls below a predetermined level).

(iii) Wrong dose error: Any dose that is the number of preformed units (e.g.tablets) or any above or below the ordered dose by a predetermined amount (e.g 20%). In case of ointments, topical solutions and sprays, an error occurs only if the medication expresses the dosage quantitatively e.g. pinch ointment or two, one second sprays.

(iv) Wrong route error: Administration of a drug by a route other than tht ordered by the physician e.g.Use of an ophthalmic ointment when eye drops are ordered. It also includes doses given by the correct route but at the wrong side (e.g. right eye instead of left).

(v) Wrong rate error: Administration of a drug by the correct route but in a different dosage form then that specified or implied by the physician e.g. use of an ophthalmic ointment when a solution was ordered. Purposeful alterations (e.g.crushing of a tablets) or substitution (e.g substituting a liqid for a tablet of an oral dosage form) to facilitate administration is not generally regarded as an error.

(vi) Wrong rater error: Administration of a drug by the correct route but in a different dosage form then that specified or implied by the physician e.g. use of an ophthalmic ointment when a solution was ordered. Purposeful alternation (e.g crushing of a tablet) or substitution (e.g. substituting a liquid for a tablet of an oral dosage form) to facilitate administration is not generally regarded as an error.

(vii) Wrong-time error: Administration of a dose of drug greater than plus or minus 'X' hours from its scheduled administration time, "X" being set by hospital policy.

(viii) Wrong preparation of a dose: Incorrect preparation of the medication dose e.g. incorrect dilution or reconstitution, not shaking suspension, using an expired drug, not keeping a light sensitive drug protected from light, and mixing drugs that are visually or chemically incompatible.

(ix) Incorrect administration technique: Situation when the drug is given via correct route, site and so forth but improper for a drug, incorrect instillation of an ophthalmic ointment and incorrect use of an administration device.

Prevention of Medication Errors

I. Labelling and Medication: General

1. Labelling of drugs should be performed by a pharmacist or under his supervision. The labels should be used only by a pharmacy.
2. The pharmacist should be consulted and should make recommendation about labelling containers and storage of housekeeping items, insecticides etc.
3. Medication labels should be typed. Labelling with pen, use of adhesive tape or marking pencils should not allowed. A label should not be superimposed upon another label.
4. The label should be legible, easily read and free from erasers or strike overs. It should be firmly affixed to the container. The stock container labels should be protected from chemical action or abrasion.
5. The label should bear the name, address and telephone number of the hospital.
6. Only one prescription should be dispensed and labeled at a time.
7. The following or similar accessory labels and cautionary statements should appear when necessary: (a) Poison (b) Not to be taken (c) Shake well before use (d) For external use only (e) For the eye (f) For nose (g) For the ear reconstitution (j) Warning-Not to be injected (k) Do not use after – (1) Not to be swallowed (m) Keep out of reach of children (n) Keep from freezing (o) Keep below freezing (p) Caution : Potent drug (q) Research Drug. (r) Contents may be used as per formulary policy, to dispense prescriptions or orders for any of the following brands of the same basic drug (Proprietary Name, Brand-Proprietary, Name-Brand etc.) (s) No change in colour size or shape. (t) Other accessory labels providing special information such as dosage, side effects, or contradictions, for investigational drugs, may be used where necessary.

8. The metric system should be given prominence on all labels. Where both metric and apothecary systems are commonly used.
9. The name of the therapeutically active ingredients should be indicated in compound mixtures.
10. Labels for medications should indicate the amount of drug or drugs in each dosage form unless otherwise indicated.
11. Drugs and chemicals for dilution or reconstitution should carry directions for doing so. Whenever possible, dilutions and labelling should be done in the pharmacy.
12. Perishable drugs e.g. antibiotics and biological should clearly indicate the date of expiry on the label.
13. The routes of administration should be indicated for parenteral medications whenever possible.
14. Numbers, letters, coined names and unofficial synonyms and abbreviations should not be used to identify medications with the exceptions of approved letter, or number codes for investigation drugs.
15. Only light resistant, tight containers meeting pharmacopoeial standards should be used.
16. Medications brought into the hospital by the patient or physician should be positively identified before use. They should be checked by the hospital pharmacist with the originating pharmacy or drug store by the prescription's serial number. An additional label should be attached in the hospital pharmacy providing information required in part II of the given guidelines. Where no pharmacist in on duty, the physician should check with the issuing pharmacy and attach a supplementary label described above.
17. Containers presenting difficulty in labelling such as small tubes, should be labeled with no less than the prescription serial, name of the drug, strength and the name of the patient, and should then be placed in a larger carton or container bearing a label with the necessary information indicated in parts II and III.
18. The label should confirm with all laws of the country.
19. Ward's floor stock medication labels should carry codes to identify source and lot number of medication.

II. Labelling and Dispensing in Patient Prescriptions.

1. In addition to the recommendations made above the inpatient prescription label bears minimum following information: (i) Patient's full name (ii) Nonproprietory and / or proprietory name of the drug actually dispensed (iii) Strength (iv) Date of issue (v) Name or initials of dispensing pharma list
2. The prescription or inpatients order should have noted theron, the time dispensed at, the source and batch, identifying number of the medication and initials of the dispenser.
3. For inpatient self-care medications label as in part-III.

III. Labelling and Dispensing Out Patient Prescriptions.

1. Medications to be dispensed to in-patients who are being discharged should be returned to the pharmacy for relabeling.

2. The out-patient prescription label should bear the following information.

   (a) Patient's full name (b) Prescription identification number (c) Specific directions for use (d) Date of Issue (e) Name or initials of dispenser (f) Name of the prescribing physician (g) Whose policy indicates, the physician requests or hospital; identify and strength should be on the label (h) A 'Keep out of reach of children label (i) Name, address and telephone number of hospital.
3. Prescription should have noted thereon, at the time dispensed, the source and batch identifying number of the medication and the initials of the dispenser.
4. An identifying check system to ensure proper identification of the out-patients should be established.

IV. Care of Drugs and Drugs Cabinets in Wards

1. Medication centers should be functional and provide :

   (a) Adequate space so that drugs can be placed and arranged in accordance with (b) Adequate space to allow all container labels to be clearly visible. (c) Adequate lighting for label to be clearly read. (d) Adequate ventilation (e) Adequate work space protected from traffic and noise (f) Hot and cold running water. (g) Sufficient equipment supplies in readily usable form (h) Refrigeration (i) Inner lockable narcotic cabinet and (j) Adequate means of security.
2. Medication should be placed in accordance with an established plan for a particular hospital and provide standardized compartments for –

   (a) Internal medications (b) Narcotics barbiturates, amphetamines (c) Poisonous and external use drugs (d) Emergency drugs (e) Ampoules and (f) Investigational drugs
3. Drugs should be arranged alphabetically within the above group as far as possible
4. Medication cabinets or room and narcotics compartments should be kept locked and the keys should be available only to the nurse incharge or her alternate.
5. Storage of drugs on mobile dressing carriages is discouraged unless properly secured.
6. Not more than one hypodermic tablets should be placed in a capsule for the purpose of protection against breakage or to facilitate counting or control.
7. Pharmacy should supply exact quantities for preparation of specific amounts of solution or should preferably supply the finished preparation. Maintenance of bulk chemicals or stock drug on the wards, nursing units for preparation of solutions should be discouraged.
8. Separate storage facilities should be provided for:

   (a) Test reagents (b) General disinfectants and antiseptics (c) Cleaning agents
9. Only drugs and equipments for preparation and administration should be stored in medication cabinets.
10. Drug cabinets should be examined weekly or more often by the nurse in charge. Drug which appear to have deteriorated or have passed their expiry

dates or are not being used should be returned to the pharmacy for proper disposal. Monthly or more frequent inspections should be made by the Chief Pharmacist and Nursing service on their delegates.

11. Controlled drug in the nursing unit shall be inventoried, recorded and inspected in accordance with an approved system.
12. Investigational drugs should be handled as directed by the organizers or personnel controlling and carrying out investigation with such drugs.
13. Reconstitution of antibiotics and other unstable drugs on the nursing unit should be kept to a minimum. They should be diluted in accordance with directions supplied by the pharmacy.
14. The above types of drugs reconstituted on the nursing unit should carry a label prepared by the nurse with essentially the following information :

    (a) Date of expiry (b) Name of the nurse or her initials (c) Dosage of strength per unit volume.
15. Empty medication containers should be returned to the pharmacy.
16. Inflammables or explosive liquids (ether or acetone) should be kept in as small supply as possible and in accordance with legal regulations.

REFERENCES

1. Joint Commission on Accreditation of Healthcare Organizations. 2005 comprehensive accreditation manual for hospitals. Oakbrook Terrace, IL: Joint Commission on Accreditation of Healthcare Organizations, 2005.
2. Larsen PD, Martin JL. Polypharmacy and elderly patients. AORN J 1999;69:619-22, 625, 627-628.
3. Stewart RB, Cooper JW. Polypharmacy in the aged. Practical solutions. Drugs Aging 1994;4:449-461.
4. Stewart RB, Hale WE. Acute confusional states in older adults and the role of polypharmacy. Annu Rev Public Health 1992; 13: 415-430.
5. Simon SR, Chan KA, Soumerai SB, Wagner AK, Andrade SE, Feldstein AC, Lafata JE, Davis RL, Gurwitz JH. Potentially inappropriate medication use by elderly persons in U.S. Healthcare Maintenance Organizations 2000-2001. J Am Geriatr Soc 2005;53:227-232.
6. Fillenbaum GG, Pieper CF, Cohen HJ, Cornoni-Huntley JC, Guralnik JM. Comorbidity of five chronic health conditions in elderly community residents: determinants and impact on mortality. J Gerontol A Biol Sci Med Sci 2000;55: M84-89.
7. Veehof LJ, Stewart R, Haaijer-Ruskamp FM, Meyboom-de Jong B. Chronic polypharmacy in one-third of the elderly in family practice. Ned Tijdschr Geneeskd 1999; 143: 93-97.
8. Veehof LJG, Stewart RE, Haaijer-Ruskamp RM, Meyboom-de Jong B. The development of polypharmacy. A longitudinal study. Family Practice 2000; 17: 261-267.
9. Kohn L, Corrigan J, Donaldson M. To err is human: Building a safer health system. Washington, DC: Institute of Medicine National Academy Press; 1999.
10. Leape LL. Error in medicine. JAMA 1994;272: 1851-1857.
11. Bates DW, Cullen DJ, Laird N, Petersen LA, Small SD, Servi D, Laffel G, Sweitzer BJ, Shea BF, Hallisey R. Incidence of adverse drug events and potential

adverse drug events. Implications for prevention. ADE Prevention Study Group. JAMA 1995; 274: 29-34.

12. Bates DW, Teich JM, Lee J, Seger D, Kuperman GJ, Ma'Luf N, Boyle D, Leape L. The impact of computerized physician order entry on medication error prevention. J Am Med Inform Assoc 1999; 6(4): 313- 321.

13. Miller RK, Nelson MS, Spurlock BW. A compendium of suggested practices for preventing and reducing medication errors. Sacramento, CA: California Institute for Health Systems Performance, 2001.

14. Lesar TS, Briceland L, Stein DS. Factor related to errors in medication prescribing. JAMA 1997; 277: 312-317.

CHAPTER 8

Drug Interactions

DEFINITION

An interaction is said to occur when the effects of one drug are changed by the presence of another drug, herbal medicine, food, drink or by some environmental chemical agent.

PREVALENCE

Among US adults older than 55, 4% are taking medication and or supplements that put them at risk of a major drug interaction. Potential drug-drug interactions have increased over time and are more common in the low educated elderly even after controlling for age, sex, place of residence, and co morbidity.

FACTORS CONTRIBUTING TO DRUG INTERACTIONS

Some of the more important risk factors that lead to drug interactions include-

1. **Multiple drug therapy:** This is very common in most acute and chronic care settings, e.g., therapy in patient suffering from hypertension and congestive heart failure includes antihypertensives as Concurrent use of non-prescription drugs, e.g. aspirin as well as herbal medications also lead to drug interactions. Theoretically, the possibility for drug interactions to occur is over 50% when a patent is receiving five medications, and the probability increases to 100% when seven drugs are used.
2. **Multiple prescribers:** Some individuals go to more than one physician, and it is common for a patient to be treated by one or more specialists in addition to family doctors. It is frequently difficult for one prescriber to become aware of all the medications that have been prescribed by others for a particular patient, and many difficulties arise for a patient while another prescribe an antihistamine having sedative properties with the possible consequence of an excessive depressant effect.
3. **Multiple pharmacological effects of drug:** Most drugs used in current therapy exhibit more than one type of pharmacological action and have the capacity to influence many physiological systems. Therefore, two concomitantly administered drugs will often affect some of the same systems, e.g. antihistamines (secondary effect is sedation) enhance the sedative effect of tranquillizers.
4. **Multiple diseases/predisposing illness:** Some patients take several drugs owing

to their suffering from more than one disease, e.g. a patient with both diabetes and hypertension. Multiple therapies in such individuals generally result in drug interactions, e.g., oral Hypoglycemics and beta-blockers can result in decreased response to anti diabetic drug resulting in elevated blood sugar levels.

5. **Poor patient compliance:** This result when a patient does not take medication in the manner intended by the doctor; which may be due to inadequate instructions from the doctor or pharmacist, confusion regarding taking several medicines, etc. all of which of may lead to either under dosing or Overdosing, and a consequent drug interaction.
6. **Advancing age patient:** Increased tendency of drug interaction episodes in elderly is generally due to decrease in liver function in such individuals.
7. **Drug-related factors:** Clinically significant interactions are most likely to occur between drugs that have potent effects, a narrow therapeutic index and a steep dose-response curve (e.g., cytotoxic, antihyper-tensive, and hypoglycemic drugs, digoxin, warfarin, etc.).

MECHANISMS OF DRUG INTERACTION

Some drugs interact together in totally unique ways, but as the many examples amply illustrate, there are certain mechanisms of interaction that are encountered time and

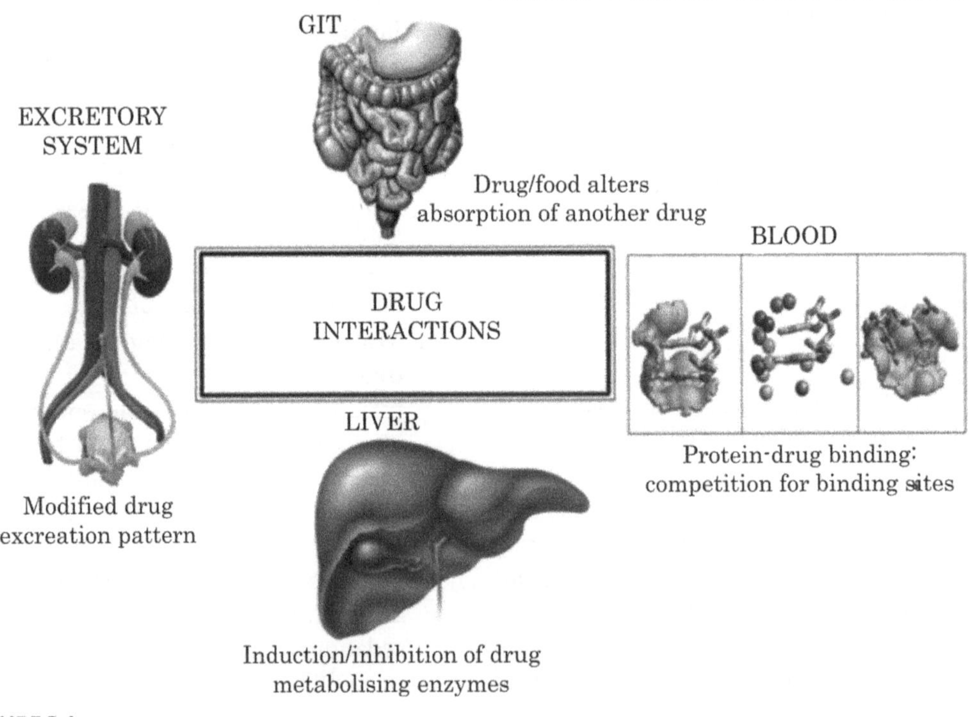

FIGURE 8.1

Pharmacokinetic interactions.

time again. Some of these common mechanisms are discussed here in greater detail. Mechanisms that are unusual or peculiar to particular pairs of drugs are detailed within the monographs. Very many drugs that interact do so, not by a single mechanism, but often by two or more mechanisms acting in concert, although for clarity most of the mechanisms are dealt with here as though they occur in isolation. For convenience, the mechanisms of interactions can be subdivided into those that involve the pharmacokinetics of a drug, and those that are pharmacodynamic.

I. Pharmacokinetic Interactions

Pharmacokinetic interactions (Fig. 8.1) are those that can affect the processes by which drugs are absorbed, distributed, metabolized and excreted (the so called ADME interactions). Table 8.1 indicates list of important pharmacokinetic interactions.

DRUG ABSORPTION INTERACTIONS

Most drugs are given orally for absorption through the mucous membranes of the gastrointestinal tract, and the majority of interactions that go on within the gut result in reduced rather than increased absorption. A clear distinction must be made between those that decrease the rate of absorption and those that alter the total amount absorbed. For drugs that are given long-term, in multiple doses (e.g. the oral anticoagulants) the rate of absorption is usually unimportant, provided the total amount of drug absorbed is not markedly altered. On the other hand for drugs that are given as single doses, intended to be absorbed rapidly (e.g. hypnotics or analgesics), where a rapidly achieved high concentration is needed, a reduction in the rate of absorption may result in failure to achieve an adequate effect.

(a) Effects of Changes in Gastrointestinal pH

The passage of drugs through mucous membranes by simple passive diffusion depends upon the extent to which they exist in the non-ionised lipid- soluble form. Absorption is therefore governed by the pKa of the drug, its lipid-solubility, the pH of the contents of the gut and various other parameters relating to the pharmaceutical formulation of the drug. Thus the absorption of salicylic acid by the stomach is much greater at low pH than at high. On theoretical grounds it might be expected that alterations in gastric pH caused by drugs such as the H2-receptor antagonists would have a marked effect on absorption, but in practice the outcome is often uncertain because a number of other mechanisms may also come into play, such as chelation, adsorption and changes in gut motility, which can considerably affect what actually happens. However, in some cases the effect can be significant. Rises in pH due to 'proton pump inhibitors', 'H2-receptor antagonists', can markedly reduce the absorption of ketoconazole.

(b) Adsorption, Chelation and Other Complexing Mechanisms

Activated charcoal is intended to act as an adsorbing agent within the gut for the treatment of drug overdose or to remove other toxic materials, but inevitably it can affect the absorption of drugs given in therapeutic doses. Antacids can also adsorb a large number of drugs, but often other mechanisms of interaction are also involved. e.g., the tetracycline antibacterials can chelate with a number of divalent and trivalent metallic ions, such as calcium, aluminum, bismuth and iron, to form complexes that are both poorly absorbed and have reduced antibacterial effects. These metallic ions are found in dairy products and antacids. Separating the dosages by 2 to 3 hours goes some way towards reducing the effects of this type of interaction. The marked reduction in the bioavailability of penicillamine caused by some antacids seems also to be due to chelation, although adsorption may have some part to play. Cholestyramine, an anionic exchange resin intended to bind bile acids and cholesterol metabolites in the gut, binds to a considerable number of drugs (e.g. digoxin, warfarin, levothyroxine), thereby reducing their absorption.

(c) Changes in Gastrointestinal Motility

Since most drugs are largely absorbed in the upper part of the small intestine, drugs that alter the rate at which the stomach empties can affect absorption. Propantheline, for example, delays gastric emptying and reduces 'paracetamol (acetaminophen)' absorption, whereas 'metoclopramide', has the opposite effect. However, the total amount of drug absorbed remains unaltered. Propantheline also increases the absorption of 'hydrochlorothiazide'. Drugs with antimuscarinic effects decrease the motility of the gut, thus the tricyclic antidepressants can increase the absorption of 'dicoumarol', probably because they increase the time available for dissolution and absorption but in the case of 'levodopa', they may reduce the absorption, possibly because the exposure time to intestinal mucosal metabolism is increased. The same reduced levodopa absorption has also been seen with 'homatropine'. These examples illustrate that what actually happens is sometimes very unpredictable because the final outcome may be the result of several different mechanisms.

(d) Malabsorption caused by Drugs

Neomycin causes a malabsorption syndrome. The effect is to impair the absorption of a number of drugs including 'digoxin', and 'methotrexate'.

DRUG DISTRIBUTION INTERACTIONS

PROTEIN-BINDING INTERACTIONS

Following absorption, drugs are rapidly distributed around the body by the circulation. Some drugs are totally dissolved in the plasma water, but many others are transported with some proportion of their molecules in solution and the rest bound to plasma proteins, particularly the albumins. The extent of this binding varies enormously but some drugs are extremely highly bound. For example, dicoumarol has only four out of every 1000 molecules remaining unbound at serum concentrations of 0.5% mg. Drugs can also become bound to albumin in the interstitial fluid, and some, such as digoxin, can bind to the heart muscle tissue. The binding of drugs to the plasma proteins is reversible, an equilibrium being established between those molecules that are bound and those that are not. Only the unbound molecules remain free and pharmacologically active, while those that are bound form a circulating but pharmacologically inactive reservoir which, in the case of drugs with a low-extraction ratio, is temporarily protected from metabolism and excretion. As the free molecules become metabolized, some of the bound molecules become unbound and pass into solution to exert their normal pharmacological actions, Depending on the concentrations and their relative affinities for the binding sites; one drug may successfully compete with another and displace it from the sites it is already occupying. The displaced (and now active) drug molecules pass into the plasma water where their concentration rises. So for example, a drug that reduces the binding from 99%-95% would increase the unbound concentration of free and active drug from 1% -5% (a fivefold increase). This displacement is only likely to raise the number of free and active molecules significantly if the majority of the drug is within the plasma rather than the tissues, so that only drugs with a low apparent volume of distribution (V_d) will be affected. Examples include the sulphonylureas, such as tolbutamide (96% bound, V_d 10 L), oral anticoagulants, such as warfarin (99% bound, V_d 9 L), and phenytoin (90% bound, V_d 35 L). However, another important factor is clearance. Clinically important protein-binding interactions are unlikely if only a small proportion of the drug is eliminated during a single-passage through the eliminating organ (low-extraction ratio drugs), since any increase in free fraction will be effectively cleared. Most drugs that are extensively bound to plasma proteins and subject to displacement reactions (e.g. warfarin, sulphonylureas, phenytoin, methotrexate, and valproate) have low extraction ratios, and drug exposure is therefore independent of protein binding. Before they, in their turn are metabolized and excreted.

DRUG METABOLISM (BIOTRANSFORMATION) INTERACTIONS

Although a few drugs are cleared from the body simply by being excreted unchanged in the urine, most are chemically altered within the body to less lipid-soluble compounds, which are more easily excreted by the kidneys. If this were not so, many drugs would persist in the body and continue to exert their effects for a long time. This chemical change is called 'metabolism', 'biotransformation', 'biochemical degradation' or sometimes 'detoxification'. Some drug metabolism goes on in the serum, the kidneys, the skin and the intestines, but the greatest proportion is carried out by enzymes that are found in the membranes of the endoplasmic reticulum of the liver cells. If liver is homogenized and then centrifuged, the reticulum breaks up into small sacs called microsomes which carry the enzymes, and it is for this reason that the metabolizing enzymes of the liver are frequently referred to as the 'liver microsomal enzymes'. Drugs are metabolized by two major types of reaction. The first, so-called phase I reactions (involving oxidation, reduction or hydrolysis), turn drugs into more polar compounds, while phase II reactions involve coupling drugs with some other substance (e.g. Glucuronic acid, known as Glucuronidation) to make usually inactive compounds. The majority of phase I oxidation reactions are carried out by the haem containing enzyme cytochrome P450. Cytochrome P450 is not a single entity, but is in fact a very large family of related isoenzymes, about 30 of which have been found in human liver tissue. However, in practice, only a few specific subfamilies seem to be responsible for most (about 90%) of the metabolism of the commonly used drugs. The most important isoenzymes are: CYP1A2, CYP2C9, CYP2C19, CYP2D6, CYP2E1 and CYP3A4. Other enzymes involved in phase I metabolism include monoamine oxidases and epoxide hydrolases. Less is known about the enzymes responsible for phase II conjugation reactions. However, UDP-glucuronyltransferases (UGT), methyltransferase, and N-acetyltransferases (NAT) are examples.

(a) Changes in First-Pass Metabolism

(i) Changes in blood flow through the liver

After absorption in the intestine, the portal circulation takes drugs directly to the liver before they are distributed by the blood flow around the rest of the body. A number of highly lipid-soluble drugs undergo substantial biotransformation during this first-pass through the gut wall and liver and there is some evidence that some drugs can have a marked effect on the extent of first pass metabolism by altering the blood flow through the liver. However, there are few clinically relevant examples of this, and many can be explained by other mechanisms, usually altered hepatic metabolism. One possible example is the increase in rate of absorption of dofetilide with 'verapamil', which has resulted in an increased incidence of torsade de pointes. Another is the increase in bioavailability of high-extraction beta blockers with 'Hydralazine', possibly caused by altered hepatic blood flow, or altered metabolism.

(ii) Inhibition or Induction of First-pass Metabolism

The gut wall contains metabolizing enzymes, principally the cytochrome P450 isoenzymes. In addition to the altered metabolism caused by changes in hepatic blood flow, there is evidence that some drugs can have a marked effect on the extent of first-pass metabolism by inhibiting or inducing the cytochrome P450 isoenzymes in the gut wall or in the liver. An example is the effect of grapefruit juice, which seems to inhibit the cytochrome P450 isoenzyme CYP3A4, mainly in the gut, and therefore reduces the metabolism of oral calcium-channel blockers. Although altering the amount of drug 'absorbed', these interactions are usually considered drug metabolism interactions. The effect of grapefruit on the metabolism of other drugs is discussed further under 'Drug-food interactions'.

(b) Enzyme Induction

When barbiturates were widely used as hypnotics it was found necessary to keep increasing the dosage as time went by to achieve the same hypnotic effect, the reason being that the barbiturates increase the activity of the microsomal enzymes so that extent of metabolism and excretion increases. This phenomenon of enzyme stimulation or 'induction' not only accounts for the need for an increased barbiturate dose but if another drug that is metabolized by the same range of enzymes is also present, its enzymatic metabolism is similarly increased and larger doses are needed to maintain the same therapeutic effect. However, note that not all enzyme-inducing drugs induce their own metabolism (a process known as auto-induction). The metabolic pathway that is most commonly induced is phase I oxidation mediated by the cytochrome P450 isoenzymes. The extent of the enzyme induction depends on the drug and its dosage, but it may take days or even 2 to 3 weeks to develop fully, and may persist for a similar length of time when the enzyme inducer is stopped. This means that enzyme induction interactions are delayed in onset and slow to resolve. Enzyme induction is a common mechanism of interaction and is not confined to drugs; it is also caused by the chlorinated hydrocarbon insecticides such as Dicophane and Lindane, and smoking tobacco. If one drug reduces the effects of another by enzyme induction, it may be possible to accommodate the interaction simply by raising the dosage of the drug affected, but this requires good monitoring, and there are obvious hazards if the inducing drug is eventually stopped without remembering to reduce the dosage again. The raised drug dosage may be an overdose when the drug metabolism has returned to normal.

(c) Enzyme Inhibition

More common than enzyme induction is the inhibition of enzymes. This results in the reduced metabolism of an affected drug, so that it may begin to accumulate within the body, the effect usually being essentially the same as when the dosage is increased. Unlike enzyme induction, which may take several days or even weeks to develop fully, enzyme inhibition can occur within 2 to 3 days, resulting in the rapid development of toxicity. The metabolic pathway that is most commonly inhibited is phase I oxidation by the cytochrome P450 isoenzymes. For example a marked increase occurred in the plasma levels of a single dose of sildenafil after Ritonavir had also been taken for 7 days, probably because Ritonavir inhibits the metabolism of sildenafil by CYP3A4. An example of inhibition of phase I hydrolytic metabolism, is the inhibition of epoxide hydrolase by valpromide, which increases the levels of 'carbamazepine', Phase II conjugative metabolism can also be inhibited. Examples are the inhibition of carbamazepine Glucuronidation by 'sodium valproate', and the inhibition of methyltransferase by aminosalicylates causing raised levels of 'azathioprine'. The clinical significance of many enzyme inhibition interactions depends on the extent to which the serum levels of the drug rise. If the serum levels remain within the therapeutic range the interaction may not be clinically important.

(d)Cytochrome P450 Isoenzymes and Predicting Drug Interactions

It is interesting to know which particular isoenzyme is responsible for the metabolism of drugs because by doing *in vitro* tests with human liver enzymes it is often possible to explain why and how some drugs interact. For example, cyclosporin is metabolized by CYP3A4, and we know that Rifampicin (rifampin) is a potent inducer of this isoenzyme, whereas ketoconazole inhibits its activity, so that it comes as no surprise that Rifampicin reduces the effects of cyclosporin and ketoconazole increases it.

What is very much more important than retrospectively finding out why two drugs interact, is the knowledge such in vitro tests can provide about forecasting which other drugs may possibly also interact. This may reduce the numbers of expensive clinical studies in subjects and patients and avoids waiting until significant drug interactions are observed in clinical use. A lot of effort is being put into this area of drug development. However, at present such prediction is, like weather forecasting, still a somewhat hit-and-miss business because we do not know all of the factors that may modify or interfere with metabolism. It is far too simplistic to think that we have all the answers just because we know which liver isoenzymes are concerned with the metabolism of a particular drug, but it is a very good start.

DRUG EXCRETION INTERACTIONS

With the exception of the inhalation anesthetics, most drugs are excreted either in the bile or in the urine. Blood entering the kidneys along the renal arteries is, first of all, delivered to the glomeruli of the tubules where molecules small enough to pass through the pores of the glomerular membrane (e.g. water, salts, some drugs) are filtered through into the lumen of the tubules. Larger molecules, such as plasma proteins, and blood cells are retained within the blood. The blood flow then passes to the remaining parts of the kidney tubules where active energy-using transport systems are able to remove drugs and their metabolites from the blood and secrete them into the tubular filtrate (Fig. 8.2). The renal tubular cells additionally possess active and passive transport systems for the re-absorption of drugs. Interference by drugs with renal tubular fluid pH, with active transport systems and with blood flow to the kidney can alter the excretion of other drugs.

(a) Changes in Urinary pH

As with drug absorption in the gut, passive reabsorption of drugs depends upon the extent to which the drug exists in the non-ionised lipid-soluble form, which in its turn depends on its pKa and the pH of the urine. Only the non-ionised form is lipid-soluble and able to diffuse back through the lipid membranes of the tubule cells. Thus at high pH values (alkaline), weakly acid drugs

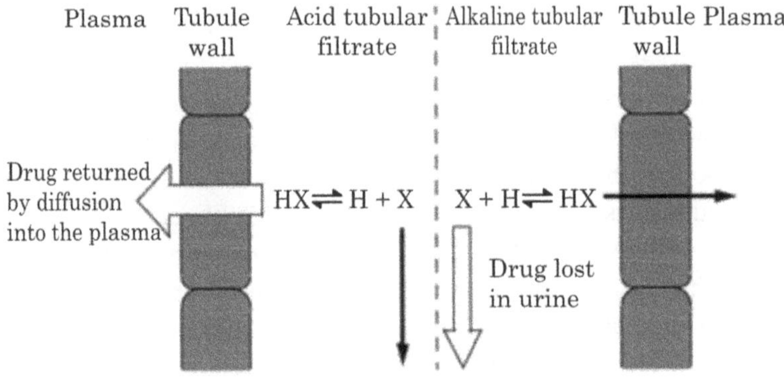

FIGURE 8.2

An excretion interaction. If the tubular filtrate is acidified, most of the molecules of weakly acid drugs (HX) exist in an un-ionised lipid-soluble form and are able to return through the lipid membranes of the tubule cells by simple diffusion. Thus they are retained. In alkaline urine most of the drug. Molecules exist in an ionised non-lipid soluble form (X). In this form the molecules are unable to diffuse freely through these membranes and are therefore lost in the urine.

(pKa 3 to 7.5) largely exist as ionised lipid-insoluble molecules, which are unable to diffuse into the tubule cells and will therefore remain in the urine and be removed from the body. The converse will be true for weak bases with pKa values of 7.5 to 10.5. Thus pH changes that increase the amount in the ionized form (alkaline urine for acidic drugs, acid urine for basic drugs) increase the loss of the drug, whereas moving the pH in the opposite direction will increase their retention.

(b) Changes in Active Renal Tubular Excretion

Drugs that use the same active transport systems in the renal tubules can compete with one another for excretion. For example, probenecid reduces the excretion of penicillin and other drugs. With the increasing understanding of drug transporter proteins in the kidneys, it is now known that probenecid inhibits the renal secretion of many other anionic drugs by organic anion transporters (OATs). Probenecid possibly also inhibits some of the ABC transporters in the kidneys. The ABC transporter, P-glycoprotein, is also present in the kidneys, and drugs that alter this may alter renal drug elimination.

(c) Changes in Renal Blood Flow

The flow of blood through the kidney is partially controlled by the production of renal vasodilatory prostaglandins. If the synthesis of these prostaglandins is inhibited the renal excretion of some drugs may be reduced. An interaction where this is the suggested mechanism is the rise in serum lithium seen with some NSAIDs.

(d) Biliary Excretion and the Entero-hepatic Shunt

(i) Enterohepatic Recirculation

A number of drugs are excreted in the bile, either unchanged or conjugated (e.g. as the Glucuronide) to make them more water soluble. Some of the conjugates are metabolised to the parent compound by the gut flora and are then reabsorbed. This recycling process prolongs the stay of the drug within the body, but if the gut flora are diminished by the presence of an antibacterial, the drug is not recycled and is lost more quickly. This may possibly explain the rare failure of the oral contraceptives that can be brought about by the concurrent use of penicillin's or Tetracyclines. Antimicrobial-induced reductions in gut bacteria may reduce the activation of 'Sulphasalazine'.

(ii) Drug Transporters

Increasing research shows that numerous drug transporter proteins (both from the ABC family and SLC family, 'Drug transporter proteins', are involved in the hepatic extraction and secretion of drugs into the bile. The relevance of many of these to drug interactions is still unclear, but the bile salt export pump (ABCB11) is known to be inhibited by a variety of drugs including cyclosporine, Glibenclamide, and Bosentan. Inhibition of this pump may increase the risk of cholestasis, and the manufacturer of Bosentan says that they should be avoided in patients taking Bosentan.

Table 8.1

List of some of the important pharmacokinetic (ADME) interactions

Object Drug (s)	Precipitant Drug (s)	Influence on Object Drug (s)
	Absorption Interactions	
1. Complexation and Adsorption		
Tetracycline, fluoroquinolones like ciprofloxacin, Penicillamine Cephalexin, sulpha-methozazole, trimethoprim, warfarin and thyroxine	Antacids, food and mineral supplements containing Al,Mg,Fe,Zn, Bi, and Ca ions Cholestyramine	Formation of poorly soluble and un-absorbable complex with such heavy metal ions Reduced absorption due to adsorption and binding
2. Alteration of GI pH		
Sulphonamides, aspirin Ferrous sulphate Ketoconazole, tetracycline, Atenolol	Antacids Sodium bicarbonate, calcium carbonate Antacids	Enhanced dissolution and absorption rate Decreased dissolution and hence absorption Decreased dissolution and bioavailability
3. Alteration of Gut Motility		
Aspirin, diazepam, levodapa, lithium carbonate, paracetamol, mexiletine.	Metoclopramide	Rapid gastric emptying; increased rate of absorption
Levodapa, lithium carbonate, mexiletine	Anticholinergic (Atropine)	Delayed gastric emptying: decreased rate of absorption
4. Alteration of GI Microflora		
Digoxin	Antibiotics (erythromycin, tetracycline)	Increased bioavailability due to destruction of bacterial flora that inactivates digoxin in lower intestine.
Oral contraceptives	Antibiotics (ampicillin)	Decreased re-absorption of drugs secreted as conjugates via bile in the intestine.
5. Malabsorption Syndrome		
Vitamin A, B12, digoxin	Neomycin (and colchicines)	Inhibition of absorption due to malabsorption/steatorrhoea caused by neomycin
	Distribution Interactions	
	Competitive Displacement Interactions	
Displaced drug(s)	**Displacer(s)**	
Anticoagulants (warfarin)	Phenylbutazone, chloral hydrate, salicylates	Increased clotting, time; increased risk of haemorrhage.
Tolbutamide	Sulphonamides	Increased hypoglycemic effect
Methotrexate	Sulphonamides, salicylic acid	Increased methotrexate toxicity
Phenytoin	Valproic acid	Phenytoin toxicity

Table 8.1 *Contd...*

Object Drug (s)	Precipitant Drug (s)	Influence on Object Drug (s)
Metabolism Interactions		
1. Enzyme Induction		
Corticosteroids, oral contraceptives, coumarins, phenytoin, tolbutamide, tricyclic antidepressants	Barbiturates	Decreased plasma levels; decreased efficacy of object drugs
Corticosteroids, oral contraceptives, theophylline, cyclosporin	Phenytoin	Decreased plasma levels; decreased efficacy of object drugs
Oral contraceptives, oral hypoglycemics, coumarins	Rifampicin	Decreased plasma levels; decreased efficacy of object drugs
2. Enzyme Inhibition		
Tyramine rich food (cheese, liver, yeast products)	MAO Inhibitors (phenelzine , pargyline)	Enhanced absorption of unmetabolised tyramine; increased pressor activity; potentially fatal risk of hypertensive crises
Drugs that undergo extensive first-pass hepatic metabolism (e.g. Propranolol, calcium channel blockers, etc.)	Grape fruit juice	Enhanced absorption of drugs; increased risk of toxicity.
Folic acid	Phenytoin	Decreased absorption of folic acid due to inhibition of an enzyme responsible for its absorption
Tricyclic antidepressants	Chlorpromazine, Haloperidol	Increased plasma half-life of tricyclics; increased risk of sudden death from cardiac disease in such patients.
Coumarins	Metronidazole, Phenylbutazone	Increased anticoagulant activity; risk of haemorrhage
Oral hypoglycemics	Phenylbutazone, sulphaphenazole, chloramphenicol	Hypoglycemia may be precipitated
Alcohol	Disulphiram, Metronidazole, Tinidazole	Disulphiram like reactions due to increase in plasma acetaldehyde levels
AZT, mercaptopurine	Xanthine oxidase inhibitors (Allopurinol)	Increased toxicity of antineoplastics
Alcohol, benzodiazepines, warfarin, phenytoin, theophylline, phenobarbital	Cimetidine	Increased blood levels of object drugs

Table 8.1 *Contd...*

Object Drug (s)	Precipitant Drug (s)	Influence on Object Drug (s)
	Excretion Interactions	
1. Changes in Active Tubular Secretion		
Penicillin, cephalosporin, Nalidixic acid, PAS, Methotrexate, Dapsone	Probenecid (acid)	Elevated plasma levels of acidic drugs; risk of toxic reactions
Procainamide	Cimetidine (base)	Increased plasma levels of basic object drugs; risk of toxicity
Acetohexamide	Phenylbutazone	Increased hypoglycemic effect
2. Changes in Urine pH		
Amphetamine, tetracycline, quinidine	Antacids, Thiazides, Acetazolamide	Increased passive reabsorption of basic drugs; increased risk of toxicity
3. Changes in Renal Blood Flow		
Lithium bicarbonate	NSAIDS (inhibitors of prostaglandin synthesis; the latter control renal blood flow partially by vasoconstriction)	Decreased renal clearance of lithium; risk of toxicity

II. Pharmacodynamic Interactions

Pharmacodynamic interactions are those where the effects of one drug are changed by the presence of another drug at its site of action. Sometimes the drugs directly compete for particular receptors (e.g. β2 agonists, such as Salbutamol, and beta blockers, such as propranolol) but often the reaction is more indirect and involves interference with physiological mechanisms. These interactions are much less easy to classify neatly than those of a pharmacokinetic type.

(a) Drugs having Similar Pharmacological Effects

An excessive response attribute to the concurrent use of drugs having similar actions is the type of interaction that occurs most often, and these potential problems warrant particular attention (Table 8.2).

CNS depressants: An excessive CNS depressant effect resulting from the concurrent use of two or more drugs exhibiting a depressant action represents one of the most dangerous drug-related problems. Older patients should be viewed as being especially susceptible to this type of response, and patients experiencing effects such as sedation and dizziness are at increased risk of falls and injuries, such as hip fractures. Patients also must be advised of the risks of operating motor vehicles or machinery. In considering multiple drug regimens, recognition must be taken of the large number of agents (e.g., sedative-hypnotics, antipsychotics, tricyclic antidepressants, opioid analgesics, and most antihistamines) than can exhibit a depressant effect that will be at least additive to the effect contributed by other drugs. If it is considered necessary to use agents with a CNS depressant action concurrently, it should be anticipated that a lower dosage of at least one of the agents should be used.

Alcohol-other CNS depressants: The increased CNS depressant effect that is experienced by individuals being treated with depressant drugs when they consume alcoholic beverages is among the best-known interactions. However, this interaction also illustrates the difficulties in trying to predict the magnitude of the response that will be experienced by a particular patient; a response will depend on many variables, including the patient's tolerance to alcohol. How then should the patient be instructed when he or she is to take a depressant medication? Certainly it would be most desirable not to consume alcoholic beverages during the period the medication is being taken. However, there should be a realistic recognition that many patients if faced with a mandate not to drink while on drug therapy will decide not to take the drug. Every patient should be alerted to the fact that the depressant effect of the drug prescribed may be increased by alcohol. If it is anticipated that a patient would not completely avoid alcoholic beverages, that patient should be urged to use them in moderation, particularly when therapy is initiated or the dosage is increased, and cautioned to observe his or her own tolerance when such combinations are employed. The fact that many individuals can take depressant drugs and consume relatively large amounts of alcoholic beverages with no apparent difficulty should not be cause to forget that such combinations have been lethal in some individuals and the cause of injury in others. Thus, there is an important need to caution all patients for whom such drugs are prescribed.

Drugs having Anti Cholinergic Activity

Drugs that differ considerably in their primary pharmacological actions may exhibit the same secondary effects. Some patients being treated with antipsychotic agents such as chlorpromazine also the given an antiparkinson agent such as trihexyphenidyl to control the extra pyramidal effects of the former. In addition, a number of these patients experience symptoms of depression, and a tricycle antidepressant such as amitriptyline might be added to the therapy. Each of these three agents possesses anticholinergic activity, and the additive effect could result in side effects such as dryness of the mouth, blurred vision, urinary retention, constipation, and elevation of intraocular pressure.

Even an effect such as dryness of the mouth, which most health professionals would consider as a minor problem, could be troublesome in certain patients. For example, persistent dryness of the mouth could make the use of dentures more difficult and also cause other dental complications. In addition, there may be increased difficulty in chewing and swallowing, an important factor with respect to the problem of malnutrition in many elderly individuals. Dryness of the mouth also may result in other problems as illustrated by a case report of a patient treated with imipramine. The patient experienced persistent dryness of the mouth and when nitroglycerin tablets were administered sublingually for the management of exertional angina, the relief of the symptoms was delayed because of the slower dissolution of the sublingual tablets.

It has been observed that an excessive anti cholinergic effect can cause an atropine-like delirium, particularly in geriatric patients. This effect could be misinterpreted as an increase in psychiatric symptoms, which might be treated by increasing the dosage of the therapeutic agents that the actually responsible for causing the problem. This example points out the difficulty that often can exist in distinguishing between the symptoms of the conditions(s) being treated and the effects of the drug(s) being employed as therapy.

Several studies call attention to other potential problems associated with the use of drugs having anticholinergic activity. In one investigation using volunteers aged 60 to 72, trihexyphenidyl was found to cause substantial memory impairment. In another study of 22 demented nursing-home patients, it was noted that those with high serum anti cholinergic concentrations had greater impairment in elf-care capacity than patients with low concentrations.

The blurring of vision, which also may be associated with the use of drugs having anticholinergic activity, may be especially distressing for older patients, particularly those whose physical activities may be limited and for whom reading is a favorite activity.

Several reports have described the development of severe hyperpyrexia in patients taking phenothaizine-antiparkinson combinations who were exposed to high environmental temperature and humidity. These investigations call attention to the ability of these combinations to interfere with the thermoregulatory system of the body and recommend that physicians treating patients in hot and humid climates should minimize outdoor exposure of patients receiving high doses of these agents.

Drugs Exhibiting Hypotensive Effects

Certain antihypertensive drugs as well as some other classes of medications e.g., tricyclic antidepressants) can cause orthostatic hypotension, resulting in symptoms such as dizziness, lightheadedness, and, in more severe cases, syncope. Older patients are most susceptible to this type of response and the associated risks such as falls and injuries, and appropriate precautions should be exercised whether these agents are given alone or in combination.

The use of sildenafil, tadalafil, and vardenafil in the treatment of erectile dysfunction is contraindicated in patients treated with nitrates because these agents may potentiate the hypotensive effect of the nitrates.

NSAIDS

Several situations exist in which a patient unknowingly may be taking several different products that contain the same NSAID. An arthritic patient whose conditions has been managed with ibuprofen obtained via prescription often at dosage levels at or near the recommended maximum may purchase an ibuprofen product available without a prescription for pain/discomfort not associated with the arthritis, without recognizing that the two products contain the same drug and that there is an increased risk of adverse effects.

Table 8.2

Additive, synergistic or summation interactions

Drugs	Result of Interaction
Antipsychotics + Antimuscarinics	Increased antimuscarinic effects; heart stroke in hot and humid conditions, toxic psychosis
Antihypertensives + drugs that cause hypotension (e.g. Phenothiazines, Sildenafil)	Increased antihypertensive effects
Beta-agonist bronchodilators + Potassium depleting drugs	Hypokalemia
CNS depressants + Alcohol + Antihistamines Benzodiazepines + Anaesthetics, general Opiods + Benzodiazepines	Impaired psychomotor skills, reduced alertness, drowsiness, stupor, respiratory depression, coma, death
Drugs that prolong the QT interval + Other drugs that prolong the QT interval Amiodarone + Disopyramide	Additive prolongation of QT interval, increased risk of torsade depointes
Methotrexate + CO-trimoxazole	Bone marrow megaloblastosis due to folic acid antagonism.
Nephrotoxic drugs + Nephrotoxic drugs (e.g.Aminoglycosides, Cyclosporin, Cisplatin, Vancomycin)	Increased nephrotoxicity
Neuromuscular blockers + Drugs with neuro-muscular blocking effects (e.g. Amino-glycosides)	Increased neuromuscular blockade; delayed recovery, prolonged apnoea.
Potassium supplements + Potassium sparing drugs (e.g. ACE inhibitors, Angiotensin II receptor antagonists, Potassium-sparing diuretics)	Hyperkalemia

(b) Drugs having Opposing Pharmacological Effects

Interactions resulting from the use of two drugs with opposing effects should be among the easiest to detect. However, these sometimes are due to the secondary effects of certain drugs and this and other factors may preclude early identification of such situations (Table 8.3).

Diuretics: The ability of the thiazides and certain other diuretics to elevate blood glucose concentrations is well known. When the diuretic is prescribed for a diabetic patient being treated with insulin or one of the oral antidiabetic agents, this action may partially counteract the glucose-lowering action of the anti-diabetic drug, necessitating an adjustment in dosage. Similarly, many diuretics may produce a hyperuricemic effect. Therapy in patients with gout should be monitored closely, as the hyperuricemic action of a diuretic may necessitate an adjustment in dosage of the agent being used in the treatment of gout.

Table 8.3

Opposing or antagonistic interactions

Drugs affected	Interacting drugs	Results of interaction
ACE inhibitors or Loop diuretics or Loop diuretics	NSAIDs	Antihypertensive effects opposed
Anticoagulants	Vitamin K	Anticoagulant effects opposed
Antidiabetics	Glucocorticoids	Blood glucose-lowering effects opposed
Antineoplastics	Megestrol	Antineoplastic effects possibly opposed
Levodopa	Antipsychotics (those with dopamine antagonist effects)	Antiparkinsonian effects opposed
Levodopa	Tacrine	Antiparkinsonian effects opposed

(c) Alteration of Electrolyte Concentrations

Several important drug interactions occur as a result of the ability of certain therapeutic agents to alter the concentration of electrolytes such as potassium and sodium. When these drugs are included in a therapeutic regimen, it is important that electrolyte concentrations be monitored periodically.

Digoxin-Diuretics

One of the problems associated with the use of most of the commonly employed diuretics (e.g., The Thiazide derivatives is that they can cause an excessive loss of potassium. Particular caution is necessary in patients also being treated with digoxin, many of whom would be candidates for diuretic therapy. If potassium depletion remains uncorrected, the heart may become more sensitive to the effects of the cardiac glycoside and arrhythmia may result.

Although potassium supplementation will be necessary in many individuals being treated with a potassium-depleting diuretic, the initiation of therapy with such a diuretic must not be viewed as a mandate also to provide potassium supplementation. This decision should be based on a consideration of the individual patient situation, and the appropriate parameters should be monitored periodically. It must be recognized that dangers also exist if hyperkalemia occurs as a result of excessive supplementation. This risk of such complications is greatest in patients with diminished renal functions.

In addition to the diuretics, other agents also can cause potassium depletion. Prolonged therapy with cathartics and corticosteroids may cause potassium depletion, although this is not likely to occur as quickly or to the same extent as with diuretics.

Interest has developed also in the clinical implications of magnesium depletion. Concern has been expressed that this condition occurs much more commonly than is recognized and that some clinical problems may continue or worsen despite seemingly adequate electrolyte therapy because magnesium deficiency has not been identified and corrected.

Diuretic therapy may lead to development of magnesium depletion, and as observed when potassium is depleted, the activity of digoxin may be increased and possibly result in toxicity. In some patients with digoxin toxicity, low serum-magnesium concentrations may coexist with normal potassium values.

Angiotensin-Converting Enzyme Inhibitors-Potassium-Sparing Diuretics

The angiotensin-converting enzyme (ACE) inhibitors (enalapril, lisinopril, ramipril) may cause an elevation of serum potassium concentrations. Potassium-sparing diuretics (amiloride, spironolactone and triamterne) or potassium supplements should be used concurrently with caution, because of the risk of hyperkalemia and associated complications. Salt substitutes containing potassium also should be used with caution.

Lithium-Diuretics

Sodium depletion is known to increase lithium toxicity, for which reason it generally has been recommended that lithium salts should not be used in patients on diuretic therapy or an a sodium-restricted diet. Even protracted sweating or diarrhea can cause sufficient depletion of sodium to result in decreased tolerance to lithium.

(d) Interactions at Receptor Sites

Monoaminooxidase inhibitors (MAOIs) - Sympathomimetic agents

Monoaminooxidase (MAO) functions to break down catecholamines such as nor epinephrine. When the enzyme is inhibited, the concentrations of nor epinephrine within adrenergic neurons increase, and a drug that can stimulate its release can bring about an exaggerated response. It is by this mechanism that interactions between MAOIs and indirectly acting sympathomimetic amines (e.g., amphetamine) develop. Thus, if amphetamine is administered to patients whose stores of norepinephrine have been increased by MAO inhibition, they may experience severe headache, hypertension (possible a hypertensive crisis), and cardiac arrhythmias. The serious consequences associated with these interactions contraindicate use of these agents in combination.

Although most sympathomimetic amines, such as amphetamine, are available only by prescription, others such as Phenylephrine, which also has been reported to interact similarly with MAOIs, are found in many nonprescription cold and allergy preparations. It is important that patients being treated with MAOIs avoid using products containing these agents.

MAOIs – tricyclic antidepressants: Cautions in the product literature, as well as case reports, warn against concurrent use of an MAOI with a tricyclic antidepressant (eg. amitriptyline, imipramine) because severe atropine-like reactions, tremors, convulsions, hyperthermia, and vascular collapse have been reported to result from such use. It is recommended in the labeling for most of these products that therapy with an MAOI or a tricyclic antidepressant should not be initiated until at least 7 to 14 days after therapy with the other has been discontinued.

Although the labeling for most MAOIs and tricyclic antidepressants notes that concurrent use is contraindicated, there is debate as to the degree of risk involved. Several studies of the combined use of these agents have revealed little evidence of interactions, and the growing impression that serious interactions are uncommon, coupled with the reports of favorable results with such combinations in selected patients who did not respond to either agent given alone, have led some to conclude that these combinations can be employed cautiously. In patients who are refractory to single antidepressants and who are not candidates for alternative therapeutic approaches, the potential benefits of combination therapy may outweigh the risks. However, such therapy should be undertaken only by those who are thoroughly familiar with the risks involved and under circumstances in which therapy can be monitored closely (Fig. 8.3).

MAOIs - selective serotonin reuptake inhibitors: Serious consequences may result from the combined use of an MAOI and a selective serotonin reuptake inhibitor (SSRI, citalopram, escitalopram, fluoxetine, fluvoxamine, paroxetine, sertaline), and concurrent use of use within 14 days before or after most of these agents is contraindicated.

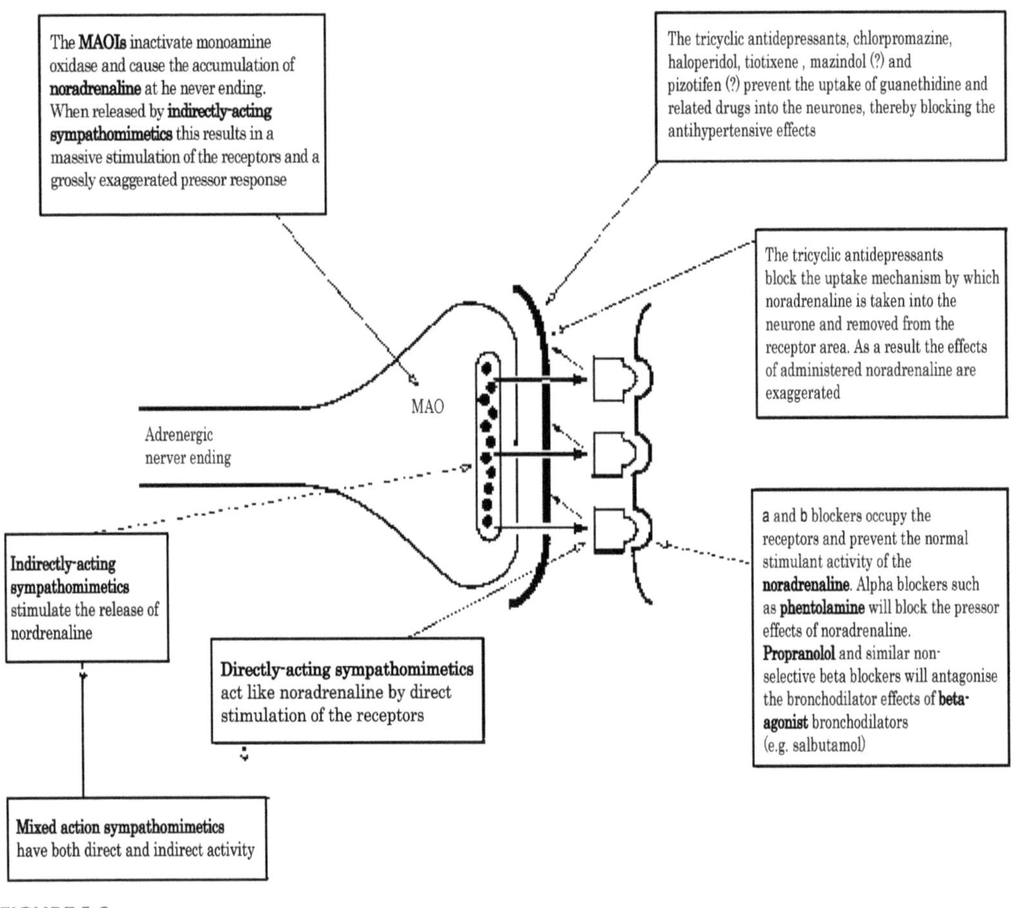

FIGURE 8.3

Interactions at adrenergic neurons. A highly simplified composite diagram of an adrenergic neuron (molecules of noradrenaline (norepinephrine) indicated as (•) contained in a single vesicle at the nerve-ending) to illustrate in outline some of the different sites where drugs can interact.

There have been several reports of deaths of patients in whom therapy with an MAOI was initiated shortly after discontinuation of fluoxetine. Because of the long half-lives of fluoxetine and its active metabolite, it is recommended that atleast 5 weeks should elapse between discontinuation of fluoxetine and initiation of therapy with an MAOI.

It should be noted that the antineoplastic procarbazine and the anti-infectives furazolidone and linezolid, also can inhibit MAO enzymes, and warnings applying to the use of other MAOIs should be heeded for these drugs also.

Guanethidine-tricyclic antidepressants: Guanethidine is transported to its site of action within adrenergic neurons by a transport system that also is responsible for uptake of nor epinephrine, as well as several indirectly acting sympathomimetic amines such as ephedrine and the amphetamines. Concentration of guanethidine in these neurons is necessary for its antihypertensive action. Tricyclic antidepressants can inhibit uptake of guanethidine into the neuron terminal, thereby preventing its concentration at these sites and reducing its activity. Other studies suggest that antipsychotic agents such as chlorpromazine and haloperidol can act similarly to the tricyclic antidepressants in reducing the antihypertensive effect of this agent.

Although other mechanisms may be involved in the development of drug interactions, the ones cited are the most important. As often stated, more than one mechanism may be responsible for certain interactions; these mechanisms may work in concert or in opposition as determinants of the resulting effect. Still other drug interactions develop by mechanisms yet to be identified.

However, an awareness of the factors predisposing to the development of drug interactions, as well as the mechanisms by which many of them occur, will be of value in the identification and prevention of potential problems.

It is evident that significant limitations still exist in trying to predict the results of combination therapy. In the following section, guidelines are provided to reduce the risk of the occurrence of drug interactions.

DRUG - FOOD INTERACTIONS

It is well established that food can cause clinically important changes in drug absorption through effects on gastrointestinal motility or by drug binding, In addition, it is well known that tyramine (present in some foodstuffs) may reach toxic concentrations in patients taking 'MAOIs'. With the growth in understanding of drug metabolism mechanisms, it has been increasingly recognized that some foods can alter drug metabolism. Currently, grapefruit juice causes the most clinically relevant of these interactions, Table 8.4 lists some food drug interactions.

(a) Cruciferous Vegetables and Charcoal-broiled Meats

Cruciferous vegetables, such as Brussels sprouts, cabbage, and broccoli, contain substances that are inducers of the cytochrome P450 isoenzyme CYP1A2. Chemicals formed by 'burning' meats additionally have these properties. These foods do not appear to cause any clinically important drug interactions in their own right,

Table 8.4

Food drug interactions

Specific Agents	Food-Drug Interaction	Comments
	Antibiotics	
Ciprofloxacin (Cipro®,Various)	• When the tablet formulation is given with food, there is a delay in the absorption of the drug, resulting in peak concentrations that occur closer to 2 hours after dosing rather than 1 hour, but bio-availability is not affected • Concurrent administration of antacids containing magnesium hydroxide or aluminum hydroxide may reduce the bioavailability by as much as 90% • Dairy products and other products containing calcium, magnesium, aluminum, iron, or zinc decrease the absorption	• Take with food or on an empty stomach and drink fluids liberally • Avoid concurrent administration with magnesium/aluminum antacids or other products containing calcium, iron, or zince • Take 2 hours before or 6 hours after taking these products • Do not take with dairy products or calcium-fortified juices • Can be taken with a meal that contains these products
Clarithromycin (Biaxin®, various) (Biaxin® XL)	• Absorption of Biaxin® XL tablets may be decreased by 30% under fasting conditions • Food delays the absorption of the immediate-release tablets, but does not affect the absorption	• Biaxin® can be taken with or without food • Take Biaxin® XL tablets with food
Erythromycin	• Food alters erythromycin concentrations • Erthromycin base and stearate are absorbed better in the fasting state	• To optimize erythromycin efficacy, take on an empty stomach, at least 30 minutes before meals • Erythromycin ethylsuccinate, erythromycin estolate, and enteric-coated erythromycin may be administered without regard to meals
	Antibiotics	
Metronidazole (Flagyl®, various)	• Concurrent administration with alcohol can cause a disulfiram-like reaction	• Avoid concurrent use with alcohol and alcohol-containing products
Nitrofurantoin monohydrate macrocrystal (Macrobid®)	• Bioavailability may be increased by 40% when given with food • Antacids containing magnesium trisilicate can decrease the rate and extent of absorption	• Take with food • Do not use antacids containing magnesium trisilicate while taking Macrobid®

Table 8.4 *Contd...*

Specific Agents	Food-Drug Interaction	Comments
	Antibiotics	
Tetracyclines **Tetracycline (Sumycin®, various)** **Demeclocycline (Declomycin®)** **Doxycycline (Vibramycin®, various)**	• Milk and other dairy products may reduce the absorption of most tetracycline derivatives by 50% or more • Absorption may be decreased when given with iron and/or food • Products/foods containing calcium, magnesium, aluminum, iron, or zinc decrease the absorption	• Take 1 hour before or 2 hours after dairy foods and/or meals • Take 2 to 3 hours before taking any products containing magnesium, aluminum, calcium, iron, or zinc
	Anticoagulants	
Warfarin (Coumadin®, various)	• Alcohol can increase or decrease PT/INR • Vitamin E can increase PT/INR • Vitamin K can decrease PT/INR	• Avoid alcohol consumption • Patients initiated on vitamin E may require dosing adjustments downward to maintain a therapeutic INR • Eat a normal, balanced diet maintaining a consistent amount of vitamin K • Avoid drastic changes in dietary habits, such as eating large amounts of green leafy vegetables • See Table 1 for foods high in vitamin K.
	Anticonvulsant Agents	
Phenytoin (Dilantin®, various)	• Absorption may increase 27% when taken with a standard meal • Serum phenytoin concentrations may be decreased by enteral feeding preparations and/or related nutritional supplements • Acute alcohol intake can increase serum levels • Chronic alcohol intake can decrease serum concentrations	• Administer phenytoin consistently with regard to meals • Do not administer phenytoin concomitantly with an enteral feeding preparation. Hold enteral feeding 2 hours before and after dosing (Dose adjustment may be necessary) • Avoid alcohol consumption or dose adjust for patients who regularly ingest ethanol
	Antifungal Agents	
Griseofulvin (Grifulvin-V®, various)	• Concurrent administration with alcohol may produce a disulfiram-like reaction • Absorption can be increased when given with a fatty meal	• Avoid alcohol and alcohol-containing products • Take after a high-fat content meal, if possible, to maximize absorption

Table 8.4 *Contd...*

Specific Agents	Food-Drug Interaction	Comments
	Antifungal Agents	
Itraconazole (Sporanox®, various)	• Bioavailability of capsule formulation is maximal when taken with a full meal • Absorption of capsule formulation can be increased after coadministration with a colabeverage (AUC may increase by 75% and C_{max} may increase by 95%) • Absorption of the solution formulation can be decreased when taken with a meal	• Take capsule formulation with a full meal • Take solution formulation on an empty stomach
Ketoconazole (Nizoral®, various)	• Concurrent administration with alcohol may produce a disulfiram-like reaction	• Avoid alcohol or alcohol-containing products
	Antineoplastic Agents	
Procarbazine (Matulane®)	• Hypertensive urgency or emergency may result when combined with foods containing tyramine • Concurrent administration with alcohol may produce a disulfiram-like reaction	• Avoid tyramine-containing foods (see MAOI section) • Avoid alcohol and alcohol-containing products
	Antipsychotic Agents	
Ziprasidone (Geodon®)	• Absorption can increase as much as 2 times with food	• Take with food
	Bronchodilators	
Theophylline	• Excessive caffeine intake can increase serum concentrations and toxicities (nausea, vomiting, palpitations, seizures) • Food may alter the bioavailability of some sustained-release preparations	• Avoid caffeine or maintain daily intake relatively constant • Take theophylline preparations consistently with regard to meals
	Gastrointestinal Stimulants	
Tegaserod (Zelnorm®)	• Food may reduce bioavailability by 40 to 65% and reduce C_{max} by 20 to 40%	• Take on an empty stomach 30 minutes before meals
	Grapefruit Juice	
Grapefruit Juice interactions with multiple drugs	**Grape juice significantly increases the bioavailability of the following medications:** • Amiodarone (Cordarone®, Pacerone®, various) • Amlodipine (Norvasc®) • Atorvastatin (Lipitor®) • Buspirone (Bupar®)	• Avoid grapefruit juice with these medications

Table 8.4 *Contd...*

Specific Agents	Food-Drug Interaction	Comments
	Grapefruit Juice	
	• Carbamazepine (Tegretol®, Carbatrol®) • Cyclosporine (Gengraf®, Neoral®, Sandimmune®) • Diazepam (Valium® various) • Digoxin (Lanoxin®, various) • Diltiazem (Cardizem®, various) • Estrogens (various) • Felodipine (Plendil®) • Itraconazole (Sporanox®) • Losartan (Diovan®) • Methylprednisolone (Medrol®) • Midazolam (Versed®) • Nicardipine (Cardene®) • Nifedipine (Adalat®, Procardia®, various) • Nimodipine (Nimotop®) • Quinidine (various) • Sildenafil (Viagra®, Revatio®) • Simvastatin (Zocor®) • Sirolimus (Rapamune®) • Tacrolimus (Prograf®) • Triazolam (Halcion®) • Verapamil (Calan®, various) • Warfarin (Coumadin®, various)	
	Non-nucleoside Reverse Transcriptase Inhibitors [NNRTI]	
Efavirenz (Sustiva®)	• High-fat/high-calorie meal can increase bioavailability by 50%	• Take on an empty stomach preferably at bedtime
	Nucleoside Reverse Transcriptase Inhibitors [NRTIS]	
Abacavir (Ziagen®)	• Alcohol can increase AUC by 41% and increase $t_{1/2}$ by 26%	• Avoid alcohol
Didanosine (Videx®)	• Food can decrease AUC by 19% and decrease C_{max} by 46%	• Take on an empty stomach 30 minutes before or 2 hours after meals
Tenofovir (Viread®)	• High-fat meal can increase bioavailability and can increase AUC by 40% and increase C_{max} by 14%	• Take with or without food, however oral bioavailability is increased following a high-fat meal

Table 8.4 *Contd...*

Specific Agents	Food-Drug Interaction	Comments
	Protease Inhibitors	
Atazanavir (Reyataz®)	• A light meal can increase AUC by 70% and C_{max} by 57%	• Take with food
Lopinavir/Ritonavir (Kaletra®)	• High-fat meal taken along with capsule formulation can increase AUC by 97% and increase C_{max} by 43% • High-fat meal taken along with solution formulation can increase AUC by 130% and increase C_{max} by 56% • No clinically significant changes have been observed following administration of the tablet formulation with food	• Capsules or oral solution may be taken with food • Tablets may be taken with or without food
Nelfinavir (Viracept®)	• High-fat meal can increase AUC by 5.1-fold and increase C_{max} by 3.8-fold	• Take with food • Increase exposure of drug by increasing fat or calorie content of food
Ritonavir (Norvir®)	• Food can increase the extent of absorption of the capsule formulation by 13%	• Take with food
	Bisphosphonates	
Alendronate (Fosamax®)	• Dairy products can reduce absorption • Food can decrease bioavailability by 40% • Orange juice or coffee can decrease bioavailability by 60% • Calcium supplements and antacids may interfere with absorption	• Take with a full glass of water upon arising for the day on an empty stomach at least 30 minutes before the first food, beverage, or medication • Avoid concurrent administration with orange juice or coffee

but their consumption may add another variable to drug interaction studies, so complicating interpretation. In drug interaction studies where alteration of CYP1A2 is a predicted mechanism, it may be better for patients to avoid these foods during the study.

(b) Grapefruit Juice

By chance, grapefruit juice was chosen to mask the taste of alcohol in a study of the effect of alcohol on felodipine, which led to the discovery that grapefruit juice itself markedly increased felodipine levels; In general, grapefruit juice inhibits intestinal CYP3A4, and only slightly affects hepatic CYP3A4. This metabolized by CYP3A4 are not much affected, whereas oral preparations of the same drugs are. These interactions result in increased drug levels. Some drugs that are not metabolized by CYP3A4 show decreased levels with grapefruit juice, such as 'fexofenadine'. The probable reason for this is that grapefruit juice is an inhibitor of some drug transporters, and possibly affects organic anion transporting polypeptides (OATPs), although inhibition of P-glycoprotein has also been suggested. The active constituent of grapefruit juice is uncertain. Grapefruit contains naringin, which degrades during processing to naringenin, a substance known to inhibit CYP3A4. Because of this, it has been assumed that whole grapefruit will not interact, but that processed grapefruit juice will. However, subsequently some reports have implicated the whole fruit. Other possible active constituents in the whole fruit include bergamottin and dihydroxybergamottin.

REDUCING THE RISK OF DRUG INTERACTIONS PRINCIPLES OF DRUG INTERACTIONS MANAGEMENT

The consequences of drug interactions may be

- Major : life threatening
- Moderate: deteriorations of patient's status
- Minor: bothersome or little effect.

The risk of drug interactions is a challenge that embraces a number of considerations. The following are guidelines to reduce and manage drug interactions.

1. Identify patient risk factors such as age, the nature of the patient's medical problem (e.g., impaired renal function), dietary habits, smoking, and problems such as alcoholism influence the effect of certain drugs.
2. Take thorough drug history and maintain complete patient medication records.
3. Impart knowledge about actions (both primary and secondary pharmacological actions) of drugs being utilized.
4. Consider therapeutic alternatives.
5. Avoid complex therapeutic regimens where possible.
6. Educate the patient to comply with instructions for administering medications. They should be encouraged to ask questions about their therapy and to report any excessive or unexpected responses.
7. Monitor therapy: Priority should be suspected as drug- related until that possibility is excluded.
8. Individualize therapy: Priority should be assigned to the needs and clinical response of the individual patient, rather than to the usual dosage recommendations, standard treatment, and monitoring guidelines.
9. Involve the patient as a partner in health care. If the optimal benefits of therapy are to be achieved with minimal risk, each participant must be knowledgeable about and diligent in fulfilling his responsibilities.
10. Probability assesment scales:

DRUG INTERACTION PROBABILITY SCALE (DIPS)			
QUESTION	YES	NO	Unknown (or) NA
1. Are there previous credible reports of this interaction in humans?	+1	-1	0
2. Is the observed interaction consistent with the known interactive properties of precipitant drug?	+1	-1	0
3. Is the observed interaction consistent with the known interactive properties of precipitant drug?	+1	-1	0
4. Is the event consistent with the known or reasonable time course of the interaction (onset and/or offset)?	+1	-1	0
5. Did the interaction remit upon dechallenge of the precipitant drug with no change in the object drug? (if there was no dechallenge, choose Unknown or Non Applicable and skip question 6)	+1	-2	0
6. Did the interaction reappear when the precipitant drug was readministered in the presence of continued use of object drug?	+2	-1	0
7. Are there reasonable alternative causes for the event? [a]	-1	+1	0
8. Was the object drug detected in the blood or other fluids in concentrations consistent with the proposed interaction?	+1	0	0
9. Was the drug interaction confirmed by any objective evidence consistent with the effects on the object drug (other than drug concentrations from question 8)?	+1	0	0
10. Was the interaction greater when the precipitant drug dose was increased or less when the precipitant drug dose was decreased?	+1	-1	0
TOTAL SCORE			

[a]Consider clinical conditions, other interacting drugs, lack of compliance, risk factors (e.g., age, inappropriate doses of object drug). A No answer presumes that enough information was presented so that one would expect any alternative causes to be mentioned. When in doubt, use Unknown or NA designation.

TOTAL SCORE	
Highly Probable	>8
Probable	5-8
Possible	2-4
Doubtful	<2

Object drug: *The one affected by the presence of another drug.*

Precipitant drug: *The one causing a change on the object drug.*

Question-1: The following are considered credible for this purpose: - prospective studies showing clear evidence supporting the interaction, or - case reports giving evidence to support the interaction, including cases in which applying the DIPS produces a result of possible or higher.

Question-2: The lists of enzyme inducers and inhibitors should be carefully pondered, since *in vitro* evidence does not always apply to *in vivo* conditions in straightforward manner.

Question-3: This calls for robust knowledge on the pharmacodynamic and pharmacokinetic characteristics of the object drug. In particular, medicines whose pharmacodynamics is affected by multiple factors may lead to false positive assessment outcomes. In the case of warfarin, for instance, the influence of dietary factors (vitamin K content) can easily be underestimated or altogether overlooked.

Question-4: The time lapse necessary for maximum inhibition to occur can be estimated from the half-life of the precipitant drug, whereas the half-life of the object drug will allow for the time of maximum change of the object drug to be estimated.

Question-5: These data are often unavailable in that both precipitant and object drug are often discontinued when a suspicion of interaction is raised. Neither can the dechallenge effect be evaluated if the doses of both drugs are changed.

Question-6: In those rare cases, usually due to unintentional rechallenge, that these data are available, the robustness of the causal relation obtained ends up being greatly reinforced.

Question-7: In this context, one of the most important limitations to causality assessment is insufficiently exploring alternative explanations for the observed reaction, other than a drug interaction.

Question-8: The answer to this question will often be "Non applicable", since pharmacodynamic interactions do not usually entail changes in the concentrations of the object drug.

Question-9: Changes in physiological (laboratory) parameters may typically be objective evidence of a drug interaction.

Question-10: In those rare cases in which a dose-response relation can be established, the causality nexus is strongly reinforced.

REFERENCES

1. Phillips KA, Veenstra DL, Oren E, Lee JK, Sadee W. Potential role of Pharmacogenomics in reducing adverse drug reactions: a systematic review. JAMA (2001) 286, 2270–79.
2. Bjornsson TD, Callaghan JT, Einolf HJ, Fischer V, Gan L, Grimm S, Kao J, King SP, MiwaG, Ni L, Kumar G, McLeod J, Obach RS, Roberts S, Roe A, Shah A, Snikeris F, Sullivan JT, Tweedie D, Vega JM, Walsh J, Wrighton SA. The conduct of in vitro and in vivo drug-drug interaction studies: a PhRMA perspective. J Clin Pharmacol (2003) 43, 443–69.
3. Bachmann KA, Ghosh R. The use of in vitro methods to predict in vivo pharmacokinetics and drug interactions. Curr Drug Metab (2001) 2, 299–314.
4. Yao C, Levy RH. Inhibition-based metabolic drug–drug interactions: predictions from in vitro data. J Pharm Sci (2002) 91, 1923–35.
5. Worboys PD, Carlile DJ. Implications and consequences of enzyme induction on preclinical and clinical drug development. Xenobiotica (2001) 31, 539–56.
6. Venkatakrishnan K, von Moltke LL, Obach RS, Greenblatt DJ. Drug metabolism and drug interactions:application and clinical value of in vitro models. Curr Drug Metab (2003) 4, 423–59.
7. Miller LG. Herbal medicinals. Selected clinical considerations focusing on known or potential drug-herb interactions. Arch Intern Med (1998) 158, 2200–11.
8. Fugh-Berman A. Herb-drug interactions. Lancet (2000) 355, 134–8. Correction. ibid. 1020.
9. Wang Z, Gorski JC, Hamman MA, Huang S-M, Lesko LJ, Hall SD. The effects of St John's wort (Hypericum perforatum) on human cytochrome P450 activity. Clin Pharmacol Ther (2001) 70, 317–26.
10. Williamson EM. Drug interactions between herbal and prescription medicines. Drug Safety (2003) 26, 1075–92.

CHAPTER 9

Adverse Drug Reactions (ADR)

ADVERSE DRUG REACTION (ADR)

An *adverse drug reaction* is a "response to a drug which is noxious and unintended and which occurs at doses normally used in man for prophylaxis, diagnosis, or therapy of disease or for the modification of physiologic function."

There is a causal link between a drug and an adverse drug reaction.

In sum, an *adverse drug reaction* is harm **directly caused by the drug at normal doses, during normal use.** Table 9.2 lists examples of adverse effects associated with specific medications.

ADVERSE DRUG EVENT (ABBREVIATED ADE)

It refers to any injury caused by the drug (at normal dosage and/or due to overdose) and any harm associated with the use of drug (e.g. discontinuation of drug therapy).

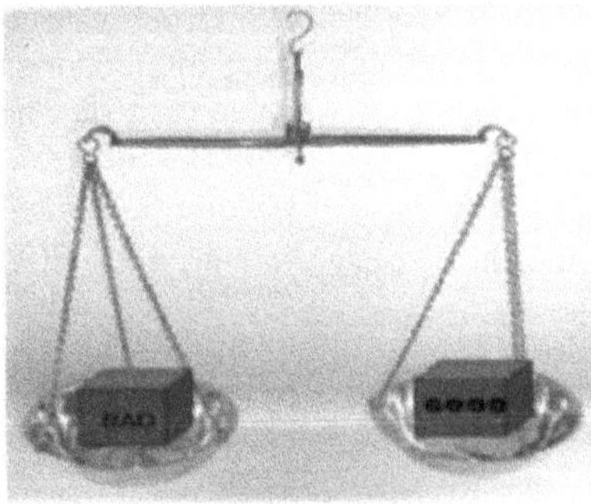

FIGURE 9.1

Adverse drug effects.

THE RISK TO BENEFIT RATIO

When prescribing drugs a doctor must assess risk to benefit ratio in the individual patient by

- Choosing an appropriate class of drug then an appropriate individual agent
- Is it effective?
- What are the chances of adverse effect?
- Are there features in this patient which affect choice ex. other drugs, organ failure, aged
- Tailoring the dose
- Considering duration of treatment

The Risks when prescribing drugs with a low therapeutic ratio are greatly increased if

1. Pharmacokinetic process is complicated e.g. high hepatic extraction, or zero order elimination
2. Wide interindividual variation in kinetics and / or response
3. Pharmacokinetics sensitive to drug interaction, disease or ageing.

CLASSIFICATION (TABLE 9.1)

PREDICTABLE REACTIONS (TYPE A)

1. Can be predicted from the known pharmacology of the drug.
2. May be common within the pharmacological groups
3. Are due either to excessive action at the target receptor or to action at a non-target receptor.
4. Are related closely to the amount of drug in the body.
5. Are determined by dose and by pharmacokinetic and pharmacodynamic factors (E.g. greatly reduced dose of Warfarin needed in liver disease).
6. Are common, accounting for 75% or more of all adverse effects.
7. Are largely avoidable with care.

UNPREDICTABLE REACTIONS (TYPE B)

1. The effect is unrelated to established pharmacological effects.
2. The effect may not be shared with in pharmacological groups
3. The effect may be serious organ damage (E.g.: Pulmonary Fibrosis with sulphasalazine)
4. There is a poor relationship to dose.
5. They are uncommon and difficult to detect in drug development.
6. They cannot be avoided if the drug is used.
7. Patient idiosyncrasy is a major factor.

Table 9.1

Classification of adverse effects

Type	Type of effect	Features	Examples
A	Augmented	Common, predictable, low mortality	Bradycardia–β-blockers
B	Bizarre	Uncommon, unpredictable, high morbidity & high mortality	Anaphylaxis - Penicillin
C	Chronic	Dose related & time related	Dyskinesia - Levodopa
D	Delayed	Time Related	Teratogenesis
E	End of use	Withdrawal of chronic therapy abruptly	Corticosteroids
F	Failure	Unexpected failure of therapy	Oral contraceptive failure - Rifampin

SERIOUSNESS AND SEVERITY

The American Food and Drug Administration define a serious adverse event as one when the patient outcome is one of the following:

- Death
- Life-threatening
- Hospitalization (initial or prolonged)
- Disability - significant, persistent, or permanent change, impairment, damage or disruption in the patient's body function/ structure, physical activities or quality of life.
- Congenital anomaly
- Requires intervention to prevent permanent impairment or damage

Severity is a point on an arbitrary scale of intensity of the adverse event in question. The terms "severe" and "serious" when applied to adverse events are technically very different. They are easily confused but cannot be used interchangeably, requiring care in usage.

A headache is severe, if it causes intense pain. There are scales like "visual analog scale" that help us assess the severity. On the other hand, a headache is not usually serious (but may be in case of subarachnoid hemorrhage, subdural bleed, even a migraine may temporally fit criteria), unless it also satisfies the criteria for seriousness listed above.

OVERALL DRUG RISK

While no official scale exists yet to communicate overall drug risk, the iGuard Drug Risk Rating System is a five color rating scale similar to the Homeland Security Advisory System:

- Red (high risk)
- Orange (elevated risk)
- Yellow (guarded risk)
- Blue (general risk)
- Green (low risk)

LOCATION

Adverse effects may be local, i.e. limited to a certain location, or systemic, where a medication has caused adverse effects throughout the systemic circulation.

For instance, some ocular anti-hypertensives cause systemic effects, although they are administered locally as eye drops, since a fraction escapes to the systemic circulation

MECHANISMS

As research better explains the biochemistry of drug use, fewer ADRs are Type B and more are Type A. Common mechanisms are:

- Abnormal pharmacokinetics due to
- genetic factors
- co-morbid disease states
- Synergistic effects between either
- A drug and a disease
- Two drugs

ABNORMAL PHARMACOKINETICS

Co-morbid disease states

Various diseases, especially those that cause renal or hepatic insufficiency, may alter drug metabolism. Resources are available that report changes in a drug's metabolism due to disease states.

Genetic factors

Abnormal drug metabolism may be due to inherited factors of either Phase I oxidation or Phase II conjugation. Pharmacogenomics is the study of the inherited basis for abnormal drug reactions.

Phase I reactions

Inheriting abnormal alleles of cytochrome P450 can alter drug metabolism. Tables are available to check for drug interactions due to P450 interactions.

Inheriting abnormal butyryl cholinesterase (pseudocholinesterase) may affect metabolism of drugs such as succinylcholine

Phase II reactions

Inheriting abnormal N-acetyltransferase which conjugated some drugs to facilitate excretion may affect the metabolism of drugs such as Isoniazid, Hydralazine, and Procainamide.

Interactions with other drugs

The risk of drug interactions is increased with polypharmacy.

Protein binding

These interactions are usually transient and mild until a new steady state is achieved. These are mainly for drugs without much first-pass liver metabolism. The principal plasma proteins for drug binding are:

1. Albumin
2. α1-acid glycoprotein
3. Lipoproteins

Some drug interactions with warfarin are due to changes in protein binding.

Cytochrome P450

Patients have abnormal metabolism by cytochrome P450 due to either inheriting abnormal alleles or due to drug interactions. Tables are available to check for drug interactions due to P450 interactions.

Synergistic effects

An example of synergism is two drugs that both prolong the QT interval.

Table 9.2

Examples of adverse effects as associated with specific medications

Condition	Substance
Abortion, miscarriage or uterine hemorrhage	Misoprostol (Cytotec), a labor-inducing drug (this is a case where the adverse effect has been used legally and illegally for performing abortions)
Addiction	Many sedatives and analgesics such as diazepam, morphine, etc.
Birth defects	Thalidomide and Accutane
Bleeding of the intestine	Aspirin therapy
Cardiovascular disease	COX-2 inhibitors (i.e. Vioxx)
Deafness and kidney failure	Gentamicin (an antibiotic)
Death, following sedation	Propofol (Diprivan)
Depression or hepatic injury	Interferon
Diabetes	Atypical antipsychotic medications (neuroleptic psychiatric drugs)

Table 9.2 *Contd...*

Condition	Substance
Diarrhea	Orlistat (Xenical)
Erectile dysfunction	Many drugs, such as antidepressants
Fever	Vaccination (in the past, imperfectly manufactured vaccines, such as BCG and poliomyelitis, have caused the very disease they intended to fight).
Glaucoma	Corticosteroid-based eye drops
Hair loss and anemia	Chemotherapy against cancer, leukemia, etc.
Headache	Spinal anesthesia
Hypertension	Ephedrine users, which prompted FDA to remove the status of dietary supplement of ephedra extracts
Insomnia	Stimulants, Ritalin, Adderall, etc.
Lactic acidosis	Stavudine (Zerit, for anti-HIV therapy) or metformin (for diabetes)
Liver failure	Paracetamol
Melasma and thrombosis	Estrogen-containing hormonal contraception such as the combined oral contraceptive pill
Irreversible Peripheral neuropathy	Fluoroquinolone medications
Rhabdomyolysis	Statins (anti-cholesterol drugs)
Seizures	Withdrawal from benzodiazepine
Drowsiness or increase in appetite	Antihistamine use. Some antihistamines are used in sleep aids explicitly because they cause drowsiness.
Stroke or heart attack	Sildenafil (Viagra) when used with nitroglycerine; COX-2 inhibitors
Suicide, increased tendency	Fluoxetine and other SSRI antidepressants
Parkinsonism	MPTP a meperidine related drug considered highly neurotoxic
Tardive dyskinesia	Long-term use of metoclopramide and many antipsychotic medications
Spontaneous Tendon rupture	Fluoroquinolone drugs even occurring as late as 6 months after treatment had been terminated.

DETECTING ADVERSE EFFECTS

- If a new drug causes a bizarre effect in 1 in 6000 patients it would need 18000 patients to use the drug for it to occur in 3 patients.
- It would take twice as many before there was any suspicion that the effect was due to the drug.
- If the effect also occurs naturally then it would take many times more patients.
- Most early trials involve about 2000 patients.
- MRHA (Medicine and Healthcare products Regulatory Agency) free phone service for reporting and information about suspected ADRs.

- Self reporting by patients and relatives using yellow cards available at pharmacies.
- Prescription event monitoring.
- New drugs – black triangles and yellow cards.

NARANJO ADVERSE DRUG REACTION PROBABILITY SCALE				
QUESTION	**YES**	**NO**	**DON'T KNOW**	**SCORE**
1. Are there previous conclusive reports on this reaction?	+1	0	0	
2. Did the adverse event appear after the suspected drug was administered?	+2	-1	0	
3. Did the adverse reaction improve when the drug was discontinued or a specific antagonist was administered?	+1	0	0	
4. Did the adverse event reappear when the drug was re-administered?	+2	-1	0	
5. Are there alternative causes (other than the drug) that could on their own have caused the reaction?	-1	+2	0	
6. Did the reaction reappear when a placebo was given?	+ 1	-1	0	
7. Was the drug detected in blood (or other fluids) in concentrations known to be toxic?	+1	0	0	
8. Was the reaction more severe when the dose was increased or less severe when the dose was decreased?	+1	0	0	
9. Did the patient have a similar reaction to the same or similar drugs in any previous exposure?	+1	0	0	
10. Was the adverse event confirmed by any objective evidence?	+1	0	0	
TOTAL SCORE				

Score	Interpretation of Scores
Total Score ≥ 9	**Definite.** The reaction (1) followed a reasonable temporal sequence after a drug or in which a toxic drug level had been established in body fluids or tissues, (2) followed a recognized response to the suspected drug, and (3) was confirmed by improvement on withdrawing the drug and reappeared on re-exposure.
Total Score 5 to 8	**Probable.** The reaction (1) followed a reasonable temporal sequence after a drug, (2) followed a recognized response to the suspected drug, (3) was confirmed by withdrawal but not by exposure to the drug, and (4) could not be reasonably explained by the known characteristics of the patient's clinical state.
Total Score 1 to 4	**Possible.** The reaction (1) followed a temporal sequence after a drug, (2) possibly followed a recognized pattern to the suspected drug, and (3) could be explained by characteristics of the patient's disease.
Total Score ≤ 0	**Doubtful.** The reaction was likely related to factors other than a drug.

PREVENTION OF ADVERSE DRUG REACTIONS

- Never use any drug unless there is good indication. If the patient is pregnant do not use the drug unless the need is imperative.
- Allergy and idiosyncrasy are important causes of ADRs. Ask if the patient had previous reactions.
- Ask if the patient is already taking other drugs including self medication
- Age, hepatic and renal disease may impair clearance of drugs so smaller doses may be needed. Genetic factors may also predispose to certain ADRs
- Prescribe as few drugs as possible and give clear instructions
- Where possible use familiar drugs. With new drugs be particularly alert for ADRs and unexpected event.
- If serious ADRs are liable to occur warn the patient.

REFERENCES

1. Nebeker JR, Barach P, Samore MH (2004). "Clarifying adverse drug events: a clinician's guide to terminology, documentation, and reporting". *Ann. Intern. Med.* **140** (10): 795–801.
2. "Adverse Drug Events, Adverse Drug Reactions and Medication Errors". VA Center for Medication Safety. Retrieved 3 February 2012.
3. Rawlins MD, Thompson JW. Pathogenesis of adverse drug reactions. In: Davies DM, ed. Textbook of adverse drug reactions. Oxford: Oxford University Press, 1977:10.
4. Aronson JK. Drug therapy. In: Haslett C, Chilvers ER, Boon NA, Colledge NR, Hunter JAA, eds. Davidson's principles and practice of medicine 19th ed. Edinburgh: Elsevier Science, 2002:147-
5. "MedWatch - What Is A Serious Adverse Event?". Archived from the original on 29 September 2007. Retrieved 2007-09-18.
6. Barriaux, Marianne (2007-10-02). "'Traffic-light' medicine risk website to launch". London: The Guardian. Retrieved 2010-04-23.
7. Rang, H. P. (2003). *Pharmacology*. Edinburgh: Churchill Livingstone. ISBN 0-443-07145-4. Page 146
8. "Clinical Drug Use". Archived from the original on 1 November 2007. Retrieved 2007-09-18.
9. Phillips KA, Veenstra DL, Oren E, Lee JK, Sadee W (2001). "Potential role of pharmacogenomics in reducing adverse drug reactions: a systematic review". *JAMA* **286** (18): 2270–9.
10. Goldstein DB (2003). "Pharmacogenetics in the laboratory and the clinic". *N. Engl. J. Med.* **348** (6): 553–6. .
11. "Drug-Interactions.com". Archived from the original on 30 August 2007. Retrieved 2007-09-18.
12. Weinshilboum R; Collins, Francis S.; Weinshilboum, Richard (2003). "Inheritance and drug response". *N. Engl. J. Med.* **348** (6): 529–37.
13. Evans WE, McLeod HL (2003). "Pharmacogenomics—drug disposition, drug targets, and side effects". *N. Engl. J. Med.* **348** (6): 538–49.
14. DeVane CL (2002). "Clinical significance of drug binding, protein binding, and binding displacement drug interactions". *Psychopharmacology bulletin.* **36** (3): 5–21.
15. Benet LZ, Hoener BA (2002). "Changes in plasma protein binding have little clinical relevance". *Clin. Pharmacol. Ther.* **71** (3): 115–21.
16. Sands CD, Chan ES, Welty TE (2002). "Revisiting the significance of warfarin protein-binding displacement interactions". *The Annals of pharmacotherapy* **36** (10): 1642–4.

17. Davies EC, Rowe PH, James S et al., (2011). "An Investigation of Disagreement in Causality Assessment of Adverse Drug Reactions". *Pharm Med* **25** (1): 17–24.
18. Aoun M, Jacquy C, Debusscher L et al., (July 1992). "Peripheral neuropathy associated with fluoroquinolones". *Lancet* **340** (8811): 127. doi:10.1016/0140-6736(92)90460-K.
19. Cohen JS (December 2001). "Peripheral neuropathy associated with fluoroquinolones". *Ann Pharmacother* **35** (12): 1540–7. doi: 10.1345/aph. 1Z429.
20. Hedenmalm K, Spigset O (April 1996). "Peripheral sensory disturbances related to treatment with fluoroquinolones". *J. Antimicrob. Chemother.* **37** (4): 831–7.
21. Jagose JT, McGregor DR, Nind GR, Bailey RR (December 1996). "Achilles tendon rupture due to ciprofloxacin". *N. Z. Med. J.* **109** (1035): 471–2.

CHAPTER 10

The Role of the Pharmacist in Disease Management

INTRODUCTION

The Pharmacy field is continuing to undergo a paradigm shift from a dispensing-focused to a patient-care-focused profession. With the advances in technology and the increased supply of pharmacy technicians, pharmacists have more time to provide clinical services. One area in which pharmacists have seized the opportunity to become involved in patient care is disease management.

DEFINITION OF DISEASE MANAGEMENT

Disease Management has been described as "it is an systematic tool that is applied to specific conditions concentrating on prevention and 'best practices' to provide high quality care at a reasonable cost with an ongoing process of monitoring and continuous improvement." In general, organizations either choose to develop and build their own DM programs or hire a vendor to perform services.

DM programs involve an intervention or series of interventions aimed at improving the patient outcomes associated with specific diseases or conditions that have a high prevalence or high treatment costs (e.g., diabetes). Although DM is applicable to all conditions, programs have typically been focused on chronic illnesses, because they account for a disproportionately high percentage of all medical expenditures. In the U.S., chronic illnesses affect over 100 million people and account for 75% of the nation's annual health care costs and are the major cause of death, disease, and disability. The intervention component of a DM program can consist of clinical practice guidelines; case management by nurses, pharmacists, or other health professionals; patient education programs; and administrative interventions aimed at avoiding duplicative services and ensuring appropriate timing of visits. The targeted outcomes of DM programs generally include clinical goals that, if achieved by a sufficient number of patients, will result in a savings that equal or exceed the financial costs of the program itself. However, from a pharmacist's perspective, it is important to note that medication use (and costs) can increase as a part of a DM program if the drug treatments are necessary to avert outpatient visits or hospitalizations. A key element of DM programs is the ability to collect and analyze data by using computerized information systems and interpret whether increased drug costs are offset by the benefits of improved patient outcomes.

Both interventions and outcomes are usually developed using the best practices that are identified through the literature, discussions with clinical experts in the disease or condition. Table 10.1 summarizes key characteristics of disease management programs.

Table 10.1

Characteristics of a Disease Management Program

- It mainly includes the specific patients suffering from a disease.
- It mainly includes the health care services that are directed toward the chosen disease by the health care system, providing an system of prevention and care.
- Involves health care services on consistent application of the best scientific information available on treatment.
- Bridges care to the outcomes of interest to consumers of health care, taking into account the multidimensional quality nature by including clinical, economic, and humanistic outcomes.

ORGANIZATIONS THAT OFFER DISEASE MANAGEMENT PROGRAMS

The growth of DM has paralleled the evolution of managed health care. The types of organizations that currently offer DM services now encompass virtually every stakeholder in the provision of health care, including health benefits supervisors, finance experts, and patients. Although managing disease has always been a part of medical care, the growth of structured DM programs did not accelerate until the early 1990s. In addition, health care purchasers, such as Medicaid have begun to use DM tools as a means to effectively manage patients. In fact, the DM industry has been among the fastest-growing investment segments in health care.

THE ROLE OF PHARMACISTS IN DISEASE MANAGEMENT

HISTORY OF PHARMACISTS' INVOLVEMENT IN PATIENT CARE

The involvement of the pharmacist in DM can be traced back to the hospital environment. In this setting, clinical pharmacy practice is believed to have begun during the 1960s. During this early period, pharmacists' interventions were reactive, as opposed to proactive; that is, the bulk of the interventions focused on correcting existing problems with drug therapy, rather than preventing them. The 1990s marked the beginning of a new paradigm within the profession, the concept of pharmaceutical care.

In practicing pharmaceutical care, a pharmacist is expected to be responsible for the patients' medication-related outcomes. However, note that the extent to which pharmacists may actually practice pharmaceutical care is highly variable. For example, a 1996 study of Virginia pharmacists found that community pharmacists who practiced in rurally located, independently owned pharmacies filled less than 150 prescriptions per day and had a good rapport. Although these findings might be attributable to geographic and patient mix differences, results suggest that higher-volume retail chains were less likely to provide pharmaceutical care. However, these findings might not be relevant currently, because recent technological advancements (e.g., electronic prescriptions) help expedite prescription processing, making it more difficult to determine whether there is an association between high prescription volume and the inability to provide pharmaceutical care. With expertise in pharmacotherapeutics and pharmaceutical care, pharmacists are uniquely qualified to participate in DM programs. Pharmacists have been involved in developing and implementing many DM programs currently existing. Some have contributed through their positions in nonclinical settings, such as PBMs, health plans, and pharmaceutical companies, whereas others have participated in clinical settings.

THE PHARMACIST'S ROLE IN PREVENTING ANTIBIOTIC RESISTANCE

THE PHARMACIST'S ROLE

In infectious diseases combating and preventing the role of pharmacist's is highly essential as vaccine and antibiotic regimens become more complex due to the evolving epidemiology of infections. There is requirement of preservation of currently available antibiotics, highlighting the pharmacist role in maximizing the utility of presently available drugs due to the marked decrease in drug development . While further training in infectious diseases may be necessary for some pharmacist roles in preventing antibiotic resistance, many others exist that all pharmacists can embrace.

ANTIBIOTIC STEWARDSHIP

Pharmacist-directed antibiotic stewardship programs (ASPs) have proliferated considerably in the past decade. After evidence emerged that these programs improve patient care, the Infectious Diseases Society of America and Society for Healthcare Epidemiology of America published a guideline for the development of ASPs specifying that an infectious diseases–trained clinical pharmacist was an essential core member. As resistance has increased and antibiotic development has lagged, ASPs have become important to improve clinical outcomes, prevent resistance, and decrease adverse events such as *Clostridium difficile* infections. ASPs take many forms, but all utilize a team approach to improve the utilization of antibiotics through means such as interventions on individual patients, guideline development, and system-wide improvement . Over time, ASPs may become a standard for all hospitals and long-term-care facilities across the nation; however, at this time only California has developed a statewide initiative to require ASPs.

Various methods may be employed for ASPs, and pharmacists are generally the key personnel members following the patients and intervening when necessary. While some of these interventions require an in-depth knowledge of infectious diseases, others are within the scope of general pharmacy practice. For example, it has been reported that dosing of vancomycin may be inadequate in obese patients. Since it has been suggested that inadequate vancomycin dosing may be associated with the promotion of resistance in *Staphylococcus aureus*, this represents an opportunity for nonspecialist pharmacists to intervene.More complex antibiotic selection or dose optimization methods may be utilized by those pharmacists with a comprehensive understanding of diagnostic tests or antibiotic pharmacokinetics and pharmacodynamics. Each intervention is an opportunity to provide feedback and education to the prescriber, which is vital to the maintenance of a stewardship program and further promotes the improvement of antibiotic utilization. Further, pharmacists frequently collect and report data about interventions and antibiotic-use patterns at hospital committees in order to assess the effectiveness of the program, identify areas for improvement, and garner continued support for stewardship.

COMMUNITY PHARMACISTS AS GATEWAY PRACTITIONERS

As gateway practitioners, community pharmacists have some of the most significant opportunities to intervene and prevent unnecessary antibiotic use, which is strongly associated with increased resistance. Patients often go to their community pharmacy first to seek advice regarding infections and OTC medications to alleviate their symptoms. Pharmacists may counsel patients on viral infections, the futility of antibacterials for them, and recommend appropriate OTC products for supportive care. Avoiding an unnecessary trip to a physician's office can prevent the pressure that physicians may feel to prescribe antibiotics that they do not believe are necessary. Of course, pharmacists should refer a patient to see a physician if a bacterial infection is suspected, the patient is severely ill or complicated by significant comorbidities, the infection is prolonged, or the pharmacist is not comfortable judging that a mild viral infection is present. A useful resource for pharmacists regarding these counseling points is the CDC Web site Get Smart: Know When Antibiotics Work.

VACCINATION

Pharmacists are crucial to promoting currently available vaccines. Vaccines can decrease the use of antibiotics directly by preventing primary infection and indirectly by preventing bacterial superinfection after a primary vaccine-preventable illness, such as influenza. Pharmacists can screen patients and identify those in need of immunizations at various time points and places: admission to a health care facility; visits to community pharmacies; at a specific age; for certain chronic conditions, medical or surgical procedures; and at certain times of the year. Pharmacists can also now administer vaccines in the community setting in every state.

EDUCATION

Preventing antibiotic resistance is the most important pharmacist role. Addressing patient and clinician concerns is most vital to increase the understanding of the appropriate use of these agents, due to many misconceptions that exist about antibiotics and vaccines,. Many of the parents are hesitant about vaccinating their children because of the concern for side effects, both real and imagined. Pharmacists can help patients to separate fact from fiction regarding immunizations.

FACTORS INFLUENCING PHARMACIST INVOLVEMENT IN DISEASE MANAGEMENT

PATIENT ACCESS

Pharmacists are uniquely positioned to become involved in DM activities for several reasons. Public opinion indicates that the

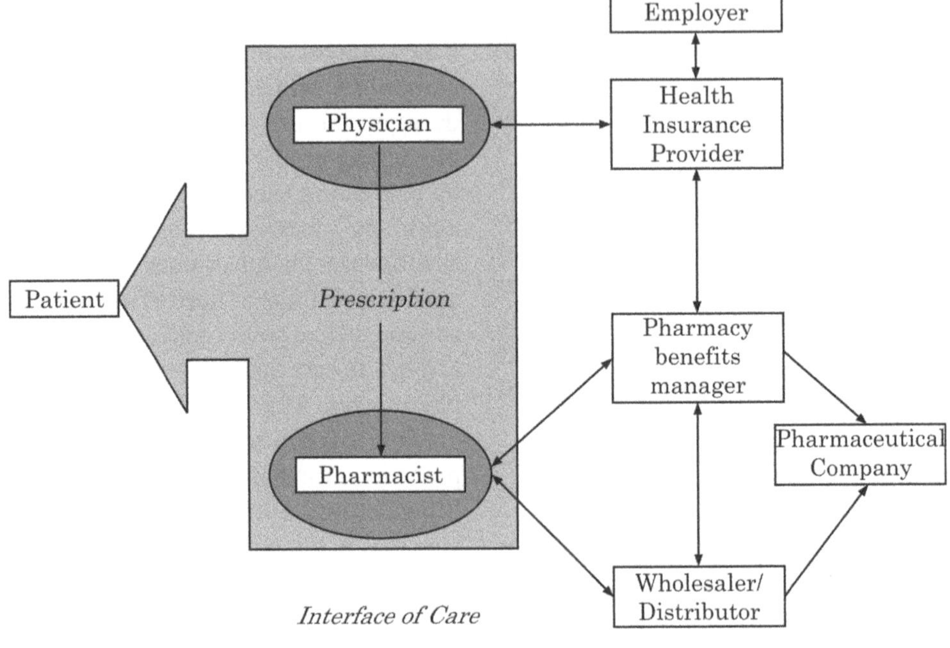

FIGURE 10.1

The prescribing process empowers pharmacists to deliver pharmaceutical DM services. Note: Circles represent the infrastructure in which pharmacists and physicians practice (e.g., group or clinic for physicians and corporate chain for pharmacists).

pharmacists are the most trusted professionals. Fig. 10.1 illustrates how the drug prescribing process places pharmacists at the interface of patient care. Because pharmacists, like physicians, have the ability to directly deliver DM services, they can serve as conduits for implementing DM programs developed by health insurance providers and employers. Community pharmacies are particularly accessible for patients: some are open 24 hours a day, 7 days a week. As of this writing, there are more than 55,000 pharmacies in the U.S. and more than 130,000 pharmacists practicing at these sites. Furthermore, no appointments or insurance preapprovals are required to receive one-on-one professional consultations with pharmacists. Finally, patients with chronic conditions are likely to visit their pharmacy regularly in order to obtain refills.

CONSISTENCY BETWEEN SITES

Another factor promoting pharmacists' involvement in DM is the organization and structure of pharmacies through pharmacists practicing at different locations. This feature, most obvious to chain pharmacies and hospital networks, provides the infrastructure required to implement programs across large or geographically dispersed patient populations. The benefits of implementing DM includes for example, outcomes data may be available through a single repository, and there is likely to be a process in place for communicating within and between the sites. For chain pharmacies, the structural layout of the stores might be similar, which could be important if a patient counseling area is required to administer DM services.

EXPANDING THE ROLE OF PHARMACY TECHNICIANS

Another factor that has fostered pharmacists' involvement in DM is the expansion of the roles of pharmacy technicians. More is the use of the technicians helps the pharmacist to devote more time to the patient.

LEGISLATIVE EFFORTS

Pharmacists' involvement in specific DM efforts has been fostered through legislative efforts. Under this legislation, the pharmacists are trained well for providing cognitive services for patients suffering with various diseases like diabetes, asthma, lipid disorders. To qualify as a provider under the waiver, pharmacists must be qualified in each of the therapeutic areas included. Table 10.2 provides the requirements for pharmacist reimbursement under this law.

Table 10.2

Requirements for Pharmacist Reimbursement
• The pharmacist must complete a qualified program which is approved by state board of pharmacy • The pharmacist should obtain a referral from the concerned patient's physician. • The pharmacy at which the credentialed pharmacist practices must have a private counseling area. • A record of services provided to the patient must be maintained in the pharmacy.

Currently, pharmacists receive Medicare reimbursement for providing education to patients with diabetes. To illustrate how this legislation could build on the experience with pharmacists in disease and drug therapy management (collective drug therapy management, CDTM) to improve the quality of care., issues surrounding atrial fibrillation and stroke will be discussed. In the future, the Centers for Medicare and Medicaid Services could mandate that in order to receive reimbursement, a pharmacist would need to be certified in anticoagulation management. Medicare could then reimburse pharmacists for the management of warfarin therapy for patients with atrial fibrillation. As a Medicare provider, pharmacists would be held to the same standards and provisions for reimbursement as other providers. By utilizing ubiquitous community-based health care professionals such as pharmacists as a means for primary stroke prevention, disease management can be delivered and the quality of care for Medicare beneficiaries will improve.

In response to this legislation and the need to qualify as DM providers, the National Association of Boards of Pharmacy (NABP) and the National Community Pharmacists Association (NCPA) was united to form the National Institute for Standards in Pharmacist Credentialing (NISPC). The NISPC currently offers pharmacists certifications in the areas of bronchial asthma, Hyperglycemia, Hyperlipidemia, and anticoagulation.

IMPACT OF THE PHARMACIST IN MANAGING SPECIFIC DISEASES

Most of the disease management efforts are concentrated on the chronic diseases that are associated with high treatment cost. Those diseases mainly include hypertension, hyperlipidemia, anticoagulation, asthma and diabetes. Research supporting these contributions is described here. Although the interventions and outcomes measured might differ considerably according to the specific disease or condition, pharmacists' have demonstrated their ability to improve patient outcomes.

ASTHMA

Asthma is a prevalent disorder affecting an estimated 15 million people in the U.S., and the total annual costs (direct and indirect) of the disease are approximately U.S.$12.7 billion.30 Pharmacists dispense more than 30.5 million prescriptions annually to treat asthma. Given these frequent patient encounters, pharmacists have a unique opportunity to provide patient care, which may lead to improved patient outcomes. The National Asthma and Education Program recognized the potential of pharmacist interventions and created a guide that describes the role of the pharmacist in asthma care. Table 10.3 presents pharmacist responsibilities delineated in this guide. An asthma DM program can assist pharmacists in providing education to patients with asthma. Hunter and Bryant developed an educational intervention administered by pharmacists and targeted at pediatric asthma patients and their parents. The educational intervention consisted of a 45-min presentation, a demonstration of drug delivery devices, and a discussion session for participants to ask questions and share experiences. All the participants indicated on a questionnaire that they had received enough information for safe and effective administration of asthma drugs. A study of a physician-directed, pharmacist-managed asthma program evaluated the impact of attending a Special asthma clinic designed for patients with frequent asthma exacerbations. The program consisted of regular telephonic conversation between the pharmacist and the patient as follow-up through the clinic. During the study period, the patients experienced fewer emergency room visits for asthma exacerbations as compared with what they did the same 6 months of the year before enrolling in the study.

Table 10.3

National Asthma Education Program Guidelines for Pharmacist responsibilities in Asthma Disease Management

- Patient should be educated about the usage of each medication
- Patients are instructed about the usage techniques for inhaling medications
- Medication use should be monitored and refill intervals to help identify patients with poorly controlled asthma.
- Patients should be encouraged regard procurement of nonprescription based asthma inhalers or tablets to seek medical care.
- Patients should be directed about the usage of peak-flow meters appropriately.

CARDIOVASCULAR DISEASE

Hypertension

Unlike asthma, hypertension is a largely asymptomatic disease. As with other asymptomatic diseases, patients with hypertension will not find problem about the treatment. This throws an challenge for health care practitioners, because chronic uncontrolled hypertension can lead to serious sequelae such as stroke, coronary disease, and cardiac failure. Pharmacists have been shown to have an impact in improving the clinical and humanistic outcomes among patients with hypertension.

A study was carried out to evaluate the clinical value of comprehensive pharmacy services for hypertensive patients in a chain pharmacy setting. Patients were enrolled into either a control or an intervention group. The patients participated in a four scheduled monthly visits, during which they received drug therapy monitoring (e.g., heart rate, blood pressure, medication history) and patient education. Control patients received traditional services used for identification of errors, prescription filling, limited patient education (i.e., drug regimen), and monitoring patient-volunteered adverse drug reactions. Both groups of patients completed quality-of-life questionnaires on entering and completing the study. Results from the study showed that blood pressure was completely improved in the control group.

A second study explored the effectiveness of the hypertension treatment in rural clinic. Before the study, the pharmacists participated in an intensive skill-development program. Patients with controlled or uncontrolled high blood pressure were randomized to either the pharmacist intervention group or the control group. Control-group patients received traditional pharmacy services, such as brief counseling and prescription review for errors. Intervention patients were scheduled to see the pharmacist every 3 to 5 weeks to have their blood pressures and heart rates measured and to be questioned regarding their compliance, adverse drug reactions, and understanding of present drug regimens and lifestyle modifications. The impact of the pharmacist intervention was positive, with blood pressure reduction and increased quality scores in physical role limitations, and bodily pain.

Another hypertension DM program at Cedars-Sinai Health System evaluated a pharmacist–physician comanagement approach at reducing both blood pressure and treatment costs. 40 Patients with uncontrolled hypertension were randomized to an alert group (primary care physicians received a letter informing them of the patient's uncontrolled status) or an intervention group (patients were enrolled in a pharmacy clinic, where a pharmacist comanaged the patients with the physicians until the patients' blood pressure goals were achieved). Interim results demonstrated that blood pressure reductions were more substantial in the intervention group, decreasing from a baseline systolic pressure of 157.7 mmHg to 148.9 mmHg and 139.6 mmHg at 6 months and 1 year, respectively. At 6 months, the total cost of treatment per member per month (PMPM) for the intervention group increased because of an increased number of patient visits. However, at 1 year, cost savings were observed in the area of laboratory tests, office visits, and medications. Results of this program demonstrated that pharmacists can contribute to containing costs within the health care system.

Hyperlipidemia

Effective management of cholesterol is known to reduce cardiovascular events. With this evidence, cholesterol treatment guidelines were developed and updated by the National Cholesterol Education Program

Expert Panel (NCEP). As a result of the new guidelines, it is estimated that the number people in the U.S. who are candidates for cholesterol-lowering medications will triple. This projection points to an increased need for pharmacist involvement in lipid management.

Several studies have evaluated the effectiveness of pharmacist-administered lipid management programs. Patients in the intervention group were used for assessment of the drug by pharmacists, whereas patients in the control group received usual medical care. Results demonstrated that the intervention group achieved a statistically significant reduction in both total cholesterol and low-density lipoprotein compared with the control group.

A smaller study by Faulkner and colleagues assessed the impact of pharmacist telephonic follow-up in patients who had recently undergone cardiac surgery and were receiving lipid-lowering therapy. Patients in the intervention group were telephoned by a pharmacist once a week for 12 weeks to emphasize the importance of lipid-lowering therapy, assess refills, and identify potential issues related to compliance (drug cost, side effects, overall well-being). Results showed that no benefit during the first twelve weeks of therapy. These results provided mixed evidence of the effectiveness of the intervention, but the authors suggest that the pharmacist telephonic follow-up might be a useful alternative when face-to-face counseling in a lipid clinic is either impractical or impossible.

The older guidelines, NCEP II, served as the basis for identifying risk factors and recommending treatment regimens. Results demonstrated that patients who received the pharmacist intervention were more likely to be prescribed lipid-lowering therapy, suggesting that pharmacist chart notes might help increase physician compliance with guidelines for prescribing lipid-lowering agents. The impact of a pharmacist–physician team on the ability to reach lipid-lowering goals. Patients in the control group received usual care, whereas the intervention group received routine pharmacist–patient consultations and pharmacist– physician interaction, including recommendations on dosage, appropriate drug treatments, and monitoring. The NCEP II guidelines were used to guide the appropriate initiation of therapy . The results indicated that twice as many intervention patients reached their lipid-lowering goals compared with patients in the usual care group.

Anticoagulation

In various settings such as the VA outpatient clinics, Kaiser Permanente outpatient services, hospital-based outpatient clinics, physician offices, and community pharmacies, pharmacists have been successfully managing patients' warfarin therapy.

Studies indicated the benefits of a pharmacist-managed anticoagulation monitoring service (AMS). Outcomes (based on number of thromboembolic and hemorrhagic events, unplanned clinic visits, emergency room visits, and hospital admissions). In addition, analysis of costs of hospital admissions, emergency room visits, and participation in the AMS indicated that a potential reduction in cost of per person year of follow up might have been possible if the control group had been followed by AMS.

A second study was conducted to evaluate clinical and economic effectiveness of a pharmacist-managed anticoagulation service. The study examined clinical and economic endpoints for 50 patients in a usual care group vs. 50 patients in a pharmacist-managed treatment group. There were no significant differences among the groups for the primary group and the group managed by the pharmacist exhibited earlier initiation of warfarin therapy and shorter hospital stay with significantly lower total hospital costs ($1594 vs. $2014). Given the complexity of titrating warfarin therapy, the severity of potential adverse events, and demonstrated benefits in terms of cost savings, pharmacist involvement in this DM area is particularly warranted.

DIABETES MELLITUS

In addition to asthma and cardiovascular conditions, pharmacists have also demonstrated a positive impact in the management of diabetes. Two studies evaluated the impact of pharmacist management on the outcomes of patients with diabetes. Few studies examined the impact of interventions that consisted of pharmacist-provided diabetes education, medication counseling, dose modification in noninsulin-dependent diabetes mellitus (NIDDM) patients. After 4 months, patients who received the interventions were found to have significant improvements in their hemoglobin A1c and fasting plasma glucose. The study did not assess the overall impact of the intervention on the total health care costs of diabetes. The second study compared a control group of patients with diabetes mellitus receiving standard pharmacist education to an intervention group receiving education via small group or individual instruction. Patients in the intervention group had significantly lower average weekly blood glucose levels, a decreased incidence of hyperglycemic events, and demonstrated a significant rise in well understanding about the antidiabetics as well as a positive difference while communicating with the pharmacist. Both studies demonstrated that intensive diabetes education involving pharmacists was associated with improved patient outcomes.

REFERENCES

1. Disease management background. Med. Market. Media (MM&M) 2002: 1.
2. MCOL Managed Care E-Dictionary: MCO Operations Terms. 2002, pp. 1–20. Available at www. mcareol.com.
3. Disease Management Association of America (DMAA). Definition of disease management. 2002, p.1.
4. John Deere Health Care, National Managed Healthcare Congress Meeting, Washington, D.C., May 1997.
5. National Pharmaceutical Council (NPC). Disease Management: Balancing Cost and Quality. An annotated bibliography of studies on the benefits of disease management services for the treatment of asthma. National Pharmaceutical Council, Reston, VA, 2002, pp. 1–51.
6. Holdford D, Kennedy D, Bernadella P, Small R. Implementing disease management in community pharmacy practice. Clin Ther. 1998; 20: 328–339.
7. Nash, D, Clark, JL. Disease management. Issue Brief 2002; 1(2): 1–23.
8. Wheatly, B. Medicaid disease management seeking to reduce spending by promoting health. State Coverage Initiatives Issue Brief; August 2001: 1–6.

9. Dezii CM. A retrospective study of persistence with single-pill combination therapy vs. concurrent two-pill therapy in patients with hypertension. Manage. Care 2000; 9 (suppl.): S2–S6.
10. Kesteloot K. Disease management: a new technology in need of critical assessment. Int. J. Technol. Assess. Hlth. Care 1999; 15: 506–519.
11. Doyle J. Health outcomes: measuring and maximizing value in disease management. In: Todd W, Nash D, Eds., Disease Management: A Systems Approach to Improving Patient Outcomes. American Hospital Publishing, New York, 2002, pp. 61–86.
12. Gurnee, MC and Da Silva, RV. Constructing disease management programs. Manage. Care Mag. 1997: 1–9. Available at www.managedcaremag.com/archives/9706/9706.disease—man.shtml, accessed August 5, 2002.
13. Zitter M. A new paradigm in health care delivery: disease management. In: Todd W, Nash D, Eds., Disease Management: A Systems Approach to Improving Patient Outcomes. American Hospital Publishing, New York, 1997, pp. 1–26.
14. Pizzi LT, Menz JM, Graber GR, Suh DC. From product dispensing to patient care: the role of the pharmacist in providing pharmaceutical care as part of an integrated disease management approach. Dis. Manage. 2001; 4: 143–154.
15. Wollschlaeger, B. Disease management: utilize the Web for healthcare delivery. Dis. Manage. 2002: 1–4. Available at www.miamimed.com/MiamiMed%20article%20archive/disease—management.htm.accessed August 23, 2002.
16. Hepler CD, Strand LM. Opportunities and responsibilities in pharmaceutical care. Am. J. Hosp. Pharm. 1990; 47: 533–543.
17. Angaran D, Hepler CD, Bjornson D, Hadsall R. Career patterns of pioneer clinical pharmacists. Am. J. Hosp. Pharm. 1988; 45: 101–108.
18. Glossary. Manag. Med. 2002. Available at www.managingmedicines.com/print.php?page=glossary, accessed August 21, 2002.

CHAPTER 11

Case Presentation

FORMAT OF CASE PRESENTATION

1. General Information at Time of Admission

   (a) Patient's initials (b) Age (c) Race (d) Sex (e) Date of admission

2. Subjective & Objective Information

   (a) Chief complaint (b) Other symptoms

3. History of Present Illness (HPI)

   (a) Briefly state in chronological order the presentation of symptoms leading to this diagnosis. Also give any pertinent negative symptomatology.

4. Past Medical History (in chronological order)

   (a) Childhood illnesses (b) Adult illnesses (c) Hospitalizations

5. Patient's Family History

   (a) Positive for what disease (b) Negative for what disease (c) Does any disease run in patient's family (d) Conditions of spouse (e) Conditions of offspring (or siblings for a child)

6. Patient's Social History

   (a) Smoking: when started, number of packs per year, when stopped (b) Alcohol: what, how much, when (c) Drug abuse (d) Occupation (e) Marital status (f) Living conditions

7. Drug History

   (a) Present Rx dose and frequency (b) OTCs (c) Any known allergies and explain reaction (d) Past Rx and OTC drugs

8. Co-morbid Conditions

   (a) primary vs. secondary (b) controlled

9. Physical Examination

   (a) Vital signs, weight (b) Any positive or pertinent negative physical findings on examination should relate to the clinical presentation.

10. Results of Pertinent Laboratory Tests

    - SMA-6
    - CBC (H & H)
    - Urinalysis
    - Serum drug levels
    - Toxicology screen
    - Drug levels
    - Any other special studies ordered on admission.

11. Patient's Hospital Course

    - Summarize the patient's hospital course, bring out pertinent +/- laboratory tests, diagnostic tests, patient symptomatology, therapy, and parameters used to monitor response to therapy.

The hospital course should be presented in a systematic chronological sequence so as to effectively convey the impact of the patient's drug therapy on his/her recovery and/or the development of complications. This can be accomplished by running, daily "diary-like" commentaries, flow diagrams, charts, graphs, tables, etc.

SUMMARIZED HOSPITAL COURSE

- Medications-dose, dose changes, dates of changes, missed doses, medications errors, duration of therapies, frequency of administration of prn meds, etc.
- Lab values with dates and times where appropriate
- Special procedures and miscellaneous therapeutic modalities
- Special test results
- Significant exam results and clinical observations
- Significant complications
- Problem list changes during hospital stay
- Assessment changes during hospital stay
- Changes in plan during hospital stay

CRITIQUE OF DRUG THERAPY

- Was drug selection appropriate?
- Was drug dosing appropriate?
- Was drug therapy appropriately monitored?
- Did complications develop due to drug therapy?
- Was drug therapy effective?
- What additional monitoring was warranted?
- What therapeutic alternatives were available
- What would you have done differently if you were in charge of the case?

12. Discharge Data
    - Final diagnosis: If expired, note the pathology findings
    - Discharge medications
    - Plan for follow-up

PRESCRIPTIVE ROLE OF CLINICAL PHARMACIST

SOAP ANALYSIS - PWDT

- Pharmacist's Work Up of Drug Therapy (PWDT)
- Desired Outcomes
- Therapeutic Endpoints
- Medication Related Problems
- Pharmacist's Interventions
- Monitoring Plans
- Patient Education

PHARMACIST'S WORK UP OF DRUG THERAPY (PWDT)

- What are reasonable outcomes for this patient?
- Based on current guidelines and literature, pharmacology, and pathophysiology, what therapeutic endpoints would be needed to achieve these outcomes?
- Are there potential medication related problems that prevent these endpoints from being achieved?
- What patient self-care behaviours and medication changes are needed to address the medication-related problems? What patient education interventions are needed to enhance achievement of these changes?
- What monitoring parameters are needed to verify achievement of goals and detect side effects and toxicity, and how often should these parameters be monitored?

REASONABLE OUTCOMES

1. Mortality outcomes

Avoid respiratory, cardiovascular, thrombo-embolic, or diabetes-related premature death.

2. Morbidity outcomes

(a) Disease-related: Reduce morbidity resulting from uncontrolled blood glucose, blood pressure, dyslipidemia, and cardio-vascular disease.

- Prevent, recognize, and treat early any complications of chronic conditions, such as Neuropathy (autonomic or peripheral), Eye disease (e.g., retinal vascular narrowing, hemorrhages), cardiac disease (e.g., LVH, CHF, MI), Nephropathy (e.g., proteinuria), and lower-leg amputation.
- Retard the progression of disease.
- Prevent chronic symptoms of asthma (e.g., coughing or breathlessness at night, in the early morning, or after exertion).
- Retain recognition of hypoglycemia symptoms.
- Maintain near-normal lung function.
- Maintain normal activity levels (including exercise and physical activity).
- Prevent recurrence of Atrial Fibrillation.

(b) Drug-related: Prevent, minimize, or manage drug-related morbidity.

- Monitor for side effects or toxicity.
- Monitor for drug-drug, drug-disease, and drug-food interactions.

3. Behavioural outcomes

(a) Obtain annual eye exams.

(b) Adhere to a medication regimen.

(c) Get routine and timely medical examinations and laboratory tests.

(d) Avoid stimulants or over-the-counter products that may affect blood glucose, blood pressure, asthma, or circulation, such as alcohol, caffeine, nicotine, and decongestants.

4. Pharmacoeconomic outcomes

(a) Keep drug and treatment costs within patient resources.

(b) Make cost-effective and efficient use of health care resources.

5. Quality-of-life outcomes

(a) Match, or minimally change, patient lifestyle and activities with treatment.

(b) Aim for no interference with work or daily activities because of disease symptoms.

(c) Work to ensure patient satisfaction with the pharmaceutical care and health care team.

THERAPEUTIC ENDPOINTS

- LDL cholesterol : <100 mg/dl
  HDL cholesterol : >55 mg/dl
- Triglycerides : <150 mg/dl
  Hb A1C : <7.0%

Self-monitoring of blood glucose: mean <140 mg/dl

- No episodes of severe hypoglycemia requiring emergency assistance
- Blood pressure: <130/80 mmHg, with minimal or no signs or symptoms of orthostatic hypotension
- Biochemical measures, such as potassium, calcium, magnesium, uric acid, serum creatinine, and blood urea nitrogen: within normal levels
- Improvement in or no worsening of peripheral edema
- Daytime asthma symptoms less than twice a week, night time symptoms no more than twice a month, and symptoms responsive to inhaled α-agonist within 15 min.
- Attain/maintain control of ventricular rate to <100 bpm

- Urinary albumin excretion: <30 g albumin/mg creatinine
- Serum digoxin: 1.5–2.0 ng/mL

MRP'S AND PI'S

MEDICATION-RELATED PROBLEMS & PROPOSED INTERVENTIONS

1. No indication for a current drug
2. Indication for a drug - but none prescribed
3. Wrong drug regimen prescribed / more efficacious choice possible
4. Too much of the correct drug
5. Too little of the correct drug
6. Adverse drug reaction/drug allergy
7. Drug-drug, drug-disease, drug-food interactions
8. Patient not receiving a prescribed drug
9. Routine monitoring (labs, screenings, exams) missing
10. Other problems, such as potential for overlap of adverse effects

MEDICATION RELATED PROBLEMS

INDICATION FOR A DRUG (OR DEVICE OR INTERVENTION) BUT NONE PRESCRIBED

✓ Peak flow meter

✓ Calcium/vitamin D/HRT supplementation

- Corticosteroid therapy
- Postmenopausal woman
- Furosemide can cause hypocalcemia.

✓ Magnesium Supplementation

- Routine Use of Magnesium in Diabetes.
- Hypomagnesemia - Risk Factor - Atrial Fibrillation, Hypertension, Insulin Resistance, Glucose Intolerance, Dyslipidemia, Increased Platelet Aggregation
- An added benefit - Constipation

✓ Angiotensin-converting enzyme (ACE) inhibitor

- Patients >55 years of age with diabetes & hypertension - ACE inhibitor - indicated
- Diltiazem - calcium-channel blocker - addresses several needs
- If additional antihypertensive, renal, or cardiac effects are indicated, an ACE inhibitor should be added to the drug regimen.

Too much of the correct drug

Patient is using excessive doses of Salmeterol & fluticasone as treatment for asthma exacerbations (at times when she can afford them).

Too little of the correct drug

✓ Potassium Chloride Supplement

Adverse drug reaction/drug allergy

✓ None

MEDICATION RELATED PROBLEMS

Drug-drug, drug-disease, drug-food - interactions

✓ Systemic Corticosteroid Therapy, Inhaled Corticosteroid Therapy, Loop Diuretics in postmenopausal woman: increased risk for development of osteoporosis

✓ Furosemide, Prednisone in diabetes, w/ Insulin, Rosiglitazone: may increase blood glucose (DOSE-RELATED RESPONSE), thus diminishing the pharmacodynamic activity of antidiabetes agents

✓ Albuterol, Salmeterol in diabetes, w/ Insulin, Rosiglitazone: sympathomimetics may increase blood glucose via stimulation of Beta 2-receptors, leading to increased glycogenolysis & diminished pharmacodynamic activity of antidiabetes agents

✓ Albuterol, Naproxen, Prednisone, Fluticasone in hypertension: may increase blood pressure (DOSE-RELATED RESPONSE)

Drug-drug, drug-disease, drug-food interactions

1. Naproxen in hypertension: INCREASE BLOOD PRESSURE
2. Naproxen in diabetes: may INCREASE RISK OF NEPHROPATHY
3. Furosemide – HYPOMAGNESEMIA/ HYPOKALEMIA
4. Furosemide, prednisone, fluticasone, salmeterol, albuterol w/DIGOXIN: - potential for DIGOXIN TOXICITY.
5. DILTIAZEM w/DIGOXIN: - ELEVATE DIGOXIN LEVELS.

Patient not receiving a prescribed drug

Salmeterol & fluticasone: not purchased because of financial constraints

Outcomes & Endpoints – Monitoring Parameters

Routine Monitoring (Labs, Screenings, Exams)

Missing

✓ Annual dilated eye exam is due

✓ Annual microalbuminuria test is due

✓ Consider screening for depression

PHARMACIST INTERVENTIONS

ASTHMA

1. Change Fluticasone & Salmeterol prescriptions to a single combination product
2. Limit use of albuterol inhaler (short-acting beta-agonist) to rescue only.
3. Consider addition of Leukotriene Inhibitor if symptoms are not controlled
4. Begin use of Peak Flow Meter every morning upon arising.
5. Develop & Implement - Asthma Action Plan

DIABETES

Algorithms

✓ Change Insulin Regimen

- Bedtime - Glargine &
- Premeal - Lispro

\- Rapid Acting

\- Long Acting

Dyslipidemia

✓ Change Fluvastatin to Atorvastatin

✓ Drug Interactions

✓ Potency – LDL lowering ability

✓ Half life

Persistent lower-extremity edema

✓ Elevate Extremities – 20 – 30 minutes, two to three times / day

✓ Wear Support Stockings - anticipating being on her feet most of the day

✓ Limit Salt Intake

✓ Minimize use - NSAIDs

Hypokalemia

✓ Increase potassium chloride supplement temporarily; reassess potassium level in 7–10 days.

✓ Titrate potassium dosage with decreasing use of Albuterol, Furosemide & Prednisone to attain & maintain potassium level of 3.5–5.0 mEq/L

OUTCOMES & ENDPOINTS

✓ **Hypertension**

- No changes at this time / consider addition or change to ACE inhibitor

✓ **Coronary artery disease**

- No changes at this time

✓ **Obesity**

- Refer - for nutrition counseling & weight loss.

✓ **Chronic pain**

- Change ongoing pain medications to ACETAMINOPHEN 500–650 mg three times a day. Minimize use of NSAIDs by limiting it to "breakthrough" pain only
- Naproxen, 250 mg, or Ibuprofen, 200 mg, as needed.

✓ **Financial Constraints**

- Apply for manufacturers' indigent drug programs and State Health Insurance Programs for combination asthma product & other expensive medications.
- Generic Equivalent
- Direct – Manufacturer
- Samples

✓ **Wellness , Preventive & Routine Monitoring Issues**

- Initiate calcium/vitamin D supplementation
- Initiate magnesium supplementation
- Reduce daily aspirin from 325 to 81 mg
- Screen for depression
- Refer for annual eye exam
- Refer for bone density scan
- Refer for nutritional counseling

PATIENT EDUCATION

✓ Asthma
✓ Diabetes
✓ Lower-extremity edema
✓ Nutrition
✓ Medication education

DISCUSSION

The flow of discussion at a case presentation is to be directed by the presenter. At the end of the discussion, the following question should have been answered.

- Did the patient receive optimal drug therapy for his disease state and symptomatology?

The presenter must decide on the best drug, dose, dosage form and dosing interval and compare the drug with other agents, to answer this question.

The student should be prepared to answer specific questions about the case. The following may serve as guidelines for information you should know about your case.

DISEASE STATE

Be prepared to relate the patient's presentation, treatment, and hospital course to the "classic" presentation, treatment, and prognosis of the disease by considering the following:

- Definition
- Etiology
- Incidence
- Prevalence
- Pathology
- Diagnostic lab./tests
- Major Symptoms
- Drug therapy -classic & investigational
- Prognosis -treated & untreated

DRUG THERAPY OF THE PATIENT

Know the pharmacokinetics, pharmacology, DDIs, and toxicology of the patient's drugs.

1. Pharmacokinetics
   - Absorption: • Comparison of sites. • Agents that may effect absorption.
   - Distribution.
   - Protein binding.
   - Biological half-life.
   - Metabolism: • Sites. • Pathway (e.g. glucuronide conjugation). • Activity of metabolites.
   - Excretion.
   - Normal times for onset, maximal activity, and duration.
2. Pharmacology
   - Major actions and mechanisms.
   - Clinical uses: Accepted and investigational.
   - Normal dosing ranges for specific clinical uses (e.g. atropine 0.2-0.3mg for drying effect; 0.4-0.6mg for preop twilight sleep effect).
3. Drug Interactions
   - Be aware of all possible interactions with this drug, including mechanisms if known (e.g. protein binding replacement).
   - Make special note of any potential drug interactions during your patient's hospital course.
4. Toxicology
   - Symptoms of overdose.
   - Antidotes, if any.
   - Potential problems in treating overdose.
   - Addiction potential (physical or psychological).
   - Teratogenicity.
5. Counseling for oral medications
   - Possible adverse reactions.
   - Optimal medication regimen.
   - Tips to improve compliance.

REFERENCES

1. Nancy Cochran, M.D., Dartmouth Medical School, Adapted in part from University of Washington School of Medicine with thanks to Dr. Steve McGee.

CHAPTER 12

Patient Counseling

PATIENT COUNSELING

Patient counseling is a key competency element of the Pharmaceutical Care process. Given the advertising for medication in the media and easy access to information on the Web, it is important for pharmacists to provide appropriate, understandable and relevant information to patients about their medication.

The pharmacist is in a highly visible and readily available position to answer patient concerns and enquiries about their medications and alternate treatments they may read about or hear from others.

Counseling may be defined as "one -to-one interaction between a pharmacist and a patient and/or caregiver. It is interactive in nature. It should include an assessment of whether or not the information was received as intended and that the patient understands how to use the information to improve the probability of positive therapeutic outcomes."

INTERPERSONAL COMMUNICATION

Because pharmacists and pharmacy technicians communicate with patients, carers and other healthcare professionals on a regularly, communication skills plays an important role.

The Ethics for Pharmacists and Pharmacy Technicians is based on seven principles. A pharmacist or technician must endeavor to:

- Make the care of patients their primary concern
- Apply professional judgment in the interests of the patients.
- Show regard for others
- Support patients to participate in decisions about their care
- Increase their professional knowledge and competence
- Be honest and trustworthy
- Take responsibility for their working practices.

Communication is a two-way process. The essence of good communication is that the message received is the same as the message sent. The well-known children's game 'Chinese Whispers' can be used to demonstrate this point effectively. To play the game, everyone sits in a circle. One person whispers a long phrase to their neighbor, who, in turn, whispers what they heard to the next person, and so on. The last person in the circle announces what they heard.

According to the famous anecdote demonstrating the massive changes that can occur, the original message 'Send reinforcements we're going to advance' finally when the chain turned into 'Send three and four-pence we're going to a dance'.

The number of people in the chain can significantly affect the final outcome as the number of opportunities for misinterpretation increases. The Chinese Whispers effect could have serious consequences in a pharmacy environment. In a worst case scenario there could be seven or eight possible interactions involved. Consider the scenario below, a not unusual occurrence in a community pharmacy:

Mrs. Sameul brings her husband's prescription into the pharmacy. The pharmacist enters the details of the patient into the computer and realizes there is a patient medication record. The prescription is for a new item that is not already there. The item ordered is timolol eye drops but there is no indication of the strength required nor are there any directions for use for the patient.

The pharmacist asks Mrs. Sameul if she knows the strength of the eye drops her husband normally uses. She replies that her husband has been to the doctor this morning but she was unable to go with him and as far as she was aware he had never been given eye drops before. The pharmacist tries to phone the surgery but the phone is engaged. The pharmacy is very busy and therefore the pharmacist explains the problem to the pharmacy technician.

The technician then phones the surgery and speaks to the receptionist, the receptionist then speaks to the doctor, the doctor tells the receptionist, the receptionist tells the technician and the technician tells the pharmacist.

The pharmacist then dispenses the item and passes on the information to the patient's wife who then in turn passes on the information to the patient.

There is plenty of opportunity for misinterpretation at any point. In the above scenario, there are at least eight possibilities for misinterpretation.

Communication involves three elements: the sender, the receiver and the message.

THE SENDER

The sender can try to make sure the message is received correctly by:

- Speaking clearly
- Speaking slowly
- Using appropriate language
- Checking understanding.

THE RECEIVER

The receiver can make sure the message is received correctly by:

- Listening carefully
- Asking for clarification
- Writing it down
- Repeating the message back in order to check the message received is the one given.

THE MESSAGE

When we communicate we send a message but what makes up the message? The message we send normally consists of factual information and 'feeling' information and this is transmitted both verbally and non-verbally. A message is sent from the sender to the receiver but there is usually some feedback from the receiver and this feedback will influence the action of the sender. This can be verbal or nonverbal

VERBAL COMMUNICATION

Verbal communication is purely the linguistic element of the message. It is affected by the vocabulary employed and the use of language. The use of appropriate vocabulary and avoidance of jargon is important. Often words that are second nature to the pharmacist may be totally alien to the patient. For example, if a pharmacist or pharmacy technician advised a patient that there is a 'PIL' enclosed with their medication, instead of saying there is a 'patient information leaflet' enclosed, it may lead to confusion. To a patient the term 'PIL' is likely to mean a pharmaceutical form (a pill) and they will probably think of a tablet or more likely the contraceptive pill.

Try to avoid what has been referred to as 'restricted language code'. This makes use of colloquial expressions, very short and simple sentences, repetitive use of conjunctions (but, because, so . . .) and the use of statements phrased as questions 'Know what I mean?', ' . . . you know?', ' . . . isn't it?', etc. In most patient interactions the use of restricted language code is undesirable; however, occasionally it may need to apply it when interacting with certain patients to ensure the information is clearly understood.

NON-VERBAL COMMUNICATION

Non-verbal communication could be defined as all forms of human communication except for the purely verbal message, i.e. the words used themselves. Vocal non-verbal communication includes the tone, pitch, volume, accent, speed, etc. and this is known as paralanguage.

A meaning of a phrase can be altered by changing the emphasis placed on the words. Consider the following phrase:

'Dr. Better told me to buy tablets' and see how the meaning changes depending on the emphasis (as indicated by the underlined word or words):

- 'Dr. Better told me to buy tablets' (i.e. he was the one who told me, no-one else).
- 'Dr. Better told me to buy tablets' (i.e. he didn't ask or request, he told me).
- 'Dr. Better told me to buy tablets' (i.e. he told me, not you or anyone else).
- 'Dr. Better told me to buy tablets' (i.e. I don't expect them for nothing; I want you to sell them to me).
- 'Dr. Better told me to buy tablets' (i.e. not capsules or liquid, but tablets).

The voice can also be used to infer emotional states and your inner feelings. The message a patient coming into the pharmacy receives can be quite different depending on the demeanour and tone of voice. For example, the greeting 'Good afternoon, I'm Jane the pharmacist. How may I help you?' accompanied by an attentive look, a smile and clear diction will give the right message. But imagine the difference if there is no eye contact, no smile and a mumbled question.

This more likely gives the message 'Not another customer, my feet are killing me and I want to go home'. Pharmacists and pharmacy technicians must be aware of how tone of voice can alter the message given out.

BODY LANGUAGE

Body language used in transmitting a message also affects communication. In fact, tone of voice and body language combined contribute more towards communication than the words in the message. There are five main areas of body language: gaze or eye contact, facial expression, proximity and orientation, posture, and touch.

GAZE OR EYE CONTACT

The presence or lack of eye contact can be significant.

In a two-way conversation:

- The speaker often looks away from the listener when talking (because they are concentrating on what they are saying) and then will look directly at the listener if trying to elicit a response
- The listener will look straight into the eye of the speaker while paying attention, but will look away if attention wanders.

It is very important when listening to look at the speaker because if the speaker looks up and notices the listener's gaze is elsewhere, he or she will assume the attention is elsewhere. Therefore when listening to a patient it is important to maintain eye contact in order to show attentiveness.

FACIAL EXPRESSION

Judgements are often made about the emotional state of someone just by the interpretation of facial expressions, particularly movements of the eyebrows and mouth, which signal different types of emotion. This has led to the popularity of 'emoticons' when conversing on-line or via mobile telephone text messages.

PROXIMITY AND ORIENTATION

The orientation and level of the individuals during a conversation is also important. Consider the differences when the patient is seated and the pharmacist is standing; or if the pharmacist is speaking from a raised dispensary down to the patient in the pharmacy (or to a patient in a wheelchair); or the patient is one side of the counter and the pharmacist is the other (a physical barrier).

Positioning can be very important if a patient is asking for recommended treatment for a rash for example. If the pharmacist moves across or out from behind the counter to examine the condition this shows interest in the patient. Similarly if a patient requests a pregnancy test and the pharmacist gets close to the patient to give the results this shows empathy with the patient; the pharmacist demonstrates sensitivity to the need for confidentiality.

POSTURE

How people sit, stand or lie can communicate feelings to others. Upright or slouched, arms crossed or not. A forward sloping stance suggests a wish to dominate. This could be made worse if accompanied by invasion of the personal space. A slouched or bent posture suggests lack of interest and conviction in what is being said, while an upright posture demonstrates assertive behavior without any hidden meanings and shows that a speaker has confidence in what they are saying. Body movements such as clenched fists, fidgeting hands, tapping feet are all indicators of stress or tension, while still, open hands suggest a relaxed frame of mind. The position of the head and shoulders further conveys non-verbal messages: tension, anger, anxiety, excitement, happiness and approachability can all be conveyed non-verbally by the posture adopted.

TOUCH

There are many different types of touch, for example:

- Social touch such as a handshake
- Consoling touch, usually on arm or hand used to calm a distressed person
- Occupational touch, such as, for a pharmacist, simple examination, minor first aid, measuring and fitting hosiery/ trusses or demonstration of use of medication or appliances (e.g. asthma inhalers).

Communication consists of three main parts, questioning, listening and explaining. All are required for successful communication to occur.

QUESTIONING

There are different styles of questioning and different question types that may be used to elicit a response, but what is a question? By definition it is a request for information. The amount and quality of information received may well be affected by the questioning style.

A number of styles of question have been identified by psychologists and linguists, but there are six basic types that will be used by pharmacists: closed, open, leading/biased, probing, prompting and multiple questions.

CLOSED QUESTIONS

Closed questions require short factual, often one-word answers. They place restrictions on the responder by closing down the number of options available. There are three categories that are useful in pharmacy:

- Selection questions – the patient is asked to choose one from two or more alternatives, e.g. 'Would you prefer tablets or capsules?'

  'Would you like aspirin or paracetamol?'
- Yes/no questions – these simply require a yes or no answer, e.g. 'Have you had this pain before?' 'Did you get on OK with the medicine I gave you last week?'
- Identification questions – the patient provides a piece of factual information as a response to the question, e.g. 'What is your name?' 'How old is your baby?'

OPEN QUESTIONS

Open questions give a patient the opportunity to give full answers and there is a greater degree of freedom in deciding how to respond. Open questions are generally broad in nature and require more than a one- or two-word answer. Words such as 'how', 'what', 'feel' and 'think' are useful for encouraging a full response, e.g. 'How did you get on at the doctor's today?' 'What exactly are the symptoms?' 'What do you think about trying to do these exercises once a day?'

LEADING/BIASED QUESTIONS

These questions always have an expectation attached to them. They indicate to the listener the answer the questioner wants to hear. Therefore the patient is led in the direction of a certain answer. They may be used in a positive manner to stimulate the flow of conversation. The idea here is that they should anticipate a likely response to show a common understanding and therefore help to develop a rapport, e.g: 'It's a lovely day today, isn't it? Leading questions may be simple in style, leading the patient in the direction that the pharmacist wants them to go or placing pressure on the patient to concur, e.g. 'You don't drive while your taking these tablets, do you?' 'You have been using the cream as we discussed, haven't you?'

More complex leads exert more pressure on a patient to reply in the expected manner. This can be a problem as it can affect the evaluation of information and eventual diagnosis. The patient may be afraid to disagree or alternatively agree in order to please you, the questioner, e.g. 'Like most conscientious parents, wouldn't you want to give your children fluoride supplements to strengthen their teeth?'

PROBING QUESTIONS

Probing questions are add-on questions or follow-up questions used to build upon an initial response. They may be open, closed or leading in nature. They are of value because they indicate attention to and interest in the patient. The problem is that they may become interrogative in nature if used too frequently. They may be used in different situations. Consider the following questions and how they differ:

- 'What do you mean?' 'Can you explain that?' 'In what way?' These questions are asking for previously received information to be clarified.
- 'Why do you say that?' Here the patient is being asked to justify a statement they have previously made.
- 'Can you remember anything else?' 'Go on?' These questions encourage the patient to give further information to extend the information they have given earlier.
- 'What type of pain?' This question asks for more detail to illustrate the meaning of previous information.
- 'Are you sure you took one twice a day?' This question reaffirms information received and checks the accuracy of information provided by the patient.

Finally there are parroting or echoing styles of questioning which are considered probing. For

Example:

Patient: I don't like tablets, I prefer syrup.

Pharmacist: You prefer syrup?

PROMPTING QUESTIONS

These are useful if a patient fails to answer the original question or gives an inadequate answer.

They may be necessary because the original question posed was not sufficiently specific. For example, following the original question and answer:

Pharmacist: How often do you take the tablets?

Patient: Fairly often. could be followed with the prompt:

Pharmacist: How many do you take each day?

Patient: Four.

Sometimes the question posed may confuse the patient or unintentionally use words with which the patient is unfamiliar. Therefore a simpler question needs to be posed. For example, the original question and answer:

Pharmacist: Do you have any gastro-intestinal symptoms?

Patient: (Perplexed silence, puzzled expression) could be followed by a simpler question:

Pharmacist: Do you have a stomach upset?

Patient: Yes I get heartburn if I eat late at night.

MULTIPLE QUESTIONS

The use of multiple questions is not recommended.

Consider the following two examples:

- 'Do you know how to take them? Would you like me to explain again?'
- 'Have you had the pain long? Is it worse in the morning? Are your joints stiff?'

The first example is not too bad but can lead to misunderstanding. The patient might just answer 'Yes' but do they mean 'Yes, I know how to take them' or 'Yes, I would like you to explain again'?

The second could result in confusion because the patient does not know which question to

answer first and will probably be unable to remember all the questions that have been fired at them.

It will not always be the pharmacist or pharmacy technician who will ask questions. You should also encourage patients to ask you questions. When patients are comfortable asking the questions, that indicates the good communication skills.

Read the following scenario and decide if the question s posed by the pharmacist are open, closed, leading, prompting or multiple.

Pharmacist: Hello, How can I help you? (Question 1)

Patient: I want something for a stomach upset.

Pharmacist: Stomach upset? (Question 2)

Patient: Yes, I've had it for over a week.

Pharmacist: How does it affect you? What are your symptoms? (Question 3)

Patient: Sickness and diarrhoea.

Pharmacist: When did it start? (Question 4)

Patient: Just after I came back from holiday with the family.

Pharmacist: Too much of the good life eating and drinking while you were away? (Question 5)

Patient: NO!

Pharmacist: How long have you been back? (Question 6)

Patient: Two weeks.

Pharmacist: It's been really bad all that time?

Have you taken anything for it or been to the doctor?

(Question 7)

Patient: Yes.

Pharmacist: What did he say? (Question 8)

Patient: No. I had kaolin and morphine in the house so I took that for diarrhoea.

Pharmacist: But have you seen the doctor?

(Question 9)

Patient: No.

Pharmacist: Is your temperature raised? (Question 10)

Patient: Yes I get hot at times.

Pharmacist: Have you had this before or is this the first time?

(Question 11)

Patient: I've had sickness and diarrhea before but never for as long as this.

Pharmacist: Do any other members of your family have gastroenteritis?

(Question 12)

Patient: Pardon. What's that?

Pharmacist: Do they have diarrhoea and vomiting as well?

(Question 13)

Patient: My wife had it but it seems to have cleared up.

The Questions Vary in Style:

- Question 1 is an open question. Almost a greeting question.
- Question 2 is a probing question, asking the patient to further explain what they mean by 'stomach upset'. This could mean different things to different people. It could indicate gastroenteritis as in this case, or it may just be sickness or just diarrhoea.
- Question 3 is a multiple question. This offers an open question and then immediately qualifies that with a probing question.

  Consider whether it would be better to just ask the one probing question. In this case the multiple question is reinforcing the information required.
- Question 4 is an open question.
- Question 5 is a leading question, perhaps suggesting that the condition was somehow selfinflicted, causing possible offence and hostility in the patient.
- Question 6 is a closed question, allowing the pharmacist to identify the duration of the problem.
- Question 7 is a multiple question. Note the patient only responds with a simple yes. The real question is 'yes' to which question? It is obvious from the next question that the response is not to the question that the pharmacist thought they had posed.
- Question 8 is a probing question trying to gain more information but, because the original question was part of a multiple question some confusion sets in as the patient tries to tie in this question with the previous one.
- Question 9 is a closed question that finally elicits the response required from question 7.
- Question 10 is a closed question obtaining specific information.
- Question 11 is a multiple question. In this case the patient was helpful. 'Yes' could easily have been the answer, which would have left the pharmacist wondering whether he meant 'Yes, I have had it before' or 'Yes, it was the first time'. An answer 'No' could have meant 'No, I have not had it before' or 'No, it was the first time'. A closed multiple question allows for misinterpretation.
- Question 12 clearly shows how the use of language must be kept simple in order not to confuse or embarrass the patient. Using the term 'gastroenteritis' in this setting assumes the patient has knowledge of the disease and will understand. This patient clearly does not understand. How will that patient feel? Stupid? How would this be likely to affect their relationship with the pharmacist?
- Question 13 is a prompting question, but the use of diarrhoea and vomiting rather than the patient's terminology of sickness and diarrhoea may serve to further alienate the patient.

Consider the following scenario: Mrs Smith is a regular customer, and she wants to give her something for indigestion. Some suggested questions have been given below. Try to think of your own questions and identify the types of questions used. Consider the strengths and weaknesses of the questions asked and the styles used.

- Question 1: 'Tell me about your symptoms.'
- Question 2: 'Do you get pain at night?'
- Question 3: 'So you want to buy some indigestion mixture?'
- Question 4: 'Would you prefer liquid or tablets.'
- Question 5: 'Is the main problem pain or are you getting wind as well?'

QUESTIONING MNEMONICS

The importance of questioning patients correctly cannot be underestimated. The information from the patient is vital when 'responding to symptoms'. Therefore the interaction needs to be structured in order to ensure all the relevant details are obtained.

How do you ensure that interview with a patient is unbiased and thorough? How it was make sure that you do not forget to ask something? The decision with regards to counter prescribing or referral to a GP will be based on the information that manage to obtain from the patient.

Because of the importance of remembering all of the information a number of mnemonics are used. These are valuable as a starting point.

All the information is valid and it can build upon the framework to obtain further information from a patient. It is important to bear in mind, however, that no mnemonic is fully comprehensive.

WWHAM

- Who is the medicine for?
- What are the symptoms?
- How long have you been ill?
- Action taken so far?
- Medicines being taken at the moment?

This system of questioning will establish the presenting complaint and will also give information about what the patient has already done about the symptoms. However it fails to consider family history, previous symptoms, general appearance or any social or lifestyle factors associated with the presenting symptoms.

For example, if these were the only questions used to differentiate between patients, a young mum presenting with indigestion/heartburn caused by hectic lifestyle with poor eating habits ('eating on the go') might be given the same treatment as an elderly man presenting with similar symptoms but with a greater chance of the symptoms being caused by a disease state rather than poor eating habits.

ENCORE

- Explore
- No medication?
- Care
- Observe
- Refer
- Explain.

Explore

This gives the opportunity to obtain information regarding the nature of the symptoms, discover any other associated symptoms or any other medication being taken by the patient and hence any other preexisting medical conditions. As a result of 'exploration' we may exclude possibility of serious disease. It also enables the questioner to obtain the identity of the patient.

No Medication

This is a reminder that medication is not always the answer and lifestyle changes may be more advisable – there is not necessarily 'a pill for all ills'.

Care

This is to remind us that different patients have different needs. Some patients' needs are greater, for example paediatric and geriatric patients may be special cases as would be pregnant or breast-feeding women. These factors may well influence the recommendations made by pharmacists or pharmacy technicians.

Observe

This is particularly important when attempting diagnosis.

Refer

This is to remind that one can refer a patient for a second opinion. Usually referral is advised if the patients are at increased risk, for example, paediatric patients, geriatric patients, etc., if the symptoms are persistent or if the symptoms suggest a potentially serious condition.

Explain

This is to remind us to fully explain decisions to patients. If a course of action is clearly explained the patient is more likely to be compliant. This system of questioning takes into account the appearance of the patient. Careful observation of a patient can reveal a lot. If a patient presenting with symptoms is seriously ill, they will rarely look well. If you define what you think are observable symptoms of ill health you could include flushing, sweating, dilated pupils or smell. 'N' and 'R', although they are relevant, do not really help towards making differential diagnosis. Once again no social or lifestyle factors are considered; nor is family history taken into account.

ASMETTHOD

- Age of the patient?
- Self or someone else?
- Medicines the patient is taking?
- Exactly what does the patient mean by the symptom?
- Time/duration of the symptom?
- Taken anything for it or seen the doctor?
- History of any disease or condition?
- Other symptoms being experienced?
- Doing anything to aggravate or alleviate the condition?

This system establishes the presenting complaint and whether or not the patient has had it before. It can be used to find the necessary information for making a diagnosis. Remember that not all questions will necessarily need to be asked and that the order of questioning is not that critical. Use the mnemonic as a checklist or aide memoir.

SIT DOWN SIR

- Site or location?
- Intensity or severity?
- Type or nature?
- Duration?
- Onset?
- With? (Other symptoms)
- N annoyed or aggravated by?
- Spread or radiation?

- Incidence or frequency pattern?
- Relieved by?

This mnemonic may help to elicit more information. It establishes severity, nature of symptoms and previous history but again the importance of social or lifestyle factors is ignored, as is the general appearance of the patient. Try using these mnemonics in the scenario above that demonstrated the use of different types of questions. Were all the points covered? While these mnemonics are a useful aid or memory jogger they are not a replacement for clinical consultation. They should aid your decision making but not constrain it.

LISTENING

Listening involves both verbal and non-verbal communication. There are different levels of listening and, as explained earlier, what we say is not always what is heard and, conversely, we do not always hear what is said to us. There are various different modes of listening:

- 'Half an ear listening' is background noise listening. We can hear the radio in the background but are we really listening to it?
- In 'passive listening', also known as 'stunned mullet listening' (an Australian term), the listener shows a vacant expression, a completely blank look and gives the speaker no feedback. This can be useful for calming people down but is not generally the type of listening we would want to see in a pharmacy.
- In 'reflective listening' the listener reflects the statements back to the speaker to encourage them to carry on with the thread of conversation.
- 'Active listening' is the main type of listening used in pharmacy when responding to symptoms.

Listening can be divided into six distinct processes:

1. Concentrating, organising and analyzing what is said. This may seem obvious but the process can be hindered in a number of ways through, for example:
   - Distractions from other demands within the pharmacy
   - Tiredness at the end of the day resulting in simple inattentiveness
   - The 'I've heard this all before' syndrome.
2. Processing the information provided. As you do this you may find you need to alter the pattern of the consultation to accommodate any new issues that arise. Words do not always paint a true picture: Listen to the underlying message that is conveyed by 'feelings'.
3. Approaching the conversation with an open mind and avoiding preconceptions. This can be difficult to achieve when dealing with regular patients who may be known at the pharmacy as 'That nice Mr Jones' or 'That nuisance Mrs Smith'. While listening to a person having already stereotyped them you are likely to only hear what to expect to hear and may therefore miss a vital piece of information.

   Remember also that patients may make snap judgements about the pharmacist that may hinder communication.
4. Listening with eyes as well as ears. Maintain eye contact as this will help to maintain interest and show interest.

More than two thirds of communication can be non-verbal . Look at the patient's facial expression and posture and be aware of the own posture.

5. Keeping quiet while the other person is speaking. Do not interrupt a patient: let them finish before you speak.
6. Acknowledging the other person and showing them that you are listening. When listening to a patient:
   - make encouraging gestures, for example, nod occasionally
   - encourage verbally by prompts: 'And . . .' , for example, and reinforce the understanding by summarising information given: 'Now let me see if I've got that right?' 'You say that . . .'
   - repeat certain significant or 'loaded' phrases or words or paraphrase some of the things the patient has said.

   If listening actively to a patient ,should be able to repeat back in own words what has been said by the patient.

   Do not necessarily have to agree with what they are saying!

   Remember, all the benefits of effective communication will be lost if the pharmacist then fails to explain the use of the recommended treatment.

EXPLANATION

When responding to symptoms in the pharmacy it is important to explain any decisions made to the patient clearly. Perhaps even more crucial is explanation of the purpose and use of prescribed or over-the-counter medicines.

Pharmacists and pharmacy technicians are the last link in the prescribing chain. The pharmacist is responsible for ensuring the correct medicine is dispensed and it is important that to make certain the patient knows how to take it correctly. Part of the pharmacist's and pharmacy technician's role is to help patients overcome any confusion they may have with respect to their medication.

It has been said that 'Good explanations, like good bikinis, should be brief, appealing, yet cover the essential features'! A mnemonic to help remember this is 'KISSER':

- Keep
- It
- Simple
- Short
- Empathetic
- Relevant.

There are three parts to a good explanation: planning, presentation and feedback.

PLANNING

Identify the information to be given and link your explanation to the individual to ensure understanding. At a basic level the information can just be provided to the patient but if the information can be linked to the individual, the relevance of the information will be understood and the information will more likely be taken on board by the patient.

PRESENTATION

This refers to the clarity of the message given, including the use of appropriate language. Tips for successful presentation include:

- Use analogies, examples and illustrations use pauses for effect, breaking down the information into bite-sized chunks
- Emphasise important points, use words or phrases such as 'important', 'essential' or 'the main thing to remember is'
- If appropriate, do not just explain verbally, demonstrate (e.g. the use of an inhaler)
- Summarise key points, e.g. 'KISSER' .

FEEDBACK

Check that the listener has understood by:

- Asking if they have any questions
- Getting them to summarise what they have been told or demonstrate their understanding
- Looking for non-verbal feedback, for example looking puzzled or confused
- Asking questions in order to check understanding.

Consider these two explanations about how to take indomethacin MR capsules:

1. 'These are the capsules for the arthritis. Take one capsule in the morning and one at night before going to bed. They should be swallowed whole and always taken with food.'
2. 'These are the capsules for the arthritis. Take one capsule in the morning and one at night before going to bed. One should find that the night time dose will help relieve the morning stiffness that have been experiencing.

It is important to take the capsules with food to help reduce or prevent any stomach upset. Also the capsules have been designed to have a long lasting effect, so they must be swallowed whole. Have any further questions? If have any concerns do not hesitate to come back and see me.' Which explanation will help the patient to remember? It is a fact that if a patient understands the reasons for doing something they are far more likely to be compliant. It is human nature. The pharmacist had planned what was to be said to the patient and the comment regarding morning stiffness showed that this pharmacist had taken the time to develop a rapport with the patient previously.

When do we use explanations in pharmacy?

- When responding to a patient's symptoms. In this case we need to explain/justify our actions.
- When dispensing prescriptions. Here we need to clearly explain the prescriber's directions and any associated cautions that apply to a particular medicine. We need to ensure that patients understand complex dosage instructions, such as a reducing dosage for a course or oral steroids, or the importance of completing a course of antibiotics.
- When demonstrating the use of a dosage form or appliance. Often it is better to explain verbally before doing the actual demonstration as the act of demonstrating may detract from the art of listening.
- When discussing side-effects and their prevalence. The rare but serious side-effects associated with some drugs need to be explained.
- When explaining possible medication and/ or food interactions, for example the importance of avoiding alcohol with certain drugs such metronidazole or cheese with monoamine oxidase inhibitors (MAOIs).
- When explaining public health issues, such as the reasons to give up smoking,

reduce cholesterol or blood pressure or the benefits of a healthy diet and lifestyle.

- When correcting mistaken beliefs. Patients often believe firmly in old wives tales, such as:
  - 'Feed a cold and starve a fever' – It is highly unlikely if a patient has a fever that they will want to eat but with the help of an antipyretic, their temperature will come down and subsequently their appetite will return.
  - 'Colds cause ear infections' – This is unlikely since colds are caused by viruses and most ear infections by bacteria, however the build up of fluids in the ears associated with a cold is a fertile breeding ground for bacteria so the two can seem to go hand in hand.
- When providing advice. Pharmacists and pharmacy technicians advise patients in response to their symptoms on a daily basis.

For example:

- Advising a patient with a blocked nose: 'Have you tried an inhalation? Karvol Capsules or Friar's Balsam can help.'
- Advising against the purchase of an old fashioned medicine and guiding towards a better, evidence-based treatment. For example liquid paraffin is not considered to be the best treatment for constipation. Lactulose is the preferred treatment nowadays.
- Advising the choice of one medicine rather than another, such as an expectorant rather than a cough suppressant for a patient requesting a cough medicine. In this case a logical explanation may be required. For example, 'An expectorant will help clear your lungs of the phlegm as it will thin the phlegm and you will be able to cough it up yourself. A suppressant, while it will stop you coughing, will leave the phlegm sitting on your lungs, which is not advised.'

EXPLAINING AND EDUCATING PATIENTS TO IMPROVE CONCORDANCE

It has been estimated that around half of patients do not take their medicines as intended. To try to improve on this, now it is for a prescriber and patient to come to joint decisions regarding their treatment and for the pharmacist, doctor and patient to become members of the same team.

Using a multidisciplinary team means that it is often easier to address the problems that cause lack of compliance (a patient is said to be compliant with their prescribed therapy if they take their medication as advised). Often the pharmacist is seen as more accessible to the patient and therefore in the best position to improve the chances of a patient complying with a medication regimen. If patients understand why they are taking a medicine and the benefits for them they are more likely to be happy to continue treatment.

When a pharmacist conducts a medicines use review (MUR), it is an ideal opportunity to find out exactly what the patient is doing with their medication and how they are complying with the regimen. By empowering the patient by giving them more involvement in decision making, allow the patient to decide themselves whether or not to take a medication. Because of the openness of the exchange, their reasons for not taking a medication can be rationally discussed and a joint decision to comply with the current dosage regimen (or if necessary an amended regimen) obtained. This is termed concordance. Compliance and concordance can be affected by the patient's perceived benefit or lack of benefit from the therapy. It can also be affected by the reason for the instigation of medication. A heart attack would be a frightening experience and brings the idea of mortality to the patient's mind and therefore, at least to begin with, the importance of taking their medication will be a priority. But with the passage of time and if no further events happen, encouragement to continue a long-term treatment may be needed. Educating patients about their conditions, particularly if they are 'symptom free' conditions such as hypertension (high blood pressure), may improve compliance. Explaining the damaging effect to the body organs of high blood pressure and the effects it can have on life expectancy can be sufficiently motivating to the patient so that they take part in the decision to take medication and understand the necessity for it. In order to make compliance easier for a patient it is often better to develop a routine. For example while the kettle is boiling for the first cup of tea of the day get into the habit of taking the first dose of medication. With complex dosage regimens a pill organiser or monitored dosage system may be of value.

These are usually seven-day organisers with a compartment for each day that is then split into sections that equate to breakfast, lunch, evening meal and bedtime. Although they have their disadvantages

- Some medicines cannot be placed in these containers (for example, soluble tablets), they need re-filling weekly, and there is no guarantee that medication has actually been taken if it is missing from the device as it may have fallen on the floor and been lost
- They are helpful if the non-compliance is unintentional and a result of forgetfulness. Similarly when completing an MUR you may find that a patient is not fully compliant because of problems of manual dexterity, either due to inflammatory conditions such as arthritis or neurological disease such as Parkinson's disease. These types of problems can make even the simplest packaging an obstacle to taking the medicine. It is often said that grandma asks the grandchildren to open her child-resistant containers.

Side-effects or the concern about side-effects listed in patient information leaflets can also be a barrier to patient compliance. What patients perceive is the probability of a side-effect listed and what the terminology used actually means is often at variance. Pharmacists can play a major part in patient compliance by talking to patients when they are first prescribed an item, giving the patient another opportunity to raise any concerns and to have an open discussion to allay their fears.

Pharmacists are also in an ideal position to review compliance with long-term medication. Often by observation and checking with the patient dosage regimens, pharmacists are able to recognise that a patient has an existing compliance problem. Once the problem is identified it may be addressed and coping strategies or managing strategies may be employed as outlined above. Pharmacists and pharmacy technicians are often the last link in the prescribing chain and if patients are to obtain the best from their medication it is up to the pharmacist to ensure compliance.

WRITTEN COMMUNICATION

When patients are counselled verbally their understanding at the time of the explanation can be checked, but the length of time the information is retained can vary from patient to patient. In the pharmacy we provide two forms of written communication to patients: the labels on dispensed medicines and the patient information leaflets contained in both prescribed medicines and over-the-counter sales.

Pharmacists may also add further cautions with regard to certain formulations. These include pharmaceutical cautions, such as 'For external use only', 'Not to be taken', 'Shake the bottle', storage conditions, such as 'Store in fridge' for items needing to be stored below room temperature, and discard dates for items which should be discarded after a particular date (e.g. reconstituted antibiotic mixtures or eye drops after opening).

The written word is no replacement for verbal communication. Many patients prefer to be told in person about their medication and often seem to feel that the purpose of the patient information leaflet is to highlight every sideeffect ever noted. After all, they probably do not have the expertise or knowledge to sort out which side-effect is serious and which are very likely or very unusual.

Some information leaflets include pictograms describing how a product should be used. These can be valuable, for example, when trying to explain the use of eye drops, pessaries, suppositories, inhalers, etc. There are also many leaflets available from the internet (for example, www.medicines.org.uk), where patient information leaflets may be down loaded in large print versions and audio versions.

COMMUNICATION WITH OTHER HEALTHCARE PROFESSIONALS

While most of the day-to-day communication will be with patients, there will also be times when pharmacists and pharmacy technicians communicate with prescribers and other healthcare professionals.

Communication with other healthcare professions will include both verbal and written communication. For example, patient referral forms would be a form of written communication from the pharmacist to the prescriber. These forms concern information that the pharmacist may have obtained:

- As a result of a 'responding to symptoms' interview with a patient
- As a result of tests perfomed in the pharmacy
- As an information provide to the GP, for example when medicines have been supplied to a patient following an emergency request from the patient.

In community pharmacy the most common form of contact with a GP is by telephone concerning a prescription that has been received in the pharmacy. As pharmacists we are problem solving all the time, so if there is a problem with a prescription we will normally try to resolve it without resorting to contacting the prescriber.

However in certain cases contact with the prescriber will be required. It is important to prepare for the consultation, as quite often you will be interrupting a busy surgery. There are two main issues: the patient and the drug. Before speaking to the prescriber you need to obtain the complete picture and formulate plans. References need to be checked, such as the British National Formulary, summary of product characteristics, other drug information, etc. The information is needed with regard to the patient, name, address, age, most of which will be available from the prescription.

The NHS number (or equivalent) for the patient should also be available. Using the references available (do not forget that the patient may also be a valuable information source) need to formulate a plan. If there is a problem regarding the supply of a drug, for example, a manufacturer's delay or something similar, need to be able to suggest alternative therapy, and it would be best to suggest an item that is stocked by the pharmacy and therefore easily obtainable.

When contacting a prescriber, introduce yourself, identify the patient and describe the concern (always have a pen and paper with you so that you can jot down information you want to give and any information you receive from the prescriber). The prescriber may suggest a plan of action or may expect to have already formulated a plan which could share and modify if necessary. Together should reach a conclusion and then need to confirm that understood the prescriber's intentions correctly, summarise what have heard and repeat the information back to the prescriber for confirmation; the strength, dosage and frequency of the medication are particularly important.

All the time listen to the information being given to you. Remember speaking to another healthcare professional. Treat them with the respect they deserve, being ever mindful of how would like to be treated if someone was querying something had done. Consider the following examples. These case studies highlight that often the problems we encounter as pharmacists are not of our own making and our role seems to be one of a negotiator.

MEDICATION COUNSELING TIPS

- Establish relationship – show interest in patient (verbal & nonverbal)
- Verify patient's name and prescriber's name
- Why the patient is being prescribed the medication (if known) or the medication's use, expected benefits and action
- Open the medication containers and show patient what the medication looks like, or demonstrate use
- How to take the medication
- When to take and how long to take the medication
- What to do if a dose is missed
- Any special precautions to follow
- Foods, alcoholic beverages or OTC's to be avoided
- How the patient will know the medication is working
- How to store the medication
- If the prescription can be refilled, and if so, when
- Verify the patients' knowledge and understanding
- Ask the patient if they have any questions
- Document the interaction

PATIENTS WHO SHOULD ALWAYS BE COUNSELED

- Confused patients, and their caregivers
- Patients who are sight or hearing impaired
- Patients with poor literacy
- Patients whose profile shows a change in medications or dosing
- New patients, or those receiving a medication for the first time (transfer prescription)
- Children, and parents receiving medication
- Patients receiving medication with special storage requirements, complicated directions, significant side effects

PATIENTS WHO SHOULD BE COUNSELED AT CERTAIN INTERVALS

- Asthmatic patients
- Diabetic patients
- Patients taking 4 or more prescribed medications
- Patients who are mentally ill
- Patients using appliances
- Epileptic patients
- Patients with skin complaints
- Patients misusing drugs
- Patients who are terminally ill

REFERENCES

1. Beardsley, RS. Review of literature: oral patient counseling by pharmacists. Proceedings of the National Symposium on Oral Counseling by Pharmacists About Prescription Medicines. 1997 Sep 19-21; Lansdowne,Virginia.
2. Harvey M. Rappaport et al. The Guidebook for Patient Counselling. Lancaster, Pennsylvania: Technomic Publishing Company, 1994.
3. Tindall, William N, Robert S. Beardsley, Carole L. Kimberlin. Communication Skills in Pharmacy Practice (fourth edition). Baltimore, Maryland and Philadelphia, Pennsylvania : Lippincott Williams & Wilkins, 2003.

CHAPTER 13

Parenteral Nutrition

DEFINITION

Parenteral nutrition (PN) is feeding a person intravenously, bypassing the usual process of eating and digestion. The person receives nutritional formulae that contain nutrients such as glucose, amino acids, lipids and added vitamins and dietary minerals. It is called Total parenteral nutrition (TPN) or Total nutrient admixture (TNA) when no food is given by other routes.

Parenteral nutrition is a means of providing protein, CHO, fat, vitamins, and minerals to those who are unable to assimilate nutrients provided via the gastrointestinal tract. Parenteral nutrition is safe and effective when delivered according to strict protocols by nutritional support team or other trained person. Total parenteral nutrition is prepared in the pharmacy and administered through a central venous catheter. TPN is usually initiated at slow rate of 25 to 50cc per hour and advanced at 12 to 24 hour intervals as metabolic status allows, till the required volume and calories are reached. When a patient is unable to receive nutrition support via the GI tract, it is necessary to choose between central or peripheral vascular access.

KEY FACTORS INFLUENCING THIS DECISION ARE

- Anticipated time frame for the use.
- Total nutrient needs.
- Capacity to handle fluid volume.
- Condition of peripheral vein.

INDICATIONS WHERE PN SHOULD BE A PART OF ROUTINE CARE

- Patients with inability to absorb nutrients via GI tract
- Massive small bowel resection, diseases of the small intestine, radiation enteritis, severe diarrhea, intractable vomiting.
- Patients undergoing high dose chemotherapy, radiation and bone-marrow transplantation
- Moderate to severe pancreatitis
- Severe malnutrition in the face of nonfunctional GI tract or catabolism when the patient is unable to eat for 5 or more days.
- Severely catabolic patients with or without malnutrition when GI tract is not useable within 5 to 7 days.

INDICATIONS WHERE PN WILL BE HELPFUL

- Major surgery: examples including patients undergoing total colectomy, esophagogastrostomy, pancreaticoduodenectomy, elective repair of an abdominal aortic aneurysm etc.

- Moderate stress: patients with moderate trauma, 30%-50% body surface area burns, moderately severe pancreatitis, neurological trauma, and other similar stress.
- Entrocutaneous fistulae
- Inflammatory bowel disease
- Hyperemesis gravidarum
- Moderately malnourished patients who require intensive medical or surgical intervention
- Patients in whom adequate enteral nutrition cannot established within 7 to 10 days period in hospitalization.
- Patients with inflammatory adhesions with small bowel obstruction.
- Patients receiving intensive cancer chemotherapy

CLINICAL SETTINGS WHERE PN IS OF LIMITED VALUE

- Minimal stress and trauma in the well-nourished patient, when the GI tract is usable within 10 days of period.
- Immediate postoperative or post stress period
- Proven or suspected untreatable disease

CLINICAL CONDITIONS WHERE PN SHOULDN'T BE USED

- Patients who have a functional and usable GI tract, capable of absorption of adequate nutrients
- When sole dependence on TPN is anticipated to be less than 5 days
- Inability to obtain venous access
- A prognosis that does not warrant aggressive nutritional support
- Patients in need of urgent operation should not have that operation delayed solely in favor of TPN
- When the risks of TPN are judged to exceed potential benefits.

NUTRIENT SOURCES IN PARENTERAL NUTRITION

PROTEIN

Commercially available standard solutions are composed of essential and nonessential crystalline amino acids in solution. Specialized formulas with adjusted amino acid profiles are available for patients with hyper metabolism, renal or liver disease. The amino acid component of TPN solution can vary in concentration as well as composition of individual amino acids. The concentration varies between 3% to 15%. Thus 10% solution of amino acid supplies 100g of protein per liter.

Requirements

For healthy adults 0.8 g/kg per day

In critical illness 1.2 to 2.5 g/kg per day

Optimal Protein Intake

- For an individual, the optimal protein intake may be measured using nitrogen balance (protein intake/6.25 – urinary urea nitrogen + 4). Protein should be given adequately to maintain a positive (2 to 4 g) nitrogen balance.
- Generally 15% - 20% of total calories should come from protein
- Excess protein administration does not result in protein accretion

- For normal individuals, about 300 non-protein calories are needed for optimal utilization of 1 g of nitrogen
- In critical illness, about 100 to 150 non-protein calories are needed for optimal utilization of 1 g of nitrogen.

CARBOHYDRATE

Carbohydrate is provided as dextrose monohydrate in concentration ranging from 5%-70%. As with amino acids, 10% solution of dextrose yields 100g of carbohydrate per liter of solution. The dextrose concentration of central venous nutrition is higher than that given peripherally because the larger central vein can rapidly dilute the infusate.

Requirements

- The minimal amount of carbohydrate a person requires is unknown but an estimate of 1 mg/kg/min (100g per day for a 70 kg individual) is usually used. Inadequate intake of carbohydrate results in utilization of protein as an energy source. 100g of carbohydrate ensures that proteins are not utilized for calorie purpose.
- The maximal amount of carbohydrate tolerated is approximately 5 mg/kg/min; excessive administration of carbohydrate has been associated with
  - Hyperglycemia – lower the concentration of dextrose
  - Glycosuria
  - Synthesis and storage of fat
  - Hepatic steatosis
  - Cholestasis
  - Increased CO_2 production causing respiratory failure – the alter respiratory quotient (RQ) ratio during respiratory failure change solution to lower dextrose and higher fat concentration.

FAT

Fat emulsions are composed of aqueous suspensions of soybean or safflower oil with egg yolk phospholipids as the emulsifier. Fat emulsions are available in 10% and 20% concentrations. A 10% emulsion provides 1.1 calorie/ml; a 20% solution provides 2 calorie/ml (9-calorie/g fat).

Requirements

- Exact fat requirements are unknown
- To prevent EFAD, 2% - 4% calorie requirement should come from lonelier acid (25 to 100 mg/kg per day)
- Ten percent of calorie from soy or safflower oil emulsion should provide adequate lonelier acid to prevent EFAD
- Maximal fat dosage should not exceed 60% of calories
- To minimize the negative effect of lonelier acid on immunity, fat intake may be restricted to less than 30% of total calories, or 1g/kg per day

Optimal Intake

- The optimal percentage of calories from is not known.
- Approximately 20% -60% of calories from fat have been administered without ill effects.
- 30% of calories from fat have been shown to reduce elevated liver function tests compared with glucose-based PN alone

Consequences of Excess Fat Administration

- Fat overload syndrome with neurologic, cardiac, pulmonary, hepatic, and renal dysfunction
- Thrombocyte adhesiveness
- Reduced pulmonary diffusion capacity has been reported, but not confirmed
- Accumulation of the lipid in the reticuloendothelial system (RES), leading to RES dysfunction
- Impaired immune response has been associated with high intake of lonelier acid

VITAMINS / MINERALS/ TRACE ELEMENTS (TABLE 13.1)

Parenteral vitamin requirements differ from enteral vitamin requirements because of differences in efficiency in absorption and utilization of nutrients administered via parenteral route and physiochemical stability in the parenteral solutions.

Parenteral vitamin supplementation is based on recommendations. Several commercial products are available that encompass these guidelines. Specific brand names will vary in their contents, according to the institution.

Vitamin K is not included in the multi-vitamin preparations and must be given either intramuscularly or as an intravenous injectable added to PN solution

Vitamin K, (2 to 4 mg per week) should also be included in PN formulations; its administration should be avoided in-patients on coumadin therapy.

Table 13.1

Recommendations for parenteral minerals intake

Mineral	Amount
Zinc	2.5 – 4.0 mg*
Copper	0.5 – 1.5 mg
Chromium	10.0 – 15.0 mg
Magnesium	0.15 – 0.8 mg

ELECTROLYTES

Electrolyte composition of a PN solution is designed to maintain normal body function and also provide for excess and deficiencies of minerals based on the underlying disease process. Commercial multiple-electrolyte solutions are available and their composition is indeed to meet the normal range of daily electrolyte requirements.

- Electrolyte requirements in parenteral nutrition vary, but representative ranges are found in Table 13.1 Individual nutrients may be altered as needed to correct electrolyte imbalance
- The need for electrolyte increased when abnormal losses occur (renal, GI, or dermal) and during refeeding of starve patients.
- The need for electrolyte decreased in situations where electrolytes are retained (congestive heart failure or renal failure). A factor that increases or decreases the need of electrolyte is shown in Table 13.2

Table 13.2

Factors that alter the electrolyte needs

	Increase	Decrease
Potassium	Potassium wasting medications Diuretics Gastrointestinal losses e.g. diarrhea, nasogastric suction, Anabolism	Potassium sparing medications Renal failure
Sodium	Gastrointestinal losses e.g. vomiting, nasogastric loss, severe diarrhea	Congestive heart failure
Phosphorus	Anabolism	Renal failure
Magnesium	Anabolism Magnesium-wasting medications, Hypokalemia	Renal failure
Calcium	Pregnancy	Hypercalcemia
Chloride	Metabolic alkalosis, nasogastric losses	Metabolic acidosis

Trace elements: several micronutrients have been identified as essential in parenteral nutrition solutions to prevent clinical deficiency

1. **Zinc:** Widely distributed in the body and the part of several enzyme systems. Required for growth, wound healing, cellular mobility
2. **Copper:** Plays role in iron absorption and transportation. Component of metalloprotein necessary for skeletal development, function, and structure of the central nervous system, taste sensation, and pigmentation
3. **Chromium:** Functions in insulin sensitivity and glucose tolerance. Difficult to detect deficiency except monitoring glucose tolerance
4. **Manganese:** Activate a number of enzyme systems. Involved in protein and energy metabolism. Excreted primarily via biliary tract. Decreased requirement in biliary obstruction.
5. **Selenium:** Component of the active site of the peroxide destroying enzyme glutathione peroxidase.

FLUIDS

Fluid requirements increased with increased renal GI, dermal or respiratory losses. Table 13.3 indicates fluid requirements.

Fluid requirements decreased with cardiac and renal insufficiency.

Fluid intake and output along with comparison of actual Vs dry weight are evaluated when considering fluid needs.

Table 13.3

Fluid intake

Method 1	Fluid (ml/kg)
For young, vigorous, previously healthy adults	40
For other adults	35
For elderly adults	25

PHYSICAL CHARACTERISTICS OF PARENTERAL FORMULAS

RENAL SOLUTE LOAD

The term is defined as the solute load presented to the kidneys for excretion in the urine.

The renal solute load determines the volume of water needed to form urine.

Inadequate water excretes waste result in Azotemia; therefore adequate fluid must be given with PN.

CALCIUM PHOSPHORUS COMPATIBILITY

The combination of calcium and phosphorus salts in excessive amounts may result in crystalline precipitate and possible catheter occlusion.

The maximum amount of calcium and phosphorus that may be added to given volume of total parenteral nutrition (TPN) is depend on several factors including the volume of fluid. The pH solution, and mixing procedures.

VITAMINS

Stability of vitamins in PN is affected by Light, Temperature, pH, Length of storage, other vitamins and minerals, Preservatives.

ROUTE OF ADMINISTRATION

PN can be delivered through peripheral or central venous lines. The limiting factor in deciding route of delivery is Osmolarity of the AA-glucose solution which is dependent on dextrose concentration. A dextrose concentration greater than 12.5% has an acidic pH and can be irritating to the peripheral veins. In addition to dextrose, electrolytes and minerals added to the solution increase the osmolarity of the solution. Hypertonic solution need to be administered through central venous line. Increasing use of peripherally inserted central catheters (PICC) has facilitated administration of PN while avoiding many potential complications of surgically inserted central lines. Short-term PN can be given through peripheral venous line. Another attractive optionin neonates is central line inserted through umbilical vein. Position of central line should be confirmed by X-ray before starting infusion through it. The venous access. Used for PN should not be interrupted for giving antibiotics or other medications. For this a separate intravenous line should be established. Peripheral access offers the advantage of a lower risk of infection due to the greater distance of the catheter from the central circulation as well as a smaller risk of mechanical complications. However, nutrition delivery is limited with peripheral lines due to constraints created by a solution's osmolarity. Osmolarity refers to the number of particles per weight of water in kilograms and is typically used to describe enteral feedings and a standard in describing blood. Osmolarity refers to the number of millimoles of liquid or solid in a liter of solution and is the preferred term for TPN. In peripheral access concentration greater than 900-1000 mOsm/ L are to be avoided. With central access, solutions greater than 1,000 mOsm/L are acceptable.

COMPLICATIONS ASSOCIATED WITH PN

COMPLICATIONS MAY BE CLASSIFIED AS FOLLOWS

- Metabolic Complications such as; hypovalemia, hyperkalemia, hypokalemia,

hypernatremia, hyponatremia, hyperglycemia, hypoglycemia, hypertriglyceridemia, hypercalcemia, hypocalcemia, hypermagnesemia, hypomagnesemia, hyperphosphatemia, prerenal azotemia, overfeeding, essential fatty acid deficiency.
- Catheter related complications such as; pneumothorax, air embolism, catheter embolization, venous thrombosis, catheter occlusion, improper tip location, phlebitis, catheter related sepsis.
- Gastrointestinal complications such as; fatty liver, cholestasis, gastrointestinal atrophy.
- Appropriate monitoring can minimize complications developed by PN.

CYCLIC TOTAL PARENTERAL NUTRITION

- Refers to intermittent infusion of solution over a specified amount of time.
- Most often used to prepare patients for home parenteral nutrition so that they have an infusion-free period to resume activity.
- For correction of fatty liver associated with prolonged infusion of hypertonic dextrose solution.
- Patient with limited central venous access, cyclic TPN may allow administration of incompatible medications during the hours that TPN is not in use.
- The length of infusion is dependent on the volume of the solution that the patient requires the maximum tolerated rate.

CONCLUSION

1. Determine if PN is truly indicated
2. Assess the patient (medical history, medication profile, anthropometric data & lab values)
3. Determine need for long-term vs. short term
   - <7–10 days
4. Confirm or establish adequate IV access
   - Peripheral or central?
5. Determine estimated kcal, protein and lipid needs
   - 20–30 kcal/kg
   - Protein 0.8–1.5 gm/kg
   - Higher levels may be needed in severe catabolic states
6. Lipid to provide d" 30% of kcals. Determine initial electrolyte, vitamin and trace element requirements; consider ongoing losses
7. Consider any additional additives to PN formulation including insulin and H_2-receptor antagonists
8. Monitor for:
   - Risk of refeeding syndrome
   - Glucose intolerance
   - Start low and advance slowly if labs stable over 24-48 hours
   - Fluid, electrolyte, metabolic, macro- and micro-nutrient changes
   - Complications – sepsis, thrombosis, abuse
9. Initiate trophic feedings or convert patient to PO or enteral feeding when feasible.

REFERENCES

1. Skipper A, Marian MJ. Parenteral nutrition. In: Gottschlich MM, Matarese LE, Shronts EP, eds. Nutrition Support Dietetics Core Curriculum. Silver Spring, Md: ASPEN; 1993:105-121.
2. Kudsk KA, Croce MA, Fabian TC, et al. Enteral versus parenteral feeding: effects

on septic morbidity following blunt and penetrating abdominal trauma. Ann Surg. 1992: 215; 503-513.

3. Anon. Midline and midclavicular catheters. J Intravenous Nurs. 1997; 20(4): 175-178.
4. Rollins CJ. Total nutrient admixtures: stability issues and theirimpact on nursing practice. J Intraven Nurs. 1997; 20: 299-304.
5. Lenssen P. Management of total parenteral nutrition. In:Skipper A, ed. Dietitian's Handbook of Enteral and Parenteral Nutrition. 2nd ed. Gaithersburg, Md: Aspen Publ; 1998: 481-513.
6. The National Advisory Group on Standards and PracticeGuidelines for Parenteral Nutrition. Safe practices for parenteral nutrition formulations. J Parenter Enteral Nutr. 1 9 9 8; 22: 49-66.
7. Fuhrman M. Management of complications of parenteral nutrition. In Contemporary NutritionSupport Practice: A Clinical Guide, eds Matarese L, Gottschlich M.Philadelphia, PA: Saunders;1998. 236-237. 249, 252-253.

CHAPTER 14

Pharmacovigilance

DEFINITION

The science and activities relating to the Detection, Assessment, Understanding and Prevention of adverse effects or any other medicine-related problem –WHO

VIGILANCE

- Vigilare = to watch
  - alert watchfulness
  - forbearance of sleep; wakefulness
  - watchfulness in respect of danger; care; caution; circumspection
  - the process of paying close and continuous attention

HISTORY

- Registration of New Chemical Entities was very much dependant on the status of products in the reference countries
- Changes to product information was mainly industry driven
- Few pre-clinical studies conducted in the region and hardly any Phase IV studies
- Adverse drug reaction reporting was very minimal and mainly involved reports submitted by health care professionals
- Most reports were for known reactions involving older drugs which were used in government-run hospitals
- Signal detection not possible as there were too few reports
- Only able to detect some quality defects of generics which manifested as adverse drug reactions (ADRs)
- Pharmacovigilance was mainly about getting ADR reports and submitting them to WHO
- No significant regulatory changes made based on these reports

CURRENT SCENARIO

- Increased awareness and interest amongst doctors and pharmacists to report ADRs as they have seen some benefit in reporting
- Increasing number of clinical trials being conducted especially in Singapore, Thailand and Malaysia
- Good clinical practice (GCP) training for investigators served to increase awareness of serious adverse event (SAE) and ADR reporting amongst health care professionals and the industry
- More hospitals and companies using on-line reporting system – less hassle than submitting hard copy reports
- Increasing involvement by hospital pharmacists in Pharmacovigilance – during clinical ward rounds and when counseling patients

MAJOR AIMS

- Early detection of unknown safety problems

- Identification of risk factors
- Quantifying risks
- Preventing patients from being affected unnecessarily
- To improve patient care and safety
- To improve public health and safety
- To contribute to the assessment of benefit, harm, effectiveness and risk of medicines
- To promote understanding, education and clinical training
- Rational and safe use of medicines

COMMON ADRS

- Constipation after Codeine; Sedation with Antihistamine;
- Nausea with Fluoxetine; GIT upset with NSAIDs
- 1959/61–Thalidomide 4.000 – 10.000 cases (Phocomelia)

"Medicines are supposed to save lives."

Dying from a disease is sometimes unavoidable; dying from a medicine is unacceptable. WHO. Geneva 2005

WHY PHARMACOVIGILANCE?

RISK

No medicinal product is entirely or absolutely safe for all people, in all places, at all times.

We must always live with some measure of uncertainty.

Humanitarian concern

- Insufficient evidence of safety from clinical trials
- Animal experiments
- Phase 1 – 3 studies prior to marketing authorization

Drug discovery and clinical trails (Fig. 14.1, 14.2) indicates stages of drug development, preclinical and clinical studies.

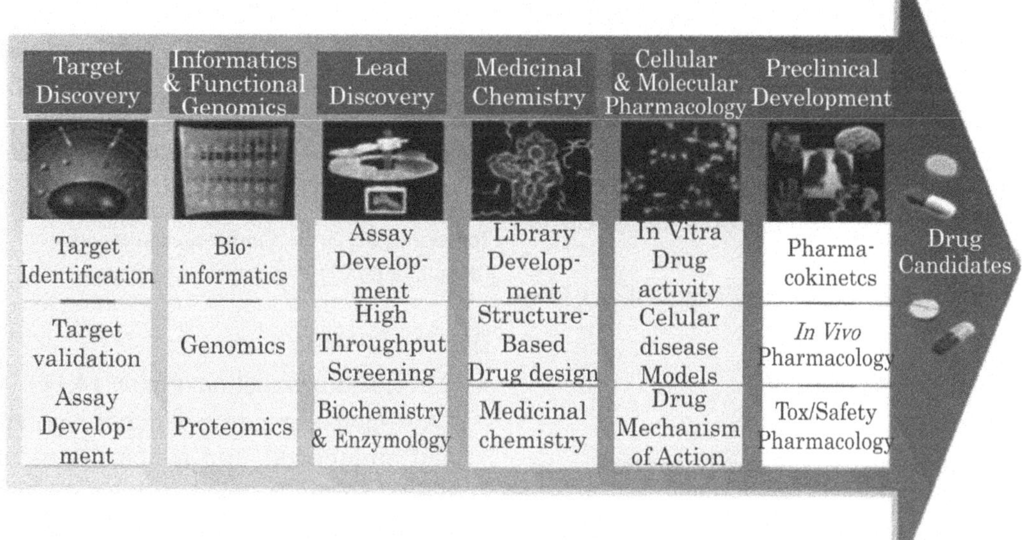

FIGURE 14.1

Drug development.

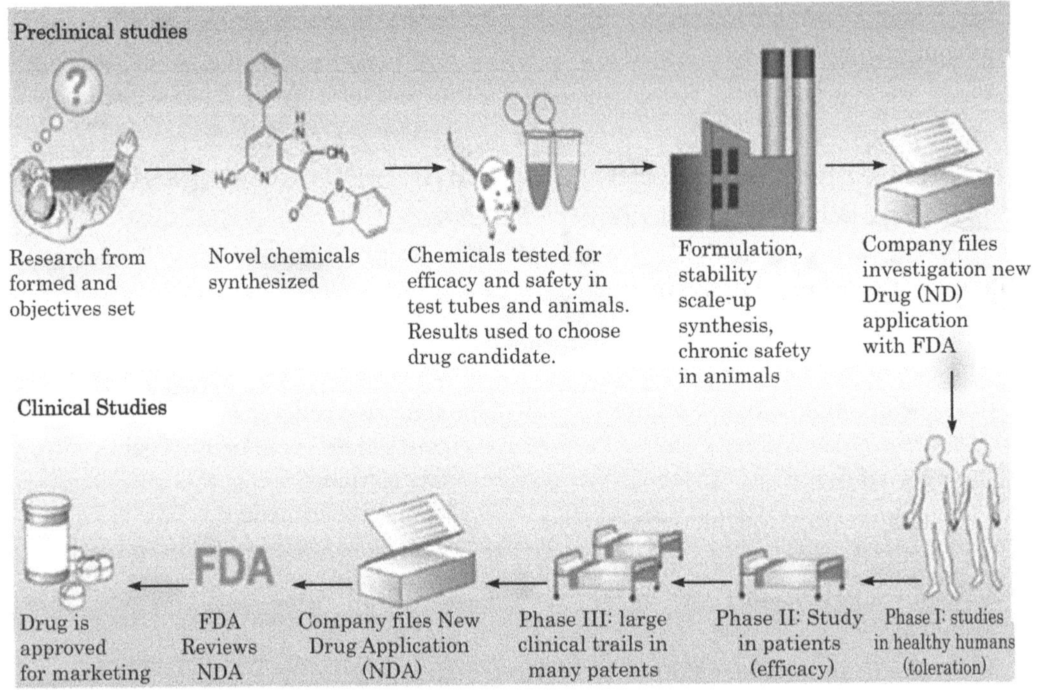

FIGURE 14.2

Preclinical and clinical studies.

LIMITATIONS OF PHASE 1-3 CLINICAL TRIALS

- Limited size: no more than 5000 and often as little as 500 volunteers
- Narrow population: age and sex specific
- Narrow indications: only the specific disease studied
- Short duration: often no longer than a few weeks

WITHDRAWN DRUGS (IN THE US, SINCE 2000)

Thalidomide (1961)	Congenital limb defects
Benoxaprofen (1982)	Hepatotoxicity
Phenformin (1982)	Lactic acidosis
Fenfluramine (1997)	Heart-valve abnormalities
Astemizole	Many drug interactions
Phenylpropanolamine (2000)	Hemorrhagic stroke
Kava kava	Liver abnormalities
Cerivastatin	Rhabdomyolysis
Cisapride	Cardiac arrhythmias
Rofecoxib (2004)	Cardiovascular events
Valdecoxib (2005)	Cardiovascular events, Serious skin reactions
Comfrey, Senecio	Nephrotoxicity
Tegaserod (2007)	Cardiovascular events
Clobutinol (2007)	Cardiac arrhythmia

DEFINITIONS

- Adverse drug reaction (Table 14.1)
  – "A response to a drug which is noxious and unintended, and which occurs at doses normally used in man for the prophylaxis, diagnosis, or therapy of disease, or for the modification of physiological function."
- Adverse event

- Any untoward medical occurrence that may present during treatment with a pharmaceutical product but which does not necessarily have a causal relationship with this treatment
- Side effect
- Any unintended effect of a pharmaceutical product occurring at doses normally used in man which is related to the pharmacological properties of the drug

OUTCOME OF PVG

- Contribute to the regulatory assessment of benefit, harm, effectiveness and risk of medicines, encouraging their safe, rational and more effective (including cost effective) use.
- Improve patient care and safety in relation to use of medicines and all medical and paramedical interventions.
- Improve public health and safety in relation to use of medicines.
- Promote understanding, education and clinical training in pharmacovigilance and its effective communication to the public.
- The results of pharmacoepidemiological studies would confirm or disprove the license.
- Effectiveness of the drug in clinical practice (confirmation of the therapeutic effect), determine whether approved uses should be expanded or restricted.

DRUG OUTCOMES

- Outcomes:
  - Effects (Pharmacological, therapeutic)
  - Side effects (Unintended)
  - Interactions (Expected, unexpected)
- Impact:
  - Beneficial
  - Harmful
- Harmful Effects
  - Mortality
  - Morbidity
  - Hospitalization
    - Prolonged stay
    - Extra treatment
- Cost

WHO PROGRAMME FOR INTERNATIONAL DRUG MONITORING

The WHO Programme, which was established in 1968, consists of a network of

- The National Centre's
- WHO Headquarters, Geneva and
- The WHO Collaborating Centre for International Drug Monitoring, the Uppsala Monitoring Centre(UMC), in Uppsala, Sweden.

WHO COLLABORATING CENTRE (UPPSALA MONITORING CENTRE)

- Collection and processing of data: maintaining and developing the international adverse drug reaction database > 4 million reports
- Regular screening of data to issue signals
- Research
  - New ADR findings, new methodology, technology, methods of communication
- Information centre
- Training centre

SUBSEQUENTLY AIMS TO

- Generate broad based ADR data on the Indian population and share the information with global health-care community through WHO-UMC
- Ensure optimum safety of drug products in the Indian market

- Provide technical expertise for evaluating statutory AE reports furnished by sponsors conducting clinical trials in India

NATIONAL PHARMACOVIGILANCE POLICY

MILESTONES

- **Short-term objectives:** To foster a culture of notification
- **Medium-term objectives:** To engage several healthcare professionals and NGOs in the drug monitoring and information dissemination processes.
- **Long-term objectives:** To achieve such operational efficiencies that would make Indian National Pharmacovigilance Programme a benchmark for global drug monitoring endeavors'.

EXPECTED AND UNEXPECTED EVENTS

Expected are those adverse events that were observed during clinical trials or post-approval observations and are mentioned in Summary of Product Characteristics (SPC)

- Unexpected are those adverse events that were not previously observed and are not documented (in SPC)
- Based on frequency of occurrence there are following categories of adverse events:

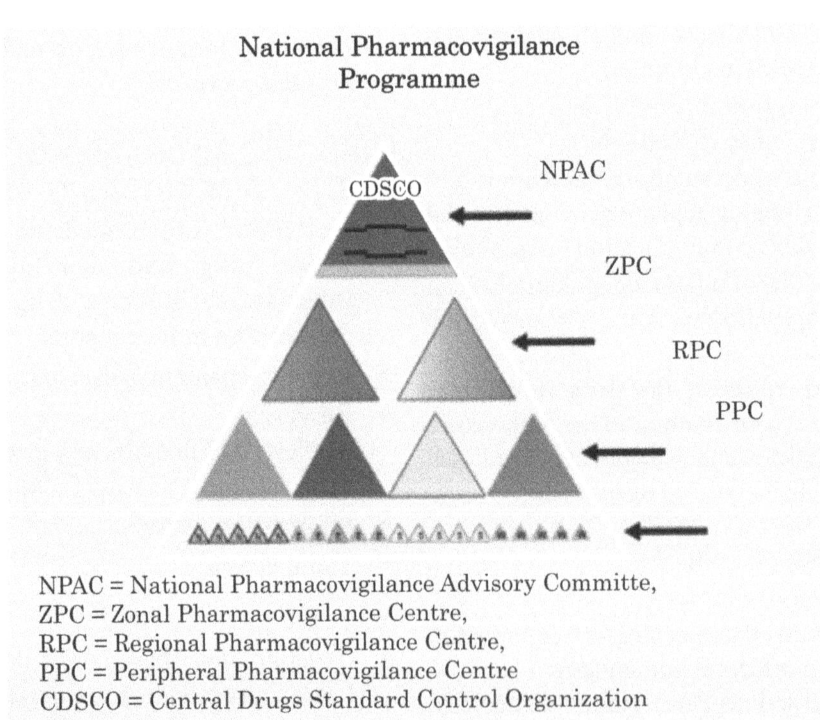

FIGURE 14.3

National pharmacovigilance programme.

Table 14.1

Types of adverse reactions (rawlins and thompson classification)

Type	Type of effect	Features	Examples
A	Augmented	Common, predictable, low mortality	Bradycardia– β-blockers
B	Bizarre	Uncommon, unpredictable, high morbidity and high mortality	Anaphylaxis - Penicillin
C	Chronic	Dose related and time related	Dyskinesia - Levodopa
D	Delayed	Time Related	Teratogenesis
E	End of use	Withdrawal of chronic therapy abruptly	Corticosteroids
F	Failure	Unexpected failure of therapy	Oral contraceptive failure - Rifampin

KEY FACTS

- No medicine is risk free. Vigilant assessment of the risks and benefits of medicines promotes patient safety.
- People in every country of the world are affected by ADRs. In some countries ADR-related costs, such as hospitalization, surgery and lost productivity, exceed the cost of the medications.
- Unintended, harmful reactions to medicines (known as adverse drug reactions) are among the leading causes of death in many countries.

The Majority of Adverse Drug Reactions (ADR) is Preventable and can be due to:

1. Wrong diagnosis of the patient's condition;
2. Prescription of the wrong drug or wrong dosage of the right drug;
3. An undetected medical, genetic or allergic condition that might cause a patient reaction;
4. Self-medication with prescription medicines;
5. Not following the instructions for taking the medication;
6. Reactions with other drugs (including traditional medicines) and certain foods;
7. Use of a sub-standard medication whose composition and ingredients do not meet the correct scientific requirements, and can be ineffective and often dangerous;
8. Use of counterfeit medicines with no active ingredients or the wrong ingredients, which can be dangerous or fatal.

Prescribing and transcription –60%;

Administration –30%;

Dispensing –10%

Causality Assessment

To determine likelihood of a causal relationship between drug exposure and adverse events it is necessary to evaluate:

- Association in time/place between drug use and event
- Pharmacology (including current knowledge of nature and frequency of adverse reactions)
- Medical or pharmacological plausibility (signs and symptoms, tests, pathological findings, mechanism)

- Likelihood or exclusion of other causes (Case reports describe suspected ADRs)

There are more than 34 types of assessment scales for causality evaluation which include:

- Karch and Lasagna scale
- Naranjo's scale
- The literature (9 points of consideration – Morges, Switzerland, 1981)
- WHO probability scale
- Aetiological – Diagnostic Systems (Bénchiou's group method)
- French imputation systems
- Kramer's scale
- Jones scale
- European ABO system
- Bayesian system.

KARCH AND LASAGNA

- Uses three categories of causality
  - A – causality is highly probable
  - B – not adequate proof of causality
  - O – data are not adequate to assess causality

THE LITERATURE (9 POINTS OF CONSIDERATION – MORGES, SWITZERLAND, 1981)

1. Drug given prior to event?
2. Reaction at site of application?
3. Drug/ADR interval compatible with the event?
4. ADR immediately follows drug administration and is of acute onset?
5. Re-challenge positive?
6. De-challenge positive?
7. Were concomitant drugs stopped the same time?
8. Same adverse reaction to this drug before?
9. Adverse reaction known with the suspected drug?

METHODS USED IN PHARMACOVIGILANCE

The activities undertaken in the name of Pharmacovigilance can be roughly divided into three groups: regulatory, industry, and academia. Regulatory Pharmacovigilance is driven by the aim to provide drugs with a positive benefit–harm profile to the public. Some of the problems related to regulatory post-marketing surveillance will be discussed in this context, followed by a description of the methods used to detect new ADRs and a discussion of the pros and cons of each method.

1. Clinical trial data insufficient to evaluate drug risk

The main method currently used to gather information on a drug in the pre-marketing phase is to conduct a clinical trial. Pre-marketing clinical trials can be divided into three phases. Phase III studies are often double blind randomized controlled trials; these are considered to be the most rigorous approach to determining whether a cause–effect relationship exists between a treatment and an outcome. However, when it comes to monitoring the safety of a drug, this study design is not optimal. Due to the limited number of patients participating, it is generally not possible to identify ADRs that occur only rarely. The relatively short duration of clinical trials makes it difficult to detect ADRs with a long latency. Another limitation of clinical trials is the population in which a drug is tested. The characteristics of the participants do not always correspond to the characteristics of the population in which it will later be used; consequently, it may be difficult to extrapolate the results obtained from clinical trials to the population at large. This is especially true for the elderly, for women or for people belonging to a minority ethnic group. In order to study rare ADRs, ADRs with a long latency and ADRs in specific populations, careful monitoring of the drug in the post-marketing phase is essential. Post-marketing studies can be descriptive or analytical. Descriptive studies generate hypotheses and attempt to describe the occurrence of events related to drug toxicity and efficacy. Analytical studies test hypotheses and seek to determine associations or causal connections between observed effects and particular drugs, and to measure the size of these effects. Descriptive studies are widely used in post-marketing surveillance because they are able to generate hypotheses that will become starting points for analytical studies. Two forms of descriptive studies—spontaneous reporting and intensive monitoring—will be discussed. Analytical studies can be conducted using a variety of approaches, including case–control studies,cohort studies and clinical trials. In order to be able to conduct retrospective cohort and case–control studies, data which have been collected in a reliable and routine manner needs to be available.

2. Spontaneous reporting

Spontaneous reporting systems (SRS) were created, and these have become the primary method of collecting post marketing information on the safety of drugs. The main function of SRS is the early detection of signals of new, rare and serious ADRs. A spontaneous reporting system enables physicians and, increasingly more often, pharmacists and patients to report suspected ADRs to a Pharmacovigilance centre. The task of the Pharmacovigilance centre is to collect and analyse the reports and to inform stakeholders of the potential risk when signals of new ADRs arise. Spontaneous reporting is also used by the pharmaceutical industry to collect information about their drugs. By means of a SRS it is possible to monitor all drugs on the market throughout their entire life cycle at a relatively low cost. The main criticism of this approach is the potential for selective reporting and under reporting.

3. Data mining in spontaneous reporting

In the past, signal detection in spontaneous reporting has mainly occurred on the basis of case-by-case analyses of reports. In recent years, however, data mining techniques have become more important. The term 'data mining' refers to the principle of analyzing data from different perspectives and extracting the relevant information. Algorithms are often used to determine hidden patterns of associations or unexpected occurrences—i.e. signal—in large databases. Although the methodology of the various data mining methods applied in Pharmacovigilance differ, they all share the characteristic that they express to what extent the number of observed cases differs from the number of expected cases. Several approaches of data mining are currently in use. Proportional reporting ratios (PPRs), compare the proportion of reports for a specific ADR reported for a drug with the proportion for that ADR in all other drugs.

4. Intensive monitoring

These intensive monitoring systems use prescription data to identify users of a certain drug. The prescriber of the drug is asked about any adverse event occurring during the use of the drug being monitored. These data are collected and analyzed for new signals. The basis of intensive monitoring is a non-interventional observational cohort, which distinguishes it from spontaneous reporting because the former only monitors selected drugs during a certain period of time. Through its non-interventional character, intensive monitoring provides real world clinical data involving neither inclusion nor exclusion criteria throughout the collection period. It is unaffected by the kind of selection and exclusion criteria that characterize clinical trials, thereby eliminating selection bias. Strength of the methodology is that it is based upon event monitoring and is therefore capable of identifying signals for events that were not necessarily suspected as being ADRs of the drug being studied. Intensive monitoring programmes also enable the incidence of adverse events to be estimated, thus enabling quantification of the risk of certain ADRs. This approach, however, also has recognized limitations. The proportion of adverse effects that go unreported to doctors is unknown. The studies also produce reported event rates rather than true incident rates. This is the same for all studies based on medical record data, including computer databases and record linkage.

5. Database studies

In order to test a hypothesis, a study has to be performed.The study can be conducted using a variety of methods, including case–control studies and cohort studies. The limitations of these methods include power considerations and study design. In order to be able to conduct retrospective cohort and case–control studies, data which have been collected in a reliable and routine fashion needs to be available. The General Practice Research Database (GPRD) and the PHARMO Record Linkage System, which will be described in further detail in the following sections, were chosen here because they represent two different types of European databases.

6. General Practice Research Database

Virtually all patient care in the UK is coordinated by the general practitioner (GP), and data from this source provide an almost complete picture of a patient, his illnesses and treatment. In any given year, GPs, who are members of the GPRD, collect data from about 3 million patients (about 5% of the UK population). These patients are broadly representative of the general UK population in terms of age, sex and geographic distribution. The data collected include demographics (age and sex), medical diagnoses that are part of routine care or resulting from hospitalizations, consultations or emergency care, along with the date and location of the event. There is also an option of adding free text, referral to hospitals and specialists, all prescriptions, including date of prescription, formulation strength, quantity and dosing instructions, indication for treatment for all new prescriptions and events leading to withdrawal of a drug or a treatment. Data on vaccinations and miscellaneous information, such as smoking, height, weight, immunizations, pregnancy, birth, death, date entering the practice, date leaving the practice and laboratory results, are also collected.

7. PHARMO

In the early 1990s, the PHARMO system of record linkage was developed in The Netherlands. PHARMO links community pharmacy and hospital data within a specific region on the basis of patient birth date, gender and GP code. The system now includes drug-dispensing records from community pharmacies and hospital discharge records of about 2 million people in the Netherlands. The data collection is longitudinal and goes back to 1987. More recently, PHARMO has also been linked to other data, such as primary care data, population surveys, laboratory and genetic data, cancer and accident registries, mortality data and economic outcomes. The system has well-defined denominator information that allows incidence and prevalence estimates and is relatively cheap because existing databases are used and linked. The PHARMO database is used for follow-up studies, case–control studies and other analytical epidemiological studies for evaluating druginduced effects. In the past the database has been used for studies on drug utilisation, persistence with treatment,economic impact and ADRs

WHO SHOULD REPORT SAFETY DATA

- Health care professional (Physicians, Pharmacists, Dentists and nurses)
- Pharmaceutical companies qualified persons – (Pharmacovigilance / Regulatory manager)
- Investigational products (clinical trials)
- Post-approval reporting – Individual Case Safety Report (ICSR), Periodic Safety Update Report (PSUR)

WHAT TO REPORT – WHO RECOMMENDATIONS

- All adverse events related to the use of a drug.
- All suspected adverse reactions
- Reactions to any other drugs which are suspected of significantly affecting a patient's management, including reactions suspected of causing:
- Death
- Life-threatening (real risk of dying)
- Hospitalization (initial or prolonged)
- Disability (significant, persistent or permanent)
- Congenital anomaly
- Required intervention to prevent permanent impairment or damage

WHERE TO REPORT

- The prescribed 'Adverse Drug Event Reporting Form' shall be used for the purpose of National Pharmacovigilance Programme (Fig. 14.4).
- After completion the form shall be returned/ forwarded to the same Pharmacovigilance Centre from where it was received.
- Only those forms which meet the following criteria shall be analyzed:
- Authenticity (including reporter's and patient's traceability)

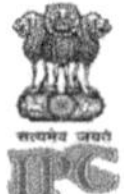

Version-1.2

SUSPECTED ADVERSE DRUG REACTION REPORTING FORM

For VOLUNTARY reporting of Adverse Drug Reactions by Healthcare Professionals

INDIAN PHARMACOPOEIA COMMISSION (National Coordination Centre-Pharmacovigilance Programme of India) Ministry of Health & Family Welfare, Government of India Sector-23, Raj Nagar, Ghaziabad-201002	FOR AMC/NCC USE ONLY AMC Report No. :
Report Type ☐ Initial ☐ Follow up	Worldwide Unique No. :
A. PATIENT INFORMATION 1. Patient Initials ______ | 2. Age at time of Event or Date of Birth ______ | 3. M ☐ F ☐ Other ☐ | 4. Weight______Kgs	12. Relevant tests/ laboratory data with dates
B. SUSPECTED ADVERSE REACTION 5. Date of reaction started (dd/mm/yyyy) 6. Date of recovery (dd/mm/yyyy) 7. Describe reaction or problem	13. Relevant medical/ medication history (e.g. allergies, race, pregnancy, smoking, alcohol use, hepatic/renal dysfunction etc.) 14. Seriousness of the reaction: No ☐ if Yes ☐ (please tick anyone) ☐ Death (dd/mm/yyyy) ☐ Congenital-anomaly ☐ Life threatening ☐ Required intervention to Prevent permanent impairment/damage ☐ Hospitalization/Prolonged ☐ Disability ☐ Other (specify) 15. Outcomes ☐ Recovered ☐ Recovering ☐ Not recovered ☐ Fatal ☐ Recovered with sequelae ☐ Unknown

C. SUSPECTED MEDICATION(S)

S.No	8. Name (Brand/Generic)	Manufacturer (if known)	Batch No. / Lot No.	Exp. Date (if known)	Dose used	Route used	Frequency (OD, BD etc.)	Therapy dates		Indication	Causality Assessment
								Date started	Date stopped		
i											
ii											
iii											
iv											

S.No as per C	9. Action Taken (please tick)						10. Reaction reappeared after reintroduction (please tick)			
	Drug withdrawn	Dose increased	Dose reduced	Dose not changed	Not applicable	Unknown	Yes	No	Effect unknown	Dose (if reintroduced)
i										
ii										
iii										
iv										

11. Concomitant medical product including self-medication and herbal remedies with therapy dates (Exclude those used to treat reaction)

S.No	Name (Brand/Generic)	Dose used	Route used	Frequency (OD, BD, etc.)	Therapy dates		Indication
					Date started	Date stopped	
i							
ii							
iii							

Additional Information:	**D. REPORTER DETAILS** 16. Name and Professional Address:______ Pin:______E-mail______ Tel. No. (with STD code)______ Occupation:______ Signature:______ 17. Date of this report (dd/mm/yyyy):

Confidentiality: The patient's identity is held in strict confidence and protected to the fullest extent. Programme staff is not expected to and will not disclose the reporter's identity in response to a request from the public. Submission of a report does not constitute an admission that medical personnel or manufacturer or the product caused or contributed to the reaction.

FIGURE 14.4 (a)

Adverse effect reporting form.

National Coordination Centre
Pharmacovigilance Programme of India
Ministry of Health & Family Welfare,
Government of India
Sector-23, Raj Nagar, Ghaziabad-201002
Tel.: 0120-2783400, 2783401, 2783392
Fax: 0120-2783311
www.ipc.nic.in

Pharmacovigilance Programme of India for Assuring Drug Safety

ADVICE ABOUT REPORTING

A. What to report

- Report serious adverse drug reactions. A reaction is serious when the patient outcome is:
    - Death
    - Life-threatening
    - Hospitalization (initial or prolonged)
    - Disability (significant, persistent or permanent)
    - Congenital anomaly
    - Required intervention to prevent permanent impairment or damage
- Report non-serious, known or unknown, frequent or rare adverse drug reactions due to Medicines, Vaccines and Herbal products.

B. Who can report

- All healthcare professionals (Clinicians, Dentists, Pharmacists and Nurses) can report adverse drug reactions

C. Where to report

- Duly filled Suspected Adverse Drug Reaction Reporting Form can be send to the nearest Adverse Drug Reaction Monitoring Centre (AMC) or directly to the National Coordination Centre (NCC).
- Call on Helpline (Toll Free) 1800 180 3024 to report ADRs.
- Or can directly mail this filled form to pvpi@ipcindia.net or pvpi.ipcindia@gmail.com
- A list of nationwide AMCs is available at:
  http://www.ipc.gov.in, http://www.ipc.gov.in/PvPI/pv_home.html

D. What happens to the submitted information

- Information provided in this form is handled in strict confidence. The causality assessment is carried out at AMCs by using WHO-UMC scale. The analyzed forms are forwarded to the NCC through ADR database. Finally the data is analyzed and forwarded to the Global Pharmacovigilance Database managed by WHO Uppsala Monitoring Centre in Sweden.
- The reports are periodically reviewed by the NCC-PvPI. The information generated on the basis of these reports helps in continuous assessment of the benefit-risk ratio of medicines.
- The information is submitted to the Steering committee of PvPI constituted by the Ministry of Health & Family Welfare. The Committee is entrusted with the responsibility to review the data and suggest any interventions that may be required.

E. Mandatory field for suspected ADR reporting form

- Patient initials, age at onset of reaction, reaction term(s), date of onset of reaction, suspected medication(s) and reporter information.

For ADRs Reporting Call on PvPI Helpline (Toll Free)

1800 180 3024

(9:00 AM to 5:30 PM, Working Days)

FIGURE 14.4 (b)

Adverse effect reporting form.

- Completeness (at least with respect to point no.'s 1, 5, 8, 11, 20 and 22 on the ADE Reporting Form)

ROLE OF NPV CENTRE

1. Shall monitor the ADRs to identify previously unexpected or indicate that certain reactions occur more commonly than previously.

- This will include the collation, review and evaluation of all spontaneous ADR reports received by the unit on a nation-wide basis.
- Information will then be keyed into the ADR database for use in aggregate analysis.
- These reports shall also be submitted to the WHO International Drug Monitoring Programme for international collaboration on drug safety.

2. Shall review Periodic Safety Update Reports (PSURs) Pharmaceutical companies are required to submit the PSURs of all new chemicals drugs and expected to be submitted every 6 monthly for the first 2 years of marketing in India, and annually for the subsequent 2 years.
3. Shall maintain contacts with international regulatory bodies working in pharmacovigilance and exchange information on drug safety.
4. Based on the available data, the Advisory Committee shall make recommendations on product label amendments, product withdrawals and suspension.
5. Shall provide information to end-users through adverse drug reaction news bulletins, drug alerts and seminars.

LIMITATIONS

- Too many patients: no time for filling the forms
- Lack of trained manpower
- Lack of responsibility regarding ADR
- Lack of institutional commitment
- Lack of pharmaceutical care service in hospital

FUTURE STRATEGIES AND PROPOSALS

- Building and maintaining a Robust Pharmacovigilance system
- Strengthen the programme with trained scientific and medical assessors for Pharmacovigilance
- Health care professionals being communicated through internet facilities
- Education and training of medical students, pharmacists and nurses in the area of Pharmacovigilance
- Collaborating with Pharmacovigilance organizations in enhancing drug safety.

SO....WHAT IS OUR ROLE?

◉ Send not Only Quantity but.... Quality Reports

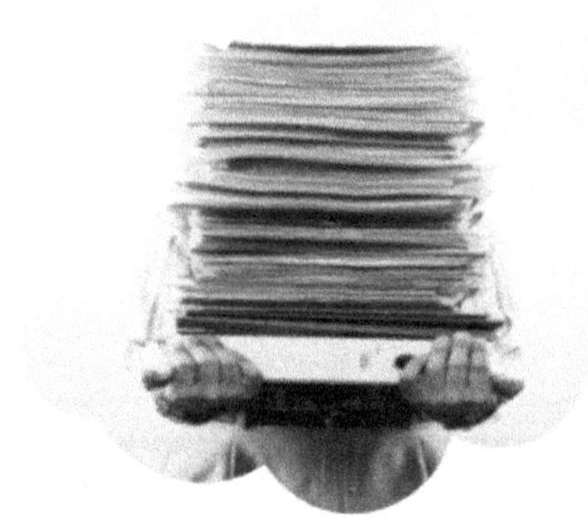

REFERENCES

1. Source: The Importance of Pharmacovigilance, WHO 2002
2. Pharmacovigilance. Mann RD, Andrews EB, eds. John Wiley and Sons Ltd, Chichester, 2002. spontaneous reports are very useful.
3. Rahman, SZ; Khan, RA; Gupta, V; Uddin, Misbah (July 2007). "Pharmacoenvironmentology – A Component of Pharmacovigilance". Environmental Health 6 (20).

4. Rahman, SZ; Khan RA, Gupta V, Misbah Uddin (2008). "Chapter 2: Pharmaco-environmentology – Ahead of Pharmaco-vigilance". In Rahman SZ, Shahid M and Gupta A. An Introduction to Environmental Pharmacology (1st ed.). Aligarh: Ibn Sina Academy. pp. 35–52.
5. Ilene Sue Ruhoy, Christian G. Daughton. Beyond the medicine cabinet: An analysis of where and why medications accumulate. Environment International 2008, Vol. 34 (8): 1157-1169.
6. WHO guidelines on safety monitoring of herbal medicines in pharmacovigilance systems, World Health Organization, Geneva, 2004.
7. S Z Rahman and K C Singhal, Problems in pharmacovigilance of medicinal products of herbal origin and means to minimize them, Uppsala Reports, WHO Collaborating Center for ADR monitoring, Uppsala Monitoring Centre, Sweden, Issue 17 January 2002: 1-4.

CHAPTER 15

Essential Drugs

In 1975, world health organization (WHO) has come to know about the drug problems faced by developing country. There is the concept of essential drugs. Each country has its own essential drug policy it is given by experts from pharmacology and other branches.

1st essential drug list prepared in 1977 and 10th – 1998.

The concept of essential medicines

A limited range of carefully selected essential medicines leads to better health care, better drug management, and lower costs.

DEFINITION

"Those drugs that satisfy the health care needs of the majority of the population; they should therefore be available at all times in adequate amounts and in appropriate dosage forms, at a price the community can afford."

HISTORY OF THE WHO MODEL LIST OF ESSENTIAL DRUGS

- 1977 First Model list published, ± 200 active substances.
- List is revised every two years by WHO Expert Committee.
- 2002 Revised procedures approved by WHO.
- April revision 2003 contains 315 active substances.

The first list was a major breakthrough in the history of medicine, pharmacy and public health.

PURPOSE

Essential medicines are intended to be available within the context of functioning health systems at all times, in adequate amounts, in the appropriate dosage forms, with assured quality, and at a price the individual and the community can afford. Fig. 15.1 shows the essential medicines target.

IMPLEMENTATION

The implementation of the concept of essential medicines is intended to be flexible and adaptable to many different situations; exactly which medicines are regarded as essential remains a national responsibility.

Clinical guidelines and a list of essential medicines lead to better prevention and care.

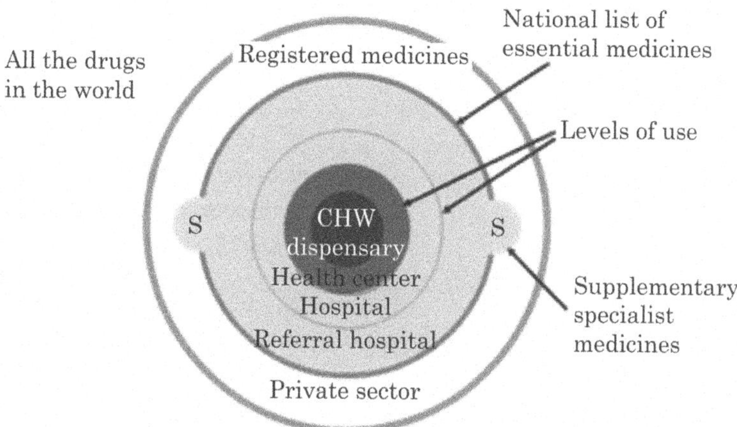

FIGURE 15.1

Essential medicines target.

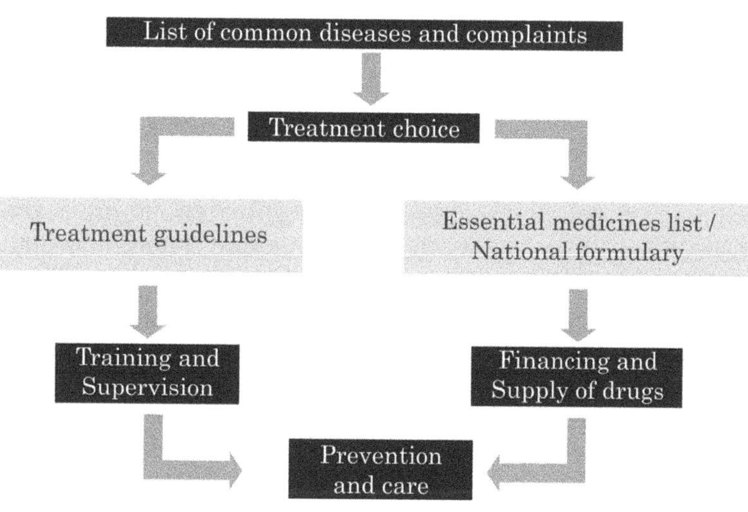

FIGURE 15.2

Clinical guidelines.

These should be available in all times in adequate amounts in appropriate dosage forms. Model list of essential drugs is of great importance due to following reasons

1. Development of treatment guidelines (Fig. 15.2).
2. Development of National formulary.
3. Measure to use drug information to patient and public.

CHOICE OF ESSENTIAL DRUG

1. Prevalence of disease in the country.
2. Treatment facilities available.
3. Financial status of the country.
4. Level of training and experience by personnel, who handle these drugs.
5. Based on genetic, environmental and demographic factors.

SEVEN STEPS TO GET A NEW MEDICINE ON

1. Identification of public-health need for a medicine
2. Development of the medicine; phase I-II-III trials
3. Regulatory approval in a number of countries
   > Effective and safe medicine on the market
4. More experience under different field circumstances; post-marketing surveillance
5. Price indication for public sector use
6. Review by WHO disease programme; define comparative effectiveness and safety in real-life situations, comparative cost-effectiveness and public health relevance
   > Medicine included in WHO treatment guideline
7. Submission to WHO Expert Committee on Essential Drugs
   > Medicine included in WHO Model List

SYSTEMATIC AND TRANSPARENT PROCESS

- Guideline development group with wide representation
- Careful consideration of conflict of interest
- Systematic computer search for evidence
- Evaluation of strength of evidence
- Systematic cost-effectiveness analysis
- For WHO: evaluation of public health considerations
- Graded recommendations with linked references
- External review of draft recommendations
- If there is insufficient evidence: consensus expert opinion

STEPS IN REVIEW OF APPLICATIONS TO THE MODEL LIST

1. Summary of application posted on WHO Medicines web site
2. Specialist assessment of comparative efficacy, safety and cost effectiveness
3. Review of assessments by Expert Committee member ("presenter"); formulation of draft
4. Recommendation
5. Review of draft recommendation by relevant Expert Advisory Panel members; and posted on WHO Medicines web site
6. Review by presenter, prepares final draft recommendation
7. Discussion of draft recommendation and proposed text for WHO Model Formulary by the Expert Committee

ROLE OF TREATMENT COST AND GLOBAL COST-EFFECTIVENESS ANALYSES

- High cost alone should not exclude an essential medicine.
- Cost-effectiveness (C/E) comparisons will be made among alternative medicines within the same therapeutic group.
- Price information from existing UN sources will be used; all information sources will be identified.

- Simple indicators will be used: cost per unit, cost per treatment/month, cost per cure, cost per case prevented.
- Emphasis on usual outcome measures, and use of existing and published comparative cost-effectiveness analyses.
- New C/E calculations will be transparent and can be adapted.

PRESENTATION OF RECOMMENDATIONS, REPORT

PRESENTATION OF RECOMMENDATIONS

- Summary of reasons for each recommendation.
- Reference to underlying evidence and systematic reviews.
- Reference to existing clinical guidelines.
- Inclusion in WHO Essential Medicines Library

REPORT, WEB SITE, TRANSLATIONS

- Report of the meeting published on WHO Medicines web site
- Report issued in WHO Technical Report Series
- List and recommendations translated into other languages

The WHO Model List of Essential Drugs (Fig. 15.3) Selection of Essential Drugs Depends on Following Factors

1. It should be evidence based, not situation based.
2. Selected drugs should have sound and adequate data on efficacy and quality based on clinical studies.
3. Performance of drug as general use in variety of medical settings.

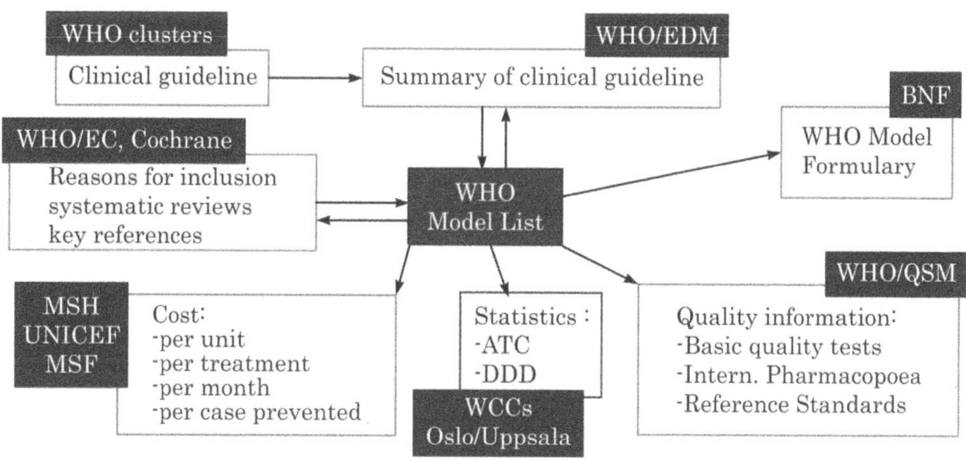

FIGURE 15.3

WHO essential medicines model list.

4. Based on bioavailability and stability of drug.
5. Whether the drug is available in particular or appropriate dosage form approved by National Drug and Therapeutics Committee (NDTC).
6. If two drugs having similarity in bioavailability stability then we go into consideration for efficacy, safety, quality and availability of drug.
7. Cost effectiveness —- cost / benefit ratio only unit cost should not be taken into consideration. The cost that will happen for entire treatment is taken into consideration. For this Pharmaco-economics come into consideration.
8. Based on pharmacokinetics of the drug.
9. Local storage is applicable (or) not and is taken into consideration. Generally single drug is preferred.
10. If combination of the drugs is taken then each ingredient should have its own efficacy, economy and patient compliance

    E.g., T.B. drugs Isoniazid, rifampicin and pyrazinamide as drugs.

PHARMACEUTICAL DOSAGE FORMS – GUIDELINES FOR IN THE LIST OF ESSENTIAL DRUGS

1. The dosage form should have general utility and wider availability
2. Tablets are having wider acceptability.
3. Establish local preference.
4. Stability under ambient temperature conditions.
5. Consideration of pharmacokinetic and bioavailability parameters.
6. Salt forms of the drug also should be taken into consideration. E.g., Chloramphenicol palmitate, Erythromycin estolate.
7. Sustained / controlled release dosage forms having low t½ should be included into this essential drug list on the basis of advice given by the expert. E.g., Theophylline

1998-10TH LIST MODEL LIST OF ESSENTIAL DRUGS SALIENT FEATURES

1. Drugs included as therapeutic need not be mentioned as pharmacological classification, there are 27 classes from anesthesia drugs to vitamins
2. Anaesthetics
    (i) Local anesthetics
    (ii) General anesthetics
    (iii) Pre-operative medication
    (iv) Cardiovascular drugs
    (v) Anti hypertensive's
    (vi) Anti arrythmics
    (vii) Thrombolytics
    (viii) Hypolipidemics
3. Dosage forms as well as dose also will be mentioned in the right hand corner
4. Most commonly used drugs having wider availability are included. Again 2-4 drugs are included in each class.
5. Some of the drugs are indicated by a square preceeding which indicates it as a therapeutic drug.
6. For some of the drugs numbers are included in parenthesis (brackets)
    (i) Drugs which are under international control narcotics and psychotropics.
    (ii) Drugs which improves patient compliance (for E.g., T.B drugs)

(iii) Drugs having renal impairment. E.g., Ethambutol

(iv) Drugs having narrow therapeutic index. E.g., Digitalis, theophylline)

(v) Drugs that require therapeutic drug monitoring. E.g., Digoxin.

Tasks that has to be carried out after preparation of essential drugs list.

1. Updating the essential drugs list: in the one year mean time it should be updated for new disease.
2. Model list of essential drugs for primary health care centers: There will not be adequate amount of medicines due to inadequate diagnostic equipments the persons. They should be educated and proper supply of drugs.
3. Specialist control for drug usage: Should have specialist for control of Antineoplastics, T.B drugs, Antiviral drugs. Educate the patients.
   (a) Antiviral drugs
   (b) Antineoplastics
   (c) Immunosuppressive drugs
   (d) T.B.drugs
4. Research and development: Consider the Q.A and research activity is done after the preparation of essential drug list.
5. Drug information and health education: Educate the patient and also the prescribes should know the knowledge of drugs.
6. List of reserves antibiotic drugs: E.g., Ampicillin, cephalexin, cephatriazone, amoxicillin. These are included in essential drug list.
7. Post registration drug studies:
   (a) In clinical trials not done on children, pregnant women and elderly people.
   (b) Some of the genetic and environmental factors
   (c) If there is any misuse or over usage of drug is not reveled in clinical trials.
   (d) Unexpected use of the drug is not revealed.
   (e) Any poor manufacturing process deviation is not revealed in clinical trials.

CONCLUSION

- The concept of essential medicines is a global concept
- WHO clinical guidelines are the foundation for the Model List of Essential Drugs; the Model List remains a strong public health tool
- The WHO Essential Medicines Library is a valuable information base for all Member States, international organisations, drugs and therapeutic committees and health insurance organisations.

REFERENCES

1. "Essential medicines". World Health Organization. Retrieved 20 January 2017.
2. "The Selection and Use of Essential Medicines (ss 4.2)". Essential Medicines and Health Products Information Portal. WHO Technical Report Series. WHO. 2003. p. 132.

CHAPTER 16

Therapeutic Drug Monitoring

Same doses of a drug produce satisfactory therapeutic activity in some persons, cause toxicity in others and have little effect in some. Hence to improve the situation, clinical pharmacokinetics and Laboratory technology were integrated with clinical medicine giving birth to "Therapeutic Drug Monitoring" (TDM). Its main aim is to maximize the benefits medically and economically.

DEFINITION

Therapeutic Drug Monitoring (TDM) can be defined as the use of drug measurements in biological fluids as an aid to the management of patients receiving drug therapy for the alleviation or prevention of diseases.

OBJECTIVES OF THERAPEUTIC DRUG MONITORING

1. To achieve optimal drug therapy.
2. To achieve desired pharmacological effect of a drug within shortest possible time with no toxicity.
3. To monitor serum drug concentration with clinical response so as to modulate the therapy.
4. To benefit the patient medically and economically by reducing hospital stay and drug related toxicity.
5. To monitor individual complicating factors like patient characteristics, diseases and drug interactions.

STAGES IN THERAPEUTIC DRUG MONITORING

Most of TDM work in carried out using plasma and measuring the total concentration of drug present, Once the steady state has been reached the size and timing of fluctuation about the mean drug concentration in blood are determined by the mode of delivery, bioavailability, the interval between dosing as well as pharmacokinetics of the drug itself.

I. Production and validation of a suitable analytical technique

Usually the validation technique used are colorimetry, spectrophotometry, spectro-flurometry, thin layer chromatography, gas chromatography, high –pressure liquid chromatography, immuno assays including enzyme-linked immunoabsorbant assay (ELISA), radiommuno assay (RIA), flame polarization immuno assay (FPIA), enzyme multiplied immuno assay test (EMIT) etc.

II. Selection of appropriate samples for analysis and their preservation

Plasma or serum samples are usually used in analysis because these samples contain fewer interfering substance than whole blood. Drugs are usually distributed between erythrocytes and plasma, the ratio varying according to the drugs. To ensure that haemolysis of erythrocytes does not interfere with analysis, plasma should be separated form erythro-cytes as soon as possible after the anticoagulant has been added.

At times urine and saliva are useful for estimation. Light, oxidation, hydrolysis, temperature etc. play an important role in decomposing the biological sample hence preservatives like sodium azide (0.1 % w/v) or sodium fluoride (1 % w/v) with possible inclusion of potassium oxalate (0.5 % w/v) in presence of anticoagulant are added.

III. To establish that the blood drug concentration correlates with therapeutic efficacy and/or toxicity of the drug

To establish this relationship a few guidelines should be considered:

- Sample should be collected after a steady state has reached because samples collected during absorption and distributions can lead to misinterpretation.
- Sample form I.V. bolus injection should be collected form the opposite arm 20 to 30 minutes after injection to ascertain peak levels.
- Peaks levels are attained after 30 to 60 minutes. of I.M. infection
- Trough concentrations are defined as serum drug concentration just prior to next dose.
- For toxicity - peak levels are preferred for all drugs expect aminoglycosides while for efficacy, through levels are preferred for all drugs except aminoglycosides.
- Most serum drug concentrations mean total drug concentration measuring both the drug bound to plasma proteins and free drug.

Therapeutic drug monitoring if performed properly, this process allows for the achievement of therapeutic concentrations of a drug more rapidly and safely than can be attained with empiric dose changes. Together with observations of the drug's clinical effects, it should provide the safest approach to optimal drug therapy.

The usefulness of plasma drug concentration data is based on the concept that pharmacologic response is closely related to drug concentration at the site of action. For certain drugs, studies in patients have provided information on the plasma concentration range that is safe and effective in treating specific diseases—the therapeutic range. Within this therapeutic range, the desired effects of the drug are observed. Below it, there is greater probability that the therapeutic benefits are not realized; above it, toxic effects may occur. No absolute boundaries divide sub therapeutic, therapeutic, and toxic drug concentrations. A gray area usually exists for most drugs in which these concentrations overlap due to variability in individual patient response.

Numerous pharmacokinetic characteristics of a drug may result in variability in the plasma concentration achieved with a given dose when administered to various patients (Figure 16.1). This interpatient variability is primarily attributed to one or more of the following:

- Variations in drug absorption
- Variations in drug distribution
- Differences in an individual's ability to metabolize and eliminate the drug (e.g., genetics)

- Disease states (renal or hepatic insufficiency) or physiologic states (e.g., extremes of age, obesity) that alter drug absorption, distribution, or elimination
- Drug interactions

Therapeutic monitoring using drug concentration data is valuable when:

1. A good correlation exists between the pharmacologic response and plasma concentration. Over at least a limited concentration range, the intensity of pharmacologic effects should increase with plasma concentration. This relationship allows us to predict pharmacologic effects with changing plasma drug concentrations.
2. Wide intersubject variation in plasma drug concentrations results from a given dose.
3. The drug has a narrow therapeutic index (i.e., the therapeutic concentration is close to the toxic concentration).
5. The drug's desired pharmacologic effects cannot be assessed readily by other simple means (e.g., blood pressure measurement for antihypertensives).

Fig. 16.1 outlines the process clinicians may choose to follow in making drug dosing decisions by using therapeutic drug monitoring. Fig. 16.2 shows the relationship of pharmacokinetic and pharmacodynamic factors.

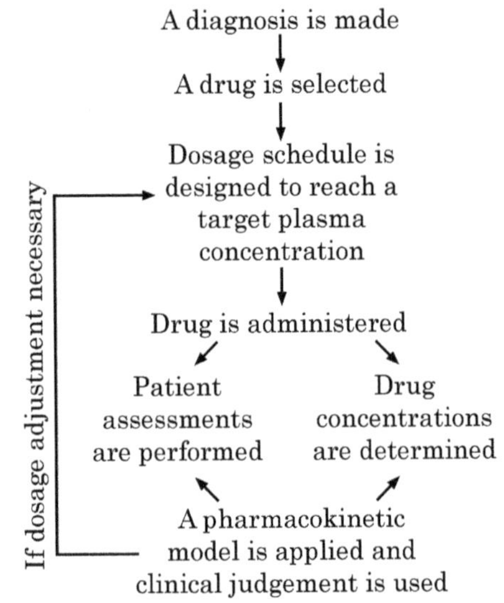

FIGURE 16.1

Process for reaching dosage decisions with therapeutic drug monitoring,

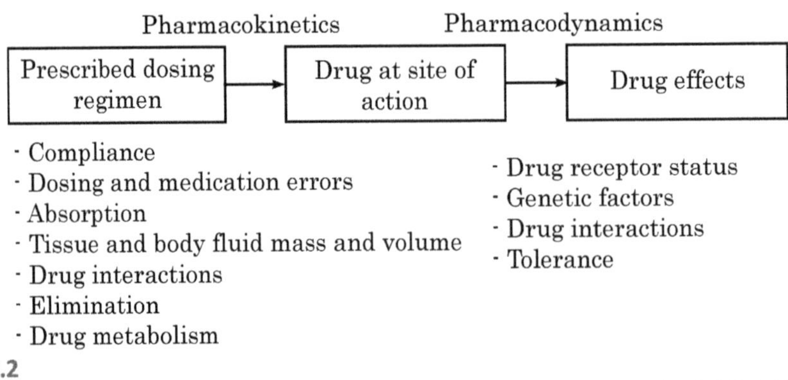

FIGURE 16.2

Relationship of pharmacokinetics and pharmacodynamics and factors that affect each.

INDICATIONS WHERE TDM IS IMPORTANT (TABLE 16.1)

1. Drug efficacy difficult to establish clinically (Phenytoin)
2. Suspected toxicity
3. Inadequate therapeutic response
4. Compliance concerns
5. Dosage change
6. Change in patient's clinical state
7. Change in co-medications (Quinidine decreases digoxin clearance)
8. Manifestations of toxicity and disease state are similar (Theophylline)

INDICATIONS WHERE TDM IS OF LESS VALUE

TDM is of limited value for these drugs:

1. Drugs which show tolerance in their effect on continuous administration, do not demonstrate predictable concentration – effect relationship like opiates, barbiturates etc.
2. Fairly safe drugs like penicillin do not require plasma concentration measurement for purpose of dosage adjustment.
3. In situation where therapeutic effect can be easily monitored like B.P., pulse rate, blood sugar etc. the cost effectiveness of plasma measurements does not work.
4. For drugs where plasma concentration does not correlate with drug effect e.g., reserpine, MAOI. These drugs are known as 'hit and run' drugs, since their biological effective half-life outlasts their plasma half – life.
5. Drugs which have better correlation of dose – effect relationship than concentration – effect relationship do not require estimation of plasma concentration e.g., Sodium valproate.
6. For drugs with an active metabolite or a prodrug it is difficult to interpret plasma concentration Vs effect relationship e.g. procainamide, Lidocaine etc.

Table 16.1

Indications where TDM is of immense value

Indications for TDM	Example	Purpose
A. Pharmacokinetic Considerations		
1. Drugs with narrow Therapeutic range	Lithium, Digoxin, Phenytoin, Gentamycin, Valproic acid	To avoid dose related toxicity
2. Drugs showing Concentration –dependent Kinetics within therapeutic range.	Phenytoin, Antibiotics	Subtle adjustments of dose
3. To check bioavailability	-	To explain nonattainment of therapeutic outcome or un-anticipated dose related toxicity following administration of standard dose of drug.

Table 16.1 *Contd...*

Indications for TDM	Example	Purpose
B. Pharmacodynamic Considerations		
1. Drugs showing wide Inter-individual variation in metabolism	Tricyclic anti-depressants (20-30 fold difference in Antiarrhythmics).	To maintain plasma concentration within Acceptable. Therapeutic range
2. Drugs used for Prophylactic purpose	Tricyclic anti-depressants (in endogenous depression Antiarrhythmics).	To replace biochemical And clinical end Points.
3. Drugs used in patients at Risks (renal failure, Liver disease metabolic Disorder, compromised Cardiovascular function etc.)	Aminoglycoside antibiotics, Theophylline and other bronchodilators Cardiovascular drugs.	To compensate for disease mediated changes in t1/2, V_d and clearance.
C. Toxicological and other Considerations		
1. To distinguish between Drug related adverse effect from disease Symptoms.	Digoxin	To assist in differential diagnosis.
2. Suspected drug – drug Interaction	Quinidine-digoxin interaction (increased plasma Digoxin concentration)	To avoid toxicity
3. To check patient compliance	-	To explain therapeutic failure with standard does of the drug.

DRUGS FOR WHICH TDM MAY BE INDICATED

The drugs for which TDM is performed in developing countries are selected on the basis of total workload, cost effectiveness and cost benefit. Anticonvulsant drugs have been monitored most extensively.

(a) TDM of Anticonvulsants

The most common indication for TDM of anticonvulsants has been non response to a standard dose of drug. This allows differentiation between noncompliance, need for a higher dose and true drug resistance requiring change over to second drug. Other common indications include suspected drug toxicity, dose adjustment in pregnancy and drug interactions (especially common with antituberculous drugs). Correlating the patients' signs and symptoms with plasma concentrations has resulted in maximum benefit to the patient. Appropriate dosage adjustment and achieving therapeutic concentrations results in over 70% of epileptic patients getting good seizure control. It was observed that nearly 20% of patients needed dose increments of only 25 or 50 et al., in 20 children receiving either phenytoin alone or in combination with phenobarbitone, showed wide inter individual variation in the steady state levels of phenytoin . A study in 108 children referred for TDM showed that at the first estimation, 3/23 on phenytoin, 20/31 on phenobarbitone and 15/25 on carbamazepine had plasma concentrations in the therapeutic range. 92% children required dosage adjustment to achieve optimal concentrations highlighting the need for greater referral for TDM in This age group.

(b) TDM of Antituberculin Drugs

Tuberculosis is highly prevalent in developing countries and there is growing concern about drug resistance. The available data suggest that selected patients with tuberculosis and mycobacterium avium complex (MAC) fail to respond to therapy because they malabsorb their medication. In particular, patients with AIDS and known gastrointestinal diseases have been shown to have problems absorbing these drugs. TDM of anti mycobacterial drugs offers the clinician a chance to ensure that the patient achieves a serum concentration above the minimum inhibitory concentration .The Madras tuberculosis centre in South India has developed a urine test to identify noncompliance with isoniazid therapy. Recently, in one charitable dispensary, where generic rifampicin was being given, several non responders were detected. The bioavailability of the generic rifampicin was found to be comparable with the standard preparation (unpublished data). TDM along with in vitro resistance testing would have probably helped in this situation. However, whether low levels are due to poor compliance, poor formulation or poor absorption needs to be investigated further. TDM for anti mycobacterial drugs is still not widely available.

(c) Serum Lithium Monitoring

As with other drugs that require TDM, there is debate about the need for, and the frequency of routine serum lithium estimations. Levels of 0.5–0.8"1 mmol /L are recommended for long-term therapy of bipolar disorder. Concentrations lower than 0.5"1 mmol /L may be effective in some elderly patients while higher than 0.8"1 may be needed in younger patients. With the widespread availability of equipment to assay lithium, lithium TDM is being done more frequently.

Lithium monitoring in developing countries has focused on aspects such as compliance, patient Education, ethnic differences, and predicting response to treatment. Shanming considered that one of the reasons for the restricted use of lithium in China may be the lack of facilities for monitoring serum lithium levels. It has been emphasized that there is an urgent need to improve available laboratory facilities in mental health institutions, to encourage research in biological psychiatry and allow for cross cultural comparisons between the developed and the developing countries. Lee [30mmol/l], in a study of 50 Chinese patients attending the first lithium clinic in Hongkong showed that a mean serum lithium level of 0.63"1 was seen. Laboratory monitoring however, was haphazard and polypharmacy abounded.

(d) TDM of Cyclosporin

The bioavailability of critical care drugs such as cyclosporin is extremely important and there may be ethnic differences in its pharmacokinetics. 30 consecutive adult patients were studied who underwent renal transplantation with regular blood cyclosporin monitoring [33mg/kg]. The patients were treated initially with 0.7"1 mg/kg and the dose titrated in response to blood levels. The cyclosporin dose was brought down to 0.1"1ng/mL. This study showed that Indian patients required a relatively lower dose than Caucasians to achieve optimum blood concentrations. The blood levels obtained were between 387 and 2120"1 and there was no evidence of rejection or irreversible nephrotoxicity.

BENEFITS OF THE TDM SERVICE

The rewards of TDM anticonvulsant service have come by way of patients who are seizure free, who are able to hold good jobs or epileptic men and women who have married and had children. Two years ago, it was observed if the service benefited patients as much. A pharmacoeconomic analysis calculated the direct and indirect costs of the service and the cost to the patient showed a significant benefit in those in whom therapeutic drug monitoring was carried out. Benefits included reduction in number of seizures, reduction in adverse drug reactions and better scholastic performance compared with those in whom TDM was not carried out. All other methods of management remained identical.

Some drug interactions, which can be anticipated and avoided from knowledge of pharmacology, were noted to be frequently occurring, e.g. calcium tablets prescribed with phenytoin and proconvulsant antibacterials such as ciprofloxacin and mefloquine prescribed to epileptic patients.

The clinical pharmacologist's copious notes on the interpretation of TDM results can (and should) form excellent educational material. It was very pleased to note a medical student who had taught was working in the emergency room and referred a convulsing patient to the neurologist. He remarked that the patient was likely to be non compliant, and that a blood sample should be sent immediately to the Clinical Pharmacology department for TDM, and the dose adjusted bearing in mind the nonlinear kinetics of phenytoin!

TDM can also be used as a useful research tool. In the early 1990s, with the resurgence of malaria in the city, chloroquine resistant strains began emerging as a major problem. The estimation of plasma levels of chloroquine and its metabolite desethyl chloroquine and were able to prove that the non responsiveness to chloroquine in these patients was due to parasite resistance and not to sub therapeutic levels. This was true both for drug resistant vivax and falciparum malaria. The Malaria Clinical Pharmacology outpatient department runs daily and monitors and treats all malaria cases. In addition, referrals for resistance testing also come from all over the city. The patients with severe life threatening drug resistant malaria who has been treated successfully when TDM of chloroquine has been used as an adjunct to therapy.

THE FUTURE

Developing countries differ from developed ones in having weak health-care structures, inadequate financial resources, unreliable supply and quality of pharmaceuticals, lack of adequate drug legislation and policy and a high rate of inappropriate self-medication. Priorities for health services are radically different from those in developed nations; for example TDM of anticonvulsants has a very low priority and may not be asked for even once during the entire treatment period in a patient with epilepsy.

Funding for drug monitoring services is hard to come by given the dedicated staff and equipment required. It is necessary to overcome the initial barrier; a questioning of the necessity and the utility of such a service. With TDM service, which began in a very small way, have been able to use the principles of clinical pharmacology as well as successfully educate physicians and medical students about them. Today TDM service includes in addition to phenytoin, phenobarbitone, Carbamazepine, lithium, cyclosporin, and Valproic acid. TDM department routinely carries out testing of generic formulations. Interestingly, the nephrologists of the hospital do not prescribe a generic cyclosporin unless its bioavailability has been tested and proven by us. At a time when cost considerations in the west have led to pooling of resources between clinical biochemistry and clinical pharmacology departments, in this country, the discipline of clinical pharmacology is still fairly new with only a few hospitals having fully-fledged departments. The ability of this discipline to be able to contribute in practically every area of medicine and add 'value' to the existing facilities remains its greatest asset. TDM particularly in a developing country forms an indispensable arm of this discipline.

REFERENCES

1. Gross AS.Best practice in Therapeutic Drug Monitoring.Br. J Clin. Pharmacol, 2001; 52: 5S-10S.
2. Nicoll D.Pocket Guide to Diagnostic Tests, Third Edition.Lange/McGraw-Hill, 2001.
3. Karande SC, Joshi MV, Kshirsagar NA, Shah PU. An analysis of epileptic patients non responsive to drugs. J Assoc Phys Ind. 1992; 40: 445-447.
4. Singh LM, Mehta S, Vohra RM, Nain CK. Monitoring of drug therapy in epileptic children. Int J Clin Pharmacol Ther Toxicol. 1987; 25: 251-254.
5. Karande SC, Dalvi SS, Kshirsagar NA. Shortcomings in the pharmacotherapy of epileptic children in Bombay, India. J Trop Ped. 1995; 41:247-249.
6. Peloquin CA. Using therapeutic drug monitoring to dose the anti mycobacterial drugs. Clin Chest Med. 1997; 18: 79-87.
7. Sarma GR, Immaneul C, Kailasam S, Kannapiran M, Nair NG, Radhakrishna S. A modified method for the estimation of acetylisoniazid in urine. Ind J Med Res. 1974; 62: 945-952.
8. Schou M. Forty years of lithium treatment. Arch Gen Psych. 1997; 54: 9-13.
9. Shanming Y. Lithium therapy in China. Brief communication. Acta Psychiat Scand. 1981; 64: 270-272.
10. Abidoun OA. The role of laboratory medicine in psychiatry. East Afr Med J. 1991; 68: 389-399.
11. Lee S. The first lithium clinic in HongKong: a Chinese profile. Aust NZ J Psych. 1992; 26: 450-453.
12. Raj DS, Somiah S, Mani K. Optimal cyclosporine therapy—an Indian experience. J Assoc Phy Ind.1996; 44: 34-36.
13. mg tablets of phenytoin. Kshirsagar NA, Joshi MV, Shah PU, Dalvi SS. Need for 25 J Assoc Phys Ind. 1991; 39: 395-396.
14. Rane CT, Gogtay NJ, Kadam VS, Powar HS, Dalvi SS, Kshirsagar NA. Subtherapeutic levels of phenytoin with standard doses in infants-need to review dosage schedule. Br J Clin Pharmacol. 1999 in press.
15. Gogtay NJ, Garg MR, Bodhe PV, Tilve GH, Kshirsagar NA. Response of vivax malaria to chloroquine in mumbai. J Assoc Phys Ind. 1998; 46: 843-845.
16. Garg MR, Gopinathan N, Bodhe PV, Kshirsagar NA. Vivax malaria resistant to chloroquine: case reports from Bombay. Trans Roy Soc Trop Med Hyg. 1995; 89: 656-657.
17. Heaney D, Josemir WAS. Anti epileptic drugs in developing countries. Lancet. 1998; 351: 1967.
18. Shenfield GM. Therapeutic drug monitoring beyond 2000. Br J Clin Pharmacol. 1998; 46: 93-94.

PART - II LIFE STAGES

17 Posology

18 Drug Therapy in Neonates and Paediatrics

19 Drug Therapy in Geriatric Patients

20 Dose and Dosage Schedule of Digoxin

21 Drug Dosing Adjustments in Patients with Renal Failure

CHAPTER 17

Posology

DEFINITION

POSOLOGY

(Derived from the Greek posos, how much, and logos, science) is the branch of medicine/ pharmacy dealing with doses.

DOSE

Dose is the quantitative amount administered or taken by a patient for the intended medicinal effect.

DOSAGE REGIMEN

- The schedule of dosing (e.g., four times a day for 10 days) is referred to as the dosage regimen.
- The proper selection of both the dose size and the frequency of administration is an important factor that influences whether a satisfactory therapeutic plasma concentration is achieved and maintained over the prescribed course of treatment.

DRUG EFFECT IN A POPULATION SAMPLE

- The idea being to produce the optimum therapeutic effect in a particular patient with the lowest possible dose.
- The familiar bell-shaped curve shows that: (Fig. 17.1)
  1. In a normal distribution of patients, a drug's usual dose will provide an average effect in the majority of individuals.
  2. In a portion of the patients, the drug will produce little effect (resistant individuals).
  3. In another group of similar size, the drug will produce an effect greater than the average effect (Sensitive individuals).

So, the drug's usual dose would be the starter dose for an individual taking the drug for the first time, then the physician may increase or decrease subsequent doses to meet the requirements of his patient.

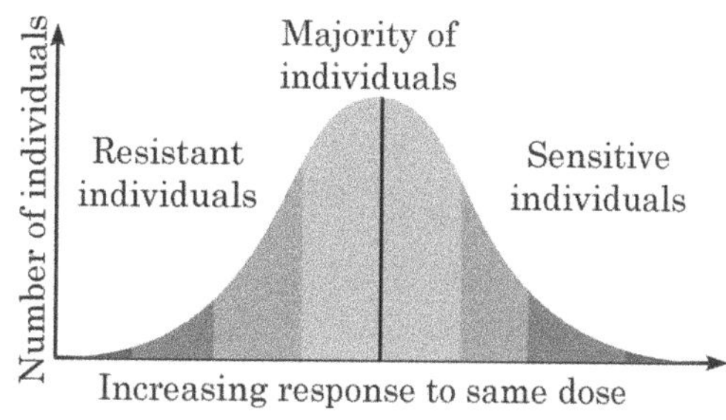

FIGURE 17.1

Drug effect in a population sample (Dose – response curve).

Factors Affecting Drug Dosage

- **Age**

- Newborn infants (pediatric) are abnormally sensitive to certain drugs because of the immature state of their hepatic and renal function by which drugs are inactivated and eliminated from the body. Failure to detoxify and eliminate drugs results in their accumulation in the tissues to a toxic level.

- The decline in renal and hepatic function in the elderly (geriatric) may slow drug clearance and increases the possibility of drug accumulation in the body and subsequent toxicity. Elderly individuals may also respond abnormally to the usual amount of a drug because of changes in drug-receptor sensitivity or because of age-related alterations in target tissues and organs.

Various rules of dosage in which the pediatric dose was a fraction of the adult dose:

- **Young's rule, based on age**

For calculating doses for children two years of age or older.

Young's formula

Child Dose =

$$\left(\frac{\text{Age in years}}{\text{Age in years} + 12}\right)\text{adult dose}$$

- **Cowling's rule**

For calculating doses for children two years of age or older.

Cowling's formula

Child Dose =

$$\frac{(\text{Age in years} + 1)}{24} \times \text{adult dose}$$

- **Fried's rule for infants**

For calculating doses for infants younger than one year of age.

Fried's formula

Child Dose =

$$\frac{\text{Age in months}}{150} \times \text{adult dose}$$

- **Body weight**

- The official usual doses for drugs are considered suitable for 70 kg (150 pounds) individuals.
- The ratio between the amount of drug administered and the size of the body influences the drug concentration at the site of action. Therefore, drug dosage may require adjustment from the usual adult dose for abnormally lean or obese patients.

To calculate the dose of a drug for children based on body weight

The determination of drug dosage for children on the basis of body weight is more dependable than that based on age.

- **Clark's rule**

$$\text{Child dose} = \frac{\text{Weight in kg}}{60} \times \text{adult dose}$$

- **Body surface area**

- A close relation exists between a large number of physiological processes and body surface area (BSA).
- The surface area of individuals may be determined from a nomogram composed of scales of height, weight and surface area.
- Two such nomograms are presented, one for adults and one for children.
- Surface area is indicated where a straight line drawn to connect the height and weight of an individual intersects the surface area column.

- To calculate the dose of a drug for children based on body surface area as related to weight:
- Many physicians believe that doses for children should be based upon body surface area, since the correct dosage of drugs seems more proportional to the surface area.

Problems based on body surface area

Child dose =

$$\frac{\text{Body surface area of child}}{\text{Body surface area of adult}} \times \text{Adult dose}$$

- **Sex**
- Women are more susceptible to the effects of certain drugs than are men.
- Pregnant women and nursing mothers should use medications only with the advise and under the guidance of their physician.
- Examples of drugs that are transported from the maternal to the fetal circulation e.g. alcohol, anesthetic gases, barbiturates, anticoagulants, etc.
- Because of the undeveloped drug detoxification and excretion mechanisms present in the fetus, concentrations of drugs may reach a higher level in the fetus than in the maternal circulation. The transfer of drugs from the mother to the nursing infant through human milk may occur with various drugs with the drug effects becoming manifest in the infant.

- **Pathological state**
- The effects of certain drugs may be modified by the pathological condition of the patient and must be considered in determining the dose.
- Warning and precautions are used in the drug labeling to alert the physician to certain restrictions in the use of a particular drug.

A-precaution: Is used to advise the prescriber of some possible problems attendant with the use of the drug. It is less restrictive than warning.

- E.g., The use of tetracycline antibiotic may result in overgrowth of fungi.
- In such a case, the physician may prescribe an alternate drug.

B-warning: It is used when the potential for patient harm is greater than in instances in which the precaution is used. e.g. If tetracycline is used in the presence of renal impairment, it may lead to accumulation of the drug and possible liver toxicity.

- **So**, lower than usual doses are indicated.
- If therapy is prolonged, blood serum levels of the drug should be taken and the patient monitored at regular intervals to assure the maintenance of non-toxic levels of the drug.

C-contraindication: A term that used to indicate an absolute prohibition to the use of a drug in the presence of certain stated conditions. It is the most restrictive of the warnings which limits the use of drugs.

- **Tolerance**

Drug tolerance: The ability to endure the influence of a drug, particularly when acquired by a continued use of the substance.

- Tolerance occurs commonly in such drugs e.g., antihistaminics, narcotic analgesics.

- Normal sensitivity may be regained by suspending the drug administration for a period of time.
- The development of tolerance can be minimized by:

I. Initiating therapy with the lowest effective dose.

II. Avoiding prolonged administration.

- **Drug-drug interactions**
- The effects of a drug may be modified by the concurrent administration of another drug.
- These drug-drug interactions are due to:

  A-chemical or physical interaction between drugs.

  B-alteration of the absorption, distribution, metabolism or excretion patterns of one of the drugs.

  The effects of drug-drug interactions may be:

I. Beneficial: E.g., probenecid causes prolongation of penicillin serum levels (as it decreases its renal excretion). So

- Reduction in penicillin dose is required.
- Decrease the frequency of its administration.

II. Detrimental: E.g., Tetracyclines can combine with the metal ions (calcium, magnesium, aluminum and iron) in the gastrointestinal tract to form complexes that are poorly absorbed.

- Many antacids drugs are rich in these metals should be:
- Avoided during tetracycline administration.
- Given alternately according to strict schedule.
- Certain calcium containing foods, as milk, cheese and other dairy products must be restricted during tetracycline administration.
- E.g., Diabetic patients who smoke heavily may require insulin dosage one-third higher than normal.
- Smoking–induced peripheral vasoconstriction reduces the rate of insulin absorption following subcutaneous absorption.
- **Time of administration**
- The time at which a drug is administered sometimes influences dosage. This is especially true for oral therapy in relation to meals.
- Absorption proceeds more rapidly if the stomach and upper portions of the intestinal tract are free of food, and an amount of a drug that is effective when taken before a meal may be ineffective if administered during or after eating. Irritating drugs are better tolerated by the patient if food is present in the stomach to dilute the drug's concentration.
- **Route of administration**
- Drugs administered intravenously enter the blood stream directly and thus the full amount administered is present in the blood.
- In contrast, drugs administered orally are rarely fully absorbed due to the various physical, chemical and biologic barriers to their absorption, including interactions with the gastric and intestinal contents. Thus, a lesser parentral dose of a drug is required than the oral dose to achieve the same blood levels of drug.

- **Pharmaceutical dosage form and drug physical state**

  E.g., Increasing the surface area of a drug by the reduction of its particle size has a significant effect on the rate of absorption, therefore, the dose can be minimized by reducing the particle size.

  - Thus, crystalline and amorphous forms of a drug shows a significant difference in the rate of absorption.

CHAPTER 18

Drug Therapy in Neonates and Paediatrics

Physiologic processes that influence pharmacokinetic variables in the infant change significantly in the first year of life, particularly during the first few months. Therefore, special attention must be paid to pharmacokinetics in this age group. Pharmacodynamic differences between pediatric and other patients have not been explored in great detail and are probably small except for those specific target tissues that mature at birth or immediately thereafter (e.g., the Ductus arteriosus).

DRUG ABSORPTION

Drug absorption in infants and children follows the same general principles as in adults. Unique factors that influence drug absorption include blood flow at the site of administration, as determined by the physiologic status of the infant or child; and, for orally administered drugs, gastrointestinal function, which changes rapidly during the first few days after birth. Age after birth also influences the regulation of drug absorption.

BLOOD FLOW AT THE SITE OF ADMINISTRATION

- Absorption after intramuscular or subcutaneous injection depends mainly, in neonates as in adults, on the rate of blood flow to the muscle or subcutaneous area injected. Physiologic conditions that might reduce blood flow to these areas are cardiovascular shock, vasoconstriction due to sympathomimetic agents, and heart failure.
- However, sick preterm infants requiring intramuscular injections may have very little muscle mass. This is further complicated by diminished peripheral perfusion to these areas. In such cases, absorption becomes irregular and difficult to predict, because the drug may remain in the muscle and absorbed more slowly than expected.
- If perfusion suddenly improves, there can be a sudden and unpredictable increase in the amount of drug entering the circulation, resulting in high and potentially toxic concentrations of drug. Examples of drugs especially hazardous in such situations are cardiac glycosides, aminoglycoside antibiotics, and anticonvulsants.

GASTROINTESTINAL FUNCTION

- Significant biochemical and physiologic changes occur in the neonatal gastrointestinal tract shortly after birth. In full-term infants, gastric acid secretion begins soon after birth and increases gradually over several hours. In preterm infants, the secretion of gastric acid occurs more slowly, with the highest concentrations appearing on the fourth day of life. Therefore, drugs that are partially or totally inactivated by the low pH of gastric contents should not be administered orally.

- Gastric emptying time is prolonged (up to 6 or 8 hours) in the first day or so after delivery. Therefore, drugs that are absorbed primarily in the stomach may be absorbed more completely than anticipated. In the case of drugs absorbed in the small intestine, therapeutic effect may be delayed. Peristalsis in the neonate is irregular and may be slow.
- The amount of drug absorbed in the small intestine may therefore be unpredictable; more than the usual amount of drug may be absorbed if peristalsis is slowed, and this could result in potential toxicity from an otherwise standard dose. Table 18.1 summarizes data on oral bioavailability of various drugs in neonates compared with older children and adults. An increase in peristalsis, as in diarrheal conditions, tends to decrease the extent of absorption, because contact time with the large absorptive surface of the intestine is decreased.

Table 18.1

Oral drug absorption (bioavailability) of various drugs in the neonate compared with older children and adults

Drug	Oral absorption
Acetaminophen	Decreased
Ampicillin	Increased
Diazepam	Normal
Digoxin	Normal
Penicillin G	Increased
Phenobarbital	Decreased
Phenytoin	Decreased
Sulphonamides	Normal

Gastrointestinal enzyme activities tend to be lower in the newborn than in the adult. Activities of a-amylase and other pancreatic enzymes in the duodenum are low in infants up to 4 months of age.

DRUG DISTRIBUTION

- As body composition changes with development, the distribution volumes of drugs are also changed. The neonate has a higher percentage of its body weight in the form of water (70%–75%) than does the adult (50%–60%). Differences can also be observed between the full-term neonate (70% of body weight as water) and the small preterm neonate (85% of body weight as water). Similarly, extracellular water is 40% of body weight in the neonate, compared with 20% in the adult. Most neonates will experience diuresis in the first 24–48 hours of life. Since many drugs are distributed throughout the extracellular water space, the size (volume) of the extracellular water compartment may be important in determining the concentration of drug at receptor sites. This is especially important for water-soluble drugs (such as aminoglycoside) and less crucial for lipid-soluble agents.
- Preterm infants have much less fat than full-term infants. Total body fat in preterm infants is about 1% of total body weight, compared with 15% in full-term neonates. Therefore, organs that generally accumulate high concentrations of lipid-soluble drugs in adults and older children may accumulate smaller amounts of these agents in less mature infants.
- Another major factor determining drug distribution is drug binding to plasma proteins. Albumin is the plasma protein

with the greatest binding capacity. In general, protein binding of drugs is reduced in the neonate. This has been seen with local anesthetic drugs, diazepam, phenytoin, Ampicillin, and phenobarbital. Therefore, the concentration of free (unbound) drug in plasma is increased initially. Because the free drug exerts the pharmacologic effect, this can result in greater drug effect or toxicity despite a normal or even low plasma concentration of total drug (bound plus unbound). Consider a therapeutic dose of a drug (e.g., diazepam) given to a patient. The concentration of total drug in the plasma is 300 mcg/L. If the drug is 98% protein-bound in an older child or adult, then 6 mcg/L is the concentration of free drug. Assume that this concentration of free drug produces the desired effect in the patient without producing toxicity. However, if this drug is given to a preterm infant in a dosage adjusted for body weight and it produces a total drug concentration of 300 mcg/L—and protein binding is only 90%—then the free drug concentration will be 30 mcg/L, or five times higher. Although the higher free concentration may result in faster elimination, this concentration may be quite toxic initially.

- Some drugs compete with serum bilirubin for binding to albumin. Drugs given to a neonate with jaundice can displace bilirubin from albumin. Because of the greater permeability of the neonatal blood-brain barrier, substantial amounts of bilirubin may enter the brain and cause kernicterus. This was in fact observed when sulphonamide antibiotics were given to preterm neonates as prophylaxis against sepsis. Conversely, as the serum bilirubin rises for physiologic reasons or because of a blood group incompatibility, bilirubin can displace a drug from albumin and substantially raise the free drug concentration. This may occur without altering the total drug concentration and would result in greater therapeutic effect or toxicity at normal concentrations. This has been shown to happen with phenytoin.

DRUG METABOLISM

- The metabolism of most drugs occurs in the liver. The drug-metabolizing activities of the cytochrome P450-dependent mixed-function oxidases and the conjugating enzymes are substantially lower (50%–70% of adult values) in early neonatal life than later. The point in development at which enzymatic activity is maximal depends upon the specific enzyme system in question. Glucuronide formation reaches adult values (per kg body weight) between the third and fourth years of life. Because of the neonate's decreased ability to metabolize drugs, many drugs have slow clearance rates and prolonged elimination half-lives.
- If drug doses and dosing schedules are not altered appropriately, this immaturity predisposes the neonate to adverse effects from drugs that are metabolized by the liver. Table 18.2 demonstrates how neonatal and adult drug elimination half-lives can differ and how the half-lives of phenobarbital and phenytoin decrease as the neonate grows older. The process of maturation must be considered when administering drugs to this age group, especially in the case of drugs administered over long periods.

Table 18.2

Comparison of elimination half-lives of various drugs in neonates and adults

Drug	Neonatal Age	Neonates $t_{1/2}$ (hours)	Adults $t_{1/2}$ (hours)
Acetaminophen		2.2–5	0.9–2.2
Diazepam		25–100	40–50
Digoxin		60–70	30–60
Phenobarbital	0–5 days	200	64–140
	5–15 days	100	
	1–30 months	50	
Phenytoin	0–2 days	80	12–18
	3–14 days	18	
	14–50 days	6	
Salicylate		4.5–11	10–15
Theophylline	Neonate	13–26	5–10
	Child	3–4	

Another consideration for the neonate is whether or not the mother was receiving drugs (e.g., Phenobarbital) that can induce early maturation of fetal hepatic enzymes. In this case, the ability of the neonate to metabolize certain drugs will be greater than expected, and one may see less therapeutic effect and lower plasma drug concentrations when the usual neonatal dose is given.

DRUG EXCRETION

- The glomerular filtration rate is much lower in newborns than in older infants, children, or adults, and this limitation persists during the first few days of life. Calculated on the basis of body surface area, glomerular filtration in the neonate is only 30%–40% of the adult value. The glomerular filtration rate is even lower in neonates born before 34 weeks of gestation. Function improves substantially during the first week of life. At the end of the first week, the glomerular filtration rate and renal plasma flow have increased 50% from the first day. By the end of the third week, glomerular filtration is 50%–60% of the adult value; by 6–12 months, it reaches adult values (per unit surface area). Therefore, drugs that depend on renal function for elimination are cleared from the body very slowly in the first weeks of life.
- Penicillin's, for example, are cleared by preterm infants at 17% of the adult rate based on comparable surface area and 34% of the adult rate when adjusted for body weight. The dosage of Ampicillin for a neonate less than 7 days old is 50–100 mg/kg/d in two doses at 12-hour intervals. The dosage for a neonate over 7 days old is 100–200 mg/kg/d in three doses at 8-hour intervals. A decreased rate of renal elimination in the neonate has also been observed with aminoglycoside antibiotics (kanamycin, Gentamicin, neomycin, and streptomycin). The dosage

of Gentamicin for a neonate less than 7 days old is 5 mg/kg/d in two doses at 12-hour intervals. The dosage for a neonate over 7 days old is 7.5 mg/kg/d in three doses at 8-hour intervals.

- Total body clearance of digoxin is directly dependent upon adequate renal function, and accumulation of digoxin can occur when glomerular filtration is decreased. Since renal function in a sick infant may not improve at the predicted rate during the first weeks and months of life, appropriate adjustments in dosage and dosing schedules may be very difficult. In this situation, adjustments are best made on the basis of plasma drug concentrations determined at intervals throughout the course of therapy.
- While great focus is naturally concentrated on the neonate, it is important to remember that toddlers may have *shorter* elimination half-lives of drugs than older children and adults, due probably to *increased* renal elimination and metabolism. For example, the dose per kg of digoxin is much higher in toddlers than in adults. The mechanisms for these developmental changes are still poorly understood.

SPECIAL PHARMACODYNAMIC FEATURES IN THE NEONATE

- The appropriate use of drugs has made possible the survival of neonates with severe abnormalities who would otherwise die within days or weeks after birth. For example, administration of indomethacin causes the rapid closure of a patent Ductus arteriosus, which would otherwise require surgical closure in an infant with a normal heart. Infusion of prostaglandin E_1, on the other hand, causes the Ductus to remain open, which can be life-saving in an infant with transposition of the great vessels or tetralogy of Fallot.

An unexpected effect of such infusion has been described. The drug caused antral hyperplasia with gastric outlet obstruction as a clinical manifestation in 6 of 74 infants who received it. This phenomenon appears to be dose-dependent.

PAEDIATRIC DOSAGE FORMS AND COMPLIANCE

- The form in which a drug is manufactured and the way in which the parent dispenses the drug to the child determines the actual dose administered. Many drugs prepared for children are in the form of elixirs or suspensions.
- **Elixirs** are alcoholic solutions in which the drug molecules are dissolved and evenly distributed. No shaking is required, and unless some of the vehicle has evaporated, the first dose from the bottle and the last dose should contain equivalent amounts of drug.
- **Suspensions** contain undissolved particles of drug that must be distributed throughout the vehicle by shaking. If shaking is not thorough each time a dose is given, the first doses from the bottle may contain less drug than the last doses, with the result that less than the expected plasma concentration or effect of the drug may be achieved early in the course of therapy. Conversely, toxicity may occur late in the course of therapy, when it is not expected. This uneven distribution is

a potential cause of inefficacy or toxicity in children taking phenytoin suspensions. It is thus essential that the prescriber know the form in which the drug will be dispensed and provide proper instructions to the pharmacist and patient or parent.

- Compliance may be more difficult to achieve in pediatric practice than otherwise, since it involves not only the parent's conscientious effort to follow directions but also such practical matters as measuring errors, spilling, and spitting out. For example, the measured volume of "teaspoons" ranges from 2.5 to 7.8 ml. The parents should obtain a calibrated medicine spoon or syringe from the pharmacy. These devices improve the accuracy of dose measurements and simplify administration of drugs to children.
- When evaluating compliance, it is often helpful to ask if an attempt has been made to give a further dose after the child has spilled half of what was offered. The parents may not always be able to say with confidence how much of a dose the child actually received.
- The parents must be told whether or not to wake the infant for its every-6-hour dose day or night. These matters should be discussed and made clear, and no assumptions should be made about what the parents may or may not do. Noncompliance frequently occurs when antibiotics are prescribed to treat Otitis media or urinary tract infections and the child feels well after 4 or 5 days of therapy. The parents may not feel there is any reason to continue giving the medicine even though it was prescribed for 10 or 14 days. This common situation should be anticipated so the parents can be told why it is important to continue giving the medicine for the prescribed period even if the child seems to be "cured."
- Practical and convenient dosage forms and dosing schedules should be chosen to the extent possible. The easier it is to administer and take the medicine and the easier the dosing schedule is to follow, the more likely it is that compliance will be achieved.
- Consistent with their ability to comprehend and cooperate, children should also be given some responsibility for their own health care and for taking medications. This should be discussed in appropriate terms both with the child and with the parents. Possible adverse effects and drug interactions with over-the-counter medicines or foods should also be discussed.
- Whenever a drug does not achieve its therapeutic effect, the possibility of noncompliance should be considered. There is ample evidence that in such cases parents' or children's reports may be grossly inaccurate. Random pill counts and measurement of serum concentrations may help disclose noncompliance.
- Because many pediatric doses are calculated e.g., using body weight-rather than simply read from a list, major dosing errors may result from incorrect calculations. Typically, tenfold errors due to incorrect placement of the decimal point have been described. In the case of digoxin, for example, an intended dose of

0.1 ml containing 5 mcg of drug, when replaced by 1.0 ml which is still a small volume can result in fatal over dosage. A good rule for avoiding such "decimal point" errors is to use a leading "0" plus decimal point when dealing with doses less than "1" and to avoid using a zero after a decimal point.

REFERENCES

1. American Heart Association (AHA) guidelines for cardiopulmonary resuscitation (CPR) and emergency cardiovascular care (ECC) of pediatric and neonatal patients: Pediatric basic life support. Circulation. 2005;112(24 Suppl):IV1.
2. Benitz WE, Tatro DS: *The Pediatric Drug Handbook,* 3rd ed. Year Book, 1995.
3. Berlin CM Jr: Advances in pediatric pharmacology and toxicology. Adv Pediatr 1997;44:545.
4. Besunder JB, Reed MD, Blumer JL: Principles of drug biodisposition in the neonate: A critical evaluation of the pharmacokinetic-pharmacodynamic interface. (Two parts.) Clin Pharmacokinet 1988; 14: 189, 261.

CHAPTER 19

Drug Therapy in Geriatric Patients

Older patients are more sensitive to drugs than younger adults. Show wider individual variations- experience more adverse drug reactions and drug-drug interactions.

PRINCIPLE UNDERLYING FACTORS

- Altered pharmacokinetics (secondary to organ system degeneration)
- Multiple and severe illnesses
- Multiple drug therapy
- Poor compliance
- Individualization of treatment is essential: each patient must be monitored for desired responses and adverse responses and the regimen must be adjusted accordingly
- Usual objective is to reduce symptoms and improve quality of life since cure is generally impossible

I. PHARMACOKINETIC CHANGES IN THE ELDERLY

There is a gradual, progressive decline in organ function which can alter the absorption, distribution, metabolism, and excretion of drugs- changes increase drug sensitivity and varies greatly among patients

A. Absorption

- Altered GI absorption is not a major factor in drug sensitivity
- The percentage of an oral dose that becomes absorbed does not change with age
- The rate of absorption may be slowed (because of delayed gastric emptying and reduced splanchnic blood flow)
- Responses may be somewhat delayed
- Gastric acidity is reduced in the elderly and may alter the absorption of certain drugs

B. Distribution

Major facts

- Increased percent body fat which provides a storage depot for lipid soluble drugs
  - Plasma levels of these drugs are reduced, causing a reduction in responses
- Decreased percent lean body mass causes water soluble drugs (e.g., ethanol) to be distributed in a smaller volume
  - Concentrations of these drugs is increased, causing their effects to be more intense
- Decreased total body water
  - Albumin levels are only slightly reduced in healthy adults but can be significantly reduced in malnourished adults

- Reduced concentration of serum albumin
- because of reduced albumin levels, protein binding of drugs decreases, causing levels of free drug to rise and effects may be more intense

C. Metabolism

- Rates of hepatic drug metabolism tend to decline with age- underlying factors include reduced hepatic blood flow, reduced liver mass, and decreased activity of some hepatic enzymes
- Because liver function is diminished, the half-lives of certain drugs may be increased, there by prolonging responses

D. Excretion

- Undergoes progressive decline
- Drug accumulation secondary to reduced renal excretion is the most important cause of adverse drug reactions in the elderly
- Decline in renal function is the result of reductions in renal blood flow, glomerular filtration rate, active tubular secretion, and number of nephrons- co-existence of renal pathology can further compromise kidney function- proper index of renal function is **creatinine clearance**
- Not serum creatinine levels- creatinine levels do not reflect kidney function in the elderly because the source of serum creatinine – lean muscle mass – declines in parallel with the decline in kidney function- as a result, creatinine levels may be normal even though renal function is greatly reduced

II. PHARMACODYNAMIC CHANGES IN THE ELDERLY

- In support of the possibility of altered pharmacodynamics is the observation that beta-adrenergic blocking agents (drugs used for cardiac disorders) are less effective in the elderly than in younger adults- possible explanation for this observation include:
- Reduction in the number of available beta receptors
- Reduction in the affinity of beta receptors for beta-receptor blocking agents.

III. ADVERSE DRUG REACTIONS (ADRs) & DRUG INTERACTIONS

ADRs are seven times more common in the elderly than in younger adults- vast majority of these reactions are dose related – not idiosyncratic - symptoms are often nonspecific (e.g., dizziness, cognitive impairment), making identification of ADRs difficult Most Important Factors:

- Drug accumulation secondary to reduced renal function
- Polypharmacy (treatment with multiple drugs)
- Greater severity of illness
- Presence of multiple pathologies
- Greater use of drugs that have a low therapeutic index
- Increased individual variation secondary to altered pharmacokinetics
- Inadequate supervision of long-term therapy
- Poor patient compliance

Measures to Reduce ADR Incidence

- Take a thorough drug history, including OTC meds
- Accounting for the pharmacokinetic and pharmacodynamic changes that occur with aging
- Initiating therapy with low doses

- Monitoring clinical responses and plasma drug levels to provide a rational basis for dosage

Adjustment

- Employing the simplest regimen possible
- Monitoring for drug-drug interactions and iatrogenic illness
- Periodically reviewing the need for continued drug therapy, and discontinuing medications as

Appropriate

- Encouraging the patient to dispose of old meds
- Taking steps to promote compliance

IV. PROMOTING COMPLIANCE

Some patient never fill their prescriptions- some fail to refill their prescriptions- some don't follow the prescribed dosing schedule- noncompliance can result in therapeutic failure (from under dosing or erratic dosing, which is the most common) or toxicity (from overdosing)

CONTRIBUTING FACTORS TO UNINTENTIONAL NONCOMPLIANCE

- Forgetfulness
- Failure to comprehend instructions (because of intellectual, visual or auditory impairment)
- Inability to pay for medications
- Use of complex regimens (several drugs taken several times a day)

CONTRIBUTING FACTORS TO INTENTIONAL NONCOMPLIANCE

- Patient's conviction that the drug was simply not needed in the dosage prescribed
- Unpleasant side effects
- Expense

STEPS TO PROMOTE COMPLIANCE

- Simplifying the regimen
- Explaining the treatment plan using clear, concise **verbal and written** instructions
- Choosing an appropriate **dosage form** (e.g., liquid if patient has difficulty swallowing)
- Labeling drug containers clearly and avoiding containers that are difficult to open
- Suggesting the use of a calendar, diary or pill counter for record of drug administration
- Asking the patient if he / she has access to a pharmacy and can afford the medication
- Enlisting the aid of a friend, relative, or visiting healthcare professional
- Monitoring for therapeutic responses, adverse reactions and plasma drug levels

REFERENCES

1. Cannon KT, Choi MM, Zuniga MA (June 2006). "Potentially inappropriate medication use in elderly patients receiving home health care: a retrospective data analysis". *Am J Geriatr Pharmacother* **4** (2): 134–43.
2. Gidal BE (January 2006). "Drug absorption in the elderly: biopharmaceutical considerations for the antiepileptic drugs". *Epilepsy Res.* **68** (Suppl 1): S65–9.
3. Hutchison LC, Jones SK, West DS, Wei JY (June 2006). "Assessment of medication management by community-living elderly persons with two standardized assessment tools: a cross-sectional study". *Am J Geriatr Pharmacother* **4** (2): 144–53.
4. Isaacs B (1965). *An introduction to geriatrics*. London: Balliere, Tindall and Cassell.

CHAPTER 20

Dose and Dosage Schedule of Digoxin

INTRODUCTION

Digoxin is one of the most commonly used drugs in medicine. Despite this widespread use and a history of over 200 years of clinical use and research, much controversy continues concerning its efficacy and safety.

Two of the most prominent features of the clinical use of digoxin are its narrow therapeutic index and an endpoint of therapy which is difficult to define and measure. Digitalis toxicity is one of the most frequently encountered drug-related causes of hospitalization. Conversely, the effect of serum digoxin concentrations below 0.8 ng/mL is clinically unimportant in most patients.

The great variability in serum digoxin concentrations in patients given the same dose has led to the development of nomograms and equations designed to estimate the optimal digoxin dosage. These methods include factors such as age, weight, sex, renal function, disease state, and concurrent drug therapy to calculate the dose and corresponding serum concentration. An accurate method could decrease the potential for drug toxicity, which can be life-threatening, and decrease the time period required to optimize therapy, which is otherwise done by trial and error.

Lalonde and Pao compared the accuracy of eighteen different digoxin dosing methods. The method of Dobbs and Koup as modified by Koda-Kimble appeared to produce the best balance of minimum bias and greatest precision. Using a target concentration of 1.2 ng/mL, the Koda-Kimble method achieves a concentration between 0.9 and 1.5 ng/mL in 80% of cases. However, some patients will have measured serum digoxin concentrations well outside this range.

An adequate loading dose is necessary for rapid attainment of therapeutic serum levels. Choosing to initiate therapy without a loading dose means that, because of digoxin's long half-life, therapeutic serum levels may not be achieved for weeks. Fig. 20.1 indicates flowchart of digoxin doing.

MONITORING PARAMETERS

1. The following patient parameters should be monitored during digoxin therapy:

- Digoxin serum level
  Obtain level within 24 hours of digitalization, weekly until stable, and at steady state.
- BUN and serum creatinine
  Measure every two days, or every day in unstable renal function.
- Weigh patient daily.
- Measure and monitor urine output daily.
  Monitor apical pulse daily.

2. Therapeutic serum concentrations the usual digoxin therapeutic range is 0.8 to 2 ng/mL.

PRECAUTIONS

1. Proper timing of serum sampling is critical.

   Serum samples should be drawn just prior to the daily dose and no sooner than six hours after administration of the drug.

2. Factors affecting digoxin pharmacokinetics

(a) Factors which predispose to digoxin toxicity: Hypokalemia, hypoma-gnesemia, coronary artery disease, uncorrected hypothyroidism, renal dysfunction, and interacting drugs which decrease digoxin clearance (quinidine, spironolactone, and verapamil).

(b) Factors which predispose to suboptimal clinical response: Hyperkalemia, uncorrected hyperthyroidism, interacting drugs which delay or prevent oral absorption (antacids, cholestyramine, metoclopramide).

DIGOXIN DOSING FLOW CHART

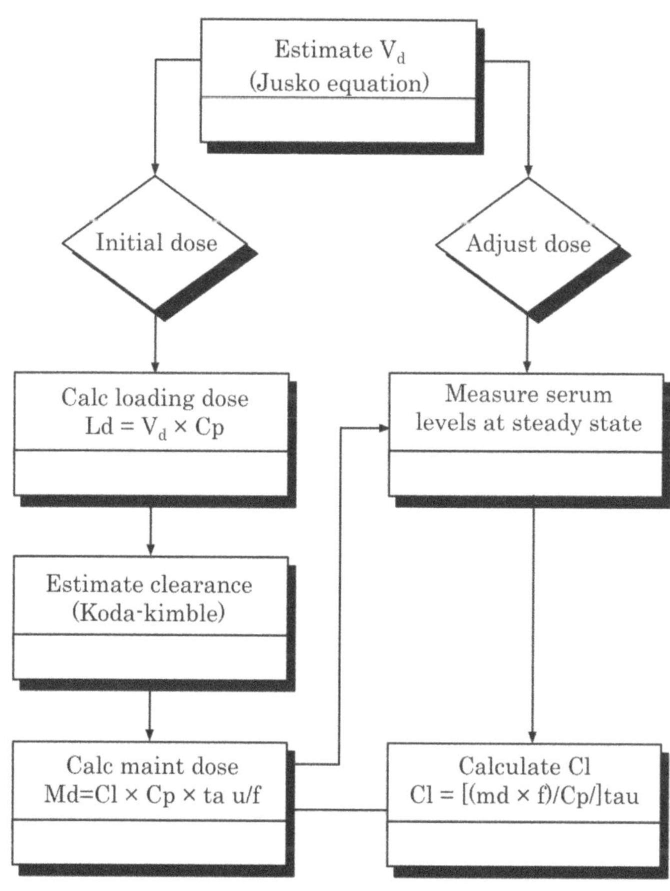

FIGURE 20.1

Dosing of digoxin flow chart.

USUAL ADULT DOSE FOR CONGESTIVE HEART FAILURE

RAPID DIGITALIZATION WITH A LOADING DOSE

Peak digoxin body stores of 8 to 12 mcg/kg generally provide a therapeutic effect with minimum risk of toxicity in most patients with heart failure and normal sinus rhythm. The loading dose should be administered in several fractions, with approximately half the total given as the first dose. Additional fractions of the total dose may be given at 6 to 8 hour intervals. Careful assessment of the patient's clinical response should be considered before each additional dose. If the patient's response necessitates a change from the calculated loading dose of digoxin, then calculation of the maintenance dose should be based upon the amount actually given.

TABLETS

Initial: 500 to 750 mcg usually produces a detectable effect in 0.5 to 2 hours with a maximal effect in 2 to 6 hours. Additional doses of 125 to 375 mcg may be given at 6 to 8 hour intervals until clinical evidence of an adequate effect is noted. The usual amount of digoxin tablets that a 70 kg patient requires to achieve 8 to 12 mcg/kg peak body stores is 750 to 1250 mcg.

CAPSULES

Initial: 400 to 600 mcg of digoxin capsules generally produces a detectable effect in 0.5 to 2 hours with a maximal effect in 2 to 6 hours. Additional doses of 100 to 300 mcg may be given cautiously at 6 to 8 hour intervals until clinical evidence of an adequate effect is noted. The usual amount of digoxin capsules that a 70 kg patient requires to achieve 8 to 12 mcg/kg peak body stores is 600 to 1000 mcg.

INJECTION

Initial: 400 to 600 mcg of digoxin intravenously usually produces a detectable effect in 5 to 30 minutes with a maximal effect in 1 to 4 hours. Additional doses of 100 to 300 mcg may be given cautiously at 6 to 8 hour intervals until clinical evidence of an adequate effect is noted. The usual amount of digoxin injection that a 70 kg patient requires to achieve 8 to 12 mcg/kg peak body stores is 600 to 1000 mcg. The injectable route is frequently used to achieve rapid digitalization, with conversion to digoxin tablets or digoxin capsules for maintenance therapy.

MAINTENANCE DOSE

The doses of digoxin tablets used in controlled trials in patients with heart failure have ranged from 125 to 500 mcg once daily. In these studies, the digoxin dose has been generally titrated according to the patient's age, lean body weight, and renal function. Therapy is generally initiated at a dose of 250 mcg once daily in patients under age 70 with good renal function.

USUAL ADULT DOSE FOR ATRIAL FIBRILLATION

Peak digoxin body stores larger than the 8 to 12 mcg/kg required for most patients with heart failure and normal sinus rhythm have been used for control of ventricular rate in patients with atrial fibrillation. Doses of digoxin used for the treatment of chronic atrial fibrillation should be titrated to the minimum dose that achieves the desired ventricular rate control without causing undesirable side effects.

USUAL PEDIATRIC DOSE FOR ATRIAL FIBRILLATION

Do not give full total digitalizing dose at once. Administer loading doses in several portions;

give roughly half the total as the first dose. Give additional fractions of the total dose at 6 to 8 hour intervals (oral) or 4 to 8 hour intervals (parenteral). Divided daily dosing is recommended for infants and young children under 10 years of age.

Parenteral administration should be used only when the need for rapid digitalization is urgent or when the drug cannot be taken orally. Intravenous administration is preferred over intramuscular injection as it can lead to severe pain at the injection site. If it is necessary to administer the drug by the intramuscular route, it should be injected deep into the muscle followed by massage. No more than 500 mcg should be injected into a single site.

CALCULATED DOSES SHOULD BE BASED ON LEAN BODY WEIGHT

Premature: Digitalizing (Loading) dose: Oral elixir: 20 to 30 mcg/kg; Intravenous: 15 to 25 mcg/kg

Maintenance dose: Oral 5 to 7.5 mcg/kg; intravenous 4 to 6 mcg/kg

Full term: Digitalizing (Loading) dose: Oral elixir: 25 to 35 mcg/kg; Intravenous: 20 to 30 mcg/kg

Maintenance dose: Oral 6 to 10 mcg/kg; intravenous 5 to 8 mcg/kg

1-24 months: Digitalizing (Loading) dose: Oral elixir: 35 to 60 mcg/kg; Intravenous: 30 to 50 mcg/kg

Maintenance dose: 10 to 15 mcg/kg oral; intravenous 7.5 to 12 mcg/kg

3 to 5 years: Digitalizing (Loading) dose: Oral elixir: 30 to 40 mcg/kg; Intravenous: 25 to 35 mcg/kg

Maintenance dose: Oral 7.5 to 10 mcg/kg; intravenous 6 to 9 mcg/kg

6 to 10 years: Digitalizing (Loading) dose: Oral elixir: 20 to 35 mcg/kg; Intravenous: 15 to 30 mcg/kg

Maintenance dose: Oral 5 to 10 mcg/kg; intravenous 4 to 8 mcg/kg

11 years and older: Digitalizing (Loading) dose: Oral elixir: 10 to 15 mcg/kg; Intravenous: 8 to 12 mcg/kg

Maintenance dose: Oral 2.5 to 5 mcg/kg; intravenous 2 to 3 mcg/kg

RENAL DOSE ADJUSTMENTS

CrCl <10 mL/min: Loading dose: Generally reduced by 50%.

Maintenance dose: Can be administered as 10%- 25% of maintenance dose or the interval increased to every 48 hours.

CrCl 10 to 50 mL/min: Total digitalizing dose: 0.5 to 1 mg (the initial dose is usually one-half of the total digitalizing dose, followed by 1/4 of the digitalizing dose in each of two subsequent doses at 6 and 12 hour intervals). Maintenance dose: 25% -75% of the normal daily dose or administer normal dose every 36 hours.

In general, a maintenance dose of 125 mcg orally once daily is recommended in patients with impaired renal function, and at a dose of 62.5 mcg is recommended in patients with marked renal impairment. Doses may be increased every 2 weeks according to clinical response.

Because of altered digoxin distribution and elimination, projected peak body stores for patients with renal insufficiency should be conservative (i.e., 6 to 10 mcg/kg).

DOSE ADJUSTMENTS

If patients are switched from intravenous to oral formulations, allowances must be made for differences in bioavailability when calculating maintenance dosages. When changing from oral formulations to IM or IV therapy, dosage should be reduced by 20%-25%.

Lanoxicaps (gelatin capsules) have greater bioavailability than standard tablets, and the recommended oral doses are only 80% of those for tablets and elixir. Therefore, the 0.2 mg capsule is equivalent to 0.25 mg tablets; the 0.1 mg capsule is equivalent to 0.125 mg tablets; and the 0.05 mg capsule is equivalent to 0.0625 mg. Divided dosage of the capsule formulation is preferred in patients that require a daily dose greater than 300 mcg, those with a previous history of digitalis toxicity, and in patients who may be more likely to become toxic.

Hyperthyroid patients generally require a slightly higher loading dose (10%). Hypothyroid patients generally require a slightly lower loading dose (10%).

REFERENCES

1. Jusko WJ, et. al. Pharmacokinetic design of digoxin dosage regimens in relation to renal function. J Clin Pharmacol 1974;14:525-35.
2. Koup JR, et. al. Digoxin pharmacokinetics: role of renal failure in dosage regimen design. Clin Pharmacol Ther 1975;18:9-21.
3. Walsh FM, Sode J. Significance of non-steady-state serum digoxin concentrations. Am J Clin Pathol 1975; 63: 446-50.
4. Dobbs SM, Mawer GE. Prediction of digoxin dose requirements. Clin Pharmacok 1977; 2:281-91.
5. Koda-Kimble MA: Congestive heart failure, in Applied Therapeutics for Clinical Pharmacists, 2nd ed, edited by MA Koda-Kimble et al, Applied Therapeutics, Inc, San Francisco 1978; pp 161-86.
6. Thomas RW, Maddox RR. The interaction of spironolactone and digoxin: a review and evaluation. Ther Drug Monit 1981; 3: 117-20.
7. Klein HO, et. al. The influence of verapamil on serum digoxin concen-tration. Circul 1982; 65: 998-1003.
8. Hyneck ML, et. al. Comparison of methods for estimating digoxin dosing regimens. AJHP 1981; 38: 69-73.
9. Bigger JT. The quinidine-digoxin interaction. Mod Con Card Dis 1982; 51: 73-78.
10. Lalonde RL, Pao D. Correlation coefficient versus prediction error in assessing the accuracy of digoxin dosing methods. Clin Pharm 1984; 3: 178-83.
11. Reuning RH, Garaets DR. "Digoxin", in Evans W, Schentag J, Jusko J (eds): Applied Pharmacokinetics. Applied Therapeutics, Inc, San Francisco 1986; pp 908-43.

CHAPTER 21

Drug Dosing Adjustments in Patients with Renal Failure

DEFINITION

Renal failure or **kidney failure** (formerly called **renal insufficiency**) describes a medical condition in which the kidneys fail to adequately filter toxins and waste products from the blood. Renal failure is described as a decrease in Glomerular Filtration Rate. Biochemically, Renal failure is typically detected by an elevated serum creatinine level. Problems frequently encountered in kidney malfunction include abnormal fluid levels in the body, deranged acid levels, abnormal levels of potassium, calcium, phosphate, and (in the longer term) anemia as well as delayed healing in broken bones. Depending on the cause, haematuria (blood loss in the urine) and proteinuria (protein loss in the urine) may occur. Long-term kidney problems have significant repercussions on other diseases, such as cardiovascular disease. Table 21.1 indicates staging system to cheonic kidney disease.

CLINICAL FEATURES

- High levels of urea in the blood, which can result in: Vomiting and/or diarrhea, which may lead to dehydration
- A build up of phosphates in the blood that diseased kidneys cannot filter out may cause: Itching, Bone damage
- Failure of kidneys to remove excess fluid may cause: Swelling of the legs, ankles, feet, face and/or hands, Shortness of breath due to extra fluid on the lungs
- Polycystic kidney disease, which causes large, fluid-filled cysts on the kidneys and sometimes the liver, can cause Pain in the back or side
- Other symptoms include: Appetite loss, a bad taste in the mouth, Difficulty sleeping.

Table 21.1

National kidney foundation K/DOQI staging system for chronic kidney disease

Stage	Description	GFR (ml per minute per 1.73 m^2)
1	Kidney damage with normal or increased GFR	≥ 90
2	Kidney damage with a mild decrease in GFR	60 to 89
3	Moderate decrease in GFR	30 to 59
4	Severe decrease in GFR	15 to 29
5	Kidney failure	< 15 (or dialysis)

DOSING ADJUSTMENTS

- Loading doses usually do not need to be adjusted in patients with chronic kidney disease.
- Published guidelines suggest methods for maintenance dosing adjustments: dose reduction, lengthening the dosing interval, or both.
- Dose reduction involves reducing each dose while maintaining the normal dosing interval. This approach maintains more constant drug concentrations, but it is associated with a higher risk of toxicities if the dosing interval is inadequate to allow for drug elimination.
- Lengthening the dosing interval has been associated with a lower risk of toxicities but a higher risk of sub therapeutic drug concentrations, especially toward the end of the dosing interval.

Table 21.2, 21.3, 21.4, 21.5, 21.6 indicates doing requirements of different categories of drugs in chronic kidney disease.

Table 21.2

Antihypertensive agents: dosing requirements in patients with chronic kidney disease

Drug	Usual dosage*	Dosage adjustment (percentage of usual dosage) based on GFR (ml per minute per 1.73 m^2)		
		> 50	10 to 50	< 10
ACE inhibitors†				
Benazepril (Lotensin)	10 mg daily	100%	50% -75%	25% -50%
Captopril (Capoten)	25 mg every 8 hours	100%	75%	50%
Enalapril (Vasotec)	5 to 10 mg every 12 hours	100%	75%- 100%	50%
Beta blockers				
Acebutolol (Sectral)	400 to 600 mg once or twice daily	100%	50%	30% - 50%
Atenolol (Tenormin)	5 to 100 mg daily	100%	50%	25%
Diuretics				
Amiloride (Midamor)	5 mg daily	100%	50%	Avoid
Bumetanide (Bumex)	No adjustment needed	—	—	—
Furosemide (Lasix)	No adjustment needed	—	—	—
Metolazone (Zaroxolyn)	No adjustment needed	—	—	—
Spironolactone (Aldactone)	50 to 100 mg daily	Every 6 to 12 hours	Every 12 to 24 hours	Avoid
Thiazides|	25 to 50 mg daily	100%	100%	Avoid

Table 21.3

Hypoglycemic agents: dosing requirements in patients with chronic kidney disease

Drug	Usual dosage*	Special considerations
Acarbose (Precose)	Maximum: 50 to 100 mg three times daily	Lack of data in patients with a serum createnine level higher than 2 mg per dl (180 μmol per L); therefore, acarbose should be avoided in these patients[18]
Glipizide (Glucotrol)	5 mg daily	Dosage adjustment not necessary in patients with renal impairment
Metformin (Glucophage)	500 mg twice daily	Avoid if serum creatinine level is higher than 1.5 mg per dl (130 μmol per L) in men or higher than 1.4 mg per dl (120 μmol per L) in women, and in patients older than 80

Table 21.4

Antimicrobial agents: dosing requirements in patients with chronic kidney disease

Drug	Usual dosage	Dosage adjustment (percentage of usual dosage) based on GFR (ml per minute per 1.73 m^2)		
		> 50	10 to 50	< 10
Antifungals				
Fluconazole (Diflucan)	200 to 400 mg every 24 hours	100%	50%	50%
Itraconazole (Sporanox)	100 to 200 mg every 12 hours	100%	100%	50% (IV form is contraindicated)
Anti virals				
Acyclovir IV (Zovirax)*	5 to 10 mg per kg every 8 hours	100%	100% every 12 to 24 hours	50% every 12 to 24 hours
Acyclovir (oral)	200 to 800 mg every 4 to 12 hours	100%	100%	200 mg every 12 hours
Carbapenems				
Ertapenem (Invanz)	1 g every 24 hours	100%	100%	50%
Imipenem	0.25 to 1 g every 6 hours	100%	50%	25%
Cephalosporins				
Cefaclor (Ceclor)	250 to 500 mg every 8 hours	100%	50 to 100%	50%
Cefadroxil (Duricef)	0.5 to 1 g every 12 hours	100%	Every 12 to 24 hours	Every 36 hours
Cefamandole (Mandol)	0.5 to 1 g every 4 to 8 hours	Every 6 hours	Every 6 to 8 hours	Every 8 to 12 hours

Table 21.4 *Contd...*

Drug	Usual dosage	Dosage adjustment (percentage of usual dosage) based on GFR (ml per minute per 1.73 m^2)		
		> 50	10 to 50	< 10
Macrolides				
Azithromycin (Zithromax)	No adjustment needed	—	—	—
Clarithromycin (Biaxin)	250 to 500 mg every 12 hours (Biaxin); 1 g daily (Biaxin XL)	100%	50 to 100%	50%
Penicillins				
Amoxicillin	250 to 500 mg every 8 hours	Every 8 hours	Every 8 to 12 hours	Every 24 hours
Ampicillin/sulbactam (Unasyn)	1 to 2 g ampicillin and 0.5 to 1 g sul-bactam every 6 to 8 hours	100% (GFR ≥ 30)	Every 12 hours (GFR 15 to 29)	Every 24 hours (GFR 5 to 14)
Quinolones				
Ciprofloxacin (Cipro)	400 mg IV or 500 to 750 mg orally every 12 hours	100%	50 to 75%	50%
Gatifloxacin (Tequin)	400 mg every 24 hours	100%	400 mg initially, then 200 mg daily	400 mg initially, then 200 mg daily
Gemifloxacin (Factive)	320 mg every 24 hours	100%	50 to 100%	50%
Sulpha drugs				
Sulphamethoxazole (Gantanol)	1 g every 8 to 12 hours	Every 12 hours	Every 18 hours	Every 24 hours
Sulphisoxazole (Gantrisin)	1 to 2 g every 6 hours	Every 6 hours	Every 8 to 12 hours	Every 12 to 24 hours
Trimethoprim (Proloprim)	100 mg every 12 hours	Every 12 hours	Every 12 hours (GFR > 30); every 18 hours (GFR 10 to 30)	Every 24 hours
Tetracyclines				
Doxycycline (Vibramycin)	No adjustment needed	—	—	—
Tetracycline	250 to 500 mg two to four times daily	Every 8 to 12 hours	Every 12 to 24 hours	Every 24 hours

Table 21.5

Statins: Dosing requirements in patients with chronic kidney disease

Drug	Usual Dosage*	Dosage adjustments based on degree of renal function
Atorvastatin (Lipitor)	10 mg daily Maximal dosage: 80 mg daily	No adjustment needed
Fluvastatin (Lescol)	20 to 80 mg daily 80 mg daily (sustained release)	50% dose reduction in patients with a GFR less than 30 mL per minute per 1.73 m^2

Table 21.6

Other common agents: dosing requirements in patients with chronic kidney disease

Drug	Usual dosage*	Dosage adjustments based on (percentage of usual dosage) GFR (ml per minute per 1.73 m^2)		
		> 50	10 to 50	< 10
Allopurinol (Zyloprim)†	300 mg daily	75%	50%	25%
Esomeprazole (Nexium)	No adjustment needed	—	—	—
Famotidine (Pepcid)	20 to 40 mg at bedtime	50%	25%	10%

REFERENCES

1. National Kidney Foundation. K/DOQI clinical practice guidelines for chronic kidney disease: evaluation, classification, and stratification. *Am J Kidney Dis.* 2002; 39 (2 suppl 1): S1–266.
2. Poggio ED, Wang X, Greene T, Van Lente F, Hall PM. Performance of the modification of diet in renal disease and Cockcroft-Gault equations in the estimation of GFR in health and in chronic kidney disease. *J Am Soc Nephrol.* 2005;16: 459–66.
3. Burkhardt H, Hahn T, Gretz N, Gladisch R. Bedside estimation of the glomerular filtration rate in hospitalized elderly patients. *Nephron Clin Pract.* 2005; 101: c1–8.
4. Aronoff GR. Drug Prescribing in Renal Failure: Dosing Guidelines for Adults. 4th ed. Philadelphia, Pa.: American College of Physicians, 1999.
5. Saseen JJ, Carter BL. Hypertension. In: DiPiro JT, Talbert RL, Yee GC, Matzke GR, Wells BG, Posey LM, eds. Pharmacotherapy. 6th ed. New York, N.Y.: McGraw-Hill, 2005:185–215.
6. Chobanian AV, Bakris GL, Black HR, Cushman WC, Green LA, Izzo JL Jr, et al. The seventh report of the Joint National Committee on Prevention, Detection, Evaluation, and Treatment of High Blood Pressure: the JNC 7 report [Published correction appears in JAMA 2003;290:197] *JAMA.* 2003; 289: 2560–72.

7. Carter BL. Dosing of antihypertensive medications in patients with renal insufficiency. *J Clin Pharmacol.* 1995;35:81–6.
8. Brater DC. Diuretic therapy. *N Engl J Med.* 1998;339:387–95.
9. Pitt B, Zannad F, Remme WJ, Cody R, Castaigne A, Perez A, et al., for the Randomized Aldactone Evaluation Study Investigators. The effect of spironolactone on morbidity and mortality in patients with severe heart failure. *N Engl J Med.* 1999;341:709–17.
10. Pitt B, Remme W, Zannad F, Neaton J, Martinez F, Roniker B, et al., for the Eplerenone Post-Acute Myocardial Infarction Heart Failure Efficacy and Survival Study Investigators. Eplerenone, a selective aldosterone blocker, in patients with left ventricular dysfunction after myocardial infarction [Published correction appears in N Engl J Med 2003; 348: 2271] *N Engl J Med.* 2003;348:1309–21.

PART - III
PHARMACOTHERAPEUTICS

GASTRO INTESTINAL DISORDERS

22 Peptic Ulcer Disease
23 Inflammatory Bowel Disease
24 Diarrhea
25 Constipation
26 Nausea and Vomiting
27 Gastro Esophageal Reflux Disorder
28 Ascites
29 Dysphagia

HEPATIC DISORDERS

30 Liver Disease
31 Alcoholic Hepatitis
32 Hepatitis
33 Drug Induced Hepatotoxicity
34 Pancreatitis

RENAL DISORDERS

35 Acute Renal Failure
36 Chronic Kidney Disease
37 Benign Prostate Hyperplasia (BPH)
38 Diabetic Nephropathy
39 Urinary Stone Disease

CARDIOVASCULAR DISORDERS

40 Hypertension
41 Heart Failure
42 Arrhythmia
43 Dyslipidemia
44 Coronary Artery Disease
45 Ischemic Heart Disease
46 Atrial Flutter
47 Hypertrophic Cardiomyopathy

RESPIRATORY DISORDERS

48 Asthma
49 Chronic Obstructive Pulmonary Disease
50 Pulmonary Hypertension
51 Cystic Fibrosis
52 Hemoptysis

NEUROLOGICAL AND PSYCHOLOGICAL DISORDERS

53 Insomnia and Anxiety
54 Schizophrenia
55 Epilepsy
56 Parkinsonism
57 Pain
58 Alzheimer's Disease
59 Anxiety Disorders
60 Major Depressive Disease
61 Headache
62 Stroke
63 Obsessive Compulsive Disorder

INFECTIONS

64 Respiratory Tract Infections
65 Urinary Tract Infections
66 Infective Meningitis
67 Tuberculosis
68 HIV Infection
69 GI Infections
70 Sexually Transmitted Diseases
71 Sepsis and Septic Shock

PROTOZOAL INFECTIONS

72 Malaria
73 Filaria

ENDOCRINE DISORDERS

74 Thyroid Disorders
75 Parathyroid Disorders
76 Diabetes Mellitus
77 Cushing's Syndrome
78 Addisons Disease
79 Pheochromocytoma

OBSTETRICS AND GYNECOLOGICAL DISORDERS

80 Menstrual Cycle Disorders
81 Menopause
82 Drug Therapy in Pregnancy
83 Drug Therapy in Lactation

MALIGNANT DISORDERS

84 Leukemia
85 Lymphoma
86 Breast Cancer
87 Prostate Cancer
88 Colorectal Cancer

RHEUMATIC DISORDERS

89 Rheumatoid Arthritis
90 Osteoarthritis
91 Gout and Hyperuricemia

EYE DISORDERS

92 Glaucoma
93 Diabetic Retinopathy

SKIN DISORDERS

94 Psoriasis
95 Skin Disorders and Cutaneous Drug Reactions
96 Acne Vulgaris

MISCELLANEOUS

97 Male Sexual Dysfunction
98 Drug Dependence and Drug Abuse
99 Nutraceuticals
100 Pharmacoeconomics
101 Pharmacogenomics

CHAPTER 22

Peptic Ulcer Disease

DEFINITION

Peptic ulcer disease (PUD) refers to a group of ulcerative disorders of the upper GI tract that require acid and pepsin for their formation. Ulcers differ from gastritis and erosions in that they extend deeper into the muscularis mucosa.

The three common forms of peptic ulcers include *Helicobacter pylori* (HP) – associated ulcers, nonsteroidal anti-inflammatory drug (NSAID)–induced ulcers, and stress-related mucosal damage (also called stress ulcers).

PREVALENCE

The lifetime risk for developing a peptic ulcer is approximately 10%. In Western countries the prevalence of *Helicobacter pylori* infections roughly matches age (i.e., 20% at age 20, 30% at age 30, 80% at age 80 etc.). Prevalence is higher in third world countries. Transmission is by food, contaminated groundwater, and through human saliva (such as from kissing or sharing food utensils). A minority of cases of *H. pylori* infection will eventually lead to an ulcer and a larger proportion of people will get non-specific discomfort, abdominal pain or gastritis. Peptic ulcer disease had a tremendous effect on morbidity and mortality until the last decades of the 20th century, when epidemiological trends started to point to an impressive fall in its incidence.

ETIOLOGY

Normally, the lining of the stomach and small intestines is protected against the irritating acids produced in your stomach. If this protective lining stops working correctly and the lining breaks down, it results in inflammation (gastritis) or an ulcer.

Most ulcers occur in the first layer of the inner lining. A hole that goes all the way through the stomach or duodenum is called a perforation. A perforation is a medical emergency.

The most common cause of such damage is infection of the stomach by bacteria called *Helicobacter pylori* (*H.pylori*). Most people with peptic ulcers have these bacteria living in their gastrointestinal (GI) tract. Yet, many people who have these bacteria in their stomach do not develop an ulcer.

The following also raise risk for peptic ulcers:

- Drinking too much alcohol
- Regular use of aspirin, ibuprofen, naproxen, or other nonsteroidal anti-inflammatory drugs (NSAIDs). Taking aspirin or NSAIDs once in a while is safe for most people.

- Smoking cigarettes or chewing tobacco
- Being very ill, such as being on a breathing machine
- Having radiation treatments

A rare condition called Zollinger-Ellison syndrome causes stomach and duodenal ulcers. Persons with this disease have a tumor in the pancreas. This tumor releases high levels of a hormone that increases stomach acid.

PATHOPHYSIOLOGY

- The pathogenesis of duodenal ulcers (DU) and gastric ulcers (GU) is multifactorial and most likely reflects a combination of pathophysiologic abnormalities and environmental and genetic factors.
- Most peptic ulcers occur in the presence of acid and pepsin when HP, NSAIDs, or other factors disrupt normal mucosal defense and healing mechanisms. Acid is an independent factor that contributes to disruption of mucosal integrity. Increased acid secretion has been observed in patients with DU and may result from HP infection. Patients with GU usually have normal or reduced rates of acid secretion.
- Alterations in mucosal defense induced by HP or NSAIDs are the most important cofactors in peptic ulcer formation (Fig. 22.1). Mucosal defense and repair mechanisms include mucus and bicarbonate secretion, intrinsic epithelial cell defense, and mucosal blood flow. Maintenance of mucosal integrity and repair is mediated by endogenous prostaglandin production.
- HP infection causes gastritis in all infected individuals and is causally linked to PUD. However, only about 20% of infected persons develop symptomatic PUD. Most non-NSAID ulcers are infected with HP, and HP eradication markedly decreases ulcer recurrence. HP may cause ulcers by direct mucosal damage, altering the immune/ inflammatory response, and by hypergastrinemia leading to increased acid secretion.
- Nonselective NSAIDs (including aspirin) cause gastric mucosal damage by two mechanisms: (1) a direct or topical irritation of the gastric epithelium, and (2) systemic inhibition of the cyclooxygenase-1 (COX-1) enzyme, which results in decreased synthesis of protective prostaglandins.
- Use of Corticosteroids alone does not increase the risk of ulcer or complications, but ulcer risk is doubled in corticosteroid users taking NSAIDs concurrently.
- Epidemiologic evidence links cigarette smoking to PUD, impaired ulcer healing, and ulcer related GI complications. The risk is proportional to the amount smoked per day.
- Although clinical observation suggests that ulcer patients are adversely affected by stressful life events, controlled studies have failed to document a cause-and-effect relationship. Coffee, tea, cola beverages, beer, milk, and spices may cause dyspepsia but do not increase PUD risk. Ethanol ingestion in high concentrations is associated with acute gastric mucosal damage and upper GI bleeding but is not clearly the cause of ulcers.

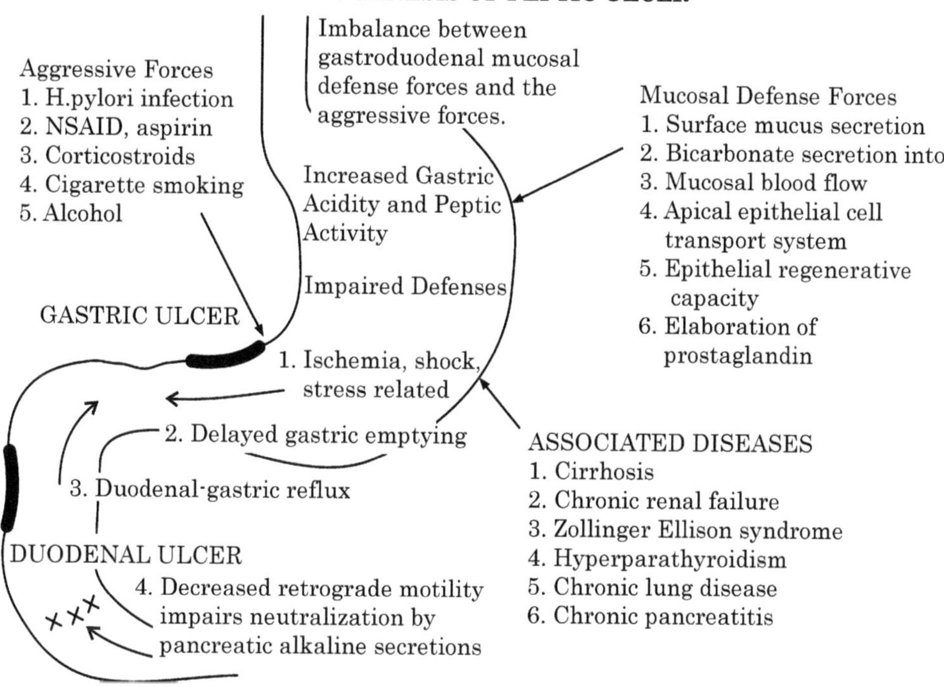

FIGURE 22.1

Pathogenesis of peptic ulcer.

CLINICAL FEATURES

- Abdominal pain is the most frequent symptom of PUD. The pain is often epigastric and described as burning but can present as vague discomfort, abdominal fullness, or cramping. A typical nocturnal pain may awaken patients from sleep, especially between 12 AM and 3 AM.
- Pain from DU often occurs 1 to 3 hours after meals and is usually relieved by food, whereas food may precipitate or accentuate ulcer pain in GU. Antacids provide rapid pain relief in most ulcer patients.
- Heartburn, belching, and bloating often accompany the pain. Nausea, vomiting, and anorexia are more common in GU than DU.
- The severity of symptoms varies from patient to patient and may be seasonal, occurring more frequently in the spring or fall.
- Pain does not always correlate with the presence of an ulcer. Asymptomatic patients may have an ulcer at endoscopy, and patients may have persistent symptoms even with endoscopically proven healed ulcers. Many patients (especially older adults) with NSAID-induced, ulcer-related complications have no prior abdominal symptoms.
- Complications of ulcers caused by HP and NSAIDs include upper GI bleeding,

perforation into the peritoneal cavity, penetration into an adjacent structure (e.g., pancreas, biliary tract, or liver), and gastric outlet obstruction. Bleeding may be occult or present as melena or hematemesis.

Perforation is associated with sudden, sharp, severe pain, beginning first in the epigastrium but quickly spreading over the entire abdomen. Symptoms of gastric outlet obstruction typically occur over several months and include early satiety, bloating, anorexia, nausea, vomiting, and weight loss.

DIAGNOSIS

- The physical examination may reveal epigastric tenderness between the umbilicus and the xiphoid process that less commonly radiates to the back.
- Routine laboratory tests are not helpful in establishing a diagnosis of uncomplicated PUD. The hematocrit, hemoglobin, and stool hemoccult tests are used to detect bleeding.
- The diagnosis of HP infection can be made using endoscopic or nonendoscopic tests. The tests that require upper endoscopy are invasive, more expensive, uncomfortable, and usually require a mucosal biopsy for histology, culture, or detection of urease activity. The nonendoscopic tests include serologic antibody detection tests, the urea breath test (UBT), and the stool antigen test. Serologic tests detect circulating immunoglobulin G directed against HP but are of limited value in evaluating post treatment eradication. The UBT is based on urease production by HP. Testing for HP is only recommended if eradication therapy is considered. If endoscopy is not planned, serologic antibody testing is reasonable to determine HP status. The UBT is the preferred nonendoscopic method to verify HP eradication after treatment.
- The diagnosis of PUD depends on visualizing the ulcer crater either by upper GI radiography or endoscopy. Radiography may be the preferred initial diagnostic procedure in patients with suspected uncomplicated PUD. Upper endoscopy should be performed if complications are thought to exist or if an accurate diagnosis is warranted. If a GU is found on radiography, malignancy should be excluded by direct endoscopic visualization and histology.

TREATMENT

NONPHARMACOLOGICAL TREATMENT

- Patients with PUD should eliminate or reduce psychological stress, cigarette smoking, and the use of nonselective NSAIDs (including aspirin). If possible, alternative agents such as **acetaminophen**, a nonacetylated salicylate (e.g., **salsalate**), or a COX-2 selective inhibitor should be used for pain relief.
- Although there is no need for a special diet, patients should avoid foods and beverages that cause dyspepsia or exacerbate ulcer symptoms (e.g., spicy foods, caffeine and alcohol).

PHARMACOLOGICAL TREATMENT

- An algorithm for the evaluation and management of a patient with dyspeptic or ulcer-like symptoms is presented in Fig. 22.2

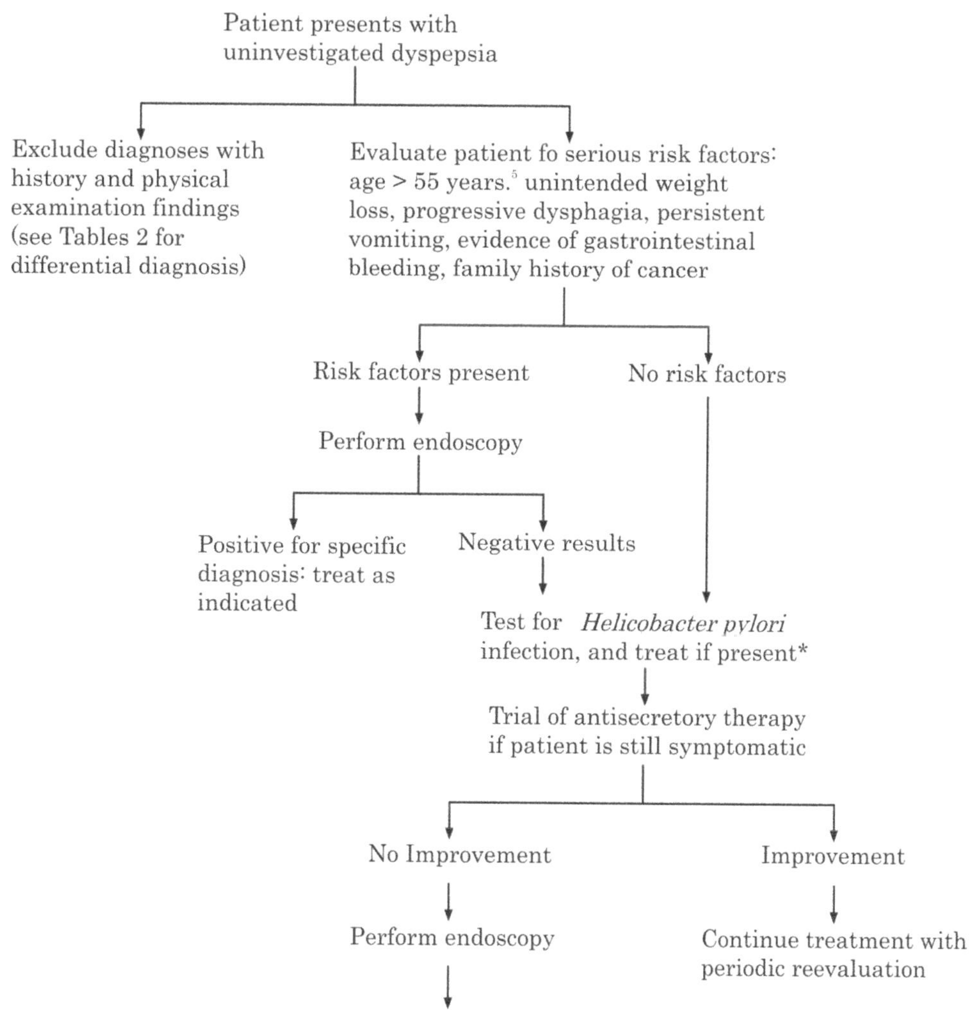

* – Physicians may prefer a trial of antisecretory therapy before testing for *Helicobacter pylori* infecction, especially when the onset of dyspepsia is relatively recent (less than three to six months)

FIGURE 22.2

Algorithm for the evaluation and management of a patient with dyspeptic or ulcer.

- Eradication of HP is recommended for HP-infected patients with GU, DU, ulcer-related complications, and in some other situations. Treatment should be effective, well tolerated, easy to comply with, and cost-effective (Table 22.1).
- First-line eradication therapy is a proton pump inhibitor (PPI)–based, three-drug regimen containing two antibiotics, usually **Clarithromycin** and **amoxicillin**, reserving **Metronidazole** for back-up therapy (e.g., Clarithromycin–

Table 22.1

Drug regimens to eradicate helicobacter pylori[a]

Drug 1	Drug 2	Drug 3	Drug 4
Proton pump inhibitor-based three-drug regimens[a]			
Omeprazole 20 mg twice daily	Clarithromycin 500mg daily	Amoxicillin 1 g twice daily **or** Metronidazole 500 mg twice daily	
or lansoprazole 30 mg twice daily			
or pantoprazole 40 mg twice daily			
or esomerprazole 40 mg daily			
or rabeproazole 20 mg daily			
Bismuth-based four-drug regimens[b]			
Omeprazole 40 mg twice daily	Bismuth sub-salicylate 525mg four times daily	Metronidazole 250-500-mg four times daily	Tetracycline 500 mg four times daily **or** amoxicillin 500 mg four times daily, **or** Clarithromycin 250-500mg four times daily
or lansoprazole 30 mg twice daily			
or pantoprazole 40 mg twice daily			
or esomerprazole 40 mg daily			
or rabeproazole 20 mg daily			
or standard ulcer-healing dosage of an histamine 2 receptor antagonist taken for 4-6 weeks			

a Although treatment is minimally effective if used for 7 days, 10–14 days of treatment is recommended. The antisecretory drug maybe continued beyond antimicrobial treatment in patients with a history of complicated ulcer (e.g., bleeding or in heavy smokers).

b In the setting of an active ulcer, acid suppression is added to hasten pain relief.

Metronidazole in penicillin-allergic patients). The PPI should be taken 30 to 60 minutes before a meal along with the two antibiotics. Although an initial 7-day course provides minimally acceptable eradication rates, longer treatment periods (10 to 14 days) are associated with higher eradication rates and less antimicrobial resistance. First-line treatment with quadruple therapy using a PPI (with **bismuth, Metronidazole,** and **tetracycline**) achieves similar eradication rates as PPI based triple therapy and permits a shorter treatment duration (7 days). However, this regimen is often recommended as second-line treatment when a Clarithromycin–amoxicillin regimen is used initially. All medications except the PPI should be taken with meals and at bedtime. Fig. 22.3 indicates drugs used to low a gastric acid.

- If the initial treatment fails to eradicate HP, second-line empiric treatment should: **1.** Use antibiotics that were not included in the initial regime **2.** Include antibiotics that do not have resistance problems; **3.** Use a drug that has a topical effect (e.g., bismuth); and **4.** Be extended to 14 days. Thus, if a PPI–amoxicillin–Clarithromycin regimen fails, therapy should be instituted with a PPI, bismuth subsalicylate, Metronidazole, and tetracycline for 14 days.
- Treatment with a conventional antiulcer drug (e.g., PPI, histamine-2 receptor antagonist [H_2 RA], or sucralfate alone is an alternative to HP eradication but is discouraged because of the high rate of ulcer recurrence and ulcer-related complications. Dual therapy (e.g., H_2 RA plus sucralfate, H_2 RA plus PPI) is not recommended because it increases cost without enhancing efficacy (Fig. 22.4).
- Maintenance therapy with a PPI or H_2 RAis recommended for high-risk patients with ulcer complications, patients who fail HP eradication, and those with HP-negative ulcers.
- For treatment of NSAID-induced ulcers, nonselective NSAIDs should be discontinued (when possible) if an active ulcer is confirmed. Most uncomplicated NSAID-induced ulcers heal with standard regimens of an H_2 RA, PPI, or sucralfate (see Table 22.2) if the NSAID is discontinued. If the NSAID must be continued, consideration should be given to reducing the NSAID dose or switching to acetaminophen, a nonacetylated salicylate, a partially selective COX-2 inhibitor, or a selective COX-2 inhibitor. PPIs are the drugs of choice when NSAIDs must be continued because potent acid suppression is required to accelerate ulcer healing. If HP is present, treatment should be initiated with an eradication regimen that contains a PPI. Patients at risk of developing serious ulcer-related complications while on NSAIDs should receive prophylactic cotherapy with misoprostol or a PPI.

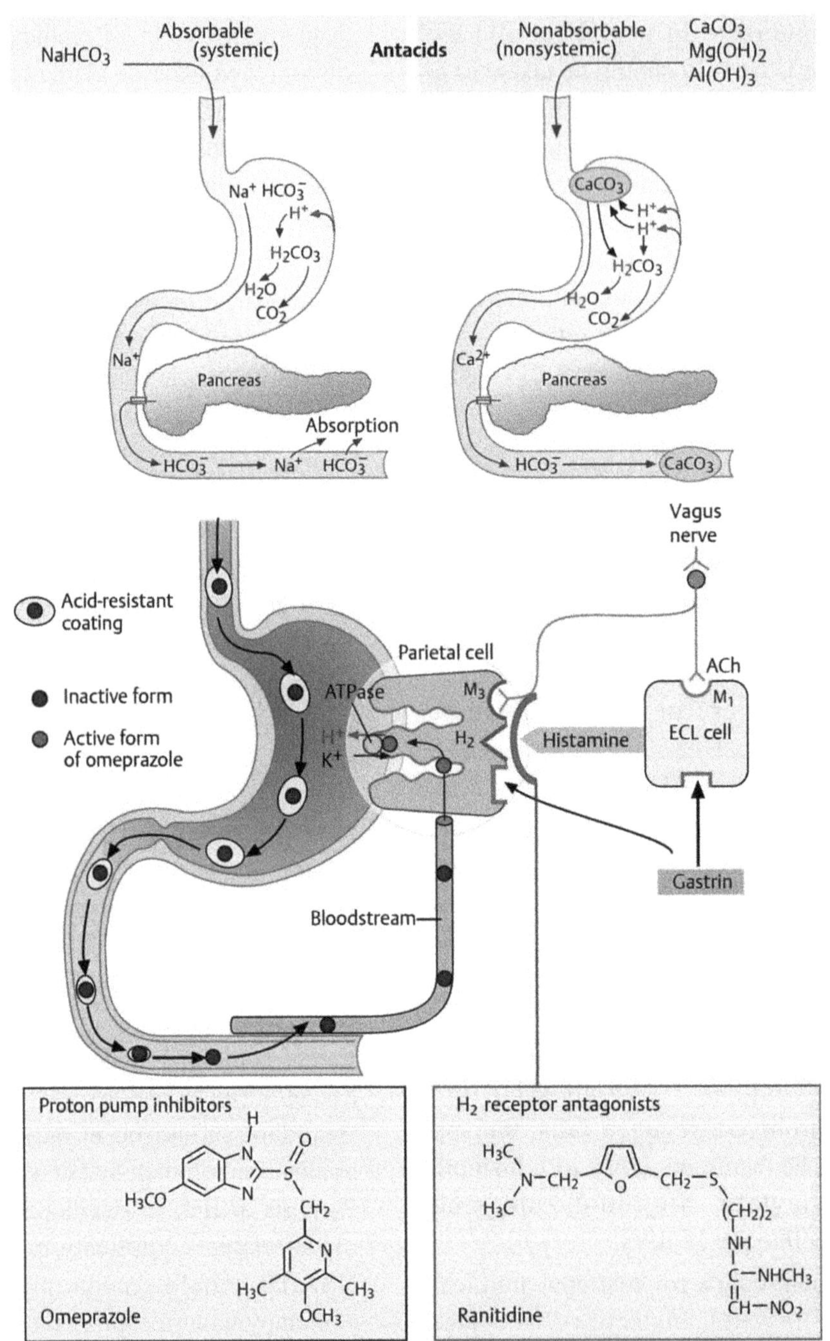

FIGURE 22.3

Drugs used to lower and neutralize gastric acid.

(Source : Colour Atlas of Pharmacology, 3rd edition, Page no.171)

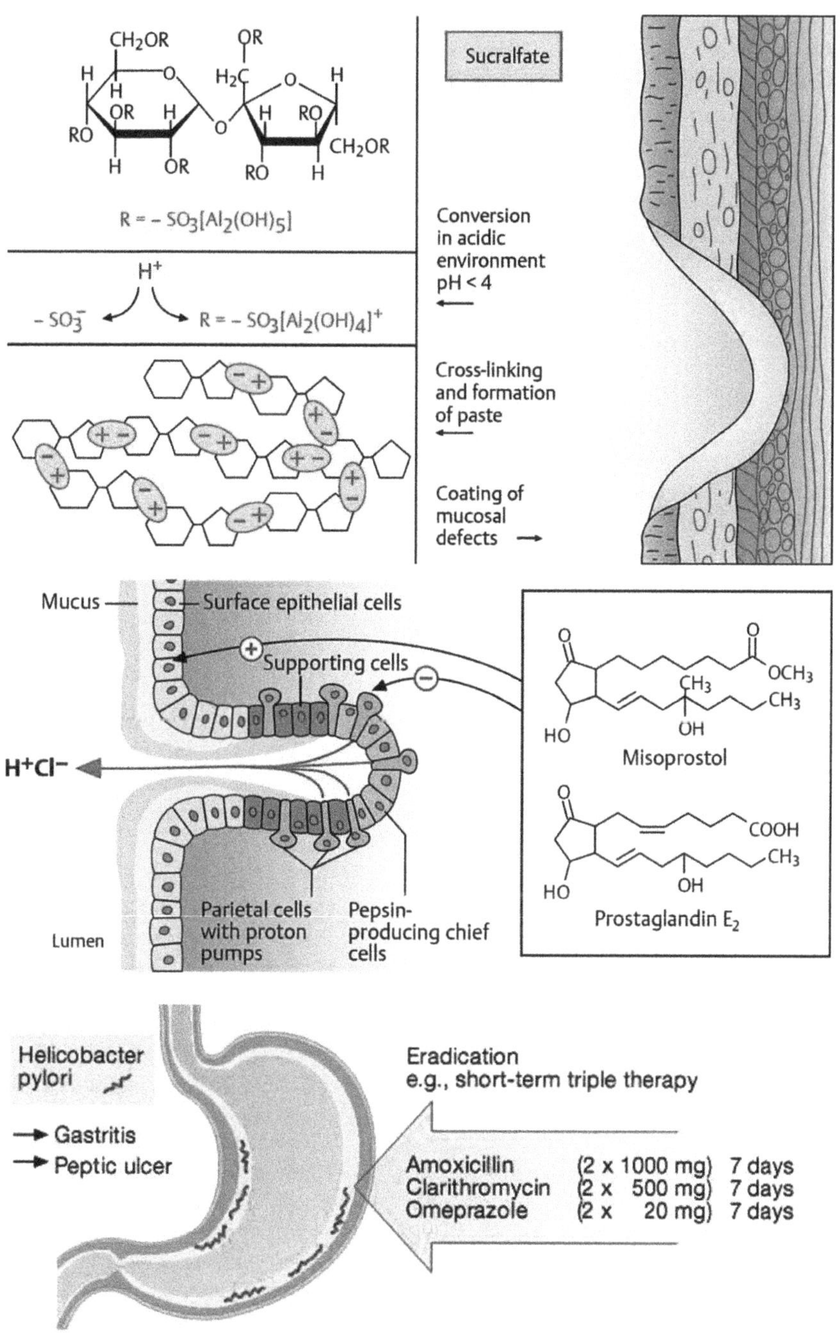

FIGURE 22.4

Protective effects of sucralfate, misoprostol and helicobacter eradication.

(Source : Colour Atlas of Pharmacology, 3rd edition, Page no.173)

Table 22.2

Oral drug regimens used to heal peptic ulcers or maintain ulcer healing

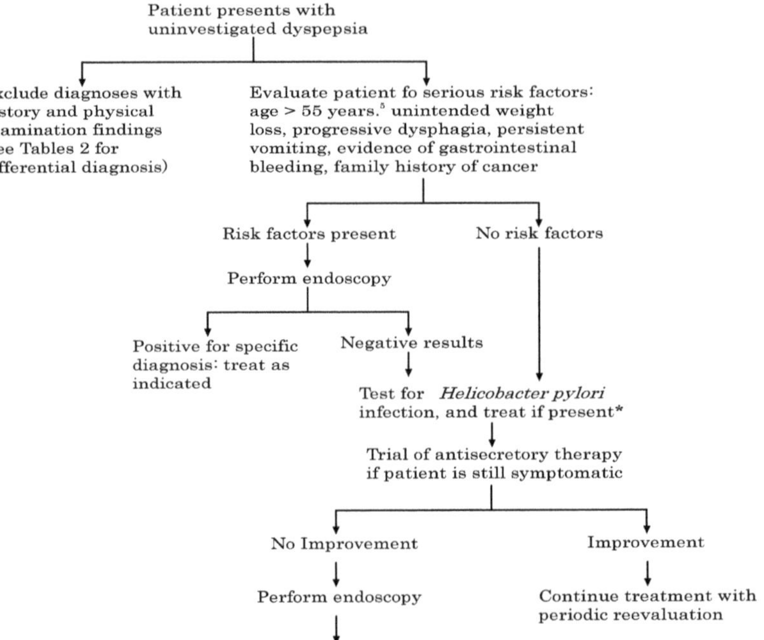

REFERENCES

1. Cullen DJ, Hawkey GM, Greenwood DC, *et al.* (1997). "Peptic ulcer bleeding in the elderly: relative roles of Helicobacter pylori and non-steroidal anti-inflammatory drugs". *Gut* **41** (4): 459–62.
2. Kato, Ikuko; Abraham M. Y. Nomura, Grant N. Stemmermann and Po-Huang Chyou (1992). "A Prospective Study of Gastric and Duodenal Ulcer and Its Relation to Smoking, Alcohol, and Diet".*American Journal of Epidemiology* **135** (5): 521 530. PMID 1570818.
3. Martin, U.S.A.F.M.C. (Major), David F.; Captain Elizabeth Montgomery, U.S.A. M.C., Arthus S, Dobek, Ph.D., Geoffrey A, Patrissi, M.A., Colonel David A, Peura, U.S.A. M.C., F.A.C.G. (28 June 2008)."Campylobacter pylori, NSAIDS, and Smoking: Risk Factors for Peptic Ulcer Disease". *American Journal of Gastroenterology* **84** (10): 1268–72. doi: 10. 1111/j.1572 0241.1989.tb06166. x.PMID 2801677. Retrieved 2010-03-18.
4. Kurata., John H.; Nogawa, Aki N. M.S. (Jan 1997). "Meta-analysis of Risk Factors for Peptic Ulcer: Nonsteroidal Antiinflammatory Drugs, *Helicobacter pylori*, and Smoking". *Journal of Clinical Gastroenterology* **24** (1): 2–17.
5. "Peptic ulcer". Retrieved 2010-06-18.
6. "Tests and diagnosis". Retrieved 2010-06-18.
7. "ATLAS OF PATHOLOGY". Retrieved 2007-08-26.

8. Rigas, Basil; Papavasassiliou, Efstathios D. (22 May 2002). "Ch. 7 John Lykoudis. The general practitioner in Greece who in 1958 discovered the etiology of, and a treatment for, peptic ulcer disease.". In Marshall, Barry J..*Helicobacter pioneers: firsthand accounts from the scientists who discovered helicobacters, 1892–1982*. John Wiley & Sons. pp. 74–88.
9. Duffull SB, Robinson BA. Clinical pharmacokinetics and dose optimisation of carboplatin. Clin Pharmacokinet 1997: 33: 161-183.
10. Winter ME. Aminoglycosides. In Basic Clinical Pharmacokinetics, Applied Therapeutics Inc, Vancouver,1994: 128.
11. Holford NHG. A size standard for pharmacokinetics. Clin Pharmacokinet 1996: 30: 329-332.
12. Lin JH, Lu AYH. Inhibition and induction of cytochrome P450 and the clinical implications. Clin Pharma-cokinet 1998: 35: 361-390.
13. Clinical Pharmacy Defined (Pharma-cotherapy 2008; 28(6): 816-817).

CHAPTER 23

Inflammatory Bowel Disease

DEFINITION

There are two forms of idiopathic inflammatory bowel disease (IBD): ulcerative colitis, a mucosal inflammatory condition confined to the rectum and colon, and Crohn's disease, a transmural inflammation of GI mucosa that may occur in any part of the GI tract. The etiologies of both conditions are unknown, but they may have a common pathogenetic mechanism.

PREVALENCE

Although the incidence and prevalence of ulcerative colitis and Crohn's disease are beginning to stabilize in high-incidence areas such as northern Europe and North America, they continue to rise in low-incidence areas such as southern Europe, Asia, and much of the developing world. As many as 1.4 million persons in the United States and 2.2 million persons in Europe suffer from these diseases. Previously noted racial and ethnic differences seem to be narrowing.

ETIOLOGY

- An unknown factor/agent (or a combination of factors) triggers the body's immune system to produce an inflammatory reaction in the intestinal tract that continues without control. As a result of the inflammatory reaction, the intestinal wall is damaged leading to bloody diarrhoea and abdominal pain.
- Genetic, infectious, immunologic, and psychological factors have all been implicated in influencing the development of IBD was presented in Table 23.1.
- There is a genetic predisposition (or perhaps susceptibility) to the development of IBD. However, the triggering factor for activation of the body's immune system has yet to be identified. Factors that can turn on the body's immune system include an infectious agent (as yet unidentified), an immune response to an antigen (e.g., protein from cow milk), or an autoimmune. As the intestines are always exposed to things that can cause immune reactions, more recent thinking is that there is a failure of the body to turn off normal immune responses.

PATHOPHYSIOLOGY

- The major theories of the cause of IBD involve a combination of infectious, genetic, and immunologic causes. The inflammatory response with IBD may indicate abnormal regulation of the normal immune response or an autoimmune reaction to self-antigens. Micro flora of the GI tract may provide a trigger to activate inflammation. Crohn's disease may involve a T lymphocyte disorder that arises in genetically susceptible individuals as a result of a breakdown in the regulatory constraints on mucosal immune responses to enteric bacteria. Proposed etiologies for IBD are found in Table 23.1.

- Smoking appears to be protective for ulcerative colitis but associated with increased frequency of Crohn's disease.
- Ulcerative colitis and Crohn's disease differ in two general respects: anatomic sites and depth of involvement within the bowel wall.

ULCERATIVE COLITIS

- Ulcerative colitis is confined to the colon and rectum and affects primarily the mucosa and the sub mucosa. The primary lesion occurs in the crypts of the mucosa (crypts of Lieberkühn) in the form of a crypt abscess.
- Local complications (involving the colon) occur in the majority of ulcerative colitis patients. Relatively minor complications include hemorrhoids, anal fissures, or perirectal abscesses.
- A major complication is toxic megacolon, a severe condition that occurs in up to 7.9% of ulcerative colitis patients admitted to hospitals. The patient with toxic megacolon usually has a high fever, tachycardia, distended abdomen, elevated white blood cell count, and a dilated colon.
- The risk of colonic carcinoma is much greater in patients with ulcerative colitis as compared with the general population.
- Approximately 11% of patients with ulcerative colitis have hepatobiliary complications including fatty liver, pericholangitis, chronic active hepatitis, cirrhosis, sclerosing cholangitis, cholangiocarcinoma, and gallstones.
- Arthritis commonly occurs in IBD patients and is typically asymptomatic and migratory. Arthritis typically involves one or a few large joints such as the knees, hips, ankles, wrists, and elbows.

Table 23.1

Proposed etiologies for inflammatory bowel disease
Infectious agents
• Viruses (e.g., measles)
• L-Forms of bacteria
• Mycobacteria
• Chlamydia
Genetics
• Metabolic defects
• Connective tissue disorders
Environmental factors
• Diet
• Smoking (Crohn's disease)
Immune defects
• Altered host susceptibility
• Immune-mediated mucosal damage
Psychological factors
Stress
Emotional or physical trauma
Occupation

Ocular complications (iritis, episcleritis, and conjunctivitis) occur in up to 10% of patients. 5% - 10% of patients experience dermatologic or mucosal complications (erythema nodosum, pyoderma gangrenosum, aphthous stomatitis).

CROHN'S DISEASE

- Crohn's disease is a transmural inflammatory process. The terminal ileum is the most common site of the disorder but it may occur in any part of the GI tract.

- About two-thirds of patients have some colonic involvement, and 15%- 25% of patients have only colonic disease.
- Patients often have normal bowel separating segments of diseased bowel; that is, the disease is often discontinuous.
- Complications of Crohn's disease may involve the intestinal tract or organs unrelated to it. Small-bowel stricture and subsequent obstruction is a complication that may require surgery. Fistula formation is common and occurs much more frequently than with ulcerative colitis.
- Systemic complications of Crohn's disease are common and similar to those found with ulcerative colitis. Arthritis, iritis, skin lesions, and liver disease often accompany Crohn's disease.
- Nutritional deficiencies are common with Crohn's disease.

CLINICAL FEATURES

ULCERATIVE COLITIS

- There are a wide range of ulcerative colitis presentations. Symptoms may range from mild abdominal cramping with frequent small-volume bowel movements to profuse diarrhea (Table 23.2). Many patients have disease confined to the rectum.
- Most patients with ulcerative colitis experience intermittent bouts of illness after varying intervals of no symptoms.
- Mild disease, which afflicts two-thirds of patients, has been defined as fewer than four stools daily, with or without blood, with no systemic disturbance and a normal erythrocyte sedimentation rate.

Table 23.2

Clinical features of ulcerative colitis

Signs and symptoms
- Abdominal cramping
- Frequent bowel movements, often with blood in the stool
- Weight loss
- Fever and tachycardia in severe disease
- Blurred vision, eye pain, and photophobia with ocular involvement
- Arthritis
- Raised, red, tender nodules that vary in size from 1 cm to several centimeters

Physical examination
- Haemorrhoids, fissures, or perirectal abscesses may be present
- Iritis, uveitis, episcleritis, and conjunctivitis with ocular involvement
- Dermatologic findings with erythema nodosum, pyoderma gangrenosum

Laboratory tests
- Decreased haematocrit haemoglobin
- Increased erythrocyte sedimentation rate
- Leukocytosis and hypoalbuminemia with severe disease

Table 23.3

Clinical features of crohn's disease

Signs and symptoms
- Malaise and fever
- Abdominal pain
- Frequent bowel movements
- Hematochezia
- Fistula
- Weight loss
- Arthritis

Physical examination
- Abdominal mass and tenderness
- Perianal fissure or fistula

Laboratory tests
- Increased white blood cell count and erythrocyte sedimentation rate

- Patients with moderate disease have more than four stools per day but with minimal systemic disturbance (Fig. 23.1).
- With severe disease, the patient has more than six stools per day with blood, with evidence of systemic disturbance as shown by fever, tachycardia, anemia, or erythrocyte sedimentation rate greater than 30.

CROHN'S DISEASE

- As with ulcerative colitis, the presentation of Crohn's disease is highly variable (Table 23.3). A single episode may not be followed by further episodes, or the patient may experience continuous, unremitting disease. A patient may present with diarrhea and abdominal pain or a perirectal or Perianal lesion.
- The course of Crohn's disease is characterized by periods of remission and exacerbation. Some patients may be free of symptoms for years, while others experience chronic problems in spite of medical therapy.

TREATMENT

GENERAL APPROACH

- Treatment of IBD centers on agents used to relieve the inflammatory process. Salicylates, glucocorticoids, anti-microbials, and immune-suppressive agents are commonly used to treat active disease and, for some agents, to lengthen the time of disease remission.
- In addition to the use of drugs, surgical procedures are sometimes performed when active disease is not adequately controlled or when the required drug dosages pose an unacceptable risk of adverse effects.

NON PHARMACOLOGICAL TREATMENT

Nutritional Support

- Patients with moderate to severe IBD are often malnourished.
- The nutritional needs of the majority of patients can be adequately addressed with enteral supplementation. Patients who have severe disease may require a course of parenteral nutrition.
- Probiotic formulas have been effective in maintaining remission in ulcerative colitis.

Surgery

- For ulcerative colitis, colectomy may be performed when the patient has disease uncontrolled by maximum medical therapy or when there are complications of the disease such as colonic perforation, toxic dilatation (megacolon), uncontrolled colonic haemorrhage, or colonic strictures.
- The indications for surgery with Crohn's disease are not as well established as they are for ulcerative colitis, and surgery is usually reserved for the complications of the disease. There is a high recurrence rate of Crohn's disease after surgery.

PHARMACOLOGICAL THERAPY

- The major types of drug therapy used in IBD include **aminosalicylates, glucocorticoids,** immunosuppressive agents (**azathioprine, mercapto-purine, cyclosporine,** and **methotrexate**), antimicrobials (**Metronidazole** and **ciprofloxacin**), and agents to inhibit tumor necrosis factor-α (TNF-α) (anti–TNF-α antibodies).

- **Sulphasalazine**, an agent that combines a sulphonamide (sulphapyridine) antibiotic and mesalamine (5-aminosalicylic acid) in the same molecule, has been used for many years to treat IBD. Mesalamine-based products are listed in Table 23.4.
- Corticosteroids and adrenocorticotropic hormone have been widely used for the treatment of ulcerative colitis and Crohn's disease and are used in moderate to severe disease. Prednisone is most commonly used. Budesonide is an oral controlled-release formulation that minimizes systemic effects.
- Immunosuppressive agents such as **azathioprine** and **mercaptopurine** (a metabolite of azathioprine) are sometimes used for the treatment of IBD. These agents are generally reserved for cases that are refractory to steroids and may be associated with serious adverse effects such as lymphomas, pancreatitis, or nephrotoxicity. Cyclosporine has been of short-term benefit in acute, severe ulcerative colitis when used in a continuous infusion.
- Methotrexate given 15 to 25 mg intramuscularly once weekly is useful for treatment and maintenance of Crohn's disease.
- Antimicrobial agents, particularly **Metronidazole**, are frequently used in attempts to control Crohn's disease, particularly when it involves the perineal area or fistulas.
- Infliximab is an anti-TNF antibody that is useful in moderate to severe active disease and steroid-dependent or fistulizing disease but the cost far exceeds that of other regimens. Adalimumab is another anti-TNF antibody that is an option for patients with moderate to severe active Crohn's disease previously treated with infliximab who have lost response.

ULCERATIVE COLITIS

MILD TO MODERATE DISEASE

- The first line of drug therapy for the patient with mild to moderate colitis is oral **Sulphasalazine** or an oral **mesalamine** derivative, or topical mesalamine or steroids for distal disease.
- When given orally, usually 4 g/day, up to 8 g/day of Sulfphasalazine is required to attain control of active inflammation. **Sulphasalazine** therapy should be instituted at 500 mg/day and increased every few days up to 4 g/day or the maximum tolerated.
- Oral **mesalamine** derivatives (such as those listed in Table 23.4) are reasonable alternatives to Sulphasalazine for treatment of ulcerative colitis but they are not more effective than Sulphasalazine.
- Steroids have a place in the treatment of moderate to severe ulcerative colitis that is unresponsive to maximal doses of oral and topical mesalamine. **Prednisone** up to 1 mg/kg/day or 40 to 60 mg daily may be used for patients who do not have an adequate response to Sulphasalazine or mesalamine.

- Steroids and Sulphasalazine appear to be equally efficacious; however, the response to steroids may be evident sooner.
- Rectally administered steroids or mesalamine can be used as initial therapy for patients with distal colitis.
- Transdermal **nicotine** improved symptoms of patients with mild to moderate active ulcerative colitis in daily doses of 15 to 25 mg.

SEVERE OR INTRACTABLE DISEASE

- Patients with uncontrolled severe colitis or incapacitating symptoms require hospitalization for effective management. Most medication is given by the parenteral route.
- With severe colitis, there is a much greater reliance on parenteral steroids and surgical procedures. Sulphasalazine or mesalamine derivatives have not been proven beneficial for treatment of severe colitis.
- Steroids have been valuable in the treatment of severe disease because the use of these agents may allow some patients to avoid colectomy. A trial of steroids is warranted in most patients before proceeding to colectomy, unless the condition is grave or rapidly deteriorating.
- Continuous IV infusion of **cyclosporine** (4 mg/kg/day) is recommended for patients with acute severe ulcerative colitis refractory to steroids.

Table 23.4

Mesalamine derivates for treatment of inflammatory bowel

Product	Formulation	Dose/Day	Site of Action
Sulphasalazine	Tablet	4-6 g	Colon
Mesalamine	Enema	1-4 g	Rectum, terminal colon
	Mesalamine tablet coated with Eudragit-S 9delayed-release acrylic resin)	2.4-4.8 g	Distal ileum and colon
	Mesalamine capsules encapsulated in ethyl cellulose microgranules	2-4 g	Small bowel and colon
	Mesalamine tablet formulated with Multi matrix System TM delayed-release technology, allows for once-daily dosing	2.4-4.8 g	Colon
	Mesalamine suppository	500-1,000 mg	Rectum
Olsalazine	Dimer of 5-aminosalicylic acid oral capsule	1.5-3 g	Colon
Balsalazide	Capsule	6.75 g	Colon

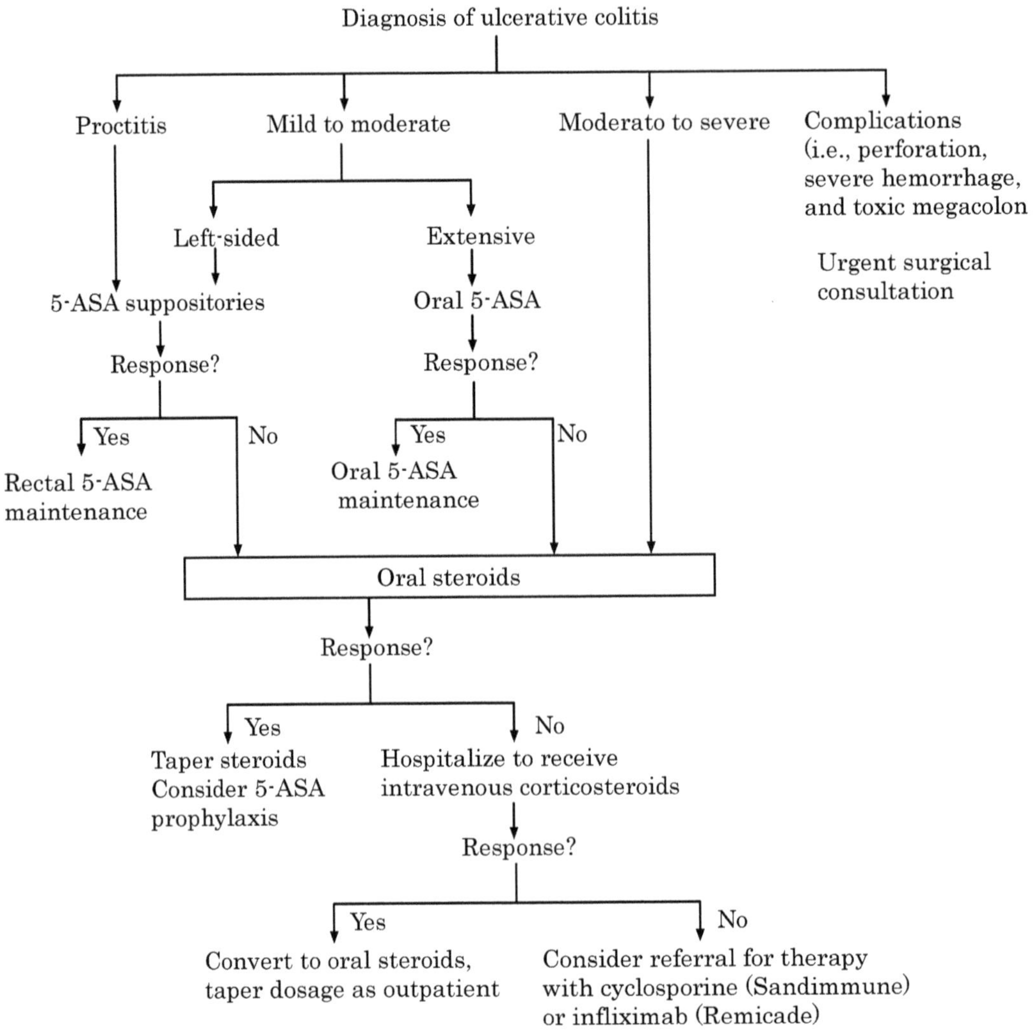

FIGURE 23.1

Diagnosis of ulcerative colitis.

MAINTENANCE OF REMISSION

- Once remission from active disease has been achieved, the goal of therapy is to maintain the remission.
- The major agents used for maintenance of remission are **Sulphasalazine** (2 g/day) and the **mesalamine** derivatives, although mesalamine is not as effective as Sulphasalazine.
- Steroids do not have a role in the maintenance of remission with ulcerative colitis because they are ineffective.

Steroids should be gradually withdrawn after remission is induced (over 3 to 4 weeks). If they are continued, the patient will be exposed to steroid side effects without likelihood of benefits.

- **Azathioprine** is effective in preventing relapse of ulcerative colitis for periods exceeding 4 years. However, 3 to 6 months may be required for beneficial effect. For patients who initially respond to infliximab, continued administration of 5 mg/kg every 8 weeks as maintenance therapy is an alternative for steroid dependent patients.

CROHN'S DISEASE (FIG 23.2)

ACTIVE CROHN'S DISEASE

- The goal of treatment for active Crohn's disease is to achieve remission; however, in many patients, reduction of symptoms so that the patient may carry out normal activities or reduction of the steroid dose required for control is a significant accomplishment.
- In the majority of patients, active Crohn's disease is treated **with Sulphasalazine, mesalamine** derivatives, or **steroids**, although **azathioprine, mercaptopurine, methotrexate, infliximab,** and **Metronidazole** are frequently used.
- **Sulphasalazine** is more effective when Crohn's disease involves the colon.
- Mesalamine derivatives (such as **Pentasa** or **Asacol**) that release mesalamine in the small bowel may be more effective than Sulphasalazine.
- **Steroids** are frequently used for the treatment of active Crohn's disease, particularly with more severe presentations, or in those patients unresponsive to aminosalicylates. Budesonide is a viable first-line option for patients with mild to moderate right-sided disease. Systemic steroids induce remission in up to 70% of patients and should be reserved for patients with moderate to severe disease who have failed aminosalicylates or Budesonide.
- **Metronidazole** (given orally up to 20 mg/kg/day) may be useful in some patients with Crohn's disease, particularly in patients with colonic or ileocolonic involvement or those with perineal disease. The combination of Metronidazole with ciprofloxacin is efficacious in some patients.
- The immunosuppressive agents (**azathioprine** and **mercaptopurine**) are generally limited to use in patients not achieving adequate response to standard medical therapy, or to reduce steroid doses when toxic doses are required. The usual dose of azathioprine is 2 to 3 mg/kg/day and 1 to 1.5 mg/kg/day for mercaptopurine. Up to 3 to 4 months may be required to observe a response. Starting doses are typically 50 mg/day and increased at 2-week intervals while monitoring complete blood count with differential.
- Patients deficient in thiopurine S-methyltransferase (TPMT) are at greater risk of bone marrow suppression from azathioprine and mercaptopurine. Determination of TPMT or TPMT genotype is recommended to guide dosage.

- **Cyclosporine** is not recommended for Crohn's disease except for patients with symptomatic and severe Perianal or cutaneous fistulas. The dose of cyclosporine is important in determining efficacy. An oral dose of 5 mg/kg/ day was not effective, whereas 7.9 mg/kg/ day was effective. However, toxic effects limit application of the higher dosage. Dosage should be guided by Cyclosporine whole-blood concentrations.
- **Methotrexate**, given as a weekly injection of 5 to 25 mg, has demonstrated efficacy for induction of remission in Crohn's disease as well as for maintenance therapy. The risks are bone marrow suppression, Hepatotoxicity, and pulmonary toxicity.
- **Infliximab** is used for moderate to severe active Crohn's disease in patients failing immunosuppressive therapy, in those who are corticosteroid dependent, and for treatment of fistulizing disease. A single, 5 mg/kg infusion is effective when given every day for 8 weeks. Additional doses at 2 and 6 weeks following the initial dose results in higher response rates.

  Adalimumab is effective in 54% of patients with moderate to severe Crohn's disease who have lost response to infliximab. The typical dosage is 160 mg subcutaneously initially, followed by 80 mg subcutaneously at week 2, with subsequent doses of 40 mg subcutaneously every other week thereafter.

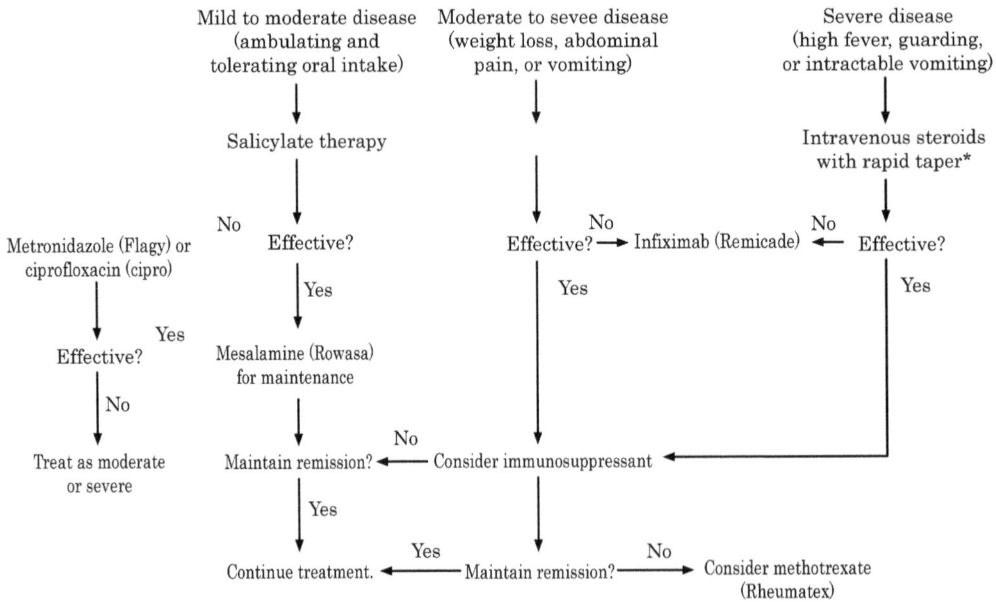

FIGURE 23.2

Treatment of crohn's disease.

MAINTENANCE OF REMISSION

- Prevention of recurrence of disease is clearly more difficult with Crohn's disease than with ulcerative colitis. **Sulphasalazine** and oral **mesalamine** derivatives are effective in preventing acute recurrences in quiescent Crohn's disease.
- **Steroids** also have no place in the prevention of recurrence of Crohn's disease; these agents do not appear to alter the long-term course of the disease.
- Although the published data are not consistent, there is evidence to suggest that **azathioprine, mercaptopurine, methotrexate, infliximab,** and **Adalimumab** are effective in maintaining remission in Crohn's disease.

SPECIAL CONSIDERATIONS

PREGNANCY

- Drug therapy for IBD is not a contraindication for pregnancy, and most pregnancies are well managed in patients with these diseases. The indications for medical and surgical treatment are similar to those in the non pregnant patient. If a patient has an initial bout of IBD during Pregnancy, a standard approach to treatment with sulphasalazine or steroids should be initiated.
- Folic acid supplementation, 1 mg twice daily, should be given.
- **Metronidazole** or **methotrexate** should not be used during pregnancy. Azathioprine and mercaptopurine may be associated with fetal deformities.

ADVERSE DRUG REACTIONS TO AGENTS USED FOR TREATMENT OF INFLAMMATORY BOWEL DISEASE

- Sulphasalazine is often associated with either dose-related or idiosyncratic adverse drug effects. Dose-related side effects usually include GI disturbances such as nausea, vomiting, diarrhea, or anorexia, but may also include headache and arthralgia.
- Patients receiving Sulphasalazine should receive oral **folic acid** supplementation since Sulphasalazine inhibits folic acid absorption.
- Non–dose-related adverse effects of Sulphasalazine include rash, fever, or hepatotoxicity most commonly, as well as relatively uncommon but serious reactions such as bone marrow suppression, thrombocytopenia, pancreatitis, pneumonitis, interstitial nephritis, and hepatitis.
- Oral mesalamine derivatives may impose a lower frequency of adverse effects compared with Sulphasalazine. Up to 90% of patients who are intolerant to Sulphasalazine will tolerate oral mesalamine derivatives. Olsalazine may cause watery diarrhea in up to 25% of patients.
- The well-appreciated adverse effects of glucocorticoids include hyperglycemia, hypertension, osteoporosis, fluid retention and electrolyte disturbances, myopathies, psychosis, and reduced resistance to infection. In addition, glucocorticoids use may cause adrenocortical suppression.
- Specific regimens for withdrawal of glucocorticoids therapy have been suggested.

- Immunosuppressant's such as azathioprine and mercaptopurine have a significant potential for adverse reactions, including bone marrow suppression, and have been associated with lymphomas (in renal transplant patients) and pancreatitis. Myelosuppression resulting in leukopenia is related to a deficiency in TPMT in some patients.
- Infliximab has been associated with infusion reactions, serum sickness, sepsis, and reactivation of latent tuberculosis. Adalimumab carries risks similar to infliximab.

REFERENCES

1. Baumgart DC, Carding SR (2007). "Inflammatory bowel disease: cause and immunobiology.". *The Lancet* **369** (9573): 1627–40.
2. Baumgart DC, Sandborn WJ (2007). "Inflammatory bowel disease: clinical aspects and established and evolving therapies.". *The Lancet* **369** (9573): 1641–57.
3. Xavier RJ, Podolsky DK (2007). "Unravelling the pathogenesis of inflammatory bowel disease." *Nature* **448** (7152): 427–34.
4. Elson, CO; Cong, Y; Weaver, CT; Schoeb, TR; McClanahan, TK; Fick, RB; Kastelein, RA (2007). "Monoclonal Anti–Interleukin 23 Reverses Active Colitis in a T Cell–Mediated Model in Mice". *Gastroenterology* **132** (7): 2359–70.
5. Hanauer, Stephen B.; William Sand born (2001-03-01). "Management of Crohn's disease in adults" (PDF). *American Journal of Gastroenterology* **96** (3): 635–43.
6. Shepherd, NA (August 2002). "Granulomas in the diagnosis of intestinal Crohn's disease: a myth exploded?". *Histopathology* **41** (2): 166–8.
7. Mahadeva, U; Martin, JP; Patel, NK; Price, AB (July 2002). "Granulomatous ulcerative colitis: a re-appraisal of the mucosal granuloma in the distinction of Crohn's disease from ulcerative colitis". *Histopathology* **41**(1): 50–5.
8. Pages 152-156 (Section: Inflammatory bowel disease(IBD)) in:Elizabeth D Agabegi; Agabegi, Steven S. (2008). *Step-Up to Medicine (Step-Up Series)*. Hagerstwon, MD: Lippincott Williams & Wilkins.
9. Section "Antibiotics and Ulcerative Colitis" in: Prantera, C.; Scribano, M. (2009). "Antibiotics and probiotics in inflammatory bowel disease: why, when, and how". *Current opinion in gastroenterology* **25** (4): 329–333.

CHAPTER 24

Diarrhea

DEFINITION

Diarrhea is an increased frequency and decreased consistency of fecal discharge as compared with an individual's normal bowel pattern. Frequency and consistency are variable within and between individuals. For example, some individuals defecate as many as three times a day, while others defecate only two or three times per week. Most cases of acute diarrhea are caused by infections with viruses, bacteria, or protozoa and are generally self-limited.

PREVALENCE

Worldwide in 2004 approximately 2.5 billion cases of diarrhea occurred which results in 1.5 million deaths among children under the age of five. Greater than half of these were in Africa and South Asia. This is down from a death rate of 5 million per year two decades ago. Diarrhea remains the second leading cause of death (16%) after pneumonia (17%) in this age group.

ETIOLOGY

Diarrhea is usually a symptom of gastroenteritis, an infection of the bowel. Gastroenteritis may be caused by:

- A virus, such as norovirus or rotavirus
- Bacteria, such as campylobacter, *Clostridium difficile* (C. difficile), *Escherichia coli* (E. coli), salmonella and shigella – these may all cause food poisoning
- Parasites, such as the *Giardia intestinalis* parasite that causes giardiasis.

Diarrhea caused by contaminated food or water from a foreign country is known as Travellers' diarrhea.

Other short-term causes

Other short-term causes of diarrhea include:

- Emotional upset or anxiety
- Drinking too much alcohol
- Drinking too much coffee
- A food allergy
- Appendicitis (swelling of the appendix)
- Damage to the lining of the intestines due to radiotherapy
- Damage to the intestines due to reduced blood supply, for example, because of a hernia

MEDICINES

Diarrhea can also be a side effect of many different medicines, including:

- Antibiotics
- Antacid medicines that contain magnesium

- Some medicines used in chemotherapy
- Non-steroidal anti-inflammatory drugs
- Selective serotonin reuptake inhibitors

Conditions that can cause persistent ***Diarrhea include***:

- Irritable bowel syndrome – a poorly understood condition where the normal functions of the bowel are disrupted
- Coeliac disease – a digestive condition where the person becomes intolerant to the protein gluten
- Crohn's disease – a condition that causes inflammation of the lining of the digestive system
- Cystic fibrosis – an inherited condition that affects the lungs and digestive system
- Diabetes – a condition caused by too much glucose in the blood
- Diverticular disease – when small pouches (diverticula) form in the large intestine, causing symptoms such as Diarrhea
- Gastrectomy – a surgical procedure to remove part of the stomach, for example, to treat stomach cancer
- Lactose intolerance – lactose is a natural sugar that is found in milk
- Microscopic colitis – a type of inflammatory bowel disease that causes watery Diarrhea

PATHOPHYSIOLOGY

- Diarrhea is an imbalance in absorption and secretion of water and electrolytes. Diarrhea may be associated with a specific disease of the GI tract or with a disease outside the GI tract.
- Four general pathophysiologic mechanisms disrupt water and electrolyte balance, leading to diarrhea. These four mechanisms are the basis of diagnosis and therapy. They are

1. A change in active ion transport by either decreased sodium absorption or increased chloride secretion;
2. A change in intestinal motility;
3. An increase in luminal osmolarity; and
4. An increase in tissue hydrostatic pressure.

These mechanisms have been related to four broad clinical diarrheal groups: secretory, osmotic, exudative, and altered intestinal transit.

- Secretory diarrhea occurs when a stimulating substance (e.g., vasoactive intestinal peptide [VIP], laxatives, or bacterial toxin) increases secretion or decreases absorption of large amounts of water and electrolytes.
- Poorly absorbed substances retain intestinal fluids, resulting in osmotic diarrhea.
- Inflammatory diseases of the GI tract can cause exudative diarrhea by discharge of mucus, proteins, or blood into the gut.
- Intestinal motility can be altered by reduced contact time in the small intestine, premature emptying of the colon, and by bacterial overgrowth.

CLINICAL FEATURES

- The clinical presentation of diarrhea is shown in Table 24.1.

Many agents, including antibiotics and other drugs, cause diarrhea (Table 24.2). Laxative abuse for weight loss may also result in diarrhea.

Table 24.1

Clinical features of diarrhea

General

- Usually, acute diarrheal episodes subside within 72 hours of onset, whereas chronic diarrhea involves frequent attacks over extended time periods.

Signs and symptoms

- Abrupt onset of nausea, vomiting, abdominal pain, headache, fever, chills, and malaise.
- Bowel movements are frequent and never bloody, and diarrhea lasts 12– 60 hours.
- Intermittent periumbilical or lower right quadrant pain with cramps and audible bowel sounds is characteristic of small intestinal disease.
- When pain is present in large intestinal diarrhea, it is a gripping, aching sensation with tenesmus (straining, ineffective and painful stooling).
  Pain localizes to the hypogastric region, right or left lower quadrant, or sacral region.
- In chronic diarrhea, a history of previous bouts, weight loss, anorexia, and chronic weakness are important findings.

Physical examination

- Typically demonstrates hyper peristalsis with generalized or local tenderness.

Laboratory tests

- Stool analysis studies include examination for microorganisms, blood, mucus, fat, osmolarity, pH, electrolyte and mineral concentration, and cultures.
- Stool test kits are useful for detecting GI viruses, particularly rotavirus.
- Antibody serologic testing shows rising titers over a 3- to 6-day period, but this test is not practical and is nonspecific.

Table 24.1 *Contd...*

- Occasionally, total daily stool volume is also determined.
- Direct endoscopic visualization and biopsy of the colon may be undertaken to assess for the presence of conditions such as colitis or cancer.
  Radiographic studies are helpful in neoplastic and inflammatory conditions.

Table 24.2

Drugs causing diarrhea

Laxatives
Antacids containing magnesium
Antineoplastics
Auranofin (gold salt)
Antibiotics

- Clindamycin
- Tetracyclines
- Sulphonamides
- Any broad-spectrum antibiotic

Antihypertensives

- Reserpine
- Guanethidine
- Methyldopa
- Guanabenz
- Guanadrel
- Angiotensin-converting enzyme inhibitors

Cholinergic

- Bethanechol
- Neostigmine

Cardiac agents

- Quinidine
- Digitalis
- Digoxin

Nonsteroidal anti-inflammatory drugs
Misoprostol
Colchicine
Proton pump inhibitors
H_2-receptor blockers

Disorders causing diarrhea. Clinicians must clearly understand that diarrhea, like a cough, may be a body defense mechanism for ridding itself of harmful substances or pathogens. The correct therapeutic response is not necessarily to stop diarrhea at all costs!

TREATMENT

GENERAL PRINCIPLES

- Management of the diet is a first priority for treatment of diarrhea (Fig. 24.1). Most clinicians recommend stopping solid foods for 24 hours and avoiding dairy products.
- When nausea or vomiting is mild, a digestible low-residue diet is administered for 24 hours.
- If vomiting is present and is uncontrollable with antiemetics, nothing is taken by mouth. As bowel movements decrease, a bland diet is begun. Feeding should continue in children with acute bacterial diarrhea.

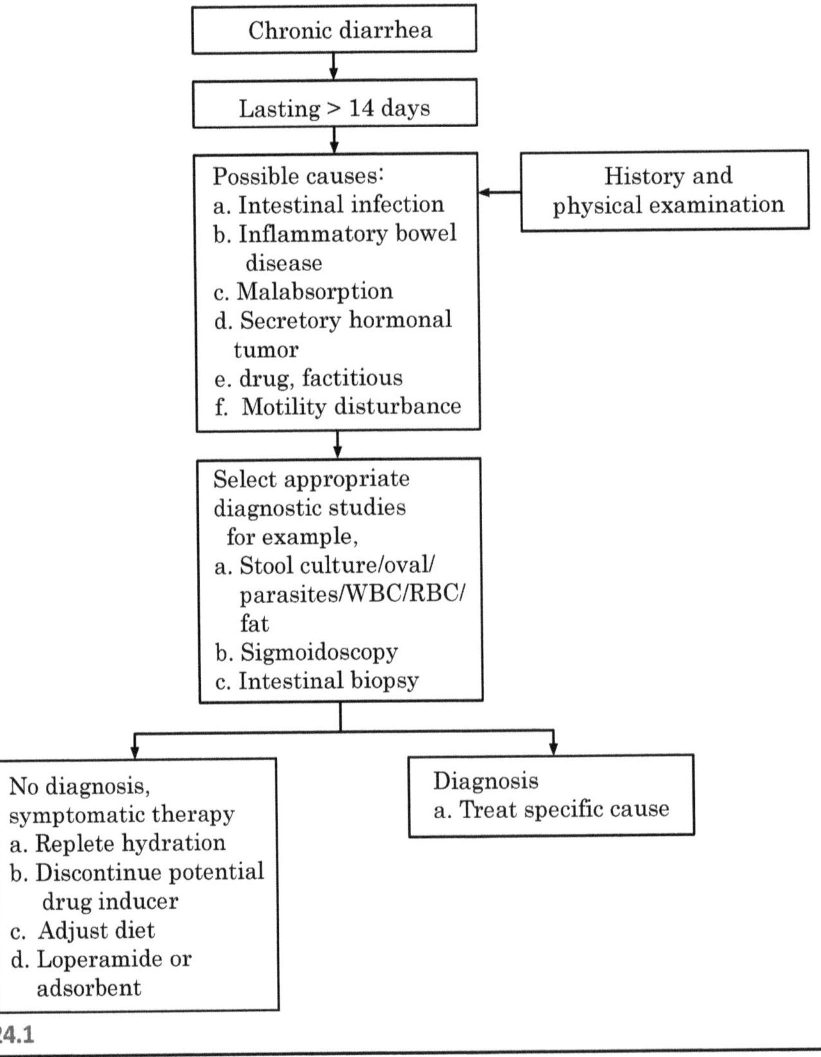

FIGURE 24.1

Treatment of diarrhea.

- Rehydration and maintenance of water and electrolytes are the primary treatment measures until the diarrheal episode ends. If vomiting and dehydration are not severe, enteral feeding is the less costly and preferred method.
- Recommendations for treating chronic diarrhea. Follow these steps:

1. Perform a careful history and physical examination.
2. The possible causes of chronic diarrhea are many.

- These can be classified into intestinal infections (bacterial or protozoal), inflammatory disease (Crohn's disease or ulcerative colitis), malabsorption (lactose intolerance), secretory hormonal tumor (intestinal carcinoid tumor or vasoactive intestinal peptide-secreting tumors), drug (antacid), factitious (laxative abuse), or motility disturbance (diabetes mellitus, irritable bowel syndrome, or hyperthyroidism).

3. If the diagnosis is uncertain, selected appropriate diagnostic studies should be ordered.
4. Once diagnosed, treatment is planned for the underlying cause with symptomatic antidiarrheal therapy.
5. If no specific cause can be identified, symptomatic therapy is prescribed. (RBC, red blood cells; WBC, white blood cells.)

PHARMACOLOGICAL THERAPY

- Various drugs have been used to treat diarrhea (Table 24.3) (Fig. 24.2). These drugs are grouped into several categories: antimotility, adsorbents, antisecretory compounds, antibiotics, enzymes, and intestinal microflora. Usually, these drugs are not curative but palliative.
- Opiates and Opioid derivatives delay the transit of intraluminal content or increase gut capacity, prolonging contact and absorption. The limitations of the opiates are addiction potential (a real concern with long-term use) and worsening of diarrhea in selected infectious diarrheas.
- **Loperamide** is often recommended for managing acute and chronic diarrhea. Diarrhea lasting 48 hours beyond initiating loperamide warrants medical attention.
- Adsorbents (such as **kaolin-pectin**) are used for symptomatic relief (see Table 24.3) Adsorbents are nonspecific in their action; they adsorb nutrients, toxins, drugs, and digestive juices. Co-administration with other drugs reduces their bioavailability.
- **Bismuth subsalicylate** is often used for treatment or prevention of diarrhea (traveler's diarrhea) and has antisecretory, anti-inflammatory, and antibacterial effects. Bismuth subsalicylate contains multiple components that might be toxic if given in excess to prevent or treat diarrhea.
- **Lactobacillus** preparation is intended to replace colonic micro flora. This supposedly restores intestinal functions and suppresses the growth of pathogenic microorganisms. However, a dairy product diet containing 200 to 400 g of lactose or dextrin is equally effective in recolonization of normal flora. Anticholinergic drugs, such as **atropine**, block vagal tone and prolong gut transit time. Their value in controlling diarrhea is questionable and limited by side effects.
- **Octreotide**, a synthetic octapeptide analog of endogenous somatostatin, is prescribed for the symptomatic treatment

of carcinoid tumors and VIP secreting tumors. Octreotide is used in selected patients with carcinoid syndrome. Octreotide blocks the release of serotonin and other active peptides and is effective in controlling diarrhea and flushing. Dosage range for managing diarrhea associated with carcinoid tumors is 100 to 600 mcg/ day in two to four divided doses, subcutaneously for 2 weeks. Octreotide is associated with adverse effects such as cholelithiasis, nausea, diarrhea, and abdominal pain.

Table 24.3

Drugs used to treat diarrhea

	Dose Form	Adult Dose
Antimotility		
Diphenoxylate	2.5 mg/tablet 2.5 mg/5 ML	5 mg four times daily; do not exceed 20 mg/ day
Loperamide	2 mg/capsule 1mg / 5 ML	Initially 4 mg, then 2 mg after each loose stool; do not exceed 16 mg/day
Paragonic	2 mg/5mL (morphine)	5-10 mL 1-4 times daily
Opium tincture	5 mg/5mL 9morphine)	0.6mL four times daily
Difenoxin	1 mg/tablet	Two tablets, then one tablet after each loose stool; up to 8 tablets/day.
Adsorbents		
Kaolin-pectin mixture	5.7 g kaolin +130.2 mg pectin /30mL	30-120mL after each loose stool
Polycarbophil	500 mg/tablet	Chew 2 tablets four times daily or after each loose stool; do not exceed 12 tablets/day
Attapulgite	750 mg/ 15 mL 300 mg/7.5 mL 750 mg/tablet 600 mg/tablet 300 mg/tablet	1,2000-1,500 mg after each loose bowel movement or every 2 hours; up to 9,000 mg/day
Antisecretory		
Bismuth subsalicylate	1,050 mg/30mL 262 mg/15mL 524 mg/15mL 262 mg/tablet	Two tablets or 30 mL every 30 minutes to 1 hour as needed up to 8 doses /day.
Enzymes (lactase)	1,250 neutral lactase units / 4 drops. 3,300 FCC lactase units per tablet	3-4 drops taken with milk or dairy product. One or two tablets as above
Octreotide	0.05 mg/mL 0.01mg/mL 0.5 mg/mL	Initial: 50 mcg subcutaneously 1-2 times per day and titrate dose based on indication up to 600 mcg/day in 2-4 divided doses.

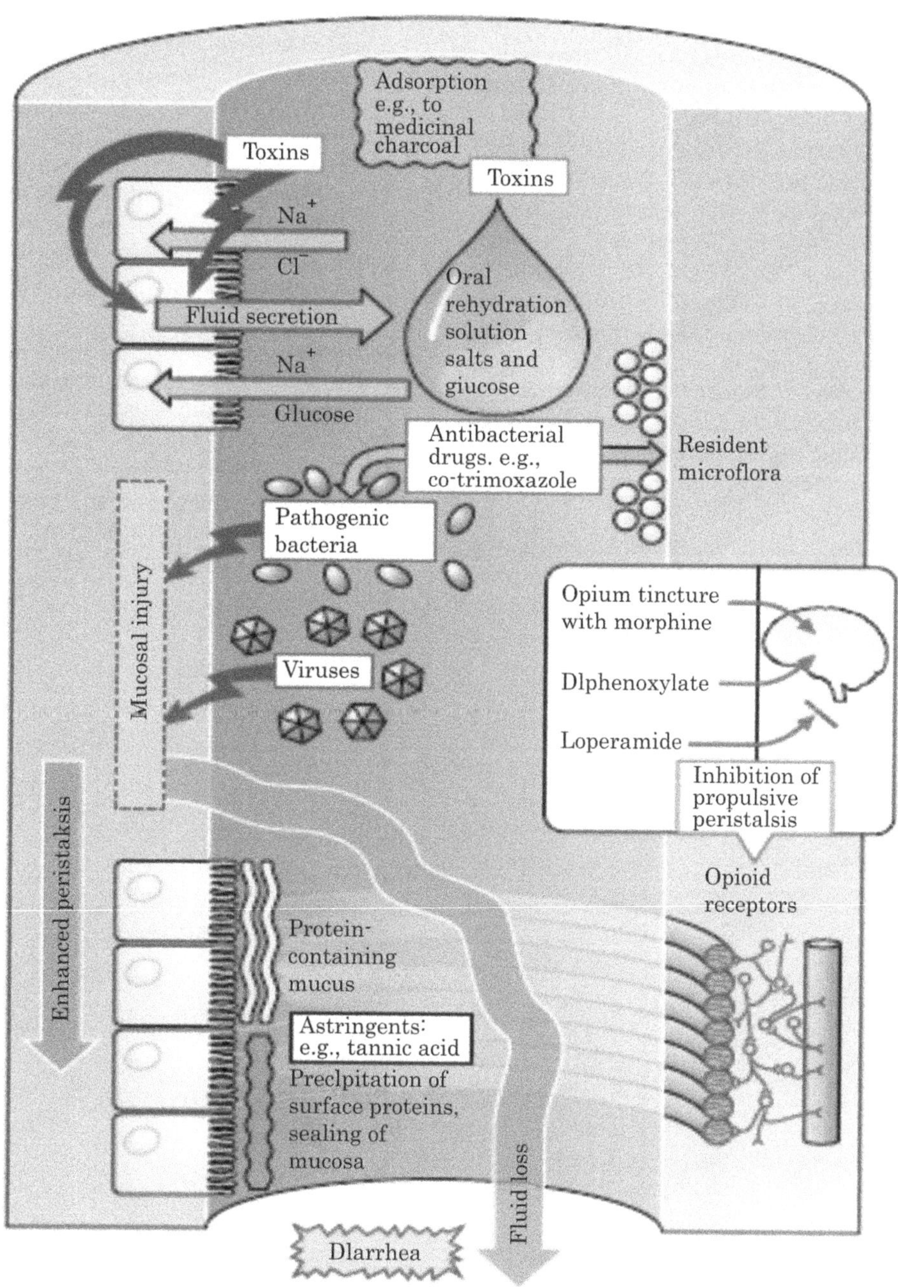

FIGURE 24.2

Anti diarrheals and their site of action.

(Source : http://intranet.tdmu.edu.ua/data/kafedra/internal/pharmakologia/classes_stud/en/pharm/prov_pharm/ptn/Pharmacology/3%20year/14%20Gastrointestinal%20agenrs%20-1..htm)

REFERENCES

1. Alam NH, Ashraf H (2003). "Treatment of infectious diarrhea in children". *Paediatr Drugs* **5** (3): 151–65.
2. Longstreth GF, Thompson WG, Chey WD, Houghton LA, Mearin F, Spiller RC (2006). "Functional bowel disorders". *Gastroenterology* **130** (5): 1480–91.
3. Wedlake, L; A'Hern, R, Russell, D, Thomas, K, Walters, JR, Andreyev, HJ (2009). "Systematic review: the prevalence of idiopathic bile acid malabsorption as diagnosed by SeHCAT scanning in patients with Diarrhea-predominant irritable bowel syndrome". *Alimentary pharmacology & therapeutics* **30** (7): 707–17.
4. Kasper DL, Braunwald E, Fauci AS, Hauser SL, Longo DL, Jameson JL.Harrison's Principles of Internal Medicine. New York: McGraw-Hill, 2005.
5. ^ Hempel, S; Newberry, SJ, Maher, AR, Wang, Z, Miles, JN, Shanman, R, Johnsen, B, Shekelle, PG (2012 May 9). "Probiotics for the prevention and treatment of antibiotic-associated diarrhea: a systematic review and meta-analysis.". *JAMA : the journal of the American Medical Association* **307** (18): 1959-69.
6. Schiller LR (2007). "Management of diarrhea in clinical practice: strategies for primary care physicians". *Rev Gastroenterol Disord* **7** (Suppl 3): S27–38.
7. Pawlowski SW, Warren CA, Guerrant R (May 2009). "Diagnosis and treatment of acute or persistent diarrhea". *Gastroenterology* **136** (6): 1874–86.

CHAPTER 25

Constipation

DEFINITION

Constipation does not have a single, generally agreed upon definition. Normal people pass at least three stools per week. Some of the definitions of constipation include: fewer than three stools per week for women and five for men despite a high-residue diet or a period of greater than 3 days without a bowel movement; straining at stool greater than 25% of the time and/or two or fewer stools per week; or straining at defecation and less than one stool daily with minimal effort.

ETIOLOGY

Theoretically, constipation can be caused by the slow passage of digesting food through any part of the intestine. More than 95% of the time, however, the slowing occurs in the colon.

MEDICATIONS THAT CAUSE CONSTIPATION (TABLE 25.1)

A frequently over-looked cause of constipation is medications. The most common offending medications include:

- Narcotic pain medications such as codeine and hydromorphone
- Antidepressants such as amitriptyline and imipramine
- Anticonvulsants such as phenytoin and carbamazepine
- Iron supplements
- Calcium channel blocking drugs such as diltiazem and nifedipine.
- Aluminium-containing antacids

PATHOPHYSIOLOGY

- Constipation is not a disease but a symptom of an underlying disease or problem.
- Disorders of the GI tract (e.g., irritable bowel syndrome or diverticulitis), metabolic disorders (e.g., diabetes), or endocrine disorders (e.g., hypothyroidism) may cause constipation.
- Constipation commonly results from a diet low in fiber or from use of constipating drugs such as opiates. Constipation may sometimes be psychogenic in origin.
- Diseases or conditions that may cause constipation are:
  - o GI disorders.
- Irritable bowel syndrome, diverticulitis, upper and lower GI tract diseases, hemorrhoids, anal fissures, tumors, hernia, syphilis, tuberculosis, lymphogranuloma venereum,
  - o Metabolic and endocrine disorders.

- Diabetes mellitus with neuropathy, hypothyroidism, panhypo-pituitarism, pheochromocytoma, hypercalcemia, enteric glucagons excess.
  - o Pregnancy.
  - o Neurogenic constipation.
- Head trauma, CNS tumors, spinal cord injury, cerebrospinal accidents, Parkinson's disease.
  - o Psychiatric disorders.
  - o Inappropriate bowel habits.
  - o Causes of drug-induced constipation are listed in Table 25.1.
  - o All opiate derivatives are associated with constipation, but the degree of intestinal inhibitory effects seems to differ between agents. Orally administered opiates appear to have greater inhibitory effect than parenterally administered agents; oral codeine is well known as a potent antimotility agent.

CLINICAL FEATURES

The laxative abuser may present with contradictory findings, sometimes diarrhea or weight loss. Laxative abusers may also have vomiting, abdominal pain, lassitude, thirst; edema, and bone pain (due to osteomalacia). With prolonged abuse, patients may have fluid and electrolyte imbalances (most commonly hypokalemia), protein-losing gastroenteropathy with hypoalbuminemia, and syndromes resembling colitis. Laxative abusers frequently deny laxative use (Table 25.2).

Table 25.1

Drugs causing constipation
Analgesics
Inhibitors of prostaglandin synthesis
Opiates
Anticholinergics
Antihistamines
Antiparkinsonian agents (e.g., benztropine or trihexyphenidyl)
Phenothiazines
Tricyclic antidepressants
Antacids containing calcium carbonate or aluminum hydroxide
Barium sulphate
Calcium channel blockers
Clonidine
Diuretics (non potassium-sparing)
Ganglionic blockers
Iron preparations
Muscle blockers (D-tubocurarine, succinylcholine)
Non steroidal anti-inflammatory agents
Polystyrene sodium sulphonate

TREATMENT

GENERAL APPROACH TO TREATMENT

- The patient should be asked about the frequency of bowel movements and the chronicity of constipation. The patient should also be carefully questioned about usual diet and laxative regimens.

Table 25.2

Clinical features of constipation
Signs and symptoms
It is important to ascertain whether the patient perceives the problem as infrequent bowel movements, stools of insufficient

Table 25.2 *Contd...*

size, a feeling of fullness, or difficulty and pain on passing stool. Signs and symptoms include hard, small or dry stools, bloated stomach, cramping abdominal pain and discomfort, straining or grunting, sensation of blockage, fatigue, headache, and nausea and vomiting.

Laboratory tests

A series of examinations, including proctoscopy, sigmoidoscopy, colonoscopy, or barium enema, may be necessary to determine the presence of colorectal pathology.

Thyroid function studies may be performed to determine the presence of metabolic or endocrine disorders.

- General measures believed to be beneficial in managing constipation include dietary modification to increase the amount of fiber consumed daily, exercise and adjustment of bowel habits so that a regular and adequate time is made to respond to the urge to defecate, and increasing fluid intake.
- If an underlying disease is recognized as the cause of constipation, attempts should be made to correct it. GI malignancies may be removed through a surgical resection. Endocrine and metabolic derangements are corrected by the appropriate methods.
- Potential drug causes of constipation should be identified. For some medications (e.g., antacids), non constipating alternatives exist. If no reasonable alternatives exist to the medication thought to be responsible for constipation, consideration should be given to lowering the dose.
- In a small percentage of patients presenting with complaints of constipation, surgical procedures (such as intestinal resection) are necessary. Surgery is usually necessary with most colonic malignancies and with GI obstruction from a number of causes.

DIETARY MODIFICATION AND BULK-FORMING AGENTS

- The most important aspect of the therapy for constipation for the majority of patients is dietary modification to increase the amount of fiber consumed. Patients should be advised to include at least 10 g of crude fiber in their daily diets. Fruits, vegetables, and cereals have thc highest fiber content.
- A trial of dietary modification with high-fiber content should be continued for at least 1 month before effects on bowel function are determined.
- The patient should be cautioned that abdominal distention and flatus may be particularly troublesome in the first few weeks, particularly with high bran consumption.

PHARMACOLOGICAL THERAPY (TABLE 25.3)

- The various types of laxatives are discussed in this section. The agents are divided into three general classifications:

1. Those causing softening of feces in 1 to 3 days (bulk-forming laxatives, **Docusates**, and **lactulose)**;
2. Those that result in soft or semi fluid stool in 6 to 12 hours (Bisacodyl and senna); and

3. Those causing water evacuation in 1 to 6 hours (**saline cathartics, castor oil,** and **polyethylene glycol-electrolyte lavage solution**).

- Dosage recommendations for laxatives and cathartics are provided in Table 25.3.

RECOMMENDATIONS

- The basis for treatment and prevention of constipation should consist of bulk-forming agents in addition to dietary modifications that increase dietary fiber.
- For most non hospitalized persons with acute constipation, the infrequent use (less than every few weeks) of most laxative products is acceptable; however, before more potent laxative or cathartics are used, relatively simple measures may be tried. For example, acute constipation may be relieved by the use of a **tap-water enema** or a **Glycerin** suppository; if neither is effective, the use of oral Sorbitol, low doses of Bisacodyl or senna, or saline laxatives (e.g., **milk of magnesia**) may provide relief.
- If laxative treatment is required for longer than 1 week, the person should be advised to consult a physician to determine if there is an underlying cause of constipation that requires treatment with agents other than laxatives.
- For some bedridden or geriatric patients, or others with chronic constipation, bulk-forming laxatives remain the first line of treatment, but the use of more potent laxatives may be required relatively frequently. Agents that may be used in these situations include **milk of magnesia** and **lactulose**.
- In the hospitalized patient without GI disease, constipation may be related to the use of general anesthesia and/or opiate substances. Most orally or rectally administered laxatives may be used. For prompt initiation of a bowel movement, a **tap-water enema** or **glycerin** suppository is recommended, or **milk of magnesia**. The approach to the treatment of constipation in infants and children should consider neurologic, metabolic, or anatomic abnormalities when constipation is a persistent problem. When not related to an underlying disease, the approach to constipation is similar to that in an adult. High fiber diet should be emphasized.

EMOLLIENT LAXATIVES (DOCUSATES)

- These surfactant agents, **Docusate** in its various salts, work by facilitating the mixing of aqueous and fatty materials within the intestinal tract. They may increase water and electrolyte secretion in the small and large bowel.
- These products result in a softening of stools within 1 to 3 days.
- Emollient laxatives are not effective in treating constipation but are used mainly to prevent constipation. They may be helpful in situations where straining at stool should be avoided, such as after recovery from myocardial infarction, with acute perianal disease, or after rectal surgery.
- It is unlikely that these agents are effective in preventing constipation if major causative factors (e.g., heavy opiate use, uncorrected pathology, inadequate dietary fiber) are not concurrently addressed.

LUBRICANTS

- **Mineral oil** is the only lubricant laxative in routine use and acts by coating stool and allowing easier passage. It inhibits colonic absorption of water, thereby increasing stool weight and decreasing stool transit time. Generally, the effect on bowel function is noted after 2 or 3 days of use.
- Mineral oil is helpful in situations similar to those suggested for docusates: to maintain a soft stool and avoid straining for relatively short periods of time (a few days to 2 weeks).
- Mineral oil may be absorbed systemically and cause a foreign-body reaction in lymphoid tissue. Also, in debilitated or recumbent patients, mineral oil may be aspirated, causing lipoid pneumonia.

LACTULOSE AND SORBITOL

- **Lactulose** is a disaccharide that causes an osmotic effect retained in the colon. It is generally not recommended as a first-line agent for the treatment of constipation because it is costly and not necessarily more effective than agents such as milk of magnesia. It may be justified as an alternative for acute constipation and has been found to be particularly useful in elderly patients.
- Occasionally, the use of lactulose may result in flatulence, cramps, diarrhea, and electrolyte imbalances.
- **Sorbitol**, a monosaccharide, has been recommended as a primary agent in the treatment of functional constipation in cognitively intact patients. It is as effective as lactulose and much less expensive.

SALINE CATHARTICS

- Saline cathartics are composed of relatively poorly absorbed ions such as magnesium, sulphate, phosphate, and citrate, which produce their effects primarily by osmotic action to retain fluid in the GI tract. These agents may be given orally or rectally.
- A bowel movement may result within a few hours of oral doses and in 1 hour or less after rectal administration.
- These agents should be used primarily for acute evacuation of the bowel, which may be necessary before diagnostic examinations, after poisonings, and in conjunction with some anthelmintics to eliminate parasites.
- Agents such as **milk of magnesia** (an 8% suspension of magnesium hydroxide) may be used Occasionally (every few weeks) to treat constipation in otherwise healthy adults.
- Saline cathartics should not be used on a routine basis to treat constipation. With fecal impactions, the enema formulations of these agents may be helpful.

CASTOR OIL

- **Castor oil** is metabolized in the GI tract to an active compound, Ricinoleic acid, which stimulates secretory processes, decreases glucose absorption, and promotes intestinal motility, primarily in the small intestine. Castor oil usually results in a bowel movement within 1 to 3 hours of administration. Because the agent has such a strong purgative action, it should not be used for the routine treatment of constipation.

GLYCERIN

- This agent is usually administered as a 3-g suppository and exerts its effect by osmotic action in the rectum. As with most agents given as suppositories, the onset of action is usually less than 30 minutes.
- **Glycerin** is considered a safe laxative, although it may occasionally cause rectal irritation. Its use is acceptable on an intermittent basis for constipation, particularly in children.

POLYETHYLENE GLYCOL-ELECTROLYTE LAVAGE SOLUTION

- Whole-bowel irrigation with **polyethylene glycol-electrolyte lavage solution** has become popular for colon cleansing before diagnostic procedures or colorectal operations.
- Four liters of this solution is administered over 3 hours to obtain complete evacuation of the GI tract. The solution is not recommended for the routine treatment of constipation, and its use should be avoided in patients with intestinal obstruction.

LUBIPROSTONE

- Lubiprostone is a chloride channel activator that acts locally on the gut to accelerate genitourinary transit time and delay gastric emptying. It is approved for chronic idiopathic constipation in adults. The dose is 24 mg capsule twice daily with food. Lubiprostone may cause headache, diarrhea, and nausea.

OTHER AGENTS

- Tap-water enemas may be used to treat simple constipation. The administration of 200 mL of water by enema to an adult often results in a bowel movement within 1.5 hours. Soapsuds are no longer recommended for use in enemas because their use may result in proctitis or colitis.

Table 25.3

Dosage recommendations for laxatives and cathartics

Agent	Recommend Dose
Agents that cause softening of feces in 1-3 days	
Bulk-forming agents/osmotic laxatives	
Methylcellulose	4-6 g/day
Polycarbophil	4-6 g/day
Psyllium	Varies with product
Emollients	
Docusate sodium	50-360 mg/day
Docusate calcium	50-360 mg/day
Docusate potassium	100-300 mg/day
Lactulose	15-30mL orally
Sorbitol	30-50g/day orally
Mineral oil	15-30mL orally
Agents that result in soft or semi fluid stool in 6-12 hours	
Bisacodyl (oral)	5-15 mg orally
Senna	Dose varies with formulation
Magnesium sulfate (low dose)	<10g orally
Agents that cause watery evacuation in 1-6 hours	
Magnesium citrate	18 g 300 mL water
Magnesium hydroxide	24-4.8g orally
Magnesium sulphate (high dose)	10-30g orally
Sodium phosphates	Varies with salt used
Bisacodyl	10mg rectally
Polyethylene glycol-electrolyte preparations	4l

REFERENCES

1. McCallum, I. J. D.; Ong, S.; Mercer-Jones, M. (2009). "Chronic constipation in adults". *BMJ* **338**: b831.

2. Emmanuel, A. V.; Tack, J.; Quigley, E. M.; Talley, N. J. (December 2009). "Pharmacological management of constipation". *Neurogastroen-terol Motil* **21**: 41–54.
3. Leung FW (February 2007). "Etiologic factors of chronic constipation: review of the scientific evidence". *Dig. Dis. Sci.* **52** (2): 313–6.
4. Arce DA, Ermocilla CA, Costa H (June 2002). "Evaluation of constipation". *Am Fam Physician* **65** (11): 2283–90.
5. Bharucha, A. (2007). "Constipation". *Best Practice & Research Clinical Gastro-enterology* **21** (4): 709–31.
6. "Is PEG (Polyethylene Glycol) a more effective laxative than Lactulose in the treatment of a child who is constipated?". *BestBETs*. 16 July 2007.
7. Candy D, Belsey J (February 2009). "Macrogol (polyethylene glycol) laxatives in children with functional constipation and faecal impaction: a systematic review". *Arch. Dis. Child.* **94** (2): 156–60.
8. Sonnenberg, A; Koch, TR (1989). "Epidemiology of constipation in the United States". *Dis Colon Rectum* **32** (1): 1–8.

CHAPTER 26

Nausea and Vomiting

DEFINITION

- Nausea is usually defined as the inclination to vomit or as a feeling in the throat or epigastric region alerting an individual that vomiting is imminent. Vomiting is defined as the ejection or expulsion of gastric contents through the mouth, often requiring a forceful event.

ETIOLOGY

- Food allergies
- Infections of the stomach or bowels, such as the "stomach flu" or food poisoning
- Leaking of stomach contents (food or liquid) upwards (also called gastroesophageal reflux or GERD)
- Medications or medical treatments, such as cancer chemotherapy or radiation treatment
- Migraine headaches
- Morning sickness during pregnancy
- Seasickness or motion sickness
- Severe pain, such as with kidney stones

Nausea and vomiting may also be early warning signs of more serious medical problems, such as:

- Appendicitis
- Blockage in the intestines
- Cancer or a tumour
- Ingesting a drug or poison, especially by children

Ulcers in the lining of the stomach or small intestine

PATHOPHYSIOLOGY

- The three consecutive phases of emesis include nausea, retching, and vomiting. Nausea, the imminent need to vomit, is associated with gastric stasis. Retching is the labored movement of abdominal and thoracic muscles before vomiting. The final phase of emesis is vomiting, the forceful expulsion of gastric contents due to GI retro peristalsis.
- Vomiting is triggered by afferent impulses to the vomiting centre, a nucleus of cells in the medulla. Impulses are received from sensory centres, such as the Chemoreceptor trigger zone (CTZ), cerebral cortex, and visceral afferents from the pharynx and GI tract. When excited, afferent impulses are integrated by the vomiting centre, resulting in efferent impulses to the salivation centre, respiratory centre, and the pharyngeal, GI, and abdominal muscles, leading to vomiting.

- The CTZ, located in the area postrema of the fourth ventricle of the brain, is a major chemosensory organ for emesis and is usually associated with chemically induced vomiting.

Numerous neurotransmitter receptors are located in the vomiting centre, CTZ, and GI tract. Examples of such receptors include cholinergic and histaminic, Dopaminergic, opiate, serotonin, neurokinin (NK), and benzodiazepine receptors. Theoretically, chemotherapeutic agents, their metabolites, or other emetic compounds trigger the process of emesis through stimulation of one or more of these receptors.

Table 26.1

Clinical features of nausea and vomiting

General
- Depending on severity of symptoms, patients may present in mild to severe distress

Symptoms
- Simple: Self-limiting, resolves spontaneously and requires only symptomatic therapy
- Complex: Not relieved after administration of antiemetics; progressive deterioration of patient secondary
- To fluid-electrolyte imbalances; usually associated with noxious agents or psychogenic events

Signs
- Simple: Patient complaint of queasiness or discomfort
- Complex: Weight loss; fever; abdominal pain

Laboratory tests
- Simple: None
- Complex: Serum electrolyte concentrations; upper/lower GI evaluation

Table 26.1 *Contd...*

Other information
- Fluid input and output
- Medication history
- Recent history of behavioural or visual changes, headache, pain, or stress
- Family history positive for psychogenic vomiting

TREATMENT

GENERAL APPROACH TO TREATMENT

- Treatment options for nausea and vomiting include drug and nondrug modalities. The treatment depends on associated medical conditions.
- For patients with simple complaints, perhaps related to food or beverage consumption, avoidance or moderation of dietary intake may be preferable.
- Nonpharmacologic interventions are classified as behavioural interventions and include relaxation, biofeedback, self-hypnosis, cognitive distraction, guided imagery, and systematic desensitization. Psychogenic vomiting may benefit from psychological interventions.

PHARMACOLOGICAL MANAGEMENT

Information concerning commonly available antiemetic preparations is compiled in Table 26.2.

For most conditions, a single-agent antiemetic is preferred; however, for those patients not responding to such therapy and those receiving highly emetogenic chemotherapy, multiple-agent regimens are usually required. The treatment of simple nausea and vomiting usually requires minimal therapy. Both non-prescription and prescription drugs useful in the treatment of simple nausea and vomiting are usually effective in small, infrequently administered doses. The management of complex nausea and vomiting, for example, in patients who are receiving cytotoxic chemotherapy, may require combination therapy.

DRUG CLASS INFORMATION

Antacids

Single or combination non-prescription antacid products, especially those containing magnesium hydroxide, aluminium hydroxide, and/or calcium carbonate, may provide sufficient relief from simple nausea or vomiting, primarily through gastric acid neutralization. Common antacid dosage regimens for the relief of nausea and vomiting

ANTIHISTAMINE–ANTICHOLINERGIC DRUGS

Antiemetic drugs from the antihistaminic–Anticholinergic category may be appropriate in the treatment of simple symptomatology. Adverse reactions that may be apparent with the use of the antihistaminic–Anticholinergic agents primarily include drowsiness or confusion, blurred vision, dry mouth, urinary retention, and possibly tachycardia, particularly in elderly patients.

PHENOTHIAZINES

Phenothiazines are most useful in patients with simple nausea and vomiting. Rectal administration is a reasonable alternative in patients in whom oral or parenteral administration is not feasible. Problems associated with these drugs include troublesome and potentially dangerous side effects, including extra pyramidal reactions, hypersensitivity reactions with possible liver dysfunction, marrow aplasia, and excessive sedation.

Corticosteroids

Dexamethasone has been used successfully in the management of chemotherapy-induced nausea and vomiting (CINV) and postoperative nausea and vomiting (PONV), either as a single agent or in combination with selective serotonin reuptake inhibitors (SSRIs). For CINV, Dexamethasone is effective in the prevention of both cisplatin-induced acute emesis and when used alone or in combination for the prevention of delayed nausea and vomiting associated with CINV.

Metoclopramide

Metoclopramide increases lower oesophageal sphincter tone, acids gastric emptying, and accelerates transit through the small bowel, possibly through the release of acetylcholine. Metoclopramide is used for its antiemetic properties in patients with diabetic gastroparesis and with Dexamethasone for prophylaxis of delayed nausea and vomiting associated with chemotherapy administration.

Cannabinoids

When compared with conventional antiemetics, oral **nabilone** and oral **dronabinol** were slightly more effective than active comparators in patients receiving moderately emetogenic chemotherapy regimens. The efficacy of Cannabinoids as compared to SSRIs for CINV has not been studied. They should be considered for the treatment of refractory nausea and vomiting in patients receiving chemotherapy.

Substance P/Neurokinin 1 Receptor Antagonists

Substance P is a peptide neurotransmitter in the NK family whose preferred receptor is the NK1 receptor. Substance P is believed to be the primary mediator of the delayed phase of CINV and one of two mediators of the acute phase of CINV.

Aprepitant is the first approved member of this class of drugs and is indicated as part of a multiple drug regimen for prophylaxis of nausea and vomiting associated with high-dose cisplatin-based chemotherapy. Numerous potential drug interactions are possible; clinically significant drug interactions with oral contraceptives, warfarin, and oral Dexamethasone have been described.

Selective Serotonin Receptor Inhibitors *(Ondansetron, Granisetron, Dolasetron, and Palonosetron)* SSRIs (**dolasetron, granisetron, ondansetron,** and **palonosetron**) act by blocking presynaptic serotonin receptors on sensory vagal fibers in the gut wall.

The most common side effects associated with these agents are constipation, headache, and asthenia

Chemotherapy-induced nausea and vomiting

Nausea and vomiting that occur within 24 hours of chemotherapy administration is defined as acute, whereas when it starts more than 24 hours after chemotherapy administration, it is defined as delayed.

Prophylaxis of chemotherapy-induced nausea and vomiting

Patients receiving chemotherapy that is classified as being of high emetic risk should receive a combination antiemetic regimen containing three drugs on the day of chemotherapy administration (day 1)—an SSRI plus Dexamethasone plus aprepitant. Patients receiving regimens that are classified as being of moderate emetic risk should receive a combination antiemetic regimen containing an SSRI plus Dexamethasone on day 1. Dexamethasone alone is recommended for prophylaxis prior to regimens of low emetic risk.

Table 26.2

Anti-nausea drugs

Anti-nausea medications					
Drug name	**Trade name**	**Dose**	**No. of days to take it**	**How it works**	**Side-effects**
Ondansetron	Zofran	4-8 mg table is orally, or wafers on the tongue, morning and night	4-5	Inhibits chemo-receptors (serotonin, or 5HT3, receptros) in gut and brain, specifically stopping the nausea reflex.	Constipation (common) Migraine headaches (uncommon)
Dolasetron	Anzemet	200 mg orally, mornings	2	As above	As above
Tropisetron	Navoban	5 mg orally on empty stomach	2	As above	As above

Table 26.2 *Contd...*

Anti-nausea medications					
Drug name	**Trade name**	**Dose**	**No. of days to take it**	**How it works**	**Side-effects**
Dexamethasone	Decadron	2-4 mg orally, mornings	4-5	Inhibits chemo-receptors in brain	Appetite stimulation. Insomnia. "Feeling high" increased energy May unsettle diabetic control Sedation.
Lorazepam	Ativan	1-2 mg orally at night	4-5	Sedative-hypnotic and relaxant. Seems also to synergise with the other drugs to improve anti-nausea control.	Don't drive after it! Don't mix with alcohol.
Prochlor-perazine tablets	Stemetil	5-10 mg orally three times daily as required	As required	Inhibits chemoreceptors in brain	Mild sedation. Muscular spasms of face muscles (rare)
Prochlor-perazine suppositories	Sitemetil Suppositories	25 mg rectally twice daily as required	As required	Inhibits chemoreceptors in brain	Mild sedation. Muscular spasms of face muscles (rare)
Aprepitant	Emend	125 mg 1 hr prechemo 80 mg daily for 2 days	3	Inhibits neurokinin-1 receptors in the brain.	minimal

TREATMENT OF CHEMOTHERAPY-INDUCED NAUSEA AND VOMITING

Chlorpromazine, prochlorperazine, promethazine, Methylprednisolone, lorazepam, metoclopramide, Dexamethasone, or dronabinol may be used for adult patients. Around the clock dosing should be considered. The choice of specific agent should base on patient specific factors, including potential for adverse drug reactions, and cost. SSRIs are effective for breakthrough nausea and vomiting but they are not superior to the less expensive antiemetics above.

Aprepitant, Dexamethasone, or metoclopramide have demonstrated efficacy in preventing CINV, whereas the results with SSRIs are inconsistent. Aprepitant and Dexamethasone can be used on the 2 days following administration of high emetic risk chemotherapy.

POSTOPERATIVE NAUSEA AND VOMITING

A variety of pharmacologic approaches is available and may be prescribed as single or combination therapy for prophylaxis of PONV. Most patients undergoing an operative procedure do not require preoperative prophylactic antiemetic therapy and universal PONV prophylaxis is not cost effective. SSRIs in doses of Dolasetron 12.5 mg, Granisetron 0.1 mg, Ondansetron 1mg, or Tropisetron 0.5 mg are recommended in patients who experience PONV despite prophylactic Dexamethasone or when no prophylactic agent was used.

RADIATION-INDUCED NAUSEA AND VOMITING

Patients receiving single-exposure, high-dose radiation therapy to the upper abdomen, or total or hemi body irradiation, should receive prophylactic antiemetics. Preventive therapy with an SSRI and Dexamethasone is recommended in patients receiving total-body irradiation

ANTIEMETIC USE DURING PREGNANCY

Initial management of nausea and vomiting of pregnancy often involves dietary changes and/or lifestyle modifications. Pyridoxine (10 to 25 mg one to four times daily) is recommended as first line therapy. If symptoms persist, addition of a histamine-1 receptor antagonist, such as Dimenhydrinate, Diphenhydramine, or Meclizine, is recommended.

REFERENCES

1. Malagelada J-R, Malagelada C. Nausea and vomiting. In: Feldman M, Friedman LS, Brandt LJ, eds. *Sleisenger & Fordtran's Gastrointestinal and Liver Disease*. 9th ed. Philadelphia, Pa: Saunders Elsevier; 2010:chap 14.
2. Mcquaid K. Approach to the patient with gastrointestinal disease. In: Goldman L, Schafer AI, eds. *Cecil Medicine*. 24th ed. Philadelphia, Pa: Saunders Elsevier; 2011:chap 134.

CHAPTER 27

Gastro Esophageal Reflux Disorder

Gastroesophageal reflux disease (GERD) results from the abnormal retrograde movement of gastric contents from the stomach to the esophagus. When the esophagus is constantly exposed to refluxed material for prolonged periods, inflammation of the esophagus occurs and in some cases it progresses to erosion of the squamous epithelium (erosive esophagitis). Severe reflux symptoms associated with normal endoscopic findings are referred to as nonerosive reflux disease, or endoscopy-negative reflux disease, "symptomatic GERD".

PATHOPHYSIOLOGY (FIG.27.1)

The main factor responsible for development of GERD is the abnormal reflux of gastric contents from the stomach to the esophagus.

- In few cases, gastroesophageal reflux is associated with defective lower esophageal sphincter (LES) pressure or function. Patients may have reduced LES pressures related to spontaneous transient LES relaxations, Increased intraabdominal pressure, or an atonic LES (Table 27.1). A variety of foods and medications may decrease LES pressure.

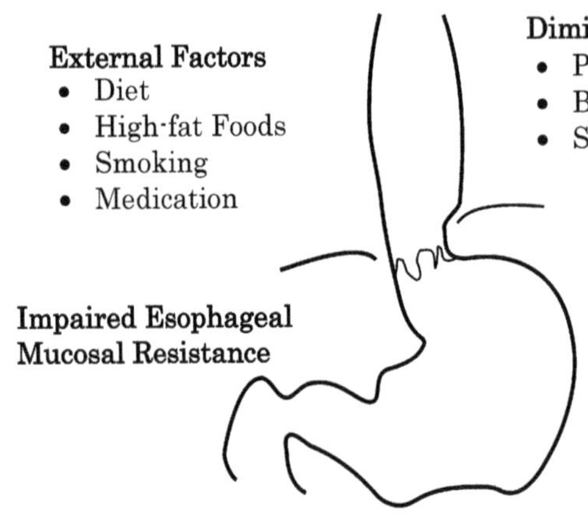

FIGURE 27.1

Pathophysiology of GERD.

(Source: http://ocw.tufts.edu/Content/48/lecturenotes/595117/595140)

- Problems related to normal mucosal defense mechanisms may also responsible for the development of GERD, including delayed gastric emptying, prolonged acid clearance time from the esophagus, and reduced mucosal resistance.
- Aggressive factors that causes esophageal damage upon reflux into the esophagus include gastric acid, bile acids, pepsin and pancreatic enzymes. The composition and volume of the refluxate and the duration of exposure are the most important factors in considering the consequences of gastroesophageal reflux.

CLINICAL FEATURES

The main symptom of gastroesophageal reflux and esophagitis is heartburn, or pyrosis. It is classically described as a sensation of warmth or burning that may radiate to the neck. It is waxing and waning in character and is often aggravated by activities that may increase the severity of gastroesophageal reflux (e.g., recumbent position, bending over, eating a high-fat meal). Other symptoms include water brash (hypersalivation), belching, and regurgitation.

- Atypical symptoms includes chronic cough, nonallergic asthma, hoarseness, dental erosions, pharyngitis, and chest pain that mimics angina.
- Inadequately treated GERD may lead to complications from long-term acid exposure such as continual pain, dysphagia, and odynophagia. Other complications includes esophageal strictures, hemorrhage, Barrett's esophagus, and esophageal adenocarcinoma.

Table 27.1

Foods and medications that may worsen gastroesophageal reflux disease symptoms

Decreased lower esophageal sphincter pressure	
Foods	
Fatty meal	Garlic
Carminatives (peppermint, spearmint)	Onions
Chocolate	Chili peppers
Coffee, cola, tea	
Medications	
Anticholinergics	Ethanol
Barbiturates	Nicotine (smoking)
Caffeine	Nitrates
Dihydropyridine calcium channel blockers	Progesterone
Dopamine	Tetracycline
Estrogen	Theophylline
Direct irritants to the esophageal mucosa	
Foods	
Spicy foods	Tomato juice
Orange juice	Coffee
Medications	
Aspirin	Iron
Bisphosphonates (e.g., alendronate)	Quinidine
Nonsteroidal antiinflammatory drugs	Potassium chloride

DIAGNOSIS

The diagnosis can be based on diagnostic tests including barium radiographs, esophagoscopy, esophageal motility testing, and/or ambulatory pH monitoring. These tests allow the clinician to demonstrate that reflux occurs and to quantitate it. When used appropriately they identify end-organ effects of reflux on the esophagus and larynx. These tests can also evaluate the effects of reflux on lower esophageal sphincter (LES) pressure and esophageal acid clearance.

- Barium radiography: Barium studies are highly inexpensive and widely available for use in diagnosis of esophageal disease. When evaluating the esophagus, a barium swallow (preferably with double contrast) should be ordered to ensure optimal evaluation. Ordering an upper GI series will often result in insufficient evaluation of esophageal function, concentrate excessively on the stomach and duodenum, and not pay careful attention to potential mucosal or motility abnormalities in the esophagus. The best use of the barium study is in evaluation of suspected complications of GERD, including motility abnormalities or peptic stricture.
- Endoscopy is the single best test to document mucosal abnormalities and establish a diagnosis of erosive esophagitis or Barrett's esophagus in the patient with suspected gastroesophageal reflux disease. When patients with heartburn and regurgitation are evaluated prospectively, endoscopy reveals erosive esophagitis in 45-60% (4) of patients, with the remainder having nonerosive disease (mucosal edema, hyperemia, or a normal-appearing esophagus).
- Laryngoscopic examination in suspected reflux-related laryngitis reveals edema and erythema of the arytenoid cartilage, posterior larynx and posterior portion of true vocal folds.
- Mucosal biopsy and cytology are of limited value in evaluation of the patient with GERD unless Barrett's esophagus or malignancy is suspected. The light microscopic signs of GERD [elongation of rete pegs and hyperplasia of the basal cell layer] do not distinguish between acute and chronic disease and do not help predict the response to therapy. It is our feeling that these findings are nonspecific and do not aid in the diagnosis of GERD.
- Ambulatory pH monitoring is the best test for quantifying esophageal reflux and determining if symptoms are due to GERD. Now a widely available technology, it is usually performed by placing a 2-mm-diameter catheter transnasally into the esophagus with the distal antimony electrode placed 5 cm above the lower esophageal sphincter, which is located by esophageal manometry.
- Esophageal manometry is useful to establish abnormality of LES pressure or esophageal motility and to obtain preoperative information for the surgeon. Decreased lower esophageal sphincter pressure is a major determinant of gastroesophageal reflux, but a single measurement of LES pressure is rarely low in patients with GERD.

TREATMENT (TABLE 27.2)

The primary goal of managing GERD with or without associated extraesophageal disease is complete symptom resolution. Additional therapeutic endpoints include healing of esophagitis when present, prevention of complications such as peptic stricture or Barrett's esophagus, and the maintenance of symptom control in patients with chronic disease. The overall management strategies can be classified as lifestyle changes, pharmacologic manipulations of gastric acid and motility.

ANTACIDS/ALGINIC ACID

Used on an as needed basis, antacids and alginic acid are the mainstay of rapid, safe, effective relief of heartburn symptoms. Antacids primarily work by neutralizing acid, albeit for relatively short periods of time. Therefore, patients need to take antacids frequently, usually 20-30 minutes after meals and bedtime, depending on the severity of symptoms. Liquid forms are preferable to tablets, although the latter are the most popular preparation of this medication. Containing antacids and alginic acid, Gaviscon is a popular over-the-counter treatment for GERD. The active component of this medication, alginic acid, interacts with saliva to form a highly viscous solution that floats on the surface of the gastric pool, acting as a mechanical barrier. The barrier reduces the number of reflux episodes and diminishes esophageal acid exposure during the day but not at night. Antacids and alginic acid are effective for relieving mild to moderate intermittent reflux symptoms. They are particularly useful in patients with situational heartburn brought on by lifestyle changes or pregnancy. Even in high doses, these agents are not effective in healing esophagitis. Excessive use of antacids may be associated with side effects. Magnesium containing antacids produce diarrhea, while aluminum-containing products are constipating. The potential for magnesium or aluminum toxicity further limits their use in patients with significant renal disease. Low-sodium antacids (e.g., magaldrate-Riopan) are preferable for individuals on salt-restricted diets. Antacids and alginic acid are the initial agents of choice for treating reflux symptoms in pregnant women since they are nontoxic. In this special situation, adverse effects are rare but include interference with iron absorption, with ingestion of sodium bicarbonate, metabolic alkalosis and fluid overload in both the fetus and mother.

H2-RECEPTOR ANTAGONISTS

The four currently available H2-receptor antagonists (H2-RAs), cimetidine, ranitidine, famotidine, and nizatidine, act competitively and reversibly to inhibit stimulation of the parietal cell by histamine. The plasma concentration of the drug correlates approximately with the degree of inhibition. These agents block nocturnal acid secretion more effectively, having minimal effect on meal-stimulated acid secretion. H2-receptor antagonists have no significant effect on gastric emptying, LES pressure, or pancreatic secretion. Overall, H2-RAs decrease acid reflux by 30–50%. Standard doses of H2-RAs given twice a day (morning and before supper) alleviate symptoms of GERD and heal mild to moderate erosive esophagitis. The typical duration for these studies ranges from 6 to 12 weeks. Some patients, failing a course of standard dose of H2-RAs, may be hypersecretors of acid; they may require higher and more frequent doses of the H2-RAs. Ranitidine is the only H2-RA approved for the maintenance healing of erosive esophagitis. The recommended dose is 150 mg twice daily, with placebo-controlled trials having been carried out for one year.

All the H2-RAs are now available over the counter, usually at 50% the prescription dose. Their use is similar to that of antacids for the treatment of intermittent heartburn, although the rapidity of relief is not as good as with antacids. The over-the-counter H2-RAs are superior to antacids in preventing reflux episodes after large meals, exercise, or other provocative situations when given 30 minutes before the refluxogenic activity.

The H2-RAs have an excellent side-effect profile and a low incidence of the following adverse reactions: central nervous system disturbances (especially cimetidine in high concentrations), headaches, diarrhea, gynecomastia, and impotence.

Drug interactions (cimetidine binds to the cytochrome P-450 system with greater affinity than does ranitidine) include those with theophylline, warfarin, phenytoin, and benzodiazepines. Neither famotidine nor nizatidine interacts with the cytochrome P-450 system. The H2-RAs cross the placental blood barrier and are excreted in breast milk. A recent large case-control study in Canada, however, found no adverse side effects in pregnant women taking this class of drugs at any stage of pregnancy. Therefore, the H2-RAs can be used in pregnant women with very severe reflux symptoms not responding to lifestyle changes or antacids.

PROMOTILITY AGENTS

The newer promotility agents, cisapride and domperidone, are effective in the treatment of mild to moderate heartburn and healing mild erosive esophagitis. This class of drugs improves GERD by augmenting lower esophageal sphincter pressure, increasing the amplitude of esophageal peristalsis and thereby improving acid clearance, and accelerating gastric emptying or modifying duodenogastric reflux, if abnormal.

The older agents, including metoclopramide and bethanechol, were not particularly effective and were frequently associated with central nervous system side effects. Recent data shows that cisapride at 10 mg four times a day (30 minutes before meals and bedtime) provides symptomatic relief and healing of esophagitis with results comparable to cimetidine 400 mg four times a day or ranitidine 150 mg twice a day and superior to placebo. Some data suggest there may be benefit combining the promotility agents with the H2-RAs. Additional data suggest that cisapride may be effective as maintenance therapy for mild GERD. Side effects are infrequent with cisapride and usually consist of abdominal pain, diarrhea, or headaches. Metoclopramide has been used safely as an antiemetic agent during pregnancy for about 30 years.

H^+/K^+-ATPASE (ACID PROTON PUMP) INHIBITORS

Acid-forming parietal cells are located in the oxyntic glands of the gastric fundus and body. Parietal cell membrane consists of three classes of receptors: histamine, paracrine receptors; gastrin, endocrine receptors; and acetylcholine, neurocrine (muscarinic) receptors. All of these receptors mediate the final step in the secretion of hydrochloric acid through the activation of the H^+/K^+-ATPase acid pump.

Antacids have no direct influence on gastric acid secretion. These agents work by neutralizing the gastric acid secreted by parietal cells, thereby increasing the intragastric pH. Both the H2-RAs and the acid proton pump inhibitors block acid secretion. The H2-RAs only block histamine receptors on the parietal cell surface, while the gastrin and acetylcholine receptors are still active and can augment acid secretion. On activation of the parietal cell, the enzyme H^+/K^+- ATPase moves from the cytoplasm of the gastric parietal cell to the permeable membrane of the secretory canaliculi . The enzyme can subsequently move hydrogen ions across the parietal cell membrane in exchange for potassium ions, thereby secreting acid with a pH of about 1.0. Both of the currently available substituted benzimidazoles, more commonly called proton pump inhibitors (omeprazole and lansoprazole), bind to the H^+/K^+-ATPase enzyme, thus blocking acid secretion. Since both nocturnal and meal-stimulated acid is inhibited, a single morning dose maintains gastric pH at 5 or more for almost 24 hours, decreases gastric volume by over 60%, and normalizes acid reflux parameters in over 80% of patients . Proton pump inhibitors have no effect on LES pressure.

In general, the proton pump inhibitors are well tolerated and easy to use with dosing either once or twice a day. Rare side effects include diarrhea, nausea, dry mouth, dizziness, weakness, headaches, and numbness. However, these side effects are no more common than with placebo in the published studies. Omeprazole inhibits selective isoenzymes of the cytochrome P-450 system, including those that metabolize phenytoin, warfarin sodium, and benzodiazepines (but not theophylline or propranolol). On the other hand, lansoprazole minimally inhibits this system and does not appear to significantly interfere with other drugs metabolized by cytochrome P-450 . The major long-term concern with using the proton pump inhibitors is their ability to produce a profound decrease in gastric acid secretion. This causes a secondary increase in gastrin production from the antral G cells resulting in serum gastrin levels usually elevated two to four times above basal values. Theoretically, the prolonged gastrin stimulation of enterochromaffin-like (ECL) cells could produce tropic changes in the gastric mucosa and was associated with increased stomach tumors in rats treated for a lifetime.

However, the human experience with the use of proton pump inhibition is over a decade, with a number of patients with severe reflux esophagitis taking the drug continuously for up to 10 years. There have not been any reported cases of gastric carcinoid-type tumors in patients receiving either omeprazole or lansoprazole, with the rare exception of subjects with the multiple endocrine adenomatosis syndrome where carcinoid tumors are commonly seen.

Table 27.2

Therapeutic approach to Gastroesophageal Reflux Disease (GERD)

Patient Presentation	Recommended Treatment	Comments
	Regimen or Proton pump inhibitors (for 4–8 weeks); all are given once daily • Rabeprazole 20 mg • Pantoprazole 40 mg • Omeprazole 20 mg • Lansoprazole 15 mg • Esomeprazole 20 mg	Patients with moderate to severe symptoms should receive a proton pump inhibitor as initial therapy.
Healing of erosive esophagitis or treatment of patients presenting with moderate to severe symptoms or complications	Lifestyle modifications plus Proton pump inhibitors for 4–16 weeks (up to twice daily) • Omeprazole 20 mg daily • Lansoprazole 30 mg daily • Esomeprazole 20–40 mg daily • Rabeprazole 20 mg daily • Pantoprazole 40 mg daily	For atypical or alarm symptoms, obtain endoscopy (if possible) to evaluate mucosa. Give a trial of a proton pump inhibitor. If symptoms are relieved, consider MT. Proton pump inhibitors are the most effective maintenance therapy in patients with atypical symptoms, complications, and erosive disease.
	High dose H_2-receptor antagonist (for 8–12 weeks) • Cimetidine 400 mg four times daily or 800 mg twice daily • Famotidine 40 mg twice daily • Nizatidine 150 mg four times daily • Ranitidine 150 mg four times daily Antireflux surgery or endoscopic therapies	Patients not responding to pharmacologic therapy, including those with persistent atypical symptoms, should be evaluated via ambulatory reflux monitoring to confirm the diagnosis of GERD (if possible).

LIFESTYLE MODIFICATIONS

Lifestyle changes include eating smaller meals and avoiding the supine position soon after meals, dietary modification to avoid certain types of foods as well as alcohol, weight reduction, smoking cessation, and elevation of the head of the bed for sleep. The lifestyle changes are intuitively appealing to physicians since they do not have side effects. These changes have other obvious medical benefits; they are within the "patient's control," and these changes are "simply the right thing to do." Although all patients could be counseled about these lifestyle changes, the reality is that probably only a small subset of patients experiences significant relief with these interventions alone.

Nocturnal acid reflux can be particularly damaging, as the normal acid clearance mechanisms are impaired. Gravity is not effective, as we usually sleep in the supine or prone position. During sleep esophageal peristalsis is minimal and saliva (pH 6.8–7.4) is not made the reason we awaken with a "cotton mouth or dry mouth" in the morning. Limited data suggest that elevating the head of the bed 6–8 inches protects the esophagus from acid reflux during sleep . Placing pillows under the head is usually not enough; the head and upper body elevation typically requires placement of a foam wedge underneath the mattress or blocks underneath the headboard to elevate the entire bed. The impact of this maneuver reduced the time of esophageal pH < 4 from 22 to 14% in one study. This recommendation should target patients with nocturnal reflux symptoms and/ or nocturnal asthma symptoms such as wheezing, chest tightness, and coughing.

Cigarette smoking through the pharmacologic effect of nicotine contributes to GERD by decreasing lower esophageal sphincter (LES) pressure, increasing the frequency of reflux episodes, and decreasing acid clearance. Smoking cessation alone can significantly improve respiratory symptoms in patients with asthma. In the only study to investigate the impact of cessation of cigarette smoking on GERD, it was found that the immediate discontinuation of smoking decreased the number of daily reflux episodes but did not affect the total esophageal acid exposure in patients without esophagitis. Therefore, the contribution of cigarette smoking to GERD may only be modest; nevertheless, it should be recommended vigorously to all patients for the other overwhelming medical benefits.

Patients who give a history of worsening reflux symptoms with certain foods should be counseled about avoiding these products. Foods can aggravate reflux symptoms by a number of mechanisms, including increased gastric volume producing gastric distention and transient LES relaxation, food contents directly lowering LES pressure, and direct irritant effects of food, possibly due to hyperosmolarity on inflamed esophageal mucosa. Fatty foods, alcohol, and chocolates are generally best avoided, especially prior to assuming the supine position. Also, a variety of medications, both prescribed and over-the-counter, can lower esophageal sphincter pressure and have direct effects by producing gastric and esophageal mucosal damage. Drugs in the former group include progesterone, theophylline, several prostaglandins, anticholinergic drugs, oral β-adrenergic agonists, β-dopamine, diazepam, meperidine, morphine, and calcium channel blockers. Medications commonly causing direct injury to the esophagus include doxycycline, slow-release potassium, ascorbic acid, ferrous sulfate, aspirin, nonsteroidal anti-inflammatory drugs, quinidine, and alendronates. It appears that inhaled α-agonists such as salbutamol do not affect esophageal function . Whether obesity actually contributes to GERD and whether weight loss has beneficial effects is unknown.

REFERENCES

1. Robinson M, Lanza F, Avner D, Haber M. Effective maintenance treatment of reflux esophagitis with low-dose lansoprazole. Ann Intern Med 1996; 124:859–867.
2. Ismail-Beigi F, Horton PF, Pope CE. Histological consequences of gastroesophageal reflux in man. Gastroenterology 1970; 58:163–174.
3. DeVault KR, Castell DO. Guidelines for the diagnosis and treatment of gastroesophageal reflux disease. Arch Intern Med 1995; 155:2165–2173.
4. Pope CE. Acid-reflux disorders. N Engl J Med 1994; 331:654–660.
5. Simpson WG. Gastroesophageal reflux disease and asthma. Arch Intern Med 1995;155:798–804.
6. Howden CW, Castell DO, Cohen S, Freston JW, Orlando RC, Robinson M. The rationale for continuous maintenance treatment of reflux disease. Arch Intern Med 1995; 155:1465–1471.
7. Richter JE, Castell DO. Gastroesophageal reflux: pathogenesis, diagnosis, and therapy. Ann Intern Med 1982; 97:93–103.

CHAPTER 28

Ascites

INTRODUCTION

Ascites is defined as accumulation of fluid in the peritoneal cavity. It is a common complication of cirrhosis, indicating portal hypertension which occurs in 80– 85% of patients with ascites. Nearly 60% of patients with compensated liver cirrhosis develop ascites within 10 years after onset of the liver disease. Once patients have developed ascites their prognosis is poor; nearly half of them die within 2– 3 years. However, other less common causes of ascites should be evaluated in the differential diagnosis of ascites. Other causes of ascites are, for example, malignancy (10%), cardiac failure (5%) and abdominal tuberculosis (2%).

ETIOLOGY

The causes of ascites may be grouped into two different pathological pathways .

The first group is not associated with peritoneal disease and consists of diseases which

(i) Cause a general flow block such as sinusoidal portal hypertension (acute alcoholic hepatitis, cirrhosis, subacute viral or toxic hepatitis, congestive heart failure, constrictive pericarditis, inferior vena cava obstruction, and hepatic venoocclusive disease, i.e. after bone marrow transplantation);
(ii) Lead to hypoalbuminemia (nephrotic syndrome, protein-losing enteropathy, and malnutrition)
(iii) Include a variety of disorders which may lead to ascites through different mechanisms such as myxedema, ovarian diseases (carcinoma, benign tumors, ovarian hyperstimulation syndrome), chronic pancreatitis, biliary tract leakage (biliary tract surgery, secondary to liver trauma, or transhepatic cholangiography), diseases affecting the lymphatic system of the splanchnic area, and chronic renal failure.

In the second group ascites is formed as a consequence of primary peritoneal disease or as a result of peritoneal involvement in systemic processes such as tuberculosis, fungal (*Candida albicans, Coccidioides immitis*) infection, parasitic and granulomatous peritonitis (sarcoidosis, Crohn's disease, peritoneal granulo-matous reaction to talc, cotton and wood fibers, starch and barium), primary or metastatic peritoneal tumors, vasculitis (systemic lupus erythematosus, Wegener's granulomatosis, Henoch–Schönlein purpura), eosinophilic gastroenteritis, and Whipple's disease.

SOME COMMON CAUSES OF ASCITES

MALIGNANT ASCITES

Approximately 50% of all malignant ascites are due to peritoneal carcinomatosis. In patients with malignancy- related ascites, serum ascites albumin gradient (SAAG) is usually low in up to 80-85% of the cases and ascites may be bloody. The ascitic cell count is generally high with normal glucose, normal LDH and elevated cholesterol levels. Cytological investigation is specific with a low sensitivity of <70%.

CARDIAC ASCITES

Ascites due to heart failure may be difficult to distinguish from ascites due to cirrhosis. Common causes are ischemic heart disease, cardiomyopathy, valvular and restrictive lung disease and constrictive pericarditis. The characteristics of cardiac ascetic fluid are high SAAG (>1.1 g/dl) with a high total protein level (>2.5 g/dl). Sometimes it is necessary to carry out a more invasive testing procedure such as measurement of the hepatic venous pressure gradient.

TUBERCULOUS PERITONITIS

The mechanism of formation of ascites is exudation of fluid from the peritoneal surface affected by the disease. The SAAG and protein is variable, the SAAG is often <1.1 g/dl and the protein value >2.5 g/dl.

The ascitic cell count is elevated between 1,000 and 3,000/mm3 with a predominance of lymphocytes. The red blood cell count in ascites could be mildly elevated. Glucose values are usually within the normal limits, and LDH levels could be high.Fluid culture and polymerase chain reaction- based analysis should be performed. A direct smear is not recommended because of a low sensitivity

HISTORY AND PHYSICAL EXAMINATION

Ascites is rarely the sole physical finding. Evidence of liver disease must be considered (jaundice, spider angiomata, palmar erythema, caput medusae, muscle wasting, splenomegaly, gynecomastia). Edema of the lower extremities or significant proteinuria may suggest a nephrotic syndrome as the cause of ascites due to, for example, glomerulonephritis, collagen diseases or diabetes. Jugular venous distention, pathologic heart sound, pulmonary crackles, dyspnea and peripheral edema imply right-side heart failure. Clinical tests for ascites include inspection for bulging flanks and flank dullness and the fluid wave test.

DIAGNOSTIC TESTS FOR ASCITES

Following diagnostic paracentesis of ascites, it has to be decided which tests should be performed and which parameters should be analyzed.

While many tests are available, it is neither useful nor cost effective to carry them all out. Further tests can be performed as indicated by the initial specimen (Tabl 28.1). As most patients with ascites have liver disease, exclusion of malignancy, tuberculosis or other less common causes is normally not required after the first paracentesis.

CELL COUNT

Cell count, as a mandatory test, may be performed in an EDTA tube using a small amount of fluid. The average normal total white blood cell count in patients with ascites due to liver disease is 100– 500/mm3. In bloody ascites, the white blood cell count could be misinterpreted: one polymorphonuclear leukocyte (PMN) count per 250 red blood cells can be taken as contamination. In SBP, the total white blood cell count as well as the absolute PMN count are elevated. A PMN count >250/mm^3 is defined as spontaneous bacterial peritonitis (SBP) and indicates initiation of an empiric antibiotic regime

In tuberculous or malignant ascites, lymphocytes dominate in the ascitic fluid . If malignant ascites is suspected, cytology should be performed. If tuberculosis is suspected, microbiological tests and a polymerase chain reaction- based method can be performed.

CYTOLOGY

Ascitic fluid cytology should be performed in suspected cases of malignancy- related ascites. The fluid should be examined rapidly after paracentesis – either fresh or fixed. The amount of ascitic fluid should be 50 – 100 ml. Cell count is often elevated in malignant ascites. However, in patients with hepatocellular carcinoma ascitic cytology is positive in <10% .

TOTAL PROTEIN

Ascites used to be divided into exudative and transudative types using a cut- off value of 2.5 g/dl total protein [9]. Ascites due to secondary abdominal processes like malignancy or abdominal tuberculosis (50%) would be exudates (>2.5 g/dl), whereas ascites due to portal hypertension would be transudates (<2.5 g/dl). However, approximately 20% of cirrhotic patients have an ascitic total protein of >2.5 g/dl and would therefore be categorized incorrectly . Furthermore, patients with cardiac ascites have a high total protein (>2.5 g/dl).

SERUM ASCITES ALBUMIN GRADIENT

Calculation of the serum ascites albumin gradient (SAAG) may differentiate the causes of ascites into two groups. It helps determine whether or not ascites is related to portal hypertension. The gradient can be calculated by measuring the albumin concentration in blood and ascitic fluid and subtracting the ascitic from the serum value. If a patient has portal hypertension, there must be a high oncotic gradient, which means a high albumin gradient between blood and ascitic fluid.

If the SAAG is > 1.1 g/dL, the cause of ascites is portal hypertension with a reliability of more than 90% [9], another cause could be cardiac disease with a high protein content in ascitic fluid.

While SAAG enables differentiation of ascites into one of two categories, it cannot replace further evaluation. A SAAG of < 1.1 g/dL indicates that the patient does not have portal hypertension, but that a process such as peritoneal carcinomatosis, abdominal tuberculosis, pancreatic ascites, nephrotic syndrome, or biliary ascites may be present.

MICROBIOLOGICAL CULTURE AND GRAM STAIN

Ascites culture is negative in approximately 40% of patients with SBP. The cultures should be collected at the bedside, including aerobic and anaerobic media with a minimum amount of 10 mL ascitic fluid. Ascitic fluid gram stain is generally a useless investigation due to the low concentration of bacteria in patients with SBP.

OTHER ASCITIC FLUID TESTS

CHOLESTEROL

No laboratory test completely distinguishes malignant ascites from ascites associated with cirrhosis. It has been suggested that a fraction of the cholesterol could be derived from a malignant cell . Measurement of total ascitic cholesterol concentration seems to be a rapid and cost- effective diagnostic test for discrimination between ascites of malignant and benign origin. A cholesterol concentration of >45 mg/dL is suspicious for malignant ascites.

LACTATE DEHYDROGENASE

Lactate dehydrogenase (LDH) as a diagnostic test has little clinical relevance in delineating the cause of ascites. An elevation of LDH is common in SBP, tuberculous peritonitis or secondary bacterial peritonitis with a fluid:serum LDH ratio >0.5, a ratio >1.0 is suspicious of abdominal tuberculosis.

GLUCOSE

The ascitic glucose concentration does not fall during intraperitoneal infection. Gut perforation seems to be one exception. Low levels of glucose in ascitic fluid compared to serum glucose levels could indicate secondary bacterial peritonitis.

AMYLASE

Ascitic amylase is increased if amylase is released into ascitic fluid, e.g. due to pancreatitis or gut perforation. In pancreatic ascites, the amylase concentration is often higher than that found in gut perforation .

TUMOR MARKERS

Measurement of tumor markers in ascitic fluid like carcinoembryonic antigen has been suggested as an aid in the diagnosis of malignancy- related ascites. However, this has achieved only little clinical relevance because of its low sensitivity.

Table 28.1

Ascitic tests

Mandatory	Optional	Rarely used
Cell count/ differential	Albumin (ascitic and blood)	Bilirubin
Total protein	Cytology	Triglycerides
	Culture	Tumor markers
	Cholesterol	LDH
		Glucose
		Amylase

TREATMENT

DIURETICS

Loop diuretics, includes furosemide, and potassium sparing diuretics, in particular aldosterone antagonists, are the drugs most commonly used in the treatment of ascites in patients with cirrhosis. Other diuretics such as thiazide diuretics and metolazone, which inhibit sodium reabsorption in the cortical diluting segment or actetazolamide, an inhibitor of carbonic anhydrase activity in the renal proximal tubule, are sometimes considered only for treatment of ascites resistant to high doses of both an aldosterone antagonist and a loop diuretic. All diuretics inhibit the absorption of $Na+$, Cl^- and water by their interaction with luminal uptake mechanisms.

Diuretics are kidney specific, not because they interfere with proteins specific for the kidney but because, with the only exception of aldosterone antagonists, they are secreted into the lumen of the tubule. This secretion, together with the water absorption along the tubule, contributes to the high free concentrations of diuretics in the tubule lumen. Furosemide and thiazides are taken across the basolateral membrane by an anion exchanger while amiloride and triamterene are taken up by a cation exchanger. The exit step into the lumen is less clear but may involve ATP-driven pumps

ALDOSTERONE ANTAGONISTS

Aldosterone exerts its action on the epithelial cells of the late distal and collecting ducts by binding the cytosolic mineralocorticoid receptor. The aldosterone- receptor complex migrates into the nucleus and it increases both the synthesis of a longlasting protein that facilitates sodium transport from the tubular lumen by amiloride- sensitive sodium channel (ASSC) and de novo synthesis of channel proteins (ASSC, Na- K- ATPase). As a result, more sodium crosses the luminal membrane through ASSC and leaves the tubular cell through the Na- K- ATPase transporter located at the basolateral membrane. The drugs acting against them compete with aldosterone at the mineralocorticoid receptor, thus blocking their effect on gene expression .

This mechanism implies clinically relevant consequences: (a) The drug dosage to achieve full antagonism is proportional to the degree of hyperaldosteronism, and (b) The effect of antagonists has a latency of at least 48 h from their administration. Thus, making a decision about their efficacy and/or increasing dosage earlier is not rational.

Spironolactone is a 17- spirolactone steroid with high selectivity and efficacy, and is the most widely used aldosterone antagonist in clinical practice. This lipophylic molecule undergoes an almost complete first-pass effect in the liver, so that its action is promoted by its metabolite canrenone that contributes to, but does not fully account for the biological activity of spironolactone . In fact, spironolactone metabolism produces a number of further and still active molecules. This, along with their reduced clearance in cirrhosis, explains the persistent anti-mineralocorticoid effect after withdrawal lasting up to a week or more. Canrenoate, a hydrophilic molecule that can be administered i.v., derives from a modification of the canrenone lateral chain.

It has no intrinsic activity, but exerts biological effects by virtue of its inter-conversion with canrenone in the plasma, thus avoiding the hepatic first-pass effect. The epoxy derivative of aldosterone eplerenone has a more selective binding affinity for the mineralocorticoid receptor. It has been widely used for treating hypertension and heart failure, but no controlled studies in advanced cirrhosis and ascites are available.

Aldosterone antagonists undergo a ready and almost complete intestinal absorption (bioavailability 75–95%) facilitated by the presence of food. Their elimination half-life is prolonged (up to 24 h), and they can be administered once daily.

Spironolactone exerts anti-androgenic effects, leading to painful gynecomastia and impotence through different mechanisms: decreased testosterone production in the adrenal gland, secondary to microsomal cytochrome P450 (CP450) depletion and inhibition of the CP450- dependent enzymes 17α-hydroxylase and desmolase, and competitive inhibition of dihydrotestosterone-receptor binding, which interferes with its nuclear translocation. K-canrenoate metabolism has much less impact on CP450, and its anti-androgenic effects are substantially attenuated. Protection from such effects also derives from a more selective binding affinity for the mineralocorticoid receptor, as reported with epleronone.

Aldosterone antagonists favor bicarbonate and reduce hydrogen ion excretions, potentially leading to metabolic acidosis, but this seldom becomes clinically significant . Instead, hyperkalemia may be severe, but this usually occurs in patients with an impaired GFR. Otherwise, if aldosterone antagonist administration is followed by natriuresis, hyperkalemia does not develop even with high dosages.

The recommended starting dosage of spironolactone or other antagonists (canrenone, K- canrenoate) is 100–200 mg/day, which should be increased by 100 (200) mg/day every third day. 400 mg/day as the maximal recommended dose for spironolactone which can be extended to canrenone and K-canrenoate.

OTHER 'POTASSIUM- SPARING' DIURETICS

Triamterene and amiloride also act at the distal nephron, somehow mimicking the effect of aldosterone antagonists by blocking the ASSC. There are no controlled clinical trials devoted to the use of triamterene in cirrhosis.

LOOP DIURETICS

These organic acids are secreted into the tubular fluid by the proximal tubule and inhibit the Na^+ $2Cl^-$ K^+ symporter located in the luminal membrane of epithelial cells lining the thick ascending limb of Henle's loop. This nephron segment reabsorbs up to 25% of the filtered sodium load. Therefore, loop diuretics can exert an intense diuretic action as the distal nephron does not have the reabsorptive capacity to compensate for this increased load; Part of the loop diuretic effect is mediated by prostaglandin E2 synthesis, and nonsteroidal anti- inflammatory agents impair their efficacy.

Loop diuretics are rapidly absorbed by the gut (30 min to 2 h); their bioavailability is variable, ranging from about 80% for bumetanide and torasemide to 40-60% for furosemide. Their action occurs promptly: it starts within 30 min after oral administration, peaks within 1-2 h, and ends in 3-4 h. Whether furosemide pharmacokinetics are altered in cirrhosis is debated: some authors reported a reduced bioavailability, but others did not.

The most widely employed loop diuretic is furosemide. Guidelines indicate an initial oral dose of 20-40 mg/day, to be progressively increased every other day up to 160 mg/day. However, such a dosage can seldom be reached because of the occurrence of even severe side effects at lower doses. Similar indications can be followed for other loop diuretics, taking into account that 40 mg of furosemide is equivalent to about 1 mg of bumetanide, 30 mg of torasemide and 50 mg of ethacrynic acid.

Otoxicity is a potential side effect of loop diuretics, namely ethacrynic acid that has been almost abandoned for this reason. Other side effects are somehow exacerbated by the peculiar pathophysiological context of advanced cirrhosis. Their brisk and potent action can induce a sudden blood volume contraction that cannot be compensated by vasoconstriction because of the blunted cardiovascular responsiveness to vasoconstrictors. Thus, effective volemia deteriorates and worsens hyperaldosteronism, impairs GFR and increases arginine-vasopressin secretion, ultimately leading to renal failure and hyponatremia.Potassium, magnesium and calcium depletions are exacerbated by secondary hyperaldosteronism if an adequate aldosterone blockade is not achieved. The inhibition of sodium and chloride reabsorption at Henle's loop impairs free water clearance and favors hyponatremia. Because of hydrogen ion, chloride and potassium depletions, along with plasma volume contraction, hypochloremic alkalosis can ensue. Alkalosis favors hydrogen ion entry into the tubular cells, where it enhances ammonia generation, and augments blood- brain barrier permeability to ammonia. Hypovolemia, alkalosis and increased ammonia production can worsen or precipitate hepatic encephalopathy, a phenomenon that is amplified by concomitant hyponatremia.

There is no scientific evidence for preferring one loop diuretic to another. The main problem with this class of diuretics is related to their violent action, and a drug exerting a longer- term effect could be better tolerated. This may be the case of torasemide, but available data do not suggest a substantial advantage over furosemide. Under appropriate clinical conditions, continuous furosemide infusion could maximize its diuretic action and minimize untoward hemodynamic effects.

LARGE VOLUME PARACENTESIS

Approximately 10% of patients with cirrhosis develop ascites refractory to medical treatment alone and hence need serial therapeutic paracentesis. In large volume paracentesis (LVP) more than 5 liters of ascitic fluid is drained. Other indications for LVP may include tense ascites, respiratory distress, and impending rupture of the umbilical hernia prior to adequate USG examination of liver and transjugular intrahepatic portosystemic shunt (TIPS) placement.

If albumin is the plasma expander being infused, using 6-8 g/L is appropriate if greater than 5 liters of ascitic fluid is removed. This is useful since in about 20% of patients LVP gets complicated by postparacentesis circulatory dysfunction (PPCD) . As opposed to LVP, in total volume paracentesis (TVP) all the ascitic fluid is drained and this can be performed safely when albumin has been used. Both LVP and TVP are associated with immediate symptomatic relief but this is short lived as there is recurrence of ascites. Hence, repeated procedures are involved without a significant increase in survival.

Transjugular intrahepatic portosystemic shunt (TIPS) is yet another modality of treatment available for the treatment of refractory ascites. TIPS is a side-to-side portocaval shunt aimed at correcting the portal hypertension. It is hence effective in not only controlling ascites but also in preventing its re-accumulation. Comparing the effect of TIPS versus LVP in cirrhotics with refractory ascites, it was concluded that TIPS was significantly better than LVP in transplant- free survival but encephalopathy occurred more in the former group as compared to the latter. TIPS improved the quality of life in all patients apart from those who developed encephalopathy.

REFERENCES

1. Karim A: Spironolactone metabolism in man revisited; in Brunner HR (ed): Contemporary Trends in Diuretic Therapy. Amsterdam, Excerpta Medica, 1986, pp 22–37.
2. Bernardi M, Servadei D, Trevisani F, Rusticali AG, Gasbarrini G: Importance of plasma aldosterone concentration on the natriuretic effect of spironolactone in patients with liver cirrhosis and ascites. Digestion 1985; 31: 189–193.
3. Cordoba J, Minguez B: Hepatic encephalopathy. Semin Liver Dis 2008; 28: 70–80.
4. Gerbes AL, Jungst D, Xie YN, Permanetter W, Paumgartner G: Ascitic fluid analysis for the differentiation of malignancy-related and nonmalignantascites: proposal of a diagnostic sequence. Cancer 1991; 68: 1808–1814.
5. Sevinc A, Sari R, Fadillioglu E: The utility of lactate dehydrogenase isoenzyme pattern in the diagnostic evaluation of malignant and nonmalignant ascites. J Natl Med Assoc 2005; 97: 79–84.
6. Runyon BA, Hoefs JC: Ascitic fluid analysis in the differentiation of spontaneous bacterial peritonitis from gastrointestinal tract perforation into ascetic fluid. Hepatology 1984; 4: 447–450.
7. Runyon BA: Amylase levels in ascitic fluid. J Clin Gastroenterol 1987; 9: 172–174.
8. Sandhu BS, Sanyal AJ: Management of ascites in cirrhosis.Clin Liver Dis 2005; 9: 715–732.

CHAPTER 29

Dysphagia

Dysphagia means difficulty in transferring food from the mouth to the stomach. The process of swallowing food consists of 2 stages.

- The *oropharyngeal stage:* In this movement of the food bolus from the mouth to the esophagus occurs voluntarily.
- The *esophageal stage:* Involuntary movement of food through the esophagus into the stomach.

SIGNS AND SYMPTOMS

Signs and symptoms of pharyngeal dysphagia includes the following:

- Coughing
- Difficulty in swallowing
- Sialorrhea
- Sudden weight loss
- Change in dietary habits
- Pneumonia
- Changes in voice or speech (wet voice)
- Nasal regurgitation

Signs and symptoms of esophageal dysphagia includes the following:

- Sensation of food sticking in the chest
- Change in dietary habits
- Pneumonia heartburn, belching, sour regurgitation, and water brash.

DIAGNOSIS

Since history and physical examination alone may not be adequate to make a diagnosis in cases of silent aspiration, additional diagnostic tests, such as the following, may be needed:

- Endoscopic examination
- Transnasal esophagoscopy: Especially useful in cases of esophageal diverticula or tumor
- Pulmonary function tests
- Imaging studies: CT scanning, MRI, chest radiography
- Esophageal pH monitoring: In this a nasogastric probe is inserted into the esophagus of the patient to record pH levels, and these values are compared with the patient's symptoms over 24 hours to know whether acid reflux is responsible.
- Blood tests: vitamin B-12, TSH and creatine kinase; may be useful in neurogenic dysphagia

ETIOLOGY

CENTRAL NERVOUS SYSTEM DISORDERS

Central nervous system (CNS) pathologies that can produce dysphagia include the following:

- Alzheimer disease
- Brain tumors
- Guillain-Barré syndrome
- Huntington disease
- CNS infections
- Stroke
- Traumatic brain injury (TBI)
- Parkinson disease
- Poliomyelitis
- Cerebral palsy
- Multiple sclerosis
- Amyotrophic lateral sclerosis (ALS)

MUSCULAR DISORDERS

Muscular disorders that can cause dysphagia include the following:

- Muscular dystrophies
- Spinal muscular atrophy
- Polymyositis
- Dermatomyositis

NEUROPATHIC DISORDERS

Dysphagia can result from sensory neuropathies affecting the laryngeal nerves.

ENDOCRINE DISORDERS

Dysphagia can result from the following:

- Secondary myopathies in Cushing syndrome, hyperthyroidism, and hypothyroidism
- Vitamin B-12 deficiency: Leading to pseudobulbar palsy secondary to corticobulbar tract dysfunction

PHARMACOLOGICAL CAUSES

Various medications, including the following, can produce dysphagia by causing a decrease in cognition or giving rise to drug-induced myopathies:

- CNS depressants
- Antipsychotics
- Corticosteroids
- Lipid-lowering agents
- Colchicine
- Aminoglycosides
- Anticholinergic drugs

Mucosal injury may be caused by the following drugs:

- Potassium chloride tablets
- Nonsteroidal anti-inflammatory drugs (NSAIDs)
- Antibiotics (eg, doxycycline, tetracycline, clindamycin, trimethoprim sulfamethoxazole)

Xerostomia may be caused by the following agents:

- Anticholinergics
- Alpha-adrenergic blockers
- Angiotensin-converting enzyme (ACE) inhibitors
- Antihistamines

SURGICAL CAUSES

Surgeries that can lead to dysphagia include the following:

- Laryngectomy
- Pharyngectomy, esophagectomy reconstructed by gastric pull-up
- Head and neck surgery (oral cavity cancer)
- Surgery involving the pharyngeal plexus during cervical fusion or carotid endarterectomy

ADDITIONAL IATROGENIC CAUSES OF DYSPHAGIA

These include the following:

- Use of a cervical brace
- Ventilator dependency

PSYCHOGENIC DYSPHAGIA

This diagnosis is one of exclusion. The condition is characterized by oral apraxia with intact speech and pharyngoesophageal and neurologic function.

Associated psychiatric conditions include anxiety, depression, somatoform disorders, hypochondriasis, conversion disorders, and eating disorders. Psychiatric evaluation and treatment often are needed.

Instances of swallowed foreign bodies do occur (bezoars), especially in patients with developmental disabilities, and this possibility also should be considered.

MOTILITY DISORDERS

Motility disorders that can produce dysphagia include the following:

- Diffuse esophageal spasms (DES)
- Achalasia (megaesophagus)
- Scleroderma
- Presbyesophagus
- Cricopharyngeal dysfunction

ESOPHAGITIS

The following may also result in dysphagia:

- Gastroesophageal reflux disease (GERD)
- Infectious esophagitis (eg, as in human immunodeficiency virus [HIV], herpes, candidiasis)
- Radiation esophagitis: Especially after radiation treatments of 4500 to 6000 radiation over 6-8 weeks
- Medication-induced esophagitis: May develop from enteric-coated nonsteroidal anti-inflammatory drugs (NSAIDs); substances such as quinidine, potassium, vitamins, and $FeSO_4$ also may produce esophageal injury

STRUCTURAL DISORDERS

These include the following:

- Zenker diverticulum at the upper esophagus or epiphrenic diverticula at the midesophagus or distal esophagus
- Esophageal strictures, webs, or rings
- Tracheoesophageal fistula
- Schatzki rings
- Plummer-Vinson or Paterson-Kelly syndromes and hypopharyngeal webs with iron deficiency anemia
- Cervical spondylosis

TREATMENT

The goals of dysphagia treatment are to maintain adequate nutritional intake for the patient and to maximize airway protection.

Disorders of oral and pharyngeal swallowing are usually amenable to rehabilitation, including dietary modification and training in swallowing techniques and maneuvers. Surgery is rarely indicated for patients with swallowing disorders, although in patients with severe disorders, bypassing the oral cavity and pharynx in their entirety and providing enteral nutrition may be necessary. Options include percutaneous endoscopic gastrostomy and intermittent oroesophageal catheterization.

Various treatments have been suggested for the treatment of oropharyngeal dysphagia in adults. Direct and indirect strategies for treating dysphagia have been described. Direct strategy usually refers to treatment that involves food, whereas indirect strategy refers to an exercise regimen performed without a food bolus. Direct techniques include modifications of food consistency; indirect techniques include stimulation of the oropharyngeal structures and the adoption of behavioral techniques, such as those involving postural changes or the swallow maneuver.

The Dietetics in Physical Medicine and Rehabilitation dietetic practice group conceived the National Dysphagia Diet project in 1996. This group became known as the National Dysphagia Diet Task Force (NDDTF). Growing frustration regarding a lack of standardization for solid-food textures, liquid consistencies, and nomenclature led to the formation of a task force to study the issue and to formulate a new diet based on scientific food properties and clinical swallowing problems. In 2002, the American Dietetic Association established the National Dysphagia Diet (NDD) to provide national guidelines and standardized terminology for texture modification for dysphagia management. The NDD contains suggested viscosity ranges for different types of modified fluids.

PHARMACOLOGICAL TREATMENT

Medications used in the treatment of dysphagia include the following:

- Botulinum toxin type A (BoNT-A): Injected endoscopically into the gastroesophageal sphincter and upper esophagus to decrease tone; this can be very useful in cricopharyngeal spasms causing dysphagia
- Diltiazem: Can aid in esophageal contractions and motility, especially in the disorder known as the nutcracker esophagus
- Glucagon: Used in disimpacting esophageal bodies; diazepam also is sometimes used; no major study has proved the effectiveness of either drug
- Cystine-depleting therapy with cysteamine: Treatment of choice for patients with dysphagia due to pretransplantation or posttransplantation cystinosis
- Nitrates: Including isosorbide dinitrate, which can especially be recommended in achalasia

DIETARY MODIFICATION

Dietary modification is the key component in the general treatment program of dysphagia. A diet of pureed foods is recommended for patients who have difficulties with the oral preparatory phase of swallowing, who pocket food in the buccal recesses, or who have significant pharyngeal retention of chewed solid foods.

As patients' swallowing function improves, their dysphagic diet may be advanced to the next level of soft and semisolid foods with regular consistencies. Recommend to patients that they alternate bites with sips, bite or sip size, and the number of swallows per size.

MEDICATION SUMMARY

The goals of pharmacotherapy are to prevent complications and reduce morbidity.

Histamine H2 Antagonists

Class Summary

These agents are used prophylactically to prevent complications.

View full drug information

CIMETIDINE

Cimetidine inhibits histamine at H2 receptors of gastric parietal cells, which results in reduced gastric acid secretion, gastric volume, and hydrogen concentrations.

RANITIDINE

Ranitidine inhibits histamine stimulation of the H2 receptor in gastric parietal cells, which, in turn, reduces gastric acid secretion, gastric volume, and hydrogen ion concentrations.

FAMOTIDINE

Famotidine competitively inhibits histamine at the H2 receptor of gastric parietal cells, resulting in reduced gastric acid secretion, gastric volume, and hydrogen ion concentrations.

NIZATIDINE

Nizatidine competitively inhibits histamine at the H2 receptor of the gastric parietal cells, resulting in reduced gastric acid secretion, gastric volume, and reduced hydrogen concentrations.

PROTON PUMP INHIBITORS

CLASS SUMMARY

Proton pump inhibitors inhibit gastric acid secretion by inhibition of the H^+-K^+-ATPase enzyme system in the gastric parietal cells. They are used prophylactically in cases not responsive to H2-antagonist therapy.

OMEPRAZOLE (PRILOSEC)

Omeprazole decreases gastric acid secretion by inhibiting the parietal cell H^+/K^+-adenosine triphosphate (ATP) pump at the secretory surface of gastric parietal cells.

LANSOPRAZOLE

Lansoprazole decreases gastric acid secretion by inhibiting the parietal cell H^+/K^+-ATP pump at the secretory surface of gastric parietal cells.

RABEPRAZOLE

Rabeprazole decreases gastric acid secretion by inhibiting the parietal cell H^+/K^+-ATP pump at the secretory surface of gastric parietal cells.

PANTOPRAZOLE

Pantoprazole decreases gastric acid secretion by inhibiting the parietal cell H^+/K^+-ATP pump at the secretory surface of gastric parietal cells.

ESOMEPRAZOLE

Esomeprazole inhibits gastric acid secretion by inhibiting the H^+/K^+-ATPase enzyme system at the secretory surface of gastric parietal cells at the secretory surface of gastric parietal cells.

REFERENCES

1. Arora AS, Yamazaki K. Eosinophiliceso-phagitis: asthma of the esophagus? Clin Gastroenterol Hepatol 2004;2:523-30.
2. Arora AS.Management strategies for dysphagia with a normalappearing esophagus. Clin Gastroenterol Hepatol 2005; 3(3): 299-302.
3. Roeder BE, Murray JA, Dierkhising RA. Patient localization of esophageal dysphagia. Dig Dis Sci 2004; 49: 697-701.
4. Spechler SJ. AGA technical review on treatment of patients with dysphagia caused by benign disorders of the distal esophagus. Gastroenterology 1999; 117: 233-54.
5. Varadarajulu S, Eloubeidi MA, Patel RS, Mulcahy HE, Barkun A, Jowell P, et al. The yield and the predictors of esophageal pathology when upper endoscopy is used for the initial evalua-tion of dysphagia Gastrointest Endosc 2005;61(7): 804-8.

CHAPTER 30

Liver Disease

DEFINITION

Liver disease is any disturbance of liver function that causes illness. The liver is responsible for many critical functions within the body and should it become diseased or injured, the loss of those functions can cause significant damage to the body. Liver disease is also referred to as hepatic disease.

CLASSIFICATION

- Hepatitis, inflammation of the liver, is caused mainly by various viruses (viral hepatitis) but also by some liver toxins (e.g. alcoholic hepatitis), autoimmunity (autoimmune hepatitis) or hereditary conditions.
- Alcoholic liver disease is a term used to describe any hepatic manifestation of alcohol over consumption, including fatty liver disease, alcoholic hepatitis, and cirrhosis. Analogous terms such as "drug-induced" or "toxic" liver disease are also used to refer to the range of disorders caused by various drugs and environmental chemicals.
- Fatty liver disease (hepatic steatosis) is a reversible condition where large vacuoles of triglyceride fat accumulate in liver cells. Non-alcoholic fatty liver disease is a spectrum of disease associated with obesity and metabolic syndrome, among other causes. Fatty liver may lead to inflammatory disease (i.e. steatohepatitis) and, eventually, cirrhosis.
- Cirrhosis is the formation of fibrous tissue (fibrosis) in the place of liver cells that have died due to a variety of causes, including viral hepatitis, alcohol overconsumption, and other forms of liver toxicity. Cirrhosis causes chronic liver failure.
- Primary liver cancer most commonly manifests as hepatocellular carcinoma and/or cholangiocarcinoma; rarer forms include angiosar-coma and hemang-iosarcoma of the liver. (Many liver malignancies are secondary lesions that have metastasized from primary cancers in the gastrointestinal tract and other organs, such as the kidneys, lungs, breast, or prostate.)
- Primary biliary cirrhosis is a serious autoimmune disease of the bile capillaries.
- Primary sclerosing cholangitis is a serious chronic inflammatory disease of the bile duct, which is believed to be autoimmune in origin.

- Budd-Chiari syndrome is the clinical picture caused by occlusion of the hepatic vein, which in some cases may lead to cirrhosis.
- Hereditary diseases that cause damage to the liver include hemochromatosis, involving accumulation of iron in the body, and Wilson's disease, which causes the body to retain copper. Liver damage is also a clinical feature of alpha 1-antitrypsin deficiency and glycogen storage disease type II.
- In transthyretin-related hereditary amyloidosis, the liver produces a mutated transthyretin protein which has severe neurodegenerative and/or cardiopathic effects. Liver transplantation can provide a curative treatment option.
- Gilbert's syndrome, a genetic disorder of bilirubin metabolism found in about 5% of the population, can cause mild jaundice.

ETIOLOGY

The liver can be damaged in a variety of ways.

- Cells can become inflamed (such as in hepatitis: hepar = liver + itis = inflammation).
- Bile flow can be obstructed (such as in cholestasis: chole = bile + stasis = standing).
- Cholesterol or triglycerides can accumulate (such as in steatosis; steat = fat + osis = accumulation).
- Blood flow to the liver may be compromised.
- Liver tissue can be damaged by chemicals and minerals, or infiltrated by abnormal cells.

ALCOHOL ABUSE

Alcohol abuse is the most common cause of liver disease in North America. Alcohol is directly toxic to liver cells and can cause liver inflammation, referred to as alcoholic hepatitis. In chronic alcohol abuse, fatty accumulation (steatosis) occurs in liver cells causing the cells to malfunction.

CIRRHOSIS

Cirrhosis is a late-stage liver disease. Scarring of the liver and loss of functioning liver cells cause the liver to fail.

DRUG-INDUCED LIVER DISEASE

Liver cells may become temporarily inflamed or permanently damaged by exposure to medications or drugs. Some medications or drugs require an overdose to cause liver injury while others may cause the damage even when taken in the appropriately prescribed dosage.

Taking excess amounts of acetaminophen (Tylenol, Panadol) can cause liver failure that is permanent. This is the reason that warning labels exist on many over-the-counter medications that contain acetaminophen and why prescription narcotic-acetaminophen combination medications (for example,Vicodin, Lortab, Norco, Tylenol #3) limit the numbers of tablets to be taken in a day.

Statin medications are commonly prescribed to control elevated blood levels of cholesterol. Even when taken in the appropriately prescribed dose, liver inflammation may occur and can be detected by blood tests that measure liver enzymes. Stopping the medication usually results in return of the liver function to normal.

Niacin is another medication used to control elevated blood levels of cholesterol, but liver inflammation for this medication is related to the dose taken. Similarly, patients with underlying liver disease may be at higher risk of developing liver disease due medications such as niacin.

There are numerous other medications that may cause liver inflammation, most of which will resolve when the medication is stopped. These include antibiotics such as nitrofurantoin (Macrodantin, Furadantin, Macrobid), amoxicillin and clavulanic acid (Augmentin, Augmentin XR), tetracycline (Sumycin), and isoniazid (INH, Nydrazid, Laniazid). Methotrexate (Rheumatrex, Trexall), a drug used to treat autoimmune disorders and cancers, has a variety of side effects including liver inflammation that can lead to cirrhosis. Disulfiram (Antabuse) used to treat alcoholics and can cause liver inflammation.

INFECTIOUS HEPATITIS

The term "hepatitis" means inflammation, and liver cells can become inflamed because of infection.

Hepatitis A is a viral infection that is caused primarily through the fecal-oral route when small amounts of infected fecal matter are inadvertently ingested. Hepatitis A causes an acute inflammation of the liver which generally resolves spontaneously. The hepatitis A vaccine can prevent this infection.

Hepatitis B is spread by exposure to body fluids (needles from drug abusers, contaminated blood, and sexual contact) and can cause an acute infection, but can also progress to cause chronic inflammation (chronic hepatitis) that can lead to cirrhosis and liver cancer. The hepatitis B vaccine prevents this infection.

Hepatitis C causes chronic hepatitis. An infected individual may not recall any acute illness. Hepatitis C is spread by exposure to body fluids (needles from drug abusers, contaminated blood, and sexual contact). Chronic hepatitis C may lead to cirrhosis and liver cancer. At present, there is no vaccine against this virus.

Hepatitis D is a virus that requires concomitant infection with hepatitis B to survive, and is spread via body fluid exposure (needles from drug abusers, contaminated blood, and sexual contact).

Hepatitis E is a virus that is spread via contaminated food and water exposure.

OTHER VIRUSES

Other viruses can also cause liver inflammation or hepatitis as part of the cluster of symptoms. Viral infections with infectious mononucleosis (Epstein Barr virus), adenovirus, and cytomegalovirus can inflame the liver. Non-viral infections such as toxoplasmosis and Rocky Mountain spotted fever are less common causes.

NON-ALCOHOLIC FATTY LIVER DISEASE

Accumulation of fat within the liver can cause gradual decrease in liver function. Also known as non-alcoholic steatohepatitis, fatty liver disease, or NASH.

HAEMOCHROMATOSIS

Haemachromatosis (iron overload) is a metabolic disorder that leads to abnormally elevated iron stores in the body. The excess iron may be found in the tissues of the liver, pancreas, and heart and can lead to inflammation, cirrhosis, liver cancer, and liver failure. Haemachromatosis is an inherited disease.

WILSON'S DISEASE

Wilson's disease is another inherited disease that affects the body's ability to metabolize copper. Wilson's disease may lead to cirrhosis and liver failure.

GILBERT'S DISEASE

In Gilbert's disease, there is an abnormality in bilirubin metabolism in the liver. It is a common disease that affects up to 7% of the North American population. There are no symptoms and it is usually diagnosed incidentally when an elevated bilirubin level is found on routine blood tests. Gilbert's disease is a benign condition and no treatment is necessary.

CANCERS

Primary cancers of the liver arise from liver structures and cells. Two examples include hepatocellular carcinoma and cholangiocarcinoma.

Metastatic cancer (secondary cancer of the liver) begins in another organ and spreads to the liver, usually through the blood stream. Common cancers that spread to the liver begin in the lung, breast, intestine, stomach, and pancreas. Leukemia and Hodgkin's lymphoma may also involve the liver.

BILE FLOW ABNORMALITIES

Normally, bile flows from the liver into the gallbladder and ultimately into the intestine to help with the digestion of food. If bile flow is obstructed, it can cause inflammation within the liver. Most commonly, gallstones can cause an obstruction of the ducts that drains bile from the liver.

Abnormalities of the opening of the bile duct into the intestine (sphincter of Oddi) can lead to abnormalities of bile flow. The sphincter of Oddi acts as a "valve" that allows bile to flow from the common bile duct into the intestine.

Primary biliary cirrhosis and primary sclerosing cholangitis can lead to progressive scarring of the bile ducts, causing them to become narrow, which results in reduced bile flow through the liver. Eventually, damage and scarring of the liver architecture causes liver failure to develop.

OTHER DISEASES AND CONDITIONS

Conditions such as portal hypertension (increased blood pressure within the portal vein), abnormal blood clotting, and hepatic encephalopathy (abnormal brain function due to elevated levels of ammonia in the blood stream).

CLINICAL FEATURES

- The symptoms related to liver dysfunction include both physical signs and a variety of symptoms related to digestive problems, blood sugar problems, immune disorders, abnormal absorption of fats, and metabolism problems.
- The malabsorption of fats may lead to symptoms that include indigestion, reflux, deficit of fat-soluble vitamins, haemorrhoids, gall stones, intolerance to fatty foods, intolerance to alcohol, nausea and vomiting attacks, abdominal bloating, and constipation.

- Nervous system disorders include depression, mood changes, especially anger and irritability, poor concentration and "foggy brain", overheating of the body, especially the face and torso, and recurrent headaches (including migraine) associated with nausea.
- The blood sugar problems include hypoglycaemia.
- Abnormalities in the level of fats in the blood stream, whether too high or too low levels of lipids in the organism. Hypercholesterolemia: elevated LDL cholesterol, reduced HDL cholesterol, elevated triglycerides, clogged arteries leading to high blood pressure, heart attacks and strokes, build up of fat in other body organs (fatty degeneration of organs), lumps of fat in the skin (lipomas and other fatty tumours), excessive weight gain (which may lead to obesity), inability to lose weight even while dieting, sluggish metabolism, protuberant abdomen (pot belly), cellulite, fatty liver, and a roll of fat around the upper abdomen (liver roll) etc. Or too low levels of lipids: hypocholesterolemia: low total cholesterol, low LDL and VLDL cholesterol, low triglyderides.

DIAGNOSIS

The precise diagnosis of liver disease involves a history and physical examination performed by the health care professional. Understanding the symptoms and the patient's risk factors for liver disease will help guide any diagnostic tests that may be considered.

Liver disease can have physical findings in almost all body systems including the heart, lungs, abdomen, skin, cognitive function, and other parts of the nervous system. The physical examination can require evaluation of the entire body.

- Blood tests are helpful in assessing liver inflammation and function.
- Specific liver function blood tests include:
- AST and ALT (transaminase chemicals released with liver cell inflammation);
- GGT and alkaline phosphatase (chemicals released by cells lining bile ducts); bilirubin; and
- Protein and albumin levels.

Other blood tests may be considered, including the following:

- Complete blood count (CBC), patients with end stage liver disease may have bone marrow suppression and low red blood cells, white blood cells and platelets;
- Electrolytes, BUN and creatinine to assess kidney function; and
- Ammonia blood level assessment is helpful in patients with mental confusion.

  Imaging studies may be used to visualize, not only the liver, but other organs nearby that may be diseased. Examples of imaging studies include:
- CT scan (computerized axial tomography),
- MRI (magnetic resonance imaging), and
- Ultrasound (sound wave imaging, which is especially helpful in assessing the gallbladder and bile ducts.

Liver biopsy may be considered to confirm a specific diagnosis for liver disease. Under local anaesthetic, a long thin needle is inserted through the chest wall into the liver, where a small sample of liver tissue is obtained for examination under a microscope.

TREATMENT

Each liver disease will have its own specific treatment regimen. For example, hepatitis A requires supportive care to maintain hydration while the body's immune system fights and resolves the infection. Patients with gallstones may require surgery to remove the gallbladder. Other diseases may need long-term medical care to control and minimize the consequences of their disease

In patients with cirrhosis and end-stage liver disease, medications may be required to control the amount of protein absorbed in the diet. The liver affected by cirrhosis may not be able to metabolize the waste products, resulting in elevated blood ammonia levels and hepatic encephalopathy. Low sodium diet and water pills (diuretics) may be required to minimize water retention.

In those with large amounts of ascites fluid, the excess fluid may have to be occasionally removed with a needle and syringe (paracentesis). Using local anaesthetic, a needle is inserted through the abdominal wall and the fluid withdrawn.

Operations may be required to treat portal hypertension and minimize the risk of bleeding. Liver is the final option for patients whose liver has failed.

The most effective way to treat alcoholic liver disease and non-alcoholic fatty liver disease is to make lifestyle changes, such as:

- Cutting out **alcohol**.
- Improving the **diet**.
- Taking **regular exercise**.

Anti-viral medications are available to treat infections such as **hepatitis B** and **hepatitis C**. This is an area of active research and drug development and today many treatments offer improved outcomes, by clearing or controlling the virus to slow any decline in the condition of your liver.

Other conditions may be managed by slowing down disease progression:

- By using steroid-based drugs in autoimmune hepatitis.
- Regularly removing a quantity of blood from a vein (venesection) in the iron overload condition, **haemochromatosis**.
- Wilson's disease, a condition where copper builds up in the body, can be managed with drugs which bind copper allowing it to be passed from the body in urine.

In cholestatic liver disease (where the flow of bile is affected) a medication called ursodeoxycholic acid (URSO, also referred to as UDCA) may be given. Made from naturally occurring bile acid, it may offer some protection for the liver from the harmful chemicals in the bile, slowing damage.

REVERSING THE DAMAGE FROM LIVER DISEASE

Fatty deposits in the liver or inflammation may be reversed once the cause of the damage is removed. Scarring such as fibrosis may also be improved. Once cirrhosis has developed, damage is more permanent, but removing the cause should prevent any further progression.

TREATING COMPLICATIONS OF LIVER DISEASE

Another aspect of treatment is to deal with the complications which occur in more advanced stages of liver damage.

PORTAL HYPERTENSION AND VARICEAL BLEEDING

Where scarring of the liver prevents blood from flowing, pressure may build-up in the portal vein (portal hypertension) and blood may be forced through more delicate veins (varices) which burst under the pressure.

Medicines including β blockers may be prescribed to reduce the risk and the severity of any bleed. If a bleed occurs, a technique known as 'banding' may be used where a small band is placed around the base of the vein to control the bleeding. Alternatively, a substance can be injected into the veins to induce clotting and scar tissue that will help stop the bleeding (injection sclerotherapy).

In some cases a tube with a balloon on the end is passed down the throat into the stomach. Once inflated, the balloon puts pressure on the varices and helps control the bleeding.

If bleeding cannot be controlled, a procedure to lower pressure in the portal vein may be needed, called a transjugular intrahepatic portosystemic stent shunt (TIPSS). A metal tube (stent) is passed through the liver to join two large veins (the portal vein and hepatic vein), creating a bypass (shunt) so the blood flows straight into the hepatic vein relieving the pressure.

ASCITES AND PERIPHERAL OEDEMA

Ascites (fluid building in your abdominal cavity, appearing like a bulge across your tummy area) and peripheral oedema (swelling in your ankles and legs) are very common in people with advanced cirrhosis. Ascites can be uncomfortable and make it hard for people to breathe and eat normally.

The main treatments are restricting the salt in the diet and the use of diuretics (fluid tablets). Fluid may also be drained from your abdomen using a tube to make more comfortable.

HEPATIC ENCEPHALOPATHY

Many people with cirrhosis experience episodes of mental confusion (known as hepatic encephalopathy). It can range from sleep disturbance, subtle personality changes and slightly poorer performances in tests, to problems in movement and speech, and can progress to a loss of consciousness, where it can be life-threatening.

The main treatment is lactulose (a sweet syrupy medicine). This acts as a laxative and also helps the body remove the toxins that build up when the liver is failing.

Most periods of encephalopathy are triggered by problems such as:

- Infection.
- Constipation.
- Dehydration.
- Medicines.
- Bleeding.

The cause of an episode will also need to be identified and treated.

BLEEDING

The liver makes products to help blood clot and when it stops working effectively, people can be at risk of severe bleeding. Vitamin K and plasma may be given as a treatment in medical emergencies.

KIDNEY PROBLEMS

People with advanced cirrhosis who are already very ill with problems such as encephalopathy, jaundice and bleeding problems, are at risk of a serious complication called hepatorenal syndrome, which is kidney failure in liver disease. For most patients, a liver transplant is needed.

LIVER CANCER

Some people with cirrhosis develop liver cancer, most commonly hepatocellular carcinoma (HCC). The aim is to detect and treat the cancer as early as possible.

Treatment can involve cutting out the part of the liver affected. Other treatments aimed at controlling the cancer include:

- Targeting the tumour cells with chemicals, heat or radiation.
- Cutting off the tumour's blood supply.

A liver transplant may be an option for some patients.

LIVER TRANSPLANTATION

If liver is very badly damaged, a liver transplant may be needed. It's a major operation and usually only recommended if other treatments are no longer helpful and your life is threatened by end stage liver disease. It's usually very successful, although in some cases it's possible for liver diseases to return and affect your new liver. Unfortunately, the numbers of transplants which can be performed are limited by the number of donor livers available.

REFERENCES

1. Fauci, Anthony S., et al. Harrison's Principles of Internal Medicine. 17th ed. United States: McGraw-Hill Professional, 2008.
2. Ergasa NV. Approach to the patient with liver disease. In: Goldman L, Ausiello D, eds. *Cecil Medicine*. 23rd ed. Philadelphia, Pa: Saunders Elsevier;2007:chap 149.
3. Roche SP, Kobos R Jaundice in the adult patient. Am Fam Physician 2004; 69:299–304.
4. Neri S, Raciti C, D'Angelo G, Ierna D, Bruno CM. Hyde's prurigo nodularis and chronic HCV hepatitis. J Hepatol 1998; 28:161–164.

CHAPTER 31

Alcoholic Hepatitis

Alcoholic hepatitis is a form of toxin-induced liver disease that runs a wide clinical spectrum. Alcoholic patients suffering with jaundice are indicated by alcoholic hepatitis. Excessive alcohol intake over a long period of time is necessary for development of alcoholic hepatitis with cirrhosis. Whereas there is considerable variation, atleast 40-60 g of ethanol per day for more than 15 yr is required for the development of alcoholic hepatitis with cirrhosis. This is equal to about six, 12-oz beers per day, 4 glasses of wine, or three, 2-oz shots of whiskey. Women may develop disease with smaller amounts due to their smaller body size, hormonal differences, and less prehepatic metabolism of ethanol by gastric alcohol dehydrogenase (ADH).

METABOLISM OF ALCOHOL

There are two predominant pathways for alcohol metabolism in the hepatocyte: the ADH pathway in the cytosol of the cell, and the microsomal ethanol oxidizing system (MEOS) located in the endoplasmic reticulum. Both pathways result in production of acetaldehyde that is the toxic intermediate in alcohol metabolism. The ADH system is the predominant mode of metabolism, and occurs mainly in the liver. ADH is also located in the stomach, to varying degrees, and metabolism that occurs here may affect liver toxicity by decreasing the amount of alcohol reaching the liver. Differences in gastric ADH may explain, in part, the observation that some individuals develop toxicity from smaller amounts of alcohol than others. For example, women tend to have lower rates of gastric alcohol metabolism than men, and may develop liver injury from alcohol at lower doses than men .

When ethanol is oxidized by ADH, acetaldehyde is produced, and reducing equivalents are transferred to nicotinamide adenine dinucleotide (NAD), converting it to a reduced form, NADH. Acetaldehyde is then metabolized to acetate by the enzyme aldehyde dehydrogenase (ALD), releasing additional reducing equivalents. The release of a large number of reducing equivalents tends to overwhelm the hepatocyte's ability to maintain a normal redox state. This results in several disorders like Metabolic acidosis, gout. The decreased *NAD/NADH* ratio also contributes to triglyceride accumulation in the hepatocytes.

The MEOS is part of an inducible P450 enzyme system that oxidizes ethanol to acetaldehyde.

This is a secondary system to the ADH system. However, the effect of alcohol on this inducible system has potentially important clinical ramifications. For example, with acute alcohol intake, there is competition between alcohol and other drugs such a phenobarbital, dilantin, and coumadin for enzyme-binding sites. This results in a decreased rate of metabolism of the medications and, thus, higher blood levels. This explains the increased toxicity of drugs taken together with alcohol during suicide attempts. During the chronic phase of alcohol intake, however, induction of this enzyme system results in increased metabolism of the drugs and, as a result, more drug is needed to maintain normal levels. This can be deleterious, in that drugs such as acetaminophen in alcoholics may be more rapidly metabolized to toxic intermediates, resulting in hepatotoxicity at lower doses.

PATHOLOGY

The hepatic injury tends to be seen first, and is most severe in the centrilobular region of the liver. Fatty infiltration is extremely common, and the term alcoholic steatohepatitis is a more accurate description of the process. Steatohepatitis is not unique, however, to alcoholic liver injury. Mallory bodies are histologically identified as a collection of purple-red material near the nucleus of the hepatocyte when viewed with hematoxylin and eosin stain. Mallory bodies are felt to be formed from collections of intermediate filaments. Mallory bodies are the product of a gene that normally is suppressed, but somehow becomes activated during the course of toxic injury to the hepatocyte. Mallory bodies were once considered diagnostic of alcoholic liver injury, but they have since been demonstrated in nonalcoholic steatohepatitis.

Cholestatic changes are also commonly seen with bile stasis, plugging, and, at times, destruction of bile ductules in the portal triads. This is most commonly due to an intrahepatic process and reflects direct toxin injury and also possibly mechanical compression of small ducts from hepatocyte swelling and fatty infiltration .

PATHOGENESIS OF ALCOHOLIC HEPATITIS

Most of the toxic effects of alcohol on the liver are felt to be mediated through production of acetaldehyde. Acetaldehyde is produced mainly through the action of ADH. However, with chronic alcohol intake, induction of the MEOS also contributes. Acetaldehyde levels are controlled by ALD located in the mitochondria. Chronic alcohol intake inhibits ALD, resulting in further elevation of acetaldehyde.

The balloon-like hepatocytes seen in alcohol-induced liver injury. This results in accumulation of lipoproteins and other proteins made by the cell. The result of this process is swelling of the cells and eventual destruction. Free radicals are also generated by parts of the MEOS. These free radicals react with unsaturated fatty acids present in cellular organelles and membranes. Unstable intermediates are produced in this way that then undergo peroxidative degeneration. This results in changes in membrane fluidity, and loss of enzyme function that ultimately leads to cell death. Acetaldehyde also probably promotes lipid peroxidation through inactivation of free radical scavengers. With chronic alcohol use, lipocytes in the liver transform into myofibroblast-like cells that produce collagen and, ultimately, cirrhosis. Acetaldehyde may further enhance this situation by up-regulating the production of collagen.

Immune mechanisms may also play a role in alcohol-related hepatotoxicity. Mallory bodies can bind to immunoglobulins and, when released from dying hepatocytes, are complexed with these immunoglobulins and with tissue and serum carbohydrates. In this form they possess chemotactic properties and may help explain the neutrophilic inflammatory infiltrate seen in alcoholic hepatitis.

Finally, alcohol and its metabolites, particularly acetaldehyde, are responsible for the significant lipid accumulation characteristic of alcoholic hepatitis. Acetaldehyde also increases fatty acid synthesis by increasing the NADH/NAD ratio and damaging mitochondria.

INCIDENCE OF ALCOHOLIC HEPATITIS

Due to the large number of individuals who have only mild symptoms, the true incidence of alcoholic hepatitis can only be estimated, as most of these cases will not be brought to medical attention and liver biopsy would be necessary to establish the diagnosis. There also appears to be a variation in incidence in different nationalities. In Denmark, a study of patients who were admitted for alcohol detoxification and treatment showed changes on liver biopsy consistent with alcoholic hepatitis in about 20%. In a United States study involving veterans with liver disease, who underwent liver biopsy, approx 35% had changes consistent with alcoholic hepatitis. These were skewed populations, however, in that these were patients seen in the hospital. Persons with mild asymptomatic disease would not be detected, and, thus, the figure of 35% likely underestimates the true incidence in the population.

FACTORS INFLUENCING ALCOHOL-INDUCED LIVER INJURY

NUTRITIONAL FACTORS

Alcoholic hepatitis was originally felt to be a nutritional problem based on the observation that most patients presenting with moderate to severe disease were malnourished. It has subsequently been shown that alcoholic hepatitis and cirrhosis could develop despite adequate nutritional support. The mechanism of malnutrition in alcoholic liver disease is multifactorial.

The heavy drinker may consume nearly half of his daily caloric intake in the form of ethanol.

Whereas the total number of calories may be nearly adequate, the ethanol provides mainly "empty" calories. Patients with this condition are often in a net catabolic state. Protein intake may be inadequate to meet the needs of cellular repair. In addition, alcohol intake produces anorexia, further complicating the situation. Lastly, the effects of alcohol on other organ systems, such as the pancreas, may result in malabsorption. It is not known, though, whether malnutrition plays a role in the liver injury or if it is simply a condition associated with alcoholism .

GENETICS

There is evidence for a genetic predisposition for alcohol-induced liver injury. Ethanol is metabolized predominantly in the liver. After ingestion, ethanol is rapidly absorbed from the stomach and small intestine. Serum levels are then determined by the rate of oxidative metabolism of ethanol by the liver. Acetaldehyde and the production of reducing agents, mainly NADH, are felt to be the primary contributors to liver injury. The two enzymes primarily involved in ethanol metabolism are ADH and ALD. Multiple isoenzymes of ADH and ALD have been discovered. These isoenzymes have a different predominance in different populations and function differently. For example, the flushing phenomenon is commonly seen in people with a particular subtype of ALD that results in slow metabolism of acetaldehyde. This is common in Asians. Variation in the metabolism of ethanol as liver function of these genetic differences may explain the higher prevalence of alcoholic liver injury in some populations.

CYTOKINES

Cytokines are a group of soluble polypeptides that act as modifiers of biologic responses by regulating gene expression, differentiation and proliferation of cells. They are secreted by cells into the microenvironment where they interact with various receptors, and the end result is often a function of a cascade of cytokines. Various cytokines have been examined for their possible role in alcoholic hepatitis. These include the interleukins, tumor necrosis factor, colony-stimulating factors, and transforming growth factor. These cytokines have been implicated in induction and continuation of the inflammatory response and stimulation of cells that lead to increased production of extracellular matrix and, ultimately, fibrosis and cirrhosis. It is not known, however, whether these agents are directly regulated by ethanol and its metabolites or whether the increased expression of these agents is a function of the underlying inflammatory response.

HEPATITIS C VIRUS

The interaction of alcohol and hepatitis C is not clear. It is known, however, that alcoholics with more severe liver disease are more likely to have concurrent infection with hepatitis C.

Histologically, the liver damage contains both alcoholic and viral features, suggesting one superimposed on the other.

DIAGNOSIS OF ALCOHOLIC HEPATITIS

Clinical signs and symptoms of alcoholic hepatitis vary from asymptomatic to acute liver failure. In asymptomatic individuals, one of the most common findings is an enlarged liver (greater than 12 cm in the mid-clavicular line). Cirrhosis is commonly seen in biopsies from patients with alcoholic hepatitis. However, unlike other processes that produce cirrhosis, the liver in alcoholic hepatitis often remains enlarged, as opposed to becoming small and shrunken.

Evidence of liver failure may be present as portal hypertension with ascites and varices, and encephalopathy. It is important to recognize that alcoholic hepatitis by itself, without cirrhosis, may produce these findings, and that this is a potentially reversible condition. Liver biopsy is the only reliable way to establish whether the patient has underlying cirrhosis. Laboratory findings are varied and reflect underlying liver damage as well as nutritional deficits, and a direct toxic effect of alcohol on the bone marrow. A macrocytic anemia is commonly seen. This may result from both the changes induced in red cell membranes, and also from folate deficiency that is common in alcoholics. Vitamin B12 levels are usually increased, reflecting release from the damaged liver. There will be cahges in Liver aspartate aminotransferase and alanine aminotransferase. The greater elevation in AST probably reflects its greater concentration in the centrilobular region of the liver where alcohol-induced liver injury is more severe. Despite a significant amount of inflammation seen histologically, it is very unusual for the AST to exceed levels greater than 200 lU/L or 5 times the upper limit of normal. Elevations greater than 300 lUlL should raise suspicion of another or concurrentprocess affecting the liver. However, AST / ALT ratio of greater than 2 is seen in only about half the patients, generally those with the most severe disease. This feature, along with the leukocytosis and fever that can be present, may present diagnostic problems trying to distinguish this entity from gallbladder and biliary tract disease. This is an important distinction, as operating on a patient with severe alcoholic hepatitis carries a significant risk of morbidity and mortality. The GGT is generally high. This is not very useful as a test, because it reflects microsomal enzyme induction as well as liver injury. Alterations in the prothrombin time and albumin may be seen reflecting both hepatic synthetic dysfunction as well as nutritional deficiency.

Imaging studies are generally not helpful in diagnosing alcoholic hepatitis. They invariably show an enlarged, fatty-appearing liver. They are more helpful in eliminating other or concurrent problems, such as biliary tract disease and pancreatitis. Even in this capacity, care must be taken in their interpretation or they may suggest an incorrect diagnosis. For example, the HIDA scan used to help confirm a diagnosis of cholecystitis. There are no specific reco-mmendations regarding the use of liver biopsy in alcoholic hepatitis. In severe alcoholic hepatitis, the biopsy may be relatively contraindicated because of a coagulopathy or thrombocytopenia. The diagnosis is often not difficult in these cases, and can generally be established by a history of long-term, heavy alcohol use, serologic tests, and noninvasive imaging studies to help rule out biliary tract obstruction. Biopsy is useful in the patient who has recovered from a bout of severe alcoholic hepatitis or in the patient with mild disease to determine if the patient has cirrhosis. It should be kept in mind that this will not significantly alter management of the patient. From the standpoint of management, liver biopsy is probably most useful in the patient who may have multiple potential causes of liver disease, such as drugs other than alcohol. Approximately 20% of alcoholic patients who have clinical and laboratory features suggesting alcoholic hepatitis will have another cause found on liver biopsy . Biopsy may also occasionally be useful in the patient who does not admit to significant drinking. Findings on the biopsy showing alcoholic hepatitis may be helpful in forcing the patient to confront a potential problem before it becomes more serious.

PROGNOSTIC FEATURES IN ALCOHOLIC HEPATITIS

Typical patients who present with severe alcoholic hepatitis have generally stopped drinking several days to a week prior to presentation. Their illness will commonly worsen over the next 10-14 d despite cessation of drinking. Most of the early mortality from alcoholic hepatitis occurs during this time period. The prognosis regarding acute 30-d mortality depends on the severity of the hepatitis at the time of admission. Various methods have been employed for evaluation. However, currently the most widely used and best predictor of severity is the so called Maddrey discriminate function. This is an objective measure of severity of alcoholic hepatitis based on two laboratory criteria, the prothrombin time and bilirubin. Prothrombin time and bilirubin were found to be the two best predictors of survival. The discriminate function is equal to 4.6 X (prothrombin time - control) + bilirubin (mg/dL). Values greater than 32 indicate severe disease with a significant 30-d mortality . Beyond the initial acute phase of alcoholic hepatitis, there is little long-term data regarding mortality. One study followed patients with serial liver biopsies. No patients that continued to drink recovered, and about a third of these progressed to cirrhosis. Of those that stopped drinking, after a year, half still had alcoholic hepatitis, a quarter had progressed to cirrhosis,and the remainder had healed.

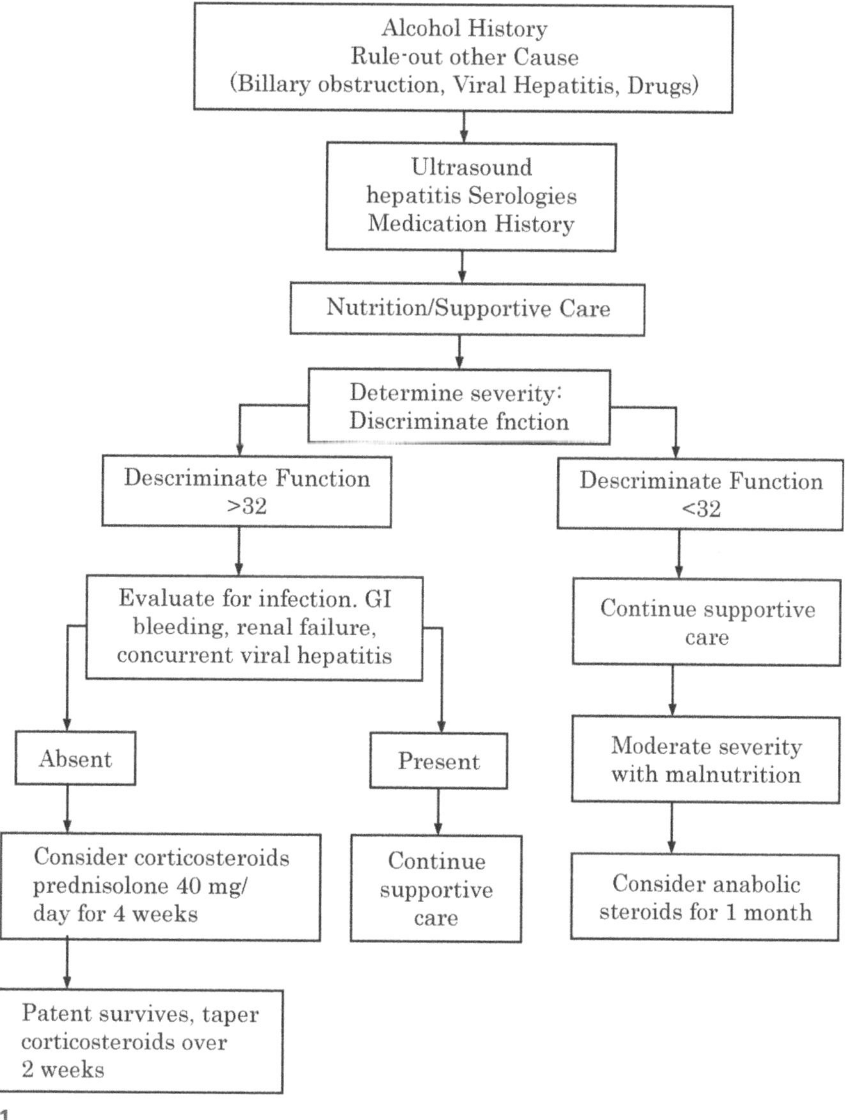

FIGURE 31.1

A scheme for the treatment of alcoholic hepatitis.

TREATMENT

Abstinence is the mainstay of treatment of alcoholic liver disease. However, in practice this may be difficult to achieve. In one study only approx 10% of chronic alcohol users were able to maintain complete abstinence over a 2 yr period. An approach to treatment is outlined in Fig. 31.1.

NUTRITION

The role of nutrition in patients with alcoholic hepatitis has been extensively studied, with the rationale being that almost all these patients are malnourished. This is particularly true in patients requiring hospitalization. In most, voluntary food intake is not adequate to meet their nutritional needs. These patients must then catabolize protein stores in order meet their basal energy requirements. This is not a desirable situation, and most of these patients will require additional nutritional support, either enterally or parenterally. Both modes have been studied with each showing the ability to establish a positive nitrogen balance. The enteral route is preferred. However, if this is not possible, parenteral alimentation should be used. The goal of nutritional therapy should be to establish a positive nitrogen balance. The approximate daily needs of the patient can be estimated at about 30 cal, and 1 g/kg body weight of protein. A common mistake is to restrict protein to avoid inducing or worsening hepatic encephalopathy. Adequate protein is necessary to establish a positive balance, and no studies have shown this to worsen encephalopathy to any significant degree. Whereas dietary supplementation will improve various clinical parameters in patients with alcoholic hepatitis, it has, however, been difficult to demonstrate any significant effect on acute mortality. Two specific nutrients that are of interest are polyunsaturated lecithin and diets high in saturated fats. Polyunsaturated lecithin can inhibit the formation of cirrhosis in animal models. This may occur by stimulation of collagenase activity that offsets the acetaldehyde-induced increase in collagen production. Of interest is one study suggesting a diet high in saturated fats may be advantageous in alcoholic hepatitis.

MEDICATIONS

Corticosteroids: There have been many trials examining the role of corticosteroids in the treatment of alcoholic hepatitis. The rationale for their use is the acute inflammatory reaction observed histologically in the liver. Corticosteroids at a dose equal to 40 mg/d prednisolone have been used in most trials. In general, corticosteroids did not affect mortality in alcoholic hepatitis. There may, however, be a subset with severe disease, defined as a discriminate function score of greater than 32, that will have an improved 30-d mortality if treated with corticosteroids. This subset is further restricted to those without sepsis, concurrent viral hepatitis, gastrointestinal bleeding, or significant renal failure. Improvement in long-term mortality has also recently been reported. For those patients with severe alcoholic hepatitis that meet the above criteria, it is reasonable to treat them with prednisolone or an equivalent at a dose of 40 mg/d for 4 wk and then taper the dose off over the next 2 wk. Most studies had the patients cut their dose to 20 mg in the fifth week, 10 mg in the sixth week, and then stop.

Anabolic Steroids: Anabolic steroids have been used with the rationale that they would increase anabolism and repair of the damaged liver. Oxandrolone in a dose of 80 mg/d is the drug that has been most used in the different studies. As with corticosteroids, in general, no effect was observed on mortality in patients with alcoholic hepatitis. One subgroup that did appear to benefit, however, was that with moderate alcoholic hepatitis and moderate malnutrition who were maintained with adequate nutritional support during therapy. These patients were treated for 1-3 month periods with Oxandrolone, and long-term survival at 6 months was demonstrated. No significant side effects were reported with the drug, even in women who were administered the drug for a few weeks. For those patients with alcoholic hepatitis who fit the above profile, it could be justified to treat them with 80 mg/d of Oxandrolone for 1 month.

Other Medical Therapies: Several other agents have been studied for their role in effecting survival in patients with alcoholic hepatitis. These include propylthiouracil, colchicine, insulin and glucagon. Although some studies have demonstrated potential promise, these therapies cannot be recommended at this time, outside of clinical trials.

LIVER TRANSPLANTATION

This is the ultimate treatment for any form of severe liver disease. Its use in alcoholic liver disease has been mainly limited to patients with end-stage cirrhosis who have been abstinent from alcohol for at least 6 months. At one point, this was the most common reason for liver transplantation. Patients transplanted with alcoholic liver disease generally do well with 2-yr survival of approx 70%. Most transplant centers, however, will not accept for transplantation a patient who has been actively drinking. This effectively excludes patients with severe alcoholic hepatitis, as they have been recently abusing alcohol. The initial concern regarding this group of patients was that they would resume drinking after their transplantation. Overall, risk of returning to active ethanol abuse remains the single most important factor in the decision of whether to transplant these patients.

REFERENCES

1. Lieber CS. Alcohol and the liver: 1994 update. Gastroenterology 1994;106:1085-1105.
2. Lieber CS. Biochemical factors in alcoholic liver disease. Seminars in Liver Dis 1993;13:136-153.
3. Pares A. Hepatitis C virus antibodies in chronic alcoholic patients: association with severity of liver injury. Hepatology 1990;12:1295-1299.
4. Arron R. Molecular biological aspects of alcohol-induced liver disease. Alcoholism: Clin Exp Res 1995; 19:247-256.
5. Goldberg S1. Veterans Administration Cooperative Study Group on Alcoholic Hepatitis IV: Describing the population with minimal hyperbilirubinemia. Am J Gastro 1986;11:1024-1037.
6. Mezey E. Treatment of alcoholic liver disease. Sem Liver Dis 1993;13:210-216.
7. Galambos JT. Alcoholic hepatitis: its therapy and prognosis. Prog Liver Dis 1972;4:567-588.
8. Orrego H. Long-term treatment of alcoholic liver disease with propylthiouracil. NEJM 1987;317: 1421-1427.
9. Morgan TR. Treatment of alcoholic hepatitis. Sem Liver Dis 1993;13:384-394.
10. Nanji AA. Dietary fatty acids: a novel treatment for alcoholic liver disease. Gastroenterology 1995; 1 09:547-554.
11. Krom RAF. Liver transplantation and alcohol: who should get transplants. Hepatology 1994;20:288-32S.

CHAPTER 32

Hepatitis

DEFINITION

Viral hepatitis refers to the clinically important hepatotropic viruses responsible for hepatitis A (HAV), hepatitis B (HBV), delta hepatitis, hepatitis C (HCV), and hepatitis E.

HEPATITIS A

- HAV infection primarily occurs through transmission by the fecal–oral route, person-to-person, or by ingestion of contaminated food or water. The incidence of HAV correlates directly with low socioeconomic status, poor sanitary conditions, and overcrowding. Rates of HAV infection have increased among international travelers, injection drug users, and men who have sex with men.
- HAV infection usually produces a self-limited disease and acute viral infection with a low case-fatality rate, and confers lifelong immunity.
- The disease exhibits three phases: incubation (averaging 28 days, with a range of 15 to 50 days), acute hepatitis (generally lasting 2 months), and convalescence. Most patients have full clinical and biochemical recovery within 12 weeks. Nearly all individuals will have clinical resolution within 6 months of the infection. HAV does not lead to chronic infections.
- The clinical presentation of HAV infection is given in Table 32.1.
- The diagnosis of acute HAV infection is based on clinical criteria of acute onset of fatigue, abdominal pain, loss of appetite, intermittent nausea and vomiting, jaundice or elevated serum aminotransferase levels, and serologic testing for immunoglobulin (Ig) G anti-HAV.

TREATMENT

No specific treatment options exist for HAV. Management of HAV infection is primarily supportive. Steroid use is not recommended.

PREVENTION

- The spread of HAV can be best controlled by avoiding exposure. The most important measures to avoid exposure include good hand-washing techniques and good personal hygiene practices.
- The current vaccination strategy in the United States includes vaccinating all children at 1 year of age. Groups who should receive HAV vaccine are shown in Table 32.2.

Table 32.1

Clinical presentation of acute hepatitis A

Signs and symptoms

- The preicteric phase brings nonspecific influenza-like symptoms consisting of anorexia, nausea, fatigue, and malaise.
- Abrupt onset of anorexia, nausea, vomiting, malaise, fever, headache, and right upper quadrant abdominal pain with acute illness.
- Icteric hepatitis is generally accompanied by dark urine, acholic (light-colored) stools, and worsening of systemic symptoms.
- Pruritus is often a major complaint of icteric patients.

Physical examination

- Icteric sclera, skin, and secretions
- Mild weight loss of 2–5 kg
- Hepatomegaly

Laboratory tests

- Positive serum immunoglobulin M anti-hepatitis A virus.
- Mild elevations of serum bilirubin, γ-globulin, and hepatic transaminase (alanine transaminase and aspartate transaminase) values to about twice normal in acute anicteric disease.
- Elevations of alkaline phosphatase, γ-glutamyl transferase, and total bilirubin in patients with cholestatic illness.

- Two inactivated virus vaccines are currently licensed in the United States, Havrix and Vaqta. Approved dosing recommendations are shown in Table 32.3. Seroconversion rates >94% are achieved with the first dose.
- IG is used when pre- or postexposure prophylaxis against HAV infection is needed. It is most effective if given during the incubation phase of infection. A single dose of IG of 0.02 mL/kg intramuscularly is recommended for travelers to high-risk areas if travel is for less than 3 months. For lengthy stays, a single dose of 0.06 mL/kg is used.
- For people recently exposed to HAV and not previously vaccinated, IG is indicated for.
- Those in close contact with an HAV-infected person, all staff and attendees of daycare centers when HAV is documented, if involved in a common source exposure (such as a food-borne outbreak), classroom contacts of an index case patient, and schools, hospitals, and work settings where close personal contact occurred with the case patient.
- Common vaccine side effects include soreness and warmth at the injection site, headache, malaise, and pain.

HEPATITIS B

- HBV is a leading cause of chronic hepatitis, cirrhosis, and hepatocellular carcinoma.
- Transmission of HBV occurs sexually, parenterally, and perinatally. In the United States, transmission occurs predominantly through sexual contact or

injection-drug use. International travel is also an important risk factor.

- Approximately 20% of patients with chronic HBV infection develop complications of decompensated cirrhosis, including hepatic insufficiency and portal hypertension. HBV is a risk factor for development of hepatocellular carcinoma.
- There are three phases of HBV infection. The incubation period for HBV is 4 to 10 weeks during which patients are highly infective. This is followed by a symptomatic phase with intermittent flares of hepatitis and marked increases in aminotransferase serum levels. The final phase is seroconversion to anti-hepatitis B core antigen (anti-HbcAg). Patients who continue to have detectable hepatitis B surface antigen (HbsAg) and HBcAg and a high serum titer of HBV DNA for more than 6 months have chronic HBV.
- The interpretation of serologic markers for HBV is given in Table 32.4.
- Clinical manifestations of acute HBV infection are age dependent. Infants infected with HBV are generally asymptomatic, while about 85% to 95% of children aged 1 to 5 years are asymptomatic.
- The clinical presentation of chronic HBV is given in Table 32.5.

Table 32.2

Recommendations for hepatitis A vaccination

All children at 1 year of age
In areas without existing hepatitis A vaccination programs, catch-up vaccination of children ages 2–18 years can be considered.
Persons traveling to or working in countries that have high or intermediate endemicity of infection.[a]
Men who have sex with men.
Illegal-drug users.
Persons who have occupational risk for infection (e.g., persons who work with HAV-infected primates or HAV in a research laboratory setting).
Persons who have clotting-factor disorders.
Persons who have chronic liver disease (e.g., persons with chronic liver disease caused by hepatitis B or C and persons awaiting liver transplants).

a: Travelers to Canada, Western Europe, Japan, Australia, or New Zealand are at no greater risk for HAV infection than they are while in the United States. All other travelers should be assessed for hepatitis A risk.

Table 32.3

Recommended dosing of havrix and vaqta

Vaccine	Vaccine's Age (years)	Dose	Volume (mL)	Number Doses	Schedule (months)
Havrix	2–18	720 ELISA units	0.5	2	0, 6–12
	≥19	1,440 ELISA units	1	2	0, 6–12
Vaqta	1–18	25 units	0.5	2	0,6–18
	≥19	50 units	1	2	0, 6–18

Table 32.4

Interpretation of serologic tests in hepatitis B virus

Tests		
HB_SAg	(–)	
Anti-HB_C	(–)	Susceptible
Anti-HB_S	(–)	
HB_SAg	(–)	
Anti-HB_C	(+)	Immune because of natural infection
Anti-HB_S	(+)	
HB_SAg	(–)	Immune because of vaccination (valid only if
Anti-HB_C	(–)	test performed 1–2 months after third
Anti-HB_S	(+)	vaccine dose)
HB_SAg	(+)	
Anti-HB_C	(+)	
1gM anti-HB_C	(+)	Acute infection
HB_SAg	(+)	
Anti-HB_S	(+)	
1gM anti-HB_C	(–)	Chronic infection
Anti-HB_S	(–)	
HB_SA	(–)	Four interpretations possible:
Anti-HB_C	(+)	1. Recovery from acute infection
Anti-HB_S	(–)	2. Distant immunity and test not sensitive enough to detect low level of HB_S in serum
		3. Susceptible with false-positive anti- HB_S
		4. May have undetectable level of HB_SAg in serum and be chronically infected

HB_C,hepatitis B core; HBsA, hepatitis B surface; HB_SA, hepatitis B surface associated; HB_SAg, hepatitis B surface antigen; IgM, immunoglobulin M. From Centers for Disease Control and Prevention: Hepatitis B Serology

PREVENTION

- Prophylaxis of HBV can be achieved by vaccination or by passive immunity in postexposure cases with hepatitis B immunoglobulin.
- Two products are available for prevention of hepatitis B infection: **hepatitis B vaccine**, which provides active immunity, and **hepatitis B immuneglobulin (HBIg)**, which provides temporary passive immunity.
- The goals of immunization against viral hepatitis include prevention of the short-term viremia that can lead to transmission of infection, clinical disease, and chronic HBV infection.
- Persons who should receive HBV vaccine are listed in Table 32.6.
- Side effects of the vaccines are soreness at the injection site, headache, fatigue, irritability, and fever.

Table 32.5

Clinical presentation of chronic hepatitis B[a]

Signs and symptoms

- Easy fatigability, anxiety, anorexia, and malaise.
- Ascites, jaundice, variceal bleeding, and hepatic encephalopathy can manifest with liver decompensation.
- Hepatic encephalopathy is associated with hyperexcitability, impaired mentation, confusion, obtundation, and eventually coma.
- Vomiting and seizures.

Physical examination

- Icteric sclera, skin, and secretions.
- Decreased bowel sounds, increased abdominal girth, and detectable fluid wave.
- Asterixis.
- Spider angiomata.

Laboratory tests

- Presence of hepatitis B surface antigen for at least 6 months.
- Intermittent elevations of hepatic transaminase (alanine transaminase and aspartate transaminase) and hepatitis B virus DNA greater than 10^5 copies/mL.
- Liver biopsies for pathologic classification as chronic persistent hepatitis, chronic active hepatitis, or cirrhosis.

[a]Chronic hepatitis B can be present even without all the signs, symptoms, and physical examination findings listed being apparent.

Table 32.6

Recommendations for hepatitis B virus (HBV) vaccination

- Infants
- Adolescents, including all previously unvaccinated children <19 years old
- All unvaccinated adults at risk for infection
- All unvaccinated adults seeking vaccination (specific risk factor not required)
- Men and women with a history of other sexually transmitted diseases and persons with a history of multiple
- sex partners (>1 partner/6 months)
- Men who have sex with men
- Injection-drug users
- Household contacts and sex partners of persons with chronic hepatitis B infection and health care and public
- safety workers with exposure to blood in the workplace
- Clients and staff of institutions for the developmentally disabled
- International travelers who plan to spend >6 months in countries with high rates of HBV infection and who
- will have close contact with the local population
- Recipients of clotting-factor concentrates
- Sexually transmitted disease clinic patients
- HIV patient/HIV-testing patients
- Drug-abuse treatment and prevention clinic patients
- Correctional facilities inmates
- Chronic dialysis/ESRD patients

ESRD, end-stage renal disease; HIV, human immunodeficiency virus.

HEPATITIS B IMMUNE GLOBULIN

- HBIg is used only for postexposure prophylaxis for HBV for perinatal exposure of infants of HBV-carrier mothers, sexual exposure to HBs Ag-positive persons, percutaneous or permucosal exposure to HBsAg-positive blood, and exposure of an infant to a caregiver who has acute hepatitis B.
- The recommended dose is 0.06 mL/kg administered intramuscularly.

TREATMENT

- The key goals of therapy are to increase the likelihood of immunoclearance of the virus, prevent disease progression to cirrhosis or hepatocellular carcinoma, and to minimize further liver injury. Successful therapy is associated with loss of HBcAg status and seroconversion to anti-HBc Ag.
- No specific therapy is available for the management of acute HBV infection. Some patients with chronic HBV infection should be treated. A suggested treatment algorithm for chronic HBV is as shown for patients without and with cirrhosis .
- All chronic HBV infection patients should avoid alcohol and be immunized against HAV.
- Drug therapy is used to suppress viral replication by immune mediating or antiviral effects.

Interferon α20b (IFN-α **2b**), **lamivudine, telbivudine, adefovir , entecavir,**and **pegylated IFN-α 2a** (PEG-IFN) are approved in the United States for first-line treatment of chronic HBV.

- Several factors correlate with improved response to IFN therapy, including increased alanine transaminases and HBV DNA levels, high histologic activity score at biopsy, and being non-Asian. Treatment for a minimum of 12 months is associated with greater sustained virologic response rates than treatment for 4 to 6 months. Conventional IFN therapy has been virtually replaced with pegylated IFN, because of the ease of administration (once-weekly injections), fewer side effects, and improved efficacy.
- Lamivudine (100 mg daily given orally) may be used alone or in combination with PEG-IFN for chronic HBV.

HEPATITIS C

- HCV is the most common blood-borne pathogen. Screening for HCV infection is recommended in selected groups who are at high risk for infection (Table 32.7).
- HCV is most often acquired through IV drug use; sexual contact; hemodialysis; or household, occupational, or perinatal exposure.
- In the vast majority of patients (up to 85%) acute HCV infection leads to chronic infection defined by persistently detectable HCV RNA for 6 months or more.
- Patients with acute HCV are often asymptomatic and undiagnosed. One third of adults will experience some mild and nonspecific symptoms, including fatigue, anorexia, weakness, jaundice, abdominal pain, or dark urine. The most common symptom of chronic HCV infection is persistent fatigue. An estimated 20% of patients with chronic HCV infection will

develop cirrhosis and half of those patients will progress to decompensated cirrhosis or hepatocellular carcinoma.

- The diagnosis of HCV infection is confirmed with a reactive enzyme immunoassay for anti-HCV. Serum transaminase values are elevated within 4 to 12 weeks after exposure.

Table 32.7

Recommendations for hepatitis C virus (HCV) screening

- Current or past injection drug use
- Coinfection with HIV
- Received blood transfusions or organ transplantations before 1992
- Received clotting factors before 1987
- Ever on chronic hemodialysis
- Patients with unexplained elevated ALT levels or evidence of liver disease
- Health care and public safety workers after an occupational exposure
- Children born to HCV-positive mothers
- Immigrants from countries with a high prevalence of HCV infection

ALT, alanine transaminase; HIV, human immunodeficiency virus.

TREATMENT

- The goal of treating HCV is to eradicate HCV infection, which prevents the development of chronic HCV infection and sequelae.
- Treatment for HCV infection is necessary because a high percentage of acutely infected patients develop chronic infections. Treatment is indicated in patients previously untreated who have chronic HCV, circulating HCV RNA, increased alanine transaminases levels, evidence on biopsy of moderate to severe hepatic grade and stage, and compensated liver disease. Contraindications to treatment include: autoimmune hepatitis, decompensated liver disease, women who are pregnant or patients whose female partners are pregnant, hemoglobinopathies, creatinine clearance <50 mL/min, hemodialysis, or ischemic cardiovascular or cerebrovascular disease. Treatment response is best in patients with HCV genotype 1 and those who take at least 80% of their medications for at least 80% of the treatment time.
- All patients with chronic HCV infection should be vaccinated for hepatitis A and B. Patients should be advised to maintain good overall health, stop smoking, and avoid alcohol and illicit drugs.
- The current standard of treatment for chronic HCV infection is a combination of once-weekly **PEG-IFN** and a daily oral dose of **ribavirin**. Sustained virologic response rates are 54% to 56%. Therapy is optimized based on genotype, patient weight, and response to therapy. Recommended treatment regimens for HCV infection are given in Table 32.8.
- Two PEG-IFNs are available, Pegasys and PEG-Intron (Table 32.9). It is unclear which is superior.
- Common side effects of peginterferon are given in Table 32.10. Common side effects of ribavirin are fatigue, flu-like symptoms, neutropenia, thrombocytopenia, and anemia.

Table 32.8

Recommended hepatitis C virus treatment dosing

Genotype		Ribavirin	Dose	Duration[a]
1,2,3	Peginterferon α_{2a} 180 mcg/wk or Peginterferon α_{2b} 1.5 mcg/wk	<75 kg[b]	1,000 mg	48 weeks
		≥75 kg	1,200 mg	
	Peginterferon α_{2a} 180 mcg/wk or Peginterferon α_{2b} 1.5 mcg/wk		800 mg	24 weeks

[a]Actual treatment duration may be reduced depending on early virologic response.
[b]Patient weight.

Table 32.9

Pegylated interferon comparison

	Pegasys	PEG-Intron
Interferon	Alpha-2a	Alpha-2b
Indications	HBV, HCV	HCV
PEG moiety (weight)	Branched (40 kDa)	Linear (12 kDa)
Distribution	8–12 L; highest concentration in liver, spleen, kidneys	Body-weight dependent: 1 L/kg; distributes throughout body
Metabolism	Liver	Liver
Excretion	Renal	Renal
Dosing	Fixed: 180 mcg/wk subcutaneously	Weight dependent: 1.5 mcg/kg/wk subcutaneously

HBV, hepatitis B virus; HCV, hepatitis C virus.

Table 32.10

Common side effects associated with peginterferon therapy (experienced by >20% of patients)

Fatigue	Arthralgia
Fever	Musculoskeletal pain
Headache	Insomnia
Nausea	Depression
Anorexia	Anxiety/emotional lability
Rigors	Alopecia
Myalgia	Injection site reactions

REFERENCES

1. From Centers for Disease Control and Prevention. A comprehensive immunization strategy to eliminate transmission of hepatitis B virus infection in the United States: Recommendations of the Advisory Committee on Immunization Practices (ACIP) Part 1: Immunization of infants, children, and adolescents. MMWR Morb Mortal Wkly Rep 2005;54(RR-16):1–31.
2. Data from Hoofnagle JH. Course and outcome of hepatitis C. Hepatology 2002;36(5 Suppl 1):S21–S29.

CHAPTER 33

Drug Induced Hepatotoxicity

Drug-induced liver disease can mimic any acute or chronic liver disorder and should always be considered in evaluating a patient with liver disease. Patients may present with fulminant hepatic failure from an intrinsic hepatotoxin, such as acetaminophen, or simply be found to have abnormal liver function tests on a laboratory screening panel. Classic drug-induced hypersensitivity is an idiosyncratic, probably immunoallergic reaction which presents with fevers, dermatitis, arthralgias, and eosinophilia. This presentation is rarely seen in its entirety. Dermatitis and eosinophilia are most specific, but least commonly seen. The time interval between starting the medication and onset of symptoms is also important in assessing a temporal relationship. Hypersensitivity hepatotoxicity usually occurs within 5-90 d of starting a medication or within 15 d of rechallenge. After withdrawal of the drug, it may take a month or more before significant resolution of liver serum enzymes is seen. Idiosyncratic metabolic reactions generally do not have a predictable time course to presentation, withdrawal or rechallenge.

Incriminating a drug may be straight forward in the example of an overdose, but more often involves a process of elimination. The most important part of the evaluation is a careful history of what medications the patient is taking, the dose, how long they have been taken, the relationship of individual drugs to the onset of hepatotoxicity, and possible external factors, such as alcohol use or the presence of underlying liver disease, that could increase the potential toxicity of an agent. For example, chronic alcohol use increases the potential for acetaminophen hepatotoxicity.

DIAGNOSTIC APPROACHES

EVALUATION OF PATIENTS WITH SUSPECTED DRUG-INDUCED HEPATOTOXICITY

Physical Examination

The examination of the patient should include a search for jaundice and features of chronic liver disease. The skin associated with a cholestatic process or rashes suggesting an allergic phenomenon also should be examined. The liver size should be measured and recorded so that future changes can be followed. The patient should be examined for signs and symptoms of encephalopathy.

Laboratory

Laboratory tests are used to help determine whether the patient has primarily a hepatocellular, cholestatic, or mixed type of pattern. The aminotransferases (ALT and AST), and alkaline phosphatase are most useful in this regard . It should be emphasized that the finding of abnormal serum liver enzymes does not necessarily imply liver damage. If available, an effort should be made to obtain previous records of liver enzyme levels. This will help determine if the process is acute or chronic.

Exclusion of Other Causes of Liver Damage

In cases in which the process is hepatitic, viral hepatitis should be excluded. If the patient's aminotransferases have been elevated for more than 6 mo, they have chronic hepatitis by definition and autoimmune and metabolic disorders should also be excluded. In patients with a cholestatic or mixed picture, obstruction of the biliary tree must be excluded. Thc presence of pain, fluctuating liver enzymes, and fever is more common with mechanical obstruction of the biliary tree. An imaging study, generally an ultrasound, should be the initial study of choice to look for the presence of gallstones and or dilatation of the biliary tree. If the ultrasound is unrevealing and evaluation still suggests biliary obstruction, an ERCP should be performed to definitively exclude this possibility. Concurrent with the above, serum levels of medications with intrinsic hepatotoxic potential, for example salicylates, should be measured.

After excluding nondrug causes, if the process appears to be resolving, and the patient asymptomatic, they may simply be monitored. This is particularly true of patients with only mild elevations in liver enzymes. Initially, obtaining weekly values would be a reasonable interval. If the patient is symptomatic or the abnormalities persist or worsen over a period of a few weeks, nonessential medications and those drugs recognized as commonly producing the particular hepatotoxicity pattern (hepatocellular or cholestatic) should be stopped. This may necessitate changing essential medications to alternative agents. If the enzyme values return to normal, no further evaluation is necessary. If not, a liver biopsy should be performed. It should be remembered that it may take several months for the abnormalities to completely resolve. However, improvement should be seen within a few weeks. To definitely incriminate a particular medication in producing liver disease, rechallenge with the drug is confirmatory but it is not performed due to adverse effects. Instead, alternative chemically unrelated agents are substituted. It should be noted that aminotransferase levels often do not correlate with toxicity. For example, methotrexate toxicity is related to the total cumulative dose of the medication. Aminotransferase levels fluctuate and may be only mildly elevated in the presence of substantial liver damage. A liver biopsy is required to fully evaluate the extent of disease. Information regarding the toxicity of individual drugs is discussed in the Tables 33.1 to 33.6.

SPECIFIC COMMONLY USED DRUGS THAT HAVE HEPATOTOXICITY

ANTIARRHYTHMICS

Amiodarone

Hepatocellular necrosis and liver failure has been associated with iv amiodarone infused at rates higher than those currently recommended. Liver enzymes are commonly elevated and often subside with continuation or reduction in dosage. The incidence of symptomatic liver disease is related to duration of exposure. Monitoring of serum liver enzymes is recommended. However, liver biopsy is needed to confirm hepatic injury.

Procainamide

Despite a high incidence of hypersensitivity reactions, hepatotoxicity is rarely seen with this drug.

Quinidine

Acute hepatocellular injury may be seen with this agent. The mechanism appears to be a hypersensitivity reaction.

ANTIHYPERTENSIVE AGENTS

Alpha-Methyldopa

Hepatic injury is variable and is probably not increased in patients with Coombs-positive hemolytic anemia. Liver enzyme abnormalities are common, and drug-induced acute hepatitis does occur. Onset of injury can be delayed. Chronic liver disease and fulminant hepatic necrosis can occur, generally in patients continued on the medication after evidence of clinical hepatotoxicity develops. Hepatotoxicity may be part of a multiorgan hypersensitivity syndrome.

Beta Blockers

Hepatocellular toxicity has been reported with acebutolol, labetalol, metoprolol, and propranolol. Cholestasis has been reported with atenolol. Fatalities have occurred. Hepatotoxicity is considered rare for propranolol.

ACE Inhibitors

Hepatotoxicity is unusual and suggests idiosyncratic hypersensitivity. Injury will typically occur 2-8 wk after starting the drug. Cross reactivity has been noted between Captopril and Enalapril. Fatalities have been noted with these drugs.

Calcium Channel Blockers

All types of hepatotoxicity have been reported, but are considered rare.

United States Trade Names as listed in the 1997 Physicians' Desk Reference are listed in capitals. *Mortalityn* +

(Generic) The generic name of the suspected component has been included immediately after the trade name in parentheses. A '+' sign indicates other ingredients in formulation present, but not known to cause drug reaction.

Generic are drugs not known to cause cholestasis, but are included because reactions noted in similar drugs.

Note: All drugs known to cause cholestasis or cholestatic hepatitis as of the publication date are listed in this table. The drug families included in this table summarize what has been seen with the entire class, but may not be true for a particular drug. Drugs known to be withdrawn from the world market were excluded from this table. This table only contains drugs associated with cholestasis and cholestatic hepatitis. Drug combinations only list component known to cause cholestasis.

Types of reaction: BD = bile duct injury, inflammation or destruction documented; C = cholestatic; CH = cholestatic hepatitis; RARE = cholestasis rarely seen but documented in commonly used drug; HB = hyperbilirubinemia.

Table 33.1

Medications associated with predominantly cholestatic injury

Name of the Drug	Reaction Type	Data	Mortality
17 alpha-Alkylated Androgenic			
Steroids	See anabolic steroids		
A/T/S	[Erythromycin base]		
Acebutolol	CH	+++	
Aceprometazine	C	+	
Acetohexamide	CH	++	
ADALAT (nifedipine)	C	+	
ADVIL (ibuprofen)	C/CH	+++	
AFLAXEN (naproxen)	C/CH	+++	
Ajmaline	C/BD	++	
ALDOCLOR	See chlorothiazide and methyldopa		
ALDOMET (methyldopa)	CH	++	
ALDORIL	See methyldopa (and hydrochlorothiazide)		
ALEVE (naproxen)	C/CH	+++	
Allopurinol	C/CH	+++	
Alpha-methyldopa (methyldopa)	CH	++	
Alprazolam	C	++1+	
Amineptime	C/CH	+++	
Aminoglutethamide	CH	+++	
Amiodarone	CH	+	
Amitriptyline	CH	+++	
Amoxacillin iclavulanic acid	C/CH	+++	+
Ampicillin	CH	+	
Anabolic steroids	C/CH	+++	+
ANAPROX (naproxen)	C/CH	+++	
ANDROID (methyltestosterone)	C/CH	+++	+
AREPSAZIDE	See hydralazine (and hydrochlorothiazide)		
APRESOLINE (hydralazine)	C	+++	
Aprindine	CH	+++	
Arsenical derivatives	C	++	
Atenolol	C	++	
A TRETOL (carbamazepine)	CH	+++	
ATROMID-S (clofibrate)	C	+	
AUGMENTIN (amoxicillin clavulanic acid)	C/CH	+++	+
Azapropazone	CH	++	
Azathioprine	C/CH/rare	+++	

Table 33.1 *Contd...*

Name of the Drug	Reaction Type	Data	Mortality
AZO-GANTANOL (sulfamethoxazole)	See sulfonamides (and phenazopyridine)		
AZULFIDINE (sulfasalazine)	C	++	+
BACTRIM	See sulfonamides (and trimethoprim)		
Barbiturates	C/CH/rare	+++	
BCNU	C	+	
Saramycin	HB	+	
BENEMID (probenecid)	C/HB	++	
BENZAMYCIN	See erythromycin (and benzoyl peroxide)		
Benzodiazepines	CH/rare	++	+
Bisantrene	C	+++	
BREVICON	See estrogens and progestins		
Busulfan	C	+	
CALAN (verapamil)	C	+	
Calcium carbimide	C/CH	++	
CAPOTEN (captopril)	C/CH	++	
CAPOZIDE	See captopril (and hydrochlorothiazide)		
Captopril	C/CH	++	
Carbamazepine	CH	+++	
Carbimazole	CH	+++	
Carbutamide	C	+ +	
CARDIZEM (diltiazem)	CH	+++	
Ceftriaxone	Biliary sludge	+	
Cephalosporins	C/CH/rare	+	
Chloramphenicol	C/rare	+	
Chlordiazepoxide	CH	+	
Chloromycetin (chloramphenicol)	C/rare	+	
Chlorothiazide	C/CH	+	
Chlorozotocin	C	+	
Chlorpromazine	CH	+++	+
Chlorpropamide	CH	+++	
Chlorthalidone	CH	+	
Chlorzoxazone	CH	+++	
Chromoglycate (cromolyn)	CH	++	
Cimetidine	C/CH/rare	+++	
Cisplatin	C	+++	
Clavulanate	See augmentin and timentin		
Clavulanic acid (clavulanate)	See augmentin and timentin		
CLIMARA	See estrogens		

Table 33.1 *Contd...*

Name of the Drug	Reaction Type	Data	Mortality
CLINORIL (sulindac)	C/CH	+++	
Clofibrate	C	+	
Clorazepate	CH	+	
Cloxacillin	CH/rare	++	
Clozapine	CH	+++	
Clozaril (clozapine)	CH	+++	
Co-trimoxazole	See sulfonamides (and trimethoprim)		
COLBENEMID	See probenecid (and colchicine)		
COMBIPRES	See chlorthalidone (and clonidine)		
COMP AZINE (prochlorperazine)	CH	++	
Conjugated estrogens	See estrogens		
CORDARONE (amiodarone)	CH	+	
COUMADIN (warfarin)	C	++	
Cromolyn	CH	++	
CUPRIMINE (penicillamine)	CH	++	
Cyclosporin A	C/CHIHB	++	
PALA (N-phosphonoacetyl-L-aspartate)	HB/C	+	
N-phosphonoacetyl-L-aspartate	HB/C	I	
Cyproheptadine	C	++	
Cyproterone	C	++	
CYT ADREN (aminoglutethamide)	CH	+++	
Cytarabine	C	+++	
CYTOSAR-U (cytarabine)	C	+++	
Cytosine arabinoside (cytarabine)	C	+++	
DALMANE (flurazepam)	C	+	
Danazol	See anabolic steroids		
DANOCRINE (danazol)	See anabolic steroids		
DANTRIUM (dantrolene)	C	+++	
Dantrolene	C	+++	
Dapsone	ch	+++	
DEMI-HYGROTON	See chlorthalidone (and reserpine)		
DEMI-REGROTON	See chlorthalidone (and reserpine)		
DEMULEN	See estrogens and progestins		
DEPEN (penicillamine)	CH	++	
Desipramine	See tricyclic antidepressants		
DESOGEN	See estrogens and progestins		
DESYREL (trazodone)	C	++	

Table 33.1 *Contd...*

Name of the Drug	Reaction Type	Data	Mortality
Dextropropoxyphene	CH	+++	
DIABENESE (chlorpropamide)	CH	+++	
DIABET A (glyburide)	C	++	
Diazepam	CH	+	
Dicloxacillin	CH/rare	++	
Diethyl stilbestrol	C	+	
DIFLUCAN (fluconazole)	C	+++	
Diflunisal	CH/rare	++	
DILACOR XR (diltiazem)	CH	+++	
DILANTIN (phenytoin)	CH	+++	
Diltiazem	CH	+++	
Disopyramide	CH	++	
DIUPRES	See chlorothiazide (and reserpine)		
DIURIL (chlorothiazide)	CICH	+	
DIZAC (diazepam)	ch	+	
DOLOBID (diflunisal)	CH/rare	++	
E-MYCIN	[erythromycin base]		
E.E.S. (erythromycin ethylsuccinate)	CH	+++	
EC-NAPROSYN (naproxen)	C/CH	+++	
ELA VIL (amitriptyline)	CH	+++	
EMGEL	(Erythromycin)		
Enalapril	CH	++	
ERY-TAB	[Erythromycin base]		
ERYC	[Erythromycin base]		
ERYCETTE	[Erythromycin base]		
ERYGEL	[Erythromycin]		
ERYMAX	[Erythromycin]		
ER YPED (erythromycin ethylsuccinate)	CH	+++	
ERYTHRA-DERM	[Erythromycin base]		
Erthrocin stearate (erythromycin stearate)	CH	+	
Erythromycin estolate	CH	+++	
Erythromycin ethylsuccinate	CH	+++	
Erythromycin propionate	CH	+++	
Erythromycin	See specific agent		
Erythromycin stearate	CH	+	
ERYZOLE (erythromycin ethylsuccinate)	CH	+++	

Table 33.1 *Contd...*

Name of the Drug	Reaction Type	Data	Mortality
ESTRACE	See estrogens		
ESTRADERM	See estrogens		
ESTRATAB (estrogens)	See estrogens		
ESTRATEST	See estrogens and methyltestosterone		
Estrogens	CICH	+++	
Estropipate	See estrogens		
Ethambutol	CHirare	+++	
ETRAFON	See amitriptyline and perphenazine		
Etretinate	CH	++	
EULEXIN (flutamide)	C	+++	
Exifone	CH	++	
FELDENE (piroxicam)	C/CH	++	
Fenoprofen	CH	+++	
Floxacillin	CH	++	
Floxuridine (FUDR)	C	++	
Flucloxacillin	C/CH/rare	+++	
Fluconazole	C	+++	
Fluorodeoxy uridine	C	++	
Fluphenazine	C	+?	
Flurazepam	C	+	
Flutamide	C	+++	
FUDR	C	++	
FUL VICIN PIG (griseofulvin)	C	+	
Furazolidone	CH	+++	
FUROXONE (furazolidone)	CH	+++	
Fusidic acid	C	++	
GANT ANOL (sulfamethoxazole)	See sulfonamides		
GASTROCROM (cromolyn)	CH	++	
GEN-XENE (clorazepate)	CH	+	
GLIBENCLAMIDE (glyburide)	C	++	
Glyburide	C	++	
GL YNASE (glyburide)	C	++	
Gold salts	CH	+++	
GRIFUL VIN V (griseofulvin)	C	+	
GRIS-PEG (griseofulvin)	C	+	
GRISACTIN (griseofulvin)	C	+	
Griseofulvin	C	+	

Table 33.1 *Contd...*

Name of the Drug	Reaction Type	Data	Mortality
H2-blockers	CH/rare	+++	
HALCION (triazolam)	C	++	
HALDOL (haloperidol)	CH	++	
Haloperidol	CH	++	
HCTZ [hydrochlorothiazide]	(No documented cholestasis)		
HYDRA-ZIDE	See hydralazine (and HCTZ)		
Hydralazine	C	+++	
Hydrochlorothiazide	(No documented cholestasis)		
HYGROTON (chlorthalidone)	CH	+	
IBU TABLETS (ibuprofen)	C/H	+++	
IBU-TAB (ibuprofen)	C/CH	+++	
Ibuprofen	C/CH	+++	
11-2 (interleukin-2)	C	+++	
ILOSONE (erythromycin estolate)	CH	+++	
ILOTYCIN gluceptate	[Erythromycin gluceptate]		
ILOTYCIN ophthalmic	[Erythromycin base]		
Imipenem/ cilastatin	C	++	
Imipramine	CH	+++	
IMURAN (azathioprine)	C/CH/rare	+++	
INDOCIN (indomethacin)	CH	+	
Indomethacin	CH	+	
INTAL ~cromol~n)	CH	++	
Interleukin-2	C	+++	
Iprindole	C	+++	
ISOPTIN (verapamil)	C	+	
Isoxicam	CH	+	
Itraconazole	C	++	
Ketoconazole	C	+++	
Labetolol	CH	++ +?	
LEVIEN	See estrogens and progestins		
LIBRAX	See chlordiazepoxide (and clidinium)		
LIBRIT ABS (chlordiazepoxide)	CH	+	
LIBRIUM (chlordiazepoxide)	CH	+	
LIMBITROL	See amitriptyline and chlordiazepoxide		
LO/OVRAL	See estrogens and progestins		
LUDIOMIL (maprotiline)	CH	+	
MACRODANTIN (nitrofurantoin)	C/CH	+++	

Table 33.1 *Contd...*

Name of the Drug	Reaction Type	Data	Mortality
Macrolide antibiotics	See erythromycins and troleandomycin		
Maprotiline	CH	+	
MELLARIL (thioridazine)	CH	++	
Menest	See estrogens		
MENRIUM	See chlordiazepoxide and estrogen		
Mercaptopurine-6	CH	+++	
Metahexamide	CH	+++	
Metandienone	See anabolic steroids		
Metaprine	C	+	
Metenolone	See anabolic steroids		
Methimazole	C	+++	
Methyldopa	CH	++	
Methy lenedianiline	CH	++	
Methyl testosterone	C/CH	+++	+
MICRONASE (glyburide)	C	++	
MICRONOR	See progestins		
MINTEZOL (thiabendazole)	C/CH	+++	+
MODICON	See estrogens and progestins		
MOTRIN (ibuprofen)	C/CH	+++	
Moxisylyte	CH	+++	
MP-6 (6-mercaptopurine)	CH	+++	
MUCOMYST (n-acetylcysteine)	C	+++	
MYAMBUTOL (ethambutol)	C/rare	+++	
MYLERAN (busulfan)	C	+	
MYOCHRYSINE (gold salts)	CH	+	++
N -Acety lcysteine	CHA	+++	
N-Phosphonoacetyl-L-aspartate	C	++	
NALFON (fenoprofen)	CH	+++	
NAPRELAN (naproxen)	C/CH	+++	
NAPROSYN (naproxen)	C/CH	+++	
Naproxen	C/CH	+++	
NASALCROM (cromolyn)	CH	++	
NECON	See estrogens and progestins		
NELOVA	See estrogens and progestins		
NEORAL (cyclosporin A)	C/CH/HB	++	
Niacin (nicotinic acid)	C	+++	
NIACIN-TIME (nicotinic acid)	C	+++	
Niclofan	CH	++	

Table 33.1 *Contd...*

Name of the Drug	Reaction Type	Data	Mortality
NICOBID (nicotinic acid)	C	+++	
NICOLAR (nicotinic acid)	C	+++	
Nicotinamide	See nicotinic acid		
Nicorinic acid	C	+++	
Nifedipine	C	+	
Nitrazepam	CH	+	
Nitrofurantoin	C/CH	+++	
Nitropropane-2	C	++	
NIZORIL (ketoconazole)	C	+++	
NOLV ADEX (tamoxifen)	C	+++	
NOR-QD See progestins			
Nor-androstenolone cyclohexylpropionate	C	++	
Nordette	See estrogens and progestins		
Norethandrolone 17-alpha-ethinyl-19-nortestosterone	C	++	
NORETHIN	See estrogens and progestins		
N orethisterone	See progestins		
Norethynodrel	See progestins		
NORINYL	See estrogens and progestins		
NORMODYNE (labetolol)	CH	++	+
NORPACE (disopyramide)	CH	++	
NORPRAMIN (desipramine)	See tricyclic antidepressants		
Novobiocin	C	+	
NSAIDS	See specific agent		
OGEN	See estrogens		
OMNIPEN (ampicillin)	CH	+	
OPTIC ROM (cromolyn)	CH	++	
Oral contraceptive	See estrogen and progestins		
ORETON (methyltestosterone)	C/CH	+++	+
ORTHO-CEPT	See estrogens and progestins		
ORTHO-CYCLEN	See estrogens and progestins		
ORTHO-EST	See estrogens		
ORTHO-NOVUM	See estrogens and progestins		
ORTHO-TRI-CYCLEN	See estrogens and progestins		
OVRON	See estrogens and progestins		
OVRAL	See estrogens and progestins		
Oxacillin	CH/rare	++	

Table 33.1 *Contd...*

Name of the Drug	Reaction Type	Data	Mortality
Oxandrolone	See anabolic steroids		
Oxazepam	CH	+	
Oxymetholone	See anabolic steroids		
Para-aminobenzoic acid	C	++	
Paracetamol	CH	+++	
P ARAFLEX (chlorzoxazone)	CH	+++	
PARAFON FORTE (chlorzoxazone)	CH	+++	
Paraquat	C/CH	+++	
PARNATE (tranylcypromine)	CH	+	
PCE	(Erythromycin base)		
Pecazine	C	+	
PEDIAZOLE (erythromycin ethylsuccinate)	CH See erythromycin ethylsuccinate and sulfonamides	+++	
Penicillamine	CH	++	
Penicillins	C/rare	+	
Pentazocine	C	+	
PERIACTIN (cyproheptadine)	C	++	
Perphenazine	CH	+	
Phenindione	C	++	+
Phenobarbitone	See barbiturates		
Phenothiazines	C/CH	++	
Phenylbutazone	CH	+++	
Phenytoin	CH	+++	
Piperazine	CH	+++	
Piroxicam	C/CH	++	
Pizotifen	C	++	
PLATINOL (cisplatin)	C	+++	
PMB 200/400	See estrogens (and meprobamate)		
POLYCILLIN (ampicillin)	CH	+	
Prajmalium	H	+++	
PREMARIN	See estrogens		
PREMPHASE	See estrogens and medroxyprogesterone		
PREMPRO	See estrogens and medroxyprogesterone		
PRIMAXIN (imipenem/cilastatin)	C	++	
Probenecid	C/HB	++	
Procainamide	C	+++	
PROCAN SR (procainamide)	C	+++	
PROCARDIA (nifedipine)	C	+	

Table 33.1 *Contd...*

Name of the Drug	Reaction Type	Data	Mortality
Prochlorperazine	CH	++	
Progestins	C	+	
PROLIXIN (fluphenazine)	C	+?	
Promazine	C	+	
Propafenone	C	+	
Propylthiouracil	CH	+++	
PROVERA	See progestins		
PTU (propylthiouracil)	CH	+++	
PURINETHOL (mercaptopurine)	CH	+++	
Pyritinol	CH	+++	
Ranitidine	C/rare	+++	
REGROTON (chlorthalidone)	CH	+	
REMULAR (chlorzoxazone)	CH	+++	
RESTORIL (temazepam)	CH	+	
RETROVIR (zidovudine)	CH	+++	
RHYMOLE (propafenone)	C	+	
Rifampicin	CH	+	
ROCEPHIN (ceftriaxone)	biliary sludge	+	
SANDIMMUNE (cyclosporin A)	C/CH/HB	++	
Saramycin	C	+	
SECTRAL (acebutolol)	CH	+++	
SEPTRA	See sulfonamides (and trimethoprim)		
SER-AP-ES	See hydralazine (and HCTZ and reserpine)		
SERAX (oxazepam)	CH	+	
SINE-AIDIB	See ibuprofen (and pseudoephedrine)		
SLO-NIACIN (nicotinic acid)	C	+++	
Spiramycin	CH	++	
SPORANOX (itraconazole)	C	++	
STANOZOLOL	See anabolic steroids		
STELAZINE (trifluoperazine)	C	+	
STILPHOSTROL (diethylstilbestrol)	C	+	
Sulfamethoxazole	See sulfonamides		
Sulfasalazine	C	++	+
Sulindac	C/CH	+++	
SULFATRIM	See sulfonamides (and trimethoprim)		
Sulfonamides	CICH	+++	
T-STAT	[Erythromycin base]		

Table 33.1 *Contd...*

Name of the Drug	Reaction Type	Data	Mortality
TAGAMET (cimetidine)	C/CH/rare	+++	
TALACEN	See pentazocine (and acetaminophen)		
TAL WIN (pentazocine)	C	+	
Tamoxifen	C	+++	
TAO CAPSULES (troleandomycin)	CH	+++	
TAPAZOLE (methimazole)	C	+++	
TEGISON (etretinate)	CH	++	
TEGRETOL (carbamazepine)	CH	+++	
Temazepam	CH	+	
TENORETIC	See atenolol and chlorthalidone		
TENORMIN (atenolol)	C	++	
TESTRED (methyltestosterone)	CICH	+++	+
THALITONE (chlorthalidone)	CH	+	
THERAMYCIN Z	(Erythromycin base)		
Thiabendazole	C/CH	+++	+
Thiazide diuretics	See specific agent		
Thioguanine-6	C	+	
Thiola (tiopronin)	C	+	
Thioridazine	CH	++	
Thioxanthenes	C	+	
THORAZINE (chlorpromazine)	CH	+++	
Tiaprofenic	CH	+++	
TIAZAC (diltiazem)	CH	+++	
Ticarcillin/clavulanate	CH	++	
TICLID (ticlopidine)	C	++	
Ticlopidine	C	++	
TIMENTIN (ticarcillinlclavulanate)	CH	++	
Tiopronin	C	+	
TMP-SMX	See sulfonamides (and trimethoprim)		
TOFRANIL (imipramine) q	CH	+++	
TOFRANIL-PM (imipramine)	CH	+++	
Tolazemide	C/CH	++	
Tolbutamide	CH	+++	+
Total parental nutrition (TPN)	C	++	
TRANSDATE (labetolol)	CH	++	
TRANXENE (clorazepate)	CH	+	
Tranylcypromine	CH	+	
Trazodone	C	++	

Table 33.1 *Contd...*

Name of the Drug	Reaction Type	Data	Mortality
TRI-LEVLEN	See estrogens and progestins		
TRI-NORUNYL	See estrogens and progestins		
Triacetyloleandomycin	CH	+++	

Data: + = anecdotal or not well described; ++ = good temporal relationship; +++ = confirmed by rechallenge.

Note: Confirmation does not imply greater frequency and most clinicians regard ++ and +++ to suggest reasonable proof. Frequency of cholestasis is difficult to estimate except with the most commonly used drugs and usually cannot be accurately obtained from the medical literature.

Mortality = "+" indicates mortality associated with medication. ? = causality unclear or only single case documented. *See* reference to drug group implies characteristic believed to be generalizable to drug class. Reference to specific drug indicates cholestasis only documented in drug indicated.

Table 33.2

Hepatotoxicity of some nonprescription drugs

Agent	*Injury*
Chaparral	Hepatocellular
leaf/creosote bush	Hepatocellular
Jin Bu	Veno-occlusive disease
Huanlgermander	Hepatocellular/cirrhosis
Pyrrolizidine alkaloids	Hepatocellular
bush tea Vitamin A	
(> 10,000 IV/d)	
Saccharin	

Generic: are in uppercase. US tradenames are in lowercase (as indicated in 1996 Physician's Desk Reference).

(Generic): The generic name of the suspected component has been included immediately after the tradename in parenthesis. A '+' sign indicates other ingredients in formulation present but not known to cause drug reaction.

[Generic]: are drugs not known to case hepatits, but are included because of reactions noted in similar drugs.

Note: All drugs known to cause hepatitis as of 1997 are listed in this table. The drug families included in this table summarize what has been seen with the entire class, but may not be true for a particular drug. Drugs known to be withdrawn from the world market were excluded from this table. This table contains only drugs associated with hepatitis. Drug combinations only list component known to cause hepatitis.

Types of reaction: H = hepatitis (aminotransferase elevations or biopsy); TOX = hepatotoxic (unspecified); H/Tox = mixed hepatitis/toxic; LFT = serum liver test abnormality (unspecified); RARE = hepatocellular reaction rarely seen.

Data: + = anecdotal or not well described; ++ = good temporal relationship; +++ = confirmed by rechallenge.

Note: Confirmation does not imply greater frequency and most clinicians regard ++ and +++ to suggest reasonable proof. Frequency of hepatitis is difficult to estimate except with the most commonly used drugs and usually cannot be accurately obtained from the medical literature.

Table 33.3

Medications associated with predominantly hepatocellular injury

Name of the drug	Reaction type	Data	Mortality
Acebutolol	H	+++	
Acitretin	H	++	
Albendazole	H	+++	
Allopurinol	H	+++	FH
Acetaminophen	TOX	+++	M
Amieptine	H	+++	
Amiodarone	H	++	
Amiodiaquine	H/TOX	++1+++	FH
Amitriptyline	H	+++	FH
AmoxicilliniClavulanic Acid	H	++	
Amoxicillin	H	+	
Ampicillin	H	+	
Aprindine	H	+++	
Aspirin	H	+++	
Azapropazone	H	++	
Azathioprine	H	+++	
BCG	H	++	
Benzarone	H	+++	
Captopril	H	+++	FH
Carbamazepine	H	+++	
Carbimazole	H	+++	
Carbutamide	H	+	
Cephalexin	H	+	
Cephalosporins	See specific agent		
Chlordiazepoxide	H	+	
Chlormezonone	H	++	FH
Chlorothiazide	H	+	
Chlorpromazine	H	+	FH
Chlorpropamide	H	+	
Chlorzoxazone	H	+++	
Cimetidine	H	+++	FH
Clindamycin	H	++	
Clofibrate	H	+	
Clometacin	H	+++	
Clomipramine	H	++	
Clonazepam	H	+++	

Table 33.3 *Contd...*

Name of the drug	Reaction type	Data	Mortality
Clotrizepam	H	++	FH
Cocaine	H	++	
Copper Salts	TOX		
Dantrolene	H	+++	FH
Dapsone	H	++	
Desipramine	H	+	
Diazepam	H	+	FH
Diclofenac	H	+++	FH
Difenamizole	H	+	
Diflunisal	H	++	
Diltiazem	H	+	
Disulfiram	H	+++	
Dothiepim	H	++	
Doxorubicin	CAH	+	
Enalapril	H	++	
Enflurane	H	+++	FH
Ethionamide	TOX	+++	
Acetaminophen	TOX	+++	FH
Aspirin	H/TOX	++	
Etretinate	H	+++	
Exifone	H	++	FH
Fenbufen	H	+++	
Fenfibrate	H	+	
Fenfluramine	H	+	
Fipexidine	H	++	FH
Flucloxacillin	H	+	
Flucytosine	H	++	
5-Fluorouracil	LFT	+	
Flutamide	H	+++	
Glafenine	H	+++	
Glyburide	H	++	
Gold Salts	H	+++	FH
Halothane	H	+++	FH
Heparin	LFT	++	
Hycanthone	TOX	+++	
Hydralazine	H	+++	

Table 33.3 *Contd...*

Name of the drug	Reaction type	Data	Mortality
Ibuprofen	H	+++	
Idarubicin	H	++	FH
Indocine N-oxide	H	++	FH
Indomethacin	H	+	FH
Iodipamide meglumine	H	++	
Iron	TOX	+++	
Isocarboxazide	H	++	
Isoniazid	H	+++	
Kanamycin	H	+	
Ketoconazole	H	+++	FH
Labetalol	H	+++	FH
Lergotrile	H	++	
Lisinopril	H	++	FH
Mebendazole	H	+++	
Meclofenamate	H	+	
Mercaptopurine-6	H/TOX	+++	
Mesalazine	H	++	
Metahexamide	H	+++	FH
Methimazole	H	+++	
Methotrexate	TOX	+++	
Methoxyflurane	H	+++	FH
N-Methylcarbamate	H	+	
Methyldopa	H	+++	FH
Metoprolol	H	++	
MINOCYCLINE	H	+++	M
Mistletoe	H	+++	
Monochlorobenzene	TOX	+++	
Moxisylyte	H	+++	
Naproxen	H	+++	
Nicotinic Acid	TOX	+++	
Niacin (Nicotinic Acid)	TOX	+++	
Nifedipine	H	++	
Niflumic Acid	H	++	
Nitrofurantoin	H	+++	FH
Norfloxacin	H	++	
Omeprazole	H	+	M
Oxacillin	H	++	
Oxyphenbutazone	H	+	

Table 33.3 *Contd...*

Name of the drug	Reaction type	Data	Mortality
Para-aminosalicylic Acid	TOX	+++	
Paracetamol	H	+++	
Paraquat	TOX	+++	
Pemoline	H	++	FH
Penicillin	H	+	
Pennyroyal oil	H	++	
Perhexiline	H	++	
Phencyclidine	H	+	
Pheniprazine	H	+	
Phenoxyproperazine	H	+	
Phenozopyridine	H	+	
Phenylbutazone	H	+++	
Phenytoin	H	+++	FH
Phosphorus	TOX	+++	
Piperazine	H	+++	
Pirprofen	H	+++	FH
Piroxicam	H	++	FH
Probenecid	H	++	
Procainamide	H	+++	
Procarbazine	H	++	
Prochlorperazine	H	++	
Progabide	H	++	
Propylthiouracil	H	+++	
Pyrazinamide	H	+++	FH
Pyricarbate	H	+++	
Quinidine	H	+++	
Quinine	H	+++	
Ranitidine	H	+++	
SEATONE	H	++	
Simvastatin	H	++	
Spironolactone	H	+++	
Sulfadioxine-pyrimethamine	H	++	FH
Sulfasalazine	H	+++	
Sulfonamides	H	+++	FH
Tetrachloroethane	TOX	+++	
Tetrahydroaminoacridine	H	+++	
Tocainide	H	+	

Mortality: M = mortality associated with medication; ? = causality unclear or only single case documented; FH = fulminant hepatitis. *See* reference to drug group implies characteristic believed to be generalizable to drug class.

Table 33.4

Medications associated with tumors and other liver pathology

Name of drug	Reaction type
Aflatoxin	C,HCC
Allopurinol	GH
Amiodarone	GH
Amoxacillin	GH
Ampicillin	GH
Androgens	P,A,HCC,AS
Arsenic	AS,HCC, C, P
Aspirin	GH
Azapropazone	GH
Azathioprine	P
BCG	GH
Beryillium	GH
Calcium carbamide	C
Carbamazepine	GH
Carbon tetrachloride	C,HCC
Carbutamide	GH
Cephalexin	GH
Chlorothiazide	GH
Chlorpromazine	GH
Chlorpropamide	GH
Clofibrate	GH
Clometacin	C,GH
Co-trimoxazole	GH
Copper salts	Gh,AS
Danazol	P,A,HCC
Dapsone	GH
Diazepam	GH
Diethylnitrosamine	C,HCC
Diethylstilbestrol	P,HCC
Diltiazem	GH
Estrogens	GH, A, AS, CHA, Others

Table 33.4 *Contd...*

Name of drug	Reaction type
Fenfluramine	GH
Flucloxacillin	GH
Glyburide	GH
Gold salts	GH
Halothane	GH
Hydralazine	GH
Hydroxyurea	P
Isoniazid	C,GH
Labetalol	C
Medroxyprogesterone	P
Methotrexate	C,HCC
Methyldopa	GH,C,CHA
Metolazone	GH
Nitrofurantoin	GH
Oxacillin	GH
Oxyphenbutazone	GH
Oxyphenisatin	C
Papaverine	GH,C
Penicillin	GH
Perhexiline	GH
Phenelzine	HCC,C
Phenylbutazone	GH
Phenytoin	GH
Polychlorinated biphenyls (PCB)	C
Procainamide	GH
Procarbazine	GH
Pyrrolizidine alkaloids	C,HCC
Quinidine	GH
Quinine	GH
Ranitidine	GH
SEATONE (herbal extract)	GH
Silica	GH
Stilbestrol	AS
Sulfadioxine-pyrimethamine	GH
Sulfasalazine	GH
Sulfonamides	GH
Talc	GH
Tamoxifen	P

Table 33.4 *Contd...*

Name of drug	Reaction type
Testosterone	P,A
Tetrachloroethane	F
Tetrahydroaminoacridine	GH
Thioguanine-6	P
Thorium dioxide	AS, P, CHA, HCC
Thorotrast (Thorium dioxide)	AS,P, CHA, HCC
Tocainide	GH
Tolbutamide	GH,HCC
Trichlormethiazide	GH
Trinitrotoluene (TNT)	C
Vinyl chloride	F, AS, P, C, Others
Vitamin A	C,P
Zimelidine	GH

A = Adenoma; AS = Angiosarcoma; C = Cirrhosis; CHA = Cholangiocarcinoma; GH = Granulomatous Hepatitis; HCC = Hepatocellular Carcinoma; P = Peliosis.

Table 33.5

Medication associated with vascular disease

Name of Drug	Reaction Type
Actinomycin-D	VOD,PH
Adriamycin (doxorubicin)	VOD
Aflatoxin	VOD
Arsenic	PH, VOD
Azathioprine	PH, VOD
BCNU	VOD
Busulfan	VOD
Carboplatin	VOD
Copper salts	PH
Cyclophosphamide	VOD
Cysteamine	VOD
Cytosine arabinoside	VOD
Dacarbazine	VOD,BC
Dactinomycin (actinomycin-D)	VOD,PH

Name of Drug	Reaction Type
Dimethylnitrosamine	VOD
Doxorubicin	VOD
Estrogens	BC
Indocine N-oxide	VOD
Medroxyprogesterone	BC
Methotrexate	PH
Mitomycin C	VOD
Nitrogen mustard	VOD
Progestin (medroxyprogesterone)	BC
Pyrrolizidine alkaloids	VOD
Thioguanine- 6	VOD, PH
Vincristine	VOD
Vitamin E (iv form only)	VOD

Table 33.5 *Contd...*

BC = Budd-Chari Syndrome; PH = Portal Hypertension (Noncirrhotic); VOD = Veno-occlusive disease

Table 33.6

Hepatotoxic drugs requiring chronic monitoring

Amiodarone (Cordarone): Periodic serum liver enzyme levels should be obtained in patients on chronic therapy, especially with high daily dosage, although effectiveness in preventing liver disease is unclear.

Anabolic steroids, androgens: Periodic serum liver enzyme levels should be obtained. If suspicion of peliosis hepatis or other tumor is suspected, the patient should be carefully evaluated.

Dantrolene (Dantrium): Hepatocellular toxicity is increased in females and patients over 35 y, serum liver enzyme levels should be obtained at intervals. The medication should be discontinued if not clear.

Doxorubicin (Adriamycin, Rubex): Dosage reduction in patients is necessary with impaired hepatic function.

Erythromycin estolate (Ilosone): Hepatic dysfunction has occurred, primarily in adults and is contraindicated in patients with pre-existing liver disease.

Etretinate (Tegison): Monitor AST, ALT and LDH at baseline, at 1-2 wk intervals for 1-2 mo, and then every 1-3 mo thereafter. Serum liver enzyme level abnormalities are common, but if fibrosis, necrosis, or cirrhosis is suspected, the medication should be discontinued and the patient should be evaluated.

Felbamate (Felbato!): Hepatic failure is definitely associated with use, but details of risk factors is limited because drug use is limited to refractory epilepsy. Serum liver enzyme levels are recommended at baseline and every 1-2 wk thereafter, with immediate withdrawal if abnormalities develop.

HMG-CoA enzyme reductase inhibitors, jluvastatin, lovastatin, simvastatin (Lescol, Mevacor, Zocor): Aminotransferase elevations >3X normal should prompt discontinuation of therapy. Serum liver enzyme levels should be taken at baseline, 6 wk, 12 wk, and periodically from the initiation of therapy and with any increase in dose.

Interferon alfa (Roferon-A, Intron A): Periodic serum liver enzyme levels are recommended may be more useful to determine effectiveness of therapy rather than monitor for hepatic failure. "Flares" with aminotransferase elevations <3X normal are common early in therapy and usually only requires monitoring.

Isoniazid (Nydrazid, Rifamate, Rifater): Risk of fatal hepatitis, (generally increased age increases risk) and is increased with daily alcohol consumption. Late reactions (after several months) can be seen. Asymptomatic, mild transient serum liver enzyme level abnormalities are common and can be followed. Clinical symptoms of hepatitis should prompt immediate withdrawal of drug with consideration of an alternative medication for TB.

Metformin (Glucophage): Lactic acidosis occurs primarily in patients with renal impairment, but patients with evidence of hepatic impairment should avoid this medication because of potential impairment in clearing lactic acid.

Methotrexate (Rheumatrex): Hepatotoxicity with fibrosis and cirrhosis can occur with prolonged therapy and are often not preceded by symptoms or abnormal serum liver enzyme levels.

Table 33.6 *Contd...*

Hepatotoxicity can only be monitored with liver biopsies. Although the frequency of liver biopsies is controversial, a reasonable approach is a baseline liver biopsy followed by biopsies every additional 1.0-1.5 g, although the exact interval, or need for every patient is controversial. Alcohol use, renal impairment, pre-existing liver disease, daily therapy, and higher total weekly dose, diabetes, obesity, and age may increase the risk of hepatic injury. Transient, asymptomatic serum liver enzyme level abnormalities do not predict or indicate methotrexate induced liver disease. Periodic serum liver enzyme levels and serum albumin is recommended, but there is no consensus in terms of frequency.

Methyldopa, methyldopate (Aldoclor, Aldomet, methyldopate): Fatal hepatic necrosis has been reported and mimics many hepatocellular and biliary processes. Periodic serum liver enzyme levels should be drawn especially during the first 6-12 wk of therapy. If a hypersensitivity pattern is seen, patients should not be rechallenged.

Minocycline (Minocine, Dynacin, Vectrin): Serum sickness, a systemic lupus erythematosus-like syndrome, and autoimmune hepatitis, the latter sometimes severe with mortality has been reported with oral administration for the treatment of acne. ANA and aminotransferases should be drawn as a baseline and followed periodically during treatment.

Tacrine (Cognex): ALT should be monitored every other week for 16 wk, then monthly for another 8 wk, and every 3 mo thereafter. Jaundiced patients with total bili >3 mg/dL should be discontinued and not rechallenged.

Valproic acid, divalproex (Depakene, Depakote): Risk of hepatic failure. Monitor serum liver enzyme levels at baseline, and frequently thereafter, especially first 6 mo. Extreme caution in patients under 2 yr of age.

DIURETICS

Hepatotoxicity is rarely seen with diuretics. Jaundice and an increased incidence of acute cholecystitis has been associated with thiazide diuretics.

ANTIEPILEPTICS

CARBAMAZEPINE

Asymptomatic aminotransferase elevations are common. Carbamazepine may induce a granulomatous hepatitis that has a classic presentation 1-16 wk after starting the medication. Fever, chills, night sweats, anorexia, and malaise are seen. Symptoms may mimic cholangitis.

BARBITURATES

Although hepatotoxicity is rare, barbiturate-induced hepatitis is often severe and can be fatal.

PHENYTOIN

Phenytoin induces elevations in GGT, which alone is not considered evidence of hepatotoxicity. Toxicity is not dose dependent. Systemic symptoms, particularly fever and rash, are common. Typically a hepatitis picture occurs, but a pseudo-mononucleosis or pseudo-lymphoma syndrome has been documented. Recovery is rapid upon withdrawal.

ANTITUBERCULOSIS AGENTS

Streptomycin, ethambutol, rifampin, and isoniazid (INH) are agents generally used in combination for treatment of tuberculosis. Streptomycin and ethambutol appear to have relatively little hepatotoxicity. Hepatotoxicity associated with rifampin has been seen mainly in patients taking it in combination with INH, but has also been documented to cause toxicity alone Oxidation of acetylated isoniazid derivatives probably plays a role. These products have been reported to bind covalently to intracellular macromolecules producing injury. Mild elevations in aminotransferases (less than 2 times normal) are common, occurring in 10-20% of cases. Generally, these elevations are not of clinical significance, and will resolve spontaneously. In approx 1 % of all individuals exposed, clinical hepatitis may develop. This percentage is higher in older persons, and is rare in individuals under the age of 35. Alcohol appears to increase the risk of hepatitis, and certain other subgroups such as black females, postpartum women, and possibly Asian men may also be at higher risk to develop INH-induced hepatitis. It was also initially considered that rapid acetylators of isoniazid were at increased risk for developing INH hepatitis. However, this has not been supported by more recent studies. There is significant potential for fulminant hepatic failure. Patients with acute INH hepatitis have up to a 10% mortality. This is much higher than that associated with viral hepatitis. INH hepatitis is rare in those who have been treated with the drug for more than 6 mo without becoming ill. Because there is also no close correlation between aminotransferase elevations and the development of clinical hepatitis, the issue of monitoring these levels is controversial. Monitoring of aminotransferase levels is not recommended for individuals under the age of 35. This younger group of patients should be instructed, however, to report immediately any symptoms out of the ordinary, such as fatigue, flu-like symptoms, or gastrointestinal complaints. In patients over the age of 35, monitoring of aminotransferases levels is recommended. It has been suggested that minor elevations <100 lUlL can be followed closely, particularly if they return to normal. If levels exceed 100 lUlL, discontinuation has been suggested. If there are any clinical symptoms or signs of hepatitis, the drug should be discontinued unless it is needed for life threatening tuberculosis.

NONSTEROIDAL ANTI-INFLAMMATORY DRUGS (NSAIDS)

The two notable exceptions are aspirin and acetaminophen. These drugs have intrinsic hepatotoxicity and cause injury in a dose-dependent manner. Salicylate toxicity is usually associated with blood levels exceeding 15-25 mg/dL. NSAIDS generallycause hepatocellular injury, but cholestatic hepatitis has been reported with diflunisal, naproxen, and sulindac.

SALICYLATES

Salicylates also deserve separate mention in relation to Reye's syndrome. Reye's syndrome is seen mainly in children who have taken salicylates for fever, and results in acute fatty degeneration of the liver. The mechanism is not understood. Reye's syndrome has been rarely reported in adults. For patients taking NSAIDS for a short period of time, monitoring is not needed. However, for patients with chronic inflammatory diseases, who will potentially be on the medication for a long period of time, monitoring may be considered, but this is controversial because hepatotoxicity is not a common problem. Most hepatotoxic reactions will occur in the first few months and only very rarely after 6 months of no ill effects. A reasonable approach would be to check a baseline ALT and then monthly for

6 months. If the patient develops ALT abnormalities, changing to an alternative agent in a different chemical class would be prudent because cross reactivity between classes has not been demonstrated. If the drug is working well for the patient and he does not want to discontinue it, the patient could be followed clinically and with serial ALTs on a weekly basis. If the levels do not increase more than 2-3 times normal or decrease, it is probably safe to continue the drug. If the ALT continues to increase, or the patient develops any clinical symptoms of hepatotoxicity, the drug must be.

ACETAMINOPHEN

Acetaminophen, or paracetamol, deserves special mention, because it is a very commonly used analgesic that may cause acute hepatitis and hepatic failure when taken in large doses. Most cases with severe liver injury involve doses greater than 15 g, but single doses of 6 g have been reported to produce severe liver injury. The best predictor of the potential severity of an ingested dose of acetaminophen is the blood level of the drug when measured 4-12 h after ingestion. Persons with acetaminophen levels less than about 150 /J.g/dL at 4 h are unlikely todevelop any significant toxicity. Levels greater than 300 /J.g/dL at 4 h predict a high likelihood of severe hepatitis.

Mechanism of Injury: Acetaminophen is primarily metabolized by conjugation to glucuronate and sulfate. It is converted slightly into Nacetyl-p-benzoquinone (NAPQI). NAPQI is considered to be the hepatotoxic intermediate. Small amounts of NAPQI are detoxified by binding to glutathione. Hepatotoxicity results when the amount of NAPQI exceeds the amount of glutathione present in the liver. This occurs when large doses of acetaminophen are ingested or when increased levels of NAPQI are produced secondary to increased activity of specific cytochrome P450 enzymes. Alcohol and other drugs such as anticonvulsants and omeprazole are known to induce these enzymes and may result in hepatotoxicity at lower doses. Alcohol abusers with chronic liver injury may additionally be at risk from lower levels of glutathione.

Treatment. Acetaminophen overdoses are treated with the glutathione precursor N-acetylcysteine. When taken within 16 h of a large dose of acetaminophen, it will prevent most of the significant liver toxicity. Treatment starts with a loading dose of 140 mg/kg and then 70 mg/kg every 4 h for a total of 17 doses. If the patient cannot drink, a nasogastric tube should be placed. In the patient that presents with a suspected acetaminophen overdose, the timing of the ingestion should be determined, blood levels should be drawn prior to treatment (4-12 h after ingestion), and treatment started immediately with acetylcysteine. If blood levels show acetaminophen in the low toxic range, the acetylcysteine can be discontinued. If borderline or higher levels, are found, the treatment should be continued and the patient's aminotransferases, bilirubin and protime monitored. The patient should be carefully followed for any signs of encephalopathy. Hepatic failure will generally occur 3-5 d following ingestion of the drug. Treatment with acetylcysteine is most effective when begun early in the course of an acetaminophen overdose. There is good data to support treatment up to 16 h following ingestion. Beyond 16 h, there is controversy regarding its efficacy, but it may be beneficial up to 24 h postoverdose. Beyond 24 h, there is little data to support its use . Recommended treatment for hepatotoxicity due to a single dose of acetaminophen does not apply to individuals who have ingested multiple doses of the drug or those chronically consuming alcohol or other drugs that induce the cytochrome P450 system.

Liver transplantation has been used successfully in patients with severe hepatotoxicity due to acetaminophen. As a general rule, if the patient shows no signs of encephalopathy, and the prothrombin time is not increasing significantly, transplantation will not be necessary. Because most acetaminophen toxicity is the result 'Of a suicide attempt, psychiatric consultation should be obtained immediately. A patient considered to be at high risk for a repeat attemptat suicide may be refused consideration for liver transplantation.

PSYCHIATRIC AGENTS

CHLORPROMAZINE/PHENOTHIAZINES

A cholestatic or mixed picture is commonly seen with chlorpromazine and is not dose related. Jaundice is seen in nearly 1% of patients and is commonly preceded by a prodromal influenza-like or gastrointestinal syndrome. Response to withdrawal is rapid, but prolonged courses are not uncommon. Cholestatic hepatitis is not rare (1 %) and not dose related. Cross reactivity with otherphenothiazines is documented but rare. Cholestasis occurs less commonly with other phenothiazines. It is unclear if chlorpromazine-induced cholestasis is immunoallergic or metabolic.

ANTIDEPRESSANTS

MAO Inhibitors. Iproniazid is associated with greater hepatotoxicity than other MAO inhibitors, but is not available in the United States. Hepatotoxicity is variable among MAO inhibitors. The relative incidence is difficult to ascertain since these drugs are less commonly used.

Tricyclic Antidepressants: Liver toxicity with tricyclics is rare, but is most commonly cholestatic when it does occur. Amineptine may be more hepatotoxic than other tricyclics. The mechanism in this class may be a combination of individual metabolic susceptibility with a hypersensitivity reaction.

Serotonin Reuptake Inhibitors: Liver enzyme abnormalities have been reported with SRIs, but this is a relatively new medication, and incidence of hepatotoxicity is still difficult to assess.

Benzodiazepines: Hepatotoxicity is considered rare, with the exception of clotiazepam. Hepatocellular injury usually responds to withdrawal and injury from rechallenge has not yet been reported. Cholestasis may be prolonged.

LIPID-LOWERING AGENTS

HMG-CoA REDUCTASE INHIBITORS

HMG-CoA reductase inhibitors may commonly produce mild aminotransferase elevations, but the incidence of true hepatotoxicity is unclear. Monitoring serum liver enzymes is recommended to detect early signs offulminant rhabdomyolysis that may be seen with the drug alone, but more commonly when used in combination with gemfibrozil.

NICOTINIC ACID

Aminotransferase elevations are common with high-dose (3g/d) nicotinic acid, but severe hepatotoxicity is rare. Jaundice is seen in up to 5% of patients. Hepatotoxicity can be delayed and has been reported up to I yr after starting high-dose nicotinic acid. Some patients who developed hepatotoxicity on sustained release nicotinic acid were subsequently able to tolerate the standard (nonsustained release) form.

ANTIBIOTICS

NITROFURANTOIN

Nitrofurantoin is associated with chronic active hepatitis and is most commonly seen in older patients and females. This may be biased by its common use in treating chronic or recurrent urinary tract infections. Symptoms within 6 months of initial exposure are uncommon. Hypoalbuminemia, hypergamm-aglobulinemia, and a positive antinuclear antibody (ANA) may often develop. A hypersensitivity reaction is suspected. Reaction to rechallenge is rapid, and intentional rechallenges are not recommended. Fulminant hepatitis and cirrhosis can occur if the medication is continued or readministered.

TETRACYCLINE

Tetracycline is a renally excreted hepatotoxin causing steatosis, especially when given in high doses and intravenously. The maximum daily doses should generally not exceed 1g intravenously or 2g orally. Pancreatitis and renal failure are common complications.

BETA-LACTAM ANTIBIOTICS (PENICILLINS/CEPHALOSPORINS)

Although hypersensitivity is common with the penicillins, hepatotoxicity is rare. Oxacillin has a greater, but still rare, propensity to cause hepatocellular injury. Other oxypenicillins may have an increased likelihood of cholestatic hepatitis such as cloxacillin, dicloxacillin, and flucloxacillin. Amoxacillin-clavulanic acid is associated with a cholestatic hepatitis. Cephalosporins are a rare cause of hepatotoxicity. Ceftriaxone has been associated with ceftriaxone-calcium microcalculi or gall stone formation that can sometimes become symptomatic, but will usually resolve when the medication is discontinued. This has mainly been reported in children.

MACROLIDES

Erythromycin and other macrolide antibiotics can cause a cholestatic hepatitis. Typically there are hyperbilirubinemia and elevations in alkaline phosphatase or GGT. Recovery is rapid upon withdrawal, and recurrence can be dramatic with rechallenge. The estolate form is mostly associated with hepatotoxicity and is age dependent.

SYNTHETIC HORMONES

Synthetic estrogens can cause a bland cholestasis or cholestatic hepatitis. The cholestasis has both genetic and dose-dependent components. Estrogens predictably decrease bile flow, although the predominant mechanism is not clear. The onset of jaundice may be delayed and may present with an initial elevation in aminotransferases that subsequently resolves. Hyperbilirubinemia is characteristic with mildly elevated alkaline phosphatase and GGT that may remain normal throughout. Prolonged cholestasis has been documented. Sinusoidal dilatation is a common histological finding, but frank peliosis hepatis is uncommon. Androgens are also associated with bland cholestasis and cholestatic hepatitis. These syndromes are dose-dependent and seen more frequently than with estrogens.

AGENTS FOR SUPPRESSION OF GASTRIC ACID PRODUCTION

H2-BLOCKERS

Idiosyncratic hepatitis and cholestasis have been reported with H2-receptor blockers, but are considered very rare. Liver enzyme abnormalities may be seen.

PROTON PUMP INHIBITORS

No significant hepatoxicity has been reported with proton pump inhibitors such as omeprazole or lansoprazole.

ANTIHYPERURICEMIC AGENTS

ALLOPURINOL

Side effects with this medication are common, but severe drug reactions are rare. Acute hepatitis can be seen and may often accompany the acute systemic hypersensitivity syndrome seen with this agent. Mortality is high in these patients (15%). The patient may continue to deteriorate after discontinuing the medication, and recovery can be delayed. Granulomas and eosinophilia are commonly seen on liver biopsies. Steroids may be beneficial in severely ill patients.

ANTIPROLIFERATIVE AGENTS

METHOTREXATE

This drug has been implicated in the development of hepatic fibrosis and cirrhosis. Toxicity is related to the total dose of the drug and also probably to the dosing interval (daily vs weekly). Toxicity appears to be more common in patients with psoriasis than rheumatoid arthritis. Liver enzymes are of little value in monitoring for toxicity. Whereas there is controversy regarding monitoring, baseline liver biopsy in patients who will be receiving long-term methotrexate is probably warranted. A cumulative dose of 1.5 g is associated with an increased risk of developing cirrhosis. It is prudent to obtain a liver biopsy then this total dose is reached. If the postmethotrexate biopsy shows increased fibrosis, (above grade 2), it is recommended that the medication be discontinued. If there is no increase in fibrosis, a repeat biopsy after each additional gram of drug is prudent .

SULFUR CONTAINING AGENTS

Although sulfonamide-induced hypersensitivity is common, hepatotoxicity is rare. Mortality is typically associated with extrahepatic hypersensitivity, but fulminant hepatitis has been reported.

Oral Hypoglycemic Agents: Hepatotoxicity with oral hypoglycemic agents is not related to the sulfa group and is uncommon. Glyburide can cause a pure cholestasis.

ANTICOAGULANTS

WARFARIN

Cholestasis has been reported with this agent, but is extremely rare.

VITAMINS

VITAMIN A

Massive intake of vitamin A can cause acute hepatotoxicity. Chronic use of vitamin A has been associated with aminotransferase abnormalities, cirrhosis, and death. Liver toxicity has been seen typically in patients taking >40,000 IU/d .

NICOTINAMIDE

NONTRADITIONAL THERAPIES

Nontraditional therapies using alternative drugs is increasing in popularity today. Whereas most of these agents taken in small doses are safe, it is important to realize that some of these medications have been associated with significant hepatotoxicity and patients should be questioned about these during the medical history.

REFERENCES

1. Zimmerman, HJ. Hepatotoxicity: the adverse effects of drugs and other chemicals on the liver. Appleton- Century-Crofts, New York, 1978.
2. Scheuer PJ. Rifampicin hepatitis: a clinical and histological study. Lancet 1974;1:421-425.
3. Mitchell JR. Isoniazid liver ~ury: clinical spectrum, pathology, and pathogenesis. Ann Int Med 1976;84: 181-192.
4. Baily WC. The effect of isoniazid on transaminases levels. Ann Int Med 1974;81:200-202.
5. Mitchell JR. Acetylation rates and monthly liver function tests during one year of isoniazid preventive therapy. Chest 1975;68:181-190.
6. KopanoffDE. Isoniazid-related hepatitis. A U.S. Public Health Service Cooperative Surveillance Study. Am Rev Respir Dis 1978;991-1001.
7. Snider DE. Isoniazid-associated hepatitis deaths: a review of available information. Am Rev Respir Dis 1992; 145 :494—497.
8. Gurumurthy P. Lack of relationship between hepatic toxicity and acetylator phenotype in three thousand South Indian patients during treatment with isoniazid for tuberculosis. Am Rev Respir Dis 1984; 129:58-61.
9. Rigas B, Spiro HM. Clinical gastro-enterology companion handbook, 4th ed. McGraw-Hill, New York, 1995, p. 574.
10. American Thoracic Society. Control of tuberculosis in the United States. Am Rev Respir Dis 1992; 146: 1623-1633.
11. Rabinovits M. Hepatotoxicity of non-steroidal anti-inflammatory drugs. Am J Gastro 1992;87: 1696-1704.
12. Zimmerman HJ, Maddrey We. Toxic and drug-induced hepatitis. In: SchiffL, SchiffER, eds. Diseases of the liver. JB Lippincott, Philadelphia, 1993, pp. 707-783.
13. Schiff E, Maddrey W. Can we prevent nonsteroidal anti-inflammatory drug-induced hepatic failure? Gastrointest Dis Today 1994;3:7-13.
14. Hamlyn AN. The spectrum of paracetamol acetaminophen overdose: clinical and epidemiologic studies. Postgrad Med 1978;54:400-404.
15. Heathcote J. Hepatotoxicity: newer aspects of pathogenesis and treatment. Gastroenterologist 1995;3: 119-29.
16. Smilkstein MJ. Efficacy of oral N-acety1cysteine in the treatment of acetaminophen overdose. N Engl J Med 1988;319: 1557-1562.
17. Cheung L. Acetaminophcn treatment nomogram. N Engl J Med 1994;330: 1907,1908.
18. Stricker NJ, Spoelstra P. Drug-induced hepatic injury: a comprehensive survey of the literature on adverse drug reactions up to January, 1985. Elsevier, Amsterdam, 1985, p. 240.
19. Stricker BH. Drug-induced hepatic injury, 2nd ed. Elsevier, Amsterdam, 1992, p. 241.
20. Farrell, Ge. Drug Induced Liver Disease. Churchill Livingstone, New York, 1994, p. 502.
21. Roenigk HH, Auerbach R, Maibach HI. Methotrexate in psoriasis: revised guidelines. J Am Acad Dermatol 1988; 19: 145-156.
22. Kremer JM. Methotrexate for rheumatoid arthritis: suggested guidelines for monitoring liver toxicity. Arth Rheum 1994;37:316-328.
23. Kowalski TE, Falestiny M, Furth E, Malet PF. Vitamin A hepatotoxicity: a cautionary note regarding 25,000 IU supplements. Am J Med 1994; 97: 523-552.

CHAPTER 34

PANCREATITIS

DEFINITION

Acute pancreatitis (AP) is an inflammatory disorder of the pancreas characterized by severe pain in the upper abdomen and increased serum concentrations of pancreatic lipase and amylase.

Chronic pancreatitis (CP) is a syndrome of destructive and inflammatory conditions resulting from long-standing pancreatic injury. It is characterized by irreversible fibrosis and destruction of exocrine and endocrine tissue but is not invariably progressive.

ACUTE PANCREATITIS

PATHOPHYSIOLOGY

- Gallstones and alcohol abuse account for most cases in the United States. A cause cannot be identified in some patients (idiopathic pancreatitis).
- Many medications have been implicated (Table 34-1), but a causal association is difficult to confirm because ethical and practical considerations prevent rechallenge.
- AP is initiated by premature activation of pancreatic zymogens (inactive enzymes) within the acinar cells, pancreatic ischemia, or pancreatic duct obstruction.
- Release of active pancreatic enzymes directly causes local or distant tissue damage. Trypsin digests cell membranes and leads to the activation of other pancreatic enzymes. Lipase damages fat cells, producing noxious substances that cause further pancreatic and peripancreatic injury.
- Release of cytokines injures acinar cells and enhances the inflammatory response. Injured acinar cells liberate chemoattractants that attract neutrophils, macrophages, and other cells to the area of inflammation, and increased vascular permeability promotes tissue edema.
- Pancreatic infection may result from increased intestinal permeability and translocation of colonic bacteria.
- Local complications in severe AP may include acute fluid collection, pancreatic necrosis, abscess, pseudocyst formation, and pancreatic ascites.
- Systemic complications may include cardiovascular, renal, pulmonary, metabolic, hemorrhagic, and CNS abnormalities.

Table 34.1

Medications associated with acute pancreatitis

Class I: Definite Association	Class II: Probable Association	Class III: Possible Association	
5-Aminosalicylic acid	Acetaminophen	Amiodarone	Indomethacin
Asparaginase	Carbamazepine	Calcium	Indinavir
Azathioprine	Cisplatin	Celecoxib	Aldesleukin
Corticosteroids	Enalapril	Clozapine	Infliximab
Cytarabine	Erythromycin	Cholestyramine	Ketoprofen
Didanosine	Hydrochlorothiazide	Cimetidine	Ketorolac
Estrogens	Interferon α_{2b}	Ciprofloxacin	Lipid emulsion
Furosemide	Lamivudine	Clarithromycin	Lisinopril
Mercaptopurine	Octreotide	Clonidine	Mefenamic acid
Opiates		Cyclosporine	Metolazone
Pentamidine		Danazol	Nitrofurantoin
Pentavalent antimonials		Diazoxide	Ondansetron
Sulfasalazine		Etanercept	Omeprazole
Sulfamethoxazole and Trimethoprim		Ethacrynic acid	Oxyphenbutazone
Sulindac		Famciclovir	Pravastatin
Tetracycline		Glyburide	Paclitaxel
Valproic acid/salts		Gold therapy	Propofol
		Granisetron	Propoxyphene
		Metformin	Rifampin
		Methyldopa	Sertraline
		Metronidazole	Zalcitabine
		Ibuprofen	

CLINICAL PRESENTATION

- The clinical presentation depends on the severity of the inflammatory process and whether damage is confined to the pancreas or involves contiguous organs.
- The initial presentation ranges from moderate abdominal discomfort to excruciating pain, shock, and respiratory distress. Abdominal pain occurs in 95% of patients and is usually epigastric, often radiating to the upper quadrants or back. The onset is usually sudden and the intensity is often described as "knife-like" or "boring." The pain usually reaches its maximum intensity within 30 minutes and may persist for hours or days. Nausea and vomiting occur in 85% of patients and usually follow the onset of pain.
- Clinical signs associated with widespread pancreatic inflammation and necrosis include marked epigastric tenderness, abdominal distention, hypotension, and low-grade fever. In severe disease, bowel sounds are diminished or absent. Dyspnea and tachypnea are signs of acute respiratory complications.

DIAGNOSIS

- A definitive diagnosis of AP is made by surgical examination of the pancreas or pancreatic histology. In the absence of these procedures, the diagnosis depends on recognition of an etiologic factor, clinical signs and symptoms, abnormal laboratory tests, and imaging techniques that predict disease severity.
- The serum amylase concentration usually rises 4 to 8 hours after symptom onset, peaks at 24 hours, and returns to normal over the next 8 to 14 days. Serum amylase concentrations greater than three times the upper limit of normal are highly suggestive of AP.
- Serum lipase is specific to the pancreas, and concentrations are usually elevated. The increases persist longer than serum amylase elevations and can be detected after the amylase has returned to normal.

AP may be associated with leukocytosis, hyperglycemia, hypoalbuminemia, mild hyperbilirubinemia, and elevations in serum alkaline phosphatase and hepatic transaminases.

- Marked hypocalcemia indicates severe necrosis and is a poor prognostic sign.
- Dehydration may lead to hemoconcentration with elevated hemoglobin, hematocrit, blood urea nitrogen, and serum creatinine.
- C-reactive protein increases by 48 hours after the onset of symptoms and may be useful in distinguishing mild from severe pancreatitis.
- Some patients with severe pancreatitis develop thrombocytopenia and a prolonged prothrombin time.
- Contrast-enhanced computed tomography (CT) is used to identify the cause of pancreatitis and confirm the diagnosis. Magnetic resonance imaging is used to grade the severity of AP and identify bile duct abnormalities not seen on CT. Ultrasonography is useful to determine pancreatic enlargement and peripancreatic fluid collections.

PHARMACOLOGICAL TREATMENT

- Medications listed in Table 34-1 should be discontinued, if possible.
- Initial treatment usually involves withholding food or liquids to minimize exocrine stimulation of the pancreas.
- Nasogastric aspiration is beneficial in patients with profound pain, severe disease, paralytic ileus, and intractable vomiting.
- Patients predicted to follow a severe course require treatment of any cardiovascular, respiratory, renal, and metabolic complications. Aggressive fluid resuscitation is essential to correct intravascular volume depletion and maintain blood pressure. **IV colloids** may be required because fluid losses are rich in protein. **Drotrecogin alfa** may benefit patients with pancreatitis and systemic inflammatory response syndrome. IV **potassium, calcium,** and **magnesium** are used to correct deficiency states. **Insulin** is used to treat hyperglycemia. Patients with necrotizing pancreatitis may require antibiotics and surgical intervention.
- Nutritional support with enteral or parenteral nutrition should be initiated if it is anticipated that oral nutrition will be withheld for more than 1 week.

- Analgesics are given to reduce abdominal pain. In the past, parenteral **meperidine** (50 to 100 mg) every 3 to 4 hours was usually used because it causes less spasm of the sphincter of Oddi than other opioids. Meperidine is used less frequently today because it is not as effective as other opioids and is contraindicated in renal failure. Parenteral **morphine** is sometimes used, but it is thought to cause spasm of the sphincter of Oddi, increases in serum amylase and, rarely, pancreatitis. **Hydromorphone** may also be used because it has a longer half-life than meperidine. Patient-controlled analgesia should be considered in patients who require frequent opioid dosing (e.g., every 2 to 3 hours).
- There is no evidence that inhibiting gastric acid secretion by antisecretory drugs prevents exacerbations of abdominal pain, but they may be used to prevent stress-related mucosal bleeding.
- **Octreotide**, 0.1 mg subcutaneously every 8 hours, may decrease sepsis, length of hospital stay, and perhaps mortality in patients with severe AP, but there are insufficient data to support its routine use in treating AP.
- Only patients with severe AP complicated by necrosis should receive infection prophylaxis with broad-spectrum antibiotics. Agents that cover the range of enteric aerobic gram-negative bacilli and anaerobic organisms should be started within the first 48 hours and continued for 2 to 3 weeks. **Imipenem–cilastatin** (500 mg every 8 hours) may be most effective; a fluoroquinolone (e.g., **ciprofloxacin, levofloxacin**) with **metronidazole** should be considered for penicillin-allergic patients.

SURGERY

- Removal of biliary tract gallstones with endoscopic retrograde cholangio pancreatography or surgery usually resolves AP and reduces the risk of recurrence. Surgery may be indicated in AP to treat pseudocyst, pancreatic abscess, and to drain the pancreatic bed if hemorrhagic or necrotic material is present.

EVALUATION OF THERAPEUTIC OUTCOMES

- In patients with mild AP, pain control, fluid and electrolyte status, and nutrition should be assessed periodically depending on the degree of abdominal pain and fluid loss.
- Patients with severe AP should be transferred to an intensive care unit for close monitoring of vital signs, fluid and electrolyte status, white blood cell count, blood glucose, lactate dehydrogenase, aspartate aminotransferase, serum albumin, hematocrit, blood urea nitrogen, serum creatinine, and international normalized ratio. Continuous hemodynamic and arterial blood gas monitoring is essential. Serum lipase, amylase, and bilirubin require less frequent monitoring. The patient should be monitored for signs of infection, relief of abdominal pain, and adequate nutritional status.

CHRONIC PANCREATITIS

PATHOPHYSIOLOGY

- In most individuals, CP is progressive and loss of pancreatic function is irreversible. Permanent destruction of pancreatic tissue usually leads to exocrine and endocrine insufficiency.

- Prolonged ethanol consumption accounts for 70% of all cases in the United States; 10% result from other causes, and 20% are idiopathic.
- Ethanol-induced pancreatitis appears to progress from inflammation to cellular necrosis, and fibrosis occurs over time. Chronic alcohol ingestion causes changes in pancreatic fluid that create intraductal protein plugs that block small ductules. This results in progressive structural damage in the ducts and acinar tissue. Calcium complexes with the protein plugs, eventually resulting in destruction of pancreatic tissue.
- Abdominal pain may be related in part to increased intraductal pressure secondary to continued pancreatic secretion, pancreatic inflammation, and abnormalities of pancreatic nerves.
- Malabsorption of protein and fat occurs when the capacity for enzyme secretion is reduced by 90%. A minority of patients develop complications including pancreatic pseudocyst, abscess, and ascites or common bile duct obstruction leading to cholangitis or secondary biliary cirrhosis.

CLINICAL PRESENTATION

- The main features are abdominal pain, malabsorption, weight loss, and diabetes. Jaundice occurs in about 10% of patients.
- Patients typically report dull epigastric or abdominal pain that radiates to the back. It may be either consistent or episodic. The pain is deep-seated, positional, frequently nocturnal, and unresponsive to medication. Nausea and vomiting often accompany the pain. Severe attacks last from several days to weeks and may be aggravated by eating and relieved by abstinence from alcohol.
- Steatorrhea (excessive loss of fat in the feces) and azotorrhea (excessive loss of protein in the feces) are seen in most patients. Steatorrhea is often associated with diarrhea and bloating. Weight loss may occur.
- Pancreatic diabetes is usually a late manifestation that is commonly associated with pancreatic calcification. Neuropathy is sometimes seen.

DIAGNOSIS

- Most patients have a history of heavy ethanol use and attacks of recurrent upper abdominal pain. The classic triad of pancreatic calcification, steatorrhea, and diabetes usually confirms the diagnosis.
- Serum amylase and lipase concentrations usually remain normal unless the pancreatic duct is blocked or a pseudocyst is present.
- The white blood cell count, fluid balance, and electrolyte concentrations usually remain normal unless fluids and electrolytes are lost due to vomiting and diarrhea.
- Malabsorption of fat can be detected by Sudan staining of the feces or a 72-hour quantitative measurement of fecal fat.
- Surgical biopsy of pancreatic tissue through laparoscopy or laparotomy is the gold standard for confirming the diagnosis of CP.

- In the absence of histologic samples, imaging techniques are helpful in detecting calcification of the pancreas and other causes of pain (ductal obstruction secondary to stones, strictures, or pseudocysts) and in differentiating CP from pancreatic cancer. Ultrasonography is the simplest and least expensive imaging technique, and abdominal CT is often used if the ultrasound examination is negative or unsatisfactory.
- Endoscopic retrograde cholangiopancreatography is the most sensitive and specific diagnostic test, but it is reserved for patients in whom the diagnosis cannot be established by imaging techniques because of the potential for complications.

PHARMACOLOGICAL TREATMENT

- In patients with ethanol-induced CP, abstinence is the most important factor in preventing abdominal pain in the early stages of the disease.
- Small and frequent meals (six meals/day) and a diet restricted in fat (50 to 75 g/day) are recommended to minimize postprandial pancreatic secretion and pain.
- Pain management should begin with nonnarcotic analgesics such as **acetaminophen** or a **nonsteroidal antiinflammatory drug** administered on a scheduled basis before meals to prevent postprandial exacerbation of pain. If pain persists, the response to exogenous non–enteric-coated pancreatic enzymes should be evaluated in patients with mild to moderate CP. If these measures fail, consideration may be given to use of **tramadol** or addition of a low-dose opioid to the regimen (e.g., **acetaminophen plus codeine**). Parenteral opioids are reserved for patients with severe pain unresponsive to oral analgesics. In patients with pain that is difficult to manage, nonnarcotic modulators of chronic pain (e.g., selective serotonin reuptake inhibitors, tricyclic antidepressants) may be considered.
- Most patients with malabsorption require pancreatic enzyme supplementation . The combination of pancreatic enzymes (lipase, amylase, and protease) and a reduction in dietary fat (to less than 25 g/meal) enhances nutritional status and reduces steatorrhea. An initial dose containing about 30,000 international units of lipase and 10,000 international units of trypsin should be given with each meal.
- Oral pancreatic enzyme supplements are available as powders, uncoated or coated tablets, capsules, enteric-coated spheres and microspheres, or enteric-coated microtablets encased in a cellulose or gelatin capsule (Table 34.2). Microencapsulated enteric-coated products are not superior to recommended doses of conventional non–enteric-coated enzyme preparations. The quantity of active lipase delivered to the duodenum appears to be a more important determinant in pancreatic enzyme replacement therapy than the dosage form. GI side effects appear to be dose related but occur less frequently with enteric-coated products. Concurrent use of an H2 receptor antagonist or proton pump inhibitor may improve the efficacy of pancreatic enzyme supplementation by both increasing pH and decreasing

intragastric volume. Antacids have little or no added effect in reducing steatorrhea. Addition of an H2 receptor antagonist may be beneficial for symptomatic patients whose steatorrhea is not corrected by enzyme replacement therapy and reducing dietary fat. A proton pump inhibitor should be considered in patients who fail to benefit from an H2 receptor antagonist.

SURGERY

- The most common indication for surgery in CP is abdominal pain refractory to medical therapy. Surgical procedures that alleviate pain include a subtotal pancreatectomy, decompression of the main pancreatic duct, or interruption of the splanchnic nerves.

EVALUATION OF THERAPEUTIC OUTCOMES

- The severity and frequency of abdominal pain should be assessed periodically to determine the efficacy of the analgesic regimen. The effectiveness of pancreatic enzyme supplementation is measured by improvement in body weight and stool

Table 34.2

Enzyme content of selected pancreatic enzyme preparations

Product	Dosage Form	Enzyme Contents (units) ∝		
		Lipase	Amylase	Protease
Creon-10	ECMS	10,000	33,200	37,500
Creon-20	ECMS	20,000	66,400	75,000
Ku-Zyme HP	C	8,000	30,000	30,000
Lipram-CR10	ECMS	10,000	33,200	37,500
Lipram-PN16	ECMS	16,000	48,000	48,000
Lipram-CR20	ECMS	20,000	66,400	75,000
Lipram-PN20	ECMS	20,000	56,000	44,000
Lipram-UL12	ECMS	12,000	39,000	39,000
Lipram-PN10	ECMS	10,000	30,000	30,000
Lipram-UL18	ECMS	18,000	58,500	58,500
Lipram-UL20	ECMS	20,000	65,000	65,000
Pancrease	ECMS	4,500	20,000	25,000
Pancrease MT-4	ECMT	4,000	12,000	12,000
Pancrease MT-10	ECMT	10,000	30,000	30,000
Pancrease MT-16	ECMT	16,000	48,000	48,000
Pancrease MT-20	ECMT	20,000	56,000	44,000
Ultrase MT-12	ECMT	12,000	39,000	39,000
Ultrase MT-18	ECMT	18,000	58,500	58,500
Ultrase MT-20	ECMT	20,000	65,000	65,000
Viokaseb	P	16,800	70,000	70,000
Viokase-8	UCT	8,000	30,000	30,000
Viokase-16	UCT	16,000	60,000	60,000

consistency or frequency. The 72- hour stool test for fecal fat may be used when the adequacy of treatment is in question.

- Serum uric acid and folic acid concentrations should be monitored yearly in patients prone to hyperuricemia or folic acid deficiency. Blood glucose must be monitored carefully in diabetic patients.

REFERENCES

1. Peter A. Banks, Center for Pancreatic Disease, Brigham and Women's Hospital, Professor of Medicine, Harvard Medical School Boston, Massachusetts.
2. Darwin L. Conwell, Center for Pancreatic Disease, Brigham and Women's Hospital, Associate Professor of Medicine, Harvard Medical School Boston, Massachusetts.
3. Phillip P. Toskes, Professor of Medicine, Division of Gastroenterology, Hepatology, and Nutrition, University of Florida College of Medicine Gainesville, Florida.

CHAPTER 35

Acute Renal Failure

DEFINITION

Acute renal failure (ARF) is broadly defined as a decrease in glomerular filtration rate (GFR) occurring over hours to weeks that is associated with an accumulation of waste products, including urea and creatinine. Clinicians use a combination of the serum creatinine (Scr) value with change in either Scr or urine output (UOP) as the primary criteria for diagnosing ARF.

PREVALENCE

Acute kidney injury is common among hospitalized patients. It affects some 3%-7% of patients admitted to the hospital and approximately 25%-30% of patients in the intensive care unit.

ETIOLOGY

The causes of acute kidney injury are commonly categorized into *prerenal*, *intrinsic*, and *postrenal*.

PRERENAL

Prerenal causes of AKI ("pre-renal azotemia") are those that decrease effective blood flow to the kidney. These include systemic causes, such as low blood volume, low blood pressure, and heart failure, as well as local changes to the blood vessels supplying the kidney. The latter include renal artery stenosis, which is a narrowing of the renal artery that supplies the kidney, and renal vein thrombosis, which is the formation of a blood clot in the renal vein that drains blood from the kidney.

INTRINSIC

Sources of damage to the kidney itself are dubbed *intrinsic*. Intrinsic AKI can be due to damage to the glomeruli, renal tubules, or interstitium. Common causes of each are glomerulonephritis, acute tubular necrosis (ATN), and acute interstitial nephritis (AIN), respectively. A cause of intrinsic acute renal failure is tumor lysis syndrome.

POSTRENAL

Postrenal AKI is a consequence of urinary tract obstruction. This may be related to benign prostatic hyperplasia, kidney stones, obstructed urinary catheter, bladder stone, ureteral or renal malignancy. It is useful to perform a bladder scan or a post void residual to rule out urinary retention. In post void residual, a catheter is inserted immediately after urinating to measure fluid still in the bladder. 50-100mL suggests neurogenic bladder. A renal ultrasound will demonstrate hydronephrosis if present. A CT scan of the abdomen will also demonstrate bladder distension or hydronephrosis, however, in case of acute renal failure; the use of IV contrast is contraindicated. On the basic metabolic panel, the ratio of blood urea nitrogen (BUN) to creatinine may indicate post renal failure.

PATHOPHYSIOLOGY

- ARF can be categorized as prerenal (resulting from decreased renal perfusion), intrinsic (resulting from structural damage to the kidney), postrenal (resulting from obstruction of urine flow from the renal tubule to the urethra), and functional (resulting from hemodynamic changes at the glomerulus independent of decreased perfusion or structural damage)

CLINICAL FEATURES

- The presentation can be subtle and depends on the setting. Outpatients often are not in acute distress; hospitalized patients may develop ARF after a catastrophic event.
- Symptoms in the outpatient setting include change in urinary habits, weight gain, or flank pain. Clinicians typically notice symptoms of ARF before they are detected by inpatients.
- Signs include edema, colored or foamy urine, and, in volume-depleted patients, orthostatic hypotension.

DIAGNOSIS

- Thorough medical and medication histories, physical examination, assessment of laboratory values and if needed, imaging studies, is important in the diagnosis of ARF.
- Scr and blood urea nitrogen cannot be used alone to diagnose ARF because they are insensitive to rapid changes in GFR and therefore may not reflect current renal function.
- Monitoring changes in UOP can help diagnose the cause of ARF. Acute anuria (less than 50 mL urine/day) is secondary to complete urinary obstruction or a catastrophic event (e.g., shock). Oliguria (400 to 500 mL urine/day) suggests prerenal azotemia. Nonoliguric renal failure (more than 400 to 500 mL urine/day) usually results from acute intrinsic renal failure or incomplete urinary obstruction.
- Urinalysis can help clarify the cause of ARF. Certain laboratory parameters are helpful in the assessment of renal function with ARF. Urine microscopy gives further information to assist with determination of the etiology of the ARF

CLASSIFICATION

STAGING (FIG. 35.1)

- The *RIFLE criteria*, proposed by the Acute Dialysis Quality Initiative (ADQI) group, aid in the staging of patients with AKI
- **Risk:** GFR decrease >25%, serum creatinine increased 1.5 times or urine production of <0.5 ml/kg/hr for 6 hours
- **Injury:** GFR decrease >50%, doubling of creatinine or urine production <0.5 mL /kg/hr for 12 hours
- **Failure:** GFR decrease >75%, tripling of creatinine or creatinine >355 μmol/L (with a rise of >44) (>4 mg/dl) OR urine output below 0.3 mL/kg/hr for 24 hours.
- **Loss:** persistent AKI or complete loss of kidney function for more than 4 weeks
- **End-stage renal disease:** complete loss of kidney function for more than 3 months

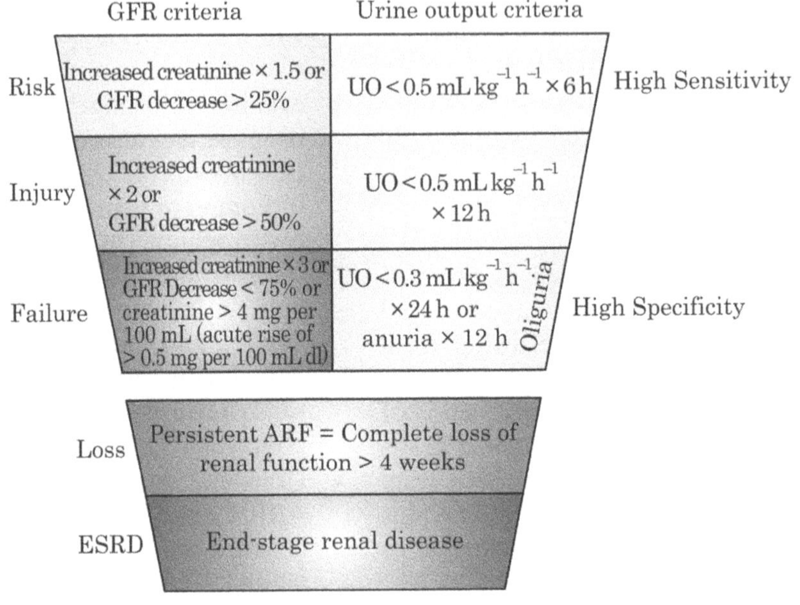

FIGURE 35.1

Staging of patients with acute renal failure.

TREATMENT

PREVENTION OF ACUTE RENAL FAILURE

- Risk factors for ARF include advanced age, acute infection, preexisting chronic respiratory or cardiovascular disease, dehydration, and chronic kidney disease (CKD). Decreased renal perfusion secondary to abdominal or coronary bypasses surgery, acute blood loss in trauma, and uric acid nephropathy also increase risk.
- Nephrotoxin administration (e.g., radiocontrast dye) should be avoided whenever possible. When patients require contrast dye and are at risk of contrast dye–induced nephropathy, renal perfusion should be maximized through strategies such as assuring adequate hydration with normal saline or sodium bicarbonate solutions and administration of **oral acetylcysteine** 600 mg every 12 hours for four doses. Strict glycemic control with **insulin, Amphotericin B** nephrotoxicity can be reduced by slowing the infusion rate to 24 hours or, in at-risk patients, substituting **liposomal Amphotericin B**
- Many other strategies are popular but *lack* supportive evidence, including **mannitol, loop diuretics, dopamine,** and **fenoldopam.**

MANAGEMENT OF ESTABLISHED ACUTE RENAL FAILURE

- No drugs have been found to accelerate ARF recovery. Therefore, patients with established ARF should be supported with nonpharmacologic and pharmacologic approaches through the period of ARF.

NONPHARMACOLOGICAL APPROACHES

- Supportive care goals include maintenance of adequate cardiac output and blood pressure to optimize tissue perfusion while restoring renal function to pre-ARF baseline.
- Medications associated with diminished renal blood flow should be stopped. Appropriate fluid replacement should be initiated. Avoidance of nephrotoxins is essential in the management of patients with ARF
- Renal replacement therapy (RRT), such as haemodialysis and peritoneal dialysis, maintains fluid and electrolyte balance while removing waste products. Intermittent and continuous options have different advantages (and disadvantages) but, after correcting for severity of illness, have similar outcomes. Consequently, hybrid approaches (e.g., sustained low-efficiency dialysis and extended Daily dialysis) are being developed to provide the advantages of both.
- Intermittent RRT (e.g., hemodialysis) has the advantage of widespread availability and the convenience of lasting only 3 to 4 hours. Disadvantages include difficult venous dialysis access in hypotensive patients and hypotension due to rapid removal of large amounts of fluid.
- Several continuous renal replacement therapy (CRRT) variants have been developed. CRRT, performed as continuous haemodialysis, continuous haemofiltration, or both, is becoming increasingly popular. CRRT gradually removes solute resulting in better tolerability by critically ill patients. Disadvantages include limited availability, need for 24-hour nursing care, high expense, and incomplete guidelines for drug dosing

PHARMACOLOGICAL APPROACHES

- Loop diuretics have not been shown to accelerate ARF recovery or improve patient outcome; however, diuretics can facilitate management of fluid overload. The most effective diuretics are mannitol and loop diuretics. **Mannitol** 20% is typically started at a dose of 12.5 to 25 g IV over 3 to 5 minutes. Disadvantages include IV administration, hyperosmolality risk, and need for monitoring because mannitol can contribute to ARF.
- Equipotent doses of loop diuretics (**furosemide, bumetanide, torsemide, ethacrynic acid**) have similar efficacy. Ethacrynic acid is reserved for sulpha allergic patients. Continuous infusions of loop diuretics appear to be more effective and to have fewer adverse effects than intermittent boluses. An initial IV loading dose (equivalent to furosemide 40 to 80 mg) should be administered before starting a continuous infusion (equivalent to furosemide 10 to 20 mg/hour).
- Agents from different pharmacologic classes, such as diuretics that work at the distal convoluted tubule (thiazides) or the collecting duct (**amiloride, triamterene, spironolactone**), may be synergistic when combined with loop diuretics. **Metolazone** is commonly used because, unlike other thiazides, it produces effective diuresis at GFR less than 20 mL/min.

ELECTROLYTE MANAGEMENT AND NUTRITION THERAPY

- Hyperkalemia is the most common and serious electrolyte abnormality in ARF. Typically, potassium must be restricted to less than 3 g/day and monitored daily.
- Hypernatremia and fluid retention commonly occur, necessitating restricting daily sodium intake to no more than 3 g. All sources of sodium, including antibiotics, need to be considered when calculating daily sodium intake.
- Phosphorus and magnesium should be monitored; neither is efficiently removed by dialysis.
- Enteral, but not parenteral, nutrition has been shown to improve patient outcomes.

DRUG-DOSING CONSIDERATIONS

- Drug therapy optimization in ARF is a challenge. Confounding variables include residual drug clearance, fluid accumulation, and use of RRTs.
- Volume of distribution for water-soluble drugs is significantly increased due to edema. Use of dosing guidelines for CKD does not reflect the clearance and volume of distribution in critically ill ARF patients.
- ARF patients may have a higher residual nonrenal clearance than CKD patients with similar creatinine clearances; this complicates drug therapy individualization, especially with RRTs.

REFERENCES

1. Webb S, Dobb G (December 2007). "ARF, ATN or AKI? It's now acute kidney injury". *Anaesthesia and Intensive Care* **35** (6): 843–4..
2. Skorecki K, Green J, Brenner BM (2005). "Chronic renal failure". In Kasper DL, Braunwald E, Fauci AS, *et al.*. *Harrison's Principles of Internal Medicine* (16th ed.). New York, NY: McGraw-Hill. pp. 1653–63. ISBN 0-071-39140-1.
3. Weisberg LS (December 2008). "Management of severe hyperkalemia". *Crit. Care Med.* **36** (12): 3246–51.
4. Tierney, Lawrence M.; Stephen J. McPhee and Maxine A. Papadakis (2004). "22". *CURRENT Medical Diagnosis and Treatment 2005* (44 ed.). McGraw-Hill. p. 871. ISBN 0071436928.
5. Brady HR, Brenner BM (2005). "Chronic renal failure". In Kasper DL, Braunwald E, Fauci AS, *et al.*. *Harrison's Principles of Internal Medicine* (16th ed.). New York, NY: McGraw-Hill. pp. 1644–53. ISBN 0-071-39140-1.
6. Bellomo R, Ronco C, Kellum JA, Mehta RL, Palevsky P (2004). "Acute renal failure - definition, outcome measures, animal models, fluid therapy and information technology needs: the Second International Consensus Conference of the Acute Dialysis Quality Initiative (ADQI) Group". *Crit Care* **8** (4): R204–12.

CHAPTER 36

Chronic Kidney Disease

DEFINITION

- Chronic kidney disease (CKD) is a progressive loss of function over several months to years, characterized by gradual replacement of normal kidney architecture with interstitial fibrosis.
- CKD is categorized by the level of kidney function, based on glomerular filtration rate (GFR), into stages 1 to 5, with each increasing number indicating a more advanced stage of the disease, as defined by a declining GFR. This classification system from the National Kidney Foundation's Kidney Dialysis Outcomes and Quality Initiative (K/DOQI) also accounts for structural evidence of kidney damage.
- CKD stage 5, previously referred to as end-stage renal disease (ESRD), occurs when the GFR falls below 15 mL/min per 1.73 m^2 body surface area. The patient with stage 5 CKD requiring chronic dialysis or renal transplantation for relief of uremic symptoms is said to have ESRD.

PREVALENCE

UK estimates suggest that 8.8% of the population of Great Britain and Northern Ireland have symptomatic CKD. Chronic kidney disease (CKD) is a major concern in African Americans, mostly due to increased prevalence of hypertension. As an example, 37% of end-stage renal disease cases in African Americans can be attributed to high blood pressure, compared with 19% among Caucasians.

ETIOLOGY

Causes of chronic kidney disease include the following:

- Diabetic kidney disease
- Hypertension
- Vascular disease
- Glomerular disease (primary or secondary)
- Tubulointerstitial disease
- Urinary tract obstruction

  Vascular diseases that can cause chronic kidney disease include the following:

- Renal artery stenosis
- Cytoplasmic pattern antineutrophil cytoplasmic antibody (C-ANCA)–positive and perinuclear pattern antineutrophil cytoplasmic antibody (P-ANCA)–positive vasculitides
- Antineutrophil cytoplasmic antibody (ANCA)–negative vasculitides
- Atheroemboli

- Hypertensive nephrosclerosis
- Renal vein thrombosis
- Unrecovered acute kidney injury

Primary glomerular diseases include the following:

- Membranous nephropathy
- Immunoglobulin A (IgA) nephropathy
- Focal and segmental glomerulosclerosis (FSGS)
- Minimal change disease
- Membranoproliferative glomerulonephritis

Rapidly progressive (crescentic) glomerulonephritis Secondary causes of glomerular disease include the following:

- Diabetes mellitus
- Systemic lupus erythematosus
- Rheumatoid arthritis
- Mixed connective tissue disease
- Scleroderma
- Good pasture syndrome
- Wegener granulomatosis
- Mixed cryoglobulinemia
- Post infectious glomerulonephritis

PATHOPHYSIOLOGY

- **Susceptibility factors** increase the risk for kidney disease but do not directly cause kidney damage. Susceptibility factors include advanced age, reduced kidney mass and low birth weight, racial or ethnic minority, family history, low income or education, systemic inflammation, and dyslipidemia.
- **Initiation factors** initiate kidney damage and can be modified by drug therapy. Initiation factors include diabetes mellitus, hypertension, autoimmune disease, polycystic kidney disease, and drug toxicity.
- **Progression factors** hasten decline in kidney function after initiation of kidney damage. Progression factors include glycemia in diabetics, hypertension, proteinuria, and smoking.
- Most progressive nephropathies share a final common pathway to irreversible renal parenchymal damage and ESRD. Key pathway elements are loss of nephron mass, glomerular capillary hypertension, and proteinuria.

CLINICAL FEATURES

- CKD development and progression is insidious. Patients with stage 1 or 2 CKD usually do not have symptoms or metabolic derangements seen with stages 3 to 5, such as anemia, secondary hyperparathyroidism, cardiovascular disease, malnutrition, and fluid and electrolyte abnormalities that are more common as kidney function deteriorates.
- Uremic symptoms (fatigue, weakness, shortness of breath, mental confusion, nausea, vomiting, bleeding, and anorexia) are generally absent in stages 1 and 2, minimal during stages 3 and 4, and common in patients with stage 5 CKD who may also experience itching, cold intolerance, weight gain, and peripheral neuropathies.

STAGES (FIG. 36.1)

All individuals with a glomerular filtration rate (GFR) <60 mL/min/1.73 m^2 for 3 months are classified as having chronic kidney disease, irrespective of the presence or absence of kidney damage. The rationale for including these individuals is that reduction in kidney function to this level or lower represents loss of half or more of the adult level of normal kidney function, which may be associated with a number of complications.

All individuals with kidney damage are classified as having chronic kidney disease, irrespective of the level of GFR. The rationale for including individuals with GFR > 60 mL/min/1.73 m^2 is that GFR may be sustained at normal or increased levels despite substantial kidney damage and that patients with kidney damage are at increased risk of the two major outcomes of chronic kidney disease: loss of kidney function and development of cardiovascular disease.

The loss of protein in the urine is regarded as an independent marker for worsening of renal function and cardiovascular disease. Hence, British guidelines append the letter "P" to the stage of chronic kidney disease if there is significant protein loss.

Stage 1: Slightly diminished function; kidney damage with normal or relatively high GFR (> 90 mL/min/1.73 m^2). Kidney damage is defined as pathological abnormalities or markers of damage, including abnormalities in blood or urine test or imaging studies.

Stage 2: Mild reduction in GFR (60–89 mL/min/1.73 m^2) with kidney damage. Kidney damage is defined as pathological abnormalities or markers of damage, including abnormalities in blood or urine test or imaging studies.

Stage 3: Moderate reduction in GFR (30–59 mL/min/1.73 m^2).British guidelines distinguish between stage 3A (GFR 45–59) and stage 3B (GFR 30–44) for purposes of screening and referral.

Stage 4: Severe reduction in GFR (15–29 mL/min/1.73m^2) Preparation for renal replacement therapy

Stage 5: Established kidney failure (GFR <15 mL/min/1.73m^2, permanent renal replacement therapy (RRT), or end stage renal disease (ESRD)

STAGES OF CKD		
Stage	Description	GFR (mL/min/ 1.73 m^2)
1	Kidney damage* with normal or increased GFR	≥90
2	Kidney damage* with mildly decreased GFR	60-89
3	Moderately decreased GFR	30-59
4	Severely decreased GFR	15-29
5	Kidney failure	<15 or dialysis

*Kidney damage: pathologic abnormalities or markers of damage, including abnormalities in blood or urine tests or imaging studies.
CKD = chronic kidney disease; GFR = glomerular filtration rate.
Adapted from reference 4.

FIGURE 36.1

Classification of chronic kidney disease.

(source : http://www.pharmacytimes.com/publications/issue/2011/february2011/p2p_ckd)

DIAGNOSIS

To determine whether person is suffering from chronic kidney failure person can undergo tests and procedures including:

- **Blood tests:** Kidney function tests look for the level of waste products, such as creatinine and urea, in patient blood.
- **Urine tests:** Analyzing a sample of urine may reveal abnormalities that point to chronic kidney failure.

- **Imaging tests:** Ultrasound is used to assess patient kidneys. Other imaging tests may be used in some cases.
- **Removing a sample of kidney tissue for testing:** Kidney biopsy was done to remove a sample of kidney tissue. The biopsy sample is sent to a laboratory for testing to help determine what's causing patient kidney problems. Kidney biopsy is often done using a long, thin needle that's inserted through the skin and into the kidney.

TREATMENTS AND DRUGS

Chronic kidney failure has no cure, but treatment can help control signs and symptoms, reduce complications, and slow the progress of the disease. If kidneys become severely damaged, patient may need treatments for end-stage kidney disease.

Treating the cause of kidney failure: Treatment will be done either to slow or reverse the disease or condition that's causing patient kidney failure. Treatment options vary depending on the cause of patient kidney failure.

Stopping the underlying condition may slow kidney damage, but sometimes kidney failure worsens despite treatment. Damage to the kidneys can cause stress on the kidneys that continues to worsen even when an underlying condition, such as high blood pressure, has been controlled.

Treating complications of kidney failure: Kidney failure complications can be controlled to make patient more comfortable. Treatments may include:

- **Treatment to control high blood pressure:** People with chronic kidney failure may experience worsening high blood pressure. Patient doctor may recommend medications to lower patient blood pressure — commonly ***Angiotensin-converting enzyme (ACE) inhibitors or Angiotensin II receptor blockers*** — and to preserve kidney function. High blood pressure medications can initially decrease Kidney function, so patient may have frequent blood tests to monitor patient condition. Patient doctor will likely also recommend a low-salt diet.
- **Medications to lower cholesterol levels:** Patient doctor may recommend medications, called ***statins***, to lower patient cholesterol. People with chronic kidney failure often experience high levels of bad cholesterol, which can increase the risk of heart disease.
- **Medications to relieve anemia:** In certain situations, patient doctor may recommend supplements of the hormone ***erythropoietin*** to induce production of more red blood cells. This may help relieve the fatigue and weakness that's associated with anemia.
- **Medications to relieve swelling:** People with chronic kidney failure may retain fluids. This can lead to swelling in patient arms and legs, as well as high blood pressure. Medications called ***diuretics*** can help maintain the balance of fluids in patient body.
- **Medications to protect patient bones:** Patient doctor may prescribe ***calcium and vitamin D*** supplements to prevent weak bones. Patient may also take a phosphate-binding medication to lower the amount of ***phosphate*** in patient blood. Lowering phosphate will increase

the amount of calcium available for patient bones so that they don't become weak and vulnerable to fracture.

- **A low-protein diet to minimize waste products in patient blood:** As patient body processes the proteins in the foods patient eat, it creates waste products that patient kidneys must filter from patient blood. To reduce the amount of work patient kidneys must do, patient doctor may recommend a low-protein diet. Patient doctor may ask patient to meet with a dietitian who can help patient assess how much protein patient eat each day and suggest ways to lower patient protein intake while still eating a healthy diet.

Treatment for end-stage kidney disease: If kidney damage continues to progress to the point where patient kidneys are functioning at less than 15 % of capacity, patient has end-stage kidney disease. Patient kidneys are no longer able to keep up with waste and fluid clearance on their own. Soon, dialysis or a kidney transplant becomes the only option to support life.

DIALYSIS

Dialysis is an artificial means of removing waste products and extra fluid from patient blood when patient kidneys aren't able to perform these functions. There are two types of dialysis. In haemodialysis, blood is pumped out of patient body to a machine that works like an artificial kidney, filtering waste out of patient blood. The blood is then pumped back into patient body. Another type of dialysis, called peritoneal dialysis, involves pumping a dialysis solution into patient abdominal cavity. Peritoneal dialysis relies on patient body's network of tiny blood vessels to carry waste products and excess fluids to patient abdominal cavity where the dialysis solution absorbs them. The dialysis solution is then pumped out of patient body, carrying the waste and excess fluids with it.

KIDNEY TRANSPLANT

If patient have no life-threatening medical conditions other than kidney failure, a kidney transplant may be an option for patient. Kidney transplant involves surgically placing a healthy kidney from a donor inside patient body. Transplanted kidneys can come from deceased donors or from living donors.

REFERENCES

1. National Kidney Foundation (2002). "K/DOQI clinical practice guidelines for chronic kidney disease". Retrieved 2008-06-29.
2. Johnson, David (2011-05-02). "Chapter 4: CKD Screening and Management: Overview". In Daugirdas, John. *Handbook of Chronic Kidney Disease Management*. Lippincott Williams and Wilkins. pp. 32–43.
3. Mitch WE. Chronic kidney disease. In: Goldman L, et al. Cecil Medicine. 23rd ed. Philadelphia, Pa.: Saunders; 2007.
4. Ferri FF. Renal failure, chronic. In: Ferri FF. Ferri's Clinical Advisor 2010. Philadelphia, Pa.: Mosby; 2009.
5. Bash LD, Erlinger TP, Coresh J, Marsh-Manzi J, Folsom AR, Astor BC. Inflammation, hemostasis, and the risk of kidney function decline in the Atherosclerosis Risk in Communities (ARIC) Study. *Am J Kidney Dis*. Apr 2009;53(4): 596-605
6. Thakar CV, Christianson A, Himmelfarb J, Leonard AC. Acute kidney injury episodes and chronic kidney disease risk in diabetes mellitus. *Clin J Am Soc Nephrol*. Nov 2011; 6(11): 2567-72.

CHAPTER 37

Benign Prostatic Hyperplasia (BPH)

DEFINITION

Benign prostatic hyperplasia (BPH), a nearly ubiquitous condition, is the most common benign neoplasm of American men and occurs as a result of androgen-driven prostate growth.

PATHOPHYSIOLOGY

- The prostate gland comprises three types of tissue: epithelial or glandular, stromal or smooth muscle, and capsule. Both stromal tissue and capsule are embedded with α1-adrenergic receptors.
- The precise pathophysiologic mechanisms that cause BPH are not clear. However, both intraprostatic dihydrotestosterone (DHT) and type II 5 α-reductase are thought to be involved.
- BPH results from static that is gradual enlargement of the prostate and also dynamic that is agents or situations that increase α-adrenergic activity and causes constriction of the gland's smooth muscle factors. Examples of drugs that can exacerbate symptoms include testosterone, α-adrenergic agonists (e.g., decongestants), and anticholinergic agents (e.g., tricyclic antidepressants, antihistamines, anticholinergic anti-spasmodics, phenothiazines and anti-cholinergics for Parkinson's disease).

CLINICAL PRESENTATION

- Patients with BPH can present with a variety of signs and symptoms categorized as obstructive or irritative. Symptoms vary over time. Mild disease may stabilize whereas other patients experience progressive disease over time.
- Obstructive signs and symptoms result when dynamic and/or static factors reduce bladder emptying. Patients experience urinary hesitancy; urine dribbles out of the penis, and the bladder feels full even after voiding.
- Irritative signs and symptoms result from long-standing obstruction at the bladder neck. Patients experience frequency, urgency, and nocturia.
- Complications include chronic kidney disease, bladder diverticula, gross hematuria, urinary incontinence, recurrent urinary tract infection, and bladder stones.

DIAGNOSIS

- Diagnosis of BPH requires a careful monitoring of the medical history, objective measures of bladder emptying (e.g., peak and average urinary flow rate, postvoid residual urine volume), physical examination, , and laboratory tests (e.g., urinalysis, blood urea nitrogen, and prostate-specific antigen [PSA]).

- Medication history should include all prescription and nonprescription medications as well as dietary supplements.
- On digital rectal examination, the prostate is usually, but not always, enlarged (more than 20 g), soft, smooth, and symmetric.

TREATMENT

- Management options for BPH include watchful waiting, drug therapy, and surgical intervention. The choice depends on the severity of signs and symptoms (Table 37.1).
- Watchful waiting is appropriate for patients with mild disease and for those with moderate disease with only mildly bothersome symptoms and without complications.
- Watchful waiting involves reassessment at yearly intervals. Patients should be educated about behavior modification such as fluid restriction before bedtime, avoiding caffeine and alcohol, frequent emptying of the bladder, and avoiding drugs that exacerbate symptoms.

PHARMACOLOGICAL THERAPY

- Pharmacological therapy is appropriate for patients with severe BPH and also moderately severe BPH and as an interim measure.
- Pharmacological therapy interferes with the stimulatory effect of testosterone on prostate gland enlargement (reduces the static factor) or relaxes prostatic smooth muscle (reduces the dynamic factor) (Table 37.2).
- Initial therapy with an α-adrenergic antagonist provides faster onset of symptom relief. A 5α-reductase inhibitor is preferred as initial therapy in patients with a prostate gland >40 g. Combination therapy should be considered for symptomatic patients with a prostate gland >40 g and PSA > 1.4 ng/mL.
- Agents that interfere with androgen stimulation of the prostate are not popular because of adverse effects. **leuprolide** and **goserelin** luteinizing hormone releasing hormone agonists mainly causes decrease in libido and can cause hot flashes, erectile dysfunction, and gynecomastia, The antiandrogens **bicalutamide** and **flutamide** cause nausea, diarrhea, and hepatotoxicity.

α-ADRENERGIC ANTAGONISTS

- The antagonists of α -Adrenergic receptors causes the relaxation of the smooth muscle in the bladder neck, thereby cause increase in urinary flow rates by 2 to 3 mL/sec in 60% to 70% of patients and reducing postvoid residual urine volumes. **Tamsulosin** and **doxazosin** produce durable responses for 6 and 10 years, respectively.
- Prostate volume is not decreased by α - Adrenergic antagonist .
- **Terazosin, doxazosin,** and **alfuzosin** are the α–adrenergic antagonists that belong to second-generation. They antagonize peripheral vascular α 1 -adrenergic receptors . Their adverse effects include orthostatic hypotension, first dose syncope, and dizziness. Alfuzosin is less likely to cause adverse effects on cardiovascular system.
- Patients should be slowly increased to a maintenance dose and should take these drugs at bedtime to minimize orthostatic hypotension and first-dose syncope with

terazosin and doxazosin. Sample titration schedules for terazosin include:

- Tamsulosin, the only third-generation α-adrenergic antagonist, is mainly selective for the prostatic α1A-receptors. Peripheral vascular smooth muscle relaxation is not caused by Tamsulosin
- Tamsulosin is the choice of drug for patients who cannot tolerate hypotension; severe orthostasis, or liver failure; have severe coronary artery disease, volume depletion, cardiac arrhythmias, or are taking multiple antihypertensives.
- **Cimetidine** and **diltiazem** metabolism is decreased by Tamsulosin. α-adrenergic antagonists **catabolism increased by Carbamazepine** and **phenytoin**.

5α-REDUCTASE INHIBITORS (DUTASTERIDE AND FINASTERIDE)

- 5α-Reductase inhibitors mainly interferes with the testosterone stimulatory effect . These agents causes slow disease progression and complications risk is decreased.
- 5α-reductase inhibitors have the disadvantages of requiring 6 months to maximally shrink an prostate which is enlarged, and less likely to induce objective improvement, and causing more sexual dysfunction compared with á-adrenergic antagonists,.
- Whether the pharmacodynamic advantages of **dutasteride** confer clinical advantages over **finasteride** is unknown. Dutasteride inhibits types I and II 5α-reductase, whereas finasteride inhibits only type II. Dutasteride more quickly and completely suppresses intraprostatic DHT (vs. 80% to 90% for finasteride) and decreases serum DHT by 90% (versus 70%).
- 5α-Reductase inhibitors are mainly preferred in patients with uncontrolled arrhythmias, poorly controlled angina, use of multiple antihypertensives, or inability to tolerate hypotensive effects of α-adrenergic antagonists.
- 5α-Reductase inhibitors reduce serum PSA levels by 50%. PSA should be measured at baseline and repeated after 6 months. If PSA does not decrease by 50% after 6 months of therapy in a compliant patient, the patient should be examined for prostate cancer.
- 5 α-Reductase inhibitors contraindicated in pregnant females as these are given FDA pregnancy category X. Pregnant and potentially pregnant women should not handle the tablets or have contact with semen from men receiving 5 α-reductase inhibitors

SURGICAL INTERVENTION

- Prostatectomy, performed transurethrally or suprapubically, is the gold standard for treatment of patients with moderate or severe symptoms of BPH and for all patients with complications.
- Retrograde ejaculation is a complication of up to 75% of transurethral prostatectomy procedures. Other complications seen in 2% to 15% of patients include bleeding, urinary incontinence, and erectile dysfunction.

PHYTOTHERAPY

- Although widely used in Europe for BPH, phytotherapy with products such as saw palmetto berry (*Serenoa repens*), stinging nettle (*Urtica dioica*), and African plum (*Pygeum africanum*) should be avoided.

Table 37.1

Categories of BPH disease severity based on symptoms and signs

Disease Severity	AUA Symptom Score	Typical Symptoms and Signs
Mild	≤ 7	Asymptomatic Peak urinary flow rate <10 mL/s Postvoid residual urine volume >25–50 mL Increased BUN and serum creatinine
Moderate	8-19	All of the above signs plus obstructive voiding symptoms and irritative voiding symptoms (signs of detrusor instability).
Severe	≤ 20	All of the above plus one or more complications of BPH

AUA, American Urological Association; BPH, Benign Prostatic Hyperplasia; BUN, Blood Urea Nitrogen.

Table 37.2

Summary of medical treatment options for benign prostatic hyperplasia

Category	Mechanism	Drug (Brand Name)
Reduces dynamic factor	Blocks α_1 -adrenergic receptors in prostatic stromal tissue	Prazosin (Minipress) Alfuzosin (Uroxatral) Terazosin (Hytrin) Doxazosin (Cardura)
Reduces static factor	Blocks α_4 receptors in the prostate Blocks 5α-reductase enzyme	Tamsulosin (Flomax) Finasteride (Proscar) Dutasteride (Avodart)
	Blocks dihydrotestosterone at its intracellular receptor	Bicalutamide (Casodex) Flutamide (Eulexin)
	Blocks pituitary release of luteinizing hormone	Leuprolide (Lupron) Nafarelin (Synarel)
	Blocks pituitary release of luteinizing hormone and blocks androgen receptor	Megestrol acetate

REFERENCES

1. Miller J, Tarter TH. Combination therapy with dutasteride and tamsulosin for the treatment of symptomatic enlarged prostate. Clin Interv Aging. 2009; 4: 251-8.
2. Curtis NJ. BPH: Costs and treatment outcomes. Am J Manag Care. 2006; 12: S141-8.
3. Berry SJ, Coffey DS, Walsh PC, Ewing LL. The development of human benign prostatic hyperplasia with age. J Urol. 1984; 132: 474-9.
4. Culig Z, Hobisch A, Cronauer MV, Radmayr C, Hittmair A, Zhang J, et al. Regulation of prostatic growth and function by peptide growth factors. Prostate. 1996; 28: 392-405.

5. Jenkins EP, Andersson S, Imperato-McGinley J, Wilson JD, Russell DW. Genetic and pharmacological evidence for more than one human steroid 5-alpha-reductase. J Clin Invest. 1992; 89: 293–300
6. Tammela T. Benign prostatic hyperplasia: Practical treatment guidelines. Drugs Aging. 1997; 10: 349–66
7. Bullock TL, Andriole GL. Emerging drug therapies for benign prostatic hyperplasia. Expert Opin Emerg Drugs. 2006; 11: 111–23.
8. Eri LM, Tveter KJ. Treatment of benign prostatic hyperplasia: A pharmacoeconomic perspective. Drugs Aging. 1997; 10: 107–18.
9. Garg G, Singh D, Saraf S. Management of benign prostate hyperplasia: An overview of á-adrenergic antagonist. Biol Pharm Bull. 2006; 29: 1554–8.
10. Blohm TR, Laughlin ME, Benson HD, Johnston JO, Wright CL, Schatzman GL. Pharmacological induction of 5-alpha reductase deficiency in rats: Separation of testosterone-mediated and 5- alpha-dihydrotestosterone-mediated effects. Endocrinology. 1986; 119: 959–66.
11. Reid P, Kantoff P, Oh W. Antiandrogens in prostate cancer. Invest New Drug. 1999; 17: 271–84.
12. Jonler M, Riehmann M, Bruskewitz RC. Benign prostatic hyperplasia: Current pharmacological treatment. Drug. 1994; 47: 66–81.
13. Wolf H, Madson PO. Treatment of benign prostatic hypertrophy with progestational agents: A preliminary report. J Urol. 1968; 99: 980–5.
14. Peters CA, Walsh PC. The effect of a nafarelinacetate luteinizing hormone releasing hormone agonist on benign prostatic hyperplasia. N Engl J Med. 1987; 317: 599–604.

CHAPTER 38

Diabetic Nephropathy

The involvement of the kidney in diabetes, known as diabetic nephropathy, is a progressive disease and is often associated with increased blood pressure.

The structural features of DN were described as a glomerulopathy with diffuse and/or nodular intercapillary glomerulosclerosis. The nodular changes are still considered specific for diabetes, although the diffuse lesions are also seen in other renal diseases. It was recognized that these ultrastructural changes were accompanied by increases in proteinuria. However, progress in the field was slow until the development of sensitive immunoassays for urinary albumin and the demonstration that increases in albuminuria are detectable several years before changes occur in total proteinuria. The major functional parameter of DN is albumin excretion rate (AER), which may increase more than 100-fold during the evolution of Diabetic nephropathy. Biphasic changes in glomerular filtration rate (GFR), consisting of an initial increase followed by progressive decline, also occur in DN, but are not routinely used to define early stages of DN. Initial increases in AER and GFR, although very sensitive, are not always sufficiently specific to diagnose DN, and should be regarded as surrogate markers for the 'hard' clinical end point of a progressive decline in GFR, which occurs 10-15 years later.

Clinically, overt DN is characterized by a persistent increase in AER above 300 mg/24 hr (>200 µg/min) in timed samples or an albumin:creatinine ratio (ACR) of >30 mg/mmol (>300 mg/g) in spot urine samples. This is equivalent to total proteinuria exceeding 0.5 g/24 hr and is detectable by conventional dipstick tests. Overt DN is related with hypertension and reduction in GFR, and is the late stage of a process that is difficult to arrest or reverse. It is now possible to diagnose nephropathy several years before progression to overt DN, by serial measurements of AER or ACR, which can monitor the transition from normoalbuminuria to microalbuminuria (AER of >20 µg/min, or ACR of >2.5 mg/mmol (>25 mg/g) for males—ACR of >3.5 mg/mmol (>35 mg/g) for females). This microalbuminuric stage is also called 'incipient nephropathy' in patients with type 1 diabetes.

Other potential contributors to an improved prognosis of DN include a focus on new targets of therapy such as AER itself, dyslipidaemia and antismoking advice (Table 38.1).

Table 38.1

Potential promoters of progression of diabetic nephropathy

Reversible	Irreversible
Glycaemic control	Age
Blood pressure	Gender
Smoking	Race
Albuminuria	Ethnicity
Dyslipidaemia	Family history
	Duration of diabetes

STAGES OF DN

The classification of Diabetic nephropathy consists of three stages: microalbuminuria (incipient DN), lasting 5–15 years; macroalbuminuria (overt DN), lasting 5–10 years; and ESRD, lasting 3–6 years without renal replacement therapy . Mogensen has suggested a five-stage classification, with two additional stages preceding microalbuminuria, for patients with type 1 diabetes. These are (stage 1) renal enlargement associated with hyperfiltration and (stage 2) a silent stage with normal AER but glomerular ultrastructural changes including mesangial expansion and basement membrane thickening (Table 38.1). Stage 1 may be present at diagnosis while stage 2 may occur within 5 years of diagnosis and persist for many years. Transient microalbuminuria may be found in both of these early stages.

CONCEPT OF MICROALBUMINURIA

Type 1 diabetic patients linked the presence of increased amounts of albumin in the urine, as measured by immunoassay, to the subsequent development of overt DN 10-14 years later. By consensus, this 'minimally raised' albumin excretion rate (AER of 30-300 mg/24 hr or 20–200 ìg/min) has been termed 'microalbuminuria', because it cannot be detected by standard bedside tests, and overt nephropathy has been termed 'macroalbuminuria' (AER of >300 mg/24 hr or >200 ìg/min). The terms 'normoalbuminuria', 'microalbuminuria' (incipient DN) and 'macroalbuminuria' do not refer to discrete.

GLYCAEMIC CONTROL AND DN

DN does not occur in the absence of hyperglycaemia, and glycaemic control is the main determinant of the onset of DN in both type 1 and type 2 diabetes. Many risk factors like hypertension, dyslipidaemia and smoking to promote the development and progression of DN. Incipient nephropathy (microalbuminuria) is closely associated with HbA1c levels over 8.0% in type 1 and also in type 2 diabetic patients.

There is a strong relationship between HbA1c and diabetic microvascular disease, both retinal and renal, without a clearcut HbA1c threshold. In addition, the DCCT data suggest that the relationship is curvilinear in type 1diabetic patients; that is, the tendency to develop microvascular disease per unit increase in HbA1c is greater at higher HbA1c levels than at lower levels. By contrast, in type 2 diabetes, there was a linear relationship between systolic blood pressure and the incidence of microvascular endpoints over the range of 120–160 mmHg.

The aetiological role of hyperglycaemia in the development and progression of DN is supported by the effects of pancreas transplantation on the morphological changes of both transplanted and native kidneys. In patients who have already received a renal transplant, a subsequent pancreatic transplant prevents any progression of the morphological changes associated with DN over a follow-up period of approximately 2 years. DN structural changes can even be reversed in native kidneys after pancreatic transplantation, but it takes 10 years of normoglycaemia to demonstrate this effect. In type 2 diabetic patients, tight glycaemic control reduced the development of overt DN. In summary, hyperglycaemia is a prerequisite for the development of DN, and two large studies have shown that intensive glycaemic control attenuates the development of DN in patients with type 1 diabetes and type 2 diabetes.

THE RELATIONSHIP OF BLOOD PRESSURE TO DN

About 80% of patients with type 1 diabetes and persistent microalbuminuria showed progressive increases in AER of 10–30% per year to the stage of overt DN over 10–15 years. The terms 'incipient' and 'overt' nephropathy have also been applied to patients with increased AER and type 2 diabetes. This presents few problems in younger patients, in whom the prognostic implications of persistent microalbuminuria are similar to those in type 1 diabetes. However, an increase in AER to the microalbuminuric range does not necessarily equate with 'incipient nephropathy' in elderly patients with type 2 diabetes. In this group of elderly patients, approximately 20% progress to overt nephropathy over 10–14 years. Microalbuminuria in the elderly is also associated with large vessel disease and may lead to fatal cardiovascular events. This lowers the predictive value of micro-albuminuria for overt DN due to survival bias. The presence of microalbuminuria in associated with retinopathy. Patients with type 2 diabetes, macroalbuminuria and retinopathy are more likely to have the typical renal ultrastructural features of DN than similar patients without retinopathy. In type 1 diabetes, the evolution of micro—to macroalbuminuria is usually accompanied by an increase in blood pressure. Some studies show that an increase in blood pressure follows the onset of microalbuminuria in patients with type 1 diabetes, while others suggest either a close association or that a rise in blood pressure precedes the onset of microalbuminuria. By contrast, in elderly patients with type 2 diabetes, a rise in blood pressure usually precedes the onset of microalbuminuria. Regardless of the sequence, the combination of hypertension and microalbuminuria promotes an accelerated increase in AER and a decline in GFR. This is likely to be mediated by dilatation of the afferent glomerular arteriole, which allows transmission of elevated systemic blood pressure to the glomerulus. Conversely, the development of DN is attenuated by renal artery stenosis, which reduces the transmission of systemic blood pressure to the glomerulus.

The increase in blood pressure during the evolution of DN is detected more sensitively by 24-hr ambulatory blood-pressure monitoring than by office blood-pressure measurements. In patients with type 1 diabetes, abnormalities in 24-hr blood pressure and autonomic function have been related to small increases in AER below the microalbuminuric range and are also seen in overt DN. Furthermore, loss of the normal nocturnal drop in blood pressure in evolving

DN may contribute to an increase in overall blood pressure load without detection by blood-pressure readings. In type 2 diabetes, the relation between blood pressure and DN differs from that in type 1 diabetes. Hypertension may precede the diagnosis of type 2 diabetes and microalbuminuria in elderly Caucasian people and in Pima Indians. In addition, microalbuminuria may precede the diagnosis of type 2 diabetes. Furthermore, progressive changes in the definition of hypertension in diabetic patients have required a reappraisal of the prevalence of hypertension, especially in type 2 DM. By contrast, less than 5% of normoalbuminuric type 1 diabetic patients are hypertensive, this rate rising to above 20% in microalbuminuric patients and above 80% in overt DN. The natural history is for blood pressure to increase by 3-4 mmHg per year in type 1 diabetic patients with microalbuminuria and approximately 6 mmHg per year in overt DN. Similar changes in blood pressure occur in type 2 diabetic patients during the evolution of DN, but are more difficult to define because most patients are already on antihypertensive treatment.

DYSLIPIDAEMIA AND DN

Type 2 diabetes is one component of the metabolic syndrome which includes impaired glucose tolerance, insulin resistance, central obesity, hypertension, combined dyslipidaemia, impaired fibrinolysis and hyperuricaemia. Microalbuminuria has also been linked to this pattern of metabolic disturbances. hypertriglyceridaemia and also low high-density lipoprotein (HDL) cholesterol are associated with Microalbuminuria. In type 1 diabetes, microalbuminuria is associated with a high prevalence of dyslipidaemia, which is more pronounced in overt nephropathy. The relationship between DN and dyslipidaemia, as well as between DN and blood pressure, is complicated by the fact that DN may be causally related to both parameters.

THE THERAPEUTIC APPROACH TO THE PATIENT WITH DIABETIC NEPHROPATHY

The therapeutic approach to patients with diabetic nephropathy is based mainly on strict control of hyperglycemia, antihypertensive treatment and low-protein diet. The lowering of serum lipids may also be advantageous in preventing progression of renal disease. There are also several potential therapeutic agents, which may play a role in the future. Moreover, with progression of diabetic nephropathy, efforts must be made to prevent and treat several comorbid conditions. In this section the approach to the diabetic patient with renal involvement is summarized (see Table 38.2 for a summary of the therapeutic approach).

The hyperfiltration that is found early in both type 1 and type 2 diabetes may be reversed by strict glucose control. However, the evidence as to the effect on renal hypertrophy is not as convincing. Two large studies have demonstrated that strict glucose control prevents the development of microalbuminuria in type 1 and proteinuria in type 2 diabetes. However, it is still not clear whether intensified glycemic control can prevent the progression from microalbuminuria to overt nephropathy, and whether it can affect the decline in glomerular filtration rate (GFR). Of importance is the observation that normalizing blood-glucose levels following pancreas transplantation resulted in improvement in the histologic changes in the kidney 10 years after transplantation, but not after 5 years. Strict control of glucose is thus of cardinal importance in prevention of overt diabetic nephropathy in patients who have signs of early renal involvement (hyperfiltration and/or microalbuminuria. However, there is no good evidence as to the effect of glucose control on the progression of renal disease in patients who have advanced nephropathy. Nevertheless, it is important even at these latter stages of the disease to maintain as near to normal blood glucose as possible in order to prevent other complications such as ketoacidosis, retinopathy, neuropathy, peripheral vascular and cardiovascular disease.

Table 38.2

Summary of the therapeutic approach to diabetic nephropathy

1. **Strict control of blood glucose**
   a. Beneficial in both type 1 and 2 diabetes
   b. Delays onset of microalbuminuria
   c. May not be as effective at slowing progression of overt renal disease
   d. Of importance in preventing other comorbid conditions such as retinopathy
2. **Treatment of hypertension**
   a. Lowering of blood pressure is the most important element in preventing progression of diabetic nephropathy
   b. The goals for treatment should be a blood pressure of 130/80 mmHg or less in all diabetic patients and 125/75 mmHg or less in patients with proteinuria greater than 1 g/day
   c. Nonpharmacologic therapeutic regimens
      i. Of major importance
         - Physical activity
         - Weight maintenance
      ii. Of moderate importance
         - Sodium restriction and potassium supplementation
         - Decreased protein diet
         - Reduction in alcohol intake
   d. Pharmacologic agents
      i. Angiotensin-converting enzyme inhibitor or angiotensin II receptor blocker—first choice
      ii. Diuretic—preferably of the thiazide group—in small dosage
      iii. Calcium-channel blocker—dihydropyridines are more effective in reducing blood pressure, while nondihydropyridines may have some specific antiproteinuric effect
      iv. Beta-blockers are mainly indicated to suppress tachycardia induced by other drugs or when a specific indication is present such as cardiovascular disease
      v. Alpha-receptor blockers are useful in reducing blood pressure
3. **Low-protein diet**
   a. A low-protein diet (about 0.8 g/kg body weight per day of high biologic value) may have a modest effect on progression of the renal disease
   b. Patients must be closely followed to prevent protein malnutrition

Table 38.2 *contd...*

4. **Control of serum lipids**
   a. Hyperlipidemia should be treated in order to prevent cardiovascular complications and possibly to slow
   b. progression of renal disease
5. **Management of the patient with mild to moderate renal involvement**
   a. Define stage of renal disease
   b. Strict glycemic control
   c. Antihypertensive treatment
   d. Lifestyle modification
6. **Management of the patient with advanced renal involvement**
   a. Antihypertensive treatment
   b. Metabolic control of hyperglycemia
   c. Stop smoking
   d. Restrict dietary protein intake
   e. Treat anemia
   f. Treat and prevent cardiovascular disease
   g. Treat hyperlipidemia
   h. Investigate and treat renal osteodystrophy
   i. Treat metabolic acidosis
   j. Adjust dosages of medications according to renal function
   k. Prepare for renal replacement therapy
7. **Treatment of patients with end-stage renal disease by dialysis**
   a. Use multidisciplinary team
   b. Decide on the mode of dialysis (hemodialysis or peritoneal dialysis)
   c. Prepare access (a-v fistula for hemodialysis or peritoneal catheter for peritoneal dialysis)
   d. Continue treating the patient as outlined in the previous section
   e. Institute dialytic therapy when the GFR is 10-15 ml/min
   f. Optimize quantity of dialysis and treat to avoid complications
8. **Treatment of patients with end-stage renal disease by transplantation**
   a. Renal transplantation
      i. Better survival than using dialysis
      ii. Living donor or cadaver donor
      iii. Early assessment for possibility of living donor
      iv. Early registration on cadaver kidney transplant waiting list
   b. Simultaneous renal and pancreas transplantation
      i. Reasonable success in type 1 diabetes
      ii. May not require insulin or may require reduced dosage
   c. Isolated pancreas transplantation
      i. Indicated in patients with brittle diabetes mellitus who have difficulty in control with insulin
   d. Pancreas islet cell transplantation
      i. Clinical trials are being conducted
      ii. Recent improvement in results
      iii. Hope for treatment of patients with type 1 diabetes

ANTIHYPERTENSIVE TREATMENT

Hypertension is often a concomitant finding in patients with diabetes. In patients with type 1 diabetes, the appearance of hypertension is linked to the appearance of microalbuminuria, whereas in type 2 diabetes, hypertension often antedates the diagnosis of diabetes. Hypertension is an important risk factor for overall mortality. Many studies have shown that reducing blood pressure can prevent the appearance of comorbid conditions and slow the progression of diabetic nephropathy. In fact, the treatment of hypertension is now considered to be the most important element in slowing progression. It has been suggested that the target values for the treatment of hypertension in diabetic patients should be 130/80 mmHg, and in patients with proteinuria greater than 1 g/day, the target should be 125/75 mmHg. Physical exercises and maintenance of a normal body weight are of primary importance in reducing blood pressure. Salt restriction and potassium supplementation, reduced protein diet and reduced alcohol intake may have a modest effect in reducing blood pressure . Angiotensin-converting enzyme inhibitors and angiotensin II receptor blockers not only reduce blood pressure, but also have additional renoprotective effects in both type 1 (ACE-I) and type 2 (AIIR) diabetic nephropathy. It is now well established that interruption of the renin-angiotensin system with either ACE-I or AIIR should be the drugs of choice for the treatment of hypertension in the diabetic patient. Both thiazide and loop diuretics may be used as ancillary drugs in the treatment of hypertension in the diabetic patient. Calcium-channel blockers, especially of the dihydropyridine group, are especially effective in reducing blood pressure, but do not reduce proteinuria and probably do not have a specific renoprotective effect. However, the members of the nondihydropyridine group of calcium-channel blockers may cause a reduction in proteinuria and are effective in combination with ACE-I. Beta blockers and alpha-receptor blockers are additional agents that may be used in the treatment of hypertension. Thus, we think that all diabetic patients with raised blood pressure should be treated initially with ACE-I or AIIR in an attempt to reach the treatment goals. Diuretics of Low-dose, calcium channel blockers, beta-blockers and alpha-receptor blockers may be subsequently added in order to achieve these goals.

LOW-PROTEIN DIET

The effects of protein restriction on the progression of renal involvement have been investigated in both types of diabetes. However, most studies were small and for a limited period of time. Protein restriction seems to have a significant, albeit small, effect on progression. A low-protein diet may be used on condition that the diet is strictly controlled in order to prevent protein malnutrition. The role of the dietitian in planning the specific diet for each patient and monitoring patient compliance is important.

CONTROL OF HYPERLIPIDEMIA

A significant correlation between the levels of serum lipids and progression of diabetic nephropathy in both type 1 and type 2 diabetes. However, interventional studies using HMG CoA reductase inhibitors have not always resulted in an improvement in progression. Lipid-lowering therapy was associated with diminished progression of renal disease. Moreover, dyslipidemia in diabetic patients has been clearly demonstrated to be an major factor for cardiovascular and other vascular diseases. Hyperlipidemia in the presence of diabetes mellitus, especially in the context of associated renal disease, should be treated both by diet and with drugs

TREATMENT OF CARDIAC COMPLICATIONS

Diabetes is associated with accelerated atherosclerosis and increased risk of coronary heart disease, congestive cardiac failure and sudden cardiac death. Indeed, it is postulated that there may be a specific cardiomyopathy in diabetes, independent of ischemic heart disease. This issue is controversial and unresolved. However, the high prevalence of cardiac dysfunction in diabetes and potential treatments for this condition have stimulated increasing basic and clinical research in this area. There is no doubt that patients with diabetic nephropathy, especially those with other risk factors, should be carefully monitored for cardiac complications and should receive prophylactic treatment.

TREATMENT OF ACID-BASE AND ELECTROLYTE DISORDERS

Pathophysiology of the many electrolyte disturbances that may occur in patients with diabetic nephropathy. The most important is hyperkalemia, which may be a result of insulin deficiency, hyporeninemic hypoaldosteronism and hyperosmolality. This problem may be further exacerbated by concomitant treatments, including agents which interrupt the reninangiotensin-aldosterone system, such as ACE-I, AIIR and spironolactone. There may also be derangements in sodium, calcium, magnesium and phosphate metabolism. Metabolic acidosis may occur even in diabetic patients with good glucose control and reasonably good renal function. This may be secondary to hyperkalemia, hypoaldosteronism or a primary tubular defect. The chapter includes an important discussion of acid-base or electrolyte disorders in diabetic patients secondary to the use of certain medications. These include lactic acidosis secondary to the use of metformin and hyperkalemia due to an array of medications. There is a discussion of water homeostasis and a description of the abnormalities in diabetic ketoacidosis.

MANAGEMENT OF THE PATIENT WITH MILD TO MODERATE RENAL INVOLVEMENT

The diabetic patient with mild to moderate renal involvement may be defined as the patient with signs of renal involvement (microalbuminuria to overt proteinuria) and/or reduced renal function (GFR of 30–90 ml/min). Good glycemic control is important during this stage of the disease. Maintenance of HbA1c below a value of 7% may reduce the rate of appearance of microalbuminuria in patients with normoalbuminuria. Strict glycemic control had been shown to prevent the progression from microalbuminuria to overt proteinuria. Nevertheless, it was suggested that strict control should be applied to prevent the progression of other microvascular complications, such as retinopathy. Similarly, there is little evidence to show that metabolic control may prevent or slow the decline in renal function. On the basis of one observational study, they suggest that strict control should be instituted if HbA1c is greater than 8%. Antihypertensive treatment, primarily with ACE-I, has not been shown reliably to prevent the development of microalbuminuria in patients with type 1 diabetes. Most of these patients are normotensive at the early stages of diabetes. However, patients with type 2 diabetes are often hypertensive at presentation, and early antihypertensive treatment may play a role in the primary prevention of microalbuminuria. The important role of treatment of hypertension with ACE-I and AIIR in the prevention of progression from microalbuminuria to overt proteinuria and in slowing progression of the disease was emphasized. The importance of treating the patients with microalbuminuria and/or hypertension with these agents, the aim being to reduce blood pressure to targets, as mentioned earlier under 'Antihypertensive treatment'. Dietary protein restriction should be reserved for patients with declining renal function. Additional factors in the treatment of these patients include cessation of smoking, careful monitoring of renal function, early referral to a nephrologist, and management of cardiovascular risk factors and cardiovascular disease.

MANAGEMENT OF THE PATIENT WITH ADVANCED RENAL INVOLVEMENT

In advanced renal disease (GFR less than 30 ml/min or nephrotic range proteinuria), treatment is aimed at slowing the rate of progression of the renal disease, preventing or treating comorbid conditions, and preparing the patient for renal replacement therapy (RRT). At this stage, it is imperative that the patients are followed in a clinic specializing in the treatment of renal failure. Control of hypertension in slowing progression of renal disease is important. Patients with advanced renal disease are likely to require several antihypertensive agents. The various medications may be associated with complications such as increased serum creatinine or hyperkalemia in patients with severely reduced renal function, and the patients must thus be closely monitored.

Strict diabetic control has not been shown to be effective in slowing progression of renal disease at this stage. However, glycemic control should be maintained in order to prevent and treat other complications of diabetes. Smoking has been shown to be associated with accelerated progression in type 2 diabetes; thus, patients should be advised to stop smoking in order potentially to retard progression and to prevent comorbid conditions. Nevertheless, there is a role for protein restriction, but care must be taken that the patient does not develop protein malnutrition. Anemia is an important complication of advanced renal disease. The degree of anemia tends to be greater in diabetic than in nondiabetic patients for the same degree of renal impairment. Anemia is one of the major factors in the clinical symptomatology of patients with renal failure and generally responds to treatment with human recombinant erythropoietin. Patients receiving erythropoietin must be closely followed and given iron supplementation according to need. The importance of hyperlipidemia and cardiovascular involvement, and their treatment in these patients. It thus imperative that all patients with advanced disease be checked for cardiovascular disease and hyperlipidemia and treated accordingly. Another possible complication of advanced renal disease is metabolic acidosis. Renal osteodystrophy is found in almost all patients with advanced renal disease and requires specific diagnostic and therapeutic measures. The doses of medications, especially those excreted by the kidney, have to be modified in order to prevent high blood levels and drug-drug interactions as the renal function decreases. Patients with advanced renal involvement should thus be carefully followed and treated with all the therapeutic measures that have been described above .

DIALYSIS IN THE TREATMENT OF DIABETIC PATIENTS WITH END-STAGE RENAL DISEASE (ESRD)

Briefly, the options include hemodialysis, peritoneal dialysis and transplantation. The decision as to the most suitable treatment for each patient will depend on many factors. It is important that the patients with ESRD are seen and treated by a multidisciplinary team, which should include an endocrinologist, a nephrologist, a cardiologist, an ophthalmologist, a social worker, a dietitian and a specialist nurse. Patients whose GFR is less than 30 mL/min should be advised of the various options, and as soon as a decision is made of the preferred option, preparation for RRT should be started. For instance, an arteriovenous fistula should be established in patients who will be undergoing hemodialysis, and a peritoneal catheter should be inserted in those who will be treated with peritoneal dialysis. The various therapeutic modalities mentioned in the previous section on advanced renal disease will be continued at this stage. It is generally accepted that when the GFR of a diabetic patient with ESRD is in the range of 10–15 mL/min, will be initiated.

THE USE OF TRANSPLANTATION IN THE TREATMENT OF DIABETIC PATIENTS ESRD

In spite of the fact that diabetic patients tend to fare less well after transplantation than nondiabetic patients, the survival of diabetic subjects who receive a kidney transplant is better than on dialysis. This is true in spite of the fact that kidney transplantation is associated with many complications as a result of the surgical procedure, the immunosuppressive therapy and the primary disease. Thus, kidney transplantation, using either a cadaver donor or living donor, is the preferred mode of treatment of ESRD due to diabetic nephropathy. Therefore, all suitable patients should be counseled about this option. Improvement in surgical technique and in the immunosuppressive therapy has made this an acceptable form of treatment. Cadaver donor pancreas transplantation can be performed simultaneously with a kidney transplant in diabetic ESRD patients, or as a solitary graft in patients who still have remnant kidney function but have brittle diabetes.

FUTURE STRATEGIES FOR THE TREATMENT OF DIABETIC NEPHROPATHY

Most of these strategies are based on various pathogenetic pathways of the disease. Some of them are in the development stage, whereas others have reached the stage of clinical trials. However, there is as yet no clinical proof of the beneficial effects of these agents.

ADVANCED GLYCATION END PRODUCTS (AGES)

These are thought to play an important role in the development of diabetic nephropathy.

The putative therapeutic strategies are prevention of the formation of AGEs, the use of cross-link breakers that can break down AGEs, and substances which block the receptors for AGEs. All these approaches to interrupt AGE dependent pathways are under current investigation.

PROTEIN KINASE C (PKC)

Protein kinase C (PKC), an important intracellular enzyme, becomes activated during the hyper glycemic condition. PKC may activate a myriad of growth factors that may be pathogenetic in diabetic nephropathy. Several PKC inhibitors have been generated and are being investigated. In particular, an inhibitor of the β2 isoform of PKC is under intensive clinical investigation.

NEWER TREATMENTS FOR HYPERTENSION

Various new inhibitors of vasoactive hormone formation are being developed and tested. One example is omapatrilat, a dual inhibitor of ACE and neutral endopeptidase. It is postulated that inhibiting these vasoactive pathways will lead not only to better blood pressure control but also superior renoprotection.

TREATMENT OF COMORBID CONDITIONS ASSOCIATED WITH DIABETES MELLITUS AND KIDNEY INVOLVEMENT

There are many complications of diabetes mellitus that are aggravated by the presence of diabetic nephropathy and the associated hypertension and cardiovascular disease.

PREGNANCY IN THE PATIENT WITH DIABETIC NEPHROPATHY

The effects of pregnancy on diabetes and renal disease in patients with diabetic nephropathy. Optimization of pregnancy outcome requires strict control of blood glucose; strict control of hypertension; avoiding medications, such as drugs acting on rennin angiotensin aldosterone system, that are contraindicated in pregnancy; regular monitoring of pregnancy; and planned delivery.

RETINOPATHY

Retinopathy is a ubiquitous complication of diabetic nephropathy and a leading cause of blindness. The risk factors for diabetic retinopathy as duration of disease, quality of metabolic control, hyperlipidemia, presence of hypertension and degree of renal involvement. The importance of careful treatment of diabetic patients on dialysis is stressed. All patients with diabetic nephropathy should be examined by an ophthalmologist annually. Treatment of hypertension, especially with ACE-I, and metabolic control are emphasized. Laser photocoagulation is indicated in patients with significant macular edema and proliferative retinopathy. Vitrectomy may need to be performed in patients showing progressive retinopathy with macular hemorrhage and retinal detachment.

REFERENCES

1. Onkamo P, Väänänen S, Karvonen M et al. Worldwide increase in incidence of type I diabetes the analysis of the data on published incidence trends, *Diabetologia* (1999) **12:** 1395–03.
2. Wiseman MJ, Saunders AJ, Keen H et al. Effect of blood glucose control on increased glomerular filtration rate and kidney size in insulin-dependent diabetes, *N Engl J Med* (1985) **312:** 617-21.

3. Vora JP, Dolben J, Williams JD et al. Impact of initial treatment on renal function in newly-diagnosed type 2 (non-insul-independent) diabetes mellitus, *Diabetologia* (1993) **36:** 734-40.
4. Mogensen CE. Microalbuminuria, blood pressure and diabetic renal disease: origin and development of ideas. *Diabetologia* (1999) **42:** 263-85.
5. Stamler J, Vaccaro O, Neaton JD et al. Diabetes, other risk factors, and 12-yr cardiovascular mortality for men screened in the Multiple Risk Factor Intervention Trial, *Diabetes Care* (1993) **16:** 434-44.
6. Bakris GL, Williams M, Dworkin L, Preserving renal function in adults with hypertension and diabetes: a consensus approach. National Kidney Foundation Hypertension and Diabetes Executive Committees Working Group, *Am J Kidney Dis* (2000) **36:** 646-61.
7. Lewis EJ, Huniscker LG, Bain RP et al. The effect of angiotensin-converting-enzyme inhibition on diabetic nephropathy, *N Engl J Med* (1993) **329:** 1456-62.
8. Brenner BM, Cooper ME, de Zeeuw D et al. Effects of losartan on renal and cardiovascular outcomes in patients with type 2 diabetes and nephropathy, *N Engl J Med* (2001) **345:** 861-9.
9. Lewis EJ, Hunsicker LG, Clarke WR et al. Renoprotective effects of the angiotensin-receptor antagonist irbesartan in patients with nephropathy due to type 2 diabetes. *N Engl J Med* (2001) **345:** 851–60.
10. Parving HH, Lehnert H, Brochner-Mortensen J et al. The effect of irbesartan on the development of diabetic nephropathy in patients with type 2 diabetes, *N Engl J Med* (2001) **345:** 870-8.
11. Bakris G, White D, Effects of an ACE inhibitor combined with a calcium channel blocker on progression of diabetic nephropathy, *J Hum Hypertens* (1997) **11:** 35-8.
12. Bakris GL, Weir MR, De Quattro V et al. Effects of an ACE inhibitor/calcium antagonist combination on proteinuria in diabetic nephropathy, *Kidney Int* (1998) **54**: 1283-9.
13. Fried LF, Orchard TJ, Kasiske BL, Effect of lipid reduction on the progression of renal disease: a meta-analysis, *Kidney Int* (2001) **59:** 260-9.

CHAPTER 39

URINARY STONE DISEASE

Urolithiasis is the medical term used to describe stones occurring in the urinary tract. Other frequently used terms are urinary tract stone disease and nephrolithiasis. Stone incidence depends on geographical, climatic, ethnic, dietary and genetic factors. The recurrence risk is basically determined by the disease or disorder causing the stone formation. Accordingly, the prevalence rates for urinary stones vary from 1% to 20%. In countries with a high standard of life such as Sweden, Canada or the US, renal stone prevalence is notably high (> 10%).

CLASSIFICATION

Stones can be classified into those caused by: infection, or non-infectious causes (infection and non-infection stones); genetic defects; or adverse drug effects (drug stones)

Table 39.1

Classification of stones

Classification of stones
Non-infection stones • Calcium oxalate • Calcium phosphate • Uric acid
Infection stones • Magnesium ammonium phosphate • Carbonate apatite • Ammonium ureate
Genetic causes • Cystine • Xanthine • 2,8-dihydroxyadenine
Drug stones

STONE COMPOSITION

RISK FACTORS FOR STONE FORMATION

- Anatomic abnormalities: medullary sponge kidney, ureteropelvic junction stenosis, pyelo-ureteral duplication, polycystic renal disease, etc.
- Epidemiological factors and genetic predisposition: dietary risk factors, climate, occupation, family history of stones.
- Excessive excretion of promoters of urinary crystallization: calcium (idiopathic hypercalciuria), oxalate (enteric hyperoxaluria), uric acid (uric acid hyperexcretion).
- Abnormalities of urinary pH: renal tubular acidosis, gouty diathesis, infection stones (struvite stones caused by urea-splitting organisms).
- Reduced excretion of inhibitors of urinary crystallization: hypocitraturia.
- Metabolic syndrome and obesity: pure uric acid stones.
- Low urine volume: reduced intake or increased loss of water.

Table 39.2

Composition of stones

Chemical name	Mineral name	Chemical formula
Calcium oxalate monohydrate	Whewellite	$CaC_2O_4.H_2O$
Calcium oxalate dihydrate	Wheddelite	$CaC_2O_4.2H_2O$
Basic calcium phosphate	Apatite	$Ca_{10}(PO_4)_6.(OH)_2$
Calcium hydroxyl phosphate	Carbonite apatite	$Ca_5(PO_3)_3(OH)$
b-tricalcium phosphate	Whitlockite	$Ca_3(PO_4)_2$
Carbonate apatite phosphate	Dahllite	$Ca_5(PO_4)_3OH$
Calcium hydrogen phosphate	Brushite	$PO_4.2H_2O$
Calcium carbonate	Aragonite	$CaCO_3$
Octacalcium phosphate	$Ca_8H_2(PO_4)_6.5H_2O$	
Uric acid	Uricite	$C_5H_4N_4O_3$
Uric acid dihydrate	Uricite	$C_5H_4O_3$-$2H_20$
Ammonium urate	$NH_4C_5H_3N_4O_3$	
Sodium acid urate monohydrate	$NaC_5H_3N_4O_3.H_2O$	
Magnesium ammonium phosphate	Struvite	$MgNH_4PO_4.6H_2O$
Magnesium acid phosphate trihydrate	Newberyite	$MgHPO_4.3H_2O$
Magnesium ammonium phosphate monohydrate	Dittmarite	$MgNH_4(PO_4).1H_2O$
Cystine	$[SCH_2CH(NH_2)COOH]_2$	
Gypsum	Calcium sulphate dihydrate Zinc phosphate tetrahydrate	$CaSO_4.2H_2O$ $Zn_3(PO_4)_2.4H_2O$
Xanthine		
2,8-Dihydroxyadenine		
Proteins		
Cholesterol		
Calcite		
Potassium urate		
Trimagnesium phosphate		
Melamine		
Matrix		
Drug stones	• Active compounds crystal-izing in urine • Substances impairing urine composition	
Foreign body calculi		

- Hypercalcemic disorders: Primary hyperparathyroidism and other disturbances of calcium metabolism.
- Lithogenic drugs: Triamterene, indinavir, sulfadiazine, uricosuric agents.
- Inflammatory bowel disease and other intestinal malabsorption states

Table 39.3

Patients who are at high risk of stone formation

General factors
• Early onset of urolithiasis (especially children and teenagers) • Familial stone formation • Uric acid and urate-containing stones • Infection stones • Solitary kidney (the kidney itself does not particularly increase the risk of stone formation, but prevention of stone recurrence is of more importance)
Diseases associated with stone formation
• Hyperparathyroidism • Metabolic syndrome • Nephrocalcinosis • Gastrointestinal diseases (i.e., jejuno-ileal bypass, intestinal resection, Crohn's disease, malabsorptive conditions, enteric hyperoxaluria after urinary diversion) and bariatric surgery • Sarcoidosis
Genetically determined stone formation
• Cystinuria (type A, B and AB) • Primary hyperoxaluria (PH) • Renal tubular acidosis (RTA) type I • 2,8-Dihydroxyadeninuria • Xanthinuria • Lesch-Nyhan syndrome • Cystic fibrosis
Anatomical abnormalities associated with stone formation
• Medullary sponge kidney (tubular ectasia) • Ureteropelvic junction (UPJ) obstruction • Calyceal diverticulum, calyceal cyst • Ureteral stricture • Vesico-uretero-renal reflux • Horseshoe kidney • Ureterocele

DIAGNOSTIC IMAGING

Standard evaluation includes a detailed medical history and physical examination. Patients with ureteral stones usually present with groin pain, vomiting, and sometimes fever, but may also be asymptomatic.

Ultrasound (US) should be used as the primary diagnostic imaging tool, although pain relief, or any other emergency measures should not be delayed by imaging assessments. US is safe (no risk of radiation), reproducible and inexpensive. It can identify stones located in the calices, pelvis, and pyeloureteric and vesicoureteric junctions, as well as in patients with upper urinary tract dilatation. US have a sensitivity of 45% and specificity of 94% for ureteric stones and a sensitivity of 45% and specificity of 88% for renal stones.

TREATMENT

THIAZIDE DIURETICS

Thiazide lowers urine calcium resulting in a fall in calcium oxalate and calcium phosphate supersaturation. Reduction of calciuria is attributed to enhanced reabsorption of calcium on the renal distal convolute tubule but very recent and compelling data show that enhanced passive Ca^{2+} transport in the proximal tubule rather than active Ca^{2+} transport in distal convolution explains thiazide-induced hypocalciuria. Doses of either chlorthalidone or hydrochlorothiazide should be no more than 25 mg/day to avoid adverse effects. Indapamide, a thiazide-like agent is also effective.

ALLOPURINOL

Allopurinol blocks uric acid production, reducing heterogeneous nucleation of calcium oxalate by both uric acid and monosodium urate. In addition, the adsorption of normally occurring macromolecular inhibitors of calcium oxalate crystallization by uric acid or monosodium urate could be possibly averted when using this drug. However, Allopurinol (100 to 300 mg/day) is indicated only when hyperuricosuria is the only metabolic abnormality. On the other hand, alkali therapy with potassium citrate may also be beneficial, since raising urinary pH will help solubilizing uric acid converting it into potassium urate.

POTASSIUM CITRATE

Potassium citrate reduces urinary saturation of calcium salts by complexing calcium and reducing ionic calcium concentration. Due to its alkalinizing effect, it also increases the dissociation of uric acid, lowers the amount of poorly soluble undissociated uric acid, reducing the propensity to form uric acid stones. The induced decline of urinary calcium during the early period of treatment represents a potential additional advantage of the drug. Therefore, potassium citrate seems to be effective in conditions of hypocitraturia, hypercalciuria, or hyperuricosuria and also in distal RTA patients, due to the need of alkalinization in the latter. Potassium citrate is preferable to sodium citrate in the prevention of urolithiasis, in doses ranging from 30 to 60 mE/day. However, adverse effects of gastrointestinal origin including epigastric pain, abdominal distention or diarrhea are common. Promising results with the use of other citrate salts such as potassium-magnesium, not yet approved by the Food and Drug Administration.

DIETARY RECOMMENDATIONS IN RENAL STONE DISEASE

1. Adequate dietary calcium intake (calcium and oxalate intakes must be in balance)
2. Reduce animal protein intake
3. Reduce salt intake
4. Increase fruits and vegetables intake (rich in potassium)
5. Increase fluid intake (at least > 2L/day)

Table 39.4

Pharmacological treatment of Nephrolithiasis according to metabolic disturbance

Hypercalciuria	Hydrochlorthiazide/Chlortalidone/Indapamide (Potassium citrate may be added)
Hypocitraturia	Potassium citrate
Hyperuricosuria	Allopurinol or Potassium citrate
Hyperoxaluria (primary)	Pyridoxine
Cystinuria	Alphamercaptoproprionylglycine (tiopronin) or D-penicillamine or angiotensin converting enzyme inhibitor
Distal Renal Tubular Acidosis	Potassium citrate
Low urinary pH	Potassium citrate
Urinary tract infection	Antibiotics

Table 39.5

Dietary recommendations in renal stone disease

Fluid intake (drinking advice)	Fluid amount: 2.5-3.0 L/day, Circadian drinking, Neutral pH beverages; Diuresis: 2.0-2.5 L/day.
Nutritional advice for a balanced diet	Balanced diet*, Rich in vegetables and fibre, Normal calcium content: 1-1.2 g/day, Limited NaCl content: 4-5 g/day, Limited animal protein content: 0.8-1.0 g/kg/day
Lifestyle advice to normalise general risk factors	BMI: retain a normal BMI level, Adequate physical activity, Balancing of excessive fluid loss

REFERENCES

1. Trinchieri A CG KS, Jun Wu K. Epidemiology. In: *Stone Disease*. C.P. Segura JW KS, Pak CY, Preminger GM, Tolley D., eds. Health Publications, Paris. 2003. p. 13-30
2. Hesse A, Brandle E, Wilbert D, et al. Study on the prevalence and incidence of urolithiasis in Germany comparing the years 1979 vs. 2000. Eur Urol 2003 Dec;44(6): 709-13
3. Wimpissinger F, Turk C, Kheyfets O, et al. The silence of the stones: asymptomatic ureteral calculi. J Urol 2007 Oct; 178 (4 Pt 1): 1341-4; discussion 1344.
4. Ray AA, Ghiculete D, Pace KT, et al. Limitations to ultrasound in the detection

and measurement of urinary tract calculi. Urology 2010 Aug; 76(2): 295-300.

5. Seitz C, Liatsikos E, Porpiglia F, et al. Medical Therapy to Facilitate the Passage of Stones: What Is the Evidence? Eur Urol 2009 Sep; 56(3): 455-71.
6. Nijenhuis T, Vallon V, van der Kemp AW, Loffing J, Hoenderop JG, Bindels RJ. Enhanced passive Ca2+ reabsorption and reduced Mg2+ channel abundance explains thiazide-induced hypocalciuria and hypomagnesemia. J Clin Invest 2005;115(6): 1651-8.
7. Goldfarb DS. Reconsideration of the 1998 NIH Consensus Statement on prevention and treatment of kidney stones: are the recommendations out of date? Rev Urol 2002; 4(2): 53-60
8. Martini LA, Cuppari L, Colugnati FAB, Sigulem DM, Szejnfeld VL, Schor N, et al. High sodium chloride intake is associated with low bone density in calcium stone forming patients. Clin Nephrol 2000;54(2): 85-93
9. Heilberg IP. Update on dietary recommendations and medical treatment of renal stone disease. Nephrol Dial Tranplant 2000; 15: 117-23.

CHAPTER 40

Hypertension

DEFINITION

- Hypertension is defined by persistent elevation of arterial blood pressure (BP) (Fig. 40.1).
- Patients with diastolic blood pressure (DBP) values <90 mm Hg and systolic blood pressure (SBP) values > 140 mm Hg have isolated systolic hypertension.
- A hypertensive crisis (BP >180/120 mm Hg) may be categorized as either a hypertensive emergency (extreme BP elevation with acute or progressing target organ damage) or a hypertensive urgency (severe BP elevation without acute or progressing target organ injury).

Blood pressure is the measurement of force applied to artery walls

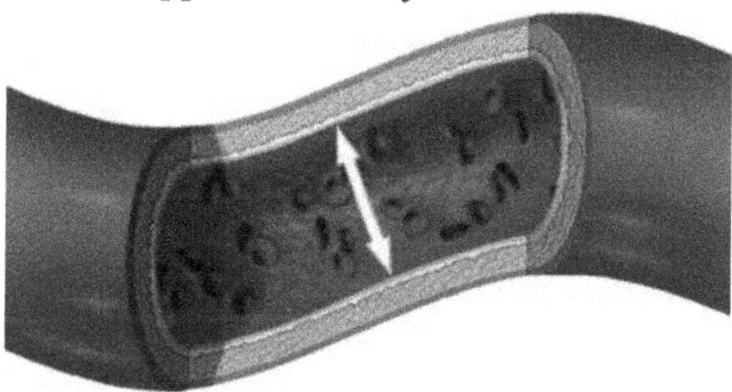

FIGURE 40.1

Blood pressure in blood vessels.

PREVALENCE

As of 2000, nearly one billion people or ~26% of the adult population of the world had hypertension. It was common in both developed (333 million) and undeveloped (639 million) countries. However rates vary markedly in different regions with rates as low as 3.4% (men) and 6.8% (women) in rural India and as high as 68.9% (men) and 72.5% (women) in Poland.

ETIOLOGY

Many factors can affect blood pressure, including:

- Water and salt taken by body
- The condition of kidneys, nervous system, or blood vessels
- The levels of different body hormones

High blood pressure increases chance of having a stroke, heart attack, heart failure, kidney disease, and early death.

Higher risk of high blood pressure if persons:

- Are African American
- Are obese
- Are often stressed or anxious
- Drink too much alcohol (more than one drink per day for women and more than two drinks per day for men)

- Eat too much salt in your diet
- Have a family history of high blood pressure
- Have diabetes
- Smoke

Most of the time, no cause of high blood pressure is found. This is called essential hypertension.

High blood pressure that is caused by another medical condition or medication is called secondary hypertension. Secondary hypertension may be due to:

- Chronic kidney disease
- Disorders of the adrenal gland (pheochromocytoma or Cushing syndrome)
- Pregnancy
- Medications such as birth control pills, diet pills, some cold medications, and migraine medications
- Narrowed artery that supplies blood to the kidney (renal artery stenosis)
- Hyperparathyroidism

PATHOPHYSIOLOGY

- Hypertension is a heterogeneous disorder that may result either from a specific cause (secondary hypertension) or from an underlying pathophysiologic mechanism of unknown etiology (primary or essential hypertension). Secondary hypertension accounts for fewer than 10% of cases, and most of these are caused by chronic kidney disease or renovascular disease. Other conditions causing secondary hypertension include pheochromocytoma, Cushing's syndrome, hyperthyroidism, hyperpa-rathyroidism, primary aldosteronism, pregnancy, obstructive sleep apnea, and coarctation of the aorta. Some drugs that may increase BP include corticosteroids, estrogens, nonsteroidal anti-inflammatory drugs (NSAIDs), amphetamines, sibutramine, cyclosporine, tacrolimus, erythropoietin, and venlafaxine.
- Multiple factors may contribute to the development of primary hypertension, including:
  - Humoral abnormalities involving the renin-angiotensin-aldosterone system, natriuretic hormone, or hyperinsulinemia;
  - A pathologic disturbance in the CNS, autonomic nerve fibers, adrenergic receptors, or baroreceptors;
  - Abnormalities in either the renal or tissue autoregulatory processes for sodium excretion, plasma volume, and arteriolar constriction;
  - A deficiency in the local synthesis of vasodilating substances in the vascular endothelium, such as prostacyclin, bradykinin, and nitric oxide, or an increase in production of vasoconstricting substances such as (Fig. 40.2) and endothelin I;
  - A high sodium intake and increased circulating natriuretic hormone inhibition of intracellular sodium transport, resulting in increased vascular reactivity and a rise in BP; and
  - Increased intracellular concentration of calcium, leading to altered vascular smooth muscle function and increased peripheral vascular resistance.
- The main causes of death in hypertensive subjects are cerebrovascular accidents, cardiovascular (CV) events, and renal failure. The probability of premature death correlates with the severity of BP elevation.

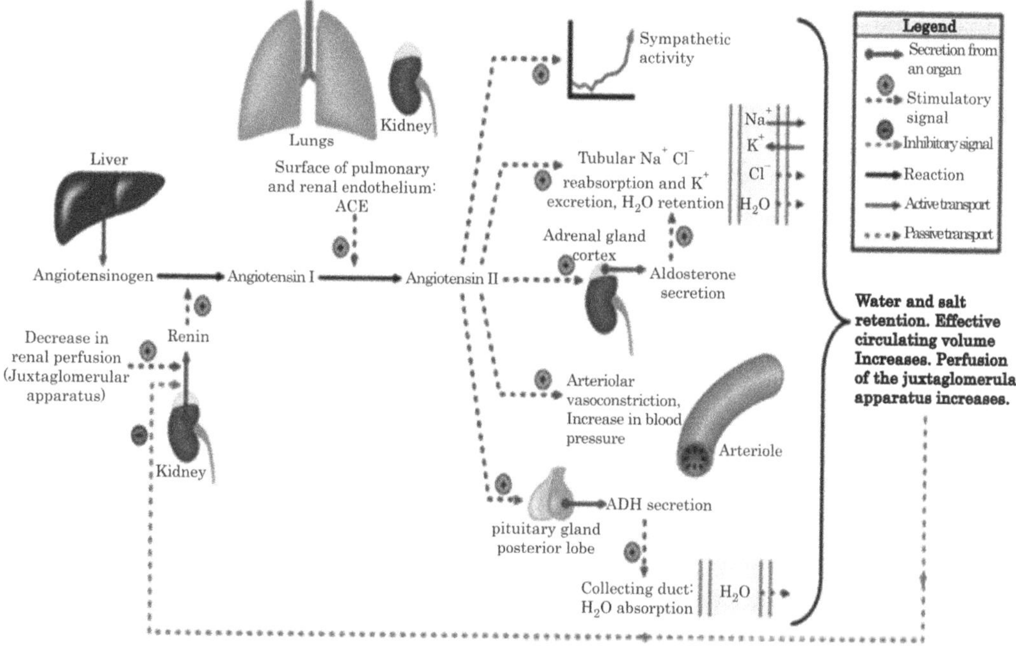

FIGURE 40.2

Rennin - angiotensin - aldosterone system.

(source: https://en.wikipedia.org/wiki/Renin%E2%80%93angiotensin_system)

CLINICAL FEATURES

- Most of the time, there are no symptoms. For most patients, high blood pressure is found when they visit their health care provider or have it checked elsewhere.
- Because there are no symptoms, people can develop heart disease and kidney problems without knowing they have high blood pressure.
- Severe headache, nausea or vomiting, confusion, changes in your vision or nosebleeds indicates a severe and dangerous form of high blood pressure called malignant hypertension.

DIAGNOSIS

- The funduscopic examination may reveal arteriolar narrowing, focal arteriolar narrowing, arteriovenous nicking, and retinal hemorrhages, exudates, and infarcts. The presence of papilledema indicates hypertensive emergency requiring rapid treatment.
- Cardiopulmonary examination may reveal an abnormal heart rate or rhythm, left ventricular (LV) hypertrophy, third and fourth heart sounds.
- Peripheral vascular examination can detect evidence of atherosclerosis, which

may present as aortic or abdominal bruits, distended veins, diminished or absent peripheral pulses, or lower extremity edema.

TREATMENT

NON PHARMACOLOGICAL THERAPY

- All patients with prehypertension and hypertension should be prescribed lifestyle modifications, including 1. Weight reduction if overweight, 2. Adoption of the Dietary Approaches to Stop Hypertension eating plan, 3. Dietary sodium restriction ideally to 1.5 g/day (3.8 g/day sodium chloride), 4. Regular aerobic physical activity, 5. Moderate alcohol consumption (two or fewer drinks per day), and 6. Smoking cessation.
- Lifestyle modification alone is appropriate therapy for patients with prehypertension. Patients diagnosed with stage 1 or 2 hypertension should be placed on lifestyle modifications and drug therapy concurrently.

PHARMACOLOGICAL THERAPY (FIG. 40.3)

- Initial drug selection depends on the degree of BP elevation and the presence of compelling indications for selected drugs.
- Most patients with stage 1 hypertension should be treated initially with a **thiazide diuretic, angiotensin-converting enzyme (ACE) inhibitor, angiotensin II receptor blocker (ARB), or calcium channel blocker (CCB).** Combination therapy is recommended for patients with stage 2 disease, with one of the agents being a thiazide-type diuretic unless contraindications exist.
- **Diuretics, ACE inhibitors, ARBs,** and **CCBs** are primary agents acceptable as first-line options based on outcome data demonstrating CV risk reduction benefits.

β-Blockers may be used either to treat a specific compelling indication or as combination therapy with a primary antihypertensive agent for patients without a compelling indication.

- **α1-Blockers, direct renin inhibitors, central α2-agonists, peripheral adrenergic antagonists,** and **direct arterial vasodilators** are alternatives that may be used in select patients after primary agents.

DIURETICS

- **Thiazides** are the preferred type of diuretic for treating hypertension, and all are equally effective in lowering BP.
- **Potassium-sparing diuretics** are weak antihypertensives when used alone but provide an additive hypotensive effect when combined with thiazide or loop diuretics. Moreover, they counteract the potassium and magnesium losing properties and perhaps glucose intolerance caused by other diuretics.
- **Aldosterone antagonists (spironolactone, eplerenone)** are also potassium- sparing diuretics but are more potent antihypertensives with a slow onset of action (up to 6 weeks with spironolactone).
- Acutely, diuretics lower BP by causing diuresis. The reduction in plasma volume and stroke volume associated with diuresis decreases cardiac output and, consequently, BP. The initial drop in cardiac output causes a compensatory increase in peripheral vascular resistance.

With chronic diuretic therapy, the extracellular fluid volume and plasma volume return almost to pretreatment levels, and peripheral vascular resistance falls below its pretreatment baseline. The reduction in peripheral vascular resistance is responsible for the long-term hypotensive effects. Thiazides lower BP by mobilizing sodium and water from arteriolar walls, which may contribute to decreased peripheral vascular resistance.

- When diuretics are combined with other antihypertensive agents, an additive hypotensive effect is usually observed because of independent mechanisms of action. Furthermore, many nondiuretic antihypertensive agents induce salt and water retention, which is counteracted by concurrent diuretic use.
- Side effects of thiazides include hypokalemia, hypomagnesemia, hypercalcemia, hyperuricemia, hyperglycemia, hyperlipidemia, and sexual dysfunction. Loop diuretics have less effect on serum lipids and glucose, but hypocalcemia may occur.
- Hypokalemia and hypomagnesemia may cause muscle fatigue or cramps. Serious cardiac arrhythmias may occur, especially in patients receiving digitalis therapy, patients with Left ventricular (LV) hypertrophy, and those with ischemic heart disease. Low-dose therapy (e.g., 25 mg **hydrochlorothiazide** or 12.5 mg **chlorthalidone** daily) rarely causes significant electrolyte disturbances.
- Potassium-sparing diuretics may cause hyperkalemia, especially in patients with chronic kidney disease or diabetes, and in patients receiving concurrent treatment with an ACE inhibitor, ARB, NSAID, or potassium supplement. **Eplerenone** has an increased risk for hyperkalemia and is contraindicated in patients with impaired renal function or type 2 diabetes with proteinuria. **Spironolactone** may cause gynecomastia in up to 10% of patients, but this effect occurs rarely with eplerenone.

ANGIOTENSIN-CONVERTING ENZYME INHIBITORS

- ACE facilitates production of angiotensin II, which has a major role in regulating arterial BP. ACE is distributed in many tissues and is present in several different cell types, but its principal location is in endothelial cells. Therefore, the major site for angiotensin II production is in the blood vessels, not the kidney. ACE inhibitors block the conversion of angiotensin I to angiotensin II, a potent vasoconstrictor and stimulator of aldosterone secretion. ACE inhibitors also block the degradation of bradykinin and stimulate the synthesis of other vasodilating substances including prostaglandin E2 and prostacyclin. The fact that ACE inhibitors lower BP in patients with normal plasma renin activity suggests that bradykinin and perhaps tissue production of ACE are important in hypertension.
- Starting doses of ACE inhibitors should be low with slow dose titration. Acute hypotension may occur at the onset of ACE inhibitor therapy, especially in patients who are sodium- or volume-depleted, in heart failure exacerbation, very elderly, or on concurrent vasodilators or diuretics. Patients with these risk factors should start with half the normal dose followed by slow dose titration (e.g., 6- week intervals).
- ACE inhibitors decrease aldosterone and can increase serum potassium

concentrations. Hyperkalemia occurs primarily in patients with chronic kidney disease or diabetes and in those also taking ARBs, NSAIDs, potassium supplements, or potassium-sparing diuretics.

- Acute renal failure is a rare but serious side effect of ACE inhibitors; preexisting kidney disease increases the risk. Bilateral renal artery stenosis or unilateral stenosis of a solitary functioning kidney renders patients dependent on the vasoconstrictive effect of angiotensin II on efferent arterioles, making these patients particularly susceptible to acute renal failure.
- Angioedema is a serious potential complication that occurs in less than 1% of patients. It may be manifested as lip and tongue were swelling and possibly difficulty breathing. Drug withdrawal is necessary for all patients with angioedema, and some patients may also require drug treatment and/or emergent intubation.
- A persistent dry cough occurs in up to 20% of patients and is thought to be due to inhibition of bradykinin breakdown.
- ACE inhibitors are absolutely contraindicated in pregnancy because of possible major congenital malformations associated with exposure in the first trimester and serious neonatal problems, including renal failure and death in the infant, from exposure during the second and third trimesters.

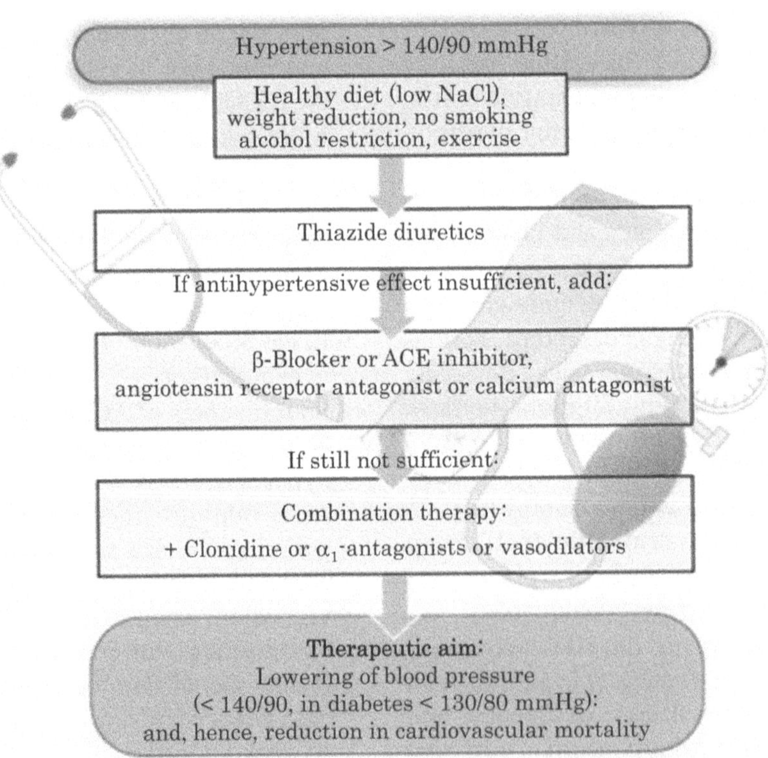

FIGURE 40.3

Therapy of hypertension.

ANGIOTENSIN II RECEPTOR BLOCKERS

- Angiotensin II is generated by the renin-angiotensin pathway (which involves ACE) and an alternative pathway that uses other enzymes such as chymases. ACE inhibitors block only the renin-angiotensin pathway, whereas ARBs antagonize angiotensin II generated by either pathway. The ARBs directly block the angiotensin type 1 receptor that mediates the known effects of angiotensin II (vasoconstriction, aldosterone release, sympathetic activation, antidiuretic hormone release, and constriction of the efferent arterioles of the glomerulus).
- Unlike ACE inhibitors, ARBs do not block the breakdown of bradykinin. While this accounts for the lack of cough as a side effect, there may be negative consequences because some of the antihypertensive effect of ACE inhibitors may be due to increased levels of bradykinin. Bradykinin may also be important for regression of myocyte hypertrophy and fibrosis, and increased levels of tissue plasminogen activator.
- All drugs in this class have similar antihypertensive efficacy and fairly flat dose-response curves. The addition of low doses of a thiazide diuretic can increase efficacy significantly.
- Like ACE inhibitors, they may cause renal insufficiency, hyperkalemia, and orthostatic hypotension. Angioedema is less likely to occur than with ACE inhibitors, but cross reactivity has been reported. ARBs should not be used in pregnancy.

CALCIUM CHANNEL BLOCKERS (CCB)

- CCBs cause relaxation of cardiac and smooth muscle by blocking voltage sensitive calcium channels, thereby reducing the entry of extracellular calcium into cells. Vascular smooth muscle relaxation leads to vasodilation and a corresponding reduction in BP. Dihydropyridine calcium channel antagonists may cause reflex sympathetic activation, and all agents (except amlodipine and felodipine) may demonstrate negative inotropic effects.
- **Verapamil** decreases heart rate, slows atrioventricular (AV) nodal conduction, and produces a negative inotropic effect that may precipitate heart failure in patients with borderline cardiac reserve. **Diltiazem** decreases AV conduction and heart rate to a lesser extent than verapamil.
- Diltiazem and verapamil can cause cardiac conduction abnormalities such as bradycardia, AV block, and heart failure. Both can cause anorexia, nausea, peripheral edema, and hypotension. Verapamil causes constipation in about 7% of patients.
- Dihydropyridine causes a baroreceptor-mediated reflex increase in heart rate because of their potent peripheral vasodilating effects. Dihydropyridine do not decrease AV node conduction and are not effective for treating supraventricular tachyarrhythmias.
- Side effects of Dihydropyridines include dizziness, flushing, headache, gingival hyperplasia, and peripheral edema. Side effects due to vasodilation such as

dizziness, flushing, headache, and peripheral edema occur more frequently with Dihydropyridines than with verapamil or Diltiazem.

β-BLOCKERS

- The exact hypotensive mechanism of β-blockers is not known but may involve decreased cardiac output through negative chronotropic and inotropic effects on the heart and inhibition of renin release from the kidney.
- Even though there are important pharmacodynamic and pharmacokinetic differences among the various β-blockers, there is no difference in clinical antihypertensive efficacy.
- **Atenolol, betaxolol, bisoprolol,** and **metoprolol** are cardioselective at low doses and bind more avidly to β1-receptors than to β2-receptors. As a result, they are less likely to provoke bronchospasm and vasoconstriction and may be safer than nonselective β-blockers in patients with asthma, chronic obstructive pulmonary disease, diabetes, and PAD. Cardio selectivity is a dose-dependent phenomenon, and the effect is lost at higher doses.
- **Acebutolol, carteolol, penbutolol,** and **pindolol** possess intrinsic sympathomimetic activity (ISA) or partial β-receptor agonist activity.
- There are pharmacokinetic differences among β-blockers in first-pass metabolism, serum half-lives, degree of lipophilicity, and route of elimination. **Propranolol** and **metoprolol** undergo extensive first-pass metabolism. **Atenolol** and **nadolol** have relatively long half-lives and are excreted renally; the dosage may need to be reduced in patients with moderate to severe renal insufficiency. Even though the half-lives of the other β-blockers are much shorter, once-daily administration still may be effective. β-Blockers vary in their lipophilic properties and thus CNS penetration.
- Side effects from β-blockade in the myocardium include bradycardia, Atrioventricular (AV) conduction abnormalities, and acute heart failure.

α1-RECEPTOR BLOCKERS

- **Prazosin, terazosin**, and **doxazosin** are selective α1-receptor blockers that inhibit catecholamine uptake in smooth muscle cells of the peripheral vasculature, resulting in vasodilation.
- A potentially severe side effect is a first-dose phenomenon characterized by orthostatic hypotension accompanied by transient dizziness or faintness, palpitations, and even syncope within 1 to 3 hours of the first dose or after later dosage increases. These episodes can be obviated by having the patient take the first dose, and subsequent first increased doses, at bedtime. Occasionally, orthostatic dizziness persists with chronic administration.
- Sodium and water retention can occur with chronic administration. These agents are most effective when given with a diuretic to maintain antihypertensive efficacy and minimize potential edema.

DIRECT RENIN INHIBITOR

- **Aliskiren** blocks the Renin-Angiotensin-Aldosterone system at its point of a activation, which results in reduced plasma renin activity and BP. It provides BP reductions comparable to an ACE inhibitor, ARB, or CCB. It also has additive antihypertensive effects when used in combination with thiazides, ACE inhibitors, ARBs, or CCBs. It is approved for monotherapy or in combination with other agents.

- Many of the cautions and adverse effects seen with ACE inhibitors and ARBs apply to Aliskiren. It is contraindicated in pregnancy.
- At this time, aliskiren should be used only as an alternative therapy because of the lack of long-term studies evaluating CV event reduction and its significant cost compared to generic agents with outcomes data.

CENTRAL 2α-AGONISTS

- **Clonidine, Guanabenz, Guanfacine,** and **Methyldopa** lower BP primarily by stimulating α2-adrenergic receptors in the brain, which reduces sympathetic outflow from the vasomotor center and increases vagal tone. Stimulation of presynaptic α2-receptors peripherally may contribute to the reduction in sympathetic tone. Consequently, there may be decreases in heart rate, cardiac output, total peripheral resistance, plasma renin activity, and baroreceptor reflexes.
- Chronic use results in sodium and fluid retention. Other side effects may include depression, orthostatic hypotension, dizziness, and Anticholinergic effects.

RESERPINE

- **Reserpine** depletes norepinephrine from sympathetic nerve endings and blocks the transport of norepinephrine into its storage granules. When the nerve is stimulated, less than the usual amount of norepinephrine is released into the synapse. This reduces sympathetic tone, decreasing peripheral vascular resistance and BP.
- Reserpine has a long half-life that allows for once-daily dosing, but it may take 2 to 6 weeks before the maximal antihypertensive effect is seen.
- Reserpine can cause significant sodium and fluid retention, and it should be given with a diuretic (preferably a thiazide).
- Reserpine's strong inhibition of sympathetic activity allows increased parasympathetic activity to occur, which is responsible for side effects of nasal stuffiness, increased gastric acid secretion, diarrhea, and bradycardia.
- The most serious side effect is dose-related mental depression resulting from CNS depletion of catecholamine's and serotonin. This can be minimized by not exceeding 0.25 mg daily.

DIRECT ARTERIAL VASODILATORS

- **Hydralazine** and **Minoxidil** cause direct arteriolar smooth muscle relaxation. Compensatory activation of baroreceptor reflexes results in increased sympathetic outflow from the vasomotor center, producing an increase in heart rate, cardiac output, and renin release. Consequently, the hypotensive effectiveness of direct vasodilators diminishes over time unless the patient is also taking a sympathetic inhibitor and a diuretic.

- All patients taking these drugs for long-term hypertension therapy should first receive both a diuretic and a β-blocker. The diuretic minimizes the side effect of sodium and water retention. Direct vasodilators can precipitate angina in patients with underlying coronary artery disease unless the baroreceptor reflex mechanism is completely blocked with a β-blocker. Nondihydropyridine CCBs can be used as an alternative to β-blockers in patients with contraindications to β-blockers.
- Hydralazine may cause a dose-related, reversible lupus-like syndrome, which is more common in slow acetylators. Lupus-like reactions can usually be avoided by using total daily doses of less than 200 mg. Other Hydralazine side effects include dermatitis, drug fever, peripheral neuropathy, hepatitis, and vascular headaches. For these reasons, Hydralazine has limited usefulness in the treatment of hypertension.
- Minoxidil is a more potent vasodilator than Hydralazine, and the compensatory increases in heart rate, cardiac output, renin release, and sodium retention are more dramatic. Severe sodium and water retention may precipitate congestive heart failure. Minoxidil also causes reversible hypertrichosis on the face, arms, back, and chest. Minoxidil is reserved for very difficult to control hypertension and in patients requiring Hydralazine who experience drug-induced lupus.

POSTGANGLIONIC SYMPATHETIC INHIBITORS

- **Guanethidine** and **Guanadrel** deplete norepinephrine from postganglionic sympathetic nerve terminals and inhibit the release of norepinephrine in response to sympathetic nerve stimulation. This reduces cardiac output and peripheral vascular resistance.
- Orthostatic hypotension is common due to blockade of reflex-mediated vasoconstriction. Other side effects include erectile dysfunction, diarrhea, and weight gain. Because of these complications, postganglionic sympathetic inhibitors have little or no role in the management of hypertension.

REFERENCES

1. Goldstein LB, Bushnell CD, Adams RJ, Appel LJ, Braun LT, Chaturvedi S, et al. Guidelines for the primary prevention of stroke: a guideline for healthcare professionals from the American Heart Association/American Stroke Association. *Stroke*. 2011 Feb;42:517-84.
2. Kaplan NM. Systemic hypertension: Treatment. In: Bonow RO, Mann DL, Zipes DP, Libby P, eds. *Braunwald's Heart Disease: A Textbook of Cardiovascular Medicine*. 9th ed. Philadelphia, Pa: Saunders Elsevier; 2011:chap 46.
3. Victor, RG. Systemic hypertension: Mechanisms and diagnosis. In: Bonow RO, Mann DL, Zipes DP, Libby P, eds.*Braunwald's Heart Disease: A Textbook of Cardiovascular Medicine*. 9th ed. Philadelphia, Pa: Saunders Elsevier; 2011:chap 45.

CHAPTER 41

Heat Failure

DEFINITION

- Heart failure (HF) is a clinical syndrome caused by the inability of the heart to pump sufficient blood to meet the metabolic needs of the body. HF can result from any disorder that reduces ventricular filling (diastolic dysfunction) and/or myocardial contractility (systolic dysfunction) (Fig. 41.1, 41.2).

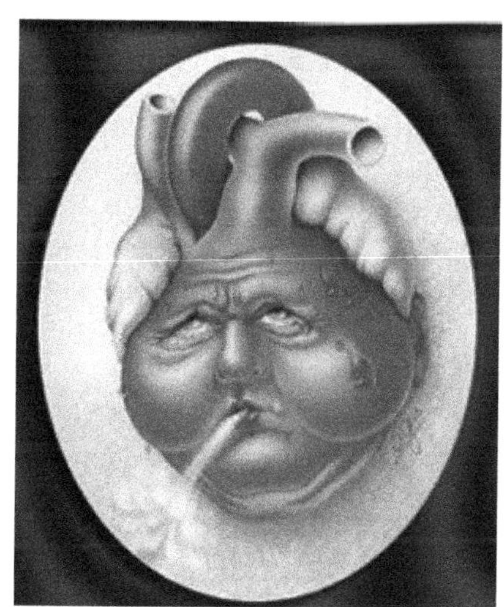

FIGURE 41.1

Heart failure.

PREVALENCE

Heart failure is the leading cause of hospitalization in people older than 65. In developed countries, the mean age of patients with heart failure is 75 years old. In developing countries, two to three percent of the population suffers from heart failure, but in those 70 to 80 years old, it occurs in 20%—30%.

Heart failure affects close to 5 million people in the USA and each year close to 500,000 new cases are diagnosed. What is of more concern is that more than 50% of patients seek re-admission within 6 months after treatment and the average duration of hospital stay is 6 days.

In tropical countries, the most common cause of HF is valvular heart disease or some type of cardiomyopathy. Moreover as underdeveloped countries become more affluent, there has also been an increase in diabetes, hypertension and obesity which has resulted in heart failure.

ETIOLOGY

Heart failure is a long-term (chronic) condition, but it can sometimes develop suddenly.

The condition may affect only the right side or only the left side of the heart. These are called right-sided heart failure or left-sided heart failure. More often, both sides of the heart are involved.

Heart failure is present when:

- Heart muscle cannot pump (eject) the blood out of the heart very well. This is called systolic heart failure.
- Heart muscles are stiff and do not fill up with blood easily. This is called diastolic heart failure.

Both of these problems mean the heart is no longer able to pump enough oxygen-rich blood out to the rest of your body, especially when you exercise or are active.

As the heart's pumping action is lost, blood may back up in other areas of the body. Fluid builds up in the lungs, liver, gastrointestinal tract, and the arms and legs. This is called congestive heart failure.

The most common cause of heart failure is coronary artery disease (CAD), a narrowing of the small blood vessels that supply blood and oxygen to the heart. For information on this condition and its risk factors, see: Heart disease - risk factors

Heart failure can also occur when an infection weakens the heart muscle. This condition is called cardiomyopathy.

Other heart problems that may cause heart failure are:

- Congenital heart disease
- Heart attack
- Heart valve disease
- Some types of abnormal heart rhythms (arrhythmias)

Other diseases that can cause or contribute to heart failure:

- Emphysema
- Overactive thyroid
- Severe anemia
- Underactive thyroid

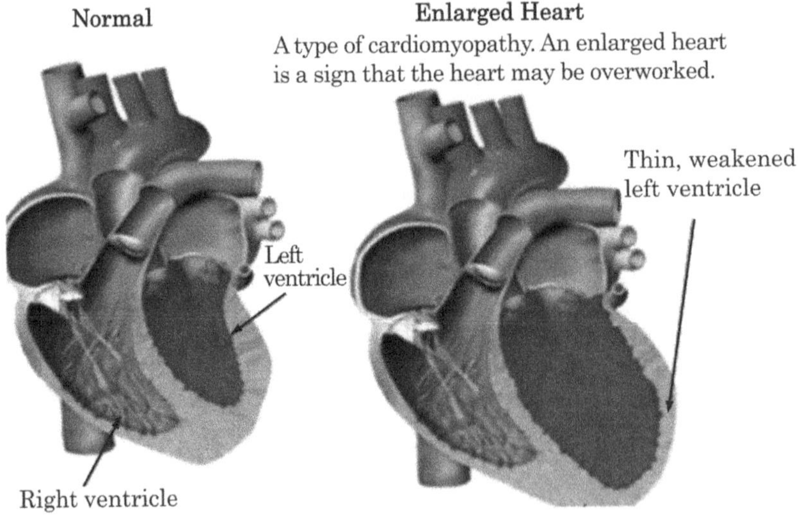

FIGURE 41.2

Normal and enlarged heart.

PATHOPHYSIOLOGY

- Causes of systolic dysfunction (decreased contractility) are reduction in muscle mass (e.g., myocardial infarction [MI]), dilated cardiomyopathies, and ventricular hypertrophy. Ventricular hypertrophy can be caused by pressure overload (e.g., systemic or pulmonary hypertension, aortic or pulmonic valve stenosis) or volume overload (e.g., valvular regurgitation, shunts and high-output states).
- Causes of diastolic dysfunction (restriction in ventricular filling) are increased ventricular stiffness, ventricular hypertrophy, infiltrative myocardial diseases, myocardial ischemia and infarction, mitral or tricuspid valve stenosis, and pericardial disease (e.g., pericarditis).
- The leading causes of HF are coronary artery disease and hypertension.
- As cardiac function decreases after myocardial injury, the heart relies on the following compensatory mechanisms: 1. Tachycardia and increased contractility through sympathetic nervous system activation; 2. The Frank-Starling mechanism, whereby increased preload increases stroke volume; 3. Vaso-constriction; and 4. Ventricular hypertrophy and remodeling. Although these compensatory mechanisms initially maintain cardiac function, they are responsible for the symptoms of HF and contribute to disease progression.
- The neurohormonal model of HF recognizes that an initiating event (e.g., acute MI) leads to decreased cardiac output but that the HF state then becomes a systemic disease whose progression is mediated largely by neurohormones and autocrine/paracrine factors. These substances include angiotensin II, norepinephrine, Aldosterone, natriuretic peptides, arginine, vasopressin, proinflammatory cytokines (e.g., tumor necrosis factor α, interleukin-6 and interleukin-1 β), and endothelin-1.
- Common precipitating factors that may cause a previously compensated patient to decompensate include noncompliance with diet or drug therapy, coronary ischemia, inappropriate medication use, cardiac events (e.g., MI, Atrial fibrillation), pulmonary infections, and anemia.
- Drugs may precipitate or exacerbate HF because of their negative inotropic, cardiotoxic, or sodium- and water-retaining properties.

CLINICAL FEATURES

- The patient presentation may range from asymptomatic to cardiogenic shock. The primary symptoms are dyspnea (particularly on exertion) and fatigue, which lead to exercise intolerance. Other pulmonary symptoms include orthopnea, paroxysmal nocturnal dyspnea, tachypnea, and cough.
- Fluid overload can result in pulmonary congestion and peripheral edema.
- Nonspecific symptoms may include fatigue, nocturia, hemoptysis, abdominal pain, anorexia, nausea, bloating, ascites,

poor appetite, ascites, mental status changes, and weight gain.

- Physical examination findings may include pulmonary crackles, cool extremities, Cheyne-Stokes respiration, tachycardia, narrow pulse pressure, cardiomegaly, symptoms of pulmonary edema (extreme breathlessness, anxiety, sometimes with coughing pink, frothy sputum), peripheral edema, jugular venous distention, hepatojugular reflux, and hepatomegaly.

DIAGNOSIS

Examine person for signs of heart failure:

- Fast or difficult breathing
- Irregular or fast heartbeat and abnormal heart sounds
- Leg swelling (edema)
- Neck veins that stick out (are distended)
- Sounds ("crackles") from fluid buildup in your lungs, heard through a stethoscope
- Swelling of the liver or abdomen

An echocardiogram (echo) is often the best test to diagnose, learn the cause of, and monitor the heart failure.

Other imaging tests are:

- Cardiac stress tests
- Heart catheterization
- MRI of the heart
- Nuclear heart scans

TREATMENT OF CHRONIC HEART FAILURE

GENERAL APPROACH

- The first step in managing chronic HF is to determine the etiology or precipitating factors. Treatment of underlying disorders (e.g., anemia, hyperthyroidism) may obviate the need for treating HF.
- Nonpharmacologic interventions include cardiac rehabilitation and restriction of fluid intake (maximum 2 L/day from all sources) and dietary sodium (approximately 2 to 3 g of sodium per day).
- **Stage A:** The emphasis is on identifying and modifying risk factors to prevent development of structural heart disease and subsequent HF. Strategies include smoking cessation and control of hypertension, diabetes mellitus, and dyslipidemia according to current treatment guidelines.

Angiotensin-converting enzyme (ACE) inhibitors (or angiotensin receptor blockers [ARBs]) should be strongly considered for antihypertensive therapy in patients with multiple vascular risk factors.

- **Stage B:** In these patients with structural heart disease but no symptoms, treatment is targeted at minimizing additional injury and preventing or slowing the remodeling process. In addition to treatment measures outlined for stage A, patients with a previous MI should receive both **ACE inhibitors** (and **ARBs** in patients intolerant of ACE inhibitors) and **α-blockers** regardless of the ejection fraction. Patients with reduced ejection fractions (less than 40%) should also receive both agents, regardless of whether they have had an MI.

- **Stage C:** Most patients with structural heart disease and previous or current HF symptoms should receive the treatments for Stages A and B as well as initiation and titration of a **diuretic** (if clinical evidence of fluid retention), **ACE inhibitor**, and **β-blocker** (if not already receiving a β-blocker for previous MI, left ventricular [LV] dysfunction or other indication). If diuresis is initiated and symptoms improve once the patient is euvolemic, long-term monitoring can begin. If symptoms do not improve, an **aldosterone receptor antagonist, ARB** (in ACE inhibitor in tolerant patients), **Digoxin**, and/or **Hydralazine/ isosorbide dinitrate** (ISDN) may be useful in carefully selected patients. Other general measures include moderate sodium restriction, daily weight measurement, immunization against influenza and pneumococcus, modest physical activity, and avoidance of medications that can exacerbate HF.
- **Stage D:** Patients with symptoms at rest despite maximal medical therapy should be considered for specialized therapies, including mechanical circulatory support, continuous intravenous positive inotropic therapy, cardiac transplantation, or hospice care.

PHARMACOLOGICAL THERAPY (FIG. 41.3)

DRUG THERAPIES FOR ROUTINE USE

Diuretics

- Compensatory mechanisms in HF stimulate excessive sodium and water retention, often leading to systemic and pulmonary congestion. Consequently, diuretic therapy (in addition to sodium restriction) is recommended in all patients with clinical evidence of fluid retention. However, because they do not alter disease progression or prolong survival, they are not considered mandatory therapy for patients without fluid retention.
- Thiazide diuretics (e.g., **hydrochlorothiazide**) are relatively weak diuretics and are used alone infrequently in HF. However, thiazide or the thiazide like diuretic **Metolazone** can be used in combination with a loop diuretic to promote effective diuresis. Thiazides may be preferred over loop diuretics in patients with only mild fluid retention and elevated blood pressure because of their more persistent antihypertensive effects.
- Loop diuretics (**furosemide, bumetanide, torsemide**) are usually necessary to restore and maintain euvolemia in HF. In addition to acting in the thick ascending limb of the loop of Henley, they induce a prostaglandin-mediated increase in renal blood flow that contributes to their natriuretic effect. Unlike thiazides, loop diuretics maintain their effectiveness in the presence of impaired renal function, although higher doses may be necessary.
- Doses of loop diuretics above the recommended ceiling doses produce no additional diuresis in HF. Thus, once those doses are reached, more frequent dosing should be used for additional effect, rather than giving progressively higher doses. Ranges of doses and ceiling doses for loop diuretics in patients with varying degrees of renal function are listed in Table 41.1.

Table 41.1

Loop diuretic use in heart failure

	Furosemide	Bumetanide	Torsemide
Usually daily dose (oral) Ceiling dose	20-160 mg/day	0.5-4 mg/day	10-80 mg/day
Normal renal function Cl cr: 20-50 mL/min Cl cr: 20 mL/min	80-160mg 160mg 400 mg	1-2mg 2 mg 8-10 mg	20-40mg 40 mg 100 mg
Bioavailability	10%-100% Average : 50%	80%-90%	80%-100%
Affected by food	Yes	Yes	No
Half-life	0.3-3.4 hours	0.3-1.5 hours	3-4 hours

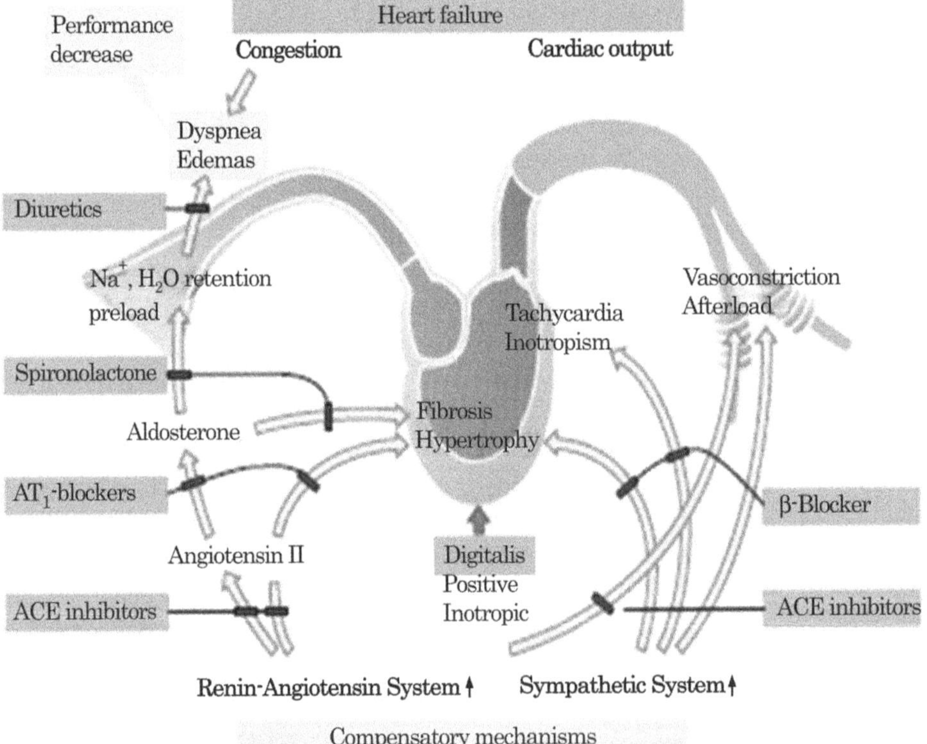

FIGURE 41.3

Congestive heart failure and its drug treatment.

ANGIOTENSIN-CONVERTING ENZYME INHIBITORS

- ACE inhibitors (Table 41.2) decrease angiotensin II and aldosterone, attenuating many of their deleterious effects, including reducing ventricular remodeling, myocardial fibrosis, myocyte apoptosis, cardiac hypertrophy, norepinephrine release, vaso constriction, and sodium and water retention.
- Clinical trials have produced unequivocal evidence that ACE inhibitors improve symptoms, slow disease progression, and decrease mortality in patients with HF and reduced LVEF (stage C). These patients should receive ACE inhibitors unless contraindications are present. ACE inhibitors should also be used to prevent the development of HF in at-risk patients (i.e., stages A and B).

β-BLOCKERS

- There is overwhelming clinical trial evidence that certain β-blockers slow disease progression, decrease hospitalizations, and reduce mortality in patients with HF.
- Beneficial effects of β-blockers may result from antiarrhythmic effects, slowing or reversing ventricular remodeling, decreasing myocyte death from catecholamine-induced necrosis or apoptosis, preventing fetal gene expression, improving LV systolic function, decreasing heart rate and ventricular wall stress and thereby reducing myocardial oxygen demand, and inhibiting plasma renin release.
- Because of their negative inotropic effects, β-blockers should be started in very low doses with slow upward dose titration to avoid symptomatic worsening or acute decompensation. Patients should be titrated to target doses when possible to provide maximal survival benefits. However, even lower doses have benefits over placebo, so any dose is likely to provide some benefit.
- Metoprolol CR/XL, Carvedilol, and Bisoprolol are the only β-blockers shown to reduce mortality in large HF trials. It

Table 41.2

ACE inhibitors routinely used for treatment of heart failure

Generic Name	Initial Dose	Target Dosing Survival Benefit
Captopril	6.25 mg three times daily	50 mg three times daily
Enalapril	2.5-5 mg twice daily	10 mg twice daily
Lisinopril	2.5-5 mg twice daily	20-40 mg daily
Quinapril	10 mg twice daily	20-40 mg twice daily
Ramipril	1.25-2.5 mg twice daily	5 mg twice daily
Fosinopril	5-10 mg daily	40 mg daily
Perindopril	2 mg daily	8-16 mg daily

cannot be assumed that immediate-release metoprolol will provide benefits equivalent to Metoprolol CR/XL. Because bisoprolol is not available in the necessary starting dose of 1.25 mg, the choice is typically limited to either carvedilol or metoprolol CR/XL. On the basis of regimens proven in large clinical trials to reduce mortality, initial and target oral doses are as follows:

- **Carvedilol,** 3.125 mg twice daily initially; target dose, 25 mg twice daily (the target dose for patients weighing more than 85 kg is 50 mg twice daily). Carvedilol CR should be considered in patients with difficulty maintaining adherence to the immediate-release formulation.
- **Metoprolol succinate CR/XL**, 12.5 to 25 mg once daily initially; target dose, 200 mg once daily.
- **Bisoprolol**, 1.25 mg once daily initially; target dose, 10 mg once daily.
- Doses should be doubled no more often than every 2 weeks, as tolerated, until the target dose or the maximally tolerated dose is reached. Patients should understand that dose up-titration is a long, gradual process and that achieving the target dose is important to maximize benefits.

DRUG THERAPIES TO CONSIDER FOR SELECTED PATIENTS

ANGIOTENSIN (AT) II RECEPTOR BLOCKERS

- The angiotensin II receptor antagonists block the angiotensin II receptor subtype AT1, preventing the deleterious effects of angiotensin II, regardless of its origin. They do not appear to affect bradykinin and are not associated with the side effect of cough that sometimes results from ACE inhibitor– induced accumulation of bradykinin. Also, direct blockade of AT1 receptors. Allows unopposed stimulation of AT2 receptors, causing vasodilation and inhibition of ventricular remodeling.
- Therapy should be initiated at low doses and then titrated to target doses:
- Candesartan, **4 to 8 mg once daily initially; target dose, 32 mg once daily.**
- Valsartan, **20 to 40 mg twice daily initially; target dose, 160 mg twice daily.**
- Blood pressure, renal function, and serum potassium should be evaluated within 1 to 2 weeks after therapy initiation and dose increases, with these endpoints used to guide subsequent dose changes. It is not necessary to reach target ARB doses before adding a β-blocker.
- Cough and angioedema are the most common causes of ACE inhibitor intolerance. Caution should be exercised when ARBs are used in patients with angioedema from ACE inhibitors because cross-reactivity has been reported.
- Combination therapy with an ARB and ACE inhibitor offers a theoretical advantage over either agent alone through more complete blockade of the deleterious effects of angiotensin II. However, clinical trial results indicate that the addition of an ARB to optimal HF therapy (e.g., ACE inhibitors, β-blockers, diuretics) offers marginal benefits at best with increased risk of adverse effects. Addition of an ARB may be considered in patients who remain symptomatic despite receiving optimal conventional therapy.

ALDOSTERONE ANTAGONISTS

- **Spironolactone and eplerenone** block the mineralocorticoid receptor, the target site for aldosterone. In the kidney, aldosterone antagonists inhibit sodium reabsorption and potassium excretion. However, diuretic effects are minimal, suggesting that their therapeutic benefits result from other actions. Effects in the heart attenuate cardiac fibrosis and ventricular remodeling. Recent evidence also suggests an important role in attenuating the systemic proinflammatory state and oxidative stress caused by aldosterone. Spironolactone also interacts with androgen and progesterone receptors, which may lead to gynecomastia and other sexual side effects; these effects are less frequent with eplerenone because of its low affinity for androgen and progesterone receptors.
- Based on clinical trial results demonstrating reduced mortality, low-dose aldosterone antagonists may be appropriate for: (1) patients with moderately severe to severe HF who are receiving standard therapy; and (2) those with LV dysfunction early after MI.
- Initial doses should be low (spironolactone 12.5 mg/day; eplerenone 25 mg/day), especially in the elderly and those with diabetes or creatinine clearance <50 mL/min. A spironolactone dose of 25 mg/day was used in one major clinical trial. The eplerenone dose should be titrated to the target dose of 50 mg once daily, preferably within 4 weeks as tolerated by the patient.

DIGOXIN

- In patients with HF and supraventricular tachyarrhythmias such as atrial fibrillation, digoxin should be considered early in therapy to help control ventricular response rate.
- For patients in normal sinus rhythm, effects on symptom reduction and quality-of-life improvement are evident in patients with mild to severe HF. Therefore, it should be used together with standard HF therapies (ACE inhibitors, β-blockers, and diuretics) in patients with symptomatic HF to reduce hospitalizations.
- Doses should be adjusted to achieve plasma digoxin concentration of 0.5 to 1 ng/mL. Higher plasma levels are not associated with additional benefits but may increase the risk of toxicity. Most patients with normal renal function can achieve this level with a dose of 0.125 mg/day. Patients with decreased renal function, the elderly, or those receiving interacting drugs (e.g., Amiodarone) should receive 0.125 mg every other day. In the absence of supraventricular tachyarrhythmia's, a loading dose is not indicated because digoxin is a mild inotropic agent that produces gradual effects over several hours, even after loading. Blood samples for measuring plasma digoxin concentrations should be collected at least 6 hours and preferably 12 hours or more, after the last dose.

NITRATES AND HYDRALAZINE

- Nitrates (e.g., **ISDN**) and **Hydralazine** were combined originally in the treatment of HF because of their complementary hemodynamic actions. Nitrates are primarily venodilators, producing reductions in preload. Hydralazine is a direct vasodilator that acts predominantly on arterial smooth muscle to reduce systemic vascular resistance (SVR) and increase stroke volume and cardiac output. Evidence also suggests that the combination may provide additional benefits by interfering with the biochemical processes associated with HF progression.

- The combination of nitrates and Hydralazine improves the composite endpoint of mortality, hospitalizations for HF, and quality of life in African Americans who receive standard therapy. A fixed-dose combination product is available that contains ISDN 20 mg and Hydralazine 37.5 mg (BiDil). Practice guidelines recommend adding ISDN and Hydralazine as part of standard therapy in African Americans with moderately severe to severe HF.

REFERENCES

1. Emanuel LL, Bonow RO. Care of patients with end-stage heart disease. In: Bonow RO, Mann DL, Zipes DP, Libby P, eds. *Braunwald's Heart Disease: A Textbook of Cardiovascular Medicine*. 9th ed. Philadelphia, Pa: Saunders Elsevier; 2011:chap 34.
2. Mann DL. Management of heart failure patients with reduced ejection fraction. In: Bo now RO, Mann DL, Zipes DP, Libby P, eds. *Braunwald's Heart Disease: A Textbook of Cardiovascular Medicine*. 9th ed. Philadelphia, Pa: Saunders Elsevier; 2011:chap 28.
3. Jessup M, Abraham WT, Casey DE, Feldman AM, Francis GS, Ganiats TG, et al. 2009 focused update: ACCF/AHA Guidelines for the Diagnosis and Management of Heart Failure in Adults: a report of the American College of Cardiology Foundation/American Heart Association Task Force on Practice Guidelines: developed in collaboration with the International Society for Heart and Lung Transplantation. Circulation. 2009 Apr 14;119(14):1977-2016. Epub 2009 Mar 26.

CHAPTER 42

Arrhythmia

DEFINITION

An arrhythmia (ah-RITH-me-ah) is a problem with the rate or rhythm of the heartbeat. During an arrhythmia, the heart can beat too fast, too slow, or with an irregular rhythm.

A heartbeat that is too fast is called tachycardia (TAK-ih-KAR-de-ah). A heartbeat that is too slow is called bradycardia (bray-de-KAR-de-ah).

Most arrhythmias are harmless, but some can be serious or even life threatening. During an arrhythmia, the heart may not be able to pump enough blood to the body. Lack of blood flow can damage the brain, heart, and other organs.

PREVALENCE

It is estimated that 3.9 million people in U.S.A have a cardiac rhythm disturbance and this results in 730000 hospital admissions each year. About 450000 death certificates cite arrhythmia as the main cause of death each year but about 500000, a quarter of all deaths, mention arrhythmias. The most common clinically significant arrhythmia is atrial fibrillation and in U.K each year about 46000 new cases are diagnosed.

PATHOPHYSIOLOGY

Regardless of the specific arrhythmia, the pathogenesis of the arrhythmias falls into one of three basic mechanisms: enhanced or suppressed automaticity, triggered activity, or re-entry. Automaticity is a natural property of all myocytes. Ischemia, scarring, electrolyte disturbances, medications, advancing age, and other factors may suppress or enhance automaticity in various areas. Suppression of automaticity of the sinoatrial (SA) node can result in sinus node dysfunction and in sick sinus syndrome (SSS), which is still the most common indication for permanent pacemaker implantation. In contrast to suppressed automaticity, enhanced automaticity can result in multiple arrhythmias, both atrial and ventricular. Triggered activity occurs when early after depolarisations and delayed after depolarisations initiate spontaneous multiple depolarisations, precipitating ventricular arrhythmias. Examples include torsades de pointes and ventricular arrhythmias caused by digitalis toxicity. Probably the most common mechanism of arrhythmogenesis results from re-entry. Requisites for re-entry include bidirectional conduction and unidirectional block. Micro level re-entry occurs with VT from conduction around the scar of myocardial infarction (MI), and macro level re-entry occurs via conduction through (Wolff-Parkinson-White [WPW] syndrome) concealed accessory pathways.

SUPRAVENTRICULAR ARRHYTHMIAS

Common supraventricular tachycardia's requiring drug treatment is atrial fibrillation (AF) or atrial flutter, paroxysmal supraventricular tachycardia (PSVT), and automatic atrial tachycardias.

ATRIAL FIBRILLATION AND ATRIAL FLUTTER

- AF is characterized as an extremely rapid (400 to 600 atrial beats/min) and disorganized atrial activation. There is a loss of atrial contraction (atrial kick), and supraventricular impulses penetrate the atrioventricular (AV) conduction system in variable degrees, resulting in irregular ventricular activation and irregularly irregular pulse (120 to 180 beats/min).
- Atrial flutter is characterized by rapid (270 to 330 atrial beats/min) but regular atrial activation. The ventricular response usually has a regular pattern and a pulse of 300 beats/min. This arrhythmia occurs less frequently than AF but has similar precipitating factors, consequences, and drug therapy.
- The predominant mechanism of AF and atrial flutter is re-entry, which is usually associated with organic heart disease that causes atrial distention (e.g., ischemia or infarction, hypertensive heart disease, valvular disorders). Additional associated disorders include acute pulmonary embolus and chronic lung disease, resulting in pulmonary hypertension; and states of high adrenergic tone such as thyrotoxicosis, alcohol withdrawal, sepsis, or excessive physical exertion.

PAROXYSMAL SUPRAVENTRICULAR TACHYCARDIA (PSVT) CAUSED BY RE-ENTRY

PSVT arising by re-entrant mechanisms includes arrhythmias caused by AV nodal re-entry, AV re-entry incorporating an anomalous AV pathway, sinoatrial (SA) nodal re-entry, and intra-arterial re-entry.

AUTOMATIC ATRIAL TACHYCARDIA'S

Automatic atrial tachycardia's such as multifocal atrial tachycardia appear to arise from supraventricular foci with enhanced automatic properties.

VENTRICULAR ARRHYTHMIAS

PREMATURE VENTRICULAR COMPLEXES

- Premature ventricular complexes (PVCs) are common ventricular rhythm disturbances that occur in patients with or without heart disease and may be elicited experimentally by abnormal automaticity, triggered activity, or re-entrant mechanisms.

VENTRICULAR TACHYCARDIA

- Ventricular tachycardia (VT) is defined by three or more repetitive PVCs occurring at a rate greater than 100 beats/min. It occurs most commonly in acute myocardial infarction (MI); other causes are severe electrolyte abnormalities (e.g., Hypokalemia), hypoxemia, and digitalis toxicity. The chronic recurrent form is almost always associated with underlying organic heart disease (e.g., idiopathic dilated cardiomyopathy or remote MI with left ventricular [LV] aneurysm).

VENTRICULAR PROARRHYTHMIA

- *Proarrhythmia* refers to development of a significant new arrhythmia (such as VT, ventricular fibrillation [VF], or TdP) or worsening of an existing arrhythmia. Proarrhythmia results from the same mechanisms that cause other arrhythmias or from an alteration in the underlying substrate due to the antiarrhythmic agent.

VENTRICULAR FIBRILLATION

- VF is electrical anarchy of the ventricle resulting in no cardiac output and cardiovascular collapse. Sudden cardiac death occurs most commonly in patients with ischemic heart disease and primary myocardial disease associated with LV dysfunction. VF associated with acute MI may be classified as either

1. Primary (an uncomplicated MI not associated with heart failure [HF]) or
2. Secondary or complicated (an MI complicated by HF).

BRADY ARRHYTHMIAS

- Asymptomatic sinus bradyarrhythmias (heart rate less than 60 beats/min) are common especially in young, athletically active individuals. However, some patients have sinus node dysfunction (sick sinus syndrome) because of underlying organic heart disease and the normal aging process, which attenuates SA nodal function.
- AV block or conduction delay may occur in any area of the AV conduction system. AV block may be found in patients without underlying heart disease (e.g., trained athletes) or during sleep when vagal tone is high. It may be transient when the underlying etiology is reversible (e.g., myocarditis, myocardial ischemia, after cardiovascular surgery, during drug therapy).

β-Blockers, digoxin, or nondihydropyridine calcium antagonists may cause AV block, primarily in the AV nodal area. Type I Antiarrhythmics may exacerbate conduction delays below the level of the AV node. AV block may be irreversible if the cause is acute MI, rare degenerative disease, primary myocardial disease, or a congenital condition.

CLINICAL FEATURES

Many arrhythmias cause no signs or symptoms. When signs or symptoms are present, the most common ones are:

- Palpitations (fluttering, or beating too hard or fast)
- A slow heartbeat
- An irregular heartbeat
- Feeling pauses between heartbeats

More serious signs and symptoms include:

- Anxiety
- Weakness, dizziness, and light-headedness
- Fainting or nearly fainting
- Sweating
- Shortness of breath
- Chest pain

DIAGNOSIS

Arrhythmias can be hard to diagnose, especially the types that only cause symptoms every once in a while. Doctors diagnose arrhythmias based on medical and family histories, a physical exam, and the results from tests and procedures.

MEDICAL AND FAMILY HISTORIES

To diagnose an arrhythmia, symptoms are observed for fluttering in chest and dizziness or light-headed.

Person family's medical history was investigated, including whether anyone in family:

- Has a history of arrhythmias
- Has ever had heart disease or high blood pressure
- Has died suddenly
- Has other illnesses or health problems

PHYSICAL EXAM

Physical examination includes

- Listening to the rate and rhythm of heartbeat
- Listening to heart for a heart murmur (an extra or unusual sound heard during heartbeat)
- Checking pulse to find out how fast heart is beating
- Checking for swelling in legs or feet, which could be a sign of an enlarged heart or heart failure
- Observing for signs of other diseases, such as thyroid disease, that could be causing the problem

DIAGNOSTIC TESTS AND PROCEDURES

EKG (ELECTROCARDIOGRAM)

An EKG is a simple, painless test that detects and records the heart's electrical activity. It's the most common test used to diagnose arrhythmias.

An EKG shows how fast the heart is beating and its rhythm (steady or irregular). It also records the strength and timing of electrical signals as they pass through the heart.

OTHER TESTS

Other tests also are used to help diagnose arrhythmias.

Blood tests: Blood tests check the level of substances in the blood, such as potassium and thyroid hormone. Abnormal levels of these substances can increase chances of having an arrhythmia.

Chest x ray: A chest x ray is a painless test that creates pictures of the structures in chest, such as heart and lungs. This test can show whether heart is enlarged.

Echocardiography: This test uses sound waves to create a moving picture of heart. Echocardiography (echo) provides information about the size and shape of heart and how well heart chambers and valves are working.

The test also can identify areas of poor blood flow to the heart, areas of heart muscle that aren't contracting normally, and previous injury to the heart muscle caused by poor blood flow.

There are several types of echo, including stress echo. This test is done both before and after a stress test (see below). A stress echo usually is done to find out whether there was an decreased blood flow to heart, a sign of coronary heart disease (CHD).

Stress test: Some heart problems are easier to diagnose when heart is working hard and beating fast. During stress testing, person exercise to make heart work hard and beat fast while heart tests are done

The heart tests done during stress testing may include nuclear heart scanning, echo, and positron emission tomography (PET) scanning of the heart.

Electrophysiology study (EPS): This test is used to assess serious arrhythmias. During an EPS, a thin, flexible wire is passed through a vein in groin (upper thigh) or arm to heart. The wire records heart's electrical signals.

Doctor uses the wire to electrically stimulate heart and trigger an arrhythmia. This allows doctor to see whether an antiarrhythmia medicine can stop the problem.

Catheter ablation, a procedure used to treat some arrhythmias, may be done during an EPS.

Tilt table testing: This test sometimes is used to help find the cause of fainting spells. People lie on a table that moves from a lying down to an upright position. The change in position may cause person to faint.

Coronary angiography: Coronary angiography uses dye and special x rays to show the inside of coronary arteries. To get the dye into coronary arteries, doctor will use a procedure called cardiac catheterization (KATH-e-ter-ih-ZA-shun).

A thin, flexible tube called a catheter is put into a blood vessel in arm, groin (upper thigh), or neck. The tube is threaded into coronary arteries, and the dye is released into bloodstream.

Special x rays are taken while the dye is flowing through coronary arteries. The dye lets doctor study the flow of blood through heart and blood vessels. This helps doctor to find blockages that can cause a heart attack.

Implantable loop recorder: This device detects abnormal heart rhythms. Minor surgery is used to place this device under the skin in the chest area.

An implantable loop recorder helps doctors figure out why a person may be having palpitations or fainting spells, especially if these symptoms don't happen very often. The device can be used for as long as 12 to 24 months.

TREATMENT

ANTIARRHYTHMIC MEDICATIONS (TABLE 42.1)

Table 42.1

Antiarrhythmic drugs

Class	Actions (Examples)
I	Sodium channel blockers
IA	Depress phase 0 of action potential; delay conduction, prolong repolarization-phase III or IV (quinidine, procainamide, disopyramide)
IB	Little effect on phase 0 of action potential in normal tissues; depress phase 0 in abnormal tissues; shorten repolarization or little effect (lidocaine, tocainide, mexiletine, diphenyl-hydantoin)
IC	Depress phase 0 of action potential; markedly slow conduction in normal tissues
II	β-Adrenergic blocking agents (acebutolol, atenolol, bisoprolol, carvedilol, metoprolol, nadolol, pindolol, propranolol)
III	Prolong action potential duration by increasing repolarization and refractoriness (amiodarone, sotalol, brethlium, dofetilide, azimilide, ibutilide)
IV	Calcium channel blockers (diltiazem, vera-pamil)
Others	Digoxin, adenosine

TREATING FAST HEARTBEATS

For fast heartbeats (tachycardia's), treatments may include one or more of the following:

- **Vagal manoeuvres:** Person may be able to stop an arrhythmia that begins above the lower half of the heart (supra-ventricular tachycardia, or SVT) by using particular manoeuvres that include holding the breath and straining, dunking the face in ice water, or coughing. The doctor may be able to recommend other manoeuvres to halt a fast heartbeat. These manoeuvres affect the nervous system that controls the heartbeat (vagus nerves), often causing the heart rate to slow.
- **Medications:** Many types of tachycardia's respond well to anti-arrhythmic medications. Though they don't cure the problem, they can reduce episodes of tachycardia or slow down the heart when an episode occurs. Some medications can slow down the heart so much that person may need a pacemaker. It's very important to take any anti-arrhythmic medication exactly as directed by the doctor, in order to avoid complications.
- **Cardioversion:** If person have a tachycardia that starts in the top half of the heart (atria), including atrial fibrillation, the doctor may use Cardioversion, which is an electrical shock used to reset the heart to its regular rhythm. Usually this is done externally in a monitored setting, and people're given medication to relax person during the procedure, so there's no pain involved.
- **Ablation therapy:** In this procedure, one or more catheters are threaded through the blood vessels to the inner heart. They're positioned on areas of the heart that the doctor believes are the sources of the arrhythmia. Electrodes at the catheter tips are heated with radiofrequency energy. Another method involves cooling the tips of the catheters, which freezes the problem tissue. Either method destroys (ablates) a small spot of heart tissue and creates an electrical block along the pathway that's causing the arrhythmia. Usually this stops the arrhythmia.

IMPLANTABLE DEVICES

Treatment for heart arrhythmias also may involve use of an implantable device:

- **Pacemaker:** A pacemaker is an implantable device that helps regulate slow heartbeats (bradycardia). A small battery-driven device is placed under the skin near the collarbone in a minor surgical procedure. An insulated wire extends from the device to the right side of the heart, where it's permanently anchored.

  If a pacemaker detects a heart rate that's too slow or no heartbeat at all, it emits electrical impulses that stimulate the heart to speed up or begin beating again. Most pacemakers have a sensing device that turns them off when the heartbeat is above a certain level. It turns back on when the heartbeat is too slow. Most people stay in the hospital one to two days after a pacemaker is implanted.
- **Implantable cardioverter-defibrillator (ICD):** The doctor may recommend this device if person're at high risk of developing a dangerously fast or quivering heartbeat in the lower half of the heart (ventricular tachycardia or ventricle fibrillation). Implantable

defibrillator units designed to treat quivering in the upper half of the heart (atrial fibrillation) also are available.

An ICD is a battery-powered unit that's implanted near the left collarbone. One or more electrode-tipped wires from the ICD run through veins to the heart. The ICD continuously monitors the heart rhythm. If it detects a rhythm that's too slow, it paces the heart as a pacemaker would. If it detects VT or VF, it sends out low- or high-energy shocks to reset the heart to a normal rhythm.

SURGICAL TREATMENTS

- **Maze procedure:** This involves making a series of surgical incisions in the upper half of the heart (atria). These heal into carefully placed scars in the atria that form boundaries that force electrical impulses in the heart to travel properly to cause the heart to beat efficiently. The procedure has a high success rate, but because it requires open-heart surgery, it's usually reserved for people who don't respond to other treatments. The surgeon may use a cryoprobe — an instrument for applying extreme cold to tissue — or a hand-held radiofrequency probe, rather than a scalpel, to create the scars.
- **Ventricular aneurysm surgery:** In some cases, a bulge (aneurysm) in a blood vessel leading to the heart is the cause of an arrhythmia. If catheter ablation and implanted ICD don't work, person may need this surgery. It involves removing the aneurysm that's causing the arrhythmia. By removing the source of the abnormal impulses, the arrhythmia often can be eliminated.
- **Coronary bypass surgery:** If person have severe coronary artery disease in addition to frequent ventricular tachycardia, the doctor may recommend coronary bypass surgery. This may improve the blood supply to the heart and reduce the frequency of the ventricular tachycardia.

REFERENCES

1. Hayes DL, Zipes DP. Cardiac pacemakers and cardioverter-defibrillators. In: Libby P, Bonow RO, Mann DL, Zipes DP, eds.*Braunwald's Heart Disease: A Textbook of Cardiovascular Medicine*. 8th ed. Philadelphia, Pa: Saunders Elsevier;2007:chap 34.
2. Zheng ZJ, Croft JB, Giles WH. State specific mortality from sudden cardiac death—United States, 1999. MMWR Morb Mortal Wkly Rep. 2002, 51: 123-126.
3. Brugada P, Brugada J, Mont L, et al. A new approach to the differential diagnosis of a regular tachycardia with a wide QRS complex. Circulation. 1991, 83: 1649-1659.
4. Crawford MH, Bernstein SJ, Deedwania PC, et al: ACC/AHA guidelines for ambulatory electrocardiography. J Am Coll Cardiol. 1999, 34: 912-948.
5. Tracy CM, Masood A, DiMarco JP, et al. ACC/AHA clinical competence statement on invasive electrophysiology studies, catheter ablation, and cardioversion. J Am Coll Cardiol. 2000, 36: 1725-1736.
6. Zipes DP, Wyse G, Friedman PL, et al. A comparison of antiarrhythmic drug therapy with implantable defibrillators in patients resuscitated from near-fatal ventricular arrhythmias. N Engl J Med. 1997, 337: 1576-1583.
7. Mushlin AI, Hall WJ, Zwanziger J, et al. The cost-effectiveness of automatic implantable cardiac defibrillators: Results of MADIT. Multicenter Automatic

Defibrillator Implantation Trial. Circulation. 1998, 97: 2129-2135.

8. Calkins H, Sousa J, El-Atassi R, et al. Diagnosis and cure of the Wolff-Parkinson-White syndrome or paroxysmal supraventricular tachycardias during a single electrophysiologic test. N Engl J Med. 1991, 324: 1612-1618.
9. Jackman W, Wang X, Friday KJ, et al. Catheter ablation of accessory atrioventricular pathways (Wolff-Parkinson-White syndrome) by radiofrequency current. N Engl J Med. 1991, 324: 1604-1611.
10. Marrouche NF, Dresing T, Cole C, et al. A circular mapping and ablation of the pulmonary vein for treatment of atrial fibrillation: Impact of different catheter technologies. J Am Coll Cardiol. 2002, 40: 464-474.
11. Chaudhry G, Muqtada MD, Haffajee CI. Antiarrhythmic agents and proarrhythmia. Crit Care Med. 2000, 28: N158-N164.
12. Bardy GH, Lee KL, Mark DB, et al. Sudden Cardiac Death in Heart Failure Trial (SCD-HeFT) Investigators: Amiodarone or an implantable cardioverter-defibrillator for congestive heart failure. N Engl J Med. 2005, 352: 225-237.
13. Kadish A, Dyer A, Daubert JP, et al. Defibrillators in Non-Ischemic Cardiomyopathy Treatment Evaluation (DEFINITE) Investigators: Prophylactic defibrillator implantation in patients with nonischemic dilated cardiomyopathy. N Engl J Med. 2004, 350: 2151-2158.
14. Wilkoff BL. Pacemaker and ICD malfunction—an incomplete picture. JAMA. 2006, 295: 1945-1946.

CHAPTER 43

Dyslipidemia

DEFINITION

Dyslipidemia or **dyslipidaemia** is an abnormal amount of lipids (e.g. cholesterol and/or fat) in the blood.

ETIOLOGY

There are many types of cholesterol. The ones talked about most are:

- Total cholesterol - all the cholesterols combined
- High density lipoprotein (HDL) cholesterol - often called "good" cholesterol
- Low density lipoprotein (LDL) cholesterol - often called "bad" cholesterol

For most people, abnormal cholesterol levels are the result of an unhealthy lifestyle — most commonly, eating a diet that is high in fat. Other lifestyle factors are:

- Being overweight
- Heavy alcohol use
- Lack of exercise and leading an inactive lifestyle

Diabetes and an underactive thyroid gland may lead to high cholesterol levels. Other illnesses that may raise cholesterol levels include polycystic ovary syndrome and kidney disease.

Higher levels of female hormones increase or change cholesterol levels. This may include women who take birth control pills or estrogen, or who are pregnant,

Medicines such as certain diuretics (water pills), beta-blockers, and some medicines used to treat depression may also raise cholesterol levels.

Several disorders that are passed down through families lead to abnormal cholesterol and triglyceride levels. They include:

- Familial combined hyperlipidemia
- Familial dysbetalipoproteinemia
- Familial hypercholesterolemia
- Familial hypertriglyceridemia

Smoking does not cause higher cholesterol levels, but it can reduce your HDL ("good") cholesterol.

PATHOPHYSIOLOGY

- Cholesterol, triglycerides, and phospholipids are transported in the bloodstream as complexes of lipid and proteins known as lipoproteins. Elevated total and LDL cholesterol and reduced HDL cholesterol are associated with the development of coronary heart disease (CHD).

- The response-to-injury hypothesis states that risk factors such as oxidized LDL, mechanical injury to the endothelium, excessive homocysteine, immunologic attack, or infection-induced changes in endothelial and intimal function lead to endothelial dysfunction and a series of cellular interactions that culminate in atherosclerosis. The eventual clinical outcomes may include angina, myocardial infarction, arrhythmias, stroke, peripheral arterial disease, abdominal aortic aneurysm, and sudden death.
- Atherosclerotic lesions are thought to arise from transport and retention of plasma LDL through the endothelial cell layer into the extracellular matrix of the sub endothelial space. Once in the artery wall, LDL is chemically modified through oxidation and nonenzymatic glycation. Mildly oxidized LDL then recruits monocytes into the artery wall. These monocytes then become transformed into macrophages that accelerate LDL oxidation.
- Oxidized LDL provokes an inflammatory response mediated by a number of chemo attractants and cytokines (e.g., monocyte colony-stimulating factor, intercellular adhesion molecule, platelet-derived growth factor, transforming growth factors, interleukin-1and interleukin-6).
- Repeated injury and repair within an atherosclerotic plaque eventually lead to a fibrous cap protecting the underlying core of lipids, collagen, calcium, and inflammatory cells such as T lymphocytes. Maintenance of the fibrous plaque is critical to prevent plaque rupture and subsequent coronary thrombosis.
- Primary or genetic lipoprotein disorders are classified into six categories for the phenotypic description of dyslipidemia. The types and corresponding lipoprotein elevations include the following: I (chylomicrons), IIa (LDL), IIb (LDL + very low density lipoprotein, or VLDL), III (intermediate-density lipoprotein), IV (VLDL), and V (VLDL + chylomicrons). Secondary forms
- Of hyperlipidemia also exist, and several drug classes may elevate lipid levels. (e.g., progestins, thiazide diuretics, glucocorticoids, β-blockers, isotretinoin, protease inhibitors, cyclosporine, mirtazapine, sirolimus).
- The primary defect in familial hypercholesterolemia is the inability to bind LDL to the LDL receptor (LDL-R) or, rarely, a defect of internalizing the LDL-R complex into the cell after normal binding. This leads to lack of LDL degradation by cells and unregulated biosynthesis of cholesterol, with total cholesterol and LDL cholesterol (LDL-C) being inversely proportional to the deficit in LDL-R.

CLINICAL FEATURES

Familial hypercholesterolemia is characterized by a selective elevation in plasma LDL and deposition of LDL-derived cholesterol in tendons (xanthomas) and arteries (atheromas).

- Familial lipoprotein lipase deficiency is characterized by a massive accumulation of chylomicrons and a corresponding increase in plasma triglycerides or a type I lipoprotein pattern. Presenting manifestations include repeated attacks of pancreatitis and abdominal pain, eruptive cutaneous xanthomatosis, and hepatosplenomegaly beginning in childhood. Symptom severity is proportional to dietary fat intake, and consequently to the elevation of chylomicrons. Accelerated atherosclerosis is not associated with this disease.

- Patients with familial type III hyperlipoproteinemia develop the following clinical features after age 20: xanthomas striata palmaris (yellow discolorations of the palmar and digital creases); tuberous or tuberoeruptive xanthomas (bulbous cutaneous xanthomas); and severe atherosclerosis involving the coronary arteries, internal carotids, and abdominal aorta.
- Type IV hyperlipoproteinemia is common and occurs in adults, primarily in patients who are obese, diabetic, and hyperuricemic and do not have xanthomas. It may be secondary to alcohol ingestion and can be aggravated by stress, progestins, oral contraceptives, thiazides, or β-blockers.
- Type V is characterized by abdominal pain, pancreatitis, eruptive xanthomas, and peripheral polyneuropathy. These patients are commonly obese, hyperuricemic, and diabetic; alcohol intake, exogenous estrogens, and renal insufficiency tend to be exacerbating factors. The risk of atherosclerosis is increased with this disorder.

DIAGNOSIS

A cholesterol test is done to diagnose a lipid disorder. Some national guidelines recommend having the first screening cholesterol test at age 20. Everyone should have their first screening test by age 35 in men, and age 45 in women.

It is important to work with the health care provider to set the cholesterol goals. General targets are:

- LDL: 70-130 mg/dl (lower numbers are better)
- HDL: more than 40-60 mg/dl (high numbers are better)
- Total cholesterol: less than 200 mg/dl (lower numbers are better)
- Triglycerides: 10-150 mg/dl (lower numbers are better)

If the cholesterol results are abnormal, the doctor may also do:

- Blood sugar (glucose) test to look for diabetes
- Thyroid function tests to look for an underactive thyroid gland.

TREATMENT

GENERAL APPROACH

- In patients with borderline-high blood cholesterol (200 to 239 mg/dl), assessment of risk factors is needed to more clearly define disease risk.
- There are four categories of risk that modify the goals and modalities of LDL-lowering therapy. The highest risk category is having known CHD or CHD risk equivalents; the risk for major coronary events is equal to or greater than that for established CHD (i.e., >20% per 10 years, or 2% per year). The next category is moderately high risk, consisting of patients with two or more risk factors in which 10-year risk for CHD is 10% to 20%. Moderate risk is

defined as two or more risk factors and a 10-year risk of > 10%. The lowest risk category is persons with zero to one risk factor, which is usually associated with a 10-year CHD risk of <10%.

- ATP III recognizes the metabolic syndrome as a secondary target of risk reduction after LDL-C has been addressed. This syndrome is characterized by abdominal obesity, atherogenic dyslipidemia (elevated triglycerides, small LDL particles, low HDL cholesterol), increased blood pressure, insulin resistance (with or without glucose intolerance), and prothrombotic and proinflammatory states. If the metabolic syndrome is present, the patient is considered to have a CHD risk equivalent.
- Other targets include non-HDL goals for patients with triglycerides >200 mg/dL. Non-HDL cholesterol is calculated by subtracting HDL from total cholesterol, and the targets are 30 mg/dL greater than for LDL at each risk stratum.

NONPHARMACOLOGICAL THERAPY

- The objectives of dietary therapy are to progressively decrease the intake of total fat, saturated fat, and cholesterol and to achieve a desirable body weight. If the total cholesterol is <200 mg/dL, then the patient has a desirable blood cholesterol level. If the HDL is also >40 mg/dL, no further follow-up is recommended for patients without known CHD and who have fewer than two risk factors .
- In patients with borderline-high blood cholesterol (200 to 239 mg/dL), assessment of risk factors is needed to more clearly define disease risk.
- There are four categories of risk that modify the goals and modalities of LDL-lowering therapy. The highest risk category is having known CHD or CHD risk equivalents; the risk for major coronary events is equal to or greater than that for established CHD (i.e., >20% per 10 years, or 2% per year). The next category is moderately high risk, consisting of patients with Excessive dietary intake of cholesterol and saturated fatty acids leads to decreased hepatic clearance of LDL and deposition of LDL and oxidized LDL in peripheral tissues.
- Increased intake of soluble fibre in the form of oat bran, pectins, certain gums, and psyllium products can result in useful adjunctive reductions in total and LDL cholesterol (5% to 20%), but these dietary alterations or supplements should not be substituted for more active forms of treatment. They have little or no effect on HDL-C or triglyceride concentrations. These products may also be useful in managing constipation associated with the bile acid resins (BARs).
- Ingestion of 2 to 3 g/day of plant sterols and stanols will reduce LDL by 6% to 15%. They are usually available in commercial margarines.
- In epidemiologic studies, ingestion of large amounts of cold-water oily fish was associated with a reduction in CHD risk. Fish oil supplementation has a fairly large effect in reducing triglycerides and VLDL cholesterol, but it either has no effect on total and LDL cholesterol or may cause elevations in these fractions. Other actions of fish oil may account for any cardioprotective effects.

- If all recommended dietary changes from the NCEP were instituted, the estimated average reduction in LDL would range from 20% to 30%.

PHARMACOLOGICAL THERAPY

BILE ACID RESINS (CHOLESTYRAMINE, COLESTIPOL, COLESEVELAM)

- The primary action of BARs is to bind bile acids in the intestinal lumen, with a concurrent interruption of enterohepatic circulation of bile acids, which decreases the bile acid pool size and stimulates hepatic synthesis of bile acids from cholesterol. Depletion of the hepatic pool of cholesterol results in an increase in cholesterol biosynthesis and an increase in the number of LDL-Rs on the hepatocyte membrane, which stimulates an enhanced rate of catabolism from plasma and lowers LDL levels. The increase in hepatic cholesterol biosynthesis may be paralleled by increased hepatic VLDL production, and, consequently, BARs may aggravate hypertriglyceridemia in patients with combined hyperlipidemia.
- BARs are useful in treating primary hypercholesterolemia (familial hypercholesterolemia, familial combined hyperlipidemia, type IIa hyperlipoproteinemia).
- GI complaints of constipation, bloating, epigastric fullness, nausea, and flatulence are most commonly reported. These adverse effects can be managed by increasing fluid intake, modifying the diet to increase bulk, and using stool softeners.
- The gritty texture and bulk may be minimized by mixing the powder with orange drink or juice. Colestipol may have better palatability than cholestyramine because it is odourless and tasteless.
- Other potential adverse effects include impaired absorption of fat-soluble vitamins A, D, E, and K; Hypernatremia and hyperchloremia; GI obstruction; and reduced bioavailability of acidic drugs such as warfarin, nicotinic acid, thyroxin, acetaminophen, hydrocortisone, hydrochlorothiazide, Loperamide, and possibly iron. Drug interactions may be avoided by alternating administration times with an interval of 6 hours or greater between the BAR and other drugs.

NIACIN

- **Niacin** (nicotinic acid) reduces the hepatic synthesis of VLDL, which in turn leads to a reduction in the synthesis of LDL. Niacin also increases HDL by reducing its catabolism.
- The principal use of niacin is for mixed hyperlipidemia or as a second-line agent in combination therapy for hypercholesterolemia. It is a first-line agent or alternative for the treatment of hypertriglyceridemia and diabetic dyslipidemia.
- Niacin has many common adverse drug reactions; most of the symptoms and bio chemical abnormalities seen do not require discontinuation of therapy.
- Cutaneous flushing and itching appear to be prostaglandin mediated and can be reduced by taking aspirin 325 mg shortly before niacin ingestion. Taking the niacin dose with meals and slowly titrating the dose upward may minimize these effects. Concomitant alcohol and hot drinks may

magnify the flushing and pruritus from niacin, and they should be avoided at the time of ingestion. GI intolerance is also a common problem.

- Potentially important laboratory abnormalities occurring with niacin therapy include elevated liver function tests, hyperuricemia, and hyperglycemia. Niacin-associated hepatitis is more common with sustained-release preparations, and their use should be restricted to patients intolerant of regular-release products. Niacin is contra-indicated in patients with active liver disease, and it may exacerbate pre-existing gout and diabetes.
- Nicotinamide should not be used in the treatment of hyperlipidemia because it does not effectively lower cholesterol or triglyceride levels.

HMG-CoA REDUCTASE INHIBITORS

(ATORVASTATIN, FLUVASTATIN, LOVASTATIN, PRAVASTATIN, ROSUVASTATIN, SIMVASTATIN)

- Statins inhibit 3-hydroxy-3-methylglutaryl coenzyme A (HMG-CoA) Reductase, interrupting the conversion of HMG-CoA to mevalonate, the rate-limiting step in de novo cholesterol biosynthesis. Reduced synthesis of LDL and enhanced catabolism of LDL mediated through LDL-Rs appear to be the principal mechanisms for lipid-lowering effects.
- When used as monotherapy, statins are the most potent total and LDL cholesterol-lowering agents and among the best tolerated. Total and LDL cholesterol are reduced in a dose-related fashion by 30% or more when added to dietary therapy.
- Combination therapy with a statin and BAR is rational because numbers of LDL-Rs are increased, leading to greater degradation of LDL cholesterol; intracellular synthesis of cholesterol is inhibited; and enterohepatic recycling of bile acids is interrupted.
- Combination therapy with a statin and ezetimibe is also rational because ezetimibe inhibits cholesterol absorption across the gut border and adds 12% to 20% further reduction when combined with a statin or other drug.
- Constipation occurs in fewer than 10% of patients taking statins. Other adverse effects include elevated serum aminotransferase levels (primarily alanine aminotransferase), elevated creatine kinase levels, myopathy, and rarely rhabdomyolysis.

FIBRIC ACIDS (GEMFIBROZIL, FENOFIBRATE, CLOFIBRATE)

- Fibrate monotherapy is effective in reducing VLDL, but a reciprocal rise in LDL may occur and total cholesterol values may remain relatively unchanged. Plasma HDL concentrations may rise 10% to 15% or more with fibrates.
- Gemfibrozil reduces the synthesis of VLDL and, to a lesser extent, apolipoprotein B with a concurrent increase in the rate of removal of triglyceride-rich lipoproteins from plasma. Clofibrate is less effective than Gemfibrozil or niacin in reducing VLDL production.
- GI complaints occur in 3% to 5% of patients, rash in 2%, dizziness in 2.4%, and transient elevations in transaminase

levels and alkaline phosphatise in 4.5% and 1.3%, respectively. Clofibrate and, less commonly, Gemfibrozil may enhance the formation of gallstones.

- A myositis syndrome of myalgia, weakness, stiffness, malaise, and elevations in creatine kinase and aspartate aminotransferase may occur and seems to be more common in patients with renal insufficiency.
- Fibrates may potentiate the effects of oral anticoagulants, and the international normalized ratio should be monitored very closely with this combination.

EZETIMIBE

Ezetimibe interferes with the absorption of cholesterol from the brush border of the intestine, a novel mechanism that makes it a good choice for adjunctive therapy. It is approved as both monotherapy and for use with a statin. The dose is 10 mg once daily, given with or without food.

FISH OIL SUPPLEMENTATION

- Diets high in omega-3 polyunsaturated fatty acids (from fish oil), most commonly eicosapentaenoic acid (EPA), reduce cholesterol, triglycerides, LDL, and VLDL and may elevate HDL cholesterol.
- **Lovaza (omega-3-acid ethyl esters)** is a prescription form of concentrated fish oil EPA 465 mg and docosahexaenoic acid 375 mg. The daily dose is 4 g/day, which can be taken as four 1-g capsules once daily or two 1-g capsules twice daily. This product lowers triglycerides by 14% to 30% and raises HDL by about 10%.
- Complications of fish oil supplementation such as thrombocytopenia and bleeding disorders have been noted, especially with high doses (EPA, 15 to 30 g/day).

TREATMENT RECOMMENDATIONS

- Treatment of type I hyperlipoproteinemia is directed toward reduction of chylomicrons derived from dietary fat with the subsequent reduction in plasma triglycerides. Total daily fat intake should be no more than 10 to 25 g/day, or approximately 15% of total calories. Secondary causes of hypertriglyceridemia should be excluded, and, if present, the underlying disorder should be treated appropriately.
- Primary hypercholesterolemia (familial hypercholesterolemia, familial combined hyperlipidemia, type IIa hyperlipoproteinemia) is treated with **BARs, statins, niacin**, or **ezetimibe**.
- Combined hyperlipoproteinemia (type IIb) may be treated with **statins, niacin**, or **Gemfibrozil** to lower LDL-C without elevating VLDL and triglycerides. Niacin is the most effective agent and may be combined with a BAR.
- Type III hyperlipoproteinemia may be treated with **fibrates** or **niacin**. Although fibrates have been suggested as the drugs of choice, niacin is a reasonable alternative because of the lack of data supporting a cardiovascular mortality benefit from fibrates and because of their potentially
- Serious adverse effects. Fish oil supplementation may be an alternative therapy.
- Type V hyperlipoproteinemia requires stringent restriction of dietary fat intake. Drug therapy with **fibrates** or **niacin** is

indicated if the response to diet alone is inadequate. **Medium-chain triglycerides**, which are absorbed without chylomicrons formation, may be used as a dietary supplement for caloric intake if needed for both types I and V.

COMBINATION DRUG THERAPY

- Combination therapy may be considered after adequate trials of monotherapy and for patients documented to be adherent to the prescribed regimen. Two or three lipoprotein profiles at 6-week intervals should confirm lack of response prior to initiation of combination therapy.
- Contraindications to and drug interactions with combined therapy should be screened carefully, and the extra cost of drug product and monitoring should be considered.
- In general, a **statin** plus a **BAR** or **niacin** plus a **BAR** provide the greatest reduction in total and LDL cholesterol.
- Regimens intended to increase HDL levels should include either **Gemfibrozil** or **niacin**, bearing in mind that **statins** combined with either of these drugs may result in a greater incidence of Hepatotoxicity or myositis.
- Familial combined hyperlipidemia may respond better to a Fibrate and a statin than to a Fibrate and a BAR4

REFERENCES

1. American Heart Association. *Drug therapy for cholesterol.* 2011 Jan 20. Accessed February 21, 2011.
2. Daniels SR, Greer FR; Committee on Nutrition. Lipid screening and cardiovascular health in childhood.*Pediatrics.* 2008;122198-208.
3. Gennest J, Libby P. Lipoprotein disorders and cardiovascular disease. In: Bonow RO, Mann DL, Zipes DP, Libby P, eds. *Braunwald's Heart Disease: A Textbook of Cardiovascular Medicine.* 9th ed. Philadelphia, Pa: Saunders Elsevier; 2011:chap 47.
4. U.S. Preventive Services Task Force. Screening for lipid disorders in adults: U.S. Preventive Services Task Force recommendation statement. Rockville (MD): Agency for Healthcare Research and Quality (AHRQ); 2008 Jun. Accessed May 19, 2011.
5. U.S. Preventive Services Task Force. Screening for lipid disorders in children. U.S. Preventive Services Task Force recommendation statement. Rockville (MD): Agency for Healthcare Research and Quality (AHRQ); 2007 Jul. Accessed May 19, 2011.

CHAPTER 44

Coronary Artery Disease

DEFINITION

Coronary artery disease (**CAD**; also **atherosclerotic heart disease**) is the result of the accumulation of athermatous plaques within the walls of the coronary arteries that supply the myocardium (the muscle of the heart) with oxygen and nutrients. It is sometimes also called w**coronary heart disease** (CHD).

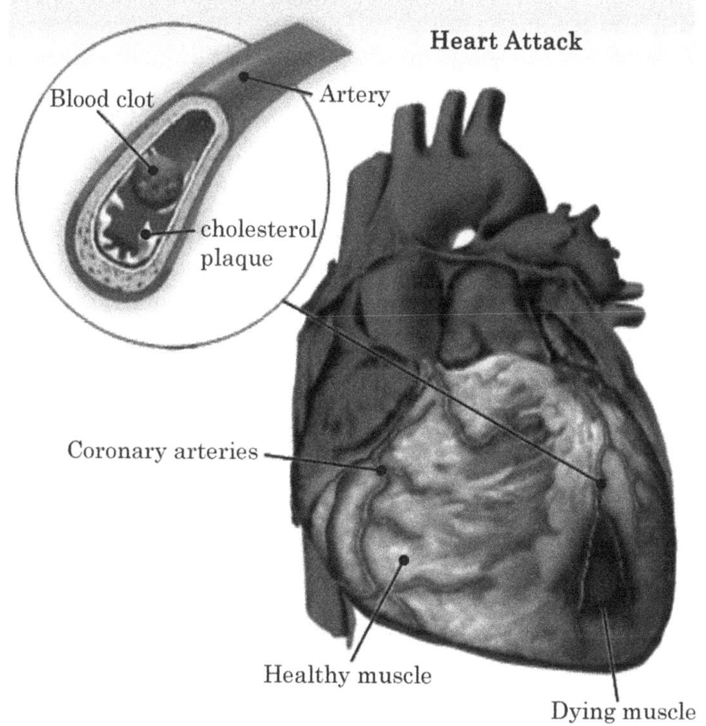

FIGURE 44.1

Heart attack.

PREVALENCE

CAD is the most common form of cardiovascular disease with an estimated prevalence of CAD in men is 6.9% and 6% among women .For people at 18 years of age and above prevalence estimates are: only 11.4% among whites. While 5.9% suffered from heart disease, 5.9% have hypertension and 2.3%have had a stroke.

ETIOLOGY

Coronary heart disease is caused by the buildup of plaque in the arteries of the heart (Fig. 44.1). This may also be called hardening of the arteries.

- Fatty material and other substances form a plaque build-up on the walls of the coronary arteries. The coronary arteries bring blood and oxygen to the heart.
- This buildup causes the arteries to get narrow.
- As a result, blood flow to the heart can slow down or stop.

The risk factors for heart disease are:

- **Age:** The risk of heart disease increases with age.
- **Gender:** Men have a higher risk of getting heart disease than women who are still getting their menstrual period. After menopause, the risk for women is closer to the risk for men.
- **Genes:** If parents or other close relatives had heart disease, there is higher risk.
- **Race:** African Americans, Mexican Americans, American Indians, Hawaiians, and some Asian Americans also have a higher risk for heart problems.

Many other risk factors for heart disease includes:

- Diabetes is a strong risk factor for heart disease.
- High blood pressure increases the risks of heart disease and heart failure.
- Extra cholesterol in the blood builds up inside the walls of the heart's arteries (blood vessels).
- Smokers have a much higher risk of heart disease.
- Chronic kidney disease can increase the risk.
- People with narrowed arteries in another part of the body (examples are stroke and poor blood flow to the legs) are more likely to have heart disease.
- Substance abuse (such as cocaine)

PATHOPHYSIOLOGY

The exact pathogenesis of CAD is not clear, and no single theory adequately explains the atherosclerotic process. Two main explanations have been proposed: the lipid hypothesis and the chronic endothelial injury hypothesis. These explanations are probably interrelated and are certainly not mutually exclusive. The lipid hypothesis speculates that elevation in lipid plasma levels promotes lipid penetration of arterial walls. In general, it is considered that this process is instigated by abnormal lipid metabolism or excessive dietary intake of cholesterol and saturated fats, particularly when coupled with a genetic predisposition. Low-density lipoproteins (LDLs) are the primary atherogenic lipid, whereas high-density lipoproteins (HDLs) have a protective effect and probably help mobilize LDLs. When LDLs undergo oxidation in the body, they become harder to mobilize and locally cytotoxic. This is where the lipid hypothesis and endothelial injury hypothesis potentially overlap. According to the latter theory, the initial step in the formation of atherosclerosis is a weakening of the arterial glycosaminoglycans (GAGs) layer. GAGs protect the internal lining of the artery (the endothelium) and promote its repair. The exposed endothelial cells of the artery are subject to free-radical damage, and damage to the endothelial lining makes those sites more permeable to plasma constituents, particularly lipoproteins. Several factors, besides oxidized LDLs, can damage endothelial cells and induce plaque formation. These factors are immunologic, inflammatory, viral, chemical, mechanical, and physical in nature. In response to cell injury, macrophages migrate from circulation into the cells that line the inside of the artery known as the sub endothelial layer of the intima. Ultimately as this process continues, smooth muscle cells of the intima join connective tissue and intracellular and extracellular lipids to form fibrous plaque. Adhesion and aggregation of platelets and release of various growth factors further augment the fibrotic process, resulting in occlusion of the blood vessel lumen and potential for plaque disruption and thrombus formation.

CLINICAL FEATURES

The most common signs and symptoms for the aspect of CAD most often seen by the clinical practitioner is angina pectoris. Other symptoms include:

- Vague, somewhat troublesome ache or severe, intense precordial crushing sensation
- Most commonly sensation is felt beneath the sternum or may radiate to the left shoulder and down the inside of the left arm; straight through to the back, into the throat, jaws, and teeth; occasionally down the inside of the right arm. Sometimes upper abdomen
- Typically precipitated by physical exertion or stress, persists for a few minutes, and subsides with rest or nitroglycerin
- Worse exertion after a meal
- Modest increase in heart rate
- Significant elevation in systolic and diastolic blood pressure, but sometimes hypotension
- Diffuse apical impulse and more distant heart sounds

DIAGNOSIS

Many tests help diagnose CHD. Usually, your doctor will order more than one test before making a diagnosis.

Tests may include:

- **Coronary angiography/arteriography** — an invasive test that evaluates the heart arteries under x-ray
- **CT angiography** — a noninvasive way to perform coronary angiography
- Echocardiogram
- Electrocardiogram (ECG)
- Electron-beam computed tomography (EBCT) to look for calcium in the lining of the arteries — the more calcium, the higher your chance for CHD
- Exercise stress test
- Heart CT scan
- Magnetic resonance angiography
- Nuclear stress test

TREATMENT

Treatment for coronary artery disease usually involves lifestyle changes and, if necessary, drugs and certain medical procedures.

LIFESTYLE CHANGES

Making a commitment to the following healthy lifestyle changes can go a long way toward promoting healthier arteries:

- Quit smoking.
- Eat healthy foods.
- Exercise regularly.
- Lose excess weight.
- Reduce stress.

DRUGS

Various drugs can be used to treat coronary artery disease, including:

- **Cholesterol-modifying medications:** By decreasing the amount of cholesterol in the blood, especially low-density lipoprotein (LDL, or "bad") cholesterol, these drugs decrease the primary material that deposits on the coronary arteries. Boosting the high-density lipoprotein (HDL, or "good") cholesterol, may help, too. The doctor can choose from a range of medications, including statins, niacin, fibrates and bile acid sequestrants.
- **Aspirin:** Doctor may recommend taking a daily aspirin or other blood thinner. This can reduce the tendency of the blood to clot, which may help prevent obstruction of the coronary arteries. If person had a heart attack, aspirin can help prevent future attacks. There are some cases where aspirin isn't appropriate, such as if person have a bleeding disorder already taking another blood thinner, so ask Doctor before starting to take aspirin.
- **Beta blockers:** These drugs slow heart rate and decrease your blood pressure, which decreases heart's demand for oxygen. If person had a heart attack, β blockers reduce the risk of future attacks.
- **Nitroglycerin:** Nitroglycerin tablets, sprays and patches can control chest pain by opening up of coronary arteries and reducing the heart's demand for blood.
- **Angiotensin-converting enzyme (ACE) inhibitors and angiotensin receptor blockers (ARBs):** These similar drugs decrease blood pressure and may help prevent progression of coronary artery disease. If the person had a heart attack, ACE inhibitors reduce the risk of future attacks.
- **Calcium channel blockers:** These medications relax the muscles that surround the coronary arteries and cause the vessels to open, increasing blood flow to the heart. They also control high blood pressure.

PROCEDURES TO RESTORE AND IMPROVE BLOOD FLOW

Sometimes more aggressive treatment is needed. Here are a few options:

- **Angioplasty and stent placement (percutaneous coronary revasculari-zation):** In this procedure, the doctor inserts a long, thin tube (catheter) into the narrowed part of the artery. A wire with a deflated balloon is passed through the catheter to the narrowed area. The balloon is then inflated, compressing the deposits against the artery walls. A stent is often left in the artery to help keep the artery open. Some stents slowly release medication to help keep the artery open.
- **Coronary arteries bypass surgery:** A surgeon creates a graft to bypass Blocked

coronary arteries using a vessel from another part of the body. This allows blood to flow around the blocked or narrowed coronary artery. Because this requires open-heart surgery, its most often reserved for cases of multiple narrowed coronary arteries.

ALTERNATIVE MEDICINE

Omega-3 fatty acids are a type of unsaturated fatty acid that's thought to reduce inflammation throughout the body. Omega-3 fatty acids can help to lower the blood pressure and may reduce the risk of heart attack.

- **Fish and fish oil** are the most effective sources of omega-3 fatty acids. Fatty fish, such as salmon, herring and to a lesser extent tuna, contain the most omega-3 fatty acids and therefore the most benefit. Fish oil supplements may offer benefit, but the evidence is strongest for dietary sources.
- **Other dietary sources of omega-3 fatty acids** include walnuts, canola oil, soybeans and soybean oil. These foods contain smaller amounts of omega-3 fatty acids than do fish and fish oil, and evidence for their benefit to heart health isn't as strong.

REFERENCES

1. Mosca L, Benjamin EJ, Berra K, Bezanson JL, Dolor RJ, Lloyd-Jones DM, et al. Effectiveness-Based Guidelines for the Prevention of Cardiovascular Disease in Women—2011 Update: a guideline from the American Heart Association. *Circulation.* 2011;123(11);1243-1262.
2. Gaziano JM, Ridker PM, Libby P. Primary and secondary prevention of coronary heart disease. In: Bonow RO, Mann DL, Zipes DP, Libby P, eds. *Braunwald's Heart Disease: A Textbook of Cardiovascular Medicine*. 9th ed. Philadelphia, Pa: Saunders Elsevier;2011: chap 49.
3. Greenland P, Alpert JS, Beller GA, Benjamin EJ, Budoff MJ, Fayad ZA, et al., 2010 ACCF/AHA guideline for assessment of cardiovascular risk in asymptomatic adults: a report of the American College of Cardiology Foundation/American Heart Association Task Force on Practice Guidelines. *Circulation.* 2010;122(25)e584-e636.
4. U.S. Preventive Services Task Force. Aspirin for the prevention of cardiovascular disease: U.S. Preventive Services Task Force recommendation statement. *Ann Intern Med.* 2009;150:396-404.

CHAPTER 45

Ischaemic Heart Disease

A recent expert consensus document redefined acute MI as the detection of a rise and/or fall in cardiac biomarkers with at least one value above the 99th percentile of the upper reference limit (URI.), together with evidence of ischemia. Ischemia was defined as any symptoms of ischemia, electrocardiographic changes suggestive of new ischemia, development of pathologic Q waves on electrocardiogram (EKG) or imaging evidence of infarction.

Acute myocardial infarction (MI) is the leading cause of death in North America and Europe. In the United States, the annual death toll from coronary heart disease is higher than 800,000. More than 1 million people each year in the United States sustain an acute MI. An additional 300,000 or more are estimated to die of acute MI before hospitalization. An American has an acute MI every 25 seconds, and someone dies of cardiovascular disease every 36 seconds. Including patients who die before hospital admission, the overall mortality rate of acute MI is >30%, although the incidence and mortality have declined over the last 30 years with the advent of the coronary care unit, fibrinolytic therapy, and catheter-based reperfusion. Although primary percutaneous coronary intervention (PCI) has been shown to lower mortality, a substantial number of patients with acute MI are not eligible for this therapy. Many patients do not have ready access to hospitals that perform 24-hour PCI for acute MI. With the elderly representing an increasing proportion of the population who have a high incidence of and mortality from acute MI and decreased eligibility for fibrinolytic therapy, it probably will remain the leading cause of death over the next several decades. Moreover, the increased incidence of diabetes and obesity stemming from a global shift to a Western diet and lifestyle will increase the sequelae of coronary artery disease in the future.

PATHOPHYSIOLOGY

Coronary **plaque fissuring or rupture** is the initiating event of acute MI. Rupture of the fibrous cap of a coronary atheroma exposes the underlying subendothelial matrix to formed elements of circulating blood, leading to activation of platelets, thrombin generation, and thrombus formation. This is a dynamic process that involves cyclical transitioning between complete vessel occlusion, partial vessel occlusion, and reperfusion. Occlusive thrombus in the absence of significant collateral vessels most often results in acute ST-segment-elevation MI (STEMI). The pathophysiology of

STEMI and non-ST-segment elevation MI (NSTEMI) is similar, and this explains the substantial overlap in acute coronary syndromes with regard to ultimate outcome, extent of necrosis, and mortality rates. However, the recognition of ST segment elevation remains important because it generally mandates the need for emergent reperfusion therapy.

Table 45.1

Clinical classification of different types of myocardial infarction

Type 1	Spontaneous MI related to ischemia from a coronary plaque rupture or dissection.
Type 2	MI due to ischemia resulting from increased oxygen demand or decreased supply.
Type 3	Sudden cardiac death with symptoms of ischemia, new ST-elevation, or LBBB or coronary thrombus.
Type 4a	MI associated with PCI.
Type 4b	MI associated with stent thrombosis.
Type 5	MI associated with CABG.

CABG - Coronary artery bypass grafting, LBBB - Left bundle-branch block, PCI- Percutaneous coronary intervention.

TREATMENT

A. Immediate management and stabilization

1. **Aspirin:** Immediate administration of aspirin is indicated for all patients with acute MI, unless there is a clear history of true aspirin allergy (not intolerance). Aspirin therapy conveys as much mortality benefit as streptokinase, and the combination provides additive benefit. The dose should be four, chewable 81-mg tablets (for more rapid absorption) or one 325-mg non chewable tablet. If oral administration is not possible, a rectal suppository can be given. If true aspirin allergy is present, clopidogrel mono-therapy is the best alternative.
2. **Thienopyridines:** Recent data indicate that clopidogrel should be added to aspirin in STEMI patients regardless of whether they undergo primary PCI or fibrinolysis. The CLARITY-TIMI 28 trial showed pretreatment with clopidogrel to be safe and effective without increased bleeding among patients treated with fibrinolytic therapy, with many receiving subsequent PCI (~57%). The composite endpoint of cardiovascular death, re infarction or revascularization was reduced from 14.1 % to 11.6% (p = 0.03) by clopidogrel pretreatment. A subsequent large randomized double-blind placebo-controlled trial (N = 22,891) called COMMIT/CCS-2 found a significant reduction in all-cause mortality (8.1 % vs. 7.5%) but no difference in major bleeding. An oral loading dose of 300 mg is given, followed by 75 mg daily. Where CABG is planned it is recommended to wait 5 to 7 days after clopidogrel administration before surgery unless urgent revascularization is needed.
3. **Oxygen:** Supplemental oxygen by means of nasal cannula should be given to all patients with suspected MI. Administration through a face mask or Endotracheal tube may be necessary for patients with severe pulmonary edema or cardiogenic shock.
4. **Nitroglycerin:** It is worthwhile to give sublingual nitroglycerin (0.4 mg) to determine whether the ST-segment elevation represents coronary artery

spasm while arrangements for reperfusion therapy are being initiated. Patients should be questioned about recent use of sildenafil (Viagra) because administration of nitroglycerin within 24 hours of sildenafil may cause life-threatening hypotension. A meta analysis performed before the age of routine reperfusion suggested a mortality benefit with intravenous nitroglycerin, although routine use of oral nitrates after MI had no benefit in two large randomized trials in the modern era. Nitroglycerin can be useful in the management of acute MI complicated by CHF, ongoing symptoms, or hypertension. A 30% reduction in systolic blood pressure can he expected with appropriately aggressive dosing (10 to 20/1g/min with 5 to 10/1g/min increases every 5 to 10 min). Intravenous therapy can be continued for 24 to 48 hours, after which time patients with heart failure or residual ischemia can convert to oral or topical therapy with an appropriate nitrate-free interval to avoid tachyphylaxis.

5. **Reperfusion therapy:** The primary goal in the management of acute MI is to institute reperfusion therapy as quickly as possible. All patients with ST-segment elevation or new LBBB MI who seek treatment within 12 to 24 hours from onset of continuous symptoms should be considered for immediate reperfusion therapy. Persistent ischemic symptoms after 12 hours may indicate a stuttering course of occlusion, spontaneous reperfusion, and reocclusion, and may indicate potential continued benefit for early therapy.

   (a) **Benefit:** The benefit of reperfusion therapy has been well documented in the management of acute MI, regardless of age, gender, and most baseline characteristics. However, the patients who derive the most benefit are those treated earliest and those at highest risk, such as those with anterior MI.

   (b) **Time to treatment is paramount:** Patients treated in the first hour have the highest morality benefit. It is unclear whether these results entirely from the prevention of myocardial damage or whether those who seek treatment early have a larger infarction and arc preselected to derive pronounced benefit. Regardless, numerous trials support an inverse relation between time to treatment and survival benefit. This relationship appears more consistent with fibrinolytic therapy than for direct PCI. After 12 hours of continuous symptoms, there is little net benefit to pharmacologic reperfusion with fibrinolytics, although recent data indicate that the benefit of primary PCI in terms of infarct-size reduction may extend even beyond 12 to 24 hours (BRAVE-2 study), even among patients without persistent chest pain.

   (c) **Fibrinolysis versus direct PCI:** After it has been determined that a patient is a candidate for reperfusion therapy, the decision to use fibrinolytic or direct PCI therapy must be made quickly.

1. If facilities for immediate coronary angiography and PCI are available within 90 minutes of first medical contact, this is the preferred therapy. Pooled data from several large trials show a significant (22%) reduction in short-term mortality for patients treated with primary angioplasty. This benefit was durable because there were significant reductions in the incidence of death, nonfatal MI, and recurrent ischemia at long-term follow-up. PCI is also associated with a reduction in the incidence of intracerebral hemorrhage compared to fibrinolytic therapy.
2. If facilities for immediate coronary angiography and direct PCI are not available, fibrinolytic therapy, unless contraindicated, should be instituted within 30 minutes of first medical contact. Anticipated prolonged transfer time to a primary PCI facility (medical contact-to-balloon time >90 minutes) is also an indication for fibrinolytic therapy. There is some controversy regarding the use of primary PCI with prolonged transfer times. Several trials, including the DANAMI-2 (Danish Multicenter Randomized Study on Thrombolytic Therapy Versus Acute Coronary Angioplasty in Acute Myocardial Infarction), AIR-PAMI (Air-Primary Angioplasty in Myocardial Infarction), and the PRAGUE (Primary Angioplasty in Patients Transferred from a General Community Hospital to Specialized PTCA Units), have investigated the benefit of on-site fibrinolysis compared with transfer to tertiary centres for direct PCI. These studies have found improved outcomes in patients randomized to a transfer strategy and direct PCI even after taking into account the increased time for patient transfer from randomization to balloon inflation of 112 minutes.
3. If a contraindication to fibrinolytic therapy exists or there is some question of the diagnosis, arrangements should be made for transfer to a PCI facility.
4. Because of the relative lack of efficacy of lytic therapy among patients with cardiogenic shock or prior bypass operations, such patients are especially well suited for primary PCI. However, if a long delay (>3 hours) is anticipated, fibrinolytic therapy may still be considered while arrangements for coronary angiography are made.

(d) **Primary PCI.** Once the decision has been made to perform reperfusion with primary PCI, the patient should he moved to the cardiac catheterization laboratory and undergo angiography as rapidly as possible. After the culprit lesion has been identified, reperfusion should be achieved with standard PCI techniques.

1. **Platelet glycoprotein IIb/IIIa inhibitors (GP IIb/IIIa):** Several clinical trials have documented the benefits of abciximab in improving clinical outcomes after primary PCI with or without stenting in patients with STEMI. Results from the RAPPORT (ReoPro and Primary PTCA Organization and Trial) showed a nearly 50% reduction in death, MI, or urgent total vascular resistance (TVR) at 30 days in patients treated with abciximab compared with placebo at the time of PCI.

2. **Aspiration devices and distal embolic protection:** Although aspiration catheters have been shown to improve ST-segment resolution and myocardial blush, they have not been shown to improve clinical outcomes. Similarly, distal embolic protection has failed to show any benefit in multiple trials and may in fact increase infarct size. The major criticism of these trials is the exclusion of patients with large thrombus burden. Regardless of this caveat, these devices are not routinely recommended for acute PCI.
3. **Coronary stenting:** The early benefit of angioplasty over thrombolytic therapy is attenuated with more extended follow-up. In the GUSTO llb (Global Use of Strategies to Open Occluded Coronary Arteries) trial in which use of accelerated tissue plasminogen activator (tPA) was compared with angioplasty alone (percutaneous transluminal coronary angioplasty, PTCA), the reduction in rates of death and nonfatal MI at 30 days (13.7% tPA vs. 9.6% PTeA) dwindled, and by 6 months, the difference (16.1 % for tPA vs. 14.1 % for PTCA) had lost statistical significance. This loss of effect may be at least partially caused by restenosis of the target lesion that was managed directly with angioplasty. Although coronary stents are known to reduce rates of restenosis during elective PCI, it was once believed that stents should not be placed in thrombus-laden lesions, such as those associated with acute MI, because of risk for in-stent thrombosis. However, clinical trials with adequate antiplatelet therapy have shown stenting to be safe.

REFERENCES

1. Qaseem A, FihnSD, Williams S, Dallas P, Owens DK, Shekelle P, for the Clinical Guidelines Committee of the American College of Physicians. Diagnosis of stable ischemic heart disease: summary of a clinical practice guideline from the American College of Physicians/American College of Cardiology Foundation/ American Heart Association/American Association for Thoracic Surgery/ Preventive Cardiovascular Nurses Association/Society of Thoracic Surgeons. Ann Intern Med. 2012; 157:729-34.
2. Fihn SD, Gardin JM, Abrams J, Berra K, Blankenship JC, Dallas P, et al. 2012 ACCF/AHA/ACP/AATS/PCNA/SCAI/STS guideline for the diagnosis and management of patients with stable ischemic heart disease: a report of the American College of Cardiology Foundation/American Heart Association Task Force on Practice Guidelines, and the American College of Physicians, American Association for Thoracic Surgery, Preventive Cardiovascular Nurses Association, Society for Cardiovascular Angiography and Interventions, and Society of Thoracic Surgeons. J Am Coll Cardiol. 2012.
3. Qaseem A, Snow V, Owens DK, Shekelle P, Clinical Guidelines Committee of the American College of Physicians. The development of clinical practice guidelines and guidance statements of the American College of Physicians: summary of methods. Ann Intern Med. 2010; 153:194-9.
4. Prevention of cardiovascular events and death with pravastatin in patients with coronary heart disease and a broad range of initial cholesterol levels. The Long-Term Intervention with Pravastatin in Ischaemic Disease (LIPID) Study Group. N Engl J Med. 1998; 339:1349-57.
5. Gottlieb SS, McCarter RJ, Vogel RA. Effect of beta-blockade on mortality among high-risk and low-risk patients after

myocardial infarction. N Engl J Med. 1998; 339:489-97.

6. Qaseem A, Fihn SD, Williams S, Dallas P, Owens DK, Shekelle P, for the Clinical Guidelines Committee of the American College of Physicians. Diagnosis of stable ischemic heart disease: summary of a clinical practice guideline from the American College of Physicians/American College of Cardiology Foundation/ American Heart Association/American Association for Thoracic Surgery/ Preventive Cardiovascular Nurses Association/Society of Thoracic Surgeons. Ann Intern Med. 2012; 157:729-34.

CHAPTER 46

Atrial Flutter

Atrial flutter is characterized by an atrial macro reentrant circuit (typically in the right atrium) leading to regular atrial depolarizations, typically at a rate of 250 to 350 beats/min. There is typically 2:1 (or less) conduction through the atrioventricular node resulting in heart rates close to 150 beats/min. The atrial impulses may be conducted at a constant rate through the atrioventricular node resulting in a regular rhythm, or the atrial impulses may be conducted at a variable rate resulting in an irregular rhythm.

Atrial flutter is less common than fibrillation. It may occur in patients with structurally normal hearts but is more commonly seen in patients with COPD, rheumatic or coronary heart disease, heart failure, ASD, or surgically repaired congenital heart disease. AF is characterized by rapid, ineffective writhing of the atrial muscle with a classic "irregularly irregular" ventricular rate. The source of the arrhythmia is one or more ectopic areas (foci) that act as independent pacemakers and fire at such a rate as to suppress normal impulse generation from the SA node. On the ECG, no identifiable P waves are present. The ECG typically demonstrates a "sawtooth" pattern of atrial activity in the inferior leads (II, III, and AVF). The reentrant circuit generates atrial rates of 250–350 beats/min, usually with transmission of every second, third, or fourth impulse through the AV node to the ventricles.

In contrast, atrial flutter is characterized by typical saw tooth atrial waves, at a rate of 280 to 320 beats/minute and a variable ventricular rate, depending on the nature of the AV block present. In most cases, the ventricular rate is approximately 150 beats/minute. Patients with atrial flutter often progress to AF. The underlying diseases and treatments of atrial flutter and AF are similar. The arrhythmogenic mechanism of AF may be due to multiple re entrant wavelets, occurring in a paroxysmal, chronic, or acute pattern. The most common presentation is paroxysmal atrial fibrillation (PAF), which can progress to chronic AF; thus, the two overlap.

CAUSES OF ATRIAL FLUTTER

CARDIAC CAUSES

1. Atrial septal defect
2. Cardiac surgery
3. Pericarditis
4. Tachycardia-bradycardia syndrome

5. Cardiomyopathy
6. Ischemic heart disease
7. Tumors,
8. lipomatous hypertrophy
9. Wolff-Parkinson-White syndrome
10. Mitral valve disease
11. Non rheumatic heart disease

SYSTEMIC CAUSES

1. Alcohol
2. Cerebrovascular accident
3. Pneumonia
4. Pulmonary embolism
5. Chronic pulmonary disease
6. Defibrillation
7. Sudden emotional or psychological-stress
8. Electrolyte abnormalities
9. Fever
10. Hypothermia
11. Trauma
12. Thyrotoxicosis

TREATMENT

Ventricular rate is controlled by using the same agents used in atrial fibrillation, but it is much more difficult with atrial flutter than with atrial fibrillation. Conversion of atrial flutter to sinus rhythm with class I antiarrhythmic agents is also difficult to achieve, and administration of these drugs has been associated with slowing of the atrial flutter rate to the point at which 1:1 AV conduction can occur at rates in excess of 200 beats/min, with subsequent hemodynamic collapse. The intravenous class III antiarrhythmic agent ibutilide has been significantly more successful in converting atrial flutter. About 50–70% of patients return to sinus rhythm within 60–90 minutes following the infusion of 1–2 mg of this agent. Electrical cardioversion is also very effective for atrial flutter, with approximately 90% of patients converting following synchronized shocks of as little as 25–50 J. Although the organization of atrial contractile function in this arrhythmia may provide some protection against thrombus formation, the risk of thromboembolism should be considered equivalent to atrial fibrillation due to the common coexistence of these arrhythmias. Precardioversion anticoagulation is not necessary for atrial flutter of less than 48 hours, duration except in the setting of mitral valve disease. As with atrial fibrillation, anticoagulation should be continued for at least 4 weeks after electrical or chemical cardioversion and long-term in patients with risk factors for thrombo-embolism.

Chronic atrial flutter is often a difficult management problem, as rate control is difficult. If pharmacologic therapy is chosen, amiodarone and dofetilide are the antiarrhythmics of choice. Dofetilide is often given in conjunction with an AV nodal blocker (other than verapamil). Atrial flutter can follow a typical or atypical re-entry circuit around the atrium. The anatomy of the typical circuit has been well defined and allows for catheter ablation within the atrium to interrupt the circuit and eliminate atrial flutter. Catheter ablation is a highly successful treatment that has become the preferred approach for recurrent typical atrial flutter. Atrial flutter and atrial fibrillation frequently coexist, and patients may require catheter ablation of both arrhythmias.

This arrhythmia occurs most often in patients with organic heart disease. Flutter may be paroxysmal, in which case there is usually a precipitating factor, such as pericarditis or acute respiratory failure, or it may be persistent. Atrial flutter (as well as AF) is very common during the first week following open-heart surgery. Atrial flutter is usually less long-lived than is AF, although on occasion it may persist for months to years. Often, if it lasts for more than a week, atrial flutter will convert to AF. Systemic embolization is less common in atrial flutter than in AF. Atrial flutter is characterized by an atrial rate between 250 and 350 beats/min. Typically, the ventricular rate is half the atrial rate, i.e., 150 beats/min because of 2:1 block in the AV node. If the atrial rate is slowed to 220 beats/min by antiarrhythmic agents such as quinidine, which also possess vagolytic properties, the ventricular rate may rise suddenly because of the development of 1:1 AV conduction. Classically, flutter waves are seen as regular sawtooth-like atrial activity, most prominent in the inferior leads. When the ventricular response is regular and not a simple fraction of the atrial rate, complete AV block is present, which may be a manifestation of digitalis toxicity. Activation mapping suggests that atrial flutter is a form of atrial reentry localized to the right atrium.

The reason for the increased risk of emboli in atrial flutter is uncertain, but the coexistence of AF is common. In patients who develop atrial flutter following open-heart surgery or recurrent flutter in the setting of acute myocardial infarction, particularly if they are being treated with digitalis, atrial pacing (using temporary pacing wires implanted at the time of operation or a pacing lead inserted into the atrium pervenously) at rates of 115 to 130% of the atrial flutter rate can usually convert the atrial flutter to sinus rhythm. Atrial pacing may also result in the conversion of atrial flutter to AF, which allows for easier control of the ventricular response. Ibutilide is a new antiarrhythmic agent that is administered intravenously and appears to be particularly effective for conversion of atrial flutter to sinus rhythm.

Quinidine, other class IA drugs, flecainide, propafenone, sotalol, dofetilide, and amiodarone (Table 46.1) may be useful in preventing recurrences of atrial flutter. Radiofrequency ablation is a highly effective treatment for patients with the most typical forms of atrial flutter, which are due to reentry around the tricuspid valve in a counter clockwise or clockwise fashion. The coronary sinus and inferior vena cava cause the wavefront of activation to pass between them and the tricuspid valve. Ablation of the narrowed isthmus using radiofrequency energy can cure flutter in 85% of cases. This is far more successful than the response to drugs. As such, ablation is considered by many to be the therapy of choice for recurrent atrial flutter.

Table 46.1

Pharmacological treatment of atrial flutter

Drug	Mode of Administration	$t_{1/2}$ (oral), h	Clinical Effects and/or Indications for Use
Digoxin	IV, 0.25–1.5 mg Oral, 0.75–1.5 mg loading dose over 12–24 h Maintenance, 0.23–0.50 mg/kg	36 hrs	Slowing of ventricular rate during AF, flutter, and other atrial tachycardias in the absence of preexcitation; slowing, termination, and/or prevention of SVT due to AV nodal reentry and AV re-entry utilizing bypass tracts; may terminate or prevent intraatrial re-entrant tachycardias; ineffective in prevention of automatic atrial tachycardias.
Adenosine	IV bolus, 6–12 mg	<10s	Acute termination of regular reentrant SVT involving the AVnode
Quinidine (class IA)	Oral, 200–400 mg q6h	8-9h	Atrial and ventricular tachyarrhythmias; all types of SVT; control of ventricular rate in patients with preexcitation and AF and flutter
Procainamide (class IA)	IV, 40–50 mg/min to total of 10–20 mg/kg Oral, 500–1000 mg q6h (sustained release forms)	3–5h	Atrial and ventricular tachyarrhythmias; all types of SVT; control of ventricular rate in patients with preexcitation and AF and flutter
Disopyramide (class IA)	Oral, 100–300 mg q6h	8-9h	Atrial and ventricular tachyarrhythmias; all types of SVT; control of ventricular rate in patients with preexcitation and AF and flutter
Lidocaine (class IB)	IV, 20–50 mg/min to total of 5 mg/kg loading dose, followed by 1–4 mg/kg	1-2h	VT and VF, especially during acute ischemia and myocardial infarction
Phenytoin (class IB)	IV, 20 mg/kg to total dose of 1000 mg Oral, 1000-mg loading dose over 24 h Maintenance, 100–400 mg/d	18-36h	Tachyarrhythmias induced by digitalis; occasionally effective for ventricular tachyarrhythmias not induced by digitalis alone or in combination with other antiarrhythmic agents; polymorphic VT associated with increased QT interval
Mexiletine (class IB)	Oral, 100–300 mg q6–8h	9–12	Ventricular tachyarrhythmias; secondary agent in combination with other class I medication
Flecainide (class IC)	Oral, begin at 50–100 mg bid, increase by 50 mg in 4-day intervals to a maximum of mg daily	7–23h	Supraventricular tachyarrhythmias including atrial fibrillation and flutter; also ventricular arrhythmias refractory to other medications or radiofrequency ablation
Propafenone (class IC)	Oral, 150–300 mg q8h	5-8h	Supraventricular tachyarrhythmias including atrial fibrillation and flutter; also ventricular arrhythmias refractory to other medications orradiofrequency ablation

Table 46.1 *contd...*

Drug	Mode of Administration	$t_{1/2}$ (oral), h	Clinical Effects and/or Indications for Use
Moricizine (class IC)	Oral, 200–400 mg q8h	2-6h	Supraventricular tachyarrhythmias including atrial fibrillation and flutter; also ventricular arrhythmias refractory to other medications orradiofrequency ablation
Beta blockers (class II) e.g., metoprolol	IV, load with 5–10 mg q5min for 3 doses, then 3 mg q6h Oral, 25–100 mg bid	3-4h	Slowing of ventricular rate during AF, atrial flutter, and other atrial tachyarrhythmias in the absence of preexcitation; SVT due to AV nodal reentry; reentry utilizing bypass tracts; arrhythmias (e.g., VT) induced by exercise or occurring in the presence of hyperthyroidism; polymorphic VT associated with congenital long QT syndrome
Bretylium (class III)	IV, 1–2 mg/kg per min to total load, 5–10 mg/kg Maintenance, 0.5–2 mg/kg	8-14h	Refractory VT and VF, especially due to acute ischemia
Amiodarone (class III)	IV, 5–10 mg/kg load over 20 min, then 1 g/24 h Oral, load 800–1600 mg/d for 1 week, then 400–600 mg/d for 3 weeks, then 200–400 mg/d thereafter AF and atrial flutter, other types of SVT, VT, VF	13-103h	Sustained VT and VF
Sotalol (class III)	Oral, 80–320 mg q12h	10-20h	Atrial and ventricular tachyarrhythmias
Ibutilide (class III)	IV, 60 kg: 0.01 mg/kg over 10 min IV, 60 kg: 1 mg over 10 min, repeat after 10 min if no effect	2-6h	AF, atrial flutter, and other SVTs including preexcitation tachycardias
Dofetilide	125–250 mg PO bid	8-12h	AF, atrial flutter, and other SVTs
Calcium channel blockers (class IV) e.g., verapamil	IV, 2.5–10 mg over 1–2 min to total of 0.15 mg/kg Oral, 240–480 qd	6-24h	Slowing of ventricular rate during AF and flutter, and other SVTs in the absence of preexcitation; idiopathic VT.
Diltiazem	IV, load with 0.25 mg/kg over 2 min; if needed, repeat after 15 min with 0.35 mg over 2 min Maintenance, 10–15 mg/h		Slowing of ventricular rate during AF and flutter, and other SVTs in the absence of preexcitation; idiopathic VT.

Note: AF, atrial fibrillation; AV, atrioventricular; SVT, supraventricular tachycardia; VF, ventricular fibrillation; VT, ventricular tachycardia.

NON PHARMACOLOGICAL THERAPY

- Valsalva maneuver or carotid sinus massage usually slows the ventricular rate (increases grade of AV block) and may make flutter waves more evident. Adenosine may be similarly helpful.
- Direct current cardioversion is the treatment of choice for acute management of atrial flutter associated with hemodynamic instability or debilitating symptoms such as angina or congestive heart failure. Electrical cardioversion is typically successful at low energy levels (20 to 25 J). Sedation of a conscious patient is highly recommended before cardioversion is performed. The use of external defbrillators with biphasic waveforms decreases the amount of energy required for cardioversion and improves cardioversion success rate.
- Overdrive pacing in the atrium may also terminate atrial flutter. This method is especially useful in patients who have recently undergone cardiac surgery and still have temporary atrial pacing wires.
- Radiofrequency ablation to interrupt the atrial ûutter is highly effective for patients with chronic or recurring atrial ûutter and is generally considered frst-line therapy in those with recurrent episodes of atrial flutter.

REFERENCES

1. Mohanty S et al. Results from a single-blind, randomized study comparing the impact of different ablation approaches on long-term procedure outcome in coexistent atrial fibrillation and flutter (APPROVAL). Circulation. 2013 May 7;127(18):1853–60. [PMID: 23572499]
2. Scheuermeyer FX et al. Emergency department management and 1-year outcomes of patients with atrial flutter. Ann Emerg Med. 2011 Jun;57(6):564–71. [PMID: 21257230.
3. Camm AJ, Lip GYH, DeCaterina R, Savelieva I, Atar D, Hohnloser SH, Hindricks G, Kirchhof P. 2012 focused update of the ESC guidelines for the management of atrial fibrillation. Eur Heart J. 2012;33:2719–47.
4. Lip GY. Stroke in atrial fibrillation: epidemiology and thromboprophylaxis. J Thromb Haemost. 2011;9 Suppl 1:344–51.
5. Olesen JB, Lip GY, Hansen ML, Tolstrup JS, Lindhardsen J, Selmer C, Ahlehoff O, Olsen AM, Gislason GH, Torp-Pedersen C. Validation of risk stratification schemes for predicting stroke and thrombo-embolism in patients with atrial fibrillation: nationwide cohort study. BMJ. 2011;342:d124.
6. Friberg L, Rosenqvist M, Lip GY. Evaluation of risk stratification schemes for ischaemic stroke and bleeding in 182,678 patients with atrial fibrillation: the Swedish atrial fibrillation cohort study. Eur Heart J. 2012;33:1500–10.
7. Connolly SJ, Ezekowitz MD, Yusuf S, et al. Dabigatran versus warfarin in patients with atrial fibrillation. N Engl J Med. 2009;361:1139–51.
8. Patel MR, Mahaffey KW, Garg J, et al. Rivaroxaban versus warfarin in nonvalvular atrial fibrillation. N Engl J Med. 2011;365(10):883–91.
9. Granger CB, Alexander JH, McMurray JJ, et al. Apixaban versus warfarin in patients with atrial fibrillation. N Engl J Med. 2011;365(11):981–92.
10. Heidbuchel H, Verhamme P, Alings M, Antz M, Hacke W, Oldgren J, Sinnaeve P, Camm AJ, Kirchhof P. European heart rhythm association practical guide on the use of new oral anticoagulants in patients with

non-valvular atrial fibrillation. Europace. 2013;15:625–51.

11. Kaseno K, Naito S, Nakamura K, Sakamoto T, Sasaki T, Tsukada N, et al. Efficacy and safety of periprocedural dabigatran in patients undergoing catheter ablation of atrial fibrillation. Circ J. 2012;76:2337–42.

12. Snipelisky D, Kauffman C, Prussak K, Johns G, Venkatachalam K, Kusumoto F. A comparison of bleeding complications post-ablation between warfarin and dabigatran. J Interv Card Electrophysiol. 2012;35:29–33.

13. Winkle RA, Mead RH, Engel G, Kong MH, Patrawala RA. The use of dabigatran immediately after atrial fibrillation ablation.J Cardiovasc Electrophysiol. 2012;23:264–8.

CHAPTER 47

Hypertrophic Cardiomyopathy

The cardiomyopathies are a group of diseases that affect the heart muscle and these are not the result of hypertension or congenital or acquired valvular, coronary, or pericardial abnormalities. When the cardiomyopathies are classified on an etiologic basis, two fundamental forms are recognized:

1. Primary type, consisting of heart muscle disease of unknown cause; and
2. Secondary type, consisting of myocardial disease of known cause or associated with a disease involving other organ systems.

Hypertropic cardiomyopathy (HCM) is a primary myocardial disorder characterized by disorganized myocyte architecture and severe thickening (hypertrophy) of the left ventricular wall out of proportion to the resistance to ventricular contraction (afterload). The interventricular septum is the most common site of enlargement, though hypertrophy may involve other focal regions or may be concentric. HCM may result in hemodynamically signifcant obstruction within the left ventricular outflow tract (LVOT) and/or impairment of the diastolic function of the left ventricle.

In the World Health Organization classification, the term *specific cardiomyopathy* is used to describe heart muscle diseases associated with certain systemic or cardiac disorders; examples include hypertensive and metabolic cardiomyopathy. In many cases, however, it is not possible to arrive at a specific etiologic diagnosis, and thus it is often more desirable to classify the cardiomyopathies into one of three types (dilated, restrictive, hypertrophic) on the basis of differences in their pathophysiology and clinical presentation.

PHYSICAL FINDINGS & CLINICAL PRESENTATION

HCM may be suspected on the basis of abnormalities found on physical examination. Classic findings include:

- Harsh, systolic, crescendo–decrescendo murmur at the left sternal border or apex. The murmur increases with maneuvers that decrease venous return or LV size (Valsalva, standing), and decreases with those that increase venous return or afterload (squatting, hand grip, post-Valsalva release).
- Paradoxic splitting of S2 (if left ventricular obstruction is present).
- Double or triple LV apical impulse ("triple ripple": atrial contraction, early rapid ejection, and late slow ejection).

- Increased obstruction can occur with: Drugs: digitalis, β-adrenergic stimulators (isoproterenol, dopamine, epinephrine), nitroglycerin, vasodilators, diuretics, alcohol
- Hypovolemia
- Tachycardia
- Valsalva maneuver
- Standing position
- Decreased obstruction is seen with: Drugs: β-adrenergic blockers, calcium channel blockers, disopyramide, α-adrenergic stimulators
- Volume expansion
- Bradycardia
- Hand-grip exercise
- Squatting position
- Release phase of the Valsalva maneuver

Clinical manifestations are as follows:

- Dyspnea
- Syncope (usually seen with exercise)
- Angina
- Palpitations

PHARMACOLOGICAL MANAGEMENT

- Beta-blocking drugs are recommended for the treatment of symptoms (angina or dyspnea) in adult patients with obstructive or nonobstructive HCM but should be used with caution in patients with sinus bradycardia or severe conduction disease. (Level of Evidence: B) If low doses of beta-blocking drugs are ineffective for controlling symptoms (angina or dyspnea) in patients with HCM, it is useful to titrate the dose to a resting heart rate of less than 60 to 65 bpm (up to generally accepted and recommended maximum doses of these drugs). (Level of Evidence: B)
- Verapamil therapy (starting in low doses and titrating up to 480 mg/d) is recommended for the treatment of symptoms (angina or dyspnea) in patients with obstructive or nonobstructive HCM who do not respond to beta-blocking drugs or who have side effects or contraindications to betablocking drugs. However, verapamil should be used with caution in patients with high gradients, advanced heart failure, or sinus bradycardia. (Level of Evidence: B)
- Intravenous phenylephrine (or another pure vasoconstricting agent) is recommended for the treatment of acute hypotension in patients with obstructive HCM who do not respond to fluid administration. (Level of Evidence: B). It is reasonable to combine disopyramide with a beta-blocking drug or verapamil in the treatment of symptoms (angina or dyspnea) in patients with obstructive HCM who do not respond to beta blocking drugs or verapamil alone. (Level of Evidence: B)
- It is reasonable to add oral diuretics in patients with nonobstructive HCM when dyspnea persists despite the use of beta blockers or verapamil or their combination. (Level of Evidence: C) Beta-blocking drugs might be useful in the treatment of symptoms (angina or dyspnea) in children or adolescents with HCM, but patients treated with these drugs should be monitored for side effects, including depression, fatigue, or impaired scholastic performance. (Level of Evidence: C)
- It may be reasonable to add oral diuretics with caution to patients with obstructive HCM when congestive symptoms persist

despite the use of beta blockers or verapamil or their combination. (Level of Evidence: C). The usefulness of angiotensin-converting enzyme inhibitors or angiotensin receptor blockers in the treatment of symptoms (angina or dyspnea) in patients with HCM with preserved systolic function is not well established, and these drugs should be used cautiously (if at all) in patients in rest. (Level of Evidence: C)

In patients with HCM who do not tolerate verapamil or in whom verapamil is contraindicated, diltiazem may be considered. (Level of Evidence: C). Nifedipine or other dihydropyridine calcium channel-blocking drugs are potentially harmful for treatment of symptoms (angina or dyspnea) in patients with HCM who are in rest. (Level of Evidence: C). Verapamil is potentially harmful in patients with obstructive. HCM in the setting of systemic hypotension or severe dyspnea at rest. (Level of Evidence: C)

- Digitalis is potentially harmful in the treatment of dyspnea in patients with HCM and in the absence of atrial fibrillation (AF). (Level of Evidence: B). The use of disopyramide alone without beta blockers or verapamil is potentially harmful in the treatment of symptoms (angina or dyspnea) in patients with HCM with AF because disopyramide may enhance atrioventricular conduction and increase the ventricular rate during episodes of AF. (Level of Evidence: B)
- Dopamine, dobutamine, norepinephrine, and other intravenous positive inotropic drugs are potentially harmful for the treatment of acute hypotension in patients with obstructive HCM. (Level of Evidence: B)

NONPHARMACOLOGIC THERAPY

- **Avoid volume depletion:** HCM patients experience decrease in stroke volume and consequent increase in left ventricular out flow gradient on exercise. This may lead to hypotension, dizziness, and syncope.
- **Exercise restriction:** The risk of sudden cardiac death is increased by exercise in HCM patients. Participation in competitive sports and intense physical activity should be avoided.
- **Advice avoidance of alcohol:** Alcohol use (even in small amounts) may result in increased obstruction of the left ventricular outflow tract.

REFERENCES

1. McMurray JJ, Adamopoulos S, Anker SD, Auricchio A, Bohm M, Dickstein K, Falk V, Filippatos G, Fonseca C, Gomez-Sanchez MA, Jaarsma T, Kober L, Lip GY, Maggioni AP, Parkhomenko A, Pieske BM, Popescu BA, Ronnevik PK, Rutten FH, Schwitter J, Seferovic P, Stepinska J, Trindade PT, Voors AA, Zannad F, Zeiher A. ESC Guidelines for the diagnosis and treatment of acute and chronic heart failure 2012: The Task Force for the Diagnosis and Treatment of Acute and Chronic Heart Failure 2012 of the European Society of Cardiology. Developed in collaboration with the Heart Failure Association (HFA) of the ESC. Eur Heart J 2012;33:1787–1847.
2. Maron BJ, Nishimura RA, McKenna WJ, Rakowski H, Josephson ME, Kieval RS. Assessment of permanent dual-chamber pacing as a treatment for drug-refractory symptomatic patients with obstructive hypertrophic cardiomyopathy. A randomized, double-blind, crossover study (M-PATHY). Circulation 1999; 99:2927–2933.

3. Thaman R, Gimeno JR, Murphy RT, Kubo T, Sachdev B, Mogensen J, Elliott PM, McKenna WJ. Prevalence and clinical significance of systolic impairment in hypertrophic cardiomyopathy. Heart 2005; 91: 920–925.
4. Harris KM, Spirito P, Maron MS, Zenovich AG, Formisano F, Lesser JR, Mackey-Bojack S, Manning WJ, Udelson JE, Maron BJ. Prevalence, clinical profile, and significance of left ventricular remodeling in the end-stage phase of hypertrophic cardiomyopathy. Circulation 2006; 114:216–225.
5. Olivotto I, Cecchi F, Poggesi C, Yacoub MH. Patterns of disease progression in hypertrophic cardiomyopathy: an individualized approach to clinical staging. Circ Heart Fail 2012; 5: 535–546
6. Olivotto I, Montereggi A, Mazzuoli F, Cecchi F. Clinical utility and safety of exercise testing in patients with hypertrophic cardiomyopathy. GItal Cardiol1999; 29: 11–19.
7. Sorajja P, Allison T, Hayes C, Nishimura RA, Lam CS, Ommen SR. Prognostic utility of metabolic exercise testing in minimally symptomatic patients with obstructive hypertrophic cardiomyopathy. Am J Cardiol 2012;109:1494–149
8. Autore C, Conte MR, Piccininno M, Bernabo P, Bonfiglio G, Bruzzi P, Spirito P. Risk associated with pregnancy in hypertrophic cardiomyopathy. J Am Coll Cardiol 2002; 40:1864–1869.

CHAPTER 48

Asthma

DEFINITION

A chronic inflammatory disorder of the airways in which many cells and cellular elements play a role. In susceptible individuals, inflammation causes recurrent episodes of wheezing, breathlessness, chest tightness, and coughing. These episodes are usually associated with airflow obstruction that is often reversible either spontaneously or with treatment. The inflammation also causes an increase in bronchial hyper responsiveness (BHR) to a variety of stimuli.

PREVALENCE

As of 2009, 300 million people worldwide were affected by asthma leading to approximately 250,000 deaths per year. It is estimated that asthma has 7%-10% prevalence worldwide. As of 1998, there was a great disparity in the prevalence of asthma across the world, with a trend toward more developed and westernized countries having higher rates of asthma, with as high as a 20 to 60-fold difference. Asthma affects approximately 7% of the population of the United States and 5% of people in the United Kingdom. Asthma causes 4,210 deaths per year in the United States. In 2005 in the United States asthma affected more than 22 million people including 6 million children. It accounted for nearly 1/2 million hospitalizations that same year. More boys have asthma than girls, but more women have it than men. In England, an estimated 261,400 people were newly diagnosed with asthma in 2005; 5.7 million people had an asthma diagnosis and were prescribed 32.6 million asthma-related prescriptions.

PATHOPHYSIOLOGY

- The major characteristics of asthma include a variable degree of airflow obstruction (related to bronchospasm, edema, and hyper secretion), BHR, and airway inflammation.
- Inhaled allergens cause an early-phase allergic reaction characterized by activation of cells bearing allergen-specific immunoglobulin E (IgE) antibodies. There is rapid activation of airway mast cells and macrophages, which release proinflammatory mediators such as histamine and eicosanoids that induce contraction of airway smooth muscle, mucus secretion, vasodilatation and exudation of plasma in the airways. Plasma protein leakage induces a thickened, engorged, edematous airway wall and a narrowing of the airway lumen with reduced mucus clearance.

- The late-phase inflammatory reaction occurs 6 to 9 hours after allergen provocation and involves recruitment and activation of eosinophils, T lymphocytes, basophils, neutrophils, and macrophages.
- Eosinophils migrate to the airways and release inflammatory mediators (leukotrienes and granule proteins), cytotoxic mediators, and cytokines.
- T-lymphocyte activation leads to release of cytokines from type 2 T-helper (TH2) cells that mediate allergic inflammation (interleukin [IL]-4, IL-5, and IL-13). Conversely, type 1 T-helper (TH1) cells produce IL-2 and interferon- α that are essential for cellular defense mechanisms. Allergic asthmatic inflammation may result from an imbalance between TH1 and TH2 cells.
- Mast cell degranulation in response to allergens results in release of mediators such as histamine; eosinophils, and neutrophils chemotactic factors; leukotrienes C4, D4, and E4; prostaglandins; and platelet-activating factor (PAF). Histamine is capable of inducing smooth muscle constriction and bronchospasm and may play a role in mucosal edema and mucus secretion.
- Alveolar macrophages release a number of inflammatory mediators, including PAF and leukotrienes B4, C4, and D4. Production of neutrophils chemotactic factor and eosinophils chemotactic factor furthers the inflammatory process.
- Neutrophils are also a source of mediators (PAFs, prostaglandins, thromboxanes, and leukotrienes) that contribute to BHR and airway inflammation.
- The 5-lipoxygenase pathway of arachidonic acid metabolism is responsible for production of cysteinyl leukotrienes. Leukotrienes C4, D4, and E4 are released during inflammatory processes in the lung and produce bronchospasm, mucus secretion, micro vascular permeability, and airway edema
- Bronchial epithelial cells participate in inflammation by releasing eicosanoids, peptidases, matrix proteins, cytokines, and nitric oxide. Epithelial shedding results in heightened airway responsiveness, altered permeability of the airway mucosa, depletion of epithelial-derived relaxant factors, and loss of enzymes responsible for degrading inflammatory neuropeptides.
- The exudative inflammatory process and sloughing of epithelial cells into the airway lumen impair mucociliary transport. The bronchial glands are increased in size, and the goblet cells are increased in size and number. Expectorated mucus from patients with asthma tends to have high viscosity.
- The airway is innervated by parasympathetic, sympathetic, and nonadrenergic inhibitory nerves. The normal resting tone of airway smooth muscle is maintained by vagal efferent activity, and bronchoconstriction can be mediated by vagal stimulation in the small bronchi. Airway smooth muscle contains non innervated β2-adrenergic receptors that produce bronchodilation. The nonadrenergic, noncholinergic nervous system in the trachea and bronchi may amplify inflammation in asthma by releasing nitric oxide.

CLINICAL FEATURES

CHRONIC ASTHMA

- Classic asthma is characterized by episodic dyspnea associated with wheezing, but the clinical presentation of asthma is diverse. Patients may also complain of episodes of dyspnea, chest tightness, coughing (particularly at night), wheezing, or a whistling sound when breathing. These often occur with exercise but may occur spontaneously or in association with known allergens.
- Signs include expiratory wheezing on auscultation, dry hacking cough, or signs of atopy (e.g., allergic rhinitis or eczema).
- Asthma can vary from chronic daily symptoms to only intermittent symptoms. The intervals between symptoms may be days, weeks, months, or years.
- The severity is determined by lung function, symptoms, nighttime awakenings, and interference with normal activity prior to therapy. Patients can present with mild intermittent symptoms that require no medications or only occasional use of short-acting inhaled β2-agonists to severe chronic asthma symptoms despite receiving multiple medications.

SEVERE ACUTE ASTHMA

- Uncontrolled asthma can progress to an acute state where inflammation, airway edema, excessive mucus accumulation, and severe bronchospasm result in profound airway narrowing that is poorly responsive to usual bronchodilator therapy.
- Patients may be anxious in acute distress and complain of severe dyspnea, shortness of breath, chest tightness, or burning. They may be able to say only a few words with each breath. Symptoms are unresponsive to usual measures.
- Signs include expiratory and inspiratory wheezing on auscultation, dry hacking cough, tachypnea, tachycardia, pallor or cyanosis, and hyperinflated chest with intercostal and supraclavicular retractions. Breath sounds may be diminished with very severe obstruction.

DIAGNOSIS

CHRONIC ASTHMA

- The diagnosis of asthma is made primarily by a history of recurrent episodes of coughing, wheezing, chest tightness, or shortness of breath and confirmatory Spirometry.
- The patient may have a family history of allergy or asthma or have symptoms of allergic rhinitis. A history of exercise or cold air precipitating dyspnea or increased symptoms during specific allergen seasons also suggests asthma.
- Spirometry demonstrates obstruction (forced expiratory volume in 1 second [FEV1]/forced vital capacity less than 80%) with reversibility after inhaled β2-agonist administration (at least a 12% improvement in FEV1). Failure of pulmonary function to improve acutely does not necessarily rule out asthma. If baseline Spirometry is normal, challenge testing with exercise, histamine, or methacholine can be used to elicit BHR.

ACUTE SEVERE ASTHMA

- Peak expiratory flow (PEF) and FEV1 are less than 50% of normal predicted values. Pulse oximetry reveals decreased arterial oxygen and O2 saturations. The best predictor of outcome is early response to treatment as measured by improvement in FEV1 at 30 minutes after inhaled β2-agonists.

- Arterial blood gases may reveal metabolic acidosis and a low PaO2.
- The history and physical examination should be obtained while initial therapy is being provided. A history of previous asthma exacerbations (e.g., hospitalizations, intubations) and complicating illnesses (e.g., cardiac disease, diabetes) should be obtained. The patient should be examined to assess hydration status; use of accessory muscles of respiration; and the presence of cyanosis, pneumonia, pneumothorax and upper airway obstruction. A complete blood count may be appropriate for patients with fever or purulent sputum.

TREATMENT (FIG. 48.3)

ACUTE SEVERE ASTHMA

- The goals of treatment include:
  1. Correction of significant hypoxemia;
  2. Rapid reversal of airway obstruction (within minutes);
  3. Reduction of the likelihood of recurrence of severe airflow obstruction; and
  4. Development of a written action plan in case of a future exacerbation.

NON PHARMACOLOGICAL THERAPY

- Patient education and the teaching of self-management skills should be the cornerstone of the treatment program. Self-management programs improve adherence to medication regimens, self-management skills, and use of healthcare services.
- Objective measurements of airflow obstruction with a home peak flow meter may not necessarily improve patient outcomes. The NAEPP advocates use of PEF monitoring only for patients with severe persistent asthma who have difficulty perceiving airway obstruction.
- Avoidance of known allergenic triggers can improve symptoms, reduce medication use, and decrease BHR. Environmental triggers (e.g., animals) should be avoided in sensitive patients, and those who smoke should be encouraged to stop.
- Patients with acute severe asthma should receive supplemental oxygen therapy to maintain arterial oxygen saturation above 90% (above 95% in pregnant women and patients with heart disease). Significant dehydration should be corrected; urine specific gravity may help guide therapy in young children, in whom assessment of hydration status may be difficult.

PHARMACOTHERAPY

β2-Agonists

- The short-acting β2-agonists (Table 30-1) are the most effective bronchodilators available.β2-Adrenergic receptor stimulation activates adenylcyclase, which produces an increase in intracellular cyclic adenosine monophosphate. This results in smooth muscle relaxation, mast cell membrane stabilization, and skeletal muscle stimulation.
- Aerosol administration enhances bronchoselectivity and provides a more

rapid response and greater protection against provocations that induce bronchospasm (e.g., exercise, allergen challenges) than does systemic administration.

- **Albuterol** and other inhaled short-acting selective β_2-agonists are indicated for treatment of intermittent episodes of bronchospasm and are the first treatment of choice for acute severe asthma and EIB. Regular treatment (four times daily) does not improve symptom control over as-needed use.
- **Formoterol** and **Salmeterol** are inhaled long-acting β_2-agonists indicated as adjunctive long-term control for patients with symptoms who are already on low to medium doses of inhaled corticosteroids prior to advancing to medium- or high-dose inhaled corticosteroids. Short-acting β_2-agonists should be continued for acute exacerbations. Long-acting agents are ineffective for acute severe asthma because it can take up to 20 minutes for onset and 1 to 4 hours for maximum bronchodilation after inhalation.
- In acute severe asthma, continuous nebulization of short-acting β_2-agonists (e.g., albuterol) is recommended for patients having an unsatisfactory response after three doses (every 20 minutes) of aerosolized β_2-agonists and potentially for patients presenting initially with PEF or FEV_1 values <30% of predicted normal. Dosing guidelines are presented in Table 48-1.
- Inhaled β_2-agonists agents are the treatment of choice for EIB. Short acting agents provide complete protection for at least 2 hours after inhalation; long-acting agents provide significant protection for 8 to 12 hours initially, but the duration decreases with chronic regular use.
- In nocturnal asthma, long-acting inhaled β_2-agonists are preferred over oral sustained-release β_2-agonists or sustained-release theophylline. However, nocturnal asthma may be an indicator of inadequate anti-inflammatory treatment.

CORTICOSTEROIDS

β_2-adrenergic receptors improve receptor responsiveness to β_2-adrenergic stimulation, thereby reducing mucus production and hyper secretion, reducing BHR, and reducing airway edema and exudation.

- Inhaled corticosteroids are the preferred long-term control therapy for persistent asthma in all patients because of their potency and consistent effectiveness; they are also the only therapy shown to reduce the risk of death from asthma. Comparative doses are included in Table 48-2. Most patients with moderate disease can be controlled with twice-daily dosing; some products have once-daily dosing indications. Patients with more severe disease require multiple daily dosing. Because the inflammatory response of asthma inhibits steroid receptor binding, patients should be started on higher and more frequent doses and then tapered down once control has been achieved. The response to inhaled corticosteroids is delayed; symptoms improve in most patients within the first 1 to 2 weeks and reach maximum improvement in 4 to 8 weeks. Maximum improvement in FEV_1 and PEF rates may require 3 to 6 weeks.

- Systemic toxicity of inhaled corticosteroids is minimal with low to moderate inhaled doses, but the risk of systemic effects increases with high doses. Local adverse effects include dose-dependent oropharyngeal candidiasis and dysphonia, which can be reduced by the use of a spacer device. The ability of spacer devices to enhance lung delivery is inconsistent and should not be relied on.

METHYLXANTHINES (FIG. 48.1)

- **Theophylline** appears to produce bronchodilation by inhibiting phosphodiesterases, which may produces bronchodilator activity through decreased mast cell mediator release, decreased eosinophils basic protein release, decreased T-lymphocyte proliferation, decreased T-cell cytokine release, and decreased plasma exudation.
- Methylxanthines are ineffective by aerosol and must be taken systemically (orally or IV). Sustained-release theophylline is the preferred oral preparation, whereas its complex with ethylenediamine (**Aminophylline**) is the preferred parenteral product due to increased solubility. IV theophylline is also available.
- Theophylline is eliminated primarily by metabolism via hepatic cytochrome P450 mixed-function oxidase microsomal enzymes (primarily CYP1A2 and CYP3A4) with 10% or less excreted unchanged in the kidney. The hepatic cytochrome P450 enzymes are susceptible to induction and inhibition by various environmental factors and drugs. Clinically significant reductions in clearance can result from co therapy with **Cimetidine, Erythromycin, Clarithromycin, Allopurinol, Propranolol, Ciprofloxacin, Interferon, Ticlopidine, Zileuton**, and other drugs. Some substances that enhance clearance include **Rifampin, Carbamazepine, Phenobarbital, Phenytoin, Charcoal-Broiled Meat**, and cigarette smoking.

Because of large interpatient variability in theophylline clearance, routine monitoring of serum theophylline concentrations is essential for safe and effective use. A steady-state range of 5 to 15 mcg/mL is effective and safe for most patients.

- Sustained-release oral preparations are favored for outpatient therapy, but each product has different release characteristics and some products are susceptible to altered absorption from food or gastric pH changes. Preparations unaffected by food that can be administered a minimum of every 12 hours in most patients are preferable.
- Adverse effects include nausea, vomiting, tachycardia, jitteriness, and difficulty sleeping; more severe toxicities include cardiac tachyarrhyth-mias and seizures.
- Sustained-release theophylline is less effective than inhaled corticosteroids and no more effective than oral sustained-release β2-agonists, cromolyn, or leukotriene antagonists.
- The addition of theophylline to optimal inhaled corticosteroids is similar to doubling the dose of the inhaled corticosteroid and is less effective overall than the long-acting β2-agonists as adjunctive therapy.

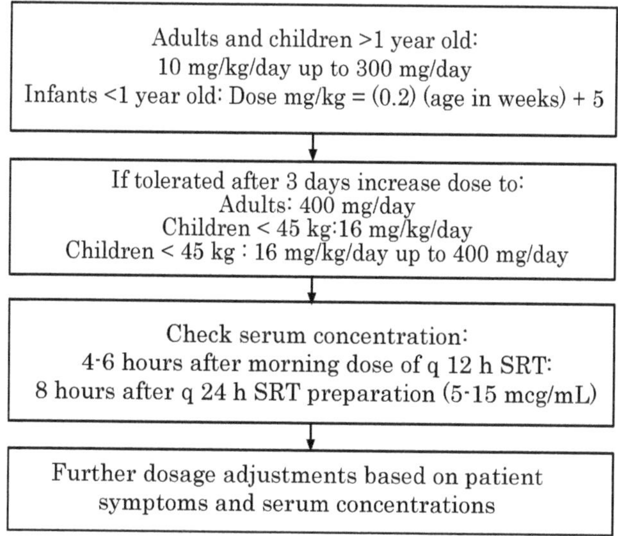

FIGURE 48.1

Algorithm for slow titration of theophylline dosage and guide for final dosage adjustment based on serum theophylline concentration measurement. For infants younger than 1 year of age, the initial daily dosage can be calculated by the following regression equation: Dose (mg/kg) = (0.2) (age in weeks) + 5. Whenever side effects occur, dosage should be reduced to a previously tolerated lower dose. (SRT, sustained-release theophylline).

ANTICHOLINERGICS

- **Ipratropium bromide** and **Tiotropium bromide** are competitive inhibitors of muscarinic receptors; they produce bronchodilation only in cholinergic mediated bronchoconstriction. Anticholinergics are effective bronchodilators but are not as potent as β2-agonists. They attenuate, but do not block, allergen- or exercise-induced asthma in a dose-dependent fashion. The time to reach maximum bronchodilation from aerosolized Ipratropium is longer than from aerosolized short-acting β2-agonists (30 to 60 minutes vs. 5 to 10 minutes). This is of little clinical consequence because some bronchodilation is seen within 30 seconds and 50% of maximum response occurs within 3 minutes. Ipratropium bromide has duration of action of 4 to 8 hours; tiotropium bromide has duration of 24 hours.
- Inhaled ipratropium bromide is only indicated as adjunctive therapy in severe acute asthma not completely responsive to β2-agonists alone because it does not improve outcomes in chronic asthma. Tiotropium bromide has not been studied in asthma.

MAST CELL STABILIZERS

- **Cromolyn sodium** and **Nedocromil sodium** have beneficial effects that are believed to result from stabilization of mast cell membranes. They inhibit the response to allergen challenge as well as EIB but do not cause bronchodilation.

- These agents are effective only by inhalation and are available as metered dose inhalers; cromolyn also comes as a nebulizer solution.
- Both drugs are remarkably nontoxic. Cough and wheezing have been reported after inhalation of each agent, and bad taste and headache after nedocromil.
- Cromolyn and nedocromil are indicated for the prophylaxis of mild persistent asthma in children and adults regardless of etiology. Their effectiveness is comparable to theophylline or leukotriene antagonists for persistent asthma. Neither agent is as effective as inhaled corticosteroids for controlling persistent asthma. Neither is as effective as the inhaled β2- agonists for preventing EIB, but they can be used in conjunction for patients not responding completely to inhaled β2-agonists.
- Most patients experience improvement in 1 to 2 weeks, but it may take longer to achieve maximum benefit. Patients should initially receive cromolyn or nedocromil four times daily; after stabilization of symptoms the frequency may be reduced to two times daily for nedocromil and three times daily for cromolyn.

LEUKOTRIENE MODIFIERS

- **Zafirlukast** (Accolate) and **Montelukast** (Singulair) are oral leukotriene receptor antagonists that reduce the proinflammatory (increased micro vascular permeability and airway edema) and bronchoconstriction effects of leukotriene D4. In adults and children with persistent asthma, they improve pulmonary function tests, decrease nocturnal awakenings and β2-agonist use, and improve asthma symptoms. However, they are less effective in asthma than low-dose inhaled corticosteroids. They are not used to treat acute exacerbations and must be taken on a regular basis, even during symptom-free periods. The adult dose of zafirlukast is 20 mg twice daily, taken at least 1 hour before or 2 hours after meals; the dose for children aged 5 through 11 years is 10 mg twice daily. For montelukast, the adult dose is 10 mg once daily, taken in the evening without regard to food; the dose for children aged 6 to 14 years is one 5-mg chewable tablet daily in the evening.
- Zafirlukast and montelukast are generally well tolerated. Rare elevations in serum aminotransferase concentrations and clinical hepatitis have been reported. An idiosyncratic syndrome similar to the Churg-Strauss syndrome, with marked circulating eosinophilia, heart failure, and associated eosinophilic vasculitis, has been reported in a small number of patients; a direct causal association has not been established.
- **Zileuton** (Zyflo) is an inhibitor of leukotriene synthesis. The dose of zileuton tablets is 600 mg four times daily with meals and at bedtime. The recommended dose of zileuton extended-release tablets is two 600-mg tablets twice daily, within 1 hour after morning and evening meals (total daily dose 2,400 mg).

  Use of zileuton is limited due to the potential for elevated hepatic enzymes (especially in the first 3 months of therapy), and inhibition of the metabolism of some drugs metabolized by CYP3A4 (e.g., theophylline, warfarin). Serum alanine aminotransferase should be monitored before treatment and then periodically thereafter.

Table 48.1

Dosages of drugs for acute severe exacerbations of asthma in the emergency department or hospital

Medications	> 6Years Old	≤ 6 Years Old	Comments
Inhaled β-agonists			
Albuterol nebulizer solution (5 mg/ml)	2.5-5mg every 20 minutes for 3 doses, then 2.5-10mg q 1-4 h as needed, or 10-15 mg/h continuously.	0.15mg/kg (minimum dose 2.5mg) every 20 minutes for three doses, then 0.15-0.3 mg/kg upto10mg q 1-4hr as needed ,or 5mg/kg/hr by continuous nebulization	Only selective β2-agonists are recommended,; for optimal delivery, dilute aerosols to minimum of 4 mL at gas flow of 6-8mL/min.
Albuterol MDI (90 mcg/puff)	4-8 puffs every 30 minutes up to 4 hours, then q 1-4 has needed	4-8 puffs every 20 minutes for three doses, then q 1-4 has needed	In patients in severe distress, nebulization is preferred; use holding-chamber-type spacer
Levalbuterol nebulizer solution	Give at one-half the mg dose of albuterol above	Give at one-half the mg dose of albuterol above	The single isomer of albuterol is likely to be twice as potent on a mg basis
Levalbuterol MDI (45mcg/puff)	Give at one-half the mg dose of albuterol above	Give at one-half the mg dose of albuterol above	
Pirbuterol MDI (200 mcg/puff)	See albuterol dose	See albuterol dose; one half as potent as albuterol on a mcg basis	Has not been studied in acute severe asthma
Systemic β-agonists Epinephrine 1:1,000 (1mg/mL)	0.3-0.5 mg every 20 minutes for three doses subcutaneously	0.01 mg/kg up to 0.5 mg every 20 minutes for three doses subcutaneously	No proven advantage of systemic therapy over aerosol
Terbutaline 91mg/mL)	0.25 mg every 20 minutes for three doses	0.01mg/kg every 20 minutes for three doses, then q 2-6hr as needed subcutaneously	Not recommended
Anticholinergics Ipratropium bromide nebulizer solution (0.25 mg/Ll)	500mcg every 30 minutes for three doses, then q 2-4 hr as needed	250 mcg every 20 minutes for three doses, then 250 mcg q 2-4 hr.	May mix in same nebulizer with albuterol; do not use as first-line therapy; only add to β2-agonist therapy.

Table 48.1 *Contd...*

Medications	> 6Years Old	≤ 6 Years Old	Comments
Inhaled β-agonists			
Ipratropium bromide MDI (17 mcg/puff)	4-8 puffs as needed q 2-4 hr	4-8 puffs as needed q 2-4 hr	Not recommended because dose in inhaler is low and has not been studied in acute asthma
Corticosteroids Prednisone, Methylprednisolone, prednisolone.	60-80 mg in 3-4 divided doses for 48 hours, then 30-40 mg/day until PEF reaches 70% of personal best	1mg/kg every 6 hours for 48 hours, then 1-2 mg/kg/day in two divided doses until PEF is 70% of normal predicted	For outpatient "burst" use 1-2 mg/kg/day, maximum 60mg, for 3-7 days;

FEV1, forced expiratory volume in the first second of expiration; MDI, metered-dose inhaler; PEF, peak expiratory flow.

Table 48.2

Available inhaled corticosteroid products and lung delivery

Inhaled Corticosteroids	Product	Lung Delivery
Betamethasone dipropionate (BDP)	40 and 80 mcg/actuation HFA MDI, 120 actuations	55%-60%
Budesonide (BUD)	200 mcg/dose DPI, Turbuhaler, 200 doses 200-and 500-mcg ampoules, 2ml each	32% (16-59) 6%
Flunisolide (FLU)	250 mcg/actuation CFC MDI, 100 actuations 80mcg/actuation HFA MDI, 120 actuations	20% 68%
Fluticasone propionate (FP)	44,110 and 220 mcg/actuation HFA MDI, 120 actuations 50mcg/dose DPI, Diskus, 60 doses	20%-25% 15%
Mometasone furoate (MF)	200 and 400 mcg/dose DPI, Twist haler, 14, 30, 60 and 120 doses	11%
Triamcinolone acetonide (TAA)	75mcg/actuation CFC MDI, 240 actuations with spacer	22%

CFC, chlorofluorocarbon; DPI, dry-powder inhaler; HFA, hydrofluoroalkane; MDI, metered-dose inhaler; UK, unknown.

COMBINATION CONTROLLER THERAPY

- The addition of a second long-term control medication to inhaled corticosteroid therapy is one recommended treatment option in moderate to severe persistent asthma.
- Single-inhaler combination products containing Fluticasone propionate and salmeterol (Advair) or Budesonide and formoterol (Symbicort) are currently available. The inhalers contain varied doses of the inhaled corticosteroid with a fixed dose of the long-acting β2-agonist.

The addition of a long-acting β2-agonist allows a 50% reduction in inhaled corticosteroid dosage in most patients with persistent asthma. Combination therapy is more effective than higher-dose inhaled corticosteroids alone in reducing asthma exacerbations in patients with persistent asthma.

- Leukotriene receptor antagonists also are successful as additive therapy in patients inadequately controlled on inhaled corticosteroids alone and as corticosteroid-sparing therapy. However, the magnitude of these benefits is less than that reported with the addition of long-acting β2-agonists.

OMALIZUMAB

- **Omalizumab** (Xolair) is an anti-IgE antibody approved for the treatment of allergic asthma not well controlled by oral or inhaled corticosteroids. The dosage is determined by the patient's baseline total serum IgE (international units/ml) and body weight (kg). Doses range from 150 to 375 mg given subcutaneously at either 2- or 4-week intervals.
- Because of its high cost, it is only indicated as step 5 or 6 care for patients who have allergies and severe persistent asthma that is inadequately controlled with the combination of high-dose inhaled corticosteroids and long-acting β2 agonists.

REFERENCES

1. Davies, S. Peak expiratory flow rate monitoring in asthma. In: UpTo Date, Rose, BD(Ed), UpToDate, Wellesley, MA, 2005.
2. Kohler, C. Metered dose inhaler techniques in adults. In: UpToDate, Rose, BD (Ed), UpToDate, Wellesley, MA, 2005.
3. Murray,J.andJ.Nadel. *Textbook of Respiratory Medicine*. Thirdedition. Philadelphia: W.B. Saunders Company, 2000.
4. Peters, et al. "Tiotropium Bromide Step-Up Therapy for Adults With Uncontrolled Asthma." *NEJM* 363(2010):1715-1726.
5. Medically reviewed by: Ellen Reich, MD, Board Certified in Allergy and Immunology, Board Certified in Pediatrics.
6. Shiber JR, Santana J (May 2006). "Dyspnea". *Med. Clin. North Am.* **90** (3): 453–79.
7. "World Health Organization Fact Sheet Fact sheet No 307: Asthma". 2009. Retrieved 2 September 2010.
8. Braman SS (July 2006). "The global burden of asthma". *Chest* **130** (Suppl): 4S-12S.
9. Lazarus SC (August 2010). "Clinical practice. Emergency treatment of asthma". *N. Engl. J. Med.* **363** (8): 755-64.

CHAPTER 49

Chronic Obstructive Pulmonary Disease

DEFINITION

- Chronic obstructive pulmonary disease (COPD) is characterized by airflow limitation that is not fully reversible. The airflow limitation is usually both progressive and associated with an abnormal inflammatory response of the lungs to noxious particles or gases. The most common conditions comprising COPD are chronic bronchitis and emphysema.
- Chronic bronchitis is associated with chronic or recurrent excess mucus secretion (Fig. 49.1) into the bronchial tree with cough that occurs on most days for at least 3 months of the year for at least 2 consecutive years when other causes of cough have been excluded.
- Emphysema is defined as abnormal, permanent enlargement of the airspaces distal to the terminal bronchioles, accompanied by destruction of their walls, but without obvious fibrosis.

PREVALENCE

COPD occurs in 34 out of 1000 greater than 65 years old. In England, an estimated 842,100 of 50 million people have a diagnosis of COPD; translating into approximately one person in 59 receiving a diagnosis of COPD at some point in their lives. In the most socioeconomically deprived parts of the country, one in 32 people were diagnosed with COPD, compared with one in 98 in the most affluent areas. In the United States, the prevalence of COPD is approximately 1 in 20 or 5%, totaling approximately 13.5 million people in USA, or possibly approximately 25 million people if undiagnosed cases are included.

ETIOLOGY

Smoking is the leading cause of COPD. The more a person smokes, the more likely that person will develop COPD. However, some people smoke for years and never get COPD.

In rare cases, nonsmokers who lack a protein called α-1 antitrypsin can develop emphysema.

Other risk factors for COPD are:

- Exposure to certain gases or fumes in the workplace
- Exposure to heavy amounts of secondhand smoke and pollution
- Frequent use of cooking fire without proper ventilation

PATHOPHYSIOLOGY

- The most common etiology is exposure to environmental tobacco smoke, but other chronic inhalational exposures can also lead to COPD. Inhalation of noxious particles and gases stimulates the activation of neutrophils, macrophages, and CD8+ lymphocytes, which release a variety of chemical mediators, including tumor necrosis factor-α, interleukin-8, and leukotriene B4. These inflammatory cells and mediators lead to widespread destructive changes in the airways, pulmonary vasculature, and lung parenchyma.
- Other pathophysiologic processes may include oxidative stress and an imbalance between aggressive plus protective defense systems in the lungs (proteases and antiprotcases). Increased oxidants generated by cigarette smoke react with and damage various proteins and lipids, leading to cell and tissue damage. Oxidants also promote inflammation directly and exacerbate the protease-antiprotease imbalance by inhibiting antiprotease activity.
- The protective antiprotease α1-antitrypsin (AAT) inhibits several protease enzymes, including neutrophil elastase. In the presence of unopposed AAT activity, elastase attacks elastin, which is a major component of alveolar walls. A hereditary deficiency of AAT results in an increased risk for premature development of emphysema. In the inherited disease, there is an absolute deficiency of AAT. In emphysema resulting from cigarette smoking, the imbalance is associated with increased protease activity or reduced activity of antiproteases.
- Activated inflammatory cells release several other proteases, including cathepsins and metalloproteinase's. In addition, oxidative stress reduces antiprotease (or protective) activity.
- An inflammatory exudate is often present in the airways that lead to an increased number and size of goblet cells and mucus glands. Mucus secretion increases, and ciliary motility is impaired. There is thickening of the smooth muscle and connective tissue in the airways. Chronic inflammation leads to scarring and fibrosis. Diffuse airway narrowing occurs and is more prominent in small peripheral airways.
- Parenchymal changes affect the gas-exchanging units of the lungs (alveoli and pulmonary capillaries). Smoking-related disease most commonly results in centrilobular emphysema that primarily affects respiratory bronchioles. Pan lobular emphysema is seen in AAT deficiency and extends to the alveolar ducts and sacs.
- Vascular changes include thickening of pulmonary vessels that may lead to endothelial dysfunction of the pulmonary arteries. Later, structural changes increase pulmonary pressures, especially during exercise. In severe COPD, secondary pulmonary hypertension leads to right-sided heart failure (cor pulmonale).

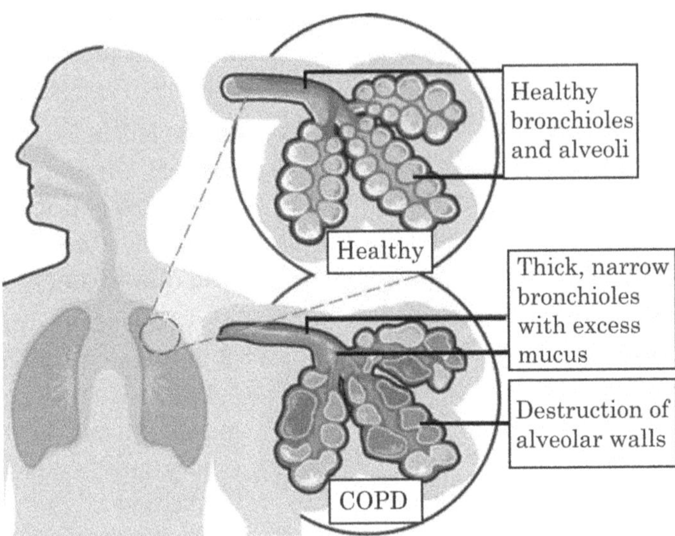

FIGURE 49.1

Alveoli with excess mucus.

(Source : Adapted from http://www.nature.com/nature/journal/v489/n7417_supp/full/489S2a.htm)

CLINICAL FEATURES

- Initial symptoms of COPD include chronic cough and sputum production; patients may have these symptoms for several years before dyspnea develops.
- The physical examination is normal in most patients who present in the milder stages of COPD. When airflow limitation becomes severe, patients may have cyanosis of mucosal membranes, development of a "barrel chest" due to hyperinflation of the lungs, an increased resting respiratory rate, shallow breathing, pursing of the lips during expiration, and use of accessory respiratory muscles.
- Patients experiencing a COPD exacerbation may have worsening dyspnea, increase in sputum volume, or increase in sputum purulence. Other common features of an exacerbation include chest tightness, increased need for bronchodilators, malaise, fatigue, and decreased exercise tolerance.

DIAGNOSIS

- The diagnosis of COPD is based in part on the patient's symptoms and a history of exposure to risk factors such as tobacco smoke and occupational exposures.

PULMONARY FUNCTION TESTS

- Assessment of airflow limitation through spirometry is the standard for diagnosing and monitoring COPD. The forced expiratory volume after 1 second (FEV1) is generally reduced except in very mild disease. The forced vital capacity (FVC) may also be decreased. The hallmark of COPD is a reduced FEV1: FVC ratio to less than 70%. A post bronchodilator

FEV1 that is less than 80% of predicted confirms the presence of airflow limitation that is not fully reversible.

- An improvement in FEV1 of less than 12% after inhalation of a rapid acting bronchodilator is considered to be evidence of irreversible airflow obstruction.
- Peak expiratory flow measurements are not adequate for diagnosis of COPD because of low specificity and a high degree of effort dependence. However, a low peak expiratory flow is consistent with COPD.

ARTERIAL BLOOD GASES

- Significant changes in arterial blood gases are not usually present until the FEV1 is less than 1 L. At this stage, hypoxemia and hypercapnia may become chronic problems. Hypoxemia usually occurs initially with exercise but develops at rest as the disease progresses.
- Patients with severe COPD can have a low arterial oxygen tension (PaO_2 45 to 60 mm Hg) and an elevated arterial carbon dioxide tension ($PaCO_2$ 50 to 60 mm Hg). Hypoxemia results from hypoventilation (V) of lung tissue relative to perfusion (Q) of the area. The low V: Q ratio progresses over several years, resulting in a consistent decline in the PaO_2.
- Some patients lose the ability to increase the rate or depth or respiration in response to persistent hypoxemia. This decreased ventilatory drive may be due to abnormal peripheral or central respiratory receptor responses. This relative hypoventilation leads to hypercapnia; in this situation the central respiratory response to a chronically increased $PaCO_2$ can be blunted. Because these changes in PaO_2 and $PaCO_2$ are subtle and progress over many years, the pH is usually near normal because the kidneys compensate by retaining bicarbonate.
- If acute respiratory distress develops (e.g., due to pneumonia or a COPD exacerbation) the $PaCO_2$ may rise sharply resulting in an uncompensated respiratory acidosis.

DIAGNOSIS OF ACUTE RESPIRATORY FAILURE IN CHRONIC OBSTRUCTIVE PULMONARY DISEASE

- The diagnosis of acute respiratory failure in COPD is made on the basis of an acute drop in PaO_2 of 10 to 15 mm Hg or any acute increase in $PaCO_2$ that decreases the serum pH to 7.3 or less.
- Additional acute clinical manifestations include restlessness, confusion, tachycardia, diaphoresis, cyanosis, hypotension, irregular breathing, miosis, and unconsciousness.
- The most common cause of acute respiratory failure in COPD is acute exacerbation of bronchitis with an increase in sputum volume and viscosity. This serves to worsen obstruction and further impair alveolar ventilation, resulting in worsening hypoxemia and hypercapnia. Additional causes are pneumonia, pulmonary embolism, left ventricular failure, pneumothorax, and CNS depressants.

TREATMENT OF CHRONIC OBSTRUCTIVE PULMONARY DISEASE

NONPHARMACOLOGICAL THERAPY

- Smoking cessation is the most effective strategy to reduce the risk of developing

COPD and the only intervention proven to affect the long term decline in FEV1 and slow the progression of COPD.

- Pulmonary rehabilitation programs include exercise training along with smoking cessation, breathing exercises, optimal medical treatment, psychosocial support, and health education. Supplemental oxygen, nutritional support, and psycho educational care (e.g., relaxation) are important adjuncts in a pulmonary rehabilitation program.
- One dose of the polyvalent pneumococcal vaccine is indicated for patients at any age with COPD; revaccination is recommended for patients older than 65 years if the first vaccination was more than 5 years earlier and the patient was younger than 65 years.

PHARMACOLOGICAL THERAPY

Bronchodilators are used to control symptoms; no single pharmacologic class has been proven to provide superior benefit over others, although inhaled therapy is generally preferred. Medication

Selection is based on likely patient adherence, individual response, and side effects. Medications can be used as needed or on a scheduled basis, and additional therapies should be added in a stepwise manner depending on response and disease severity. Clinical benefits of bronchodilators include increased exercise capacity, decreased air trapping, and relief of symptoms such as dyspnea. However, significant improvements in pulmonary function measurements such as FEV1 may not be observed.

SYMPATHOMIMETICS

- β2-Selective sympathomimetics cause relaxation of bronchial smooth muscle and bronchodilation by stimulating the enzyme adenylcyclase to increase the formation of cyclic adenosine monophosphate. They may also improve mucociliary clearance.
- Administration via metered-dose inhaler (MDI) or dry-powder inhaler is at least as effective as nebulization therapy and is usually favored for reasons of cost and convenience.
- **Albuterol, Levalbuterol, Bitolterol, Pirbuterol,** and **Terbutaline** are the preferred short-acting agents because they have greater β2 selectivity and longer durations of action than other short-acting agents **(Isoproterenol, Metapro-terenol, And Isoetharine)**. The inhalation route is preferred to the oral and parenteral routes in terms of both efficacy and adverse effects. Short-acting agents can be used for acute relief of symptoms or on a scheduled basis to prevent or reduce symptoms.
- **Formoterol** and **Salmeterol** are long-acting inhaled β2-agonists that are dosed every 12 hours on a scheduled basis and provide bronchodilation throughout the dosing interval. In 2007, Formoterol and **Arformoterol** became available in the United States as nebulized solutions. Long-acting inhaled β2-agonists should be considered when patients demonstrate a frequent need for short-acting agents. They are also useful to decrease nocturnal symptoms and improve quality of life. They are not indicated for acute relief of symptoms.

ANTICHOLINERGICS

- When given by inhalation, Anticholinergic agents produce broncho-dilation by competitively inhibiting cholinergic receptors in bronchial smooth muscle. This activity blocks acetylcholine, with the net effect being a reduction in cyclic guanosine monophosphate, which normally acts to constrict bronchial smooth muscle.
- **Ipratropium bromide** has a slower onset of action than short-acting β2-agonists (15 to 20 minutes vs. 5 minutes for albuterol). For this reason, it may be less suitable for as needed use, but it is often prescribed in this manner. Ipratropium has a more prolonged bronchodilator effect than short-acting β2-agonists. Its peak effect occurs in 1.5 to 2 hours and its duration is 4 to 6 hours. The recommended dose via MDI is two puffs four times a day with upward titration often to 24 puffs/day. It is also available as a solution for nebulization. The most frequent patient complaints are dry mouth, nausea, and, occasionally, metallic taste. Because it is poorly absorbed systemically, Anticholinergic side effects are uncommon (e.g., blurred vision, urinary retention, nausea, and tachycardia).
- **Tiotropium bromide** is a long-acting agent that protects against cholinergic bronchoconstriction for more than 24 hours. Its onset of effect is within 30 minutes with a peak effect in 3 hours.

COMBINATION OF ANTICHOLINERGICS AND SYMPATHOMIMETICS

- The combination of an inhaled Anticholinergic and β2-agonist is often used, especially as the disease progresses and symptoms worsen over time. Combining bronchodilators with different mechanisms of action allows the lowest effective doses to be used and reduces adverse effects from individual agents. Combination of both short- and long-acting β2-agonists with ipratropium has been shown to provide added symptomatic relief and improvements in pulmonary function.
- A combination product containing **Albuterol** and **Ipratropium (Combivent)** is available as an MDI for chronic maintenance therapy of COPD. Other similar combination products may become available in the future **Methylxanthines**
- **Theophylline** and **aminophylline** may produce bronchodilation by inhibition of phosphodiesterase (thereby increasing cyclic adenosine monophosphate levels), inhibition of calcium ion influx into smooth muscle, prostaglandin antagonism, stimulation of endogenous catecholamine's, adenosine receptor antagonism, and inhibition of release of mediators from mast cells and leukocytes.
- Chronic theophylline use in COPD has been shown to produce improvements in lung function, including vital capacity and FEV1. Subjectively, theophylline has been shown to reduce dyspnea, increase exercise tolerance, and improve respiratory drive. Nonpulmonary effects that may contribute to better functional capacity include improved cardiac function and decreased pulmonary artery pressure.
- Methylxanthines are no longer considered first-line therapy for COPD. Inhaled

bronchodilator therapy is preferred over theophylline for COPD because of theophylline risk for drug interactions and the interpatient variability in dosage requirements. Theophylline may be considered in patients who are intolerant or unable to use an inhaled bronchodilator. A Methylxanthines may also be added to the regimen of patients who have not achieved an optimal clinical response to an inhaled Anticholinergic and β_2- agonist.

- As with other bronchodilators in COPD, parameters other than objective measurements such as FEV1 should be monitored to assess efficacy. Subjective parameters, such as perceived improvements in dyspnea and exercise tolerance, are important in assessing the acceptability of Methylxanthines for COPD patients.
- Sustained-release theophylline preparations improve patient compliance and achieve more consistent serum concentrations than rapid-release theophylline and aminophylline preparations.
- The role of theophylline in COPD is as maintenance therapy in non–acutely ill patients. Therapy can be initiated at 200 mg twice daily and titrated upward every 3 to 5 days to the target dose; most patients require daily doses of 400 to 900 mg.
- The most common side effects of theophylline include dyspepsia, nausea, vomiting, diarrhea, headache, dizziness, and tachycardia. Arrhythmias and seizures may occur, especially at toxic concentrations.
- Factors that may decrease theophylline clearance and lead to reduced dosage requirements include advanced age, bacterial or viral pneumonia, heart failure, liver dysfunction, hypoxemia from acute decompensation, and use of drugs such as cimetidine, Macrolides, and fluoroquinolone antibiotics. Factors that may enhance theophylline clearance and result in the need for higher doses include tobacco and marijuana smoking, hyperthyroidism, and use of drugs such as phenytoin, phenobarbital, and rifampin.

CORTICOSTEROIDS

- The anti-inflammatory mechanisms whereby corticosteroids exert their beneficial effect in COPD include reduction in capillary permeability to decrease mucus, inhibition of release of proteolytic enzymes from leukocytes, and inhibition of prostaglandins.
- The clinical benefits of systemic corticosteroid therapy in the chronic management of COPD are often not evident, and there is a high risk of toxicity. Consequently, chronic, systemic corticosteroids should be avoided if possible.
- Appropriate situations to consider corticosteroids in COPD include (1) Short-term systemic use for acute exacerbations; and (2) Inhalation therapy for chronic stable COPD.
- The role of inhaled corticosteroids in COPD is controversial. Major clinical trials have failed to demonstrate any benefit from chronic treatment in modifying long-term decline in lung function. However, other important benefits have been observed in some patients, including a decrease in exacerbation frequency and improvements in overall health status.

- Consensus guidelines indicate that inhaled corticosteroid therapy should be considered for symptomatic patients with stage III or IV disease (FEV1 less than 50%) who experience repeated exacerbations despite bronchodilator therapy.
- Side effects of inhaled corticosteroids are relatively mild and include hoarseness, sore throat, oral candidiasis, and skin bruising. Severe side effects such as adrenal suppression, osteoporosis, and cataract formation are reported less frequently than with systemic corticosteroids, but clinicians should monitor patients receiving high-dose chronic inhaled therapy.
- Several studies have shown an additive effect with the combination of inhaled corticosteroids and long-acting bronchodilators. Combination therapy with salmeterol plus Fluticasone or Formoterol plus Budesonide is associated with greater improvements in FEV1, health status, and exacerbation frequency than either agent alone. The availability of combination inhalers makes administration of both drugs convenient and decreases the total number of inhalations needed daily.

REFERENCES

1. Agarwal R, Aggarwal AN, Gupta D, Jindal SK. Inhaled corticosteroids vs placebo for preventing COPD exacerbations: a systematic review and metaregression of randomized controlled trials. *Chest.* 2010; 137(2):318-325.
2. Shapiro SD, Reilly JJ Jr., Rennard SI. Chronic bronchitis and emphysema. In: Mason RJ, Broaddus VC, Martin TR, et al.*Murray & Nadel's Textbook of Respiratory Medicine*. 5th ed. Philadelphia, Pa: Saunders Elsevier; 2010:chap 39.
3. "What is COPD?". *National Heart Lung and Blood Institute*. U.S. National Institutes of Health. June 1, 2010.
4. COPD (Chronic Obstructive Pulmonary Disease)
5. "2007 NHLBI Morbidity and Mortality Chart Book" (PDF). Retrieved 2008-06-06.
6. Kitaguchi Y, Fujimoto K, Kubo K, Honda T (October 2006). "Characteristics of COPD phenotypes classified according to the findings of HRCT". *Respir Med* **100** (10): 1742–52.
7. Paoletti M, Camiciottoli G, Meoni E, et al. (December 2009). "Explorative data analysis techniques and unsupervised clustering methods to support clinical assessment of Chronic Obstructive Pulmonary Disease (COPD) phenotypes". *J Biomed Inform* **42** (6): 1013–21.
8. Badgett RG, Tanaka DJ, Hunt DK, et al. (1994). "The clinical evaluation for diagnosing obstructive airways disease in high-risk patients". *Chest* **106** (5): 1427–31.

CHAPTER 50

Pulmonary Hypertension

PULMONARY ARTERIAL PRESSURE

Pulmonary arterial pressure is generated by the right ventricle ejecting blood into the pulmonary circulation, which acts as a resistance to the output from the right ventricle. With each ejection of blood during ventricular systole, the pulmonary arterial blood volume increases, this stretches the wall of the artery. As the heart relaxes (ventricular diastole), blood continues to flow from the pulmonary artery into the pulmonary circulation. The smaller arteries and arterioles serve as the chief resistance vessels, and through changes in their diameter, regulate pulmonary vascular resistance.

In hemodynamic terms, the mean pulmonary arterial pressure (PAP) can be described by the following Equation:

$$PAP = (CO \times PVR) + PVP$$

Where,

CO = cardiac output,

PVR = pulmonary vascular resistance, and

PVP = pulmonary venous pressure.

The pulmonary venous pressure (PVP) is essentially the same as left atrial pressure. Therefore, increases in cardiac output (CO), pulmonary vascular resistance (PVR) or pulmonary venous pressure (PVP) will lead to increases in pulmonary arterial pressure (PAP). Normally, mean pulmonary arterial pressure is about 15 mmHg, and the pulmonary arterial systolic and diastolic pressures are about 25 and 10 mmHg, respectively.

PULMONARY ARTERIAL HYPERTENSION - TYPES & CAUSES

Pulmonary arterial hypertension (PAH) is defined as a mean pulmonary arterial pressure greater than 25 mmHg at rest, or greater than 30 mmHg during exercise. One older way to classify PAH is as two broad categories:

- Primary PAH
- Secondary PAH

- **Primary PAH** has no known precipitating cause (i.e., it is idiopathic) and appears to be hereditary in some individuals. This is a progressive disease that has a poor prognosis and no known cure.
- **Secondary PAH** results from an identifiable cause or condition. The most common cause of secondary PAH is chronic obstructive pulmonary disease. Chronic hypoxia associated with this

condition results in pulmonary vasoconstriction (hypoxic vasoconstriction). Other causes include obstructive sleep apnea, congenital heart disease, chronic hypoxemia, pulmonary thrombosis (blood clots), or left ventricular failure.

More recently, the World Health Organization developed a classification scheme that is based on the underlying mechanism/cause of PAH. Hemodynamically, PAH can be caused by:

- ✓ Increased right ventricular output
- ✓ Increased pulmonary systemic vascular resistance, (or)
- ✓ Increased pulmonary venous pressure.

Because the pulmonary vasculature is normally very compliant, large increases in right ventricular output do not normally cause PAH. However, if the pulmonary vasculature loses its compliance due to disease, then increased right ventricular output can lead to PAH during exercise, for example. Most individuals with primary or secondary PAH have increased pulmonary vascular resistance, which can be caused by structural changes in the vasculature or by increased smooth contraction. Patients who have left ventricular systolic or diastolic failure, or who have severe mitral valve stenosis or regurgitation, can also have secondary pulmonary hypertension because of an increase in pulmonary venous pressure.

RATIONALE FOR PHARMACOLOGIC TREATMENT

If pulmonary arterial hypertension (PAH) has an identifiable cause, then measures can be taken to correct the underlying problem. If the diagnosis is primary PAH, or treating the cause of the secondary PAH does not restore normal pulmonary artery pressure, then pharmacologic intervention is required to reduce the pressure. This is done by using vasodilator drugs to decrease pulmonary vascular resistance and thereby lower the pressure. Adjunctive therapy may include diuretics to reduce blood volume, which will reduce central venous pressure and right ventricular stroke volume, as wellas reduce some of the signs and symptoms of edema and shortness of breath associated with PAH. Anticoagulants are administered to prevent the formation of pulmonary thrombi.

TREATMENT

DIURETICS (Pulmonary & Systemic Oedema): Capillary hydrostatic pressure and therefore capillary fluid filtration is strongly influenced by venous pressure. Therefore, diuretics, by reducing blood volume and venous pressure, lower capillary hydrostatic pressure, which reduces net capillary fluid filtration and tissue edema.

CALCIUM CHANNEL BLOCKERS

For those patients who had a positive vasodilator response and relatively well preserved RV function, CCB therapy should be considered. The mechanism of action for vaso-relaxation is enhanced endothelial intracellular calcium release. CCB options include nifedipine, amlodipine, or diltiazem. Verapamil is avoided since it exhibits negative inotropic effects. It may also be best to start with short acting agents in the monitored setting to insure tolerability before converting to long-acting preparations. Close clinical follow-up of patients on CCB treatment is critical as acuter esponse may not guarantee long-term benefit.

Table 50.1

Functional assessment of pulmonary arterial hypertension

A. New York Heart Association functional classification	
Class 1:	No symptoms with ordinary physical activity.
Class 2:	Symptoms with ordinary activity. Slight limitation of activity.
Class 3:	Symptoms with less than ordinary activity. Marked limitation of activity.
Class 4:	Symptoms with any activity or even at rest.
B. World Health Organization functional assessment classification	
Class 1:	Patients with PH but without resulting limitation of physical activity. Ordinary physical activity does not cause undue dyspnea or fatigue, chest pain, or near syncope.
Class 2:	Patients with PH resulting in slight limitation of physical activity. They are comfortable at rest. Ordinary physical activity causes undue dyspnea or fatigue, chest pain, or near syncope.
Class 3:	Patients with PH resulting in marked limitation of physical activity. They are comfortable at rest. Less than ordinary activity causes undue dyspnea or fatigue, chest pain, or near syncope.
Class 4:	Patients with PH with inability to carry out any physical activity without symptoms. These patients manifest signs of right-heart failure. Dyspnea and/or fatigue may even be present at rest. Discomfort is increased by any physical activity.

Indeed, a long-term prospective study indicated that long-term response occurs in less than 10% of patients with idiopathic PAH. Side effects associated with the use of CCB include dizziness, hypotension, and fluid retention.

Table 50.2

Dosage of calcium channel blockers used in pulmonary arterial hypertension

Medication	Starting Dose	Range
Nifedipine (long-acting)	30 mg/day	30 - 240 mg/day
Amlodipine	2.5 mg/day	2.5 - 20 mg/day
Diltiazem (long-acting)	120 mg/day	120 - 900 mg/day

Calcium channel blockers and typical doses that are utilized in patients who have a positive acute vasodilator response with preserved right ventricular function. When initiating calcium channel blockers, starting doses are used initially, often with short-acting preparations, and increased as tolerated.

ENDOTHELIN RECEPTOR ANTAGONISTS

Endothelin-1 (ET-1) is a 21 amino acid peptide that is produced by the vascular endothelium. It is a very potent vasoconstrictor that binds to smooth muscle endothelin receptors, of which there are two subtypes: ETA and ETB receptors. These receptors are coupled to a Gq-protein and receptor activation leads to the formation of

IP3, which causes the release of calcium by the sarcoplasmic reticulum (SR) and increased smooth muscle contraction and vasoconstriction. There are also ETB receptors located on the endothelium that stimulate the formation of nitric oxide, which produces vasodilation in the absence of smooth muscle ETA and ETB receptor activation. This receptor distribution helps to explain the phenomenon that ET-1 administration causes transient vasodilation (initial endothelial ETB activation) and hypotension, followed by prolong vasoconstriction (smooth muscle ETA and ETB activation) and hypertension. ET-1 receptors in the heart are also linked to the Gq-protein and IP3 signal transduction pathway. Therefore, ET-1 in the heart causes SR release of calcium, which increases contractility. ET-1 also increases heart rate.

THERAPEUTIC INDICATIONS

Because of its powerful vasoconstrictor properties, and its effects on intracellular calcium, ET-1 has been implicated in the pathogenesis of hypertension, coronary vasospasm, and heart failure. A number of studies suggest a role for ET-1 in pulmonary hypertension, as well as in systemic hypertension. ET-1 has been shown to be released by the failing myocardium where it can contribute to cardiac calcium overload and hypertrophy. Endothelin receptor antagonists, by blocking the vasoconstrictor and cardiotonic effects of ET-1, produce vasodilation and cardiac inhibition. Endothelin receptor antagonists have been shown to decrease mortality and improve hemodynamics in experimental models of heart failure. At present, the one approved indication for endothelin antagonists is pulmonary hypertension.

Specific Drugs: Blockade of the endothelin receptor has been used in the treatment of PAH. Several endothelin receptor antagonists (ERAs) have been identified and differ in their selectivity toward the ET-A and ETB receptors. Currently, both selective and nonselective ERAs are approved and available for treating PAH.

- BOSENTAN (Tracleer) shows 20:1 ET-A /ET-B selectivity
- AMBRISENTAN (Letairis) 100:1 ET-A /ET-B selectivity and
- SITAXSENTAN (Thelin) has 6500:1 ET-A /ET-B selectivity

BOSENTAN TRIAL OF ENDOTHELIN ANTAGONIST THERAPY (BREATHE-1):

Thc Bosentan Trial of Endothelin Antagonist Therapy (BREATHE-1) study revealed the ability of oral bosentan in patients with PAH to improve 6 min walk test distance, improve dyspnea scores and time to clinical worsening as early as 16 weeks after initiating therapy.

The recommended treatment dosage is 125mg twice daily after careful uptitration. Bosentan can increase transaminase levels in a reversible pattern. As a result of the potential for elevated transaminases, patients receiving bosentan require monthly monitoring of liver function during continuous therapy. It is recommended that if the transaminase levels are increased to at least three times the upper limit of normal, the dosage either needs to be held or decreased until the transaminase levels return to a normal range before resuming therapy.

AMBRISENTAN, RANDOMIZED, DOUBLE-BLINDED, MULTICENTER, EFFICACY STUDY (ARIES I &II)

Ambrisentan is a more selective ET-A receptor antagonist and is currently clinically available. The Ambrisentan in Pulmonary Artery Hypertension, Randomized, Double-Blinded, Placebo-Controlled, Multicenter, Efficacy Study I and II (ARIES I and II) demonstrated the efficacy of ambrisentan in improving 6 min walk test distance and time to clinical worsening. Although ambrisentan is in the same pharmacologic class as bosentan and its use requires transaminase monitoring, elevation of transaminases was not seen in any patient treated with ambrisentan. Side effects more commonly seen were nasal congestion, peripheral edema, and headaches.

SITAXSENTAN TO RELIEVE IMPAIRED EXERCISE TRIALS (STRIDE 1 AND 2)

Sitaxsentan, is the most selective ET-A receptor antagonist clinically available. The Sitaxsentan to Relieve Impaired Exercise trials (STRIDE 1 & 2) did show 6 min walk test distance improvement and functional class improvement, there had been reported prior cases of fatal hepatitis at higher doses in the STRIDE 2 patient population comparable with placebo.

Note: All three drugs are contraindicated in conjunction with cyclosporine A and glyburide

- Bosentan induces warfarin metabolism and requires an increase in the warfarin dose
- Sitaxsentan decreases warfarin metabolism, requiring a drop in the warfarin dose
- There are no known interactions between ambrisentan and warfarin.

It is important to mention that a clinically meaningful difference between the three approved ERAs with respect to their endothelin receptor selectivity has not been demonstrated to date. In clinical practice, therefore, other features are likely to be of greater relevance when considering treatment, such as the potential for serious

Table 50.3

Dosage of endothelin receptor antagonists used in pulmonary arterial hypertension

Endothelin receptor antagonist	Oral dose	Information
Bosentan	Starting: 62.5 mg Twice daily Maintenance: 125 mg twice daily	FDA approved for use in WHO functional class II/III/IV PAH
Ambrisentan	Starting: 5 mg daily Maintenance: 5 or 10 mg daily	FDA approved for the once-daily treatment of WHO functional class II/III PAH.
Sitaxsentan	100 mg daily	Approved for the once-daily treat-ment of WHO functional class III PAH. Current status: the manufacturer voluntarily removed sitaxsentan from the market and halted clinical trials due to concerns about liver toxicity.

drug– drug interactions, convenience of the dosing schedule, and rates of limiting side effects. These characteristics bear more relation to the chemical or pharmacologic properties of the drug than to receptor selectivity itself.

A recently published robust meta-analysis confirmed the therapeutic benefit of ERAs but concluded that they have no proven effect on mortality. It is important, however, to highlight that there has been no definitive study proving a survival benefit for any ERA, owing to the fact that long-term, placebo controlled studies are perceived as ethically unjustifiable and randomized, controlled trials are not powered to detect a mortality benefit.

PHOSPHODIESTERASE-5 INHIBITORS

Sildenafil (Revatio) is a PDE-5 inhibitor initially approved for erectile dysfunction but subsequently shown to have effects on the pulmonary vasculature. Sildenafil increases the effects of locally produced nitric oxide (NO) by inhibiting the breakdown of NO's second messenger, cyclic guanosine monophosphate. This results in pulmonary vasodilation and inhibition of smooth muscle cell growth. Sildenafil is currently approved for the treatment of WHO class II and III patients.

SILDENAFIL Use in Pulmonary Arterial Hypertension (SUPER-1)

The Sildenafil Use in Pulmonary Arterial Hypertension (SUPER-1) trial showed improvement in 6 min walk test distances in patients receiving sildenafil at 20, 40, or 80mg three times daily compared with patients receiving placebo as early as 4 weeks and extending to 12 weeks. No significant improvements were noted at dosages above 20mg three times daily in the short-term trial. Therefore, it is recommended that only the lower dose be used in clinical practice.

Tadalafil (Adcirca) is the second PDE-5 inhibitor that has recently been approved by the FDA. The results of the Pulmonary Arterial Hypertension and Response to Tadalafil (PHIRST-1) study showed a improvement in 6 min walk test distance adjusted for placebo at 16 weeks in naïve treatment plus combined therapy with bosentan, and a improvement in patients also on monotherapy. Tadalafil has a longer half-life than sildenafil, thus allowing once daily dosing. The recommended daily dose is 40mg.

Vardenfil (Levitra) is a new PDE-5 inhibitor that has shown some efficacy in the treatment of PAH. A recently published randomized, double-blind, placebo-controlled study confirmed that vardenafil is effective and well tolerated in patients with PAH at a dose of 5mg twice daily. Like ERAs, PDE-5 inhibitors have no proven effect on mortality.

Prostanoids: Prostacyclin synthase levels are low in patients with PAH; the production of prostacyclin is diminished, preventing adequate vasodilation and loss of the antiproliferative effects on the smooth muscle cells in the vascular wall. Through their actions as potent pulmonary artery vasodilators, prostanoid medications have been used in the treatment of PAH.

Epoprostenol (Flolan) was the first FDA approved therapy for PAH. Because of its short half-life, it requires delivery through a continuous portable infusion pump and an indwelling central venous catheter. Epoprostenol remains the treatment of choice for patients with the most advanced disease and leads to improvements in

Table 50.4

Dosage of phosphodiesterase-5 inhibitors used in pulmonary arterial hypertension

Medication	Dose	Special Consideration
Sildenafil (Revatio)	20mg three times daily	t½=4hours. Administer doses 4-6 hours apart with or without food. Patients may have poor compliance with midday dose. Metabolized by CYP3A
Tadalafil (Adcirca)	40mg (two 20 mg tablets) daily	t½=35hours. Metabolized by CYP3A 2 tablets should be taken together once daily which can sometimes be confusing for patients.

exercise capacity, hemodynamics, and quality of life. Epoprostenol is the most comprehensively studied of all the prostanoids. It has been shown to have favourable hemodynamic effects, including lowering mean pulmonary artery pressure and pulmonary vascular resistance and increasing cardiac output.

Difficulties in administration include the need for permanent intravenous access, resulting in infected catheters, flushing, thrombocytopenia, gastrointestinal disturbances, headaches, and pain on mastication. Longer-acting prostacyclin analogs have also been developed for intravenous, inhaled, and oral use, with variable effectiveness and tolerability. These analogs include:

- Treprostinil (Remodulin), approved for subcutaneous and intravenous use
- Iloprost (Ventavis), approved for inhaled, intravenous and inhaled use
- Beraprost an oral medication approved in Japan

Iloprost is available as an inhaled prostanoid agent through a nebulizer device. The aerosolized delivery route and low incidence of adverse events are positive attributes of inhaled iloprost, while the frequency of administration and lack of comparative data limit its role in PAH. Common side effects include flushing, cough, headache, and jaw pain on mastication. Iloprost is currently FDA approved for functional class II and III patients.

Treprostinil has the pharmacologic profile of epoprostenol with a much longer half life, permitting subcutaneous rather than intravenous administration. Side effects are similar to those of other prostanoid agents.

Beraprost is absorbed rapidly after the administration of an oral dose of tablets under fasting conditions; it reaches a peak concentration within 30 min and has an elimination half life of 35–40 min. Of all the currently available therapeutic options for PAH, epoprostenol is the only drug that has a significant mortality benefit.

Table 50.5

Dosage of prostanoids used in pulmonary arterial hypertension

Medication	Dose	Route	Special Considerations
EPOPROSTENOL (Flolan)	2ng/kg/min titrated to desired clinical response in 2ng/kg/min increments; usual long term dose is 20-40 ng/kg/ min range	IV	t½=3-5minutes Continuous infusion Obtain from Specialty Pharmacy
TREPROSTINIL (Remodulin)	1.25-2.5 ng/kg/min; usual dose 30-80 ng/kg/min. 6mcg/ inhalation, 9 inhalations four times daily during waking hours	IV/SQ Inhaled	t½=4hours Continuous infusion Site pain for SQ Obtain from Specialty Pharmacy Inhalation System Respiratory tract symptoms Obtain from Specialty Pharmacy
ILOPROST (Ventavis)	2.5-5mcg, 6-9 inhalations daily during waking hours	Inhaled	t½=20-30minutes Frequent administration Respiratory tract symptoms Obtain from Specialty Pharmacy

SOLUBLE GUANYLATE CYCLASE STIMULATOR RIOCIGUAT

Riociguat was approved by the USFDA in 2013 to treat adults with two forms of PH: PAH & Chronic thromboembolic pulmonary hypertension (CTEPH). Riociguat represents a different mechanism of action compared to other currently available PAH specific therapy. It is a soluble guanylate cyclase (sGC) stimulator that produces vasodilation. Specifically, riociguat sensitizes sGC to endogenous NO by stabilizing NO-sGC binding and also acts in synergy with NO by directly stimulating sGC independently of NO availability.

Table 50.6

Dosage of soluble guanylate cyclase stimulator riociguat used in pulmonary arterial hypertension

Medication	Dose	Special Comments
Riociguat (Adempas)	0.5-1mg three times a day, increase dose at 0.5mg intervals no greater than 2 weeks as tolerated to max 2.5mg three times a day	t½= 12 hours Female patients can only obtain medication through a special program **Contraindications:** Pregnancy Concomitant nitrates or nitric oxide donors, phosphodiesterase inhibitors

REFERENCES

1. Galie' N, Ussia G, Passarelli P, Parlangeli R, Branzi A, Magnani B. Role of pharmacologic tests in the treatment of primary pulmonary hypertension. Am J Cardiol 1995; 75: 55A–62A.
2. Rich S, Kaufmann E, Levy PS. The effect of high doses of calcium-channel blockers on survival in primary pulmonary hypertension. N Engl J Med 1992; 327: 76–81.
3. Jing ZC, Jiang X, Han ZY, Xu XQ, Wang Y, Wu Y, Lv H, Ma CR, Yang YJ, Pu JL. Iloprost for pulmonary vasodilator testing in idiopathic pulmonary arterial hypertension. Eur Respir J 2009; 33: 1354–1360.
4. Barst RJ, McGoon M, Torbicki A, Sitbon O, Krowka MJ, Olschewski H, Gaine S. Diagnosis and differential assessment of pulmonary arterial hypertension. J Am Coll Cardiol 2004; 43(Suppl 1): S40–S47.
5. Galie' N, Olschewski H, Oudiz RJ, Torres F, Frost A, Ghofrani HA, Badesch DB, McGoon MD, McLaughlin VV, Roecker EB, Gerber MJ, Dufton C, Wiens BL, Rubin LJ. Ambrisentan for the treatment of pulmonary arterial hypertension. Results of the ambrisentan in pulmonary arterial hypertension, randomized, double-blind, placebo-controlled, multicenter, efficacy (ARIES) study 1 and 2. Circulation 2008; 117: 3010–3019.
6. Matura LA, McDonough A, Carroll DL. Health-related quality of life and psychological states in patients with pulmonary arterial hypertension. J Cardiovasc Nurs 2014; 29: 178–184
7. Cenedese E, Speich R, Dorschner L, Ulrich S, Maggiorini M, Jenni R, Fischler M. Measurement of quality of life in pulmonary hypertension and its significance. Eur Respir J 2006; 28: 808–815.
8. Pulido T, Adzerikho I, Channick RN, Delcroix M, Galie' N, Ghofrani HA, Jansa P, Jing ZC, Le Brun FO, Mehta S, Mittelholzer CM, Perchenet L, Sastry BKS, Sitbon O, Souza R, Torbicki A, Zeng X, Rubin LJ, Simonneau G. Macitentan and morbidity and mortality in pulmonary arterial hypertension. New Engl J Med 2013; 369: 809–818.

Cystic Fibrosis

Cystic fibrosis (CF) is a severe, complex, hereditary disease that affects 1 of every 3,200 live births, or approximately 30,000 children and adults in the United States. The course and severity of cystic fibrosis are variable and unpredictable. The median life expectancy (i.e., about 40 years) for a child born with CF in 1990 was about double what would have been expected for a child diagnosed with CF 20 years earlier because of advances in the management of this disorder. Although therapy continues to rely on treatment of symptoms rather than the underlying pathologic causes, continuing improved understanding of CF is likely to result in better control and perhaps a cure. CF is still a lethal disease, but aggressive therapy can decrease the morbidity of this disease and increase the life expectancy of the patient.

CLINICAL MANIFESTATIONS

Genotype, environmental factors, and modifier gene status all contribute to the highly variable clinical course of CF. The linking of the loss of Cystic Fibrosis Transmembrane Conductance Regulator (CFTR) function to clinical manifestations of the disease, however, has been central to gaining an understanding of the disease and in the discovery of new therapies. Normally, CFTR is highly expressed on the membranes of epithelial cells of the lungs, sweat glands, salivary glands, and male genital ducts as well as the pancreas, kidney tubules, and digestive tract.

SWEAT GLANDS

Fluid secreted by the sweat glands in patients with CF is normal, but a defect in the reabsorption of electrolytes leads to sweat with a high salt content. CFTR, in the apical membrane of the resorptive area of the sweat gland, functions as an ion channel for chloride transport and also activates an associated epithelial sodium channel (ENaC). Normally, these channels efficiently reabsorb sodium chloride from sweat. In patients with CF, loss of these functioning channels blocks the ability of the sweat ducts to reabsorb salt, leading to sweat sodium chloride (NaCl) concentrations of >100 mM. The loss of these sodium and chloride ion channels serves as the basis for the diagnostic sweat chloride test and as the scientific basis for the "infant who tastes of salt" in folklore.

SINUS INVOLVEMENT

Nasal polyps, which are outgrowths of normal sinus epidermis, can be found in up to 20% of older patients with CF and may become sufficiently large to block nasal passages. The pathogenesis of these polyps is unknown, but the obstruction of nasal passages can lead to infection. The faulty ionic transport of chloride across the apical membrane of epithelial cells lining exocrine glands leads to dehydration of extracellular fluids and the development of thickened inspissated mucus in nasal and sinus passages. Most patients with CF develop sinus disease with pan-opacification of the sinuses in 90% to 100% of patients >8 months of age. On radiographic examination, >90% of adult-age patients have pansinusitis, which can contribute to pulmonary exacerbations. The impact of sinusitis on the CF population is significant.

PANCREATIC INVOLVEMENT

The exocrine and ultimately the endocrine function of the pancreas are affected in CF. Pancreatic enzymes normally are secreted into bicarbonate-rich fluid from the pancreatic duct, and CFTR is needed to secrete the bicarbonate into the lumen. The loss of CFTR function inhibits secretion of digestive enzymes and bicarbonate into the duodenum, and the enzymes are trapped in the pancreas by ductal obstruction. Over time, these enzymes (lipase, protease, amylase) accumulate and eventually begin to digest the pancreatic tissue. The term *cystic fibrosis* arises from the fibrotic scar tissue that replaces the destroyed pancreas. Without these enzymes, there is poor digestion of fats and, to a lesser extent, proteins and carbohydrates are absorbed poorly. As a result, 90% of patients with CF experience pancreatic insufficiency characterized by steatorrhea (fatty stools), decreased absorption of the fat-soluble vitamins (A, D, E, and K), malnutrition, and failure to thrive. Early in life, serum concentrations of amylase and lipase are increased secondary to pancreatic auto digestion. This destructive process can result in either painful or asymptomatic chronic pancreatitis. Eventually, the progressive destruction of the pancreas affects its endocrine function, leading to glucose intolerance in about 17% of children and 75% of adults. Diabetes mellitus occurs in approximately 40% of adult patients with CF. The additional diagnosis of diabetes in CF is associated with significantly increased morbidity and mortality, and a decrease in insulin sensitivity is associated with pulmonary exacerbations. Early aggressive insulin therapy can result in improved clinical outcomes.

INTESTINAL INVOLVEMENT

Meconium ileus, an intestinal obstruction at birth, occurring in 20% of newborns with CF, is an inheritable trait of this disease. Outside the neonatal period, distal intestinal obstruction syndrome (DIOS, also called *meconium ileus equivalent*) can occur at any age and results from the complete or partial obstruction of the intestine. Intestinal obstruction occurs in 10% to 20% of patients and results from the inspissation of intestinal secretions and incompletely digested intestinal contents. A right lower quadrant mass, abdominal distention, failure to pass stools, and vomiting can accompany DIOS. Gastrointestinal reflux disease (GERD) is common in both children and adults with CF. Children with CF should be screened for GERD and treated, if diagnosed. Other intestinal complications include rectal prolapse, intussusception, and appendiceal abscesses.

HEPATIC INVOLVEMENT

Located on the apical surfaces of the cells lining the intrahepatic and extrahepatic bile ducts and the gallbladder, CFTR functions to facilitate ion transport. In patients with CF, the abnormal chloride efflux across the cells results in the reduction in water and sodium movement into the bile. The resulting decrease in the volume and flow of bile leads to stasis and obstruction of the biliary tree. With chronic obstruction, there is inflammation, giving rise to the characteristic lesion of focal biliary cirrhosis. Liver disease develops in the first decade of life. Significant liver disease is seen in 13% to 25% of children with CF. Prevalence rates may be underestimated. Progressive cirrhosis is associated with portal hypertension, hypersplenism, esophageal varices, ascites, and, in a small number of patients, complete hepatic failure requiring transplantation. Approximately 30% of adult patients with CF have abnormal gallbladder function and size (absent or small gallbladder) with 5% to 10% of patients developing gallstones.

GENITOURINARY INVOLVEMENT

Approximately 98% of males with CF are infertile secondary to *in utero* obstruction of the vas deferens or related structures. Hormonal secretion and secondary sexual characteristics are normal. In a small number of patients, infertility can be the only manifestation of disease, and CF may go undiagnosed until fertility testing is performed. The prevalence of infertility is higher in women with CF and hypothesized to be related to the production of thick and tenacious cervical mucus. Hundreds of pregnancies have been carried successfully to term, but these are not without risk, especially for patients with moderate to severe pulmonary disease.

BONE AND JOINT INVOLVEMENT

Patients with CF have low bone mineral density, slower rate of bone formation, high rate of bone loss, accelerated rate of bone loss, and arthritis. Osteoclastic precursors are elevated during acute pulmonary exacerbation. Although early, aggressive treatment of pulmonary exacerbations can improve bone health, sufficient intake and absorption of the fat-soluble vitamins, D and K, are important, and oral bisphosphonates may also be indicated. Patients with CF often suffer from intermittent arthritis symptoms, but only about 2% of patients have persistent symptoms. The three types of intermittent CF arthritis are

(a) hypertrophic osteoarthropathy,

(b) immunoreactive, and

(c) CF arthropathy.

PULMONARY INVOLVEMENT

The relationship of ion-channel disruption (resulting from CFTR dysfunction) to lung tissue destruction has yet to be firmly established. Presently, the CF gene mutation is believed to cause CFTR dysfunction, which in turn causes ion transporter defects, and subsequent changes in the airway secretions. The changes in airway secretions promote the infection-inflammation-tissue damage cycle. Chronic infection combined with inflammation has been the hallmark of lung disease in CF. The cycle of unchecked inflammation and infection has been the focus of much investigation and ongoing debate to "Which came first—infection or inflammation." Although the inflammatory response appears to set up bacterial colonization in the airways, infection also can stimulate an inflammatory response. In either case, the cycle of inflammation and infection eventually leads to lung tissue damage and bronchiectasis. This pattern of inflammation and infection has not been observed in any other tissue where CFTR is expressed. Differences in the airway surface liquid, mucus, and other protective mechanisms in the lung of the patient with CF are being studied, and some of these differences may help explain the inflammation–infection cycle.

Infection: Despite repeated courses of aggressive antibiotic therapy, patients with CF eventually develop endobronchial bacterial colonization and infection. Understanding why bacteria seldom are eradicated is important to treating this disease. The lower airways of a normal lung are always maintained free of pathogens through various lung defense mechanisms.

For example, a thin film of liquid on the airway surfaces called the *airway surface layer* (ASL) contains antimicrobials, antioxidants, proteases, and other substances that work to eliminate pathogens. The ASL also signals molecules to turn on the cellular immune system by recruiting neutrophils and macrophages to the site of microbe invasion. In addition, the ASL can remove invading microbes from the lung by moving a mucous gel toward the mouth through ciliary motion. Mucociliary clearance of microbes and debris is aided by the cough reflex to keep the airways clean. Because coughing is an important defense mechanism necessary for patients with CF, cough suppressants should not be prescribed or taken by them.

Inflammation: Inflammation is the lung's response to chronic infection. Neutrophils (PMN) are "called" to the site of an infection by interleukin-1 (IL-1), interleukin-8 (IL-8), leukotriene (LTB4), endotoxin, and tumor necrosis factor (TNF-α). IL-8 is a major chemoattractant, and when bound to heparan sulfatecontaining proteoglycans, its activity is prolonged. When neutrophils arrive at the site, they release proteases, oxidants, elastases, and cytokines. Antiproteases and interleukin- 10 (IL-10), an anti-inflammatory cytokine, subsequently are released in an effort to counterbalance the inflammatory system. Platelets also are dysfunctional and can contribute to inflammation through nitric oxide pathway. Anti-inflammatory compounds are relatively low in patients with CF, and levels of neutrophils, proteases, elastases, oxidants, and cytokines all are increased. These abnormalities lead to a sustained and destructive cycle of unchecked inflammation that begins at a very early age. Arachidonic acid (AA), an agonist in the inflammation pathway, is increased, and docosahexaenoic acid (DHA), a down regulator of AA, is decreased in the bronchial lavage fluid in patients with CF. This imbalance of fatty acids favors the inflammatory and mucus-producing AA, and, therefore, provides an explanation for the role of CFTR in causing inflammation and increased mucus production in the airways.

SYMPTOMS AND SIGNS

Cystic fibrosis should be suspected in a young adult with a history of chronic lung disease (especially bronchiectasis), pancreatitis, or infertility. Cough, sputum production, decreased exercise tolerance, and recurrent hemoptysis are typical complaints. Patients also often complain of chronic rhinosinusitis symptoms, steatorrhea, diarrhea, and abdominal pain. Patients with cystic fibrosis are often malnourished with low body mass index. Digital clubbing, increased anteroposterior chest diameter, hyperresonance to percussion, and apical crackles are noted on physical examination. Sinus tenderness, purulent nasal secretions, and nasal polyps may also be seen. Nearly all men with cystic fibrosis have congenital bilateral absence of the vas deferens with azoospermia. Biliary cirrhosis and gallstones may occur.

TREATMENT

Early recognition and comprehensive multidisciplinary therapy improve symptom control and the chances of survival. Referral to a regional cystic fibrosis center is strongly recommended. Conventional treatment programs focus on the following areas:

1. Clearance and reduction of lower airway secretions
2. Reversal of bronchoconstriction
3. Treatment of respiratory tract infections and airway bacterial burden
4. Pancreatic enzyme replacement and
5. Nutritional and psychosocial support (including genetic and occupational counseling).

The Pulmonary Therapies Committee, established by the Cystic Fibrosis Foundation, has issued evidenced-based recommendations regarding long-term use of medications for maintenance of lung function and reduction of exacerbations in patients with cystic fibrosis. Clearance of lower airway secretions can be promoted by postural drainage, chest percussion or vibration techniques, positive expiratory pressure (PEP) or flutter valve breathing devices, directed cough, and other breathing techniques; these approaches require detailed patient instruction by experienced personnel. Inhaled recombinant human deoxyribonuclease (rhDNase, dornase alpha) cleaves extracellular DNA in sputum, decreasing sputum viscosity; when administered long-term at a daily nebulized dose of 2.5 mg, this therapy leads to improved FEV1 and reduces the risk of cystic fibrosis–related respiratory exacerbations and the need for intravenous antibiotics. Inhalation of hypertonic saline twice daily has been associated with small improvements in pulmonary function and fewer pulmonary exacerbations. The beneficial effects of hypertonic saline may derive from improved airway mucous clearance.

Short-term antibiotics are used to treat active airway infections based on results of culture and susceptibility testing of sputum. *S aureus* (including methicillinresistant strains) and a mucoid variant of *P aeruginosa* are commonly present. *H influenzae, Stenotrophomonas maltophilia*, and *B cepacia* (a highly drug-resistant organism) are occasionally isolated.

Long-term antibiotic therapy is helpful in slowing disease progression and reducing exacerbations in patients with sputum cultures positive for *P aeruginosa*. These antibiotics include azithromycin 500 mg orally three times a week, which has immunomodulatory properties, and various inhaled antibiotics (e.g, tobramycin, aztreonam, colistin, and levofloxacin) taken two to three times a day. The length of therapy depends on the persistent presence of *P aeruginosa* in the sputum. The incidence of atypical mycobacterial colonization is higher in cystic fibrosis patients, and directed antibiotic treatment is recommended for frequent exacerbations, progressive decline in lung function, or failure to thrive. Yearly screening with sputum acidfast bacilli cultures is advised.

Inhaled bronchodilators (eg, albuterol, two puffs every 4 hours as needed) should be considered in patients who demonstrate an increase of at least 12% in FEV 1 after an inhaled bronchodilator. An inhaled corticosteroid should be added to the treatment regimen for patients who have cystic fibrosis with persistent asthma or allergic bronchopulmonary mycosis.

Ivacaftor is an oral medication, available for the 5% of cystic fibrosis patients with a G551D mutation. Ivacaftor is a potentiator of the CFTR channel that works by increasing the time the channel remains open after being activated; it has been found to improve lung function by 10% within 2 weeks of treatment, decrease pulmonary exacerbations by 55%, and decrease sweat chloride into the indeterminate range. CFTR corrector therapy for the most common mutation (DeltaF508) is under trial.

Lung transplantation is the only definitive treatment for advanced cystic fibrosis. Double-lung or heart-lung transplantation is required. A few transplant centers offer living lobar lung transplantation to selected patients. The 3-year survival rate following transplantation for cystic fibrosis is about 55%.

Vaccination against pneumococcal infection and annual influenza vaccination are advised.

Screening of family members and genetic counseling are suggested.

NON- PHARMACOLOGICAL TREATMENT

CF patients should be managed by multidisciplinary specialized teams. The overall care involves education to improve their quality of life, good nutrition and the prompt treatment of exacerbations to avoid hospitalization.

- General care should include stopping smoking, vaccination with influenza and pneumococcal vaccines and pulmonary rehabilitation.
- Oxygen therapy should be given as necessary.
- Seventy per cent of adults with CF have Pseudomonas infection in their sputum. Nebulized anti-pseudomonal antibiotic therapy improves lung function and decreases the risk of infective exacerbations and hospitalization in these patients.
- Drug therapy includes β2 agonists and inhaled corticosteroids. These produce symptomatic relief but have no effect on long-term survival.
- Airway clearance. Inhalation of recombinant DNAse (dornase alfa 2.5 mg daily) has been shown to improve FEV1 by 20% in some patients. Hypertonic saline by inhalation (in concentrations of up to 7%) gives shortterm benefit.

Amiloride, which inhibits sodium transport, has been used but no overall benefit has been shown in meta-analysis. N-acetylcysteine has been shown in vitro to liquefy CF sputum by cleaving disulfide bonds in mucus glycoproteins but clinical studies have been disappointing.

- Non-invasive ventilation improves symptoms in chronic respiratory failure but there is no evidence of a survival benefit. It acts as a bridge to lung transplantation
- Treatment for pancreatic insufficiency and malnutrition.
- Human experimental studies have been conducted on the delivery to the epithelium of the normal CFTR gene using, as a vector, a replication-deficient adenovirus containing normal human CFTR complementary DNA which is trophic for epithelial cells. Gentamicin can suppress premature termination codons, and nasal administration has been shown to correct the physiological abnormality. These studies are in their early stages.

REFERENCES

1. Henneman L et al. Evaluation of cystic fibrosis carrier screening programs according to genetic screening criteria. Genet Med 4: 241, 2002.
2. Matsui H et al. Evidence for periciliary liquid layer depletion, not abnormal ion composition, in the pathogenesis of cystic fibrosis airways disease. Cell 95:1005, 1998.
3. Prince AS: Biofilms, antimicrobial resistance, and airway infection. NEngl J Med 347: 1110, 2002.
4. Worlitsch D et al. Effects of reduced mucus oxygen concentration in airway pseudomonas infections of cystic fibrosis patients. J Clin Invest 109:317, 2002.
5. Flume PA et al. Cystic Fibrosis Foundation Pulmonary Therapies Committee. Cystic fibrosis pulmonary guidelines: pulmonary complications: hemoptysis and pneumothorax. Am J Respir Crit Care Med. 2010 Aug 1; 182(3): 298–306.
6. Mogayzel PJ Jr et al; Pulmonary Clinical Practice Guidelines Committee. Cystic fibrosis pulmonary guidelines. Chronic medications for maintenance of lung health. Am J Respir Crit Care Med. 2013 Apr 1; 187(7): 680–9.
7. Flume PA et al; Cystic Fibrosis Foundation Pulmonary Therapies Committee. Cystic fibrosis pulmonary guidelines: treatment of pulmonary exacerbations. Am J Respir Crit Care Med. 2009 Nov 1; 180(9): 802–8.

CHAPTER 52

Hemoptysis

Hemoptysis is defined as the spitting of blood derived from the lungs or bronchial tubes as a result of pulmonary or bronchial hemorrhage. Hemoptysis is classified as nonmassive or massive based on the volume of blood loss; however, there are no uniform definitions for these categories. In this article, hemoptysis is considered nonmassive if blood loss is less than 200 mL per day. The lungs receive blood from the pulmonary and bronchial arterial systems. The low-pressure pulmonary system tends to produce small-volume hemoptysis, whereas bleeding from the bronchial system, which is at systemic pressure, tends to be profuse. Blood loss volume is more useful in directing management than in reaching a diagnosis. After confirming the presence of blood, an initial task is differentiating between hemoptysis, pseudohemoptysis (i.e., the spitting of blood that does not come from the lungs or bronchial tubes), and hematemesis (i.e., the vomiting of blood).

CAUSES OF HEMOPTYSIS

In the primary care setting, the most common causes of hemoptysis are acute and chronic bronchitis, pneumonia, tuberculosis, and lung cancer.

INFECTION

Infection is the most common cause of hemoptysis, accounting for 60 to 70 percent of cases. Infection causes superficial mucosal inflammation and edema that can lead to the rupture of the superficial blood vessels. In a retrospective study of inpatient and outpatient hemoptysis in the United States, bronchitis caused 26 percent of cases, pneumonia caused 10 percent, and tuberculosis accounted for 8 percent. Invasive bacteria (e.g., Staphylococcus aureus, Pseudomonas aeruginosa) or fungi (e.g., Aspergillus species) are the most common infectious causes of hemoptysis. Viruses such as influenza also may cause severe hemoptysis. Human immunodeficiency virus (HIV) infection predisposes patients to several conditions that may produce hemoptysis, including pulmonary Kaposi's sarcoma.

CANCER

Primary lung cancers account for 23 percent of cases of hemoptysis in the United States. Bronchogenic carcinoma is a common lung cancer responsible for hemoptysis in 5 to 44 percent of all cases. Bleeding from malignant or benign tumors can be secondary to superficial mucosal invasion, erosion into blood vessels, or highly vascular lesions. Breast, renal, and colon cancers have a predilection for lung metastasis; however, metastatic lung carcinoma rarely results in bleeding. Obstructive lesions may cause a secondary infection, resulting in hemoptysis.

PULMONARY VENOUS HYPERTENSION

Cardiovascular conditions that result in pulmonary venous hypertension can cause cardiac hemoptysis. The most common of these is left ventricular systolic heart failure. Other cardiovascular causes include severe mitral stenosis and pulmonary embolism. Although hemoptysis is a recognized pulmonary embolism symptom, pulmonary embolism is an uncommon cause of hemoptysis. For example, in a patient without underlying cardiopulmonary disease, the positive and negative likelihood ratios for hemoptysis in pulmonary embolism are 1.6 and 0.95, respectively. Therefore, the presence or absence of hemoptysis alone has no significant effect on the likelihood of pulmonary embolism.

IDIOPATHY

Idiopathic hemoptysis is a diagnosis of exclusion. In 7 to 34 percent of patients with hemoptysis, no identifiable cause can be found after careful evaluation. Prognosis for idiopathic hemoptysis usually is good, and the majority of patients have resolution of bleeding within six months of evaluation. However, results from one study found an increasing incidence of lung cancer in smokers older than 40 years with idiopathic hemoptysis, and suggested that these patients may warrant close monitoring.

HAEMOPTYSIS IN CHILDREN

The major cause of hemoptysis in children is lower respiratory tract infection. The second most common cause is foreign body aspiration, with most cases occurring in children younger than four years. Another important cause is bronchiectasis, which often is secondary to cystic fibrosis. Primary pulmonary tuberculosis is a rare cause estimated to occur in less than 1 percent of cases. Although uncommon, trauma is another possible cause. Blunt-force trauma may result in hemoptysis secondary to pulmonary contusion and hemorrhage. Bleeding caused by suffocation, deliberate or accidental, also should be considered.

Table 52.1

Causes of haemoptysis.
1. Tracheobronchial source
2. Bronchiectasis
3. Airway trauma
4. Foreign body Pulmonary parenchymal source
5. Lung abscess
6. Pneumonia
7. Tuberculosis
8. Mycetoma ('fungus ball')
9. Goodpasture's syndrome
10. Idiopathic pulmonary haemosiderosis
11. Wegener's granulomatosis
12. Lupus pneumonitis
13. Lung contusion Primary vascular source
14. Arterio-venous malformation
15. Pulmonary embolism
16. Elevated pulmonary venous pressure (mitral stenosis)
17. Pulmonary artery rupture secondary to balloon-tip pulmonary artery catheter manipulation
18. Pulmonary endometriosis

Systemic coagulopathy or use of anticoagulants or thrombolytic agents.

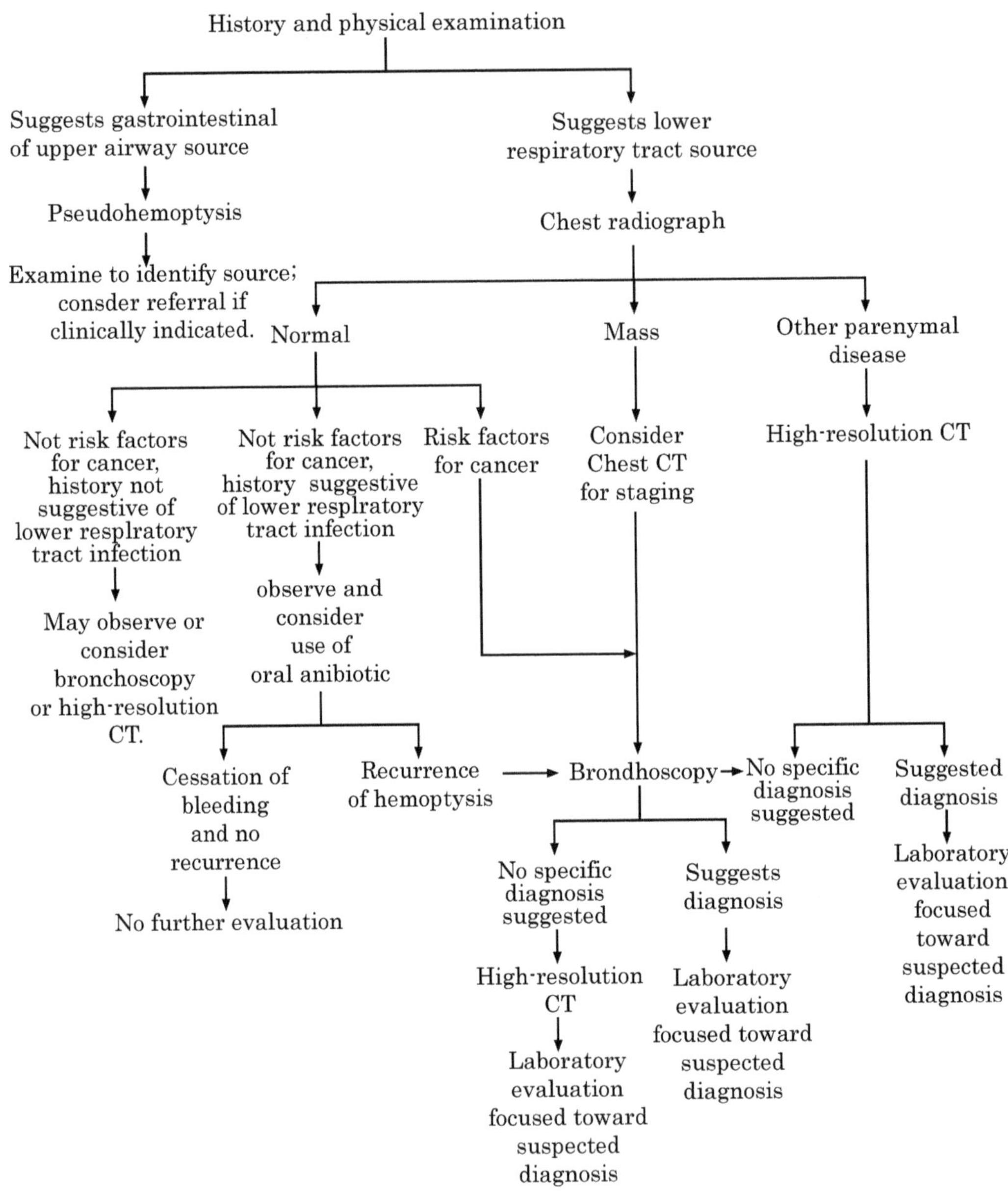

FIGURE 52.1

Algorithm for diagnosing nonmassive hemoptysis. (CT = computed tomography).

(source : Adapted with permission from Harrison TR, Braunwald E. Cough and hemoptysis. In: Harrison's Principles of internal medicine. 15th ed. New York: McGraw-Hill, 2001:208.)

MANAGEMENT

NONMASSIVE HEMOPTYSIS

The overall goals of management of the patient with hemoptysis are threefold: bleeding cessation, aspiration prevention, and treatment of the underlying cause. As with any potentially serious condition, evaluation of the "ABCs" (i.e., airway, breathing, and circulation) is the initial step.

Patients with hemoptysis should be managed based on the rate and severity of bleeding (massive or nonmassive) and the clinical condition of the patient. In case of massive bleeding in unstable patients, resuscitation is mandatory before any other diagnostic investigation. The most common presentation is acute, mild hemoptysis caused by bronchitis. Low-risk patients with normal chest radiographs can be treated on an outpatient basis with close monitoring and appropriate oral antibiotics, if clinically indicated. If hemoptysis persists or remains unexplained, an outpatient evaluation by a pulmonologist should be considered.

An abnormal mass on a chest radiograph warrants an outpatient bronchoscopic examination. For patients with a normal chest radiograph and risk factors for lung cancer or recurrent hemoptysis, outpatient fiberoptic bronchoscopy also is indicated to rule out neoplasm. High-resolution CT is indicated when clinical suspicion for malignancy exists and sputum and bronchoscopy do not yield any pathology. High-resolution CT also is indicated when chest radiography reveals peripheral or other parenchymal disease.

MASSIVE HEMOPTYSIS

A Chest radiography (CXR) should always be performed as a first instance exam. If the underlying parenchymal or pleural abnormalities causing hemoptysis (i.e., pneumonia, mass, etc.) are identified, the diagnostic and therapeutic management for the detected lesion should follow (i.e., antibiotic treatment for a young patient with fever and a pulmonary opacity on CXR; further investigation in case of a middle-aged, smoker patient with a pulmonary opacity on CXR). If hemoptysis does not resolve or recurs, further treatment (medical, endovascular, and surgical) should be considered. On the other hand, it is advised to perform a Multidetector Computed Tomography Angiography (MDCTA) in case of a negative or non localizing CXR, particularly when a lung cancer cannot be excluded.

If MDCTA reveals the cause of hemoptysis, the standard diagnostic and therapeutic management for the underlying condition should be performed. If MDCTA is negative and the episode of hemoptysis is resolving, it is possible to stop the investigation, whereas further examination such as bronchoscopy is warranted if the hemoptysis is persistent. In case of a positive result at bronchoscopy, the flowchart follows the same indication as for the above-mentioned positive diagnostic tests. If a cause cannot be identified even at bronchoscopy, a cryptogenic hemoptysis should be considered. Clinicians should wait for a spontaneous resolution of bleeding in the first instance; however, in cases of recurrent bleeding an endovascular treatment could be advised.

The mortality rate from massive hemoptysis depends on the bleeding rate and etiology. Hemoptysis greater than 1,000 mL per 24 hours in the presence of malignancy carries a mortality rate of 80 percent; therefore, massive hemoptysis warrants a more aggressive, expedient approach. These patients require intensive care and early consultation with a pulmonologist. In cases of massive or life-threatening hemoptysis, diagnosis and therapy must occur simultaneously. Supplemental oxygen and fluid resuscitation are essential. Assistance by a cardiothoracic surgeon should be considered because emergency surgical intervention may be needed.

REFERENCES

1. Stedman TL. Stedman's Medical dictionary. 27th ed. Philidelphia: Lipincott Williams & Wilkins, 2000.
2. Thompson AB, Teschler H, Rennard SI. Pathogenesis, evaluation, and therapy for massive hemoptysis. *Clin Chest Med.* 1992; 13: 69–82.
3. Knott-Craig CJ, Oostuizen JG, Rossouw G, Joubert JR, Barnard PM. Management and prognosis of massive hemoptysis. Recent experience with 120 patients. *J Thorac Cardiovasc Surg.* 1993; 105: 394-7.
4. Cahill BC, Ingbar DH. Massive hemoptysis. Assessment and management. *Clin Chest Med.* 1994; 15: 147–67.
5. Harrison TR, Braunwald E. Hemoptysis. In: Harrison's Principles of internal medicine. 15th ed. New York: McGraw-Hill, 2001: 203–6.
6. Reisz G, Stevens D, Boutwell C, Nair V. The causes of hemoptysis revisited. A review of the etiologies of hemoptysis between 1986 and 1995. *Mo Med.* 1997; 94: 633–5.
7. Bond D, Vyas H. Viral pneumonia and hemoptysis. *Crit Care Med.* 2001; 29: 2040–1.
8. Nelson JE, Forman M. Hemoptysis in HIV-infected patients. *Chest.* 1996; 110: 737–43.
9. Santiago S, Tobias J, Williams AJ. A reappraisal of the causes of hemoptysis. *Arch Intern Med.* 1991; 151: 2449–51.
10. Hirshberg B, Biran I, Glazer M, Kramer MR. Hemoptysis: etiology, evaluation, and outcome in a tertiary referral hospital. *Chest.* 1997; 112: 440–4.
11. Anish EJ, Mayewski RJ. Pulmonary embolism. In: Black ER, ed. Diagnostic strategies for common medical problems. Philadelphia: American College of Physicians, 1999: 325–37.
12. Set PA, Flower CD, Smith IE, Chan AP, Twentyman OP, Shneerson JM. Hemoptysis: comparative study of the role of CT and fiberoptic broncho-scopy. *Radiology.* 1993; 189: 677–80.
13. Herth F, Ernst A, Becker HD. Long-term outcome and lung cancer incidence in patients with hemoptysis of unknown origin. *Chest.* 2001; 120: 1592–4.
14. Jean-Baptiste E. Clinical assessment and management of massive hemoptysis. Crit Care Med. 2000; 28: 1642–7.

CHAPTER 53

Insomnia and Anxiety

INSOMNIA

DEFINITION

Insomnia is trouble falling asleep or staying asleep through the night. Episodes may come and go (episodic), last up to 3 weeks (short-term), or be long-lasting (chronic).

PREVALENCE

The National Sleep Foundation's 2002 *Sleep in America* poll showed that 58% of adults in the U.S. experienced symptoms of insomnia a few nights a week or more. Although insomnia was the most common sleep problem among about one half of older adults (48%), they were less likely to experience frequent symptoms of insomnia than their younger counterparts (45% vs. 62%), and their symptoms were more likely to be associated with medical conditions, according to the poll of adults between the ages of 55 and 84.

ETIOLOGY

Sleep habits learnt at childhood may affect sleep behaviours as adults. When these behaviours are repeated over many years, they become habits.

Poor sleep or lifestyle habits that may cause insomnia or make it worse:

- Going to bed at different times each night
- Daytime napping
- Poor sleeping environment, such as too much noise or light
- Spending too much time in bed while awake
- Working evening or night shifts
- Not getting enough exercise

The use of some medications and drugs may also affect sleep:

- Alcohol or other drugs
- Heavy smoking
- Too much caffeine, especially late in the day
- Getting used to certain types of sleep medications
- Some cold medications and diet pills

Physical, social, and mental health issues can affect sleep patterns, including:

- Anxiety disorders
- Bipolar disorder
- Certain medical conditions, such as thyroid disease
- Feeling sad or depressed. Often, insomnia is the symptom that causes people with depression to seek medical help.
- Physical pain or discomfort

- Stress, whether it is short-term or long-term. For some people, the stress caused by the insomnia makes it even harder to fall asleep.

SLEEP PHYSIOLOGY

- Humans typically have four to six cycles of non–rapid eye movement (NREM) and rapid eye movement (REM) sleep each night, each cycle lasting 70 to 120 minutes. Usually there is progression through the four stages of NREM sleep before the first REM period.
- Stage 1 of NREM is the stage between wakefulness and sleep. Stage 3 and 4 sleep is called *delta sleep* (i.e., slow-wave sleep).
- In REM sleep, there is a low-amplitude, mixed-frequency electroence-phalogram, increased electric and metabolic activity, increased cerebral blood flow, muscle atonia, poikilothermia, vivid dreaming, and fluctuations in respiratory and cardiac rate.
- In the elderly, sleep is lighter and more fragmented with more arousals and a gradual reduction in slow-wave sleep.
- Sleep is reduced when there is decreased serotonin activity or destruction of the dorsal raphe nucleus.
- REM sleep is turned on by cholinergic cells.
- Dopamine has an alerting effect. Neurochemicals involved in wakefulness include norepinephrine and acetylcholine in the cortex and histamine and
- Neuropeptides (e.g., substance P and corticotrophin-releasing factor) in the hypothalamus.
- Polysomnography (PSG) is a procedure that measures multiple electrophysiologic parameters simultaneously during sleep (e.g., electroencephalogram, electro-oculogram, and electromyogram to characterize sleep and diagnose sleep disorders.

CLINICAL FEATURES

The most common complaints or symptoms in people with insomnia are:

- Trouble falling asleep on most nights
- Feeling tired during the day or falling asleep during the day
- Not feeling refreshed when you wake up
- Waking up several times during sleep

People who have insomnia sometimes keep thinking about getting enough sleep. The more they try to sleep, the more frustrated and upset they get, and the harder sleep becomes.

DIAGNOSIS

Polysomnography, an overnight sleep study, can help rule out other types of sleep disorders (such as sleep apnea).

TREATMENT

NONPHARMACOLOGICAL THERAPY

- Behavioural and educational interventions that may help include short term cognitive behavioural therapy, relaxation therapy, stimulus control therapy, cognitive therapy, sleep restriction, paradoxical intention, and sleep hygiene education.

PHARMACOLOGICAL THERAPY

NONBENZODIAZEPINE HYPNOTICS

- Antihistamines (e.g., **Diphenhydramine, Doxylamine,** and **Pyrilamine**) are less effective than benzodiazepines, but side effects are usually minimal. Their Anticholinergic side effects may be problematic, especially in the elderly.
- **Amitriptyline, Doxepin,** and **Nortriptyline** are effective, but side effects include Anticholinergic effects, adrenergic blockade, and cardiac conduction prolongation. **Trazodone,** 25 to 100 mg, is often used for insomnia induced by selective serotonin reuptake inhibitors or Bupropion. Side effects include serotonin syndrome (when used with other serotonergic drugs), over sedation, α-adrenergic blockade, dizziness.
- **Ramelteon** is a melatonin receptor agonist selective for the MT1 and MT2 receptors. The dose is 8 mg at bedtime. It is well tolerated, but side effects include headache, dizziness, and somnolence. It is not a controlled substance.
- **Zolpidem**, chemically unrelated to benzodiazepines or barbiturates, acts selectively at the γ-aminobutyric acid A (GABAA)-receptor and has minimal anxiolytic and no muscle relaxant or anticonvulsant effects. It is comparable in effectiveness to benzodiazepine hypnotics, and it has little effect on sleep stages. Its duration is approximately 6 to 8 hours, and it is metabolized to Inactive metabolites. Common side effects are drowsiness, amnesia, dizziness, headache, and GI complaints. The usual dose is 10 mg (5 mg in the elderly or those with liver impairment), which can be increased up to 20 mg nightly. Cases of psychotic reactions and sleep-eating have been reported.
- **Zaleplon** also binds to the GABAA receptor. It has a rapid onset, a half-life of about 1 hour, and no active metabolites. It may be best used for middle of- the-night awakenings. It does not appear to cause significant rebound insomnia or next-day psychomotor impairment. The most common side effects are dizziness, headache, and somnolence. The recommended dose is 10 mg (5 mg in the elderly).
- **Eszopiclone** has a rapid onset and duration of action of up to 6 hours. The most common adverse effects are somnolence, unpleasant taste, headache, and dry mouth. It may be taken nightly for up to 6 months.
- **Valerian**, an herbal product, is also available without a prescription. The recommended dose is 300 to 600 mg.

BENZODIAZEPINE HYPNOTICS

Benzodiazines bind to GABAA receptors, and they have sedative, anxiolytic, muscle relaxant, and anticonvulsant properties. They increase stage 2 sleep and decrease REM and delta sleep.

- Overdose fatalities are rare unless benzodiazepines are taken with other CNS depressants.
- **Triazolam** is distributed quickly because of its high lipophilicity, and thus it has a short duration of effect. **Erythromycin, Nefazodone, Fluvoxamine,** and **ketoconazole** reduce the clearance of

Triazolam and increase plasma concentrations.

- **Estazolam** and **Temazepam** are intermediate in their duration of action.
- The effects of **Flurazepam** and **Quazepam** are long because of active metabolites. With the exception of **Temazepam**, which is eliminated by conjugation, all benzodiazepine hypnotics are metabolized by microsomal oxidation followed by Glucuronide conjugation.
- N–**desalkylflurazepam** accounts for most of **Flurazepam's** pharmacologic effects. This metabolite may help when daytime anxiety or early morning awakening is present, but daytime sedation with impaired psychomotor performance may occur.

Benzodiazepine adverse effects

- Side effects include drowsiness, psychomotor in coordination, decreased concentration, and cognitive deficits.
- Tolerance to the daytime CNS effects (e.g., drowsiness, psychomotor impairment, decreased concentration) may develop in some individuals.
- Tolerance to hypnotic effects develops after 2 weeks of continuous use of **Triazolam.** Efficacy of **Flurazepam, Quazepam,** and **Temazepam** lasts for at least 1 month of continuous nightly use.
- **Estazolam** reportedly maintains efficacy at maximum dosage (2 mg nightly) for up to 12 weeks.
- Rebound insomnia can be minimized by utilizing the lowest effective dose and tapering the dose upon discontinuation.
- There is an association between falls and hip fractures and the use of long elimination half-life benzodiazepines; thus, **Flurazepam** and **Quazepam** should be avoided in the elderly.

GENERALIZED ANXIETY DISORDER (GAD)

DEFINITION

Generalized anxiety disorder (GAD) is a pattern of frequent, constant worry and anxiety over many different activities and events.

PREVALENCE

In the United States, the lifetime prevalence of anxiety disorders is about 29%.

ETIOLOGY

Generalized anxiety disorder (GAD) is a common condition. Genes may play a role. Stress may also contribute to the development of GAD.

Anyone can develop this disorder, even kids. Most people with the disorder report that they have been anxious for as long as they can remember. GAD occurs somewhat more often in women than in men.

PATHOPHYSIOLOGY

- **Noradrenergic Model**

  This model suggests that the autonomic nervous system of anxious patients is hypersensitive and overreacts to various stimuli. The locus ceruleus may have a role in regulating anxiety, as it activates norepinephrine release and stimulates the sympathetic and parasympathetic nervous systems. Chronic noradrenergic over activity down regulates α2-

adrenoreceptors in patients with generalized anxiety disorder (GAD) and posttraumatic stress disorder (PTSD). Patients with social anxiety disorder (SAD) appear to have a hyper responsive adrenocortical response to psychological stress.

- **γ-Aminobutyric Acid (GABA) Receptor Model**
  GABA is the major inhibitory neurotransmitter in the CNS. Many antianxiety drugs target the GABA A receptor. **Benzodiazepines** (BZs) enhance the inhibitory effects of GABA, which has a strong regulatory or inhibitory effect on serotonin (5-HT), norepinephrine, and dopamine systems. Anxiety symptoms may be linked to under activity of GABA systems or down regulated central BZ receptors. In patients with GAD, BZ binding in the left temporal lobe is reduced. Abnormal sensitivity to antagonism of the BZ binding site and decreased binding was demonstrated in panic disorder. Growth hormone response to Baclofen in patients with generalized SAD suggests an abnormality of central GABA B receptor function. Abnormalities of GABA inhibition may lead to increased response to stress in PTSD patients.
- **5-HT Model**
  GAD symptoms may reflect excessive 5-HT transmission or over activity of the stimulatory 5-HT pathways. Patients with SAD have greater prolactin response to **Buspirone** challenge, indicating an enhanced central serotonergic response. The role of 5-HT in panic disorder is unclear, but it may have a role in development of anticipatory anxiety. Preliminary data suggest that the 5-HT and 5-HT2 antagonist *meta*-chlorophenyl-piperazine causes increased anxiety in PTSD patients.
- Patients with PTSD have a hypersecretion of corticotrophin-releasing factor but demonstrate subnormal levels of cortisol at the time of trauma and chronically. Dysregulation of the hypothalamic-pituitary-adrenal axis may be a risk factor for eventual development of PTSD.
- Functional neuroimaging studies suggest that frontal and occipital brain areas are integral to the anxiety response. Patients with panic disorder may have abnormal activation of the parahippocampal region and prefrontal cortex at rest. Panic anxiety is associated with activation of brain stem and basal ganglia regions. GAD patients have an abnormal increase in cortical activity and a decrease in basal ganglia activity.

CLINICAL FEATURES

The main symptom is the almost constant presence of worry or tension, even when there is little or no cause. Worries seem to float from one problem to another, such as family or relationship problems, work issues, money, health, and other problems.

Even when aware that their worries or fears are stronger than needed, a person with GAD still has difficulty controlling them.

Other symptoms include:

- Difficulty concentrating
- Fatigue
- Irritability

- Problems falling or staying asleep, and sleep that is often restless and unsatisfying
- Restlessness, and often becoming startled very easily

Along with the worries and anxieties, a number of physical symptoms may also be present, including muscle tension (shakiness, headaches) and stomach problems, such as nausea or diarrhoea.

DIAGNOSIS

The health care provider will perform a physical and mental health exam. Tests will be done to rule out other conditions and behaviours that cause similar symptoms.

TREATMENT

- For patients with GAD, nonpharmacologic modalities include short-term counselling, stress management, cognitive therapy, meditation, supportive therapy, and exercise. GAD patients should be educated to avoid caffeine, stimulants, excessive alcohol, and diet pills. Cognitive behavioural therapy (CBT) is the most effective psychological therapy for GAD patients, and most patients with GAD should have psychological therapy, alone or in combination with antianxiety drugs.
- Non-BZ antianxiety agents for GAD are shown in Table 53.1.
- **Hydroxyzine** was effective in 88% of patients for duration of 3 months.
- **Pregabalin** produced anxiolytic effects similar to **Lorazepam, Alprazolam,** and **Venlafaxine**

In acute trials. Sedation and dizziness were the most common adverse effects, and the dose should be tapered over 1 week upon discontinuation.

Table 53.1

Non benzodiazepine antianxiety agents for generalized anxiety disorder

Generic Name	Starting Dose	Dosage Range (mg/day)[a]
	Antidepressants	
Duloxetine	30 or 60 mg per day	60-120
Escitalopram[b]	10 mg per day	10-20
Imipramine[c]	50 mg per day	75-200
Paroxetine[b,c]	20 mg per day	20-50
Venlafaxine[b]	37.5 or 75 mg per day	75-225[d]
	Azapirones	
Buspirone[b,c]	7.5 mg twice per day	15-60[d]
	Diphenylmethane	
Hydroxyzine[b,c,e]	25 or 50 mg four times daily	200-400
	Anticonvulsant	
Pregabalin	50 mg three times daily	150-600

XR, extended-release

[a]Elderly patients are usually treated with approximately one-half of the dose listed [b]FDA approved for generalized anxiety disorder [c]Available generically [d]No dosage adjustment is required in elderly patients

ANTIDEPRESSANTS

- Antidepressants are efficacious for acute and long-term management of GAD. They are considered the treatment of choice for long-term management of chronic anxiety, especially in the presence of depressive symptoms. Antianxiety response requires 2 to 4 weeks.
- **Venlafaxine extended release, Duloxetine, Paroxetine,** and **Escitalopram** are FDA approved for treatment of GAD. **Sertraline** is also effective. Acute response and remission rates are approximately 65% and 30%, respectively. **Imipramine** may be used when patients fail to respond to selective serotonin reuptake inhibitors (**SSRIs**). In one trial, **Diazepam, Trazodone,** and **Imipramine** had greater anxiolytic activity than placebo.
- Common side effects of the **SSRIs** are somnolence, nausea, ejaculation disorders, decreased libido, dry mouth, insomnia, and fatigue. **Tricyclic antidepressants (TCAs)** commonly cause Sedation, orthostatic hypotension, Anti cholinergic effects, and weight gain. TCAs are very toxic on overdose.

BENZODIAZEPINE THERAPY

- The BZs are the most frequently prescribed drugs for the treatment of acute anxiety (Table 53.2). All BZs are equally effective anxiolytic, and most of the improvement occurs in the first 2 weeks of therapy. They are considered to be more effective for somatic and autonomic symptoms of GAD, while antidepressants are considered more effective for the psychic symptoms (e.g., apprehension and worry). It is theorized that BZs ameliorate anxiety through potentiation of GABA activity.
- The dose must be individualized. Some patients require longer treatment.
- The elderly have an enhanced sensitivity to BZs and may experience falls when on BZ therapy.

PHARMACOKINETICS

- **Diazepam** and **Clorazepate** have high lipophilicity and are rapidly absorbed and distributed into the CNS. They have a shorter duration of effect after a single dose than would be predicted on the basis of half-life, as they are rapidly distributed to the periphery.

Table 53.2

Benzodiazepine antianxiety agents

Generic Name	Approved Dosage Range (mg/day)[a]	Approximate Equivalent Dose (mg)
Alprazolam	0.75-4	0.5
Chlordiazepoxide[b]	25-100	10
Clorazepate[b]	7.5-60	7.5
Diazepam[b]	2-40	5
Lorazepam[b]	0.5-10	1
Oxazepam[b]	30-120	15

XR, extended-release. [a]Elderly patients are usually treated with approximately one-half of the dose lsited. [b]Available generically. [c]Orally disintegrating formulation.

- **Lorazepam** and **Oxazepam** are less lipophilic and have a slower onset but a longer duration of action. They are not recommended for immediate relief of anxiety.
- **IM diazepam** and **Chlordiazepoxide** should be avoided because of variability in rate and extent of absorption. **IM lorazepam** provides rapid and complete absorption.
- **Clorazepate**, a prodrug, is converted to **Desmethyldiazepam** in the stomach through a pH-dependent process that may be impaired by concurrent antacid use. Several other BZs are also converted to desmethyldiazepam, which has a long half-life and can accumulate, especially in the elderly and those with impaired oxidation.
- Intermediate- or short-acting BZs are preferred for chronic use in the elderly and those with liver disorders because of minimal accumulation and achievement of steady state within 1 to 3 days.

ADVERSE EVENTS

- The most common side effect of BZs is CNS depression. Tolerance usually develops to this effect. Other side effects are disorientation, psychomotor impairment, confusion, aggression, excitement, and anterograde amnesia *Abuse, Dependence, Withdrawal, and Tolerance*
- Those with a history of drug abuse are at the greatest risk for becoming BZ abusers.
- BZ dependence is defined by the appearance of a predictable withdrawal syndrome (i.e., anxiety, insomnia, agitation, muscle tension, irritability, nausea, malaise, diaphoresis, nightmares, depression, hyperreflexia, tinnitus, delusions, hallucinations, and seizures) upon abrupt discontinuation.

BENZODIAZEPINE DISCONTINUATION

- After BZs are abruptly discontinued, three events can occur:

  Rebound symptoms are an immediate, but transient, return of original symptoms with an increased intensity compared with baseline.
  - Recurrence or relapse is the return of original symptoms at the same intensity as before treatment.
  - Withdrawal is the emergence of new symptoms and a worsening of pre-existing symptoms.
- The onset of withdrawal symptoms is within 24 to 48 hours after discontinuation of short elimination half-life BZs and 3 to 8 days after discontinuation of long elimination half-life drugs.
- Discontinuation strategies include the following:
  - A 25% per week reduction in dosage until 50% of the dose is reached, then dosage reduction by one-eighth every 4 to 7 days. If therapy exceeds 8 weeks, a taper over 2 to 3 weeks is recommended, but if duration of treatment is 6 months, a taper over 4 to 8 weeks should ensue. Longer durations of treatment may require a 2 to 4 month taper.
  - A BZ with a long elimination half-life (t1/2) (e.g., **Diazepam, Clonazepam**) may be substituted for a drug with a short $t_{1/2}$ (e.g., **Lorazepam, Oxazepam, Alprazolam**). The substituted drug should be given for

several weeks before gradual tapering begins.

- o Adjunctive use of **Imipramine, Valproic acid,** or **Buspirone** can help to reduce withdrawal symptoms during the BZ taper.

DRUG INTERACTIONS

- The combination of **BZs** with **alcohol** or other **CNS depressants** may be fatal.
- **Alprazolam** dose should be reduced by 50% if **Nefazodone** (Serzone) or **Fluvoxamine** is added.

DOSING AND ADMINISTRATION

- Treatment of acute anxiety generally should not exceed 4 weeks. BZs can be given as needed, and if several acute courses are necessary, a BZ-free period of 2 to 4 weeks should be implemented between courses. Persistent symptoms should be managed with antidepressants.
- BZs with a long t1/2 may be dosed once daily at bedtime and may provide night time hypnotic and anxiolytic effects the next day. In the elderly, doses should be low and short-elimination half-life agents prescribed.

BUSPIRONE THERAPY

- **Buspirone** is a 5-HT 1A partial agonist that lacks anticonvulsant, muscle relaxant, sedative-hypnotic, motor impairment, and dependence-producing properties.
- It is considered a second-line agent for GAD because of inconsistent reports of efficacy, delayed onset of effect, and lack of efficacy for comorbid depressive and anxiety disorders (e.g., panic disorder or SAD). It is the agent of choice in patients who fail other anxiolytic therapies or in patients with a history of alcohol or substance abuse. It is not useful for situations requiring.
- Rapid antianxiety effects or as-needed therapy.
- It has a mean $t_{1/2}$ of 2.5 hours, and it is dosed two to three times daily.
- Side effects include dizziness, nausea, and headaches.

DRUG INTERACTIONS

- **Buspirone** may increase **Haloperidol** levels and elevate blood pressure in patients taking a monoamine oxidase inhibitor (MAOI).
- **Verapamil, Itraconazole,** and **Fluvoxamine** can increase buspirone levels, and **Rifampin** reduces buspirone blood levels by 10-fold.

DOSING AND ADMINISTRATION

- Buspirone doses can be titrated in increments of 5 mg/day every 2 or 3 days as needed. The onset of anxiolytic effects requires 2 weeks or more; maximum benefit may require 4 to 6 weeks.
- When switching from a BZ to buspirone, the BZ should be tapered slowly.

REFERENCES

1. Wickwire EM, Collop NA. Insomnia and sleep-related breathing disorders. *Chest.* 2010;137: 1449-1463.
2. Morgenthaler T, Kramer M, Alessi C, Friedman L, Boehlecke B, Brown T, et al. Practice parameters for the psychological and behavioral treatment of insomnia: an update. An American Academy of Sleep Medicine report. *Sleep.* 2006; 29: 1415-1419.
3. Vitiello MV, Rybarczyk B, Von Korff M, Stepanski EJ. Cognitive behavioral therapy for insomnia improves sleep and

decreases pain in older adults with co-morbid insomnia and osteoarthritis. *J Clin Sleep Med*. 2009 Aug 15; 5: 355-362.

4. Anxiety Disorders. National Institute of Mental Health. U.S. Department of Health and Human Services. Accessed February 5, 2010.
5. Hoffmann SG, Smits JA. Cognitive-behavioral therapy for adult anxiety disorders: a meta-analysis of randomized placebo-controlled trials. *J Clin Psychiatry*. 2008; 69: 621-632.
6. Pollack MH, Kinrys G, Delong H, Vasconcelos e Sá D, Simon NM. The pharmacotherapy of anxiety disorders. In: Stern TA, Rosenbaum JF, Fava M, Biederman J, Rauch SL, eds. *Massachusetts General Hospital Comprehensive Clinical Psychiatry*. 1st ed. Philadelphia, Pa: Mosby Elsevier; 2008: chap 41.
7. Connolly SD, Bernstein GA. Work Group on Quality Issues. Practice parameter for the assessment and treatmetn of children and adolescents with anxiety disorders. *J Am Acad Child Adolesc Psychiatry*. 2007; 46: 267-283.

CHAPTER 54

Schizophrenia

DEFINITION

Schizophrenia is a chronic heterogeneous syndrome of disorganized and bizarre thoughts, delusions, hallucinations, inappropriate affect, cognitive deficits, and impaired psychosocial functioning.

PREVALENCE

Schizophrenia affects around 0.3%–0.7% of people at some point in their life, or 24 million people worldwide as of 2011. It occurs 1.4 times more frequently in males than females and typically appears earlier in men the peak ages of onset are 20–28 years for males and 26–32 years for females. Onset in childhood is much rarer, as is onset in middle- or old age. Despite the received wisdom that schizophrenia occurs at similar rates worldwide, its prevalence varies across the world, within countries, and at the local and neighbourhood level.

ETIOLOGY

Schizophrenia is a complex illness. Mental health experts are not sure what causes it. However, genetic factors appear to play a role.

- Certain environmental events may trigger schizophrenia in people who are genetically at risk for it.
- People are more likely to develop schizophrenia if have a family member with the disease.

Schizophrenia affects both men and women equally. It usually begins in the teen years or young adulthood, but may begin later in life. It tends to begin later in women, and is more mild.

PATHOPHYSIOLOGY

Multiple etiologies likely exist.

- Increased ventricular size, decreased brain size, and brain asymmetry have been reported. Lower hippocampal volume may correspond to impairment in neuropsychological testing and poorer response to first-generation antipsychotics (FGAs).
- Dopaminergic hypothesis. Psychosis may result from hyper- or hypoactivity of dopaminergic processes in specific brain regions. This may include the presence of a dopamine (DA) receptor defect.
- Positive symptoms may be more closely associated with DA receptor hyperactivity in the mesocaudate, while negative symptoms and cognitive symptoms may be most closely related to DA receptor hypofunction in the prefrontal cortex.

- Glutamatergic dysfunction. A deficiency of Glutamatergic activity produces symptoms similar to those of dopaminergic hyperactivity and possibly symptoms seen in schizophrenia.
- Serotonin (5-HT) abnormalities. Schizophrenic patients with abnormal brain scans have higher whole blood 5-HT concentrations, and these concentrations correlate with increased ventricular size.

CLINICAL FEATURES

Schizophrenia symptoms usually develop slowly over months or years. Sometimes the person may have many symptoms, and at other times you may only have a few.

At first, the following symptoms may appear:

- Irritable or tense feeling
- Difficulty sleeping
- Difficulty concentrating

As the illness continues, problems with thinking, emotions and behaviour develop, including:

- Lack of emotion (flat affect)
- Strongly held beliefs that are not based in reality (delusions)
- Hearing or seeing things that are not there (hallucinations)
- Problems paying attention
- Thoughts "jump" between unrelated topics ("loose associations")
- Bizarre behaviours
- Social isolation

Paranoid schizophrenia symptoms may include:

- Anxious
- Angry or argumentative
- False believes that others are trying to harm you or your loved ones.

Disorganized schizophrenia symptoms may include:

- Problems with thinking and expressing ideas clearly
- Childlike behaviour
- Showing little emotion

Catatonic schizophrenia symptoms may include:

- Lack of activity
- Muscles and posture may be rigid
- Grimaces or other odd expressions on the face
- Does not respond much to other people

DIAGNOSIS

There are no medical tests to diagnose schizophrenia. A psychiatrist should examine the patient to make the diagnosis. The diagnosis is made based on a thorough interview of the person and family members. The person will be questioned about:

- How long the symptoms have lasted
- How the person's ability to function has changed
- Developmental background
- Genetic and family history
- How well medications have worked

Brain scans (such as CT or MRI) and blood tests may help to rule out other disorders that have similar symptoms to schizophrenia.

TREATMENT

NEUROLEPTICS

After neuroleptic treatment of a psychotic episode is initiated, the antipsychotic effect proper manifests following a latent period. Acutely, psychomotor damping with anxiolytics and distancing is noted. Tormenting paranoid ideas and hallucinations lose their subjective importance (**A**, dimming of flashy colours); initially, however, the psychotic process persists but then wanes gradually over the course of several weeks. Complete normalization often cannot be achieved. Even though a "cure" is unrealizable, these changes signify success because

(a) The patient obtains relief from the torment of psychotic personality changes;
(b) Care of the patient is facilitated; and
(c) Return into a familiar community environment is accelerated.

Neuroleptic therapy utilizes different drug classes, namely Phenothiazines, butyrophenones, and the atypical neuroleptics.

The **Phenothiazines** were developed from the H1-antihistamine promethazine: prototype chlorpromazine and congeners with a tricyclic ring system and a side chain containing a protonatable nitrogen atom. Phenothiazines exhibit affinity for various receptors and exert corresponding antagonistic actions. Blockade of dopamine receptors, specifically in the mesolimbic prefrontal system, appears important for the antipsychotic effect. The latency of the antipsychotic effect suggests that adaptive processes induced by receptor blockade play a role in the therapeutic response. Besides affinity for D2 dopamine receptors, neuroleptics also exhibit varying affinity to other receptors, including M-ACh receptors, α1-adrenoceptors, and histamine H1 and 5-HT receptors. Antagonism at these receptors contributes to the adverse effects. Affinity profiles of "classical" neuroleptics (Phenothiazines and butyrophenones derivatives) differ significantly from those of newer atypical drugs, in which Affinity for 5-HT receptors predominates. Neuroleptics *do not have anticonvulsant* activity. Because they *inhibit the thermoregulatory center*, neuroleptics can be employed for controlled hypothermia ("artificial hibernation"). Chronic use of neuroleptics can on occasion give rise to *hepatic damage* associated with cholestasis. A very rare, but dramatic, adverse effect is the *malignant neuroleptic syndrome* (skeletal muscle rigidity, hyperthermia, Stupor), which can have a fatal outcome in the absence of intensive counter measures (including treatment with Dantrolene). With other Phenothiazines (e. g., Fluphenazine with a Piperazine side chain substituent), antagonism at other receptor types tends to recede into the background vis-àvis the blockade of D2 dopamine receptors. The D2 receptor Affinity of the drugs concerned is defined as ++, while the differences in absolute affinity for the other receptors are ignored.

The **Butyrophenones** (prototype haloperidol) were introduced after the Phenothiazines.

With these agents, blockade of D2 receptors predominates entirely. Antimuscarinic and antiadrenergic effects are attenuated. The "extrapyramidal" motor disturbances that result from D2 receptor blockade are, however, preserved and constitute the clinically most important adverse Early dyskinesias occur immediately after neuroleptization and are manifested by involuntary abnormal movements in the head neck and shoulder region. After treatment of several weeks to months, a *parkinsonian syndrome* (pseudo parkinsonism) or *akathisia* (motor restlessness) may develop. All these disturbances can be treated by administration of antiparkinsonian drugs of the Anticholinergic type, such as Biperiden. As a rule, these disturbances disappear after withdrawal of neuroleptic medication. *Tardive dyskinesia* may become evident after chronic neuroleptization for several years, particularly when the drug is discontinued. Its postulated cause is a hypersensitivity of the dopamine receptor system. The condition is exacerbated by administration of Anticholinergics. The butyrophenones carry an increased risk of adverse motor reactions because they lack Anticholinergic activity and, hence, are prone to upset the balance between striatal cholinergic and dopaminergic activity.

Atypical neuroleptics differ in structure and pharmacological properties from the aforementioned drug groups. Extrapyramidal motor reactions are absent or less prevalent. The antipsychotic effect involves not only the positive but also the negative symptoms. In the case of *clozapine*, it was assumed at first that the drug acted as a selective antagonist at D4 dopamine receptors. Subsequently, however, the drug was recognized as a high-affinity ligand and antagonist at other receptors. Clozapine can be used when other neuroleptics have to be discontinued because of extrapyramidal motor reactions. Clozapine may cause agranulocytosis,

Necessitating close haematological monitoring. It produces marked *sedation.*

Olanzapine is structurally related to clozapine; thus far the risk of agranulocytosis appears to be low or absent.

Risperidone differs in structure from the aforementioned drugs; it possesses relatively lower affinity for all "non–D2-receptors."

Ziprasidone shows high affinity for 5-HT2A receptors. Remarkably, this new substance also stimulates 5-HT 1A receptors, which translates into an anti-depressant effect. Ziprasidone particularly influences negative symptoms, its effect on positive symptoms reportedly being equivalent to that of classical neuroleptics. Adverse effects due to blockade of M-ACh, H1 and á1-receptors are comparatively weak. Central disturbances (giddiness, ataxia, etc.) may occur. Moreover, QT interval prolongation has been observed; concurrent administration of QT-prolonging drugs must therefore be avoided.

Uses Management of acute psychotic phases requires high-potency neuroleptics. In highly agitated patients, i.v. injection of haloperidol may be necessary. The earlier therapy is started, the better is the clinical outcome. Most schizophrenic patients require maintenance therapy for which a low dosage can be selected. For stabilization and prevention of relapse, atypical neuroleptics are especially suited since they improve negative symptoms in responsive patients. The patients need good care and, if possible, integration into a suitable milieu. Difficulties arise because patients do not take their prescribed medication (N.B.: counselling of both Patient and caregivers). To circumvent lack of compliance, depot preparations have been Developed, e.g., Fluphenazine decanoate (i.m. every 2 weeks) and haloperidol decanoate (I.m. every 4 weeks), which yield stable blood levels for the period indicated. Psychopharmacological reactions that often limit therapy.

PSYCHOSOCIAL TREATMENTS FOR SCHIZOPHRENIA

While modern antipsychotic drugs have proven to be crucial in relieving the psychotic symptoms of schizophrenia – hallucinations, delusions, and incoherence, they don't always help as much with the other symptoms of the disorder. Even when people with schizophrenia are relatively free of psychotic symptoms, many still have extraordinary difficulty with communication, motivation, self-care, and establishing and maintaining relationships with others. Moreover, because patients with schizophrenia frequently become ill during the critical career-forming years of life (e.g., ages 18 to 35), they are less likely to complete the training required for skilled work. As a result, many with schizophrenia not only suffer thinking and emotional difficulties, but lack social and work skills and experience as well.

It is with these psychological, social, and occupational problems that psychosocial treatments may help most. While psychosocial approaches have limited value for acutely psychotic patients (those who are out of touch with reality or have prominent hallucinations or delusions), they may be useful for patients with less severe symptoms or for patients whose psychotic symptoms are under control. Numerous forms of psychosocial therapy are available for people with schizophrenia, and most focus on improving the patient's social functioning – whether in the hospital or community, at home, or on the job. Some of these approaches are described here. Unfortunately, the availability of different forms of treatment varies greatly from place to place.

REHABILITATION

Broadly defined, rehabilitation includes a wide array of non-medical interventions for those with schizophrenia. Rehabilitation programs emphasize social and vocational training to help patients and former patients overcome difficulties in these areas. Programs may include vocational counselling, job training, problem-solving and money management skills, use of public transportation, and social skills training. These approaches are important for the success of the community-centered treatment of schizophrenia, because they provide discharged patients with the skills necessary to lead productive lives outside the sheltered confines of a mental hospital.

INDIVIDUAL PSYCHOTHERAPY

Psychotherapy or other forms of talk therapy may be offered, with cognitive behavioural therapy being the most frequently used. This may focus on the direct reduction of the symptoms, or on related aspects, such as issues of self-esteem, social functioning, and insight. Although the results of early trials with cognitive behavioural therapy (CBT) were inconclusive, more recent reviews suggest that CBT can be an effective treatment for the psychotic symptoms of schizophrenia.

Individual psychotherapy involves regularly scheduled talks between the patient and a mental health professional such as a psychiatrist, psychologist, psychiatric social worker, or nurse. The sessions may focus on current or past problems, experiences, thoughts, feelings, or relationships. By sharing experiences with a trained empathic person – talking about their world with someone outside it – individuals with schizophrenia may gradually come to understand more about themselves and their problems. They can also learn to sort out the real from the unreal and distorted. Recent studies indicate that supportive, reality-oriented, individual psychotherapy, and cognitive-behavioural approaches that teach coping and problem-solving skills, can be beneficial for outpatients with schizophrenia. However, psychotherapy is not a substitute for antipsychotic medication, and it is most helpful once drug treatment first has relieved a patient's psychotic symptoms.

FAMILY EDUCATION

Very often, patients with schizophrenia are discharged from the hospital into the care of their family; so it is important that family members learn all they can about schizophrenia and understand the difficulties and problems associated with the illness. It is also helpful for family members to learn ways to minimize the patient's chance of relapse – for example, by using different treatment adherence strategies – and to be aware of the various kinds of outpatient and family services available in the period after hospitalization. Family "psychoeducation," which includes teaching various coping strategies and problem-solving skills, may help families deal more effectively with their ill relative and may contribute to an improved outcome for the patient.

REFERENCES

1. Leucht S, Corves C, Arbter D, Engel RR, Li C, Davis JM. Second-generation versus first-generation antipsychotic drugs for schizophrenia: a meta-analysis. *Lancet*. 2009;373:31-41. Epub 2008 Dec 6.
2. Freudenreich O, Weiss AP, Goff DC. Psychosis and schizophrenia. In: Stern TA, Rosenbaum JF, Fava M, Biederman J, Rauch SL, eds. *Massachusetts General Hospital Comprehensive Clinical Psychiatry*. 1st ed. Philadelphia, Pa: Mosby Elsevier;2008:chap 28.

CHAPTER 55

Epilepsy

DEFINITION

Epilepsy is a brain disorder in which a person has repeated seizures (convulsions) over time. Seizures are episodes of disturbed brain activity that cause changes in attention or behavior.

PREVALENCE

Epilepsy is one of the most common of the serious neurological disorders. About 3% of people will be diagnosed with epilepsy at some time in their lives. Genetic, congenital, and developmental conditions are mostly associated with it among younger patients; tumors are more likely over age 40; head trauma and central nervous system infections may occur at any age. The prevalence of active epilepsy is roughly in the range 5–10 per 1000 people. Up to 5% of people experience non febrile seizures at some point in life; epilepsy's lifetime prevalence is relatively high because most patients either stop having seizures or (less commonly) die of it.

ETIOLOGY

Epilepsy occurs when permanent changes in brain tissue cause the brain to be too excitable or jumpy. The brain sends out abnormal signals. This results in repeated, unpredictable seizures. (A single seizure that does not happen again is not epilepsy.)

Epilepsy may be due to a medical condition or injury that affects the brain, or the cause may be unknown (idiopathic).

Common causes of epilepsy include:

- Stroke or transient ischemic attack (TIA)
- Dementia, such as Alzheimer's disease
- Traumatic brain injury
- Infections, including brain abscess, meningitis, encephalitis, and AIDS
- Brain problems that are present at birth (congenital brain defect)
- Metabolism disorders that a child may be born with (such as phenylketonuria)

Epilepsy seizures usually begin between ages 5 and 20, but they can happen at any age. There may be a family history of seizures or epilepsy.

CLASSIFICATION OF SEIZURES (TABLE 55.1)

- Seizures are classified into *partial* and *generalized*
- Partial seizures are divided into
    - o Simple partial - Consciousness is not impaired
    - o Complex partial - Consciousness is impaired

- o About 2/3 of people with epilepsy have complex partial seizures
- Generalized seizures - Can be convulsive or non-convulsive
- Absence seizures - Typical vs. Atypical
- o Typical absence seizures - Non-convulsive with muscle tone preserved. The seizure usually lasts less than 10 seconds.
- o Atypical absence seizures - Convulsive, longer in duration, loss in muscle tone, and tonic/clonic movements are observed.
- Tonic-clonic seizures (Grand mal) - Generalized convulsion occurring in the tonic phase and the clonic phase. Often this is preceded by an aura.
- Tonic phase - Muscles stiffen up, person loses consciousness, body grows rigid.
- Clonic phase - Body extremities jerk and twitch.

Secondary generalized tonic-clonic seizures begins locally with partial seizures

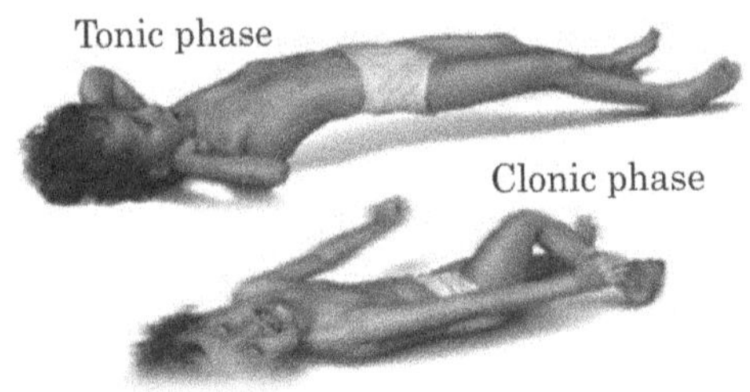

FIGURE 55.1

Tonic and clonic phase.

DIFFERENT TYPES OF SEIZURES

- Photosensitive seizures - These are very rare, even for people with epilepsy (<5%). A light related stimulus may trigger this seizure, hence the warning labels on electronic devices, theme park rides, and even video games.
- Atonic seizures - Sudden lack of muscle tone, causing the inability to sit and stand. They are also called akinetic seizures. These are very rare in adults.

PATHOPHYSIOLOGY

Epilepsy is a term which is used to define a disorder characterized by recurrent, usually transient seizures having a sudden onset and a spontaneous resolution. Actually it's not a disease but rather a condition in which a patient suffers from a complex set of symptoms. Epilepsy due to unknown cause is called primary or idiopathic epilepsy, whereas secondary or organic epilepsy exist along with an identifiable precipitating factor.

Nerve impulse propagates in the brain in a synchronous manner and for that the electrical potential reaches to zero. Any type of process which damages or cause irritation to the grey matter of the brain may cause activation or inactivation of neurons causes by unknown mechanism. This leads to sudden, excessive, synchronous discharge which results in an electrical potential. If the discharge remains localized it results in partial seizures or it may spread and involve the entire cerebrum causing generalized seizures.

Imbalance of excitatory transmitters such as γ-amino butyric acid and selective central nervous system, calcium channel blockers may be involved in the seizure disorders. The excessive neuronal disorderly discharge involving in the entire brain results in loss of consciousness, disturbances in sensation and conclusive movements. After peak of seizures there is decrease in frequency of neuronal discharge. It leads to the end of seizures. The seizure may be ending due to loss of cerebral energy reserves, local tissue

Table 55.1

Classification of epileptic seizures

Seizure Type	Features	Conventional Antiseizure Drugs	Recently Developed Antiseizure Drugs
Simple partial	Diverse manifestations determined by the region of cortex activated by the seizure (e.g. if motor cortex representing left thumb, clonic jerking of left thumb results; if somatosensory cortex representing left thumb, paresthesia of left thumb results), lasting approximately for 20 to 60 seconds. Key feature is preservation of consciousness.	Carbamazepine, phenytoin, valproate	Gabapentin, lamotrigine, levetiracetam, tiagabine, topiramate, zonisamide
Complex partial	Impaired consciousness lasting 30 seconds to 2 minutes, often associated with purposeless movements such as lip smacking or hand wringing.	Carbamazepine, phenytoin, valproate	Gabapentin, lamotrigine, levetiracetam, tiagabine, topiramate, zonisamide
Partial with secondarily generalized tonic clonic seizure	Simple or complex partial seizure evolves into a tonic-clonic seizure with loss of consciousness and sustained contractions (tonic) of muscles throughout the body followed by periods of muscle contractions alternating with periods of relaxation (clonic), typically lasting 1 to 2 minutes	Carbamazepine, phenoba rbital, phenytoin, primidone, valproate	Gabapentin, lamotrigine, levetiracetam, tiagabine, topiramate, zonisamide
Generalized seizures			
Absence seizure	Abrupt onset of impaired consciousness associated with staring and cessation of ongoing activities typically lasting less than 30 seconds.	Ethosuximide, valproate	Lamotrigine
Myoclonic seizure	A brief (perhaps a second), shock-like contraction of muscles which may be restricted to part of one extremity or may be generalized.	Valproate	Lamotrigine, topiramate
Tonic-clonic seizure	As described above for partial with secondarily generalized tonic-clonic seizures except that it is not preceded by a partial seizure.	Carbamazepine, phenobarbital, phenytoin, primidone, valproate	Lamotrigine, topiramate

anoxia, accumulation of toxic metabolites of neuronal metabolism and inhibitory neuronal feedback mechanisms.

CLINICAL FEATURES

- Signs and symptoms of epilepsy differ with the type. The generalized seizures involves in cerebral cortex. These may be Grand mal and Petit mal. In Grand mal epilepsy there is sudden loss of consciousness, clonic movement of muscles and incontinence of sphincters. Patient may remain unconscious for a long time. After awaking the patient has no recollection of the preceding events. He usually complains about light headache. The loss of consciousness is for about half an hour.

- In Petit Mal the loss of consciousness is for few seconds with no much facial expressions, only blinking of eye and jerking of arm may occur.
- The partial seizures involves convulsions of voluntary muscles, mainly clonic in nature, it generally last for a few minutes, it may spread like a old fashion manner to the adjacent muscle group called as jacksonian seizures. Sometimes it may become generalized.
- The electroencephalogram is characteristically abnormal during a seizure but may show normalcy in between seizures.

DIAGNOSIS

- **Routine investigation:**
  - o Haematology, biochemistry (electrolytes, urea and calcium), chest X-ray, electroencephalogram (EEG). Neuroimaging (CT/MRI) should be performed in all persons aged 25 or more presenting with first seizure and in those pts. with focal epilepsy irrespective of age.
- **Specialised neurophysiological investigations:** Sleep deprived EEG, video-EEG monitoring.
- **Advanced investigations** (in pts. with intractable focal epilepsy where surgery is considered): Neuropsychology, Semi-invasive or invasive EEG recordings, MR Spectroscopy, Positron emission tomography (PET) and Single photon emission computed tomography (SPECT).

TREATMENT (TABLE 55.2)

DRUGS USED IN PARTIAL SEIZURES AND GENERALIZED TONIC-CLONIC SEIZURES

The classic major drugs for partial and generalized tonic-clonic seizures are phenytoin (and congeners), carbamazepine, valproate, and the barbiturates. However, the availability of newer drugs **Lamotrigine, Levetiracetam, Gabapentin, Oxcarbazepine, Pregabalin, Topiramate, Vigabatrin, And Zonisamide** is altering clinical practice in countries where these compounds are available.

PHENYTOIN

Phenytoin has major effects on several physiologic systems. It alters Na^+, K^+, and Ca^{2+} conductance, membrane potentials, and the concentrations of amino acids and the neurotransmitters nor epinephrine, acetylcholine, and γ-aminobutyric acid (GABA). Studies with neurons in cell culture show that phenytoin blocks sustained high-frequency repetitive firing of action potentials .This effect is seen at therapeutically relevant concentrations. It is a use-dependent effect on Na^+ conductance, arising from preferential binding to and prolongation of the inactivated state of the Na^+ channel. This effect is also seen with therapeutically relevant concentrations of carbamazepine, lamotrigine, and valproate and probably contributes to their Anti seizure action in the electroshock model and in partial seizures.

When oral therapy is started, it is common to begin adults at a dosage of 300 mg/dL, regardless of body weight. This may be acceptable in some patients, but it frequently yields steady-state blood levels below

10 mcg/mL, which is the minimum therapeutic level for most patients. If seizures continue, higher doses are usually necessary to achieve plasma levels in the upper therapeutic range.

Dose-related adverse effects caused by phenytoin are unfortunately similar to other Anti seizure drugs in this group, making differentiation difficult in patients receiving multiple drugs. Diplopia and ataxia are the most common dose-related adverse effects requiring dosage adjustment; sedation usually occurs only at considerably higher levels. Gingival hyperplasia and hirsutism occur to some degree in most patients; the latter can be especially unpleasant in women. Long-term use is associated in some patients with coarsening of facial features and with mild peripheral neuropathy, usually manifested by diminished deep tendon reflexes in the lower extremities. Idiosyncratic reactions to phenytoin are relatively rare. A skin rash may indicate hypersensitivity of the patient to the drug.

MEPHENYTOIN, ETHOTOIN AND PHENACEMIDE

Many congeners of phenytoin have been synthesized, Mephenytoin and Ethotoin, like phenytoin, appear to be most effective against generalized tonic-clonic seizures and partial seizures. The incidence of severe reactions such as dermatitis, Agranulocytosis, or hepatitis is higher for mephenytoin than for phenytoin.

CARBAMAZEPINE

Closely related to Imipramine and other antidepressants, carbamazepine is a tricyclic compound effective in treatment of bipolar depression.

MECHANISM OF ACTION

The mechanism of action of carbamazepine appears to be similar to that of phenytoin. Like phenytoin, carbamazepine shows activity against maximal electroshock seizures. Carbamazepine, like phenytoin, blocks sodium channels at therapeutic concentrations and inhibits high-frequency repetitive firing in neurons in culture.

Carbamazepine is available only in oral form. The drug is effective in children, in whom a dosage of 15–25 mg/kg/dL is appropriate. In adults, daily doses of 1 g or even 2 g are tolerated. Higher dosage is achieved by giving multiple divided doses daily. Extended-release preparations permit twice-daily dosing for most patients. In patients in whom the blood is drawn just before the morning dose (trough level), the therapeutic level is usually 4–8 mcg/mL.

The most common dose-related adverse effects of carbamazepine are Diplopia and ataxia. The Diplopia often occurs first and may last less than an hour during a particular time of day. Rearrangement of the divided daily dose can often remedy this complaint.

OXCARBAZEPINE

Oxcarbazepine is closely related to carbamazepine and useful in the same seizure types, but it may have an improved toxicity profile. Oxcarbazepine has a half-life of only 1–2 hours. Its activity, therefore, resides almost exclusively in the 10-hydroxy metabolite, to which it is rapidly converted and which has a half-life similar to that of carbamazepine, i.e., 8–12 hours. The drug is mostly excreted as the Glucuronide of the 10-hydroxy metabolite. Oxcarbazepine is less potent than carbamazepine, both in animal models of epilepsy and in epileptic patients;

clinical doses of oxcarbazepine may need to be 50% higher than those of carbamazepine to obtain equivalent seizure control.

PHENOBARBITAL

The exact mechanism of action of phenobarbital is unknown, but enhancement of inhibitory processes and diminution of excitatory transmission probably contribute significantly. Recent data indicate that phenobarbital may selectively suppress abnormal neurons, inhibiting the spread and suppressing firing from the foci. Like phenytoin, phenobarbital suppresses high-frequency repetitive firing in neurons in culture through an action on Na^+ conductance, but only at high concentrations. Also at high concentrations, barbiturates block some Ca^{2+} currents (L-type and N-type). Phenobarbital binds to an allosteric regulatory site on the $GABA_A$ receptor, and it enhances the GABA receptor-mediated current by prolonging the openings of the chloride channels.

Table 55.2

Antiepileptic medications

Antiepileptic drug	Mechanism of action	Clinical efficacy
Standard drugs:		
Carbemazepine (Tegretol)	Na^+ channel blockade	Broad spectrum
Clonazepam (Klonopin)	Allosteric modulation of $GABA_A$ receptor	Broad spectrum, SE
Divalproex sodium (Depakote)	GABA synthesis	Broad spectrum
Ethosuximide (Zarontin)	T-type Ca^{2+} channel blockade	Absence seizures
Ethotoin (Peganone)	Inhibition of voltage-gated Na^+ channels	Partial/generalized
Methsuximide (Celontin)	T-type Ca^{2+} channel blockade	Absence seizures
Nitrazepam (Mogadon)	Allosteric modulation of $GABA_A$ receptor	Absence, IS
Phenobarbital (Gardenal)	Allosteric modulation of $GABA_A$ receptor	Partial/generalized
Phenytoin (Dilantin)	Inhibition of voltage-gated Na^+ channels	Partial/generalized
Primidone (Mysoline)	Allosteric modulation of $GABA_A$ receptor	Partial/generalized
Valproic acid (Depakene)	GABA synthesis and Na^+ channel blockade	Broad spectrum
Newer drugs:		
Acetazolamide (Diamox)	Inhibits brain carbonic anhydrase activity	Partial/generalized
Felbamate (Felbatol)	Na^+, Ca^{2+} and NMDA blockade	Broad spectrum/LGS
Fosphenytoin (Cerebyx)	Prodrug of phenytoin	Status epilepticus
Gabapentin (Neurontin)	GABA turnover and Ca^{2+} channel inhibition	Partial (add-on)
Lamotrigint (Lamictal)	Na^+ channel blockade	Broad spectrum
Levetiracetam (Keppra)	Inhibits N-type Ca^{2+} and conserves $GABA_A$ channels	Partial/generalized
Oxcarbazepine (Trileptal)	Na^+ and Ca^{2+} channel blockade	Partial/generalized
Tiagabine (Gabitril)	Blockade of GABA uptake	Partial (add-on)
Topiramate (Topamax)	Increases GABA and inhibits Na^+ channels	Broad spectrum
Vigabatrin (Sabril)	Inhibition of GABA transaminase	Partial (add-on), IS
Zonlsamide (Zonegran)	Na^+ and ca^{2+} channel blockade	Partial/generalized

Board spectrum = partial/generalized, absence, myoclonic; SE = status epilepticus; IS = infantile spasms; LGS = Lennox-Gastaut syndrome.

PRIMIDONE

Primidone is most efficacious when plasma levels are in the range of 8–12 mcg/mL. Concomitant levels of its metabolite, phenobarbital, at steady state usually vary from 15 mcg/mL to 30 mcg/mL. Dosages of 10–20 mg/kg/d are necessary to obtain these levels. It is very important, however, to start primidone at low doses and gradually increase over days to a few weeks to avoid prominent sedation and gastrointestinal complaints. When adjusting doses of the drug, it is important to remember that the parent drug reaches steady state rapidly (30–40 hours), but the active metabolites phenobarbital (20 days) and PEMA (3–4 days) reach steady state much more slowly.

The dose-related adverse effects of primidone are similar to those of its metabolite, phenobarbital, except that drowsiness occurs early in treatment and may be prominent if the initial dose is too large. Gradual increments are indicated when starting the drug in either children or adults.

VIGABATRIN

Vigabatrin is an irreversible inhibitor of GABA aminotransferase (GABA-T), the enzyme responsible for the degradation of GABA. It apparently acts by increasing the amount of GABA released at synaptic sites, thereby enhancing inhibitory effects. A decrease in brain glutamine synthetase activity is probably secondary to the increased GABA concentrations. It is effective in a wide range of seizure models. Vigabatrin is marketed as a race mate; the *S*(+) enantiomer is active and the *R*(–) enantiomer appears to be inactive.

Typical toxicities include drowsiness, dizziness, and weight gain. Less common but more troublesome adverse reactions are agitation, confusion, and psychosis; pre-existing mental illness is a relative contraindication

LAMOTRIGINE

Lamotrigine, like phenytoin, suppresses sustained rapid firing of neurons and produces a voltage- and use-dependent inactivation of sodium channels. This action probably explains lamotrigine efficacy in focal epilepsy. It appears likely that lamotrigine has another mechanism of action to account for its efficacy in primary generalized seizures in childhood, including absence attacks; this mechanism may involve actions on voltage-activated Ca^{2+} channels. Lamotrigine also decreases the synaptic release of glutamate.

Lamotrigine is effective against partial seizures in adults, with dosages typically between 100 and 300 mg/d and with a therapeutic blood level near 3 mcg/mL. Valproate causes a twofold increase in the drug's half-life; in patients receiving valproate, the initial dosage of lamotrigine must be reduced to 25 mg every other day.

FELBAMATE

Felbamate has been approved and marketed in the USA and in some European countries. Although it is effective in some patients with partial seizures, the drug causes aplastic anaemia and severe hepatitis at unexpectedly high rates and has been relegated to the status of a third-line drug for refractory cases.

Felbamate appears to have multiple mechanisms of action. It produces a use-dependent block of the NMDA receptor, with selectivity for the NR1-2B subtype. It also potentiates $GABA_A$ receptor responses. Felbamate has a half-life of 20 hours (somewhat shorter when administered with either phenytoin or carbamazepine) and is metabolized by hydroxylation and conjugation; a significant percentage of the drug is excreted unchanged in the urine. When added to treatment with other Antiseizure drugs, felbamate increases plasma phenytoin and Valproic acid levels but decreases levels of carbamazepine.

In spite of the seriousness of the adverse effects, thousands of patients worldwide remain on the medication. Usual dosages are 2000-4000 mg/d in adults, and effective plasma levels range from 30 mcg/mL to 100 mcg/mL. In addition to its usefulness in partial seizures, felbamate has proved effective against the seizures that occur in Lennox-Gastaut syndrome.

GABAPENTIN AND PREGABALIN

Gabapentin is an amino acid, an analogue of GABA that is effective against partial seizures.

In spite of their close structural resemblance to GABA, Gabapentin and Pregabalin do not act directly on GABA receptors. They may, however, modify the synaptic or nonsynaptic release of GABA. An increase in brain GABA concentration is observed in patients receiving Gabapentin. Gabapentin is transported into the brain by the L-amino acid transporter. Gabapentin and Pregabalin bind avidly to the subunit of voltage-gated Ca^{2+} channels. Gabapentin and Pregabalin also act presynaptically to decrease the release of glutamate; this effect is probably dependent on reduced presynaptic entry of Ca^{2+} via voltage-activated channels.

Gabapentin is effective as an adjunct against partial seizures and generalized tonic-clonic seizures at dosages that range up to 2400 mg/d in controlled clinical trials. Open follow-on studies permitted dosages up to 4800 mg/d, but data are inconclusive on the effectiveness or tolerability of such doses. The most common adverse effects are somnolence, dizziness, ataxia, headache, and tremor.

LEVETIRACETAM

Levetiracetam binds selectively to a synaptic vesicular protein SV2A. The function of this protein is not understood but it is likely that levetiracetam modifies the synaptic release of glutamate and GABA through an action on vesicular function.

The drug is marketed for the treatment of partial seizures. Oral absorption is nearly complete; it is rapid and unaffected by food, with peak plasma concentrations in 1.3 hours. Kinetics are linear. Protein binding is less than 10%. The plasma half-life is 6–8 hours and may be longer in the elderly. Two thirds of the drug is excreted unchanged in the urine. Drug interactions are minimal; levetiracetam is not metabolized by cytochrome P450. Dosing can begin with 500 mg orally twice daily; some patients require up to 3000 mg/d. Adverse effects include somnolence, asthenia, and dizziness. Idiosyncratic reactions are rare.

TIAGABINE

Tiagabine is an inhibitor of GABA uptake in both neurons and glial cells. It preferentially inhibits the transporter isoform 1 (GAT-1) rather than GAT-2 or GAT-3 and increases extracellular GABA levels in the forebrain and hippocampus. It prolongs the inhibitory action of synaptically released GABA. In rodents, it is potent against kindled seizures but weak against the maximum electroshock model.

TOPIRAMATE

Topiramate blocks repetitive firing of cultured spinal cord neurons, as do phenytoin and carbamazepine. Its mechanism of action, therefore, is likely to involve blocking of voltage-gated sodium channels. Topiramate also appears to potentiate the inhibitory effect of GABA, acting at a site different from the benzodiazepine or barbiturate sites. Topiramate also depresses the excitatory action of kainite on glutamate receptors. It is possible that all three of these actions contribute to topiramate's anticonvulsant effect.

ZONISAMIDE

Zonisamide is a sulphonamide derivative. Its primary site of action appears to be the sodium channel; it may also act on voltage-gated calcium channels. The drug is effective against partial and generalized tonic-clonic seizures and may also be useful against infantile spasms and certain myoclonias. It has good bioavailability, linear kinetics, low protein-binding, renal excretion, and a half-life of 1–3 days. Doses range from 100 mg/d to 600 mg/d in adults and from 4 mg/d to 12 mg/d in children. Adverse effects include drowsiness, cognitive impairment, and potentially serious skin rashes. Zonisamide does not interact with other Anti seizure drugs.

DRUGS USED IN GENERALIZED SEIZURES

Ethosuximide

Ethosuximide has an important effect on Ca^{2+} currents, reducing the low-threshold (T-type) current. This effect is seen at therapeutically relevant concentrations in thalamic neurons. The T-type calcium currents are thought to provide a pacemaker current in thalamic neurons responsible for generating the rhythmic cortical discharge of an absence attack. Inhibition of this current could therefore account for the specific therapeutic action of Ethosuximide.

Therapeutic Levels and Dosage

Therapeutic levels of 60–100 mcg/mL can be achieved in adults with dosages of 750–1500 mg/d, although lower or higher dosages and blood levels may be necessary and tolerated (up to 125 mcg/mL) in some patients. Ethosuximide has a linear relationship between dose and steady-state plasma levels. The drug might be administered as single daily doses were it not for its adverse gastrointestinal effects; twice-a-day dosage is common.

The most common dose-related adverse effect of ethosuximide is gastric distress, including pain, nausea, and vomiting. When an adverse effect does occur, temporary dosage reductions may allow adaptation. Ethosuximide is a highly efficacious and safe drug for absence seizures; the appearance of relatively mild, dose-related adverse effects should not immediately call for its abandonment. Other dose-related adverse effects include transient lethargy or fatigue and, much less commonly, headache, dizziness, hiccup, and euphoria. Behavioural changes are usually in the direction of improvement.

Phensuximide and methsuximide

Phensuximide and methsuximide are phenylsuccinimides that were developed and marketed before Ethosuximide. They are used primarily as anti-absence drugs. Methsuximide is generally considered more toxic and phensuximide less effective, than Ethosuximide.

Valproic acid and sodium valproate

Valproate is active against both pentylenetetrazol and maximal electroshock seizures. Like phenytoin and carbamazepine, valproate blocks sustained high-frequency repetitive firing of neurons in culture at therapeutically relevant concentrations. Its action against partial seizures may be a consequence of this effect on Na^+ currents. Blockade of NMDA receptor-mediated excitation may also be important. Much attention has been paid to the effects of valproate on GABA. Several studies have shown increased levels of GABA in the brain after administration of valproate, although the mechanism for this increase remains unclear. An effect of valproate to facilitate glutamic acid decarboxylase (GAD), the enzyme responsible for GABA synthesis, has been described. An inhibitory effect on the GABA transporter GAT-1 may contribute. At very high concentrations, valproate inhibits GABA transaminase in the brain, thus blocking degradation of SGABA. However, at the relatively low doses of valproate needed to abolish pentylenetetrazol seizures, brain GABA levels may remain unchanged. Dosages of 25–30 mg/kg/d may be adequate in some patients, but others may require 60 mg/kg/d or even more. Therapeutic levels of valproate range from 50 mcg/ML to 100 mcg/mL.

Oxazolidinediones

Trimethadione, the first Oxazolidinediones, was introduced as an Anti seizure drug in 1945 and remained the drug of choice for absence seizures until the introduction of succinimides in the 1950s. The use of the Oxazolidinediones **(Trimethadione, Paramethadione, And Dimethadione)** is now very limited.

These compounds are active against pentylenetetrazol-induced seizures. Trimethadione raises the threshold for seizure discharges following repetitive thalamic stimulation. It or, more notably, its active metabolite dimethadione has the same effect on thalamic Ca^{2+} currents as Ethosuximide (reducing the T-type calcium current). Thus, suppression of absence seizures is likely to depend on inhibiting the pacemaker action of thalamic neurons.

The therapeutic plasma level range for trimethadione has never been established, although trimethadione blood levels above 20 mcg/mL and dimethadione levels above 700 mcg/mL have been suggested. A dosage of 30 mg/kg/d of trimethadione is necessary to achieve these levels in adults.

OTHER DRUGS USED IN MANAGEMENT OF EPILEPSY

BENZODIAZEPINES

Six benzodiazepines play prominent roles in the therapy of epilepsy. Although many benzodiazepines are similar chemically, subtle structural alterations result in differences in activity.

Diazepam given intravenously or rectally is highly effective for stopping continuous seizure activity, especially generalized tonic-clonic status epilepticus (see below). The drug is occasionally given orally on a long-term basis, although it is not considered very effective in this application, probably because of the rapid development of tolerance.

Lorazepam appears in some studies to be more effective and longer-acting than diazepam in the treatment of status epilepticus and is preferred by some experts.

Clonazepam is a long-acting drug with documented efficacy against absence seizures; on a milligram basis, it is one of the most potent Antiseizure agents known. It is also effective in some cases of Myoclonic seizures and has been tried in infantile spasms. Sedation is prominent, especially on initiation of therapy; starting doses should be small. Maximal tolerated doses are usually in the range of 0.1–0.2 mg/kg, but many weeks of gradually increasing daily doses may be needed to achieve these dosages in some patients. **Clorazepate dipotassium** is approved in the USA as an adjunct to treatment of complex partial seizures in adults. Drowsiness and lethargy are common adverse effects, but as long as the drug is increased gradually, dosages as high as 45 mg/dl can be given.

Clobazam is not available in the USA but is marketed in most countries and is widely used in a variety of seizure types. It is a 1, 5-benzo-diazepine (other marketed benzodiazepines are 1, 4-benzodiazepines) and reportedly has less sedative potential than benzodiazepines marketed in the USA. Whether the drug has significant clinical advantages is not clear. It has a half-life of 18 hours and is effective at dosages of 0.5–1 mg/kg/d.

ACETAZOLAMIDE

Acetazolamide is a diuretic whose main action is the inhibition of carbonic anhydrase. Mild acidosis in the brain may be the mechanism by which the drug exerts its Antiseizure activity; alternatively, the depolarizing action of bicarbonate ions moving out of neurons via GABA receptor ion channels may be diminished by carbonic anhydrase inhibition. The drug may have a special role in epileptic women who experience seizure exacerbations at the time of menses; seizure control may be improved and tolerance may not develop because the drug is not administered continuously. The usual dosage is approximately 10 mg/kg/d to a maximum of 1000 mg/dl.

REFERENCES

1. Duvivier EH, Pollack Jr CV. Seizures. In: Marx, JA, ed. *Rosen's Emergency Medicine: Concepts and Clinical Practice.* 7th ed. Philadelphia, Pa: Mosby Elsevier; 2009: chap 100.
2. French JA, Pedley TA. Clinical practice. Initial management of epilepsy. *N Engl J Med.* 2008;359(2):166-76.
3. Kornblau DH, Conway Jr EE, Caplen SM. Neurologic Disorders. In: Marx JA, ed. *Rosen's Emergency Medicine: Concepts and Clinical Practice.* 7th ed. Philadelphia, PA: Mosby Elsevier; 2009: chap 173.
4. Krumholz A, Wiebe S, Gronseth G, et al. Practice parameter: evaluating an apparent unprovoked first seizure in adults (an evidence-based review): report of the Quality Standards Subcommittee of the American Academy of Neurology and the American Epilepsy Society. *Neurology.* 2007; 69: 1991-2007.
5. C. L. Harden, J. Hopp, T. Y. Ting, et al. Practice Parameter update: Management issues for women with epilepsy —Focus on pregnancy (an evidence-based review). Neurology 2009; 73; 126.

CHAPTER 56

Parkinson's Disease

DEFINITION

Parkinson's disease (PD) has highly characteristic neuropathologic findings and clinical presentation, including motor deficits and, in some cases, mental deterioration.

PREVALENCE

Parkinson's disease ranks among the most common late-life neurodegenerative diseases, affecting approximately 1.5% to 2.0% of the population older than age 60 years.

ETIOLOGY

Parkinson's disease most often develops after age 50. It is one of the most common nervous system disorders of the elderly. Sometimes Parkinson's disease occurs in younger adults. It affects both men and women.

In some cases, Parkinson's disease runs in families. When a young person is affected, it is usually because of a form of the disease that runs in families.

Nerve cells use a brain chemical called dopamine to help control muscle movement. Parkinson's disease occurs when the nerve cells in the brain that make dopamine are slowly destroyed. Without dopamine, the nerve cells in that part of the brain cannot properly send messages. This leads to the loss of muscle function. The damage gets worse with time. Exactly why these brain cells waste away is unknown.

Parkinson's is rare in children. It may occur because the nerves are not as sensitive to dopamine.

The term "parkinsonism" refers to any condition that involves the types of movement changes seen in Parkinson's disease. Parkinsonism may be caused by other disorders (called secondary Parkinsonism) or certain medications.

PATHOPHYSIOLOGY

- The two hallmark features in the substantia nigra pars compacta are loss of neurons and the presence of Lewy bodies. There is a positive correlation between the degree of nigrostriatal dopamine loss and severity of motor symptoms. PD is relatively asymptomatic until profound depletion (70% to 80%) of substantia nigra pars compacta neurons has occurred.
- Reduced activation of dopamine-1 and dopamine-2 receptors results in greater inhibition of the thalamus. Clinical improvement may be more tied to restoring activity at the dopamine-2 receptor than at the dopamine-1 receptor.

Loss of presynaptic nigrostriatal dopamine neurons results in inhibition of thalamic activity and activity in the motor cortex.

- Degeneration of nigrostriatal dopamine neurons results in a relative increase of striatal cholinergic activity, which contributes to the tremor of PD.

CLINICAL FEATURES

- PD develops insidiously and progresses slowly. Clinical features are summarized in Table 56.1. Initial symptoms may be sensory, but as the disease progresses, one or more classic primary features presents (e.g., resting tremor, rigidity, bradykinesia, postural instability that may lead to falls).
- Resting tremor is often the sole presenting complaint. However, only two thirds of PD patients have tremor on diagnosis, and some never develop this sign. Tremor is present most commonly in the hands, often begins unilaterally, and sometimes has a characteristic "pill-rolling" quality. Resting tremor is usually abolished by volitional movement and is absent during sleep.
- Muscular rigidity involves increased muscular resistance to passive range of motion and can be cogwheel in nature.

Table 56.1

Presentation of Parkinson's disease (PD)

For clinically probable PD, the patient exhibits at least two of the following: resting tremor, rigidity, or bradykinesia. Asymmetric onset (unilaterality) of these features is usual.
Postural instability (difficulty with maintaining balance) is more common in advanced PD.
Motor symptoms
The patient experiences decreased manual dexterity, difficulty arising from a seated position, diminished arm swing during ambulation, dysarthria (slurred speech), dysphagia (difficulty with swallowing), festinating gait (tendency to pass from a walking to a running pace), flexed posture (axial, upper/lower extremities), "freezing" at initiation of movement, hypomimia (reduced facial animation), hypophonia (reduced voice volume), and micrographia (diminution of handwritten letters/symbols).
Autonomic and sensory symptoms
The patient experiences bladder and anal sphincter disturbances, constipation, diaphoresis, fatigue, olfactory disturbance, orthostatic blood pressure changes, pain, paresthesia, paroxysmal vascular flushing, seborrhea, sexual dysfunction, and sialorrhea (drooling).
Mental status changes
The patient experiences anxiety, apathy, bradyphrenia (slowness of thought processes), confusional state, dementia, depression, hallucinosis/psychosis (typically drug-induced), and sleep disorders (excessive daytime sleepiness, insomnia, obstructive sleep apnea, and rapid eye movement sleep behavior disorder).
Laboratory tests
No laboratory tests are available to diagnose PD.
Other diagnostic tests
Genetic testing is not routinely helpful.
Neuroimaging may be useful for excluding other causes of PD.
Medication history should be obtained to rule out drug-induced parkinsonism.

- Intellectual deterioration is not inevitable, but some patients deteriorate in a manner indistinguishable from Alzheimer's disease.

DIAGNOSIS

- Clinically probably PD is diagnosed when at least two of the following are present: limb muscle rigidity, resting tremor (at 3 to 6 Hz and abolished by movement), or bradykinesia. Definite PD is diagnosed when there is at least two of the following: resting tremor, rigidity, bradykinesia, and a positive response to antiparkinsonian medication.
- A number of other conditions must also be excluded, such as medication induced Parkinsonism (e.g., induced by antipsychotics, phenothiazine antiemetics, or metoclopramide). Other diagnostic criteria include lack of other neurologic impairment.

PHARMACOLOGICAL THERAPY

- Monotherapy usually begins with a monoamine oxidase-B (MAO-B) inhibitor, or if the patient is physiologically young, a dopamine agonist.
- When additional relief is needed, the addition of **levodopa (L-dopa)** should be considered. With the development of motor fluctuations, addition of a catechol-*O*-methyltransferase (COMT) inhibitor should be considered to extend L-dopa duration of activity.
- For management of L-dopa–induced dyskinesias, the addition of **Amantadine** should be considered.

ANTICHOLINERGIC MEDICATIONS

- Anticholinergic drugs can be effective for tremor and dystonic features in some patients but rarely show substantial benefit for bradykinesia or other disabilities. They can be used as monotherapy or in conjunction with other antiparkinsonian drugs. They differ little from each other in therapeutic potential or adverse effects.
- Anticholinergic side effects include dry mouth, blurred vision, constipation, and urinary retention. More serious reactions include forgetfulness, sedation, depression, and anxiety.

AMANTADINE

- Amantadine is often effective for mild symptoms, especially tremor. It may also decrease dyskinesia at relatively high doses (400 mg/day). Adverse effects include sedation, vivid dreams, dry mouth, depression, hallucinations, anxiety, dizziness, psychosis, and confusion. Livedo reticularis (a diffuse mottling of the skin in upper or lower extremities) is a common but reversible side effect.
- Doses should be reduced in patients with renal dysfunction.

CARBIDOPA/LEVODOPA

- **L-dopa**, the most effective drug available, is the immediate precursor of dopamine. It crosses the blood–brain barrier, whereas dopamine does not. Ultimately, all PD patients will require L-dopa.
- In the CNS and elsewhere, L-dopa is converted by L-amino acid decarboxylase (L-AAD) to dopamine. In the periphery, L-AAD can be blocked by administering **Carbidopa** Or **Benserazide**, which does not cross the blood– "Delayed-on" or "no-on" can result from delayed gastric

emptying or decreased absorption in the duodenum. Crushing the tablet of Carbidopa/L-dopa and taking with a glass of water or using the orally disintegrating tablet formulation on an empty stomach can help. Subcutaneous apomorphine may also be used as rescue therapy.

- "Freezing," a sudden, episodic inhibition of lower extremity motor function may be worsened by anxiety and may increase the risk of falls.
- Dyskinesias are involuntary choreiform movements, usually involving the neck, trunk, and extremities. They are usually associated with peak striatal dopamine levels. Less commonly, dyskinesias also can develop during the rise and fall of L-dopa effects (the dyskinesias-improvement-dyskinesias or diphasic pattern of response).

MONOAMINE OXIDASE B INHIBITORS

- At therapeutic doses, **Selegiline** and **Rasagiline** are unlikely to induce a "cheese reaction" (hypertension, headache) unless excessive amounts of dietary tyramine (400 mg or greater) are ingested. However, concomitant MAO-B inhibitors with Meperidine and other selected analgesics is contraindicated. Selegiline and Rasagiline may be neuroprotective.
- Selegiline (deprenyl; Eldepryl) is an irreversible MAO-B inhibitor that blocks dopamine breakdown and can modestly extend the duration of action of L-dopa (up to 1 hour). It often permits reduction of L-dopa dose by as much as one-half.
- Selegiline also increases the peak effects of L-dopa and can worsen preexisting dyskinesias or psychiatric symptoms such as delusions and hallucinations. Other adverse effects include insomnia.
- Metabolites of selegiline are l-methamphetamine and l-amphetamine.
- Rasagiline, another MAO-B inhibitor, has similar effects as selegiline in enhancing L-dopa effects and modest beneficial effect as monotherapy.

CATECHOL-*O*-METHYLTRANSFERASE INHIBITORS

- **Tolcapone** (Tasmar) and **Entacapone** (Comtan) are used only in conjunction with Carbidopa/L-dopa to prevent the peripheral conversion of L-dopa to dopamine (increasing the area under the curve of L-dopa by approximately 35%). Thus, "on" time is increased by about 1 hour. These agents significantly decrease "off" time and decrease L-dopa requirements. Concomitant use of nonselective MAO inhibitors should be avoided to prevent inhibition of the pathways for normal catecholamine metabolism. COMT inhibition is more effective than controlled-release Carbidopa/L-dopa in providing consistent extension of effect and avoids the delay in time to maximal effect seen with controlled-release L-dopa products.
- The starting and recommended dose of Tolcapone is 100 mg three times daily as an adjunct to Carbidopa/L-dopa. Its use is limited by the potential for fatal liver toxicity.
- Because entacapone has a shorter half-life, 200 mg is given with each dose of Carbidopa/L-dopa up to eight times a day. Dopaminergic adverse effects may occur and are managed easily by reducing the

Carbidopa/L-dopa dose. Brownish-orange urine discoloration may occur (as with tolcapone), but there is no evidence of Hepatotoxicity from entacapone.

DOPAMINE AGONISTS

- The ergot derivative **Bromocriptine** (Parlodel) and the non ergots **Pramipexole** (Mirapex), **Rotigotine** (Neupro), and **Ropinirole** (Requip) are beneficial adjuncts in patients with deteriorating response to L-dopa, those experiencing fluctuation in response to L-dopa, and those with limited clinical response to L-dopa due to inability to tolerate higher doses. They decrease the frequency of "off" periods and provide an L-dopa-sparing effect.
- The dose of dopamine agonists is best determined by slow titration to enhance tolerance and to find the least dose that provides optimal benefit.
- The nonergots are safer and are effective as monotherapy in mild-moderate PD as well as adjuncts to L-dopa.
- Bromocriptine is not commonly used because of an increased risk of pulmonary fibrosis and reduced efficacy compared to the other agonists.
- There is less risk of developing motor complications from monotherapy with dopamine agonists than from L-dopa. Because younger patients are more likely to develop motor fluctuations, dopamine agonists are preferred in this population. Older patients are more likely to experience psychosis from dopamine agonists; therefore, Carbidopa/L-dopa may be the best initial medication in elderly patients, particularly if cognitive problems or dementia is present.
- Common side effects of dopamine agonists are nausea, confusion, hallucinations, lightheadedness, lower-extremity edema, postural hypotension, sedation, and vivid dreams. Less common are compulsive behaviors, psychosis, and sleep attacks.
- **Pramipexole** is initiated at a dose of 0.125 mg three times daily and increased every 5 to 7 days as tolerated. It is primarily renally excreted, and the initial dose must be adjusted in renal insufficiency.
- **Rotigotine** is available as a Transdermal patch for once-daily admini-stration, initiated at 2 mg/day and increased by 2 mg/day on a weekly basis to a maximum of 6 mg for early PD.
- **Ropinirole** is initiated at 0.25 mg three times daily and increased by 0.25 mg three times daily on a weekly basis to a maximum of 24 mg/day. It is metabolized by cytochrome P450 1A2; fluoro-quinolones and smoking may alter ropinirole clearance.
- **Apo morphine** is a non ergot dopamine agonist given as a subcutaneous "rescue" injection. For patients with advanced PD with intermittent off episodes despite optimized therapy, subcutaneous apomorphine triggers an "on" response within 20 minutes, and duration of effect is up to 100 minutes. Most patients require 0.06 mg/kg. Prior to injection, patients should be premedicated with the antiemetic trimethobenzamide. It is contraindicated with the serotonin-3-receptor blockers (e.g., ondansetron).

STEPWISE APPROACH TO MANAGEMENT OF DRUG-INDUCED HALLUCINOSIS AND PSYCHOSIS IN PARKINSON'S DISEASE

1. General measures such as evaluating for electrolyte disturbance (especially hypercalcemia or hyponatremia), hypoxemia, or infection (especially encephalitis, sepsis, or urinary tract infection).
2. Simplify the antiparkinsonian regimen as much as possible by discontinuing or reducing the dosage of medications with the highest risk-to-benefit ratio first.
   (a) Discontinue Anticholinergics, including other nonparkinsonian medications with Anticholinergic activity such as antihistamines or tricyclic antide-pressants.
   (b) Taper and discontinue Amantadine.
   (c) Discontinue monoamine oxidase-B inhibitor.
   (d) Taper and discontinue dopamine agonist.
   (e) Consider reduction of L-dopa (especially at the end of day) and discontinuation of catechol-*O* methyltransferase inhibitors.
3. Consider atypical antipsychotic medication if disruptive hallucinosis or psychosis persists.
   (a) Quetiapine 12.5–25 mg at bedtime; gradually increase by 25 mg each week if necessary, until hallucinosis or psychosis improves *or*
   (b) Clozapine 12.5–50 mg at bedtime; gradually increase by 25 mg each week if necessary until hallucinosis or psychosis improves (requires frequent monitoring for leucopenia).

REFERENCES

1. Fearnley JM, Lees AJ. Ageing and Parkinson's disease: Substantia nigra regional selectivity. Brain. 1991, 114: 2283-2301.
2. Wood N. Genes and Parkinsonism. J Neurol Neurosurg Psychiatry. 1997, 62: 305-309.
3. Polymerop1023.
4. oulos MH, Lavedan C, Leroy E, et al. Mutation in the á-synuclein gene identified in families with Parkinson's disease. Science. 1997, 276: 2045-2047.
5. Rajput AH, Rozdilsky B, Rajput A. Accuracy of clinical diagnosis in parkinsonism—a prospective study. Can J Neurol Sci. 1991, 18: 275-278.
6. Olanow CW, Watts RL, Koller WC. An algorithm (decision tree) for the management of Parkinson's disease. Neurology. 2001, 56: (Suppl 5): S1-S88.
7. Yahr MD, Duvoisin RC. Drug therapy of parkinsonism. N Engl J Med. 1972, 287: 20-24.
8. Calne DB. Treatment of Parkinson's disease. N Engl J Med. 1993, 329: 1021-1027.
9. Lang AE, Lozano AM. Parkinson's disease. N Engl J Med. 1998, 339: 1044-1053.

CHAPTER 57

Pain

DEFINITION

Pain is an unpleasant, subjective, sensory, and emotional experience associated with actual or potential tissue damage or described in terms of such damage.

PREVALENCE

Pain is the main reason for visiting the emergency department in more than 50% of cases and is present in 30% of family practice visits. Several epidemiological studies from different countries have reported widely varying prevalence rates for chronic pain, ranging from 12%-80% of the population. It becomes more common as people approach death. A study of 4,703 patients found that 26% had pain in the last two years of life, increasing to 46% in the last month.

PATHOPHYSIOLOGY

NOCICEPTIVE PAIN

- Nociceptive (acute) pain is somatic (arising from skin, bone, joint, muscle, or connective tissue) or visceral (arising from internal organs such, as the large intestine or pancreas).

  Stimulation of free nerve endings known as *nociceptors* is the first step leading to the sensation of pain. These receptors are found in both somatic and visceral structures and are activated by mechanical, thermal, and chemical factors. Release of bradykinins, K+, prostaglandins, histamine, leukotrienes, serotonin, and substance P may sensitize and/or activate nociceptors. Receptor activation leads to action potentials that are transmitted along afferent nerve fibers to the spinal cord.
- Action potentials continue from the site of noxious stimuli to the dorsal horn of the spinal cord and then ascend to higher centres. The thalamus acts as a relay station and passes the impulses to central structures where pain is processed further.
- The body modulates pain through several processes. The endogenous opiate system consists of neurotransmitters (e.g., enkephalins, dynorphins, and β-endorphins) and receptors (e.g., μ, β, κ) that are found throughout the CNS. Endogenous opioids bind to Opioid receptors and modulate the transmission of pain impulses.
- The CNS also contains a descending system for control of pain transmission. This system originates in the brain and can inhibit synaptic pain transmission at the dorsal horn. Important neuro-

transmitters here include endogenous opioids, serotonin, nor epinephrine, ψ-aminobutyric acid, and neurotensin.

NEUROPATHIC PAIN/FUNCTIONAL PAIN

- Neuropathic and functional pain is often described in terms of chronic pain. Neuropathic pain (e.g., post herpetic neuralgia, diabetic neuropathy) is a result of nerve damage, but functional pain (e.g., fibromyalgia, irritable bowel syndrome, tension-type headache) refers to abnormal operation of the nervous system. Pain circuits may rewire themselves and produce Spontaneous nerve stimulation.
- Acute pain (e.g., surgery, trauma, labour, medical procedures) usually is Nociceptive, but it can be neuropathic. Chronic pain can be Nociceptive, neuropathic/functional, or both (e.g., pain that persists after the healing of the acute injury, pain related to a chronic disease, pain without an identifiable cause, and pain associated with cancer).

CLINICAL FEATURES

- Acute pain can be described as sharp or dull, burning, shock-like, tingling, shooting, radiating, fluctuating in intensity, varying in location, and occurring in a timely relationship with an obvious noxious stimulus. Chronic pain can present similarly, and often occurs without a timely relationship with a noxious stimulus.
- Over time, the chronic pain presentation may change (e.g., sharp to dull, obvious to vague).
- Acute pain can cause hypertension, tachycardia, diaphoresis, mydriasis, and pallor, but these signs are not diagnostic. These signs are seldom present in chronic pain.
- In acute pain, comorbid conditions are usually not present, and outcomes of treatment are generally predictable. In chronic pain, comorbid conditions are often present, and outcomes of treatment are often unpredictable.
- Pain is always subjective; thus pain is best diagnosed based on patient description, history, and physical exam. A baseline description of pain can be obtained by assessing PQRST characteristics (palliative and provocative factors, quality, radiation, severity, and temporal factors). Attention should be given to mental factors that may lower the pain threshold (anxiety, depression, fatigue, anger, fear). Behavioural, cognitive, social, and cultural factors may also affect the pain experience.
- Neuropathic pain is often chronic, not well described, and not easily treated with conventional analgesics. There may be exaggerated painful responses to normally noxious stimuli (hyperalgesia); or painful responses to normally non noxious stimuli (allodynia).

TREATMENT

- The elderly and the young are at a higher risk for under treatment of pain because of misunderstanding about the Pathophysiology of their pain.

NONOPIOID AGENTS

- The Nonopioids are preferred over the opioids for mild to moderate pain (see Table 57.1). The salicylate and non steroidal anti inflammatory drugs (NSAIDs) reduce prostaglandins produced by the arachidonic acid cascade, thereby decreasing the number of pain impulses received by the CNS.

- NSAIDs may be particularly useful for management of cancer-related bone pain.
- NSAIDs are more likely to cause GI side effects. The salicylate salts cause fewer GI side effects than aspirin and do not inhibit platelet aggregation.
- Aspirin-like compounds should not be given to children or teenagers with influenza or chickenpox, as Reye's syndrome may result.
- Acetaminophen has analgesic and antipyretic activity but little anti-inflammatory action. It is highly hepatotoxic on overdose.

Table 57.1

Nonopioid agents

Generic Name	Approx. half-life (hrs)	Dosing Schedule (hrs)	Starting dose (mgs/day)[2] Adults ≥ 50kgs	Maximum dose (mg/day)	Excretion
Para-aminophenol derivatives					
Acetaminophen (Tylenol®)	2-4	q 4-6	3750	6000	85% renal
Salicylates					
Acetylsalicylic acid[3]	3-12	q 4-6	3750	6000	100% renal
Choline magnesium trisalicylate (Trilisate®)	8-12	8-12	Initial dose; 1500 mgs; then 1000-1500 mgs q 8-12	4500	100% renal
Difunisal (Dolobid®)	8-12	12	Initial dose; 1000 mgs; then 500 mgs q 12	1000	90% renal <5% fecal
Salsalate (Disalcid®)	8-12	12	Initial dose; 1500 mgs; then 1500 mgs q 12	3000	100% renal
Propionic Acids					
Fenoprofen calcium (Nalfon®)	2-3	6	300-600 q 6-8	3200	98% renal
Flurbiprofen (Ansaid®)	5-6	8-12	100	300	65-85% renal
Lbuprofen (Motrin®, Advil® Nuprin®)	2-4	4-8	400-600 mg q 6	2400	50-75% renal
Ketoprofen (Orudus®)	2-4	6-8	25-50 mg q 8 with mild renal impairment & elderly. 75 mgs q 8 or 50 mgs q 6	300	50-90% renal 1-8% fecal

Table 57.1 *Contd...*

Generic Name	Approx. half-life (hrs)	Dosing Schedule (hrs)	Starting dose (mgs/day)[2] Adults $\geq$ 50kgs	Maximum dose (mg/day)	Excretion
Propionic Acids					
Naproxen (Naproxen®, Naprosyn®)	13	12	500	1000	95% renal
Naproxen sodium (Anaprox®, Aleve®)	13	12	550	1100	95% renal
Oxaprozin (Daypro®)	50-60; 40 with repeated dosing	24	1200	1200	60% renal 30-35% feces
Acetic Acids					
Diclofenac (Volttaren®)	2	6	75	200	50-70% renal 30-35% fecal
Indomethacin (Indocin®, Indocide®, Indomethine®)	4-5	8-12	75	200	60% renal 30% fecal
Bromfenac (Duract)	1-2	6-8	25-150	150	
Sulindac (Clinoril®)	8-16	12	Initial dose 150 mg q 12 then according to response! 400 mgs/day	400	50 % renal 25 % fecal
Tolemetin (Tolectin®)	1	8	Initial 400 mg q 8; then titirate to response	1800	100% renal
Oxicam					
Piroxicam (Feldene®)	50	24	20	40	67% renal 33% fecal
Fenamates					
Meclofenamic acid (Meclomen®)	50 mins. – 3.3 hours	4-6	50-100	400	67% renal 20-25% fecal
Mefenamic acid (Ponstel®)	2	6	Loading dose; 500 mgs; then 250 mgs	1000	67% renal 33% fecal
Pyrrolo-pyrrole					
Ketorolac (Toradol®)	4-6	4-6	IV/IM 30-60 mgs loading dose; then ½ loading dose q 6 hrs, PO 10 mgs q 6 hrs.	DI < 150 mgs IV/IM; qd. PO<40 mgs.	91% renal 6% fecal

OPIOID AGENTS (TABLE 57.2)

- With oral opioids, the onset of action usually takes about 45 minutes, and peak effect usually is seen in about 1 to 2 hours.
- Partial agonists and antagonists compete with agonists for Opioid receptor sites and exhibit mixed agonist-antagonist activity. They may have selectivity for analgesic receptor sites and cause fewer side effects.
- In the initial stages of acute pain treatment, analgesics should be given around the clock. As the painful state subsides, as-needed schedules can be used. Around-the-clock administration is also useful for management of chronic pain.
- Patients with severe pain may receive very high doses of opioids with no unwanted side effects, but as pain subsides, patients may not tolerate even low doses.
- Most of the itching or rash reported with the opioids is due to histamine release and mast cell degranulation, not to a true allergic response.
- When allergies occur with one Opioid, a drug from a different structural class of opioids may be tried with caution. For these purposes, the mixed agonist/antagonist class behaves most like the morphine-like agonists. With patient-controlled analgesia, patients self-administer preset amounts of IV opioids via a syringe pump electronically interfaced with a timing device; thus, patients can balance pain control with sedation.
- Naloxone is used to reverse respiratory depression, but continuous infusion may be required.
- Intrathecal and epidural opioids are often administered by continuous infusion or patient-controlled analgesia. They are safe and effective when given simultaneously with Intrathecal or epidural local anaesthetics' such as **Bupivacaine**. All agents administered directly into the CNS should be preservative-free.

MORPHINE AND CONGENERS (PHENANTHRENES)

- **Morphine** is considered by many clinicians to be the first-line agent for moderate to severe pain. Nausea and vomiting are more likely in ambulatory patients and with the initial dose.
- Respiratory depression increases progressively as doses are increased. It often manifests as a decrease in respiratory rate, and the cough reflex is also depressed. Patients with underlying pulmonary dysfunction are at risk for increased respiratory compromise. Respiratory depression can be reversed by **Naloxone**.
- The combination of Opioid analgesics with alcohol or other CNS depressants amplifies CNS depression and is potentially harmful and possibly lethal. **Morphine** produces venous and arteriolar dilation, which may result in orthostatic hypotension. Hypovolemic patients are more susceptible to morphine-induced hypotension. Morphine is often considered the Opioid of choice to treat pain associated with myocardial infarction, as it decreases myocardial oxygen demand.
- Morphine can cause constipation, spasms of the sphincter of Oddi, urinary retention, and pruritus (secondary to histamine release).

MEPERIDINE AND CONGENERS (PHENYLPIPERIDINES)

- **Meperidine** is less potent and has a shorter duration of action than morphine.
  - o With high doses or in patients with renal failure, the metabolite normeperidine accumulates, causing tremor, muscle twitching, and possibly seizures. In most settings, it offers no advantages over morphine, and it should not be used long term. It should be avoided in the elderly and those with renal dysfunction.
- **Fentanyl** is a synthetic Opioid structurally related to meperidine. It is often used in anaesthesiology as an adjunct to general anaesthesia. It is more potent and shorter acting than meperidine. Transdermal fentanyl can be used for treatment of chronic pain requiring Opioid analgesics. After a patch is applied, it takes 12 to 24 hours to obtain optimal analgesic effect, and analgesia may last 72 hours. It may take 6 days after increasing a dose before new steady-state levels are achieved. Thus, the fentanyl patch should not be used for acute pain. a fentanyl lozenge and a buccal dosage form are available for treatment of breakthrough cancer pain.

METHADONE AND CONGENERS (DIPHENYLHEPTANES)

- **Methadone** has oral efficacy, extended duration of action, and ability to suppress withdrawal symptoms in heroin addicts. With repeated doses, the analgesic duration of action of methadone is prolonged, but excessive sedation may also result. Although effective for acute pain, it is usually used for chronic cancer pain.

OPIOID AGONIST–ANTAGONIST DERIVATIVES

- This class produces analgesia and has a ceiling effect on respiratory depression and lower abuse potential than morphine. However, psychotomimetic responses (e.g., hallucinations and dysphoria with **Pentazocine**), a ceiling analgesic effect, and the propensity to initiate withdrawal in opioid-dependent patients have limited their widespread use.

OPIOID ANTAGONISTS

- **Naloxone** is a pure Opioid antagonist that binds competitively to Opioid receptors but does not produce an analgesic response. It is used to reverse the toxic effects of agonist and agonist antagonist opioids.

CENTRAL ANALGESIC

- **Tramadol**, a centrally acting analgesic for moderate to moderately severe pain, binds to ì opiate receptors and weakly inhibits nor epinephrine and serotonin reuptake.
- Tramadol has a side-effect profile similar to that of other opioid analgesics. It may also enhance the risk of seizures. It may be useful for treating chronic pain, especially neuropathic pain, but it has little advantage over other Opioid analgesics for acute pain.

COMBINATION THERAPY

- The combination of an Opioid and Nonopioid oral analgesic often results in analgesia superior to monotherapy and may allow for lower doses of each agent. An NSAID with a scheduled Opioid dose is often effective for painful bone metastases.

Table 57.2

Opioid analgesics

Drug	Equianalgesic dose to 10 mg of IV morphine		Half-life (h)	Comments
	Oral	Parenteral		
Fentanyl, oral transmucosal	See[a]	NA	See note[a]	For breakthrough cancer pain
Fentanyl, transdermal	NA	NA	–	[b,c]Patch sizes of 12, 25, 50, 75, 100 μg/h; slow onset to effect, necessitating "breakthrough" analgesics
Hydromorphone	7.5 mg	1.5 mg	2-3	See note[b]
Levorphanol	4 mg	2 mg	12-16	See note[b]
Methadone	3-20 mg	10 mg	15-50	[b,d]Risk of delayed toxicity due to accumulation; reduce dose or lengthen dose interval if oversedation occurs after 4-5 days; may schedule as prn initially
Morphine sulfate, controlled release	30 mg	NA	3	[b]Mg-for-mg-conversion from immediate-release form; do not crush or chew tables
Morphine sulfate, immediate release	30 mg	10 mg	3	See note[b]
Oxycodone, controlled release	15 mg	NA	–	See notes[b.a]
Oxycodone, immediate release	15 mg	NA	2-3	See note[b]
Oxymorphone	10 mg	1 mg	2-3	See note[b]
Oxymorphone, controlled release	10 mg	NA	–	

IV = intravenous; NA = not available; prn = as needed; [a]See package insert for dosing instructions. Available in lozenge and effervescent tablets. [b]Common side effect include constipation, nausea, and sedation. Uncommon side effects include itching, dry mouth, and urinary retention. Rare side effects are hypotension and inappropriate antidiuretic hormone secretion. [c]Patch duration = 72 hours, but may be 48 hours for some patients.

Equianalgesic conversion for fentanyl:

Parenteral morphine dose (mg/24 h)	Transdermal fentanyl (μg/h)
8-22	25
23-37	50
38-52	75
53-67	100
68-82	125
83-97	150

[d]Consult pain expert if converting to/from methadone in high-dose patients. Unique cardiac toxicity. [a]Available alone and in combination with aspirin or acetaminophen; at higher doses, use as a single agent.

REFERENCES

1. Acute Pain Management Guideline Panel. Acute pain management: operative or medical
(a) Procedures and trauma: clinical practice guidelines. Rockville (MD): Agency for Healthcare
(b) Policy and Research, Public Health Service, US Department of Health and Human Services; 1992.
2. Carr D, Goudas L. Acute pain. Lancet 1999; 353: 2051–8.
3. Zuckerman L, Ferrante F. Nonopioid and opioid analgesics. In: Ashburn M, Rice L, editors.
   (a) The management of pain. Philadelphia (PA): Churchill-Livingstone; 1998. p. 111–40.
4. McCormack K. Non-steroidal anti-inûammatory drugs and spinal nociceptive processing.
   (a) Pain 1994;59:9–43.
5. Vane J. Inhibition of prostaglandin synthesis as a mechanism of action for aspirin-like drugs. Nature 1971; 234: 231–8.
6. Chandrasekharan N, Dai H, Roos K, et al. COX-3, a cyclooxygenase-1 variant inhibited by acetaminophen and other analgesic/antipyretic drugs: cloning, structure, and expression. Proc Natl Acad Sci U S A 2002; 99: 13926–31
7. Codeine Sulfate; RxList 2008.
8. Bandolier; Oxford league table of analgesics in acute pain
9. Moore RA, McQuay HJ; Single-patient data meta-analysis of 3453 postoperative patients: oral tramadol versus placebo, codeine and combination analgesics.; *Pain.* 1997 Feb; 69(3): 287-94. [abstract]
10. Jones JG; The respiratory effects of meptazinol.; *Postgrad Med J.*1983; 59 Suppl 1: 72-7.
11. Frater RA, Moores MA, Parry P, et al; Analgesia-induced respiratory depression: comparison of meptazinol and morphine in the postoperative period.; *Br J Anaesth.* 1989 Sep; 63(3): 260-5.

CHAPTER 58

Alzheimer's Disease (AD)

Alzheimer's disease (AD) is a progressive dementia affecting cognition, behavior, and functional status with no known cause or cure. Patients eventually loose cognitive, analytical, and physical functioning, and the disease is ultimately fatal.

PATHOPHYSIOLOGY

- The signature findings are intracellular neurofibrillary tangles (NFTs), extracellular neuritic plaques, degeneration of neurons and synapses, and cortical atrophy.
- Mechanisms proposed for these changes are:

✓ β-Amyloid protein aggregation, leading to formation of plaques

✓ Hyperphosphorylation of tau protein, leading to intracellular NFT development and collapse of microtubules

✓ Inflammatory processes levels of multiple cytokines and chemokines are elevated in AD brains

✓ Neurovasculature dysfunction

✓ Oxidative stress

✓ Mitochondrial dysfunction

- Neuritic plaques are lesions found in brain and cerebral vasculature.
- Whether genetic variations promote a primary β-amyloidosis in the majority of AD patients is unresolved.
- Density of NFTs correlates with severity of dementia.
- While there is a variety of neurotransmitter deficits, loss of cholinergic activity is most prominent and correlates with AD severity.
- It is clear that replacement of acetylcholine activity cannot compensate for all the changes that take place in AD.
- Deficits that exist in other pathways are:

✓ Serotonergic neurons of the raphe nuclei and noradrenergic cells of the locus ceruleus are lost

✓ Monoamine oxidase type B activity is increased

✓ Glutamate pathways of the cortex and limbic structures are abnormal

- Excitatory neurotransmitters, including glutamate, have been implicated as potential neurotoxins in AD.
- Risk factors for AD are hypertension, elevated low-density lipoprotein cholesterol, low high-density lipoprotein cholesterol, and diabetes

CLINICAL PRESENTATION

- The onset of AD is almost imperceptible, but deficits progress over time. Cognitive decline is gradual, and behavioral disturbances may be present in moderate stages. Table 58.1 shows the stages of AD.

SYMPTOMS

Table 58.2 Shows the clinical presentation of AD and recommended laboratory and diagnostic tests.

Table 58.1

Stages of alzheimer's disease

Mild (MMSE score 26–18)	Patient has difficulty remembering recent events. Ability to manage finances, prepare food, and carry out other household activities declines. May get lost while driving. Begins to withdraw from difficult tasks and to give up hobbies. May deny memory problems.
Moderate (MMSE score 17–10)	Patient requires assistance with activities of daily living. Frequently disoriented with regard to time (date, year, season). Recall for recent events is severely impaired. May forget some details of past life and names of family and friends. Functioning may fluctuate from day to day. Patient generally denies problems. May become suspicious or tearful. Loses ability to drive safely. Agitation, paranoia, and delusions are common.
Severe (MMSE score 9–0)	Patient loses ability to speak, walk, and feed self. Incontinent of urine and feces. Requires care 24 hours a day, 7 days a week.

Table 58.2

Clinical presentation of alzheimer's disease

General
The patient may have vague memory complaints initially, or the patient's significant other may report that the patient is "forgetful." Cognitive decline is gradual over the course of illness. Behavioral disturbances may be present in moderate stages. Loss of daily function is common in advanced stages.
Symptoms
Cognitive
Memory loss (poor recall and losing items)
Aphasia (circumlocution and anomia)
Apraxia
Agnosia
Disorientation (impaired perception of time and unable to recognize familiar people)
Impaired executive function
Non-cognitive
Depression, psychotic symptoms (hallucinations and delusions)
Behavioral disturbances (physical and verbal aggression, motor hyperactivity, uncooperativeness, wandering, repetitive mannerisms and activities, and combativeness)

Table 58.2 *Contd...*

Functional
Inability to care for self (dressing, bathing, toileting, and eating)
Laboratory tests
Rule out vitamin B 12 and folate deficiency
Rule out hypothyroidism with thyroid function tests
Blood cell counts, serum electrolytes, liver function tests
Other diagnostic tests
CT or MRI scans may aid diagnosis

DIAGNOSIS

- Patients with suspected AD should have a history and physical examination with appropriate laboratory and other diagnostic tests, neurologic and psychiatric examinations, standardized rating assessments, functional evaluation, and a caregiver interview.
- Information about prescription drug use; alcohol or other substance use; family medical history; and history of trauma, depression, or head injury should be obtained. It is important to rule out medication use as a contributor or cause of symptoms (e.g., anticholinergics, sedatives, hypnotics, opioids, antipsychotics, and anticonvulsants) as contributors to dementia symptoms. Other medications may contribute to delirium, e.g., digoxin, nonsteroidal antiinflammatory drugs, histamine 2 receptor antagonists, amiodarone, antihypertensives, and corticosteroids.
- The Folstein Mini-Mental State Examination (MMSE) can help to establish baseline against which to evaluate change in severity. The average expected decline in an untreated patient is 2 to 4 points per year.

NON PHARMACOLOGICAL THERAPY

Sleep disturbances, wandering, urinary incontinence, agitation, and aggression should be managed with behavioural interventions whenever possible. On initial diagnosis, the patient and caregiver should be educated on the course of illness, available treatments, legal decisions, changes in lifestyle that will be necessary with disease progression, and other quality of life issues.

Treatment Options for Cognitive Symptoms in Alzheimer's Disease

- In mild–moderate disease, consider therapy with a cholinesterase inhibitor.
- Donepezil, or
- Rivastigmine, or
- Galantamine
- Titrate to recommended maintenance dose as tolerated.
- In moderate to severe disease, consider adding antiglutamatergic therapy.
- Memantine
- Titrate to recommended maintenance dose as tolerated.
- Alternatively, consider memantine or cholinesterase inhibitor therapy alone.
- Behavioral symptoms may require additional pharmacologic approaches.
- The Alzheimer's Association recommends staying physically, mentally, and socially active, adopting a low-fat/low-cholesterol diet rich in dark vegetables and fruit, and managing body weight.

Pharmacotherapy of Cognitive Symptoms

- Managing blood pressure, cholesterol, and blood sugar may reduce the risk of developing AD and may prevent the worsening of dementia in patients with AD.
- Current pharmacotherapeutic interventions are primarily symptomatic attempts to improve or maintain cognition. Table 58.3 may be used as an algorithm for managing cognitive symptoms in AD.
- Successful treatment reflects a decline of less than 2 points each year on the MMSE score.

Table 58.3

Treatment options for cognitive symptoms in alzheimer's disease

• In mild–moderate disease, consider therapy with a cholinesterase inhibitor.
• Donepezil, or
• Rivastigmine, or
• Galantamine
• Titrate to recommended maintenance dose as tolerated.
• In moderate to severe disease, consider adding antiglutamatergic therapy.
• Memantine
• Titrate to recommended maintenance dose as tolerated.
• Alternatively, consider memantine or cholinesterase inhibitor therapy alone.
• Behavioral symptoms may require additional pharmacologic approaches.

Cholinesterase Inhibitors

- Table 58.4 summarizes the clinical pharmacology of the cholinesterase inhibitors.
- No direct comparative trials have assessed the effectiveness of one agent over another.

Donepezil, rivastigmine, and **galantamine** are indicated in mild to moderate AD, while donepezil is also indicated in severe AD.

- If the decline in MMSE score is more than 2 to 4 points after treatment for 1 year with the initial agent, it is reasonable to change to a different cholinesterase inhibitor. Otherwise, treatment should be continued with the initial medication throughout the course of the illness.
- The most frequent adverse effects are mild to moderate GI symptoms (nausea, vomiting, and diarrhea), urinary incontinence, dizziness, headache, syncope, bradycardia, muscle weakness, salivation, and sweating. Abrupt discontinuation can cause worsening of cognition and behavior in some patients.

Donepezil (Aricept) is a piperidine derivative with specificity for inhibition of acetylcholinesterase rather than butyrylcholinesterase.

- **Rivastigmine** has central activity at acetylcholinesterase and butyrylcholinesterase sites, but low activity at these sites in the periphery.

Galantamine is a cholinesterase inhibitor that also has activity as a nicotinic receptor agonist.

Tacrine was the first cholinesterase inhibitor approved for the treatment of AD, but it has been replaced by safer drugs which are better tolerated.

Table 58.4

Clinical pharmacology of the cholinesterase inhibitors

	Donepezil	Rivastigmine	Galantamine
Brand name	Aricept	Exelon	Razadyne
Dosage forms	Tablet	Capsule	Tablet
	Orally disintegrating tablet	Oral solution	Oral Solution
		Patch	Extended-release (ER) Capsule
Starting dose	5 mg daily at bedtime	1.5 mg twice a day	4 mg twice a day
		4.6 mg/day (patch)	(8 mg daily for ER)
Maintenance dose	5–10 mg daily	3–6 mg twice a day	8–12 mg twice a day
		9.5 mg/day (patch)	(16–24 mg daily for ER)
Meals	No effect of food	Take with food	Take with food
Half-life	7 hours	1.5 hours	7 hours
Protein binding	6%	40%	18%
Metabolism	Substrate (minor) of CYP2D6 and 3A4	Cholinesterase-mediated hydrolysis	Substrate (minor) of CYP2D6 and 3A4
	Glucuronidation	—	Glucuronidation
Renal elimination	Yes	Major pathway	Yes

CYP, cytochrome P450.

OTHER DRUGS

Memantine (Namenda) blocks glutamatergic neurotransmission by antagonizing *N*-methyl-D-aspartate receptors, which may prevent excitotoxic reactions.

It is used as monotherapy, and data suggest that when it is combined with a cholinesterase inhibitor, there is improvement in cognition and activities of daily living.

- It is indicated for treatment of moderate to severe AD.
- It is not metabolized by the liver, but is primarily excreted unchanged in the urine (half-life of elimination = 60 to 80 hours).
- It is usually well tolerated, and side effects include constipation, confusion, dizziness, hallucinations, headache, cough, and hypertension.
- It is initiated at 5 mg/day and increased weekly by 5 mg/day to the effective dose of 10 mg twice daily. Dosing must be adjusted in patients with renal impairment.
- Recent trials do not support the use of **estrogen** to prevent or treat cognitive decline.
- Evidence related to the role of **vitamin E** in preventing AD is mixed, and conclusions cannot be drawn at this time.
- Because of a significant incidence of side effects and a lack of compelling evidence, **Nonsteroidal antiinflammatory drugs** are not recommended for treatment or prevention of AD.

- There is interest in the use of lipid-lowering agents, especially the 3hydroxy-3-methylglutaryl coenzyme A–reductase inhibitors, to prevent AD.

Pravastatin and **lovastatin**, but not **simvastatin**, were associated with a lower prevalence of AD. Further study is needed before these agents can be recommended for this use.

- A metaanalysis indicated that EGb 761 (an extract of **ginkgo biloba**) may have some therapeutic effect at doses of 120 to 240 mg of the standard leaf extract twice daily. Because of limited efficacy data, the potential for adverse effects (e.g., nausea, vomiting, diarrhea, headache, dizziness, weakness, and hemorrhage), and the poor standardization of herbal products, it is recommended that ginkgo biloba be used only with caution.

✓ Ginkgo biloba should not be used in individuals taking anticoagulants or antiplatelet drugs, and should be use cautiously in those taking **nonsteroidal antiinflammatory drugs**.

- Although initial studies suggest potential effectiveness of **huperzine A**, it has not been adequately evaluated for treatment of AD.

Pharmacotherapy of Noncognitive Symptoms

- Pharmacotherapy is aimed at treating psychotic symptoms, inappropriate or disruptive behavior, and depression. Medications and recommended doses for noncognitive symptoms are shown in Table 58.5.
- General guidelines are as follows: (1) use reduced doses, (2) monitor closely, (3) titrate dosage slowly, (4) document carefully, and (5) periodically attempt to reduce medication in minimally symptomatic patients.
- Psychotropic medications with anticholinergic effects should be avoided because they may worsen cognition.

Cholinesterase Inhibitors and Memantine

- **Cholinesterase inhibitors** and **memantine** are first-line therapy in early management of behavioral symptoms. Modest improvement may be achieved.

ANTIPSYCHOTICS

- Antipsychotic medications have traditionally been used to treat disruptive behaviors and psychosis in AD patients.
- A metaanalysis showed that 17% to 18% of dementia patients showed a modest treatment response to atypical antipsychotics. Adverse events included somnolence, extrapyramidal symptoms, abnormal gait, worsening cognition, cerebrovascular events, and increased risk of death.
- Typical antipsychotics may also be associated with a small increased risk of death, as well as more severe extrapyramidal effects and hypotension.

ANTIDEPRESSANTS

- Depression and dementia have many symptoms in common, and the diagnosis of depression can be difficult, especially later in the course of AD.
- Treatment with a selective serotonin reuptake inhibitor is usually initiated in depressed patients with AD. **Paroxetine** causes more anticholinergic side effects than the other **selective serotonin**

reuptake inhibitors Venlafaxine may also be used.

- Although probably equally effective, the **tricyclic antidepressants** are usually avoided because of anticholinergic side effects.

MISCELLANEOUS THERAPIES

- **Carbamazepine**, mean dose 300 mg/day, may improve psychosis and behavioral disturbance in AD patients.
- **Oxazepam** and other benzodiazepines have been used to treat anxiety, agitation, and aggression, but they generally show inferior efficacy compared with antipsychotics. They can also worsen cognition, cause disinhibition, and increase the risk of falls.

REFERENCES

1. Cupples LA, Farrer LA, Sadovnick AD, Relkin N, Whitehouse P, Green RC. Estimating risk curves for first-degree relatives of patients with Alzheimer's disease: the REVEAL study. Genet Med. 2004; 6: 192–6.
2. Del-Aguila JL, Koboldt DC, Black K, Chasse R, Norton J, Wilson RK, Cruchaga C. Alzheimer's disease: rare variants with large effect sizes. Curr Opin Genet Dev. 2015; 33: 49–55.
3. Farrer LA, O'Sullivan DM, Cupples LA, Growdon JH, Myers RH. Assessment of genetic risk for Alzheimer's disease among first-degree relatives. Ann Neurol. 1989;25:485–93.
4. Feldman H, Gauthier S, Hecker J, Vellas B, Hux M, Xu Y, Schwam EM, Shah S, Mastey V. Economic evaluation of donepezil in moderate to severe Alzheimer disease. Neurology. 2004; 63: 644–50.
5. Feldman HH, Lane R., Study 304 Group. Rivastigmine: a placebo controlled trial of twice daily and three times daily regimens in patients with Alzheimer's disease. J Neurol Neurosurg Psychiatry. 2007; 2007; 78: 1056–63.
6. Ferrer I, Boada Rovira M, Sanchez Guerra ML, Rey MJ, Costa-Jussa F. Neuropathology and pathogenesis of encephalitis following amyloid-beta immunization in Alzheimer's disease. Brain Pathol. 2004; 14: 11–20.
7. Gatz M, Reynolds CA, Fratiglioni L, Johansson B, Mortimer JA, Berg S, Fiske A, Pedersen NL. Role of genes and environments for explaining Alzheimer disease. Arch Gen Psychiatry. 2006; 63: 168–74.
8. Green RC, Roberts JS, Cupples LA, Relkin NR, Whitehouse PJ, Brown T, Eckert SL, Butson M, Sadovnick AD, Quaid KA, Chen C, Cook-Deegan R, Farrer LA., REVEAL Study Group. Disclosure of APOE genotype for risk of Alzheimer's disease. N Engl J Med. 2009; 361: 245–54.
9. Griciuc A, Serrano-Pozo A, Parrado AR, Lesinski AN, Asselin CN, Mullin K, Hooli B, Choi SH, Hyman BT, Tanzi RE. Alzheimer's disease risk gene CD33 inhibits microglial uptake of amyloid beta. Neuron. 2013; 78: 631–43.
10. Guerreiro R, Wojtas A, Bras J, Carrasquillo M, Rogaeva E, Majounie E, Cruchaga C, Sassi C, Kauwe JS, Younkin S, Hazrati L, Collinge J, Pocock J, Lashley T, Williams J, Lambert JC, Amouyel P, Goate A, Rademakers R, Morgan K, Powell J, St George-Hyslop P, Singleton A, Hardy J., Alzheimer Genetic Analysis Group. TREM2 Variants in Alzheimer's Disease. N Engl J Med. 2013; 368: 117–27.
11. Heston LL, Mastri AR, Anderson VE, White J. Dementia of the Alzheimer type. Clinical genetics, natural history, and associated conditions. Arch Gen Psychiatry. 1981; 38: 1085–90.
12. Holmes C, Boche D, Wilkinson D, Yadegarfar G, Hopkins V, Bayer A, Jones RW, Bullock R, Love S, Neal JW, Zotova E, Nicoll JA. Long-term effects of Abeta42 immunisation in Alzheimer's disease: follow-up of a randomised, placebo-controlled phase I trial. Lancet. 2008; 372: 216–23.

13. International Genomics of Alzheimer's Disease Consortium. Convergent genetic and expression data implicate immunity in Alzheimer's disease. Alzheimers Dement. 2015; 11: 658–71.
14. Janssen JC, Beck JA, Campbell TA, Dickinson A, Fox NC, Harvey RJ, Houlden H, Rossor MN, Collinge J. Early onset familial Alzheimer's disease: Mutation frequency in 31 families. Neurology. 2003; 60: 235–9.
15. Jarvik G, Larson EB, Goddard K, Schellenberg GD, Wijsman EM. Influence of apolipoprotein E genotype on the transmission of Alzheimer disease in a community-based sample. Am J Hum Genet. 1996; 58: 191–200.
16. Jayadev S, Steinbart EJ, Chi YY, Kukull WA, Schellenberg GD, Bid TD. Conjugal Alzheimer disease: risk in children when both parents have Alzheimer disease. Arch Neurol. 2008; 65: 373–378.

CHAPTER 59

Anxiety Disorders

DEFINITION

Anxiety disorders include a constellation of disorders in which anxiety and associated symptoms are irrational or experienced at a level of severity that impairs functioning. The characteristic features are anxiety and avoidance.

PATHOPHYSIOLOGY

- ***Noradrenergic model:*** This model suggests that the autonomic nervous system of anxious patients is hypersensitive and overreacts to various stimuli. The locus ceruleus may have a role in regulating anxiety, as it activates norepinephrine release and stimulates the sympathetic and parasympathetic nervous systems. Chronic noradrenergic overactivity down regulates $\alpha 2$-adrenoreceptors in patients with generalized anxiety disorder (GAD) and post traumatic stress disorder (PTSD). Patients with social anxiety disorder (SAD) appear to have a hyperresponsive adrenocortical response to psychological stress.
- ***γ-Aminobutyric acid (GABA) receptor model:*** GABA is the major inhibitory neurotransmitter in the CNS. Many antianxiety drugs target the GABAA receptor. **Benzodiazepines** (BZs) enhance the inhibitory effects of GABA, which has a strong regulatory or inhibitory effect on serotonin (5-HT), norepinephrine, and dopamine systems. Anxiety symptoms may be linked to underactivity of GABA systems or downregulated central BZ receptors. In patients with GAD, BZ binding in the left temporal lobe is reduced. Abnormal sensitivity to antagonism of the BZ binding site and decreased binding was demonstrated in panic disorder. Growth hormone response to baclofen in patients with generalized SAD suggests an abnormality of central GABAB receptor function. Abnormalities of GABA inhibition may lead to increased response to stress in PTSD patients.
- ***5-HT model:*** GAD symptoms may reflect excessive 5-HT transmission or overactivity of the stimulatory 5-HT pathways. Patients with SAD have greater prolactin response to **buspirone** challenge, indicating an enhanced central serotonergic response. The role of 5-HT in panic disorder is unclear, but it may have a role in development of anticipatory anxiety. Preliminary data suggest that the 5-HT and 5-HT2 antagonist *meta*chlorophenylpiperazine causes increased anxiety in PTSD patients.

- Patients with PTSD have a hypersecretion of corticotropin-releasing factor but demonstrate subnormal levels of cortisol at the time of trauma and chronically. Dysregulation of the hypothalamic-pituitary-adrenal axis may be a risk factor for eventual development of PTSD.
- Functional neuroimaging studies suggest that frontal and occipital brain areas are integral to the anxiety response. Patients with panic disorder may have abnormal activation of the para hippocampal region and prefrontal cortex at rest. Panic anxiety is associated with activation of brain stem and basal ganglia regions. GAD patients have an abnormal increase in cortical activity and a decrease in basal ganglia activity. In patients with SAD, there may be abnormalities in the amygdala, hippocampus, and various cortical regions. Lower hippocampal volumes in patients with PTSD may be a precursor for subsequent development of PTSD.

CLINICAL PRESENTATION

GENERALIZED ANXIETY DISORDER

- The clinical presentation of GAD is shown in Table 59.1. The diagnostic criteria require persistent symptoms most days for at least 6 months. The anxiety or worry must be about a number of matters and is accompanied by at least three psychological or physiologic symptoms. The illness has a gradual onset at an average age of 21 years. The course of illness is chronic, with multiple spontaneous exacerbations and remissions. There is a high percentage of relapse and a low rate of recovery.

Table 59.1

Presentation of generalized anxiety disorder

Psychological and cognitive symptoms
• Excessive anxiety
• Worries that are difficult to control
• Feeling keyed up or on edge
• Poor concentration or mind going blank
Physical symptoms
• Restlessness
• Fatigue
• Muscle tension
• Sleep disturbance
• Irritability
Impairment
• Social, occupational, or other important functional areas
• Poor coping abilities

PANIC DISORDER

- Symptoms usually begin as a series of unexpected panic attacks. These are followed by at least 1 month of persistent concern about having another panic attack.
- Symptoms of a panic attack are shown in Table 59.2. During an attack, there must be at least four physical symptoms in addition to psychological symptoms. Symptoms reach a peak within 10 minutes and usually last no more than 20 or 30 minutes.
- Many patients eventually develop agoraphobia, which is avoidance of specific situations (e.g., crowded places, bridges) where they fear a panic attack might occur. Patients may become homebound.

Table 59.2

Symptoms of a panic attack

Psychological symptoms
• Depersonalization
• Derealization
• Fear of losing control
• Fear of going crazy
• Fear of dying
Physical symptoms
• Abdominal distress
• Chest pain or discomfort
• Chills
• Dizziness or lightheadedness
• Feeling of choking
• Hot flushes
• Palpitations
• Nausea
• Paresthesias
• Shortness of breath
• Sweating
• Tachycardia
• Trembling or shaking

SOCIAL ANXIETY DISORDER

- The essential feature of SAD is an intense, irrational, and persistent fear of being negatively evaluated in a social or performance situation. Exposure to the feared situation usually provokes a panic attack. Symptoms of SAD are shown in Table 59.3. The fear and avoidance of the situation must interfere with daily routine or social/occupational functioning. It is a chronic disorder with a mean age of onset in the teens.
- In the generalized subtype, fear is of many social situations where embarrassment may occur. In the discrete or specific subtype, fear is limited to one or two situations (e.g., performing, public speaking).

Table 59.3

Presentation of social anxiety disorder

Fears
• Being scrutinized by others
• Being embarrassed
• Being humiliated
Some feared situations
• Addressing a group of people
• Eating or writing in front of others
• Interacting with authority figures
• Speaking in public
• Talking with strangers
• Use of public toilets
Physical symptoms
• Blushing
• "Butterflies in the stomach"
• Diarrhea
• Sweating
• Tachycardia
• Trembling
Types
• Generalized type: fear and avoidance extend to a wide range of social situations
• Nongeneralized type: fear is limited to one or two situations

POST TRAUMATIC STRESS DISORDER

- In PTSD, exposure to a traumatic event causes immediate intense fear, helplessness, or horror.
- The clinical presentation of PTSD is shown in Table 59.4. Patients must have at least one reexperiencing symptom, three signs or symptoms of persistent avoidance of stimuli, and at least two symptoms of increased arousal. Symptoms from each category must be present longer than 1 month and cause significant distress or impairment. PTSD can occur at any age, and the course is variable.

Table 59.4

Presentation of post traumatic stress disorder

Reexperiencing symptoms
• Recurrent, intrusive distressing memories of the trauma
• Recurrent, disturbing dreams of the event
• Feeling that the traumatic event is recurring (e.g., dissociative flashbacks)
• Physiologic reaction to reminders of the trauma
Avoidance symptoms
• Avoidance of conversations about the trauma
• Avoidance of thoughts or feelings about the trauma
• Avoidance of activities that are reminders of the event
• Avoidance of people or places that arouse recollections of the trauma
• Inability to recall an important aspect of the trauma
• Anhedonia
• Estrangement from others
• Restricted affect
• Sense of a foreshortened future (e.g., does not expect to have a career, marriage)
Hyperarousal symptoms
• Decreased concentration
• Easily startled
• Hypervigilance
• Insomnia
• Irritability or angry outbursts
Subtypes
• Acute: duration of symptoms is less than 3 months
• Chronic: symptoms last for longer than 3 months
• With delayed onset: onset of symptoms is at least 6 months posttrauma

- One-third of patients with PTSD have a poor prognosis, and about 80% have a concurrent depression or anxiety disorder. Over half of men with PTSD have comorbid alcohol abuse or dependence, and about 20% of patients attempt suicide.

DIAGNOSIS

- The diagnosis is based on complete examination of physical and mental status; relevant laboratory tests; and a series of medical, psychiatric tests and previous drug history.
- Anxiety symptoms may be associated with medical illnesses (Table 59.5) or drug therapy (Table 59.6). About 50% of patients with GAD have irritable bowel syndrome.
- The symptoms of anxiety may be present in several major psychiatric illnesses (e.g., schizophrenia, organic mental syndromes, mood disorders,and substance withdrawal).

Table 59.5

Common medical illnesses associated with anxiety symptoms

Cardiovascular
Angina, arrhythmias, congestive heart failure, ischemic heart disease, myocardial infarction
Endocrine and metabolic
Cushing's disease, hyperparathyroidism, hyperthyroidism, hypothyroidism, hypoglycemia, hyponatremia, hyperkalemia, pheochromocytoma, vitamin B
Neurologic
Dementia, migraine, Parkinson's disease, seizures, stroke, neoplasms, poor pain control
Respiratory system
Asthma, chronic obstructive pulmonary disease, pulmonary embolism, pneumonia
Others
Anemias, systemic lupus erythematosus, vestibular dysfunction

Table 59.6

Drugs associated with anxiety symptoms

Anticonvulsants: Carbamazepine
Antidepressants: Selective serotonin reuptake inhibitors, tricyclic antidepressants
Antihypertensives: Felodipine
Antibiotics: Quinolones, isoniazid
Bronchodilators: Albuterol, theophylline
Corticosteroids: Prednisone
Dopa agonists: Levodopa
Herbals: Ma huang, ginseng, ephedra
Nonsteroidal antiinflammatory drugs: Ibuprofen
Stimulants: Amphetamines, methylphenidate, caffeine, cocaine
Sympathomimetics: Pseudoephedrine
Thyroid hormones: Levothyroxine
Toxicity: Anticholinergics, antihistamines, digoxin
Withdrawal: Alcohol, sedatives

TREATMENT

GENERALIZED ANXIETY DISORDER

- Patients suffering with GAD, nonpharmacological modalities include short-term counseling, management of stress, intellectual therapy, meditation, and exercise are recommended. GAD patients are advised to avoid caffeine, CNS stimulants, excessive alcohol, and diet control pills. Cognitive behavioral therapy (CBT) is the highly effective psychological therapy for GAD patients, and most patients suffering with GAD should be given cerebral therapy along with or without antianxiety drugs.
- The drugs of choice for anxiety disorders are shown in Table 59.7, and non-BZ antianxiety agents for GAD are shown in Table 59.8.
- Anxiolytic like Kava kava is not recommended because of its lack of efficacy and hepatotoxicity.
- **Hydroxyzine** was effective in majority of patients for a duration of 3 months.
- **Pregabalin** produced anxiolytic effects that are similar to **alprazolam, lorazepam,** and **venlafaxine** . Sedation and dizziness were the most common adverse effects, and the tapering of dose should be done over 1 week upon discontinuation.
- Relation between antidepressant use and suicidality (suicidal thinking and behaviors) in children, adolescents, and young adults 18 to 24 years old has been established by the FDA. All antidepressants carry a black box warning advising caution in the use of all antidepressants in this population, and the FDA also recommends specific monitoring parameters.

Table 59.7

Drug choices for anxiety disorders

Anxiety Disorder	First-Line Drugs	Second-Line Drugs	Alternatives
Generalized anxiety	Duloxetine	Benzodiazepines	Hydroxyzine
	Escitalopram Paroxetine	Buspirone	Pregabalin
	Venlafaxine XR	Imipramine	
		Sertraline	
Panic disorder	SSRIs	Alprazolam	Phenelzine
	Venlafaxine XR	Clomipramine	
		Clonazepam Imipramine	
Social anxiety disorder	Escitalopram	Citalopram	Buspirone
	Fluvoxamine	Clonazepam	Gabapentin
	Paroxetine		Mirtazapine
	Sertraline		Phenelzine
	Venlafaxine XR		Pregabalin

SSRI, selective serotonin reuptake inhibitor; XR, extended-release.

Table 59.8

Nonbenzodiazepine antianxiety agents for generalized anxiety disorder

Generic Name	Trade Name	Starting Dose	Dosage Range (mg/day)[a]
Antidepressants			
Duloxetine	Cymbalta	30 or 60 mg per day	60–120
Escitalopram[b]	Lexapro	10 mg per day	10–20
Imipramine[c]	Tofranil	50 mg per day	75–200
Paroxetine[b,c]	Paxil	20 mg per day	20–50
Venlafaxine[b]	Effexor XR	37.5 or 75 mg per day	75–225[d]
Azapirones			
Buspirone[b,c]	BuSpar	7.5 mg twice per day	15–60 [d]
Diphenylmethane			
Hydroxyzine [b,c,e]	Vistaril, Atarax	25 or 50 mg four times daily	200–400
Anticonvulsant			
Pregabalin	Lyrica	50 mg three times daily	150–600

XR, extended-release. [a]Elderly patients are usually treated with approximately one-half of the dose listed. [b]FDA approved for generalized anxiety disorder. [c]Available generically. [d]No dosage adjustment is required in elderly patients. [e]FDA approved for anxiety and tension in children in divided daily doses of 50–100 mg.

ANTIDEPRESSANTS

- Antidepressants are highly efficacious for short and long-term management of GAD. They are the drugs of choice for long-term management of chronic anxiety, especially in the presence of depressive symptoms. Antianxiety response requires 2 to 4 weeks.
- **Venlafaxine extended release, duloxetine, paroxetine,** and **escitalopram** are FDA approved for treatment of GAD. **Sertraline** is also effective. Acute response and remission rates are approximately 65% and 30%, respectively. **Imipramine** may be used when patients fail to respond to selective serotonin reuptake inhibitors (**SSRIs**). In one trial, **diazepam, trazodone,** and **imipramine** had greater anxiolytic activity than placebo.
- Common side effects of the **SSRIs** are vomiting, ejaculation disorders, decreased libido, somnolence, dry mouth, insomnia, and fatigue. **Tricyclic antidepressants (TCAs)** may commonly cause sedation, orthostatic hypotension, anticholinergic effects, and weight gain. TCAs are very toxic on overdose.

BENZODIAZEPINE THERAPY

- The BZs are the most frequently prescribed drugs for the treatment of acute anxiety (Table 59.9). All BZs are significantly effective anxiolytics, and most of the improvement occurs in the first 2 weeks of therapy. They are considered as the most effective therapy for somatic and autonomic symptoms of GAD, while antidepressants are considered highly effective for the psychic symptoms (e.g., worry and apprehension)
- It is theorized that BZs ameliorate anxiety through potentiating the GABA activity.
- The dose must be individualized and monitored. Some patients require treatment for longer duration of time.
- The elderly have an enhanced sensitivity to BZs and may experience falls when on BZ therapy.

Table 59.9

Benzodiazepine anti anxiety agents

Generic Name	Brand Name	Approved Dosage Range (mg/day)[a]	Approximate Equivalent Dose (mg)
Alprazolam[b]	Niravamc, Xanax	0.75–4	0.5
	Xanax XR	1–10[d]	
Chlordiazepoxide[b]	Librium	25–100d	10
Clonazepam[b]	Klonopin	1–4[d]	0.25
	Klonopin Wafers[c]		
Clorazepate[b]	Tranxene	7.5–60	7.5
Diazepam[b]	Valium	2–40	5
Lorazepam[b]	Ativan	0.5–10	1
Oxazepam[b]	Serax	30–120	15

XR, extended-release. [a]Elderly patients are usually treated with approximately one-half of the dose listed, [b]Available generically, [c]Orally disintegrating formulation, [d]Panic disorder dose

Table 59.10

Pharmacokinetics of benzodiazepine anti anxiety agents

Generic Name	Time to Peak Plasma Level (hours)	Elimination Half-Life, Parent (hours)	Metabolic Pathway	Clinically Significant Metabolites	Binding (%)
Alprazolam	1–2	12–15	Oxidation	—	80
Chlordiazepoxide	1–4	5–30	N-Dealkylation	Desmethyl-chlordiazepoxide	96
			Oxidation	Demoxepam	—
				DMDZ[a]	—
Clonazepam	1–4	30–40	Nitroreduction	—	85
Clorazepate	1–2	Prodrug	Oxidation	DMDZ	97
Diazepam	0.5–2	20–80	Oxidation	DMDZ	98
				Oxazepam	
Lorazepam	2–4	10-20	Conjugation	—	85
Oxazepam	2–4	05-20	Conjugation	—	97

[a]Desmethyldiazepam (DMDZ) half-life 50–100 hours.

PHARMACOKINETICS

- BZ pharmacokinetic properties are shown in Table 59.10.
- **Diazepam** and **clorazepate** have more lipophilicity and are rapidly absorbed , distributed into the CNS. They have a shorter duration of effect after a single dose.
- The less lipophilic drugs like **Lorazepam** and **oxazepam** have a slower onset but a longer duration of action.
- Due to variability in rate and extent of absorption **IM diazepam** and **chlordiazepoxide** should be avoided. **IM lorazepam** provides rapid and complete absorption.
- **Clorazepate**, is converted to **desmethyldiazepam** in the stomach by a pH-dependent process that may be impaired by concurrent use of antacids.

Adverse Events

- The most common side effect of BZs are drowsiness, excessive sedation, impaired motor coordination, confusion, and memory loss. These effects are most troublesome during the initial week or two of treatment.

Abuse, Dependence, Withdrawal, and Tolerance

Usage of benzodiazepines causes Tolerance and dependence. Discontinuation of drug administration, particularly abrupt withdrawal, can be associated with a variety of symptoms, including rebound insomnia and rebound anxiety. More severe symptoms may occur when an individual withdraws from a supratherapeutic dose, particularly if the drug has been taken for months or years. These symptoms can include, in addition to those already mentioned, muscle weakness, tremor, hyperalgesia, nausea, vomiting, weight loss, and possibly convulsions.

Drug Interactions

- The Drug interactions with the BZs are generally pharmacodynamic or pharmacokinetic (Table 62.11).

Table 59.11

Pharmacokinetic drug interactions with the benzodiazepines

Drug	Effect
Carbamazepine	Decreased Cl of alprazolam
Ciprofloxacin	Decreased Cl of diazepam and increased $t_{1/2}$
Erythromycin	Decreased Cl of alprazolam
Fluoxetine	Decreased Cl of diazepam
Fluvoxamine	Decreased Cl of alprazolam and diazepam and prolonged $t_{1/2}$
Isoniazid	Decreased Cl of diazepam and increased $t_{1/2}$
Ketoconazole	Decreased Cl and Vd of chlordiazepoxide; increased AUC of alprazolam
Nefazodone	Decreased Cl of alprazolam, AUC doubled, and $t_{1/2}$ prolonged
Omeprazole	Decreased Cl of diazepam and prolonged $t_{1/2}$
Oral contraceptives	Decreased Cl and increased $t_{1/2}$ of diazepam and chlordia-zepoxide; decreased $t_{1/2}$ of lorazepam and oxazepam
Paroxetine	Decreased Cl of alprazolam
Phenytoin	Increased Cl of clonazepam and reduced $t_{1/2}$
Propoxyphene	Decreased Cl of alprazolam and prolonged $t_{1/2}$
Propranolol	Decreased Cl of diazepam and prolonged $t_{1/2}$
Rifampin	Increased metabolism of diazepam
St. John's wort	Decreased AUC of alprazolam
Valproate	Decreased Cl of lorazepam

AUC, area under the plasma concentration curve; BZ, benzodiazepine; Cl, clearance; $t_{1/2}$, elimination half-life; Vd, volume of distribution.

DOSING AND ADMINISTRATION

- The initial dosage of benzodiazepines should be low and adjustments are made based on the requirement. (see Table 59.9).
- Treatment of acute anxiety generally should not exceed 4 weeks. BZs can be given as needed, and if several acute courses are necessary, a BZ-free period of 2 to 4 weeks should be implemented between courses.
- BZs with a long half life should be administered once daily at bedtime and they may provide nighttime hypnotic and anxiolytic effects the next day.
- In the case of elderly, dosage should be low, and short-elimination half-life agents are prescribed.

BUSPIRONE THERAPY

- Buspirone (*BuSpar*) is the first example of a class of anxiolytic agents that can relieve some symptoms of anxiety .
- It is the second line choice of drug for the treatment of GAD because of its poor efficacy, slow onset of action and lack of efficacy against depressive and anxiety disorders (ex : panic disorder or SAD).
- It has half life of 2.5 hours and given two to three times a day.

- The side effects includes dizziness,nausea and headache.

DRUG INTERACTIONS

- Buspirone causes increase in blood pressure in patients taking monoamine oxidase inhibitor (MAOI).
- Buspirone levels are increased by Verapamil, itraconazole, and fluvoxamine and decreased to 10-fold by rifampin .

DOSING AND ADMINISTRATION

- An increments of 5 mg/day of buspirone was done every 2 or 3 days as needed.
- 2 weeks or more are required for the onset of anxiolytic effects and maximum benefit requires 4 to 6 weeks.
- When BZ to buspirone,is changed the BZ should be tapered slowly.

PANIC DISORDER

GENERAL THERAPEUTIC PRINCIPLES

- Antipanic drugs are shown in Table 59.12.
- **SSRIs, TCAs,** and CBT (Cognitive Behavioral Therapy) are equally effective in treatment of panic disorder. **Alprazolam, clonazepam, sertraline, paroxetine,** and **venlafaxine** are FDA approved for this indication.
- The first line agents for the treatment of panic disorder are SSRIs , but BZs are the most commonly used agents for panic disorder.
- Patients treated with CBT are less likely to relapse than those treated with **imipramine** alone. For patients who cannot or will not take medications, CBT alone is indicated, as it is associated with improvement in 80% to 90% of patients short-term and 75% of patients at 6-month follow-up.
- Patients must be educated to avoid **caffeine**, stimulants and drugs of abuse.
- Antidepressants, especially the SSRIs, are preferred in elderly patients and children. The BZs are second line in these patients because of potential problems with disinhibition.

ANTIDEPRESSANTS

- Stimulatory side effects (e.g., insomnia, jitteriness, irritability, anxiety) can occur in **TCA**- and **SSRI**-treated patients. This may affect the compliance and hinder dose increases. Initial doses and gradual dose titration may eliminate these effects (see Table 59.12).
- **Imipramine** blocks panic attacks within 4 weeks, but maximal improvement, including reduced antiphobic response and anticipatory anxiety, requircs 8 to 12 weeks.
- About 25% of panic patients causes side effects because of **TCAs**.
- All **SSRIs** eliminate panic attacks in 60% to 80% of patients. The antipanic effect requires 4 weeks to respond, but some patients do not respond until 8 to 12 weeks.
- Low initial doses of **SSRIs** and gradual titration and to avoid stimulatory side effects antipanic dose is required.
- **MAOIs** are reserved for the most difficult or refractory panic disorder patients. Side effects and dietary and drug restrictions affect patient acceptance . **Fluoxetine** must be stopped 5 weeks before **phenelzine** (or another MAOI) is started. Other antidepressants should be stopped 2 weeks before phenelzine is started.

- Approximately 54% to 60% of patients are panic-free on venlafaxine extended release 75 mg or 150 mg.

BENZODIAZEPINES

- **BZs** are second-line agents have rapid response which is essential. They should not be used as monotherapy in panic disorder patients with a history of depression or drug abuse or **alcohol**. BZs are often used concomitantly with antidepressants to offset the delay in onset of antipanic effects in the first week.
- About 60% to 80% of panic patients respond to BZs, but relapse rates of 50% or higher are common despite slow drug tapering.
- **Alprazolam** and **clonazepam** are the most frequently used drugs in the BZs and are well accepted by patients. Therapeutic response typically occurs in 1 to 2 weeks. With alprazolam, the duration of action may be as little as 4 to 6 hours with breakthrough symptoms between dosing. The use of extended release of alprazolam or clonazepam avoids this problem.

DOSING AND ADMINISTRATION

- The starting dose of **clonazepam** is 0.25 mg twice daily, with a dose increase to 1 mg by the third day. Increases by 0.25 to 0.5 mg every 3 days to 4 mg/day can be made if needed.
- The starting dose of **alprazolam** is 0.25 to 0.5 mg three times daily (or 0.5 mg once daily of alprazolam extended release), slowly increasing over several weeks to an ideal dose. Most patients require 3 to 6 mg/day.
- Usually patients are treated for 12 to 24 months before discontinuation (over 4 to 6 months) is attempted. Many patients require long-term therapy. Successful maintenance with single weekly doses of **fluoxetine** has been described.

SOCIAL ANXIETY DISORDER

- Social anxiety disorder patients respond very slowly than patients with other anxiety disorders.
- Minimum of One year maintenance therapy is recommended to cause improvement and decrease the rate of relapse. Long-term treatment is needed for patients with comorbidity, unresolved symptoms, an early onset of disease, or a prior history of relapse.
- CBT (Cognitive Behavioural Therapy includes cognitive restructuring, relaxation training, exposure therapy and social skills training) and pharmacotherapy is considered effective in SAD, but CBT can lead to a greater likelihood of maintaining response after treatment termination. Even after response, most patients experience more than minimal residual symptoms.
- Drugs used in treatment of SAD are shown in Table 59.13.

POST TRAUMATIC STRESS DISORDER

- Patients should receive treatment individualized according to the symptoms exhibited by the patients. (e.g., **non-BZ hypnotic**, short courses of CBT) immediately after the trauma.
- The patients should be recommended for the treatment with drugs or the psychotherapy or both based on persistence of symptoms that lasts from three to four weeks.

- stress-inoculation training, relaxation training, biofeedback, distraction techniques, CBT, group therapy, hypnosis, psychodynamic therapies, and psychoeducation are the various types of psychotherapies used for the treatment of the post traumatic stress syndrome.
- Table 59.14 shows antidepressants used in the treatment of PTSD (Post Traumatic Stress Disorder).
- Remission can be monitored with the Treatment Outcome PTSD Scale (score less than or equal to 5) and the Sheehan Disability Scale (score less than or equal to 1 on each item).

Table 59.12

Drugs used in the treatment of panic disorder.

Class/Generic Name	Brand Name	Starting Dose	Antipanic Dosage[a] Range (mg)
Selective serotonin reuptake inhibitors			
Citalopram[b]	Celexa	10 mg per day	20–60
Escitalopram	Lexapro	5 mg per day	10–20
Fluoxetine[b]	Prozac	5 mg per day	10–30
Fluvoxamine[b]	Luvox	25 mg per day	100–300
Paroxetine[b]	Paxil	10 mg per day	20–60[c]
	Paxil CR	12.5 mg per day	25–75[c]
Sertraline[b]	Zoloft	25 mg per day	50–200[c]
Serotonin norepinephrine reuptake inhibitors			
Venlafaxine XR	Effexor XR	37.5 mg per day	75–225[c]
Benzodiazepines			
Alprazolam[b]	Xanax	0.25 mg three times a day	4–10[c]
	Xanax XR	0.5–1 mg per day	1–10[c]
Clonazepam[b]	Klonopin	0.25 mg once or twice per day	1–4[c]
Diazepam[b]	Valium	2–5 mg three times a day	5–20
Lorazepam[b]	Ativan	0.5–1 mg three times a day	2–8
Tricyclic antidepressant[b]			
Imipramine[b]	Tofranil	10 mg per day	75–250
Monoamine oxidase inhibitor			
Phenelzine	Nardil	15 mg per day	45–90

CR, controlled-release; XR, extended-release.

[a]Dosage used in clinical trials but not FDA approved. [b]Available generically. [c]Dosage is FDA approved.

Table 59.13

Drugs used in the treatment of generalized social anxiety disorder

Class/Generic Name	Brand Name	Starting Dose	Dosage Range[a] (mg/day)
Selective serotonin reuptake inhibitors			
Citalopram[b]	Celexa	20 mg per day	20–40
Escitalopram	Lexapro	5 mg per day	10–20
Fluvoxamine[b]	Luvox	50 mg per day	150–300
Paroxetine[b]	Paxil	10 mg per day	10–60[c]
Paroxetine CR	Paxil CR	12.5 mg per day	12.5–37.5[c]
Sertraline[b]	Zoloft	25–50 mg per day	50–200[c]
Serotonin-norepinephrine reuptake inhibitor			
Venlafaxine XR	Effexor XR	75 mg per day	75–225[c]
Benzodiazepine			
Clonazepam[b,d]	Klonopin	0.25 mg per day	1-4
Monoamine oxidase inhibitor			
Phenelzine	Nardil	15 mg at bedtime	60–90
Alternate agents			
Buspirone[b,d]	BuSpar	10 mg twice per day	45–60
Gabapentin[b]	Neurontin	100 mg three times a day	900–3,600
Mirtazapine[a,b]	Remeron	15 mg at bedtime	30
Pregabalin	Lyrica	100 mg three times a day	600

CR, controlled-release; XR, extended-release.

[a]Dosage used in clinical trials but not FDA approved. [b]Available generically. [c]Dosage is FDA approved. [d]Used as augmenting agent.

Table 59.14

Antidepressants used in the treatment of post traumatic stress disorder

Class/Generic Name	Starting Dose	Dosage Range[a] (mg/day)
Selective serotonin reuptake inhibitors		
Citalopram[c]	20 mg per day	20–60
Escitalopram	10 mg per day	10–20
Fluoxetine[c]	10–20 mg per day	10–80
Fluvoxamine[c]	50 mg per day	100–250
Paroxetine[c]	10–20 mg per day	20–50[b]
Sertraline[c]	25–50 mg per day	50–200[b]
Other agents		
Amitriptyline[c]	25–50 mg per day	50–300
Imipramine[c]	25–50 mg per day	50–300
Mirtazapine[c]	15 mg at bedtime	15–45
Phenelzine	15 mg every night	15–90
Venlafaxine extended-release	37.5 mg per day	37.5–225

[a]Dosage used in clinical trials but not FDA approved.

[d]osage is FDA approved. [a]vailable generically.

REFERENCES

1. Baldwin DS., Polkinghorn C. Evidence-based pharmacotherapy of generalised anxiety disorder. *Int J Neuropsychopharmacolf Official Scientific Journal Of The Collegium Internationale Neuivpsychopharmacologicum (CINP).* 2005; 8: 293–302.
2. Kapczinski F., Lima MS., Souza IS., Schmitt R. Antidepressants for generalized anxiety disorder. *Cochrane Database Syst Rev.* 2003; CD003592.
3. Baldwin D., Buis C., Mayers A. Selective serotonin reuptake inhibitors in the treatment of generalised anxiety disorder. *Exp Rev Neurotherapeutics.* 2002; 2: 717–724.
4. Dell'Osso B., Buoli M., Baldwin DS., Altamura AC. Serotonin norepinephrine reuptake inhibitors (SNRIs) in anxiety disorders: a comprehensive review of their clinical efficacy. *Hum Psychopharmacol: Clin Exp.* 2010; 25: 17–29.
5. Baldwin D., Woods R., Taylor D. Efficacy of drug treatments for generalised anxiety disorder: systematic review and meta-analysis. *BMJ.* 2011; 324: 1–11.
6. Bandelow B., Zohar J., Hollander E., Kasper S., Moller HJ. World Federation of Societies of Biological Psychiatry (WFSBP) guidelines for the pharmacological treatment of anxiety, obsessive-compulsive and posttraumatic stress disorders -first revision. *World J Biol Psychiatry.* 2008; 9: 248–312.
7. Ballenger JC., Davidson JRT., Lecrubier Y., et al. Consensus statement on generalised anxiety disorder from the International Consensus Group on Depression and Anxiety. *J Clin Psychiatry.* 2001; 62(suppl 11): 53–58.
8. Swinson RP., Antony MM., Bleau PB., et al. Clinical practice guidelines: management of anxiety disorders. *Can J Psychiatry.* 2006; 51(suppl 2): 1–92.
9. Kaplan GB., Moore KA. The use of cognitive enhancers in animal models of fear extinction. *Pharmacol Biochem Behav.* 2011; 99: 217–228.
10. Steckler T. Developing small molecule nonpeptidergic drugs for the treatment of anxiety disorders: is the challenge still ahead? *Curr Top Behav Neurosci.* 2010; 2: 415–428.
11. Spooren W., Lesage A., Lavreysen H., Gasparini F., Steckler T. Metabotropic glutamate receptors: their therapeutic potential in anxiety. *Curr Top Behav Neurosci.* 2010; 2: 391–413.
12. Ravindran LN., Stein MB. The pharmacologic treatment of anxiety disorders: a review of progress. *J Clin Psychiatry.* 2010; 71: 839–854.
13. Rynn MA., Brawman-Mintzer O. Generalised anxiety disorder: acute and chronic treatment. *CNS Spectrums.* 2004; 9: 716–723.
14. Nicolini H., Bakish D., Duenas H., et al. Improvement of psychic and somatic symptoms in adult patients with generalized anxiety disorder: examination from a duloxetine, venlafaxine extended-release and placebocontrolled trial. *Psychol Med.* 2009; 39: 267–276.
15. Martin JLR., Sainz-Pardo M., Furukawa TA., et al. Review: benzodiazepines in generalized anxiety disorder: heterogeneity of outcomes based on a systematic review and meta-analysis of clinical trials. *J Psychopharmacol.* 2007; 21: 774–782.
16. Hidalgo RB., Tupler LA., Davidson JR. An effect-size analysis of pharmacologic treatments for generalised anxiety disorder. *J Psychopharmacol.* 2007; 21: 864–872.
17. Hoehn-Saric R., McLeod DR., Zimmerli WD. Differential effects of alprazolam and imipramine in generalised anxiety disorder: somatic versus psychic symptoms. *J Clin Psychiatry.* 1988; 49: 293–301.
18. Tyrer P., Baldwin D. Generalised anxiety disorder. *Lancet.* 2006; 368: 2156–2166.
19. Coplan JD., Tiffon L., Gorman JM. Therapeutic strategies for the patient with treatment-resistant anxiety. *J Clin Psychiatry.* 1993; 54(suppl): 69–74.

20. Baldwin DS., Ajel K. Role of pregabalin in the treatment of generalized anxiety disorder. *Neuropsyschiatr Dis Treat.* 2007; 3: 185–191.
21. Montgomery S., Chatmara K., Pauer L., Whalen E., Baldinetti F. Efficacy and safety of pregabalin in elderly people with generalised anxiety disorder. *Br JPsychiatry.* 2008;193: 389–394.
22. LaLonde CD., Van Lieshout RJ. Treating generalized anxiety disorder with second-generation anti-psychotics: a systematic review and meta-analysis. *J Clin Psychopharmacol.* 2011; 31: 326–333.

CHAPTER 60

Major Depressive Disease

DEFINITION

The essential feature of major depressive disorder is a clinical course that is characterized by one or more major depressive episodes without a history of manic, mixed, or hypomanic episodes. Dysthymic disorder is a chronic disturbance of mood involving depressed mood and at least two other symptoms, and it is generally less severe than major depressive disorder. This chapter focuses exclusively on the diagnosis and treatment of major depressive disorder.

PATHOPHYSIOLOGY

- ***Biogenic amine hypothesis:*** Depression may be caused by decreased brain levels of the neurotransmitters norepinephrine (NE), serotonin (5-HT), and dopamine (DA).
- ***Postsynaptic changes in receptor sensitivity:*** Studies of many antidepressants have demonstrated that desensitization or downregulation of NE or 5HT receptors may relate to onset of antidepressant effects.
- ***Dysregulation hypothesis:*** This theory emphasizes a failure of homeostatic 1A regulation of neurotransmitter systems, rather than absolute increases or decreases in their activities. Effective antidepressants are theorized to restore efficient regulation to these systems.
- ***5-HT/NE link hypothesis:*** This theory suggests that there is a link between 5-HT and NE activity, and that both the serotonergic and noradrenergic systems are involved in the antidepressant response.
- ***The role of DA:*** Several reviews suggest that increased DA neurotransmission in the mesolimbic pathway may be related to the mechanism of action of antidepressants.

CLINICAL PRESENTATION

- Emotional symptoms may include diminished ability to experience pleasure, loss of interest in usual activities, sadness, pessimistic outlook, crying spells, hopelessness, anxiety (present in almost 90% of depressed outpatients), feelings of guilt, and psychotic features (e.g., auditory hallucinations, delusions).
- Physical symptoms may include fatigue, pain (especially headache), sleep disturbance, appetite disturbance (decreased or increased), loss of sexual interest, and GI and cardiovascular complaints (especially palpitations).

- Intellectual or cognitive symptoms may include decreased ability to concentrate or slowed thinking, poor memory for recent events, confusion, and indecisiveness.
- Psychomotor disturbances may include psychomotor retardation (slowed physical movements, thought processes, and speech) or psychomotor agitation.

DIAGNOSIS

- Major depression is characterized by one or more episodes of major depression, (Table 60-1). Symptoms must have been present nearly every day for at least 2 weeks. Patients with major depressive disorder may have one or more recurrent episodes of major depression during their lifetime.
- When a patient presents with depressive symptoms, it is necessary to investigate the possibility of a medical-, psychiatric-, and/or drug-induced (Table 60.2).
- Depressed patients should have a medication review, physical examination, mental status examination, a complete blood count with differential, thyroid function tests, and electrolyte determinations.

Table 60.1

DSM-IV-TR criteria for major depressive episode

A. Five (or more) of the following symptoms have been present during the same 2-week period and represent a change from previous functioning; at least one of the symptoms is either (1) depressed mood or (2) loss of interest or pleasure.

Note: Do not include symptoms that are clearly caused by a general medical condition or mood incongruent delusions or hallucinations.

1. Depressed mood most of the day nearly every day
2. Markedly diminished interest or pleasure in all, or almost all, activities most of the day nearly every day
3. Significant weight loss when not dieting or weight gain (e.g., a change of more than 5% of body weight
4. in a month), or decrease or increase in appetite nearly every day
5. Insomnia or hypersomnia nearly every day
6. Psychomotor agitation or retardation nearly every day (observable by others, not merely subjective
7. feelings of restlessness or being slowed down).
8. Fatigue or loss of energy nearly every day
9. Feelings of worthlessness or excessive or inappropriate guilt nearly every day
10. Diminished ability to think or concentrate, or indecisiveness, nearly every day
11. Recurrent thoughts of death (not just fear of dying), recurrent suicidal ideation without a specific plan, or a suicide attempt or a specific plan for committing suicide

B. The symptoms cause clinically significant distress or impairment in social, occupational, or other important areas of functioning.

C. The symptoms are not due to the direct physiologic effects of a substance (e.g., a drug of abuse, a medication) or a general medical condition (e.g., hypothyroidism).

D. The symptoms are not better accounted for by bereavement (i.e., after the loss of a loved one), the symptoms persist for longer than 2 months or are characterized by marked functional impairment, morbid preoccupation with worthlessness, suicidal ideation, psychotic symptoms, or psychomotor retardation.

Table 60.2

Common medical conditions, substance use disorders, and medications associated with depressive symptoms

General medical conditions	Cardiovascular disease	Drug therapy
Endocrine diseases	Coronary artery disease	Antihypertensives
Hypothyroidism	Congestive heart failure	Clonidine
Addison's or Cushing's disease	Myocardial infarction	Diuretics
Deficiency states	Neurologic disorders	Guanethidine sulfate
Pernicious anemia	Alzheimer's disease	Hydralazine hydrochloride
Wernicke encephalopathy	Epilepsy	Methyldopa
Severe anemia	Huntington's disease	Propranolol
Infections	Multiple sclerosis	Reserpine
AIDS	Pain	**Hormonal therapy**
Encephalitis	Parkinson's disease	Oral contraceptives
Human immunodeficiency virus		Steroids/adrenocorticotropic hormone
Mononucleosis	Poststroke	
Sexually transmitted diseases		**Acne therapy**
Tuberculosis	Malignant disease	Isotretinoin
Collagen disorder	**Substance use disorders (including intoxication and withdrawal)**	
Systemic lupus erythematosus	Alcoholism	Other
Metabolic disorders	Marijuana abuse and Dependence	Interferon- β_{1a}
Electrolyte imbalance	Nicotine dependence	
Hypokalemia	Opiate abuse and dependence (e.g., heroin)	
Hyponatremia	Psychostimulant abuse and dependence (e.g., cocaine)	
Hepatic encephalopathy		

DESIRED OUTCOME

- The goals of treatment of the acute depressive episode are to eliminate or reduce the symptoms of depression, minimize adverse effects, ensure compliance with the therapeutic regimen, facilitate a return to a premorbid level of functioning, and prevent further episodes of depression.

TREATMENT

NON PHARMACOLOGICAL TREATMENT

- The efficacy of psychotherapy and antidepressants is considered to be additive. Psychotherapy alone is not recommended for the acute treatment of patients with severe and/or psychotic major depressive disorders. For uncomplicated nonchronic major depressive disorder, combined treatment may provide no unique advantage. Cognitive therapy, behavioural therapy, and interpersonal psychotherapy appear to be equal in efficacy.
- Electroconvulsive therapy (ECT) is a safe and effective treatment for major depressive disorder. It is considered when a rapid response is needed, risks of other

treatments outweigh potential benefits, there has been a poor response to drugs, and the patient expresses a preference for ECT. A rapid therapeutic response (10 to 14 days) has been reported. Relative contraindications include increased intracranial pressure, cerebral lesions, recent myocardial infarction, recent intracerebral hemorrhage, bleeding, and otherwise unstable vascular conditions. Adverse effects of ECT include confusion, memory impairment (retrograde and anterograde), prolonged apnea, treatment emergent mania, headache, nausea, muscle aches, and cardiovascular dysfunction. Relapse rates during the year following ECT are high unless maintenance antidepressants are prescribed.

- Bright light therapy (i.e., the patient looking into a 10,000-lux intensity light box for about 30 min/day) may be used for patients with seasonal affective disorder and as adjunctive use for major depression.

PHARMACOLOGICAL THERAPY GENERAL

THERAPEUTIC PRINCIPLES

- Table 60-3 shows adult doses of antidepressants.
- In general, antidepressants are equal in efficacy in groups of patients when administered in comparable doses.
- Factors that influence the choice of antidepressant include the patient's history of response, history of familial response, concurrent medical conditions, presenting symptoms, potential for drug–drug interactions, comparative side-effect profiles of various drugs, patient preference, and drug cost.
- Between 65% and 70% of patients with major depression improve with drug therapy.
- Psychotically depressed individuals generally require either ECT or combination therapy with an antidepressant and an antipsychotic agent.
- The acute phase of treatment lasts 6 to 10 weeks, and the goal is remission (i.e., absence of symptoms).
- The continuation phase lasts 4 to 9 months after remission. The goal is to eliminate residual symptoms or prevent relapse.
- The maintenance phase lasts at least 12 to 36 months, and the goal is to prevent recurrence of a separate episode of depression.
- Some clinicians recommend lifelong maintenance therapy for persons at greatest risk for recurrence (i.e., persons younger than 40 years with two or more prior episodes and persons of any age with three or more prior episodes).
- Educating the patients and their support systems regarding the delay in antidepressant effects (typically 2 to 4 weeks) and the importance of adherence should occur before therapy is started and throughout treatment.

DRUG CLASSIFICATION

- Table 60-3 shows the commonly accepted classification of available antidepressants.
- Table 60-4 shows the relative potency and selectivity of the antidepressants and relative side-effect profiles.

Table 60.3

Adult dosages for currently available antidepressant medications[a]

Generic Name	Trade Name	Suggested Therapeutic Plasma Concentration (ng/mL)	Initial Dose (mg/day)	Usual Dosage Range (mg/day)
Selective serotonin reuptake inhibitors				
Citalopram	Celexa		20	20–60
Escitalopram	Lexapro		10	10–20
Fluoxetine	Prozac		20	20–60
Fluvoxamine	Luvox		50	50–30
Paroxetine	Paxil		20	020–60
Sertraline	Zoloft		50	50–200
Serotonin/norepinephrine reuptake inhibitors				
Venlafaxine	Effexor		37.5–75	75–225
Duloxetine	Cymbalta		30	30–90
Aminoketone				
Bupropion	Wellbutrin		150	150-300
Triazolopyridines				
Nefazodone	Serzone		100	200-600
Trazodone	Desyrel		150	150-300
Tetracyclics				
Mirtazapine	Remeron	120–250[b]	15	15-45
Tricyclics				
Tertiary amines				
Amitriptyline	Elavil		25	100-300
Clomipramine	Anafranil	200–350[b]	25	100-250
Doxepin	Sinequan		25	100-300
Imipramine	Tofranil		25	100-300
Secondary amines		100–300[c]		
Desipramine	Norpramin	50–150	25	100-300
Nortriptyline	Pamelor		25	50-200
Monoamine oxidase inhibitors				
Phenelzine	Nardil		15	30-90
Selegiline (transdermal)	Emsam		6[d]	6-12[d]
Tranylcypromine	Parnate		10	20-60

[a]Doses listed are total daily doses; elderly patients are usually treated with approximately one-half of the dose listed. [b]Parent drug plus metabolite. [c]It has been suggested that combined imipramine + desipramine concentrations should fall between 150–240 ng/mL. [d]Transdermal delivery system designed to deliver stated dose continuously over a 24-hour period.

- The **selective serotonin reuptake inhibitors** (SSRIs) inhibit the reuptake of 5-HT into the presynaptic neuron. They are generally chosen as first line antidepressants because of their safety in overdose and improved tolerability compared to earlier agents.
- **Tricyclic antidepressants** (TCAs) are effective for all depressive subtypes, but their use has diminished because of the availability of equally effective therapies that are safer on overdose and better tolerated. In addition to inhibiting the reuptake of NE and 5-HT, they also block adrenergic, cholinergic, and histaminergic receptors.
- The monoamine oxidase inhibitors (MAOIs) **phenelzine, tranylcypromine** increase the concentrations of NE, 5-HT, and DA within the neuronal synapse through inhibition of the monoamine oxidase (MAO) enzyme system. Both drugs are nonselective inhibitors of MAO-A and MAO-B. **Selegiline** is available as a transdermal patch for treatment of major depression. It inhibits MAO-A and MAO-B in the brain, but has reduced effects on MAO-A in the gut.
- The triazolopyridines **trazodone** and **nefazodone** are antagonists at the 5HT2 receptor and inhibit the reuptake of 5-HT. They can also enhance 5HT1A neurotransmission. They have negligible affinity for cholinergic and histaminergic receptors.
- **Bupropion's** most potent neurochemical action is blockade of DA reuptake; it blocks the reuptake of NE to a lesser extent.
- The serotonin-norepinephrine reuptake inhibitors include **venlafaxine** and **duloxetine**. Venlafaxine is an inhibitor of 5-HT and NE reuptake and a weak inhibitor of DA reuptake. **Desvenlafaxine** (Pristiq) was recently approved by the FDA. The dose is 50 mg once daily.
- **Maprotiline** and **amoxapine** are inhibitors of NE reuptake, with less effect on 5-HT reuptake.
- **Mirtazapine** enhances central noradrenergic and serotonergic activity through the antagonism of central presynaptic alpha -adrenergic autoreceptors and heteroreceptors. It also antagonizes 5-HT2 and 5-HT3 receptors. It also blocks histamine receptors.
- **St. John's wort**, an herbal nonprescription medication containing hypericum, may be effective for mild to moderate depression, but it is associated with several drug–drug interactions. Its potency, purity, and manufacture are not regulated by the FDA. As depression is a potentially life-threatening disease, all antidepressant treatments should be overseen by a trained healthcare professional.

ADVERSE EFFECTS

Adverse-effect profiles of the various antidepressants are summarized in Table 60.4.

Tricyclic Antidepressants and Other Heterocyclics

- Anticholinergic side effects (e.g., dry mouth, blurred vision, constipation, urinary retention, tachycardia, memory impairment, and delirium) and sedation are more likely to occur with the tertiary

Table 60.4

Relative potencies and side-effect profile of antidepressant drugs

	Reuptake Antagonism						
	Norepine-phrine	Sero-tonin	Anti-cholinergic Effects	Sedation	Orthostatic Hypotension	Seizures[a]	Conduction[a] Abnormalities
Tricyclics							
Tertiary Amines							
Amitriptyline	+++	++++	++++	++++	+++	+++	+++
Clomipramine	++	+++	++++	++++	++	++++	+++
Doxepin	++	++	+++	++++	++	+++	++
Imipramine	+++	+++	+++	+++	++++	+++	+++
Secondary amines							
Desipramine	++	+	++	++	++	++	++
Nortriptyline	++++	++++	++	++	++	++	++
Monoamine oxidase inhibitors							
Phenelzine	++	++	+	++	++	+	
Selegiline	0	0	0	+	++	0	0
Tranylcypromine	++	++	+	++	++	+	+

++++, high; +++, moderate; ++, low; +, very low; 0, absent.

amine **TCAs** than with the secondary amine TCAs.

- Orthostatic hypotension and resultant syncope, a common and potentially serious adverse effect of the **TCAs**, occurs as a result of α–adrenergic antagonism. Additional side effects include cardiac conduction delays and heart block, especially in patients with preexisting conduction disease.
- Other side effects that may lead to noncompliance include weight gain and sexual dysfunction.
- Abrupt withdrawal of **TCAs** (especially high doses) may result in symptoms of cholinergic rebound (e.g., dizziness, nausea, diarrhea, insomnia, restlessness).
- **Amoxapine** is a demethylated metabolite of loxapine and, as a result of its postsynaptic receptor DA-blocking effects, may be associated with extrapyramidal side effects.
- **Maprotiline**, a tetracyclic drug, causes seizures at a higher incidence than do standard TCAs and is contraindicated in patients with a history of seizure disorder. The ceiling dose is considered to be 225 mg/day.

VENLAFAXINE

- **Venlafaxine** may cause a dose-related increase in diastolic blood pressure. Dosage reduction or discontinuation may be necessary if sustained hypertension occurs. Other side effects are similar to those associated with the SSRIs (e.g., nausea and sexual dysfunction).

DULOXETINE

- The most common side effects are nausea, dry mouth, constipation, decreased appetite, insomnia, and increased sweating.

SELECTIVE SEROTONIN REUPTAKE INHIBITORS

- The SSRIs produce fewer sedative, anticholinergic, and cardiovascular adverse effects than the TCAs and are less likely to cause weight gain than the TCAs. The primary adverse effects include nausea, vomiting, diarrhea, headache, insomnia, fatigue, and sexual dysfunction. Very few patients have anxiety symptoms early in treatment.

TRIAZOLOPYRIDINES

- **Trazodone** and **nefazodone** cause minimal anticholinergic effects. sedation, dizziness, and orthostatic hypotension are the most frequent dose limiting side effects.
- Priapism occurs rarely with trazodone use (1 in 6,000 male patients). Surgical intervention may be required, and impotence may result.
- A black box warning for life-threatening liver failure was added to the prescribing information for nefazodone. Treatment with nefazodone should not be initiated in individuals with active liver disease or with elevated baseline serum transaminases.

AMINOKETONE

- The occurrence of seizures with **bupropion** is dose related and may be increased by predisposing factors (e.g., history of head trauma or CNS tumor). At the ceiling dose (450 mg/day), the incidence of seizures is 0.4%. Other side effects include nausea, vomiting, tremor, insomnia, dry mouth, and skin reactions. It is contraindicated in patients with bulimia or anorexia nervosa.

MIXED SEROTONIN-NOREPINEPHRINE EFFECTS

- **Mirtazapine's** most common adverse effects are somnolence, weight gain, dry mouth, and constipation.

MONOAMINE OXIDASE INHIBITORS

- The most common adverse effect of MAOIs is postural hypotension (more likely with **phenelzine** than **tranylcypromine**), which can be minimized by divided-daily dosing. Anticholinergic side effects are common but less severe than with the TCAs. Phenelzine causes mild to moderate sedating effects, but tranylcypromine is often stimulating, and the last dose of the day is administered in early afternoon. Sexual dysfunction in both genders is common. Phenelzine has been associated with hepatocellular damage and weight gain.
- Hypertensive crisis is a potentially fatal adverse reaction that can occur when MAOIs are taken concurrently with certain foods, especially those high in tyramine (Table 60.5), and with certain drugs (Table 60.6). Symptoms of hypertensive crisis include occipital headache, stiff neck, nausea, vomiting, sweating, and sharply elevated blood pressure. Hypertensive crisis may be treated with agents, such as captopril. Education of patients taking MAOIs regarding dietary and medication restrictions is critical.

Table 60.5

Dietary restrictions for patients taking monoamine oxidase inhibitors[a]

Aged cheeses[b]
Sour cream[c]
Yogurt[c]
Cottage cheese[c]
American cheese[c]
Mild Swiss cheese[d]
Wine[d] (especially Chianti and sherry)
Beer
Herring (pickled, salted, dry)
Sardines
Snails
Anchovies
Canned, aged, or processed meats
Monosodium glutamate
Liver (chicken or beef, more than 2 days old)
Fermented foods
Canned figs
Raisins
Pods of broad beans (fava beans)
Yeast extract and other yeast products
Meat extract (Marmite)
Soy sauce
Chocolate[e]
Coffee[e]
Ripe avocado
Sauerkraut
Licorice

[a]According to the FDA-approved prescribing information for the transdermal selegiline patch, patients receiving the 6 mg/24 hourdose are not required to modify their diet. However, patients receiving the 9 or 12 mg/24 hour dose are still required to follow the dietary restrictions similar to the other monoamine oxidase inhibitors (MAOIs). [b]Clearly warrants absolute prohibition (e.g., English Stilton, blue, Camembert, cheddar). [c]Up to 56 g (2 oz) daily is acceptable. [d]An 88 mL (3 oz) white wine or a single cocktail is acceptable. [e]Up to 56 g (2 oz) daily is acceptable: larger amounts of decaffeinated coffee are acceptable.

Table 60.6

Medication restrictions for patients taking monoamine oxidase inhibitors (MAOIs)

Amphetamines	Levodopa
Appetite suppressants	Local anesthetics containing sympathomimetic vaso-constrictors
Asthma inhalants	Meperidine
Buspirone	Methyldopa
Carbamazepine	Methylphenidate
Cocaine	Other antidepressants[a]
Cyclobenzaprine	Other MAOIs
Decongestants (topical and systemic)	Reserpine
Dextromethorphan	Rizatriptan
Dopamine	Stimulants
Ephedrine	Sumatriptan
Epinephrine	Sympathomimetics
Guanethidine	Tryptophan

[a]Tricyclic antidepressants can be used with caution by experienced clinicians in treatment-resistant populations.

PHARMACOKINETICS

- The major metabolic pathways of the **TCAs** are demethylation, hydroxylation, and glucuronide conjugation. Metabolism of the TCAs appears to be linear within the usual dosage range, but dose-related kinetics cannot be ruled out in the elderly.
- The SSRIs, with the possible exception of **citalopram** and **sertraline**, may have a nonlinear pattern of drug accumulation with chronic dosing.
- **Mirtazapine** is primarily eliminated in the urine.
- Factors reported to influence **TCA** plasma concentrations include disease

states (e.g., renal or hepatic dysfunction), genetics, age, cigarette smoking, and concurrent drug administration. Similarly, hepatic impairment, renal impairment, and age have been reported to influence the pharmacokinetics of **SSRIs**.

- In acutely depressed patients, there is a correlation between antidepressant effect and plasma concentrations for some **TCAs**. Table 60.3 shows suggested therapeutic plasma concentration ranges. The best-established therapeutic range is for **nortriptyline**, and data suggest a therapeutic window.
- Some indications for plasma level monitoring include inadequate response, relapse, serious or persistent adverse effects, use of higher than standard doses, suspected toxicity, elderly patients, children and adolescents, pregnant patients, patients of African or Asian descent (because of slower metabolism), cardiac disease, suspected non-compliance, suspected pharmacokinetic drug interactions, and changing brands.
- Plasma concentrations should be obtained at steady state, usually after a minimum of 1 week at constant dosage. Sampling should be done during the elimination phase, usually in the morning, 12 hours after the last dose. Samples collected in this manner are comparable for patients on once daily, twice-daily, or thrice-daily regimens.

DRUG–DRUG INTERACTIONS

- Drug interactions of the **TCAs** are summarized in Tables 60.7 and 60.8. Table 60.9 summarizes the drug interactions of non-TCAs.
- The very slow elimination of **fluoxetine** and **norfluoxetine** makes it critical to ensure a 5-week washout after fluoxetine discontinuation before starting an **MAOI**. Potentially fatal reactions may occur when any **SSRI** or **TCA** is coadministered with an MAOI.
- Increased plasma concentrations of **TCAs** and symptoms of toxicity may occur when **fluoxetine** and **paroxetine** are added to a TCA regimen.
- The combination of an SSRI with another 5-HT augmenting agent can lead to the serotonin syndrome, which is characterized by symptoms such as clonus, hyperthermia, and mental status changes.
- The ability of an SSRI, or any antidepressant, to inhibit or induce the activity of the cytochrome P450 (CYP450) enzymes can be a significant contributory factor in determining its capability to cause a pharmacokinetic drug–drug interaction.
- Table 60.10 compares second- and third-generation antidepressants for their effects on the enzymes of the CYP450 system.
- The drug interaction literature should be consulted for detailed information concerning any real or potential drug interaction involving any psychotherapeutic agent.

Table 60.7

Pharmacokinetic drug interactions involving tricyclic antidepressants (TCAs)

Elevates plasma concentrations of TCAs
Cimetidine
Diltiazem
Ethanol, acute ingestion
SSRIs
Haloperidol
Labetalol
Methylphenidate
Oral contraceptives
Phenothiazines
Propoxyphene
Quinidine
Verapamil
Lowers plasma concentrations of TCAs
Barbiturates
Carbamazepine
Ethanol, chronic ingestion
Phenytoin
Elevates plasma concentrations of interacting drug
Hydantoins
Oral anticoagulants
Lowers plasma concentrations of interacting drug
Levodopa

SSRI, selective serotonin reuptake inhibitor.

SPECIAL POPULATIONS

ELDERLY PATIENTS

- Prominent symptoms of depression in the elderly are loss of appetite, cognitive impairment, sleeplessness, anergia, fatigue, and loss of interest in and enjoyment of the normal pursuits of life.
- The **SSRIs** are often selected as first-choice antidepressants in elderly patients.
- In healthy elderly patients, cautious use of a secondary amine **TCA** (**desipramine** or **nortriptyline**) may be appropriate because of their defined therapeutic plasma concentration ranges, well-established efficacy, and well known adverse-effect profiles.
- **Bupropion** and **venlafaxine** may also be chosen because of their milder anticholinergic and less frequent cardiovascular side effects.

CHILDREN AND ADOLESCENTS

- Symptoms of depression in childhood include boredom, anxiety, failing adjustment, and sleep disturbance.
- Data supporting efficacy of antidepressants in children and adolescents are sparse. **Fluoxetine** is the only antidepressant that is FDA approved for treatment of depression in patients less than 18 years of age.
- The FDA has established a link between antidepressant use and suicidality (suicidal thinking and behaviors) in children, adolescents, and young adults 18 to 24 years old. All antidepressants carry a black box warning providing cautions in the use of all antidepressants in this population, and the FDA also recommends specific monitoring parameters. The clinician should consult the FDA-approved labeling or the FDA website for additional information. However, several retrospective longitudinal reviews of the use of antidepressants in children found no significant increase in the risk of suicide attempts or deaths.
- Several cases of sudden death have been reported in children and adolescents taking **desipramine**. A baseline electrocardiogram (ECG) is recommended

before initiating a TCA in children and adolescents, and an additional ECG is advised when steady-state plasma concentrations are achieved. TCA plasma concentration monitoring is critical to ensure safety.

PREGNANCY

- As a general rule, if effective, non drug approaches are preferred when treating depressed pregnant patients.
- One study showed that pregnant women who discontinued antidepressants were five times more likely to relapse during their pregnancy than were women who continued treatment.
- No major teratogenic effects have been identified with the **SSRIs** or **TCAs**. However, evaluations to date suggest a possible association of **fluoxetine** with low birth weight and respiratory distress.

Table 60.8

Pharmacodynamic drug interactions involving tricyclic antidepressants

Interacting Drug	Effect
Alcohol	Increased CNS depressant effects
Amphetamines	Increased effect of amphetamines
Androgens	Delusions, hostility
Anticholinergic agents	Excessive anticholinergic effects
Bepridil	Increased antiarrhythmic effect
Clonidine	Decreased antihypertensive efficacy
Disulfiram	Acute organic brain syndrome
Estrogens	Increased or decreased anti-depressant response; increased toxicity
Guanadrel	Decreased antihypertensive efficacy
Guanethidine	Decreased antihypertensive efficacy
Insulin	Increased hypoglycemic effects
Lithium	Possible additive lowering of seizure threshold
Methyldopa	Decreased antihypertensive efficacy; tachycardia; CNS stimulation
Monoamine oxidase inhibitors	Increased therapeutic and possibly toxic effects of both drugs; hypertensive crisis; delirium; seizures; hyperpyrexia; serotonin syndrome
Oral hypoglycemic	Increased hypoglycemic effects
Phenytoin	Possible lowering of seizure threshold and reduced antidepressant response
Sedatives	Increased CNS depressant effects
Sympathomimetics	Increased pharmacologic effects of direct-acting sympathomimetics; decreased effects of indirect acting sympathomimetics
Thyroid hormones	Increased therapeutic and possibly toxic effects of both drugs; CNS stimulation; tachycardia

Table 60.9

Selected drug interactions of newer-generation antidepressants

Antidepressant Class	Interacting Drug/ Drug	Effect
Serotonin/norepinephrine reuptake inhibitors		
Venlafaxine	MAOIs	Potential for hypertensive crisis, serotonin syndrome, delirium
	Sibutramine	Serotonin syndrome
	Triptans	Serotonin syndrome
Duloxetine	MAOIs	Potential for hypertensive crisis, serotonin syndrome, delirium
	Sibutramine	Serotonin syndrome
	Thioridazine	Thioridazine C_{max} increased; longed QTc interval
Selective serotonin reuptake inhibitors		
Citalopram & Escitalopram	MAOIs	Potential for hypertensive crisis, serotonin syndrome, delirium
	Linezolid (MAOI effects)	Serotonin syndrome
	Sibutramine	Serotonin syndrome
	Triptans	Serotonin syndrome
Fluoxetine	Alprazolam	Increased plasma concentrations and half-life of alprazolam; increased psychomotor impairment
	Antipsychotics (e.g., haloperidol and risperidone)	Increased antipsychotic concentr-ations; increased extrapyramidal side effects
	ß-Adrenergic blockers	Increased metoprolol serum con-centrations; increased bradycardia; possible heart block
	Carbamazepine	Increased plasma concentrations of carbamazepine; symptoms of carbamazepine toxicity
	Linezolid (MAOI effects)	Serotonin syndrome
	MAOIs	Potential for hypertensive crisis, serotonin syndrome, delirium
	Phenytoin	Increased plasma concentrations of phenytoin; symptoms of phenytoin toxicity
	TCAs	Markedly increased TCA plasma concentrations; symptoms of TCA toxicity
	Sibutramine	Serotonin syndrome
	Triptans	Serotonin syndrome
	Thioridazine	Thioridazine C_{max} increased; prolonged QTc interval

Table 60.9 *Contd...*

Antidepressant Class	Interacting Drug/ Drug	Effect
Fluvoxamine	Alosetron	Increased alosetron AUC (sixfold) and half-life (threefold)
	Alprazolam	Increased AUC of alprazolam by 96%, increased alprazolam half-life by 71%; increased psycho-motor impairment.
	ß-Adrenergic blockers	Fivefold increase in propranolol serum concentration; bradycardia and hypotension
	Carbamazepine	Increased plasma concentrations of carbamazepine; symptoms of carbamazepine toxicity
	Clozapine	Increased clozapine serum concentrations; increased risk for seizures and orthostatic hypotension
	Diltiazem	Bradycardia
	MAOIs	Potential for hypertensive crisis, serotonin syndrome, delirium
	Methadone	Increased methadone plasma concentrations; symptoms of methadone toxicity
	Ramelteon	Increased AUC (190-fold) and C_{max} (70-fold)
Fluvoxamine	SibutramineTCAs	Serotonin syndrome Increased TCA plasma concentration; symptoms of TCA toxicity
	Theophylline & caffeine	Increased serum concentrations of theophylline or caffeine; symptoms of theophylline or caffeine toxicity
	Thioridazine	Thioridazine C_{max} increased; prolonged QTc interval
	Warfarin	Increased hypoprothrombinemic response to warfarin
Paroxetine	Antipsychotics (e.g., haloperidol, perphenazine, and risperidone)	Increased antipsychotic concentr-ations; perphenazine, and risperi-done) increased CNS and extrapyra-midal side effects
	ß-Adrenergic blockers	Increased metoprolol serum con-centrations; increased bradycardia; possible heart block
	Linezolid (MAOI effects)	Serotonin syndrome
	MAOIs	Potential for hypertensive crisis, serotonin syndrome, delirium
	TCAs	Markedly increased TCA plasma concentrations; symptoms of TCA toxicity

Table 60.9 *Contd...*

Antidepressant Class	Interacting Drug/ Drug	Effect
Paroxetine	Sibutramine	Serotonin syndrome
	Triptans	Serotonin syndrome
	Thioridazine	Thioridazine C_{max} increased; prolonged QTc interval
Sertraline	Linezolid (MAOI effects)	Serotonin syndrome
	MAOIs	Potential for hypertensive crisis, serotonin syndrome, delirium
	Sibutramine	Serotonin syndrome
	Triptans	Serotonin syndrome
Tetracyclics		
Mirtazapine	Carbamazepine	Mirtazapine concentration decrease (60%)
	MAOIs	Theoretically central serotonin syndrome could occur
Aminoketone		
Bupropion	MAOIs	Potential for hypertensive crisis
	Medications that lower seizure threshold	Increased incidence of seizures

AUC, area under the curve, Cmax , maximum concentration; MAOI, monoamine oxidase inhibitor; TCA, tricyclic antidepressant.

Table 60.10

Second- and third-generation antidepressants and cytochrome (CYP) P450 enzyme inhibitory potential

	CYP Enzyme			
Drug	**1A2**	**2C**	**2D6**	**3A4**
Bupropion	0	0	+	0
Citalopram	0	0	+	
Escitalopram	0	0	+	0
Fluoxetine	0	++	++++	++
Fluvoxamine	++++	++	0	+++
Mirtazapine	0	0	0	0
Nefazodone	0	0	0	++++
Paroxetine	0	0	++++	0
Sertraline	0	++	+	+
Venlafaxine	0	0	0/+	0

++++, high; +++, moderate; ++, low; +, very low; 0, absent.

Another study reported a sixfold greater likelihood of the occurrence of persistent pulmonary hypertension of newborn infants exposed to an SSRI after the twentieth week of gestation.

- The risks of untreated depression in pregnancy should be considered. These included low birth weight, maternal suicidality, potential for hospitalization or marital discord, poor prenatal care, and difficulty caring for other children.

DOSING

- The usual initial adult dose of most **TCAs** is 50 mg at bedtime, and the dose may be increased by 25 to 50 mg every third day (see Table 60.3).

- **Bupropion** is usually initiated at 100 mg twice daily, and this dose may be increased to 100 mg three times daily after 3 days. An increase to 450 mg/day (the ceiling dose), given as 150 mg three times daily, may be considered in patients with no clinical response after several weeks at 300 mg/day.
- A 6-week antidepressant trial at a maximum dosage is considered an adequate trial. Patients must be told about the expected lag time of 2 to 4 weeks before the onset of antidepressant effect.
- Elderly patients should receive one-half the initial dose given to younger adults, and the dose is increased at a slower rate. The elderly may require 6 to 12 weeks of treatment to achieve the desired antidepressant response.
- To prevent relapse, antidepressants should be continued at full therapeutic doses for 4 to 9 months after remission.

REFERENCES

1. M. Fava and K. S. Kendler, "Major depressive disorder," Neuron, vol. 28, no. 2, pp. 335–341, 2000.
2 R. S. Duman, "Pathophysiology of depression: the concept of synaptic plasticity," European Psychiatry, vol. 17, no. 3, pp. 306–310, 2002.

CHAPTER 61

Headache

DEFINITION

Migraine is a common, recurrent, primary headache of moderate to severe intensity that interferes with normal functioning and is associated with GI, neurologic, and autonomic symptoms. In migraine with aura, a complex of focal neurologic symptoms which accompanies the attack.

PATHOPHYSIOLOGY

- Replacing previous neuronal and vascular theories of migraine pathophysiology, a combined theory has emerged. Activity in the trigeminovascular system may be regulated partly by serotonergic neurons within the brainstem. Pathogenesis may be related to a defect in the activity of neuronal calcium channels linking the release of the neurotransmitter in the brainstem areas that modulate cerebral vascular tone and nociception. The result may be vasodilation of intracranial extracerebral blood vessels with activation of the trigeminovascular system.
- Twin studies suggest 50% heritability of migraine, with a multifactorial polygenic basis. Migraine triggers may be modulators of the genetic set point that predisposes to migraine headache.
- Serotonin (5-hydroxytryptamine [5-HT]) receptors receiving persons may be involved in the pathophysiology and treatment of migraine headache. Acute antimigraine drugs such as ergot derivatives and triptan derivatives are agonists of vascular and neuronal 5HT1 receptor subtypes, causes vaso-constriction and vasoactive neuropeptide release inhibition and pain signal transmission.

CLINICAL FEATURES

Migraine with or without aura is a common recurrent headache syndrome in children and adolescents. The criteria established by the International Headache Society (IHS)1 were developed primarily for headache disorders in adults.

In the IHS system, migraine is defined on the basis of symptom profiles and the pattern of attack. The general medical examination and neurological evaluation, as well as diagnostic tests, serve primarily to exclude secondary headache.

Migraine is a heterogeneous disorder having exacerbations or remissions in children and often vary by sex and age of the individual. In children aged 4-7, migraine is more frequent in boys than in girls.

Between the ages of 7 and 11 the prevalence is equal. From about 11–12 on, the ratio changes to the classic three girls to one boy.

MIGRAINE IN CHILDREN

Migraine is characterized by recurrent episodes of throbbing head pain of variable intensity, duration and frequency, with associated nausea and vomiting, along with phonophobia or photophobia . In 1988, the IHS proposed a new set of criteria for childhood migraine based on international expert consensus. Before this, Vahlquist was one of the first to define childhood migraine as a paroxysmal headache separated by pain-free intervals and accompanied by at least two of the following four features: vomiting, visual aura, unilateral pain and a family history of migraine. Prensky redefined migraine as paroxysmal headache, with three of six associated symptoms: aura, abdominal pain, unilateral pain, throbbing quality, relief with sleep and family history of migraine.

Unilateral pain is much more characteristic of adult migraine than childhood migraine. Although bilateral location (frontal/temporal) is common in children, unilateral headache has a high positive predictive value for migraine at 85%. These pain features should remain part of the IHS definition in children. The visual aura of migraine is reported in 14–30% of children and adolescents as disturbances, distortions, or obscuration before or as the headache begins. Children will present with complaints of seeing spots, colours or rainbows, but usually the symptoms need to be elicited by asking pointed questions. It was reported that children's visual symptomatology included three dominant visual phenomena: binocular visual impairment with scotoma (77%), monocular visual impairment or scotoma (7%), distortion or hallucinations (16%). The diagnosis of migraine with aura requires two or more fully reversible symptoms, including visual, motor or sensory symptoms. The aura should develop gradually over at least 4 min, and usually lasts 20–30 min but may last as long as 60 min. In an aura that is short in duration or rapid in onset, an alternative paroxysmal event may be the aetiology. An atypical and/or prolonged event (> 60 min) may signal an organic disorder that requires further diagnostic assessment.

MIGRAINE VARIANTS

Migraine presents with dramatic neurological signs such as hemiparesis, ataxia, acute confusional states, ophthalmoparesis and vertigo. These clinical entities are often termed 'migraine variants'. The abrupt appearance of such focal and ominous neurological signs, accompanying an excruciating headache with vomiting, will initially raise concerns of a life-threatening neurological aetiology such as a brain tumour, intracranial haemorrhage, hydrocephalus, CNS infection or intoxication. The transient deficits of the migraine variants are thought to result from a wave of depolarization migrating across the visual cortex and/or from regional oligaemia caused by a neuropeptide-mediated, sterile, neurogenic inflammation. There are frequently shared or overlapping clinical features with many of the migraine variants, and this observation suggests a common pathophysiology. Still incompletely explained are the cranial nerve signs associated with ophthalmoplegic and basilar migraine. Some of the migraine variants are represented as part of the classification system of the IHS . Inclusion of hemiplegic and basilar migraine variants within the spectrum of migraine *with aura* reflects the contemporary view of their pathogenesis. The IHS system fails to include the clinical entities confusional migraine and cyclical vomiting, but both are reviewed. Also omitted is the Alice-in-Wonderland syndrome, which most probably represents an unusual form of visual aura with distortions, illusions, micropsia and macropsia.

DIAGNOSIS

- A comprehensive headache history is the most important element in establishing the diagnosis of migraine.
- In the evaluation of the headache, diagnostic alarms should be observed. They includes mainly immediate onset of the extremes of headache ever, with increased pattern of headache following subacute onset, onset of headache after age 50 years, headache associated with systemic illness (e.g., fever, nausea, vomiting, stiff neck, and rash), headache with papilledema, and new-onset headache in a patient with cancer or human immunodeficiency virus infection.
- A stable pattern of headaches, absence of daily headache, family history for migraine, neurological examination, food triggers presence, menstrual related, long-term history, are signs indicative of migraine headache. migraine headache is not diagnosed based on aura.
- General medical and neurologic physical examinations were performed. Observation of following signs like important signs (Pyrexia, elevated blood pressure), funduscopy (papilledema, hemorrhage, and exudates), palpation and auscultation of the head and neck and neurologic examination .
- Imagining studies like computed tomography or magnetic resonance imaging are considered in patients with unexplained findings on the neurologic exam, those with additional risk factors, or those with an atypical headache history.

TREATMENT

NONSTEROIDAL ANTI-INFLAMMATORY DRUGS (NSAIDS)

NSAIDs taken daily can prevent migraine. Many of them are in Group 2, including fenoprofen (Nalfon), flurbiprofen (Ansaid), ketoprofen (Orudis, Oruvail), mefanamic acid (Ponstel), naproxen (Naprosyn), and naproxen sodium (Anaprox, Aleve, Naprelan). Ibuprofen (Advil, Motrin), which people report sometimes works, is in Group 3a.

NSAIDs block prostaglandin synthesis via cyclo-oxygenase (COX). There are two major cyclo-oxygenases—COX-1 and COX-2. COX-1 has important functions in the stomach, kidney, and platelets, while COX-2 is associated with inflammation. The older NSAIDs block both, preventing inflammation mediated by prostaglandins, but also setting up potential for adverse events in the stomach, kidneys, and platelets. If part of the mechanism of migraine pain is inflammation around the blood vessels of the meninges (see chapter 4), taking a chronic anti-inflammatory may prevent the inflammation from developing.

The problem with taking the older "two-pathway blocking" NSAIDs is their potential for side effects such as elevated blood pressure, heartburn and indigestion, gastroesophageal reflux disease (GERD), stomach ulcers, excess bleeding, and kidney disease. Some NSAIDs have a particularly high risk for producing ulcers, specifically ketorolac (Toradol), and the development of ulcers can be without symptoms until the ulcer bleeds.

Some doctors attempt to prevent stomach ulcers by simultaneously prescribing a proton pump inhibitor stomach-protecting medication omeprazole [Prilosec] is the most widely used or the histamine H2 blocker mild stomach protectors also available over the counter, such as ranitidine (Zantac), cimetidine (Tagamet), famotidine (Pepcid), and nizatidine (Axid), all of which work by interfering with the stomach's ability to produce acid.

The risk of kidney dysfunction in people taking daily NSAIDs merits renal monitoring. Because most NSAIDs inhibit platelet function, increasing the risk for bleeding, their use must be discontinued before surgery.

The last major problem in taking daily NSAIDs is that the antiinflammatories can actually cause daily headache via the habituation and rebound phenomenon (see chapter 8). In that situation, not only do they not work in preventing migraine, they can transform occasional migraine into chronic daily headache. Because of the potential for gastrointestinal problems, kidney problems, and rebound daily headache, some headache specialists recommend against using NSAIDs at all as daily preventive medications.

There are many groups of NSAIDs, and little evidence favoring one group or particular NSAID over another in the prevention of migraine. Conventionally, we tend to use the NSAIDs from Group 2 first; most headache specialists use naproxen or naproxen sodium first, although indomethacin (which is in Group 5), ketoprofen, and flurbiprofen are often used as well.

All anti-inflammatories inhibit cyclo-oxygenase, but the COX-2 inhibitors inhibit only those associated with inflammation. The three available at the time of this writing are celecoxib (Celebrex), rofecoxib (Vioxx), and valdecoxib (Bextra). The advantage of COX-2 inhibitors is that, because they do not usually cause ulcers or gastrointestinal upset, they can be used with greater safety.

Aspirin is the granddaddy of all nonsteroidal anti-inflammatories, and carries with it the same risks of daily use. Scientific studies have shown it to be effective in preventing migraine, but there is no agreement what dose will prevent migraine.

There is agreement that, if daily aspirin to prevent migraine is going to be tried, aspirin should be taken alone and not mixed with caffeine (Anacin) or caffeine plus acetaminophen (Excedrin). Those combination drugs should be used to get rid of a mild, non-disabling migraine, not to prevent migraine on a daily basis.

Some studies suggest taking a regular aspirin daily (300–325 mg), others one every other day. Another suggestion is to take a "baby aspirin" (81 mg) daily.

These doses are low enough that they will not usually cause rebound or daily headache to develop. However, it may take several months for the aspirin to reduce the frequency of migraines—if it has any effect at all.

INDOLE AND INDENE ACETIC ACIDS

Indometacin is a methylated indole derivative, with analgesic but mainly anti-inflammatory action. The peak concentration in the plasma is reached within 2h, but may be delayed when the drug is taken after meals. The half-life in the plasma is variable but is around 2h. The agent is metabolized in the liver and eliminated mostly with the urine, but also with the bile and faeces. The FDA has not approved its use in children.

HETEROARYLACETIC ACIDS

Ketorolac is a potent analgesic and a weak anti-inflammatory agent. Ketorolac is rapidly absorbed when given orally or intramuscularly, achieving the peak plasma concentration in 30–50 min. Its half-life ranges from 4 to 6 h and it is about 90% eliminated in the wine. The FDA has not approved this agent for the treatment of pain in children. Diclofenac is a phenylacetic acid derivative with three properties like anti-inflammatory, analgesic and antipyretic activities. It is rapidly absorbed when given orally and intramuscularly, achieving the peak plasma concentration in 30–50 min. The drug has a half-life of 4–6 h and is eliminated through the kidneys. The FDA has not approved this agent for the treatment of pain in children.

ARYLPROPIONIC ACIDS

Ibuprofen is the main member of the propionic class of NSAIDs. It is rapidly absorbed when given orally. The peak in plasma levels is observed after 1–2 h, with a half-life of about 2 h. The biotransformation occurs in the liver and the excretion is renal. The efficacy of this agent was evaluated compared with acetaminophen in a doublemasked, randomized controlled, crossover study performed in a group of 106 children aged 4–16 years who had migraine. The dose of ibuprofen suggested in children aged under 12 is from a quarter to half the adult dose.1 Naproxen Peak plasma concentration occurs in 2–4 h. Naproxen is also absorbed rectally with a half-life in the plasma of about 14 h. The drug is metabolized by the liver and almost entirely excreted in the urine. The FDA has approved the agent for paediatric use at the age of 12 years or over, in the abortive treatment of migraine.6 Ketoprofen shares the pharmacological properties of other propionic acid derivatives.

It is rapidly absorbed after oral administration, its maximal concentration in the plasma is achieved within 1–2 h and its half-life is about 2 h. The drug is biotransformed in the liver and excreted with urine. This agent is not approved for paediatric use in the treatment of pain.

OTHER THERAPIES

Several authors suggest that children should be given a gastrokinetic antiemetic before administration of analgesics, especially if nausea and vomiting are severe. The gastrokinetic antiemetics are domperidone and metoclopramide. Metoclopramide is also prepared as a suspension at the concentration of 5mg/5ml. It can determine adverse effects such as restlessness and extrapyramidal effects, as a result of antagonism with dopaminergic receptors in the central nervous system. *Anti-migraine drugs* Specific acute anti-migraine drugs include sumatriptan, the 'second generation of triptans' and the ergot alkaloids.

TRIPTANS

Triptans are 5-hydroxytryptamine (5HT or serotonin) derivatives; they are selective agonists for vascular 5HT receptor subtypes such as 5HT1D, 5HT1B, 5HT1F and 5HT1A, although they possess low affinity for adrenergic and dopaminergic receptors. The anti-migraine effect seems to occur through different mechanisms:

1. Inhibition of dural neurogenic inflammation
2. Direct attenuation of excitability of cells in trigeminal nuclei via stimulation of 5HT1B receptors
3. Vasoconstriction of meningeal, dural, cerebral or pial vessels mediated via stimulation of 5HT1B receptors.

Sumatriptan is a 5HT1 receptor agonist, with a high affinity for 5HT1D and 5-HT1B receptors and lower interaction with 5HT1A and 5HT1E receptors. Sumatriptan is rapidly absorbed after oral administration, with a bioavailability of 14%, as a result of an extensive first-pass metabolism and a half-life of 2.5 h. The second generation of triptans include zolmitriptan, naratriptan, rizatriptan, eletriptan and frovatriptan. This new class of agents differs from sumatriptan in their interactions with 5HT receptors and their bioavailability. Zolmitriptan is a 5HT1B/D-selective agonist with a bioavailability of 40% and a half-life of 2.5–3hrs. The FDA has approved the drug only for use in adults. Rizatriptan is a selective 5HT1B/D receptor agonist with no or very low activity at other 5HT receptor subtypes, or adrenergic, dopaminergic and histaminergic receptors. This agent is rapidly absorbed after oral administration, with a bioavailability of 40–45% and a plasma half-life of 2–3 h. It is metabolized in the liver by monoamine oxidase. A and excreted with its metabolites mostly in the urine. At the present time, several studies are being carried out that evaluate the use of this agent in children and adolescents. The FDA approved the use of this agent only in adults. Naratriptan is a selective 5HT1B and 5HT1D agonist. Absorbed when given orally, it presents a bioavailability of 70%. Metabolized in the liver, it is excreted in the urine.

ERGOTAMINE

Ergotamine belongs to the class of ergot alkaloids, derivatives of the tetracyclic compound 6-methylergoline. They are non-selective pharmacological agents which interact with various receptors, such as 5HT1 and 5HT2, adrenergic and dopaminergic receptors. The absorption of the drug when given orally is changeable as a result of an extensive first-pass metabolism. The peak plasma concentration is reached in about 70 min. Ergotamine is metabolized in the liver and excreted mostly in the bile. Only traces of unmetabolized drug are found in the urine and faeces. Ergotamine preparations are available in a variety of preparations and combinations with other agents. Ergotamine is no longer used to treat migraine and is not indicated in children.

PROPHYLACTIC TREATMENT OF MIGRAINE

Migraine is considered to be a disorder of multifactorial aetiology which can be triggered by external and internal factors. Each attack is characterized by headache combined with autonomic disturbances, mostly nausea, vomiting, photophobia and phonophobia. Migraine prophylaxis is requested in the presence of more than three attacks per month, when attacks do not respond to acute treatment or when the adverse events of acute treatments are severe. The aim of preventive treatment is to reduce the frequency and severity of attacks while keeping the side effects to a minimum. Many medications studied as preventive treatments of migraine have not been adequately evaluated in children; others were involved in clinical trials carried out before the establishment of the International Headache Society (IHS) migraine classification. In children, drugs such as β blockers, calcium channel blockers, anti-serotoninergic agents, antidepressant agents and clonidine have been widely studied.

β-*blockers*

β-Receptors include β1, β2 and β3, all of which are Gs protein coupled and differ with regard to their location. β1-Receptors are located in the heart, kidney and central nervous system (CNS), β2-receptors in the smooth muscles and CNS and β3-receptors in fat. β Blockers include propranolol, nadolol, atenolol and timolol; only propranolol and timolol are used clinically in the treatment of migraine. β Blockers are having more affinity towards beta1 & 2 receptors. relative affinity for β1- and β2-receptors, intrinsic activity, blockade of β-adrenergic receptors, differences in lipid solubility and pharmacokinetic properties. These agents are not indicated for use in patients with asthma, cardiac failure, diabetes and renal insufficiency. Side effects, including hypotension, exercise intolerance, bradycardia and bradyarrhythmias in patients with atrioventricular conduction defects, are seldom severe and are manifested as a consequence of the β-receptor blockade. The clinical efficacy of β blockers in the prevention of migraine is still unknown and their pharmacological properties do not provide sufficient explanation for the same. Propranolol interacts with an equal affinity for β1- and β2-receptors; Propranolol is mostly metabolized by the liver during the first passage through the portal circulation; only 25% reaches the systemic circulation. The bioavailability of this agent may be increased by the concomitant ingestion of food. The efficacy of propranolol in adult and childhood migraine has been suggested; administration should commence at a low dose (1–2 mg/kg per day) and continue for at least 12 weeks. The FDA has approved the use of propranolol in migraine prophylaxis in adults. Timolol is a potent, non-subtype-selective, β adrenergic antagonist, possessing no intrinsic sympathomimetic activity. It is well absorbed in the gastrointestinal tract when given orally .

CALCIUM CHANNEL BLOCKERS

Voltage-sensitive channels have been divided into various subtypes on the basis of their kinetic and functional properties. According to their kinetic characteristics, they are differentiated into 'low-threshold' and 'high-threshold' channels. The former, also called 'T' channels, can be opened by short depolarizations and play a key role in the control of the excitability and activity of some nervous cells. The latter can be opened by using high depolarizations and include L, N, P and Q channels, which are also represented in the CNS. High threshold channels are reportedly responsible for the high increases of the cytosolic Ca^{2+} and the release of intracellular calcium necessary for its action as a second messenger. Calcium Channel Blockers (CaCB) inhibit voltage-sensitive calcium by channels blocking the entry of extracellular Ca^{2+} and the release of intracellular Ca^{2+} into vascular smooth muscles, causing vasodilatation. This group of drugs includes compounds such as flunarizine, nimodipine, verapamil and diltiazem. Flunarizine is considered as a wide-spectrum CaCB: it acts on T- and L-type calcium channels by binding the receptor site at the extracellular surface of the calcium channels of the cardiac muscle, vascular smooth muscles, CNS neurons and chromaffin cells. The mechanism of action of flunarizine in the prevention of migraine is not clear; it is thought to be the result of the blockade of different pathways of intracellular calcium elevation. Several authors have suggested that the antimigraine effect is related to its ability to interfere with the dopaminergic system blocking D2-receptors. The importance of the role played by the dopaminergic system is based on the evidence that this drug is able to cause extrapyramidal side effects and/or depression. Flunarizine also seems to interfere with the cholinergic system, which is reportedly involved in the mechanisms of pain regulation, determining a decrease in the release of hippocampal acetylcholine in rats . Flunarizine appears to be effective in the prophylaxis of adult and childhood migraine at a dose of 0.1–0.3 mg/kg per day for 12 weeks. Verapamil, an L-type CaCB, acts on vascular smooth muscle and cardiac cells, inducing a negative inotropic effect on sinoatrial (SA) and atrioventricular (AV) nodes; therefore it should not be used in patients with ventricular or nodal conduction dysfunctions. When given orally, calcium channel blockers are almost completely absorbed, although their bioavailability is reduced. The most common side effects observed with this group of agents are caused by excessive vasodilatation. The FDA has not approved the use of this drug for migraine in children.

ANTI-SEROTONINERGIC DRUGS

The evidence linking 5HT to migraine is circumstantial. During a migraine attack, platelet 5HT decreases, urinary 5HT increases in some patients and 5-hydroxyindole acetic acid (5A), a major metabolite of 5HT, may increase. This class of agents includes methysergide, a congener of methylergonovine, which blocks 5HT2A, 5HT 2B and 5HT 2C receptors. Methysergide is a 5HT 1 receptor agonist and its therapeutic effect is dependent on 5HT 2 blockade and vasoconstriction of the carotid vascular bed. It was speculated that the activation of 5HT 2B and 5HT 2C receptors by endogenous 5HT could dilate cerebral vessels, resulting in the release of endothelium-derived nitric oxide (NO), which can activate sensory trigeminovascular fibres. Various side effects are manifested with this compound, although they are usually mild and of a transient nature; the most common are diarrhoea, nausea and vomiting. Central disturbances include drowsiness, weakness, nervousness, excitement and psychotic episodes. The onset of inflammatory fibrosis represents a rare but potentially severe complication of prolonged treatment. This condition can develop in different sites, giving rise to retroperitoneal fibrosis, pleuropulmonary fibrosis, and coronary and endocardial fibrosis. Fibrosis usually reverses after drug withdrawal, although persistent damage to cardiac valves has been observed in 1 of 5000 treated patients. Consistently, therapy should be interrupted after 6 months of continuous treatment. In adults, the efficacy of methysergide in the prophylaxis of migraine headache is well documented.

ANTIDEPRESSANTS

This class of drugs includes tricyclic agents such as amitriptyline, imipramine, nortriptyline, trazodone and selective serotonin reuptake inhibitors. It is used for the prophylaxis of migraine in adults. It causes a potent inhibition of 5HT reuptake and antagonizes 5HT 2 receptors. The prophylactic effect is independent of its antidepressant action and occurs due to alteration of serotoninergic. Side effects are related to the anticholinergic properties of this drug and include dry mouth, dizziness, urinary retention, cardiac arrhythmia and orthostatic hypotension. When given orally, amitriptyline reaches a peak serum level after 4 h, with a half-life of 2-25 h. The hepatic metabolism converts the drug into nortriptyline, an active derivative. The drug is excreted through the kidney. The dose of oral amitriptyline may range from 0.1 to 2 mg/kg per day.

DOPAMINE AGONISTS

Lisuride is a semi-synthetic ergot derivative capable of stimulating D1 and D2 dopamine receptor subtypes. Lisuride is characterized by potent antihistaminic, central dopaminergic and anti-serotoninergic activity. Hypotension caused by the stimulation of 5HT 7 receptors is blocked by lisuride in anaesthetized rats. A hypotensive action has been described at high doses of this drug in adults, as a result of its activity on dopamine receptors. When given orally, lisuride reaches a peak concentration after 40 min, with a half-life of 2 h. It may cause cardiovascular side effects such as orthostatic hypotension, nausea and vomiting. The use of lisuride as a prophylactic agent is based on the hypothesis of hypersensitivity of the dopaminergic system in migraineurs. Several clinical studies performed in the past with apomorphine, a dopaminergic agonist, showed the presence of a hyper-responsiveness of dopaminergic receptors in migraineurs, compared with controls.

MISCELLANEOUS

Several drugs used in the prevention of migraine have not yet been studied adequately and are therefore not used in the management of the disease. These include trazodone, clonidine, antihistamines and several anticonvulsants, such as valproate. The action of valproate as an anticonvulsant agent appears to be mediated by a prolonged recovery of voltage-activated Na^+ channels from inactivation. The mechanism of action of this compound in the treatment of migraine is still unknown. The FDA has approved use of this compound for the treatment of migraine in subjects aged over 16 years. It is administered as 15–30 mg/kg per day divided into two doses. Clonidine, an imidazoline, is an α2-selective adrenergic agonist acting on the CNS.

Table 61.1

Acute migraine therapies[a]

Medication	Dosage	Comments
Analgesics		
Acetaminophen	1,000 mg at onset; repeat every 4–6 hours as needed	Maximum daily dose is 4 g
Acetaminophen 250 mg/aspirin 250 mg/caffeine 65 mg	2 tablets at onset and every 6 hours	Available over-the-counter as Excedrin Migraine
Aspirin or acetaminophen with butalbital, caffeine	1–2 tablets every 4–6 hours	Limit dose to 4 tablets/day and usage to 2 days/week
Isometheptene 65mg/dichlor-alphenazone 100 mg/aceta-minophen 325 mg (Midrin)	2 capsules at onset; repeat 1 capsule every hour as needed	Maximum of 6 capsules/day and 20 capsules/month
Nonsteroidal antiinflammatory drugs		
Aspirin	500–1,000 mg every 4–6 hours	Maximum daily dose is 4 g
Ibuprofen	200–800 mg every 6 hours	Avoid doses >2.4 g/day
Naproxen sodium	550–825 mg at onset; can repeat 220 mg in 3–4 hours	Avoid doses >1.375 g/day
Diclofenac potassium	50–100 mg at onset; can repeat 50 mg in 8 hours	Avoid doses >150 mg/day Maximum dose is 6 mg/day or 10 mg/week; consider pre-treatment with an antiemetic
Ergotamine tartrate-		
Oral tablet (1 mg) with caffeine 100 mg, Rectal suppository (2 mg) with caffeine 100 mg	2 mg at onset; then 1–2 mg every 30 minutes as needed	Maximum dose is 4 mg/day or 10 mg/week; consider pre-treatment with an antiemetic
Sublingual tablet (2 mg)	---	---
Rectal suppository (2 mg) with caffeine 100 mg	Insert ½ to 1 suppository at onset; repeat after 1 hour as needed	Maximum dose is 4 mg/day or 10 mg/week; consider pre-treatment with an antiemetic
Dihydroergotamine		
Injection 1 mg/mL	0.25–1 mg at onset IM or subcutaneous; repeat every hour as needed	Maximum dose is 3 mg/day or 6 mg/week
Nasal spray	One spray (0.5 mg) in each nostril at onset; repeat sequence 15 minutes later (total dose is 2 mg or 4 sprays)	Maximum dose is 3 mg/day; prime sprayer four times before using; do not tilt head back or inhale through nose while spraying; discard open ampules after 8 hours
Serotonin agonists (triptans)		
Sumatriptan Injection	6 mg subcutaneous at onset; can repeat after 1 hour if needed	Maximum daily dose is 12 mg

Table 61.1 *Contd...*

Medication	Dosage	Comments
Medication		
Oral tablets	25, 50, or 100 mg at onset; can repeat after 2 hours if needed	Optimal dose is 50–100 mg; maximum daily dose is 200 mg
Nasal spray	5, 10, or 20 mg at onset; can repeat after 2 hours if needed	Optimal dose is 20 mg; maximum daily dose is 40 mg; single-dose device delivering 5 or 20 mg; administer one spray in one nostril form
Zolmitriptan		
Oral tablets	2.5 or 5 mg at onset as regular or orally disintegrating tablet; can repeat after 2 hours if needed	Optimal dose is 2.5 mg; maximum dose is 10 mg/day Do not divide ODT dosage form
Nasal spray	5 mg (one spray) at onset; can repeat after 2 hours if needed	Maximum daily dose is 10 mg/day
Naratriptan	1 or 2.5 mg at onset; can repeat after 4 hours if needed	Optimal dose is 2.5 mg; maximum daily dose is 5 mg
Rizatriptan	5 or 10 mg at onset as regular or orally disintegrating tablet; can repeat after 2 hours if needed	Optimal dose is 10 mg; maximum daily dose is 30 mg; onset of effect is similar with standard and orally disinter-grating tablets; use 5-mg dose (15 mg/day max) in patients receiving propranolol
Almotriptan	6.25 or 12.5 mg at onset; can repeat after 2 hours if needed	Optimal dose is 12.5 mg; maximum daily dose is 25 mg
Frovatriptan	2.5 or 5 mg at onset; can repeat in 2 hours if needed	Optimal dose 2.5–5 mg; maximum daily dose is 7.5 mg (3 tablets)
Eletriptan	20 or 40 mg at onset; can repeat after 2 hours if needed	Maximum single dose is 40 mg; maximum daily dose is 80 mg
Miscellaneous		
Butorphanol nasal spray	1 spray in 1 nostril (1 mg) at onset; repeat in 1 hour if needed	Limit to 4 sprays/day; consider use only when nonopioid therapies are ineffective or not tolerated
Metoclopramide	10 mg IV at onset	Useful for acute relief in the office or emergency department setting
Prochlorperazine	10 mg IV or IM at onset	Useful for acute relief in the office or emergency department setting

ODT, orally disintegrating tablet.

[a]Limit use of symptomatic medications to 2 or 3 days/week when possible to avoid medication-misuse headache.

Table 61.2

Pharmacokinetic characteristics of triptans

Drug	Half-Life (hours)	Time to Maximal Concentration (t_{max})	Bioavailability (%)	Elimination
Almotriptan	3–4	1.4–3.8 hours	70	MAO-A, CYP3A4, CYP2D6 CYP3A4
Eletriptan	5	1.4–2.8 hours	50	
Frovatriptan	25	2–4 hours	24–30	CYP1A2
Naratriptan	5–6	2–3 hours	63–74	CYP450 (various isoenzymes)
Rizatriptan	2–3		40–45	MAO-A
Oral tablets	2			
Disintegrating		1–1.5 hours		
Sumatriptan		1.6–2.5 hours		
SC injection		12–15 minutes	97	MAO-A
Oral tablets		2.5 hours	14	
Nasal spray		1–2.5 hours	17	
			40	
Zolmitriptan				
Oral	3	1.5 hours		CYP1A2, MAO-A
Disintegrating		3 hours		
Nasal		4 hours		

CYP, cytochrome P450; MAO-A, monoamine oxidase type A.

Table 61-3

Prophylactic migraine therapies

Medication	Dose
β-Adrenergic antagonists	
Atenolol	25–100 mg/day
Metoprolola	50–300 mg/day in divided doses
Nadolol	80–240 mg/day
Propranolol a,b	80–240 mg/day in divided doses
Timololb	20–60 mg/day in divided doses
Antidepressants	
Amitriptyline	25–150 mg at bedtime
Doxepin	10–200 mg at bedtime
Imipramine	10–200 mg at bedtime
Nortriptyline	10–150 mg at bedtime
Protriptyline	5–30 mg at bedtime
Fluoxetine	10–80 mg/day
Phenelzine[c]	15–60 mg/day in divided doses

Table 61.3 *Contd...*

Medication	Dose
Gabapentin	
Topiramate[b]	900–2,400 mg/day in divided doses
Valproic acid	100 mg/day in divided doses
divalproex sodium[b]	500–1,500 mg/day in divided doses
Verapamil[a]	240–360 mg/day in divided doses
Methysergide[bc]	2–8 mg/day in divided doses with food
Nonsteroidal antiinflammatory drugs[c]	
Aspirin	1,300 mg/day in divided doses
Ketoprofen[a]	150 mg/day in divided doses
Naproxen sodium[a]	550–1,100 mg/day in divided doses
Vitamin B[2]	400 mg/day

[a]Sustained-release formulation available. [b]FDA approved for prevention of migraine. [c]Daily or prolonged use limited by potential toxicity.

TENSION-TYPE HEADACHE

In adults, tension-type headache represents the most common type of primary headache. Children also have tension-type headaches but astonishingly there are few data on the prevalence, features and prognosis of this headache type in children. Before the classification by the International Headache Society (IHS), several different terms were used for tension type headache, such as muscle contraction headache, idiopathic headache, tension headache and psychogenic headache. The heterogeneity of the terminology indicates the unknown, and possibly also the heterogeneous aetiology of tension-type headache and the vague limits to other types of primary and secondary headaches. The reasons for the lack of research work on tension-type headache in children could be the difficulty in defining it, and also that it is commonly considered to be less severe and disabling than migraine. However, because a tension-type headache presents a frequent problem in adults and some patients with an episodic tension-type headache become patients with a chronic headache, it would be important to know which factors contribute to the pathogenesis of tension-type headache in children, which factors provoke and sustain the episodes, and which factors contribute to continuation of this disorder into adulthood and to the increasingly chronic nature of this disorder.

CLASSIFICATION

Before the IHS classification of headaches was published in 1988, there were no universally accepted and strict criteria for tension-type headache. In the definition by the Ad Hoc Committee on Classification of Headache, tension-type headache or muscle contraction headache is an 'ache or tightness, constriction. In the headache classification by the IHS,1 tension-type headache is defined by its typical characteristics and subdivided into episodic (180 days per year and 15 days per month) and chronic tension-type headache, and further into tension-type headache associated or unassociated with a disorder of the pericranial muscles. In addition, several possible causative factors are listed, including oromandibular dysfunction, psychosocial stress, anxiety and depression, muscular stress and drug overuse. The pericranial disorder should be detected by manual palpation, a pressure algometer or an increased electromyographic (EMG) level of pericranial muscles at rest or during physiological tests. However, manual palpation seems to be the most specific and sensitive test for pericranial muscular disorders.

In contrast to migraine, even according to the diagnostic criteria, tension-type headache is considered to be more of a symptom initiated by many different causes, rather than a separate disease or disorder. The criteria for tension-type headache have not been evaluated in population-based studies in children. It seems that the present criteria apply to children, but it is not known how reproducibly and reliably these criteria define a separate and identifiable entity of headaches in children. In the studies using the IHS criteria for tension-type headache, several children were included in the group of tension-type headache that did not quite fulfil the criteria. The proportion of these children is 26–33% of all patients with tension-type headache in clinic-based studies and 4% in a population-based study of 12-year-old children.

Nor do all adults totally fulfil the criteria of tension-type headache in population-based studies. The most specific criteria for tension-type headache in this study were mild intensity of pain and absence of nausea, and the most sensitive diagnostic criterion for tension-type headache was absence of vomiting. The IHS criteria for tension-type headache will probably be revised and the division into subclasses will be more accurate as research work in this field expands. Certain revisions for childhood tension-type headache, as well as for childhood migraine, may be adequate.

EPIDEMIOLOGY

In adults the life-time prevalence of episodic tension-type headache, according to the HIS criteria, is 40–70% and the prevalence of chronic tension-type headache is 2–3%.Tension-type headache, both episodic and chronic, seems to be more prevalent in females and the prevalence decreases in elderly adults, even though these trends are clearer with migraine. In children, tension-type headache occurs in clinic patients, representing about 35% of patients in specialized headache clinics. In clinic-based studies, the proportion of chronic tension-type headache out of all tension-type headache in children is 15–20%. Population- based prevalence data on tension-type headache in children is sparse. Some guidelines have provided thorough studies on nonmigrainous primary headache. Even when the IHS criteria have been applied, the results of different studies are not comparable. The prevalence of tension-type headache was 0.9% in 5- to 15-year-old-children , most probably representing the chronic tension-type headache with a psychogenic background. Their tension-type headache group also included children with tension-type headache that did not quite fulfil the criteria.

CLINICAL FEATURES

The typical features of tension-type headache according to the IHS criteria are mild or moderate intensity, a pressing or tightening quality and bilateral pain, the absence of vomiting and nausea, and the absence of photophobia and phonophobia. The pain was described to be occipital in the Ad Hoc Definition of tension-type headache, but is more often frontal or temporal in children. In clinic-based material with an age range of 3-19 years, episodic tension-type headache was unilateral in 22%, non-pulsating in 74%, mild in 83%, and associated with photophobia in 8% and with phonophobia in 12%. The mean duration of episodic tension-type headache was 7.9-15.0 hours. Of those who did not fulfil the criteria for tension-type headache, 30% had a duration of the headache episode of less than 30 min, which indicates the limitating role of the minimum duration limit for tension-type headache. The mean frequency of episodes was 1.5/week. Chronic tension-type headache episodes were longer than the episodic tension-type headache episodes and were sometimes associated with nausea. Those who did not quite fulfil the criteria of tension-type headache more frequently had migrainous features in their headache than those who fulfilled the criteria. The most typical duration of tension headache episodes was, however, 30 min to 2 h. The pain was described as pressing or tightening by 74%, pulsating by 16%, piercing by 5% and burning by 1% of their patients. The intensity of the pain was moderate in 49%, mild in 26%, severe in 24% and bilateral in 87% of their participants. Nausea was reported by 24%, photophobia by 30% and phonophobia by 29% of the patients.

AETIOPATHOGENETIC THEORIES

Genetic factors do not seem to be as important for tension-type headache as for migraine. However, there is an increased risk of chronic tension-type headache among first-degree relatives of chronic tension-type headache patients. The aetiology of tension-type headache is most probably multifactorial with a genetic predisposition. The exact aetiopathogenesis of tension-type headache is not known. Most probably both peripheral and central mechanisms are involved, including pericranial muscular tension, peripheral nociception, and trigeminal tract and supraspinal pain-modulation systems. It has been proposed, especially with the increasingly chronic nature of tension-type headache, that central mechanisms apply. The previously used expression for tension type headache – muscle contraction headache – as well as several clinical findings indicate that muscle tension in the pericranial musculature might be of importance in the pathogenesis. The pain in tension-type headache resembles pain from myofascial tissues, being dull, pressing and difficult to localize. Muscle spasm of the pericranial muscles is a clinical finding in many adults and children with tension-type headache. However, there is not a muscular disorder in all patients with tension type headache and such a disorder does not seem to be an important factor in defining the response to therapy. The pericranial muscular disorder can be studied by palpation or EMG. Standardized palpation points are used to evaluate the tenderness in pericranial muscles in research work. Furthermore, to increase the reliability of the tenderness evaluation, pressurecontrolled palpation equipment has been developed, as well as a method of measuring muscle hardness. Increased tenderness in the pericranial muscles, on manual palpation, is found in adults with episodic and even more often in those with chronic tension-type headache. Tenderness is also found in several patients with migraine and especially during a migraine attack. Tenderness of the pericranial muscles seems to be influenced by the recent occurrence of the headache episode. As the tenderness of muscles outlasts the headache, it cannot be the only source of pain in tension-type headache. Normal as well as increased activity in pericranial muscle EMG has been found in the resting state in patients with tension-type headache. Increased amplitudes of EMG have been found, particularly in patients with chronic tension-type headache. Decreased activation was noticed during maximal voluntary activation in patients with chronic headache and those with current headache. There is some evidence for an association of tension-type headache with altered perception of pain. The children with headache are more prone to other types of pain and to other somatic symptoms. Thermal pain detection and thermal pain tolerance thresholds are decreased during a tension-type headache episode and unaltered interictally. The peripheral myofascial pain sensitivity is measured as the pressure pain threshold and pressure pain tolerance with standardized algometers. In these studies, no consistent results have been obtained in adults with tension-type headache. In some studies, the participants with tension headache had decreased thresholds in comparison to healthy controls and others with headache, but in other studies no differences between headache groups or between headache groups and controls were observed. Any headache present seems to have no importance in pressure pain thresholds. In humans, the exteroceptive silent period of temporalis muscle activity was shortened in patients with chronic tension-type headache. Tension-type headache has been initiated experimentally by sustained tooth clenching. After the clenching those who developed headache had increased tenderness pericranially.

DIFFERENTIAL DIAGNOSIS

Tension-type headache does not have specific features and this headache requires careful exclusion of possible causative or related factors. A thorough evaluation of the psychosocial environment and functioning of the child is also recommended because disorders in these can be provoking factors for tension-type headache.

PSYCHOLOGICAL FACTORS

In adults, episodic tension-type headache is not connected with either anxiety or depression, in contrast to patients with migraine who have both of these disorders more often than people with no headache. Few studies analyse particularly the association of tension type headache with psychological disorders in children. Most of the existing studies deal with overall headache or separate migraine and non-migrainous headache; this group, however, includes a highly heterogeneous population of children with tension-type headache, migrainous headache and miscellaneous headaches, with different associations with psychological factors. Stress, anxiety and depression have been reported to occur more often in children with any headache, in comparison to children with no headache. Psychiatric co-morbidity was higher in children with chronic daily headache, in comparison with children with migraine .

TREATMENT OF TENSION-TYPE HEADACHE

Episodic tension-type headaches are treated with acute medications. If the headaches are more frequent or become chronic, preventive medication is used in conjunction with counseling, stress management, relaxation therapy, and/or biofeedback. Medication To stop or reduce the severity of the individual attack, includes aspirin, acetaminophen (Tylenol®), or ibuprofen, alone or in combination with caffeine, sedatives, or codeine, and nonsteroidal anti-inflammatory drugs (NSAIDs). Some doctors use muscle relaxants as well. The choice depends on the severity and frequency of the headaches, the associated symptoms, the presence of other medical illness, and the person's previous responses to medicine. Oral pain medications, NSAIDs, or caffeine-containing medications are useful for persons with mild-to-moderate headaches. When prescription drugs are indicated, your doctor may add butalbital or Midrin®, the adjunctive medications found in the prescription drug. Because of the risk of dependency, abuse, and daily headache, analgesic overuse must be avoided. The major side effects of NSAIDs, including aspirin, are stomach bleeding, nausea, vomiting, constipation, ulcers, epigastric pain, and diarrhea. Be sure to tell your doctor if you have a history of hypersensitivity to aspirin or any NSAID, peptic ulcers, bleeding tendency, or severe renal, cardiac, or liver impairment, or if you are being treated with anticoagulants. People with kidney failure should avoid these medications.

If the frequency and severity of your headache attacks warrant it, your doctor may suggest preventive medication.

ACUPUNCTURE

An analysis of traditional acupuncture, while suggesting that acupuncture had a role in the treatment of headache, found that the evidence was unconvincing. Among recent studies, three showed no benefit and one showed benefit comparable to medication. Some people benefit from acupuncture.

Physical Therapy: Physical therapy consists of heat, cold packs, ultrasound, and electrical stimulation; improvement of posture through stretching, exercise, and traction; and trigger point injections, or occipital nerve blocks. Eating a balanced diet, adequate sleep, and regular exercise and stretching make sense for all of us. Physical therapy may be warranted for people who have tension-type headache associated with muscle spasm or tightness.

Psychological Factors: The psychological health may also be addressed, because depression, anxiety, or both may accompany or aggravate tension-type headache. Treatments may include counseling, stress management, relaxation therapy, biofeedback, or medication. Biofeedback electromyogram: biofeedback enables people to control muscle tension by providing continuous information about the tension in one or more of the muscles. The feedback can be auditory—for example, clicks that vary in rate, or visual, such as bars that vary in length. Sessions last about one hour. The treatment starts to work when people learn to either increase or decrease their head EMG activity.

RELAXATION TRAINING

Progressive relaxation training and autogenic training are both helpful for people with tension-type headaches. Progressive relaxation training helps people recognize tension and relax by sequentially tensing and then releasing (relaxing) various groups of muscles throughout the body. Relaxation training is practiced daily at home and audiotapes are usually provided for assistance. Autogenic training is based on autosuggestion. It seeks to simultaneously regulate mental and body functions by passively concentrating on a positive phrase such as, "My forehead is cool. Cognitive behavioral interventions, such as stress management programs, may effectively reduce tension-type headaches, but they usually work best in conjunction with biofeedback or relaxation therapies, particularly for people who experience a high level of daily stress. These treatments have been shown to be effective and often improve the results of drug treatment.

CHRONIC DAILY HEADACHE (CDH)

Chronic daily headache (CDH) is a diagnostic term describing a patient who has recurrent headache, with an average frequency of 15 days/month without an underlying serious medical condition. It was described in adults by Mathew et al in 1987. Nevertheless, the prevalence rate for severe or recurrent headache in children and adolescents has been reported as 0.2%, 0.8% and 2.5% . For the sufferers and their families, this condition is a source of concern and disability. It may mask depression, and may cause a tremendous amount of dysfunction for the youngster and his or her family.

CLASSIFICATION

CDH as chronic recurrent headache that transformed from either episodic migraine or tension-type headache. Headache duration would be more than 4 hours/day, and this progression with increasing frequency and decreasing severity occurred over at least 3 months. In chronic tension-type headache, the patient would have an average headache frequency of 15 days/month (180 days/year) for 6 months. The headache would have two of the following pain characteristics: pressing/ tightening quality, bilateral location, mild or moderate severity, aggravated by walking up or down stairs or similar routine physical activity, and no autonomic characteristics. There would also be a history of episodic tension-type headache. Again there would be a transformation period of at least 3 months. In new persistent daily headache, headache lasts more than 4 hours/day for more than 1 month.There is no history of episodic migraine or tension-type headache. In hemicrania continua, headaches present for at least 1 month. It is strictly unilateral, and responds to indomethacin. Pain is continuous but fluctuating, of moderate severity and lacks precipitating mechanisms.

HISTORY

For patients with chronic headache, a skilled and careful history is the most important step in making the diagnosis and preparing an appropriate treatment plan. To arrive at the diagnosis of CDH, one must rule out serious medical diseases. While obtaining a careful headache history to rule out chronic illness or tumor, we should explore coping mechanisms and disability. For adolescent headache sufferers, it is critical to interview the youngster and parent(s) together and separately. By starting the interview together, we gain critical information about how they interact with each other. Does the mother answer all the questions for the teenager? Is there a lot of conflict? By separating them later, we learn about what each person perceives to be the problem and the disability, and show all involved the practitioner's endorsement of their views. If the youngster will not separate, or if the parent will not let go, we learn a lot about the problem. By bringing the parties together at the end of the session, we can then summarize the situation, while not betraying anyone's confidence. This approach takes time, so patients with chronic headache often require increased scheduling time by office staff. While obtaining the history, it is necessary to discuss symptoms and disability, and rule out the possibility of infections, sinus disease, trauma, hypertension, cerebrospinal pressure abnormalities and ocular disorders, as well as the possibility of factitious disorders or somatization. A careful look at psychosocial factors is also crucial. Dietary, sleep and medication histories may help to pinpoint aggravating factors. A family history of headache and/or psychiatric disease may shed additional light on to the problem. Psychiatric co-morbidity of depression or anxiety disorders has been reported to occur more frequently in patients with CDH than in patients with migraine or tension-type headaches alone. The presence or absence of daily medication overuse plays a big part in treatment options. Assessing disability for a youngster can be measured by days of school missed, days of school requiring early dismissal, visits to the nurses for medication, a drop in grades, and/or the inability to participate in afterschool activities. A disparity between parent- and patient-endorsed severity is suspicious for either child–parental conflict or parental overestimation of symptoms. In the younger child, we can glean helpful information from a careful description of how the parents react to the child when a headache is acknowledged. 'Is all OK at home?' and 'What is your home like?' are openended questions that can be answered by the youngster and the parents separately.

PHYSICAL EXAMINATION

The approach to the youngster with chronic headache demands a thorough physical examination to convince both the practitioner and the patient of benign aetiology, before proceeding with a treatment plan. Having the patient undressed facilitates a good dermatological examination, and the ability to assess Tanner staging in the adolescent. Vital signs help to rule out increased intracranial pressure as well as hypertension. Skin examination helps rule out neurofibromatosis as well as tuberous sclerosis. Palpation of the sinuses and the jaw help to rule out sinusitis and temporomandibular jaw (TMJ) dysfunction, respectively. A careful neurological examination goes without saying, stressing visual fields and fundoscopic examination. By emphasizing normalcy along the way, the examination can be made into a teaching experience for the youngster. A thorough mental status examination may help to diagnose depression or somatization. When there is mood incongruence, a patient may describe horrific symptoms, but show 'labelle indifférence'.

PHYSIOLOGY

There is a great deal of literature about the physiology of migraine; however, studies related to the aetiology and physiology of tension-type headache have been more sparse. There are no studies that look at the physiology of CDH as an entity in itself; studies focus on recurrent migraine or tension-type headache. Nevertheless, in tension-type headache, patients have been shown to respond to stress with stronger muscle contraction than patients with no headaches.

AETIOLOGICAL FACTORS

Stress has been shown to be more common in headache sufferers than in matched controls. Stress-induced headaches are gone in the summertime. Anxiety, depression and chronic somatic complaints are more common in headache sufferers; however, that various psychological symptoms are elevated only when a patient had a headache at the time of measurement, so data interpretation of such studies may be biased by the intensity of pain. Familial patterns of headache do exist, especially for recurrent migraine. Familial aggregation is lower in tension-type headache. More important than family history, the response of the family to headache behaviour may influence the transformation from acute to chronic conditions.

DIAGNOSTIC WORK-UP

Patients with suspicious histories or patients with growth delay, or pubertal delay or arrest, medical work-up is indicated. For patients with dermatological examinations that are suspicious of a neurocutaneous disorder. Sinus tenderness (computed tomography [CT] of the sinuses) or painful, limited jaw opening may warrant further dental investigation. Most patients with CDH have been imaged at some point, as their headache progression went from acute to chronic. The exception would be those patients with new persistent daily headache, where chronic headache started at the onset. Studies of children with recurrent headache with no significant change in severity or frequency over the previous 4 months, and an absence of physical examination abnormalities, do not require further imaging. The role of EEGs is similarly not helpful in the vast majority of cases, unless there is a history of an atypical aura or concern over a paroxysmal event.

TREATMENT

A rational approach based on a careful consideration of headache type, the presence or absence of medication overuse, and a consideration of functional disability will assure that patients get judicious use of medications. Assessment of the youngster's ability to comply with relaxation training will help optimize outcome, because only those who will practise will succeed. For patients with daily headache, it is important to find out whether there are intermittent migraine-like headaches superimposed on chronic tension-type headache (mixed headache). These migraine-like headaches can be treated with appropriate acute management. Careful instruction in the use of acute medications will aim to prevent inappropriate use of these agents. The presence of daily medication overuse makes treatment more complicated. Abrupt withdrawal of these medications may briefly precipitate more severe headache symptoms. Therefore we must be cautious about recommending cessation of medication until some preventive measure is in place. Although there are many studies demonstrating efficacy of preventive agents in adults, few well-designed controlled studies have been performed specifically in children. Even fewer have been done with CDH. Nevertheless, there are studies of children or combinations of adults and adolescent that use β blockers, tricyclic antidepressants, calcium channel blockers, and valproate. Studies on this subject do not rigorously define chronic headache. Nevertheless, practitioners have been using these medications for years. Behavioural treatment shows promise for patients with chronic headache. Obvious advantages include the absence of medication with side effects, and helping youngsters gain control of their chronic pain. Disadvantages are in patient selection, because it does not work if it is not practised regularly. For both behavioural and pharmacological prevention of recurrent headache, no study has used rigorous definitions of headache type. Do patients with chronic tension-type headache respond differently from patients with transformed migraine (chronic migraine) or comorbid headache (mixed headache).

REFERENCES

1. Welborn CA, Pediatric migraine. *Emerg Med Clin North Am* 1997; **15:** 625–36.
2. Welch KMA, Drug therapy of migraine. *N Engl J Med* 1993; **329:** 1476–83.
3. Spierings ELH, *Management of Migraine.* Oxford: Butterworth-Heinemann, 1996.
4. Frolich JC, A classification of NSAIDs according to the relative inhibition of cyclooxygenase isoenzymes. *Trends Pharmacol Sci* 1997; **18:** 30–4.
5. Hawkey CJ, COX-2 inhibitors. *Lancet* 1999; **353:** 307–14.
6. Micromedex: database informatic system for drug and toxicology information. 1974-1999. Micromedex Inc., vol 101.
7. Hamalainen ML, Hoppu K, Valkeila E, Santavuori P, Ibuprofen or acetaminophen for the acute treatment of migraine in children: a double-blind, randomized, placebo-controlled, crossover study. *Neurology* 1997; **48:** 103–7.
8. Ferrari MD, Migraine. *Lancet* 1998; **351:** 1043–51.
9. McDonald JT, Treatment of juvenile migraine with subcutaneous sumatriptan. *Headache* 1994; **34:** 581-2.
10. Hamalainen ML, Hoppu K, Santavuori P, Sumatriptan for migraine attacks in children: a randomized, placebo-controlled study. *Neurology* 1997; **48:** 1100-3

CHAPTER 62

Stroke

DEFINITION

Stroke is a term used to describe an abrupt onset of focal neurologic deficit that lasts at least 24 hours and is presumed to be of vascular origin. Stroke can be either ischemic or hemorrhagic in origin. Transient ischemic attacks (TIAs) are focal ischemic neurologic deficits lasting less than 24 hours and usually less than 30 minutes.

PATHOPHYSIOLOGY

RISK FACTORS FOR STROKE

- Nonmodifiable risk factors for stroke include increased age, male gender, race (African American, Asian, Hispanic), family history of stroke, and low birth weight.
- The major modifiable risk factors include hypertension and cardiac disease (especially atrial fibrillation).
- Other major risk factors include diabetes mellitus, dyslipidemia, and cigarette smoking.

ISCHEMIC STROKE

- Ischemic strokes account for 88% of all strokes and are due either to local thrombus formation or to emboli that occlude a cerebral artery. Cerebral atherosclerosis is a causative factor in most cases of ischemic stroke, although 30% are of unknown etiology. Emboli can arise either from intra- or extracranial arteries. Twenty percent of embolic strokes arise from the heart.
- In carotid atherosclerosis, plaques may rupture, resulting in collagen exposure, platelet aggregation, and thrombus formation. The clot may cause local occlusion or may dislodge and travel distally, eventually occluding a cerebral vessel.
- In the case of cardiogenic embolism, stasis of blood flow in the atria or ventricles leads to formation of local clots that can dislodge and travel through the aorta to the cerebral circulation.
- The final result of both thrombus formation and embolism is arterial occlusion, decreasing cerebral blood flow and causing ischemia and ultimately infarction distal to the occlusion.

HEMORRHAGIC STROKE

- Hemorrhagic strokes account for 12% of strokes and include subarachnoid hemorrhage, intracerebral hemorrhage, and subdural hematomas. Subarachnoid hemorrhage may result from trauma or rupture of an intracranial aneurysm or arteriovenous malformation. Intracerebral hemorrhage occurs when a ruptured blood vessel within the brain parenchyma causes formation of a hematoma. Subdural hematomas are most often caused by trauma.

- The presence of blood in the brain parenchyma causes damage to surrounding tissue through a mass effect and the neurotoxicity of blood components and their degradation products. Compression of tissue surrounding hematomas may lead to secondary ischemia. Much of the early mortality of hemorrhagic stroke is due to an abrupt increase in intracranial pressure that can lead to herniation and death.

CLINICAL PRESENTATION

- The patient may not be able to give a reliable history because of cognitive or language deficits. This information may need to be obtained from family members or other witnesses.
- The patient may experience weakness on one side of the body, inability to speak, loss of vision, vertigo, or falling. Ischemic stroke is not usually painful, but headache may occur and may be severe in hemorrhagic stroke.
- Patients usually have multiple signs of neurologic dysfunction on physical examination. The specific deficits observed depend upon the area of the brain involved. Hemi- or monoparesis and hemisensory deficits are common. Patients with posterior circulation involvement may present with vertigo and diplopia. Anterior circulation strokes commonly result in aphasia. Patients may also experience dysarthria, visual field defects, and altered levels of consciousness.

DIAGNOSIS

- Laboratory tests for hypercoagulable states should be done only when the cause of the stroke cannot be determined based on the presence of well known risk factors. Protein C, protein S, and antithrombin III are best measured in steady state rather than in the acute stage. Antiphospholipid antibodies are of higher yield but should be reserved for patients aged less than 50 years and those who have had multiple venous or arterial thrombotic events or livedo reticularis.
- Computed tomography (CT) head scan will reveal an area of hyperintensity (white) in an area of hemorrhage and will be normal or hypointense (dark) in an area of infarction. The area of infarction may not be visible on CT scan for 24 hours (and rarely longer).
- Magnetic resonance imaging of the head will reveal areas of ischemia with higher resolution and earlier than the CT scan. Diffusion-weighted imaging will reveal an evolving infarct within minutes.
- Carotid Doppler studies will determine whether there is a high degree of stenosis in the carotid arteries.
- The electrocardiogram will determine whether atrial fibrillation is present.
- A transthoracic echocardiogram can detect valve or wall motion abnormalities that are sources of emboli to the brain.
- A transesophageal echocardiogram is a more sensitive test for left atrial thrombus. It is also effective in examining the aortic arch for atheroma, another potential source of emboli.
- Transcranial Doppler can determine the presence of intracranial sclerosis (e.g., middle cerebral artery stenosis).

TREATMENT

GENERAL APPROACH

- The initial approach is to ensure adequate respiratory and cardiac support and to determine quickly whether the lesion is ischemic or hemorrhagic based on a CT scan.
- Ischemic stroke patients presenting within hours of symptom onset should be evaluated for reperfusion therapy.
- Elevated blood pressure should remain untreated in the acute period (first 7 days) after ischemic stroke because of the risk of decreasing cerebral blood flow and worsening symptoms. The pressure should be lowered if it exceeds 220/120 mm Hg or there is evidence of aortic dissection, acute myocardial infarction, pulmonary edema, or hypertensive encephalopathy. If blood pressure is treated in the acute phase, short-acting parenteral agents (e.g., labetalol, nicardipine, nitroprusside) are preferred.
- Patients with hemorrhagic stroke should be assessed to determine whether they are candidates for surgical intervention via an endovascular or craniotomy approach.
- After the hyperacute phase has passed, attention is focused on preventing progressive deficits, minimizing complications, and instituting appropriate secondary prevention strategies.

NON PHARMACOLOGICAL THERAPY

- In acute ischemic stroke, surgical interventions are limited. However, surgical decompression can be lifesaving in cases of significant swelling associated with cerebral infarction. An inter-disciplinary approach to stroke care that includes early rehabilitation is very effective in reducing long term disability. In secondary prevention, carotid endarterectomy is effective in reducing stroke incidence and recurrence in appropriate patients. Carotid stenting may be effective in reducing recurrent stroke risk in patients at high risk of complications during endarterectomy.
- In subarachnoid hemorrhage due to a ruptured intracranial aneurysm or arteriovenous malformation, surgical intervention to clip or ablate the vascular abnormality substantially reduces mortality from rebleeding. The benefits of surgery are less well documented in cases of primary intracerebral hemorrhage. In patients with intracerebral hematomas, insertion of an intraventricular drain with monitoring of intracranial pressure iscommonly performed. Surgical decompression of a hematoma is controversial except when it is a last resort in a life-threatening situation.

PHARMACOLOGICAL THERAPY OF ISCHEMIC STROKE

- The American Heart Association/ American Stroke Association (AHA/ ASA) Stroke Council guidelines for the management of acute ischemic stroke give grade A recommendations (i.e., evidence supported by data from randomized trials) to only two pharmacologic therapies: (1) IV Tissue plasminogen activator (alteplase) within 3 hours of onset; and (2) Aspirin within 48 hours of onset. Evidence-based recommendations for pharmacotherapy of ischemic stroke are given in Table 62.1.

- **Alteplase** initiated within 3 hours of symptom onset has been shown to reduce the ultimate disability due to ischemic stroke. A head CT scan must be obtained to rule out hemorrhage before beginning therapy. The patient must also meet specific inclusion criteria and no exclusionary criteria (Table 62.2). The dose is 0.9 mg/kg (maximum 90 mg) infused IV over 1 hour after a bolus of 10% of the total dose given over 1 minute. Anticoagulant and antiplatelet therapy should be avoided for 24 hours, and the patient should be monitored closely for hemorrhage.
- **Aspirin** 50 to 325 mg/day started between 24 and 48 hours after completion of alteplase has also been shown to reduce long-term death and disability.
- The AHA/ASA guidelines recommend that antiplatelet therapy as the cornerstone of antithrombotic therapy for the secondary prevention of ischemic stroke and should be used in noncardioembolic strokes. **Aspirin, clopidogrel,** and **extended-release dipyridamole plus aspirin** are all considered first-line antiplatelet agents (see Table 62.1). The combination of aspirin and clopidogrel can only be recommended in patients with ischemic stroke and a recent history of myocardial infarction or coronary stent placement and then only with ultra-low-dose aspirin to minimize bleeding risk.
- **Warfarin** is the antithrombotic agent of first choice for secondary prevention in patients with atrial fibrillation and a presumed cardiac source of embolism.
- Elevated blood pressure is common after ischemic stroke, and its treatment is associated with a decreased risk of stroke recurrence. The Joint National Committee and AHA/ASA guidelines recommend an **angiotensin-converting enzyme inhibitor and a diuretic** for reduction of blood pressure in patients with stroke or TIA after the acute period (first 7 days).

  Angiotensin II receptor blockers have also been shown to reduce the risk of stroke and should be considered in patients unable to tolerate angiotensin converting enzyme inhibitors after acute ischemic stroke.
- The National Cholesterol Education Program considers ischemic stroke or TIA to be a coronary risk equivalent and recommends the use of statins in ischemic stroke patients to achieve a low-density lipoprotein cholesterol concentration of less than 100 mg/dL.
- **Low-molecular-weight heparin** or **low-dose subcutaneous unfractionated heparin** (5,000 units twice daily) is recommended for prevention of deep venous thrombosis in hospitalized patients with decreased mobility due to stroke and should be used in all but the most minor strokes.
- The use of **full-dose unfractionated heparin** in the acute stroke period has not been proven to positively affect stroke outcome, and it significantly increases the risk of intracerebral hemorrhage. Trials of low-molecular weight heparins and heparinoids have been largely negative and do not support their routine use in stroke patients.

Table 62.1

Recommendations for pharmacotherapy of ischemic stroke

	Recommendation	Recommendation Grades[a]
Acute treatment	Alteplase 0.9 mg/kg IV (maximum 90 mg) over 1 hour in selected patients within 3 hours of onset	Class I, Level A
	Aspirin 160–325 mg daily started within 48 hours of onset	Class I, Level A
Secondary prevention		
Noncardioembolic	Antiplatelet therapy	Class I, Level A
	Aspirin 50–325 mg daily	Class IIa, Level A
	Clopidogrel 75 mg daily	Class IIb, Level B
	Aspirin 25 mg + extended-release dipyridamole 200 mg twice daily	Class IIa, Level A
Cardioembolic (esp. atrial fibrillation)	Warfarin (INR = 2.5)	Class I, Level A
All patients	Antihypertensive treatment	Class I, Level A
Previously hypertensive	ACE inhibitor + diuretic	Class I, Level A
Previously normotensive	ACE inhibitor + diuretic	Class IIa, Level B
Dyslipidemic	Statin	Class I, Level A
Normal lipids	Statin	Class IIa, Level B

ACE, angiotensin-converting enzyme; INR, international normalized ratio. [a]American Stroke Association Evidence Grading System.

RECOMMENDATION CLASS

I = Conditions for which there is evidence or general agreement that a procedure or treatment is useful and effective.

II = Conditions for which there is conflicting evidence or a divergence of opinion about the usefulness/efficacy of a procedure or treatment. IIa = Weight of evidence/opinion is in favor of usefulness or efficacy. IIb = Usefulness/efficacy is less well established by evidence/opinion.

III = Conditions for which there is evidence or general agreement that a procedure or treatment is not useful/effective and in some cases may be harmful.

LEVEL OF EVIDENCE

A = Data derived from multiple randomized clinical trials.

B = Data derived from a single randomized trial or nonrandomized studies.

C = Expert consensus or case studies.

Table 62.2

Inclusion and exclusion criteria for alteplase use in acute ischemic stroke

Inclusion Criteria (all YES boxes must be checked before treatment)

YES

- Age 18 years or older
- Clinical diagnosis of ischemic stroke causing a measurable neurologic deficit
- Time of symptom onset well established to be less than 180 minutes before treatment would begin

Exclusion Criteria (all NO boxes must be checked before treatment)

NO

- Evidence of intracranial hemorrhage on noncontrast head CT
- Only minor or rapidly improving stroke symptoms
- High clinical suspicion of subarachnoid hemorrhage even with normal CT
- Active internal bleeding (e.g., GI/GU bleeding within 21 days)
- Known bleeding diathesis, including but not limited to platelet count <100,000/mm
- Patient has received heparin within 48 hours and had an elevated a PTT
- Recent use of anticoagulant (e.g., warfarin) and elevated PT (>15 seconds)/INR
- Intracranial surgery, serious head trauma, or previous stroke within 3 months
- Major surgery or serious trauma within 14 days
- Recent arterial puncture at noncompressible site
- Lumbar puncture within 7 days
- History of intracranial hemorrhage, arteriovenous malformation, or aneurysm
- Witnessed seizure at stroke onset
- Recent acute myocardial infarction
- SBP >185 mm Hg or DBP >110 mm Hg at time of treatment

aPTT, activated partial thromboplastin time; CT, computed tomography; DBP, diastolic blood pressure; GU, genitourinary; INR, international normalized ratio; PT, prothrombin time; SBP, systolic blood pressure.

PHARMACOLOGICAL THERAPY OF HEMORRHAGIC STROKE

- There are currently no standard pharmacologic strategies for treating intracerebral hemorrhage. Medical guidelines for managing blood pressure, increased intracranial pressure, and other medical complications in acutely ill patients in neurointensive care units should be followed.
- Subarachnoid hemorrhage due to aneurysm rupture is associated with a high incidence of delayed cerebral ischemia in the 2 weeks after the bleeding episode. Vasospasm of the cerebral vasculature is thought to be responsible for the delayed ischemia and occurs between 4 and 21 days after the bleed. The calcium channel blocker **nimodipine** is recommended to reduce the incidence and severity of neurologic deficits resulting from delayed ischemia. Nimodipine 60 mg every 4 hours should be initiated on diagnosis and continued for 21 days in all subarachnoid hemorrhage patients. If hypotension occurs, it can be managed by reducing the dosing interval to 30 mg every 2 hours (same daily dose), reducing the total daily dose (30 mg every 4 hours), and maintaining intravascular volume and pressor therapy.

Table 62.3

Monitoring hospitalized acute stroke patients

Ischemic stroke	Treatment	Parameter(s)	Frequency
Ischemic stroke	Alteplase	BP, neurologic function, bleeding	Every 15 minutes × 1 hour; every 0.5 hour × 6 hours; every 1 hour × 17 hours; every shift after
	Aspirin	Bleeding	Daily
	Clopidogre	Bleeding	Daily
	IERDP/ASA	Headache, bleeding	Daily
	Warfarin	Bleeding, INR, Hb/Hct	INR daily × 3 days; weekly until stable; monthly
Hemorrhagic stroke	Nimodipine (for SAH)	BP, neurologic function, ICP	Temp. every 8 hours; CBC daily Every 8 hours Up to daily
		BP, neurologic function, fluid status	
All patients	Heparins for DVT prophylaxis	Temperature, CBC Pain (calf or chest).	Bleeding daily, platelets if suspected thrombocytopenia
		Electrolytes and ECG	
		Bleeding, platelets	

EVALUATION OF THERAPEUTIC OUTCOMES

- Patients with acute stroke should be monitored intensely for the development of neurologic worsening, complications, and adverse effects from treatments. The most common reasons for clinical deterioration in stroke patients are: (1) Extension of the original lesion in the brain; (2) Development of cerebral edema and raised intracranial pressure; (3) Hypertensive emergency; (4) Infection (e.g., urinary and respiratory tract); (5) Venous thromboembolism; (6) Electrolyte abnormalities and rhythm disturbances; and (7) Recurrent stroke. The approach to monitoring stroke patients is summarized in Table 62.3.

REFERENCES

1. American Association of Neuroscience Nurses. (2004). *Guide to the care of the patient with ischemic stroke*. Glenview, IL: Author.
2. American Stroke Association. (2000). *Every second counts*. Dallas: Author.
3. APASS Investigators. (2004). Antiphospholipid antibodies and subsequent thrombo-occlusive events in patients with ischemic stroke. *Journal of the American Medical Association, 291*(5), 576–584.
4. Bader, M. K., & Littlejohns, L. R. (Eds.). (2004). *AANN core curriculum for neuroscience nursing* (4th ed.). St. Louis: Elsevier.
5. Blank-Reid, C. (1996). How to have a stroke at an early age: The effects of crack, cocaine and other illicit drugs. *Journal of Neuroscience Nursing, 28*(1), 19–27.

6. Bonnono, C., Criddle, L. M., Lutsep, H. L., Stevens, P., Kearns, K., & Norton, R. (2000). Emergi-paths and stroke teams: An emergency department approach to acute ischemic stroke. *Journal of Neuroscience Nursing, 32*(6), 298–305.
7. Demchuk, A. M., & Buchan, A. M. (2000). Predictors of stroke outcome. *Neurologic Clinics, 19*(2), 455–473.
8. Felton, R. P., Ogden, N. R. P., Pena, C., Provost, C., Schlosser, M. J., & Witten, C. M. (2005). The Food and Drug Administration medical device review process: Clearance of a clot retriever for use in ischemic stroke. *Stroke, 36*(2), 404–406.
9. Goldstein, L. B., Bertels, C., & Davis, J. N. (1989). Interrater reliability of the NIH Stroke Scale. *Archives of Neurology, 46*, 660–662.
10. Goldstein, L. B., & Samsa, G. P. (1997). Reliability of the National Institutes of Health Stroke Scale. *Stroke, 28*(2), 307–310.
11. Goldstein, M., Barnett, H. J. M., Orgogozo, J. M., Sartorius, N., Symon, L., & Vereshchagin, N. V. (1989). Stroke—1989: Recommendations on stroke prevention, diagnosis, and therapy. Report of the WHO Task Force on Stroke and other Cerebrovascular Disorders. *Stroke, 20*(10), 1407–1431.
12. Harbison, J., Hossain, O., Jenkinson, D., Davis, J., Louw, S., & Ford, G. A. (2003). Diagnostic accuracy of stroke referral from primary care, emergency room physicians, and ambulance staff using the face arm speech test. *Stroke, 34*(1), 71–76.
13. Hickey, J. V. (2003). *The clinical practice of neurological and neurosurgical nursing* (5th ed.). Philadelphia: Lippincott, Williams & Wilkins.
14 Hinkle, J. L., & Bowman, L. (2003). Neuroprotection for ischemic stroke. *Journal of Neuroscience Nursing, 35*(2), 114–118.
15. Holloway, R. G., Vickrey, B. G., Benesch, C., Hinchey, J., & Bieber, J. (2001). Development of performance measures for acute ischemic stroke. *Stroke, 32*(9), 2058–2074.
16. Joshipura, K. J., Hung, H., Rimm, E., Willett, W., & Ascherio, A. (2003). Periodontal disease, tooth loss, and incidence of ischemic stroke. *Stroke, 34*(1), 47–52.
17 Kongable, G. (1997). Code Stroke: Using t-pa to prevent ischemic brain injury. *American Journal of Nursing, 97*(11), 16bb–16hh.
18. LaMonte, M., Bahouth, M. N., Hu, P., Pathan, M. Y., Yarbrough, K. L., Gunawardane, R., et al. (2003). Telemedicine for acute stroke triumphs and pitfalls. *Stroke, 34*(3), 725–728.
19. Lees, K. R., Zivin, J. A., Ashwood, T., Davalos, A., Davis, S. M., Diener, H. C., et al. (2006). NXY-059 for acute ischemic stroke. *New England Journal of Medicine, 354*(6), 588–600.
20. Miller, E. T., & Spilker, J. (2003). Readiness to change and brief educational interventions: Successful strategies to reduce stroke risk. *Journal of Neuroscience Nursing, 35*(4), 215–222.
21. Moore, K. (2001). Managing TIA: A nursing perspective. *Transient ischemic attack (TIA) disease management guide.* Montvale, NJ: Medical Economics Company.
22. Warlow, C., Dennis, M., van Gign, J., Hankey, G. J., Sandercock, P., Bamford, J., et al. (2001). *Stroke: A practical guide to management* (2nd ed.). London: Blackwell Science.

CHAPTER 63

Obsessive Compulsive Disorder

DEFINITION

Obsessive–compulsive disorder (OCD) is a mental disorder where people feel the need to check things repeatedly, perform certain routines repeatedly, or have certain thoughts repeatedly.

EPIDEMIOLOGY: PREVALENCE, COMORBIDITY

Childhood OCD appears to occur in 1% to 3% of children and adolescents, a rate similar to that of adults. The modal age of onset in the pediatric population is < 10 years. Because children often are secretive about their symptoms, childhood OCD frequently goes unrecognized for a long period of time. Children and adolescents who have OCD frequently have additional psychiatric disorders. Only 26% of sample of children who have OCD studied at the National Institutes of Health were free of comorbid psychiatric diagnoses. Patterns of comorbidity include high rates of tic disorders, other anxiety disorders such as generalized anxiety disorder and specific phobias, depression, attention-deficit/hyperactivity disorder, and oppositional defiant disorder.

CLINICAL DESCRIPTION

In children, adolescents, and adults, obsessive-compulsive disorder (OCD) is a mental illness characterized by intensely driven, seemingly pointless repetitive behaviors or mental acts (compulsions), along with recurrent disturbing irrational thoughts, urges, images, and worries (obsessions). Patients who have these patterns of behavior and mental activity usually recognize them to be irrational; however, children tend to be less insightful. Whether or not there is insight, the compulsive behavior and obsessive thoughts seem irresistible and necessary.

There is a wide spectrum of severity and disability associated with childhood OCD, including patients who are completely unable to function appropriately and are experiencing a profound degree of suffering with anxiety and frustration. Although defined by the presence of obsessions and compulsions, OCD is classified as an anxiety disorder. Obsessions are associated commonly with feelings of anxiety or other disturbing emotional experiences such as guilt, worry, or dread related to expectations of catastrophic, disgraceful, or tragic outcomes. Compulsions usually are linked to obsessions in that the individual considers them necessary to neutralize the obsessive thoughts and to prevent a feared outcome.

Compulsive behaviors or mental acts may be repetitive and rule-bound, needing to be performed an exact number of times, or repeated until it feels perfect or "just right." Whatever relief or satisfaction is provided by the compulsive behavior is short-lived. The obsession soon returns, renewing another cycle of compulsive behavior. Patients who have OCD often become imprisoned within these cycles and devote increasing proportions of their time and attention to them. Paradoxically, patients such as Joseph, who have obsessions and compulsions related to concerns about cleanliness, often neglect other aspects of their personal hygiene and functioning, such as schoolwork and peer relationships.

The diagnosis of OCD is made through the application of clinical criteria (Table 63.1). The diagnostic criteria (1) include the presence of obsessions or compulsions that cause significant distress, consume substantial amounts of time, or result in impairment in functioning. The diagnosis is excluded if the obsessive or compulsive symptoms are limited to preoccupations associated with other disorders such as anorexia nervosa, body dysmorphic disorder, and substance abuse disorders. The disorder is excluded also if the obsessive and compulsive symptoms are considered to be the direct result of intoxication or a medical condition.

Table 63.1

Diagnostic criteria for obsessive compulsive disorder

A. Presence of either obsessions or compulsions

Obsessions are defined by:

- Recurrent and persistent thoughts, impulses, or images that are experienced at some time during the disturbance as intrusive and inappropriate and that cause marked anxiety or distress
- The thoughts, impulses, or images are not simply excessive worries about real-life problems
- The person attempts to ignore or suppress such thoughts, impulses, or images, or to neutralize them with some other thought or action
- The person recognizes that the obsessional thoughts, impulses, or images are a product of his or her own mind (not imposed from without as in thought insertion)

Compulsions are defined by:

- Repetitive behaviors (eg, hand-washing, ordering, checking) or mental acts (eg, praying, counting, repeating words silently) that the person feels driven to perform in response to an obsession, or according to rules that must be applied rigidly
- The behaviors or mental acts are aimed at preventing or reducing distress or preventing some dreaded event or situation; however, these behaviors or mental acts either are not connected in a realistic way with what they are designed to neutralize or prevent or are clearly excessive

B. At some point during the course of the disorder, the person has recognized that the obsessions or compulsions are excessive or unreasonable. Note: This does not apply to children.

C. The obsessions or compulsions cause marked distress, are time consuming (take >1 h/d), or significantly interfere with the person's normal routine, occupational (or academic) functioning, or usual social activities or relationships.

Table 63.1 *Contd...*

D. If another Axis I disorder is present, the content of the obsessions or compulsions is not restricted to it (eg, preoccupation with food in the presence of an Eating Disorder; hair pulling in the presence of Trichotillomania; concern with appearance in the presence of Body Dysmorphic Disorder; preoccupation with drugs in the presence of a Substance Use Disorder; preoccupation with having a serious illness in the presence of Hypochondriasis; preoccupation with sexual urges or fantasies in the presence of a Paraphilia; or guilty ruminations in the presence of Major Depressive Disorder).

E. The disturbance is not due to the direct physiological effects of a substance (eg, a drug of abuse, a medication) or a general medical condition.

This last criterion is difficult to apply in the context of recent evidence implicating streptococcal infection in the etiology of some cases of OCD. Although the putative syndrome pediatric autoimmune neuropsychiatric disorders associated with streptococcal infection (PANDAS), could be interpreted to fall under these exclusion criteria, these patients currently are eligible for the diagnosis of OCD if they meet the criteria otherwise.

Childhood-onset OCD is more likely to be associated with tic disorders and disruptive behavior disorders such as attention-deficit/hyperactivity disorder. Individuals who have childhood-onset OCD are more likely to have first-degree relatives who have OCD. Although there is a male:female predominance in childhood-onset OCD, the opposite is true for adult-onset OCD. Finally, patients who have childhood-onset OCD appear to have a more favorable prognosis; a recent study showed that 44% of a sample of patients who had childhood-onset OCD had subclinical levels of symptom severity (considered to be in remission) by early adulthood. This incidence is in contrast to data indicating adult-onset OCD to have a prolonged chronic course.

There is a great deal of heterogeneity in OCD symptom patterns for individual patients. For example, one child who has OCD may have compulsive hand-washing and recurrent fears that his body is contaminated with germs, whereas another child who has OCD may walk in and out of every doorway a precise number of times and repeatedly tap things with both hands to make sure that they have done so evenly on both sides. Yet another child who has OCD may spend hours throughout the day worrying that he might kill his parents, confess to this thought repeatedly, and recite elaborate prayers asking God to protect his parents every night. Despite this heterogeneity, OCD symptoms tend to fall into one or more of the following groups: symmetry, hoarding, forbidden thoughts, and cleaning (Table 63.2).

ETIOLOGY AND PATHOPHYSIOLOGY

Evidence for neurobiologic factors in the etiology of OCD has been accumulating during the past several decades. Structural and functional brain-imaging studies in both adults and children point consistently to dysregulation of frontal corticostriatal-thalamic circuits in the pathophysiology of OCD. These circuits are modulated by serotonergic, dopaminergic, and glutamatergic neurons. It is assumed that any

Table 63.2

Obsessive-compulsive symptom groups: clinical examples

Group	Obsessions	Compulsions
Symmetry	Worrying about alignment of bilateral objects in environment	Lining up rows of objects
		Straightening position of objects
		Repetitive touching of objects same number of times with both hands
		Counting in repetitive patterns
Hoarding	Worry about losing objects that could be needed in future	Accumulating objects in home or work environment by retaining objects that are ordinarily discarded or by acquiring excessive quantities of objects
	Urges to save things	
		As a result, spaces become nonfunctional or unsanitary
Forbidden thoughts	Images of violent behavior	Confessions of violent or sexual impulses
	Images of sexual behavior that the individual considers to be deviant	Repetitive checking and securing doors and windows
	Worries about having inadvertently neglected to perform a vital safety procedure	Prayers and rituals for purification and absolution
	Worries about having inadvertently hurt a loved one	Checking to ensure the safety of a loved one
Cleaning	Excessive worry about becoming contaminated or infected with germs	Repetitive hand-washing, showering, rinsing, wiping with clean towels
	Fear of contact with surfaces thought to have germs	Wearing gloves
	Worries about transmission of infectious disease through casual contact with people	Avoidance of touching surfaces such as door handles
		Elaborate rules related to eating and preparing food

factor affecting the functioning of these circuits could contribute to the pathogenesis of OCD. Accordingly, symptoms of OCD have been shown to be associated with brain lesions affecting these circuits. Similarly, obsessive-compulsive symptoms have been observed to be associated with other diseases of the basal ganglia such as Tourette's syndrome, Huntington chorea, Sydenham chorea, and postencephalitic Parkinson disease. These latter two conditions, along with the proposed syndrome PANDAS, have led to the suggestion of an immunoreactive cause for some cases of OCD.

Genetic factors in the etiology of OCD have been implicated by studies of familial patterns of inheritance, twin studies, and genetic segregation and linkage analyses.

Twin studies estimate heritability to be in the range of 45% to 65% on the basis of genetic factors. No specific genes have been conclusively identified yet; however, studies implicating two candidate genes involving glutamate neurotransmission (GRIN2B, SLC1A1) have been replicated recently.

Given the lack of 100% concordance rates for OCD in monozygotic twins, the interaction of nongenetic factors with constitutional genetic variables also must play a significant role in the causation of OCD. Cognitive behavioral models of the role of family interactions in the reinforcement of obsessive-compulsive symptoms have generated fruitful avenues for treatment. Evidence that cognitive behavioral therapy (CBT) brings about correction of functional magnetic resonance imaging abnormalities associated with OCD points to a complex interaction of psychosocial and biological factors in the pathophysiology of OCD.

DIFFERENTIAL DIAGNOSIS

Many of the symptoms of OCD in children overlap with those of other conditions. The nature and context of symptoms must always be considered carefully in order for correct application of DSM-IV criteria. For example, patients who have depression often have repetitive negative ruminations. These thoughts could be confused with obsessive thoughts in OCD. If the repetitive thoughts are occurring primarily in the context of a depressed mood and are not associated with compensatory behaviors such as repetitive reassurance seeking and rituals, they are likely to be signs of a depressive disorder rather than OCD.

Patients who have bipolar disorder may have symptoms of hyperreligiosity in the context of a manic episode. Similarly, children who have OCD may be preoccupied with spirituality and exhibit compulsive praying and religious rituals. If the hyperreligiosity is associated primarily with elevated or mixed mood states and does not represent a compensatory behavior in response to intrusive forbidden thoughts, it is likely a sign of a manic state rather than OCD.

At times, children who have OCD experience intrusive forbidden thoughts and confess them to their parents or other responsible adults to relieve feelings of guilt. These thoughts may include suicidal, homicidal, and sexually inappropriate or aggressive ideation, and could be misunderstood to indicate actual risk of these dangerous behaviors. In these circumstances, clinicians should screen patients carefully for other disorders that may manifest this type of ideation, such as mood disorders, conduct disorder, posttraumatic stress disorder, or paraphilias (atypical sexual arousal).

If there is no evidence of these other disorders, and if the expression of these urges is understood to serve a confessional function to relieve guilt and is associated with repetitive safety checking rituals, it is likely that these symptoms are indicative of OCD. Unless there are other risk factors and comorbid conditions associated with high-risk behavior in addition to the OCD, the risk of these patients acting upon these thoughts is minimal.

Eating disorders overlap significantly with OCD, having extremely rigid adherence to rules about eating, repetitive and ritualistic exercise behavior, and obsessions related to body image. According to current classification standards, if patients who have eating disorders have obsessive-compulsive symptoms limited to the issues of body image and eating, they would not be considered to have the additional diagnosis of OCD.

Other disorders, such as the newly proposed hoarding disorder and body dysmorphic disorder, are syndromes defined by specific types of obsessive and compulsive symptoms. Patients who have the proposed hoarding disorder have compulsive tendencies to accumulate items that they do not objectively need and experience intense distress and fears associated with letting go of these items. Body dysmorphic disorder is associated with obsessive thoughts related to perceived imperfections in appearance, leading to compulsive efforts to change their appearance. Although these conditions have been identified to be on a spectrum with OCD, substantial evidence of their distinct difference from OCD on the basis of clinical characteristics, neurobiologic correlates, and treatment response supports their being separated from OCD at this time.

Pediatric Autoimmune Neuropsychiatric Disorders Associated With Streptococcal Infection

It was reported that a group of children who had OCD and tic disorders whose illnesses appeared to be temporally related to infections with group A β-hemolytic *Streptococcus* (GABHS). The proposed syndrome PANDAS is theorized to be caused by anti-GABHS antibodies cross-reacting with neurons in the basal ganglia. The following clinical characteristics are proposed to be indicative of PANDAS: (1) Onset of OCD or tic disorder before puberty, (2) Sudden onset with episodic course characterized by abrupt relapse and remission of symptoms, (3) Abnormal neurologic symptoms and signs during symptom exacerbations, and (4) Apparent temporal correlation of relapses with GABHS infections.

Although large-scale studies have supported the theorized etiologic role of GABHS in cases of OCD and tic disorders, the validity of the PANDAS as a syndrome continues to be the subject of ongoing controversy. Immunomodulatory treatments, such as intravenous immune globulin G and plasma exchange therapy, have not been proven to be beneficial and are associated with significant medical risk. Furthermore, there is insufficient evidence to support the use of prophylactic antibiotics to prevent symptom exacerbation in patients meeting criteria for PANDAS. Current approaches to the management of patients believed to have PANDAS include usual treatments for the underlying neuropsychiatric symptoms along with timely antibiotic treatment for known streptococcal infections.

TREATMENT

PSYCHOTHERAPY

The most rigorously studied and efficacious treatment to date for childhood OCD is CBT, notably CBT protocols applying the principle of exposure and response prevention (ERP). ERP is based upon the principle that compulsive symptoms occur as a response to feelings of anxiety and distress associated with obsessive thoughts. The compulsive symptoms, supported by irrational beliefs, are intended to neutralize this anxiety and distress. The compulsive symptoms provide immediate relief and thereby become strongly reinforced, ultimately becoming repetitive and habitual. When the individual attempts to resist the performance of the compulsive symptom, the anxiety and distress return, along with associated obsessive thoughts, thereby perpetuating a cycle of obsessive and compulsive symptoms.

The general approach of ERP is for children to be taught to identify triggers of obsessive thoughts, to voluntarily practice exposing themselves to these triggers, and subsequently to refrain from performing the compulsive behaviors. The treatment relies upon the principle of desensitization, in which the anxiety and distress associated with the obsessive thoughts is diminished gradually through repetitive exposure. In order for the exposure and desensitization to occur, patients must resist performing their compulsive rituals and tolerate the resulting distress.

The most challenging and important aspect of this therapy with children involves helping the child to develop insight and to come to see the obsessive-compulsive symptoms as oppressive and separate from their own motives and interests. Otherwise, the child may be extremely resistant and view the therapist as an adversary. The therapist also works with the child to reduce irrational beliefs and cognitive distortions associated with the obsessive and compulsive symptoms. The CBT helps build metacognitive skills, or the ability to think about thought, and thereby to develop a sense of empowerment over his or her thoughts rather than feeling oppressed by them. Children also learn how to manage anxiety without avoidance through cognitive and behavioral relaxation techniques.

MEDICATION

The effectiveness of serotonergic medication for treating childhood OCD has been replicated in numerous randomized controlled trials. In these studies, rates of remission defined by 25% or greater improvement in symptom severity typically range from 40% to 50%. The efficacy of these medications, including sertraline, fluoxetine, fluvoxamine, paroxetine, and clomipramine, is statistically significant and consistently demonstrated.

There was no evidence to support the superiority of any one selective serotonin reuptake inhibitor (SSRI) over another. On the other hand, a larger effect size was noted for clomipramine, a non-SSRI. This advantage is offset by other significant advantages of SSRIs, including improved tolerability and safety. Clomipramine is a tricyclic antidepressant and requires blood level monitoring because of a relatively low therapeutic index and potential arrhythmogenic effects. Adverse effects include dizziness, tremors, dry mouth, and sweating. Although not recommended for first-line treatment, clomipramine may be a useful alternative for treatment-refractory patients.

In prescribing SSRI medication for children who have OCD, clinicians should be cautious, monitoring patients carefully for adverse reactions, including suicidal ideation and other adverse behavioral effects. Mood disturbance after initial exposure to SSRI medication ranges from mild behavioral activation to frank mania. Children who have nonbipolar mood disorder or anxiety disorders appear to be at elevated risk for the development of mania when they are treated with antidepressant medication. Despite recent publicity regarding the risk of suicidal ideation in children treated with antidepressant medication, a recent meta-analysis failed to show an increased risk of suicidal ideation in children who have OCD treated with antidepressant medication.

Although it is advisable for dosage to begin at the lowest levels and to be titrated slowly while the patient is being monitored for adverse reactions, studies suggest that relatively high doses may be necessary to obtain the optimal benefit of the medications: for example, 60 to 80 mg per day of fluoxetine or 200 mg per day of sertraline. It is notable also that the effectiveness of medication may take more than 8 weeks to become established.

Patients whose symptoms remain clinically significant despite combined treatment with CBT and SSRI medication of adequate dose and duration or a trial of clomipramine may be considered for augmentation of SSRI therapy with an additional medication. Unfortunately, the evidence for these treatments is limited to uncontrolled case reports and series in children as well as studies with adults. One of these strategies is the addition of a benzodiazepine anxiolytic medication (ie, clonazepam, lorazepam, alprazolam). The risk of adverse behavioral effects, such as disinhibition and paradoxical overarousal, from these medications must be considered. Another augmentation strategy is the addition of an atypical or conventional antipsychotic medication. This approach is especially appropriate for patients for whom this medication would otherwise be indicated, such as those with comorbid tic disorders or autism spectrum disorders. Antipsychotic medication also may be considered for those patients whose obsessions and cognitive distortions are associated with impairment in reality testing.

Patients treated with antipsychotic medication should be monitored for symptoms of the metabolic syndrome, such as weight gain, impaired glucose tolerance, and hyperlipidemia. A more recent discovery of the role of the glutamate in the pathophysiology of OCD has led to the consideration of glutamatergic medications such as *N*-acetyl cysteine, riluzole, and memantine as augmenting medications. Although there is preliminary evidence that these agents may be beneficial, their use in children is considered experimental at this time.

OVERALL TREATMENT RECOMMENDATIONS

Planning treatment for OCD can be relatively complex, given the high prevalence of comorbid psychiatric disorders and the likelihood of a chronic course. A comprehensive treatment plan addressing both OCD and comorbid disorders will be necessary, and a strong treatment alliance will be needed to maintain engagement over the long-term course of the illness.

Most effective treatments in psychiatry begin with thorough education about the nature of the condition and the rationale for the various treatments. This education process is especially important for children who have OCD, who are less likely to have insight into their symptoms. Without patients having an understanding of the nature of obsessions and compulsions, the idea that treatment is going to help them to stop performing their rituals may seem threatening and provoke an adversarial relationship. Similarly, parents especially need help understanding OCD, because they will be asked to resist deeply rooted protective instincts as they help the child follow through with anxiety-provoking exposure practices.

Although CBT alone, combined CBT plus SSRI medication, and SSRI medication alone all are considered acceptable initial treatments for children who have OCD, CBT alone is an appropriate initial treatment for children who have conditions of mild-to-moderate severity. In comparison with medication, CBT is notable for having a more robust and longer-lasting symptom reduction effect. For children who have more severe symptoms, less insight, and resistance to psychotherapy, combined treatment with medication and CBT may be most effective. Similarly, for patients who have comorbid depression or other anxiety disorders, it is appropriate to provide combined treatment if possible. Although medication alone generally has a more modest and less durable effect on OCD symptom severity, it is also an acceptable initial treatment, especially when psychotherapy is not available or impractical.

OCD IN THE PRIMARY CARE SETTING

Given that OCD has a relatively high prevalence in children, and that the majority of children afflicted with OCD are unrecognized and untreated, primary care providers (PCPs) have a challenge and opportunity before them to help children who may be experiencing this disorder in silence. Children who have OCD often are secretive about their symptoms; the only external signs may be nonspecific functional impairment, such as a decrease in school performance, loss of interest in activities and peer relationships, and the emergence of unusual habits. To find out about OCD symptoms, direct questioning of the parent and child usually is necessary.

An excellent method for identifying children who have mental health needs in the primary care setting is to administer a general mental health screening instrument, such as the Pediatric Symptom Checklist. Although not capturing specific symptoms of OCD, general mental health screening can detect signs of distress and functional impairment in children that are likely to indicate the presence of psychiatric illnesses such as OCD. All children who have positive results from general mental health screening should receive further assessment by the PCP to identify areas of concern and to decide if a more detailed mental health assessment is needed.

REFERENCES

1. Hanna GL. Demographic and clinical features of obsessive-compulsive disorder in children and adolescents. J Am Acad Child Adolesc Psychiatry. 1995; 34(1): 19–27
2. Geller DA, Biederman J, Faraone S, et al. Developmental aspects of obsessive compulsive disorder: findings in children, adolescents, and adults. J Nerv Ment Dis. 2001; 189(7): 471–477
3. Bloch MH, Craiglow BG, Landeros-Weisenberger A, et al. Predictors of early adult outcomes in pediatric-onset obsessive-compulsive disorder. Pediatrics. 2009; 124(4): 1085–1093

4. Flament MF, Whitaker A, Rapoport JL, et al. Obsessive compulsive disorder in adolescence: an epidemiological study. J Am Acad Child Adolesc Psychiatry. 1988; 27(6): 764–771.
5. Swedo SE, Leonard HL, Garvey M, et al. Pediatric autoimmune neuropsychiatric disorders associated with streptococcal infections: clinical description of the first 50 cases. Am J Psychiatry. 1998; 155(2): 264–271
6. van Grootheest DS, Cath DC, Beekman AT, Boomsma DI. Twin studies on obsessive-compulsive disorder: a review. Twin Res Hum Genet. 2005; 8(5): 450–458
7. Piacentini J, Bergman RL, Chang Set al. Controlled comparison of family cognitive behavioral therapy and psychoeducation/ relaxation training for child obsessive-compulsive disorder. J Am Acad Child Adolesc Psychiatry. 2011; 50(11): 1149–1161
8. Saxena S, Gorbis E, O'Neill J, et al . Rapid effects of brief intensive cognitive-behavioral therapy on brain glucose metabolism in obsessive-compulsive disorder. Mol Psychiatry. 2009; 14(2): 197-205.

CHAPTER 64

Respiratory Tract Infections

RESPIRATORY TRACT INFECTIONS, UPPER

PREVALENCE

Transmission is via respiratory droplets or by virus-contaminated hands. Upper respiratory tract (nose, throat, sinuses) mucosa inflammation causes increased secretions, rhinorrhea and results in sneezing, and coughing facilitating the spread. In United States URIs are the most common infectious illness in the general population. URIs are the leading reasons for people missing work and school.

OTITIS MEDIA

DEFINITION

- Otitis media is an inflammation of the middle ear. Acute Otitis media involves the rapid onset of signs and symptoms of inflammation in the middle ear that manifests clinically as one or more of the following: otalgia (denoted by pulling of the ear in some infants), hearing loss, fever, or irritability. Otitis media with effusion (accumulation of liquid in the middle ear cavity) differs from acute Otitis media in that signs and symptoms of an acute infection are absent.
- Otitis media is most common in infants and children.

ETIOLOGY

Factors contributing to increased incidence of Otitis media include the winter season, attendance at a daycare center, non–breast-feeding in infants, aboriginal or Inuit origin, early age at first infection, and nasopharyngeal colonization with middle ear pathogens.

PATHOPHYSIOLOGY

- Acute bacterial Otitis media usually follows a viral upper respiratory tract infection that causes Eustachian tube dysfunction and mucosal swelling in the middle ear.
- *Streptococcus pneumonia* is the most common cause of acute Otitis media (20% - 35%). strains of *Haemophilus influenza* and *Moraxella catarrhalis* are each responsible for 20% -30% and 20% of cases, respectively. In 44% of cases, a viral etiology is found with or without concomitant bacteria.
- *Streptococcus pneumonia* isolates are often intermediate resistant to penicillin (8%- 34%) and some are highly penicillin

resistant (12%-21%). Penicillin-resistant isolates are often resistant to multiple antibiotics. β-Lactam resistance occurs in about 23%-35% of *Haemophilus. influenza* and in up to 100% of *Moraxella catarrhalis*.

CLINICAL FEATURES

- Acute Otitis media presents as an acute onset of signs and symptoms of middle ear infection such as otalgia, irritability, and tugging on the ear, accompanied by signs such as a gray, bulging, nonmotile tympanic membrane. These often follow cold symptoms of runny nose, nasal congestion, or cough Table 64.1.

Table 64.1

Clinical features of acute otitis media

General
The acute onset of signs and symptoms of middle ear infection following cold symptoms of runny nose, nasal congestion, or cough.
Signs and symptoms
• Pain that can be severe (>75% of patients).
• Children may be irritable, tug on the involved ear, and have difficulty sleeping.
• Fever is present in less than 25% of patients and, when present, is more often in younger children.
• Examination shows a discolored, thickened, bulging eardrum.
• Pneumatic otoscopy or tympanometry demonstrates an immobile eardrum; 50% of cases are bilateral.
• Draining middle ear fluid occurs (<3% of patients) that usually reveals a bacterial etiology.
Laboratory tests
Gram stain, culture, and sensitivities of draining fluid or aspirated fluid if tympanocentesis is performed.

- Resolution of acute Otitis media occurs over 1 week. Pain and fever tend to resolve over 2 to 3 days, with most children becoming asymptomatic at 7 days. Effusions resolve slowly, 90% have disappeared by 3 months.

TREATMENT

- Antimicrobial therapy is used to treat Otitis media; however, a high percentage of children will be cured with symptomatic treatment alone. Antibiotic use reduces the duration of symptoms by about 1 day.
- Delayed antibiotic treatment (48 to 72 hours) may be considered in children 6 months to 2 years of age if symptoms are not severe, as it decreases antibiotic adverse effects and minimizes bacterial resistance.
- It is difficult to identify who will benefit from antimicrobial therapy. With or without treatment, about 60% of children who have acute Otitis media are symptom-free within 24 hours.
- **Acetaminophen** or a nonsteroidal anti-inflammatory agent, such as **Ibuprofen**, can be used to relieve pain and malaise in acute Otitis media. Decongestants, antihistamines, topical corticosteroids, or expectorants have not been proven effective for acute Otitis media.
- Surgical insertion of tympanostomy tubes (T tubes) is an effective method for the prevention of recurrent Otitis media.
- Amoxicillin is the drug of choice for acute Otitis media. High-dose amoxicillin (80 to 90 mg/kg/day) is recommended. Treatment recommendations for acute Otitis media are found in Table 64.2.

Table 64.2

Acute otitis media treatment recommendations

First Line	Penicillin Allergy	Treatment Failure
Amoxicillin high dose 80-90mg /kg/day divided twice daily	Non-type 1:	Amoxicillin clavulanate
	Cefdinir 14mg/kg/day once or twice daily Cefuroxime 30 mg/kg/day divided twice daily Cefprozil 30mg/kg/day divided twice daily	
	Type 1: Azithromycin 10mg/kg/day 1, then 5 mg/kg/day for days 2-5 Clarithromycin 15mg/kg/day divided twice daily	Ceftriazone 50mg/kg/day IM/IV for 3 days
If severe symptoms (severe otalgia and temperature above 39°C (102.2°F)		Alternatives: Clindamycin 30-40 mg/kg/day in 3 divided doses
Amoxicillin clavulanate		Tympanocentesis

- If treatment failure occurs with amoxicillin, an agent should be chosen with activity against
- B-lactamase–producing *H. influenza* and *M. catarrhalis* as well as drug-resistant *S. pneumonia* (such as high-dose amoxicillin- clavulanate (recommended), or, cefuroxime, cefdinir, cefpodoxime, cefprozil, or intramuscular Ceftriaxone).
- A metaanalysis reported no difference in cure rates with short (less than 7 days) and usual durations (at least 7 days) of antibiotic therapy in children. 5 to 7 days of therapy may be used in children at least 6 years old who have mild to moderate acute Otitis media.

ANTIBIOTIC PROPHYLAXIS OF RECURRENT INFECTIONS

- Recurrent Otitis media is defined as at least three episodes in 6 months or at least four episodes in 12 months. Recurrent infections are of concern because patients younger than 3 years of age are at high risk for hearing loss and language and learning disabilities. Data from studies generally do not favor prophylaxis.
- Vaccination against influenza and pneumococcus may decrease risk of acute Otitis media, especially in those with recurrent episodes. Immunization with the influenza vaccine reduces the incidence of acute Otitis media by 36%.

PHARYNGITIS

Pharyngitis is an acute infection of the oropharynx or nasopharynx that results in 1%-2% of all outpatient visits. While viral causes are most common, Group A β–haemolytic *Streptococcus*, or *Streptococcus pyogenes*, is the primary bacterial cause.

- Viruses (such as rhinovirus, corona virus, and adenovirus) cause most of the cases of acute Pharyngitis. A bacterial etiology for acute Pharyngitis is far less likely. Of all of the bacterial causes, Group A *Streptococcus* is the most common

(15%-30% of persons of all ages with Pharyngitis), and it is the only commonly occurring form of acute Pharyngitis for which antimicrobial therapy is indicated.

- Non suppurative complications such as acute rheumatic fever, acute glomerulonephritis, and reactive arthritis may occur as a result of pharyngitis with Group A *Streptococcus*.

CLINICAL FEATURES

- The incubation period is 2 to 5 days, and the illness often occurs in clusters. The clinical presentation of Group A streptococcal pharyngitis is presented in Table 64.3.

Table 64.3

Clinical features and diagnosis of group a streptococcal pharyngitis

General
A sore throat of sudden onset that is mostly self-limited.
Fever and constitutional symptoms resolving in about 3–5 days.
Clinical signs and symptoms are similar for viral causes as well as non streptococcal bacterial causes.
Signs and symptoms
Sore throat.
Pain on swallowing.
Fever.
Headache, nausea, vomiting, and abdominal pain (especially children).
Erythema/inflammation of the tonsils and pharynx with or without patchy exudates.
Enlarged, tender lymph nodes.
Red swollen uvula, petechiae on the soft palate, and a scarlatiniform rash.
Several symptoms that are not suggestive of Group A
Streptococcus are cough, conjunctivitis, coryza, and diarrhea.
Laboratory tests
Throat swab and culture or rapid antigen detection testing.

- Guidelines from the Infectious Disease Society of America, American Academy of Pediatrics, and the American Heart Association suggest that testing for Group A *Streptococcus* be done in all patients with signs and symptoms. Only those with a positive test for Group A *Streptococcus* requires antibiotic treatment.

TREATMENT

- The goals of treatment of pharyngitis are to improve clinical signs and symptoms, minimize adverse drug reactions, prevent transmission to close contacts, and prevent acute rheumatic fever and suppurative complications such as peritonsillar abscess, cervical lymphadenitis, and mastoiditis.
- Antimicrobial therapy should be limited to those who have clinical and epidemiologic features of Group A streptococcal pharyngitis with a positive laboratory test.
- As pain is often the primary reason for visiting a physician, emphasis on analgesics such as acetaminophen and nonsteroidal anti-inflammatory drugs to aid in pain relief is strongly recommended. However, acetaminophen is a better option because there is some concern that nonsteroidal anti-inflammatory drugs may increase the risk for necrotizing fasciitis or toxic shock syndrome. Either systemic or topical analgesics can be used, as well as antipyretics and other supportive care including rest, fluids, lozenges, and saltwater gargles.

Table 64.4

Dosing guidelines for pharyngitis

Drug	Adult Dose	Pediatric Dosage	Duration
Penicillin V K	250 mg three to four times daily or 500 mg twice day 500 mg twice daily	50mg/kg/day divided in three doses	10days
Penicillin benzathine	1.2 million units intramuscularly	0.6 million units for under 27 kg (50,000 units/kg)	One dose
Penicillin G procaine and benzathine mixture	Not recommended in adolescents and adults	1.2 million units (benzathine 0.9 million units, procaine 0.3 million units)	One dose
Amoxicillin	500mg three times daily	4.-50 mg/kg/day divided in three doses	10 days
Erythromycin Estolate	20-40mg/kg/day divided two to four times daily (maximum: 1g/day)	Same as adults	--
Stearate	1 g daily divided two to four times daily (adolescents, adults)	--	--
Ethylsuccinate	40 mg/kg/day divided two to four times daily (maximum : 1 g/day)	Same as adults	
Cephalexin	250-500mg orally four times daily	25-50 mg/kg/day divided in four doses	10 days

- Antimicrobial treatment should be limited to those who have clinical and epidemiologic features of Group A streptococcal pharyngitis with a positive laboratory test. **Penicillin** is the drug of choice in the treatment of Group A streptococcal pharyngitis (Table 64.4). Table 64.5 presents dosing guidelines for recurrent infections.
- In patients allergic to penicillin, a macrolide such as **Erythromycin** or a first-generation cephalosporin such **Cephalexin** (if the reaction is non immunoglobulin E–mediated hyper-sensitivity) can be used. Newer macrolides such as Azithromycin and clarithromycin are as effective as erythromycin and cause fewer GI adverse effects.
- If patients are unable to take oral medications, intramuscular **benzathine penicillin** can be given although it is painful and no longer available in Canada.
- The duration of therapy for Group A streptococcal pharyngitis is 10 days to maximize bacterial eradication.

SINUSITIS

- Sinusitis is an inflammation and/or infection of the paranasal sinus mucosa. The term *Rhinosinusitis* is used by some specialists, because sinusitis typically also involves the nasal mucosa. The majority of these infections are viral in origin. It is important to differentiate between viral and bacterial sinusitis to aid in optimizing treatment decisions.

- Bacterial sinusitis can be categorized into acute and chronic disease. Acute disease lasts less than 30 days with complete resolution of symptoms. Chronic sinusitis is defined as episodes of inflammation lasting more than 3 months with persistence of respiratory symptoms.
- Acute bacterial sinusitis is most often caused by the same bacteria implicated in acute Otitis media: *S. pneumonia* And *H. influenza*. These organisms are responsible for about 70% of bacterial causes of acute sinusitis in both adults and children. Chronic sinusitis can be polymicrobial, with an increased prevalence of anaerobes as well as less common pathogens including gram-negative bacilli and fungi.

CLINICAL FEATURES

The typical clinical presentation of bacterial sinusitis is presented in Table 64.5.

TREATMENT

The goals of treatment of acute sinusitis are the reduction in signs and symptoms, achieving and maintaining patency of the ostia, limiting antimicrobial treatment to those who may benefit eradication of bacterial infection with appropriate antimicrobial therapy, minimizing the duration of illness, prevention of complications, and prevention of progression from acute disease to chronic disease.

Approximately 65% of patients with acute sinusitis will recover spontaneously (these are likely patients with viral sinusitis).

Table 64.5

Clinical features and diagnosis of bacterial sinusitis

General
A nonspecific upper respiratory tract infection that persists beyond 7–14 days.
Signs and symptoms
Acute
Adults:
Nasal discharge/congestion.
Maxillary tooth pain, facial or sinus pain that may radiate (unilateral in particular) as well as deterioration after initial improvement.
Severe or persistent (beyond 7 days) signs and symptoms are most likely bacterial and should be treated with antimicrobials.
Children:
Nasal discharge and cough for greater than 10–14 days or severe signs and symptoms such as temperature 39°C (102.2°F) or facial swelling or pain are indications for antimicrobial therapy.
Chronic Symptoms are similar to those of acute sinusitis but more nonspecific.
Rhinorrhea is associated with acute exacerbations.
Chronic unproductive cough, laryngitis, and headache may occur.
Chronic/recurrent infections occur three to four times a year and are unresponsive to steam and decongestants.

Nasal decongestant sprays such as **Phenylephrine** and **Oxymetazoline** that reduce inflammation by vasoconstriction are often used in sinusitis. Use should be limited to the recommended duration of the product to prevent rebound congestion. Oral decongestants may also aid in nasal or sinus patency. To reduce mucociliary function, irrigation of the nasal cavity with saline and steam inhalation may be used to increase mucosal moisture, and mucolytics (e.g.,

Guaifenesin) may be used to decrease the viscosity of nasal secretions. Antihistamines should not be used for acute bacterial sinusitis in view of their anticholinergic effects that can dry mucosa and disturb clearance of mucosal secretions.

- Antimicrobial therapy is superior to placebo in reducing or eliminating symptoms, although the benefit is small.
- **Amoxicillin** is first-line treatment for acute bacterial sinusitis. It is cost effective in acute uncomplicated disease, and initial use of newer broad spectrum agents is not justified. The approach to treating acute bacterial sinusitis is given in Table 64.6. Dosing guidelines are given in Table 64.7.

Table 64.6

Approach to treatment of acute bacterial sinusitis

Uncomplicated Sinusitis	Amoxicillin
Uncomplicated sinusitis, penicillin allergic patient	Immediate-type hypersensitivity: Clarithromycin or Azithromycin or t respiratory fluoroquinolone (levofloxacin or Gatifloxacin). Nonimmediate-type hypersensitivity: β-Lactamase-stable cephalosporin
Treatment failure or prior antibiotic therapy in past 4-6 weeks	High-dose amoxicillin with clavulanate or β-Lactamase-stable cephalosporin. Second choice: respiratory fluoroquinolone.
High suspicion of penicillin-resistant Streptococcus pneumonia	High dose amoxicillin or clindamycin. Second choice respiratory fluoroquinolone.

Table 64.7

Dosing guidelines for acute bacterial sinusitis

Drug	Adult Dosage	Pediatric Dosage
Amoxicillin	500 mg three times daily High dose: 1g three times daily	Low dose: 40-50 mg/kg/day divided in three doses High dose: 80-100 mg/kg/day divided in three doses
Amoxicillin-clavulanate	500/125mg three times daily. High dose: 2g/125mg twice daily	40-50mg/kg/day divided in three doses High dose: Can add 40-50mg/kg/day amoxicillin
Cefuroxime	250-500 mg twice daily	15mg/kg/day divided in two doses
Cefixime	200 -400mg twice daily	8mg/kg/day in one dose or divided in two doses
Clindamycin	150-450mg every 6 hours	30-40 mg/kg/day divided in three doses
Azithromycin	500 mg day 1 then 250mg/day for days 2-5	10mg/kg/day 1 then 5 mg/kg/day for days 2-5
Ceftriaxone	1 g daily	50-75 mg/kg/day divided every 12-24 hours

The current recommendations are 10 to 14 days, or at least 7 days, of antimicrobial therapy after signs and symptoms are under control.

RESPIRATORY TRACT INFECTIONS, LOWER

Lower respiratory tract infections include infectious processes of the lungs and bronchi, pneumonia, bronchitis, bronchiolitis, and lung abscess.

PREVALENCE

Two to three million cases of pneumonia are reported each year in the United States. Patients with pneumonia are responsible for over 10 million patient visits, 500,000 hospitalizations, and 45,000 deaths annually. Together, influenza and pneumonia are the eight leading causc of death in the U.S (in 2006; 56,326 deaths).

ACUTE BRONCHITIS

- *Bronchitis* refers to an inflammatory condition of the large elements of the tracheobronchial tree that is usually associated with a generalized respiratory infection. The inflammatory process does not extend to include the alveoli. The disease entity is frequently classified as either acute or chronic. Acute bronchitis occurs in all ages, whereas chronic bronchitis primarily affects adults.
- Acute bronchitis most commonly occurs during the winter months. Cold, damp climates and/or the presence of high concentrations of irritating substances such as air pollution or cigarette smoke may precipitate attacks.

PATHOPHYSHIOLOGY

- Respiratory viruses are by far the most common infectious agents associated with acute bronchitis. The common cold viruses, rhinovirus and corona virus, and lower respiratory tract pathogens, including influenza virus, adenovirus, and respiratory syncytial virus, account for the majority of cases. *Mycoplasma pneumonia* also appears to be a frequent cause of acute bronchitis. Other bacterial causes include *Chlamydia pneumonia* and *Bordetella pertussis*.
- Infection of the trachea and bronchi causes hyperemic and edematous mucous membranes and an increase in bronchial secretions. Destruction of respiratory epithelium can range from mild to extensive and may affect bronchial mucociliary function. In addition, the increase in bronchial secretions, which can become thick and tenacious, further impair mucociliary activity. Recurrent acute respiratory infections may be associated with increased airway hyper reactivity and possibly the pathogenesis of chronic obstructive lung disease.

CLINICAL FEATURES

- Bronchitis is primarily a self-limiting illness and rarely a cause of death. Acute bronchitis usually begins as an upper respiratory infection. The patient typically has nonspecific complaints such as malaise and headache, coryza, and sore throat.
- Cough is the hallmark of acute bronchitis. It occurs early and will persist despite the resolution of nasal or nasopharyngeal

complaints. Frequently, the cough is initially non productive but progresses, yielding mucopurulent sputum.

- Chest examination may reveal rhonchi and coarse, moist rales bilaterally. Chest radiographs, when performed, are usually normal. Bacterial cultures of expectorated sputum are generally of limited utility because of the inability to avoid normal nasopharyngeal flora by the sampling technique. Viral antigen detection tests can be used when a specific diagnosis is necessary. Cultures or serologic diagnosis of *M. pneumonia* and culture or direct fluorescent antibody detection for *B. Pertussis* should be obtained in prolonged or severe cases when epidemiologic considerations would suggest their involvement.

TREATMENT

- The treatment of acute bronchitis is symptomatic and supportive in nature. Reassurance and antipyretics alone are often sufficient. Bed rest and mild analgesic-antipyretic therapy are often helpful in relieving the associated lethargy, malaise, and fever. Patients should be encouraged to drink fluids to prevent dehydration and possibly decrease the viscosity of respiratory secretions.
- **Aspirin** or **acetaminophen** (650 mg in adults or 10 to 15 mg/kg per dose in children with a maximum daily adult dose of 4 g and 60 mg/kg for children) or **Ibuprofen** (200 to 800 mg in adults or 10 mg/kg per dose in children with a maximum daily dose of 3.2 g for adults and 40 mg/kg for Children) is administered.
- In children, aspirin should be avoided and acetaminophen used as the preferred agent because of the possible association between aspirin use and the development of Reye's syndrome.
- Mist therapy and/or the use of a vaporizer may further promote the thinning and loosening of respiratory secretions.
- Persistent, mild cough, which may be bothersome, may be treated with **Dextromethorphan**; more severe coughs may require intermittent **codeine** or other similar agents.
- When possible, antibiotic therapy is directed toward anticipated respiratory pathogen(s) (i.e., *Streptococcus pneumoniae*, *Haemophilus influenza*) and/or those demonstrating a predominant growth upon throat culture.
- *M. pneumoniae*, if suspected by history or positive cold agglutinins (titers greater than or equal to 1:32) or if confirmed by culture or serology, may be treated with **Azithromycin**. Also, a fluoroquinolone with activity against these pathogens (**levofloxacin**) may be used in adults.
- During known epidemics involving the influenza A virus, **Amantadine** or **Rimantadine** may be effective in minimizing associated symptomatology if administered early.

CHRONIC BRONCHITIS

PATHOPHYSIOLOGY

- Chronic bronchitis is a result of several contributing factors, including cigarette smoking; exposure to occupational dusts, fumes, and environmental pollution; and bacterial (and possibly viral) infection.

- In chronic bronchitis, the bronchial wall is thickened and the number of mucus-secreting goblet cells in the surface epithelium of both larger and smaller bronchi is markedly increased. Hypertrophy of the mucus glands and dilatation of the mucus gland ducts are also observed. As a result of these changes, patients with chronic bronchitis have substantially more mucus in their peripheral airways, further impairing normal lung defenses and causing mucus plugging of the smaller airways.
- Continued progression of this pathology can result in residual scarring of small bronchi, augmenting airway obstruction and the weakening of bronchial walls.

CLINICAL FEATURES

- The most common clinical signs of chronic bronchitis are listed in Table 64.8. The hallmark of chronic bronchitis is cough that may range from a mild "smoker's" cough to severe incessant coughing productive of purulent sputum. Expectoration of the largest quantity of sputum usually occurs upon arising in the morning, although many patients expectorate sputum throughout the day. The expectorated sputum is usually tenacious and can vary in color from white to yellow-green.
- The diagnosis of chronic bronchitis is based primarily on clinical assessment and history. By definition, any patient who reports coughing up sputum on most days for at least 3 consecutive months each year for 2 consecutive years suffers from chronic bronchitis.
- With the exception of pulmonary findings, the physical examination of patients with mild to moderate chronic bronchitis is usually unremarkable.
- An increased number of polymorphonuclear granulocytes in sputum often suggest continual bronchial irritation, whereas an increased number of eosinophils may suggest an allergic component.

TREATMENT

GENERAL PRINCIPLES

- A complete occupational/environmental history for the determination of exposure to noxious, irritating gases, as well as cigarette smoking, must be assessed. Exposure to bronchial irritants should be reduced.
- Attempts should be made with the patient to reduce or eliminate cigarette smoking.
- Humidification of inspired air may promote the hydration (liquefaction) of tenacious secretions, allowing for more effective sputum production. The use of mucolytic aerosols (e.g., *N*-acetylcysteine; deoxyribonuclease) is of questionable therapeutic value. Mucolytics may have the greatest benefit in patients with moderate or severe chronic obstructive pulmonary disease who are not receiving inhaled corticosteroids.
- Postural drainage may assist in promoting clearance of pulmonary secretions.

PHARMACOLOGICAL THERAPY

- Oral or aerosolized bronchodilators (e.g., **Albuterol** aerosol) may be of benefit to some patients during acute pulmonary exacerbations. For patients who consistently demonstrate limitations in airflow, a therapeutic change of bronchodilators should be considered.

- Long-term inhalation of ipratropium decreases the frequency of cough, severity of cough, and the volume of expectorated sputum.
- The use of antimicrobials has been controversial, although antibiotics are an important component of treatment. Agents should be selected that are effective against likely pathogens, have the lowest risk of drug interactions, and can be administered in a manner that promotes compliance.
- Selection of antibiotics should consider that up to 30%-40% of *H.influenzae* and 95% of *M. pneumoniae* are β-lactamase producers, and up to 30% of *S. pneumoniae* are at least moderately penicillin resistant.
- Antibiotics commonly used in the treatment of these patients and their .Duration of symptom-free periods may be enhanced by antibiotic regimens using the upper limit of the recommended daily dose for 5 to 7 days.
- In patients whose history suggests recurrent exacerbations of their disease that might be attributable to certain specific events (i.e., seasonal, winter months), a trial of prophylactic antibiotics might be beneficial. If no clinical improvement is noted over an appropriate period (e.g., 2 to 3 months per year for 2 to 3 years), prophylactic therapy could be discontinued.

Table 64.8

Clinical features of chronic bronchitis

Clinical features
Signs and symptoms
Cyanosis (advanced disease)
Obesity
Physical examination
Chest auscultation usually reveals inspiratory and expiratory rales, rhonchi, and mild wheezing with an expiratory phase that is frequently prolonged. There is hyper resonance on percussion with obliteration of the area of cardiac dullness.
Normal vesicular breathing sounds are diminished.
Clubbing of digits (advanced disease).
Chest radiograph
Increase in the anteroposterior diameter of the thoracic cage (observed as a barrel chest)
Depressed diaphragm with limited mobility
Laboratory tests
Erythrocytosis (advanced disease)
Pulmonary function tests
Decreased vital capacity
Prolonged expiratory flow

BRONCHIOLITIS

- Bronchiolitis is an acute viral infection of the lower respiratory tract of infants that affects approximately 50% of children during the first year of life and 100% by 3 years.
- Respiratory syncytial virus is the most common cause of bronchiolitis, accounting for up to 70% of all cases. Para influenza viruses are the second most common cause. Bacteria serve as secondary pathogens in only a small minority of cases.

CLINICAL PRESENTATION

- The most common clinical signs of bronchiolitis are found in Table 64.9. A prodrome suggesting an upper respiratory tract infection, usually lasting from 2 to 8 days, precedes the onset of clinical symptoms.

- As a result of limited oral intake due to coughing combined with fever, vomiting, and diarrhea, infants are frequently dehydrated.
- The diagnosis of bronchiolitis is based primarily on history and clinical findings. The isolation of a viral pathogen in the respiratory secretions of a wheezing child establishes a presumptive diagnosis of infectious bronchiolitis.

TREATMENT

- Bronchiolitis is a self-limiting illness and usually requires no therapy (other than reassurance and antipyretics) unless the infant is hypoxic or dehydrated. Otherwise healthy infants can be treated for fever, provided generous amounts of oral fluids, and observed closely.
- In severely affected children, the mainstays of therapy for bronchiolitis are oxygen therapy and IV fluids. Aerosolized β-adrenergic therapy appears to offer little benefit for the majority of patients but may be useful in the child with a predisposition toward bronchospasm.
- Because bacteria do not represent primary pathogens in the etiology of bronchiolitis, antibiotics should not be routinely administered. However, many clinicians frequently administer antibiotics initially while awaiting culture results because the clinical and radiographic findings in bronchiolitis
- Are often suggestive of a possible bacterial pneumonia. ***Ribavirin*** may be considered for bronchiolitis caused by respiratory syncytial virus in a subset of patients (those with underlying pulmonary or cardiac disease or with severe acute infection). Use of the drug requires special equipment (small-particle aerosol generator) and specifically trained personnel for administration via oxygen hood or mist tent.

Table 64.9

Clinical features of bronchiolitis

Signs and symptoms
Prodrome with irritability, restlessness, and mild fever
Cough and coryza
Vomiting, diarrhea, noisy breathing, and an increase in respiratory rate as symptoms progress
Labored breathing with retractions of the chest wall, nasal flaring, and grunting
Physical examination
Tachycardia and respiratory rate of 40-80/min in hospitalized infants
Wheezing and inspiratory rales
Mild conjunctivitis in one-third of patients
Otitis media in 5%–10% of patients
Laboratory examinations
Peripheral white blood cell count normal or slightly elevated
Abnormal arterial blood gases (hypoxemia and, rarely, hypercarbia)

PNEUMONIA

Pneumonia is the most common infectious cause of death in the United States. It occurs in persons of all ages, although the clinical manifestations are most severe in the very young, the elderly, and the chronically ill.

PATHOPHYSIOLOGY

- Microorganisms gain access to the lower respiratory tract by three routes: they may be inhaled as aerosolized particles; they may enter the lung via the bloodstream from an extra pulmonary site of infection; or aspiration of oropharyngeal contents may occur.

- Lung infections with viruses suppress the bacterial clearing activity of the lung by impairing alveolar macrophage function and mucociliary clearance, thus setting the stage for secondary bacterial pneumonia.
- The vast majority of pneumonia cases acquired in the community by otherwise healthy adults are due to *S. pneumonia* (pneumococcus) (up to 75% of all acute bacterial pneumonias in the United States). Other common bacterial causes include *Mycoplasma pneumonia*, *Legionella*, and *Chlamydophila pneumonia* which are referred to as "atypical" pathogens. Community-acquired pneumonias caused by *Staphylococcus aureus* and gram-negative rods are observed primarily in the elderly, especially those residing in nursing homes, and in association with alcoholism and other debilitating conditions.
- Gram-negative aerobic bacilli and *Staphylococcus aureus* are also the leading causative agents in hospital-acquired pneumonia.
- Anaerobic bacteria are the most common etiologic agents in pneumonia that follows the gross aspiration of gastric or oropharyngeal contents.
- In the pediatric age group, most pneumonia are due to viruses, especially respiratory syncytial virus, parainfluenza, and adenovirus. Pneumococcus is the most common bacterial cause, followed by Group A *Streptococcus* and *Streptococcus aureus*.

CLINICAL FEATURES

GRAM-POSITIVE AND GRAM-NEGATIVE BACTERIAL PNEUMONIA

- The clinical presentation of pneumonia is found in Table 64.10

Table 64.10

Clinical features of pneumonia

Signs and symptoms
Abrupt onset of fever, chills, dyspnea, and productive cough
Rust-colored sputum or hemoptysis
Pleuritic chest pain
Physical examination
Tachypnea and tachycardia
Dullness to percussion
Increased tactile fremitus, whispered pectoriloquy, and egophony
Chest wall retractions and grunting respirations
Diminished breath sounds over the affected area
Inspiratory crackles during lung expansion
Chest radiograph
Dense lobar or segmental infiltrate
Laboratory examination
Leukocytosis with a predominance of polymorphonuclear cells
Low oxygen saturation on arterial blood gas or pulse oximetry

- Infection with *Legionella pneumophila* is characterized by multisystem involvement, including rapidly progressive pneumonia. It has a gradual onset, with prominent constitutional symptoms such as malaise, lethargy, weakness, and anorexia ocurs. A dry, nonproductive cough is initially present that over several days becomes productive of mucoid or purulent sputum. Fevers exceed 40°C (104°F) and are typically unremitting and associated with a relative bradycardia. Pleuritic chest pain and progressive dyspnea may be seen, and fine rales are found on lung examination. Extrapulmonary manifestations remain evident throughout the illness and include diarrhea, nausea, vomiting, myalgias, and arthralgias.

- Substantial changes in a patient's mental status, often out of proportion to the degree of fever, are seen.
- Laboratory findings include leukocytosis with predominance of mature and immature granulocytes in 50% to 75% of patients. Because *Legionella pneumophila* stains poorly with commonly used stains, routine microscopic examination of sputum is of little diagnostic value. Fluorescent antibody testing can be performed to diagnose Legionnaires' disease.

ANAEROBIC PNEUMONIA

Anaerobic pneumonia is typically indolent with cough, low-grade fever, and weight loss, although an acute presentation may occur. Putrid sputum, when present, is highly suggestive of the diagnosis. Chest radiographs reveal infiltrates typically located in dependent lung segments, and lung abscesses develop in 20% of patients 1 to 2 weeks.

MYCOPLASMA PNEUMONIAE

- *M. pneumonia* pneumonia presents with a gradual onset of fever, headache, and malaise, with the appearance 3 to 5 days after the onset of illness of a persistent, hacking cough that initially is nonproductive. Sore throat, ear pain, and rhinorrhea are often present. Lung findings are generally
- Limited to rales and rhonchi; findings of consolidation are rarely present.
- Nonpulmonary manifestations are extremely common and include nausea, vomiting, diarrhea, myalgias, arthralgias, polyarticular arthritis, skin rashes, myocarditis and pericarditis, hemolytic anemia, meningoencephalitis, cranial neuropathies, and Guillain-Barré syndrome. Systemic symptoms generally clear in 1 to 2 weeks, whereas respiratory symptoms may persist up to 4 Weeks.
- Radiographic findings include patchy or interstitial infiltrates, which are most commonly seen in the lower lobes.
- Sputum Gram stain may reveal mononuclear or polymorphonuclear leukocytes, with no predominant organism. Although *M. pneumoniae* can be cultured from respiratory secretions using specialized medium, 2 to 3 weeks may be necessary for culture identification.

VIRAL PNEUMONIA

- The clinical pictures produced by respiratory viruses are sufficiently variable and overlap to such a degree that an etiologic diagnosis cannot confidently be made on clinical grounds alone. Serologic tests for virus specific antibodies are often used in the diagnosis of viral infections. The diagnostic the fold rise in titer between acute and convalescent phase sera may require 2 to 3 weeks to develop; however, same-day diagnosis of viral infections is now possible through the use of indirect immunofluorescence tests on exfoliated cells from the respiratory tract.

- Radiographic findings are nonspecific and include bronchial wall thickening and perihilar and diffuse interstitial infiltrates.

NOSOCOMIAL PNEUMONIA

The strongest predisposing factor for nosocomial pneumonia is mechanical ventilation. Risk is increased by prior antibiotic use, use of H2-receptor antagonists, and severe illness. The diagnosis of nosocomial pneumonia is usually established by presence of a new infiltrate on chest radiograph, fever, worsening respiratory status, and the appearance of thick, neutrophil-laden respiratory secretions.

TREATMENT

- The first priority on assessing the patient with pneumonia is to evaluate the adequacy of respiratory function and to determine whether there are signs of systemic illness, specifically dehydration or sepsis with resulting circulatory collapse.
- The supportive care of the patient with pneumonia includes the use of humidified oxygen for hypoxemia, fluid resuscitation, administration of bronchodilators when bronchospasm is present, and chest physiotherapy with postural drainage if there is evidence of retained secretions. Important therapeutic adjuncts include adequate hydration (by IV route if necessary), optimal nutritional support, and fever control.
- The treatment of bacterial pneumonia initially involves the empiric use of a relatively broad-spectrum antibiotic (or antibiotics) effective against probable pathogens after appropriate cultures and specimens for laboratory evaluation have been obtained. Therapy should be narrowed to cover
- Specific pathogens once the results of cultures are known.
- Antibiotic concentrations in respiratory secretions in excess of the pathogen minimum inhibitory concentration (MIC) are necessary for successful treatment of pulmonary infections.
- For treatment of bacterial pneumonia with concentration-independent antimicrobials (e.g., β-lactams and carbapenems), a plasma drug concentration exceeding the pathogen MIC for more than 50% of the dosing interval correlates with bacteriologic cure. For concentration-dependent antimicrobials (e.g., Aminoglycosides and fluoroquinolones) a peak drug concentration to pathogen MIC ratio >8 to 10 or a ratio of pathogen MIC to antibiotic area under the curve >25 to 40 for gram-positive pathogens and >100 for gram-negative pathogens correlates with bacteriologic cure.

REFERENCES

1. "Mortality and Burden of Disease Estimates for WHO Member States in 2002" (xls). *World Health Organization*. 2002.
2. Cherry DK, Hing E, Woodwell DA, Rechtsteiner EA. National Ambulatory Medical Care Survey: 2006 Summary.

Hyattsville, MD: National Center for Health Statistics; 2008. National health statistics reports.

3. Cooper RJ, Hoffman JR, Bartlett JG, et al: Principles of appropriate antibiotic use for acute pharyngitis in adults: Background. Ann Intern Med. 2001, 134: 509-517.
4. Poole MD, Portugal LG. Treatment of rhinosinusitis in the outpatient setting. Am J Med. 2005, 118: 45S-50S.
5. McGinn TG, Deluca J, Ahlawat SK, et al: Validation and modification of strepto-coccal pharyngitis prediction rules. Mayo Clin Proc. 2003, 78: 289-293.
6. Piccirillo JF. Acute bacterial sinusitis. N Engl J Med. 2004, 351: 902-910.
7. Batra PS. Radiologic imaging in rhinosinusitis. Cleve Clin J Med. 2004, 71: 886-888.

CHAPTER 65

Urinary Tract Infections

DEFINITION

- Infections of the urinary tract represent a wide variety of clinical syndromes, including urethritis, cystitis, prostatitis, and pyelonephritis.
- A urinary tract infection (UTI) is defined as the presence of microorganisms in the urine that cannot be accounted for by contamination. The organisms have the potential to invade the tissues of the urinary tract and adjacent structures.
- Lower tract infections include **cystitis** (bladder), **urethritis** (urethra), **prostatitis** (prostate gland), and epididymitis. Upper tract infections (such as **pyelonephritis**) involve the kidney and are referred to as *pyelonephritis*.
- Uncomplicated UTIs are not associated with structural or neurologic abnormalities that may interfere with the normal flow of urine or the voiding mechanism. Complicated UTIs are the result of a predisposing lesion of the urinary tract such as a congenital abnormality or distortion of the urinary tract, a stone, indwelling catheter, prostatic hypertrophy, obstruction, or neurologic deficit that interferes with the normal flow of urine and urinary tract defenses.
- Recurrent UTIs are characterized by multiple symptomatic episodes with asymptomatic periods occurring between these episodes. These infections are either due to reinfection or to relapse.
- Reinfections are caused by a different organism and account for the majority of recurrent UTIs.
- Relapse represents the development of repeated infections caused by the same initial organism.

PREVALENCE

Urinary tract infections are the most frequent bacterial infection in women. They occur most frequently between the ages of 16 and 35 years, with 10% of women getting an infection yearly and 60% having an infection at some point in their lives. Recurrences are common, with nearly half of people getting a second infection within a year. Urinary tract infections occur four times more frequently in females than males. Pyelonephritis occurs between 20–30 times less frequently. They are the most common cause of hospital acquired infections accounting for approximately 40%. Rates of asymptomatic bacteria in the urine increase with age from two to seven percent in women of child bearing age to as high as 50% in elderly women in care homes. Rates of asymptomatic bacteria in the urine among men over 75 are between 7-10%.

ETIOLOGY

- The most common cause of uncomplicated UTIs is *E. coli* , accounting for more than 85% of community-acquired infections, followed by *Staphylococcus saprophyticus* (coagulase-negative staphylococcus), accounting for 5% to 15%.
- The urinary pathogens in complicated or nosocomial infections may include *E. coli*, which accounts for less than 50% of these infections, *Proteus* spp., *Klebsiella pneumoniae*, *Enterobacter* spp., *Pseudomonas aeruginosa*, staphylococci, and enterococci. *Candida* spp. has become common causes of urinary infection in the critically ill and chronically catheterized patient.
- The majority of UTIs are caused by a single organism; however, in patients with stones, indwelling urinary catheters, or chronic renal abscesses, multiple organisms may be isolated.

PATHOPHYSIOLOGY

- The bacteria causing UTIs usually originate from bowel flora of the host.
- UTIs can be acquired via three possible routes: the ascending, hematogenous, or lymphatic pathways.
- In females, the short length of the urethra and proximity to the perirectal area make colonization of the urethra likely. Bacteria are then believed to enter the bladder from the urethra. Once in the bladder, the organisms multiply quickly and can ascend the ureters to the kidney.
- Three factors determine the development of UTI: the size of the inoculum, virulence of the microorganism, and competency of the natural host defense mechanisms.
- Patients who are unable to void urine completely are at greater risk of developing UTIs and frequently have recurrent infections.
- An important virulence factor of bacteria is their ability to adhere to urinary epithelial cells by fimbriae, resulting in colonization of the urinary tract, bladder infections, and pyelonephritis. Other virulence factors include hemolysin, a cytotoxic protein produced by bacteria that lyses a wide range of cells including erythrocytes, polymorphonuclear leukocytes, and monocytes; and aerobactin, which facilitates the binding and uptake of iron by *Escherichia coli*.

CLINICAL FEATURES

- The typical symptoms of lower and upper UTIs are presented in Table 65.1.
- Symptoms alone are unreliable for the diagnosis of bacterial UTIs. The key to the diagnosis of a UTI is the ability to demonstrate significant numbers of microorganisms present in an appropriate urine specimen to distinguish contamination from infection.
- Elderly patients frequently do not experience specific urinary symptoms, but they will present with altered mental status, change in eating habits, or GI symptoms.
- A standard urinalysis should be obtained in the initial assessment of a patient. Microscopic examination of the urine should be performed by preparation of a

Gram stain of centrifuged urine. The presence of at least one organism per oil-immersion field in a properly collected uncentrifuged specimen correlates with more than 100,000 bacteria/mL of urine.

Table 65.1

Clinical features of urinary tract infections (UTIs) in adults

Signs and symptoms
Lower UTI: Dysuria, urgency, frequency, nocturia, suprapubic heaviness, Gross haematuria
Upper UTI: Flank pain, fever, nausea, vomiting, malaise
Physical examination
Upper UTI: Costovertebral tenderness
Laboratory tests
Bacteriuria
Pyuria (white blood cell count >10/mm^3)
Nitrite-positive urine (with nitrite reducers)
Leukocyte esterase-positive urine

- The presence of pyuria (more than 10 white blood cells/mm^3) in a symptomatic patient correlates with significant Bacteriuria.

✓ The nitrite test can be used to detect the presence of nitrate-reducing bacteria in the urine (such as *E. coli*). The leukocyte esterase test is a rapid dipstick test to detect pyuria.

✓ The most reliable method of diagnosing UTIs is by quantitative urine culture. Patients with infection usually have more than 105 bacteria/mL of urine, although as many as one-third of women with symptomatic infection have less than 105 bacteria/mL.

✓ A method to detect upper UTI is the antibody-coated bacteria test, an immunofluorescent method that detects bacteria coated with immunoglobulin in freshly voided urine.

TREATMENT

GENERAL PRINCIPLES

- The management of a patient with a UTI includes initial evaluation, selection of an antibacterial agent and duration of therapy, and follow-up evaluation.
- The initial selection of an antimicrobial agent for the treatment of UTI is primarily based on the severity of the presenting signs and symptoms, the site of infection, and whether the infection is determined to be complicated or uncomplicated.

PHARMACOLOGICAL TREATMENT

- The ability to eradicate bacteria from the urinary tract is directly related to the sensitivity of the organism and the achievable concentration of the antimicrobial agent in the urine.
- The therapeutic management of UTIs is best accomplished by first categorizing the type of infection: acute uncomplicated cystitis, symptomatic abacteriuria, asymptomatic Bacteriuria, complicated UTIs, recurrent infections, or prostatitis.
- Table 65.2 lists the most common agents used in the treatment of UTIs, along with comments concerning their general use.

ACUTE UNCOMPLICATED CYSTITIS

- These infections are predominantly caused by *E. coli*, and antimicrobial therapy should be directed against this organism initially. Other causes include *Staphylococcus saprophyticus* and occasionally *Klebsiella pneumoniae* and *Proteus mirabilis*.

- Because the causative organisms and their susceptibilities are generally known, a cost-effective approach to management is recommended that includes a urinalysis and initiation of empiric therapy without a urine culture.
- Short-course therapy (3-day therapy) with **Trimethoprim–sulphamethoxazole** or a **fluoroquinolone** (e.g., **Ciprofloxacin, Levofloxacin,** or **Norfloxacin**) is superior to single-dose therapy for uncomplicated infection and should be the treatment of choice. Amoxicillin or sulphonamides are not recommended because of the high incidence of resistant *E. coli*. Follow-up urine cultures are not necessary in patients who respond.

Table 65.2

Lists the most common agents used in the treatment of UTIs

	Drug of Choice[1]	Second Line Therapy[1]	Third Line Therapy[1]	Comments
Cystitis				
Acute Uncomplicated Cystitis (AUC)	TMP/SMX (x3d) TMP (x3d) Nitrofurantoin (x7d)	Fosfomycin Amoxicillin (x7d) Cephalexin (x7d) Ciprofloxacin (x3d) Norfloxacin (x3d)	Gatifloxacin (x3d) Levofloxacin (x3d)	- Use longer courses in diabetes and if symptomatic > 7day (and In older women?)[1] - Due to increasing E.coil resistance, amoxi may not be suitable for empiric therapy; reserved for UTIs caused by strep or enterococci or if organism is known to be susceptible[1]
	Fluoroquinolones are not 1st line in cystis because of the threat of increasing fluoro-quinolone resistance			
Recurrent (<1 mt) Treat: 10-14d	TMP/SMX TMP Nitrofurantoin	Amox/Clav Norfloxcin Ciprofloxacin	Gatifloxaxin Levofloxacin	- Some references classify infections as *recurrent* if it is within 2 weeks of stopping antibiotic and as a reinfection if >2 weeks since antibiotic is stopped[4,8]
Complicated **Treat: 10-14 days**	TMP/SMX TMP Nitrofurantoin Gentamycin +/-	Amox/Clav Ceftriaxone Cefotaxime Norfloxacin	Imipenem (IV) Ceftazidime (IV)	- Definition of "complicated UTT" varies but usually includes urinary tract

Table 65.2 *Contd...*

	Drug of Choice[1]	Second Line Therapy[1]	Third Line Therapy[1]	Comments
	Ampicillin (IV) Tobramycin + Ampicillin (IV)	Ciprofloxacin (IV/po) Tobramycin (IV)	Imipenem Ceftazidime Piperacillin/ Tazobactam (IV)	Structural abnormalities (ie. Catheters) and specific populations (men, pregnant women, patients with diabetes, patients taking immunosup presants, and patients who have received a renal transplant)[4] - IV antibiotics used in severe UTIs should be switch to oral as soon as possible
Pyelonephritis				
Pyelonephritis (out patients)	TMP/SMX TMP Norfloxacin Ciprofloxacin	Amox/Clav	Gatifloxacin Levofloxacin Ceftriaxone (IV) Cefotaxime (IV) Gentamycin +/- Ampicillin (IV)	- Symptoms of pyelonephritis typically includes frequency, urgency, dysuria, fever and flank pain[4] - Effective antibiotic therapy should stabilize patients in 24 hours, significantly reduce urinary bacteria within 48 hours and within 72 hours, most patients should be afebrile and experiencing fewer symptoms[4]
Pyelonephritis (in patient)	Ampicillin + Tobramycin (IV) Gentamycin +/- Ampicillin (IV)	Ceftriaxone Cefotaxime	Imipenem Norfloxacin Ciprofloxacin	
Prostatitis				
Prostatitis[1] Acute: treat 2-4 weeks	TMP/SMX Ciprofloxacin Norfloxacin Ampicillin + Tobramycin (IV) Gentamycin +/- Ampicillin (IV)	Tobramycin (IV)	Ciprofloxacin Gatifloxacin Levofloxacin	- Chronic prostatitis may need longer treatment[1] - Chronic may not caused by bacteria, so if patient has not responded to antibiotic in 4-6 weeks, refer or try another option (ie. alpha-blocker)[1]

SYMPTOMATIC ABACTERIURIA

- Single-dose or short-course therapy with **trimethoprim–sulphamethoxazole** has been used effectively, and prolonged courses of therapy are not necessary for the majority of patients.
- If the patient reports recent sexual activity, therapy for *Chlamydia trachomatis* should be considered (Azithromycin 1 g as a single dose or Doxycycline 100 mg twice daily for 7 days).

ASYMPTOMATIC BACTERIURIA

- The management of asymptomatic Bacteriuria depends on the age of the patient and, if female, whether she is pregnant. In children, treatment should consist of conventional courses of therapy, as described for symptomatic infections.
- In the nonpregnant female, therapy is controversial; however, it appears that treatment has little effect on the natural course of infections.
- Most clinicians feel that asymptomatic Bacteriuria in the elderly is a benign disease and may not warrant treatment. The presence of Bacteriuria can be confirmed by culture if treatment is considered.

COMPLICATED URINARY TRACT INFECTIONS

Acute Pyelonephritis: The presentation of high-grade fever (greater than 38.3°C [100.9°F]) and Severe flank pain should be treated as acute pyelonephritis, and aggressive management is warranted. Severely ill patients with pyelonephritis should be hospitalized and IV drugs administered initially. Milder cases may be managed with oral antibiotics in an outpatient setting.

- At the time of presentation, a Gram stain of the urine should be performed, along with urinalysis, culture, and sensitivities.
- In the mild to moderately symptomatic patient for whom oral therapy is considered, an effective agent should be administered for at least a 2-week period, although use of highly active agents for 7 to 10 days may be sufficient. Oral antibiotics that have shown efficacy in this setting include

Trimethoprim–sulfamethoxazole or fluoroquinolones: If a Gram stain reveals gram-positive cocci, *Streptococcus faecalis* should be considered and treatment directed against this pathogen (**Ampicillin**).

- In the seriously ill patient, the traditional initial therapy has included an IV **fluoroquinolone**, an **aminogly coside** with or without **Ampicillin**, or an extended-Spectrum **cephalosporin** with or without an aminoglycoside.
- If the patient has been hospitalized in the last 6 months, has a urinary catheter, or is in a nursing home, the possibility of *Pseudomonas aeruginosa* and *enterococci* infection, as well as multiply-resistant organisms, should be considered. In this setting, **Ceftazidime, Ticarcillin-Clavulanic Acid, Piperacillin, Aztreonam, Meropenem,** Or **Imipenem,** in combination with an **aminoglycoside**, is recommended. If the patient responds to initial combination therapy, the aminoglycoside may be discontinued after 3 days.

URINARY TRACT INFECTIONS IN MALES

- A urine culture should be obtained before treatment, because the cause of infection in men is not as predictable as in women.
- If gram-negative bacteria are presumed, **trimethoprim–sulphamethoxazole** or a **fluoroquinolone** is a preferred agent. Initial therapy is for 10 to 14 days. For recurrent infections in males, cure rates are much higher with a 6-week regimen of **trimethoprim**–sulphamethoxazole.

RECURRENT INFECTIONS

- Recurrent episodes of UTI (reinfections and relapses) account for a significant portion of all UTIs.
- These patients are most commonly women and can be divided into two groups: those with fewer than two or three episodes per year and those who develop more frequent infections.
- In patients with infrequent infections (i.e., fewer than three infections per year), each episode should be treated as a separately occurring infection. Short-course therapy should be used in symptomatic female patients with lower tract infection.
- In patients who have frequent symptomatic infections, long-term prophylactic antimicrobial therapy may be instituted .Therapy is generally given for 6 months, with urine cultures followed periodically.
- In women who experience symptomatic reinfections in association with sexual activity, voiding after intercourse may help prevent infection. Also, self-administered, single-dose prophylactic therapy with **trimethoprim– sulphamethoxazole** taken after intercourse has been found to significantly reduce the incidence of recurrent infection in these patients.
- Women who relapse after short-course therapy should receive a 2-week course of therapy. In patients who relapse after 2 weeks, therapy should be continued for another 2 to 4 weeks. If relapse occurs after 6 weeks of treatment, urologic examination should be performed, and therapy for 6 Months or even longer may be considered.

SPECIAL CONDITIONS

URINARY TRACT INFECTION IN PREGNANCY

- In patients with significant bacteriuria, symptomatic or asymptomatic, treatment is recommended in order to avoid possible complications during the pregnancy. Therapy should consist of an agent with a relatively low adverse-effect potential (a **sulphonamide, cephalexin, amoxicillin, amoxicillin/clavulanate, nitrofurantoin**) administered for 7 days.
- Tetracyclines should be avoided because of teratogenic effects, and sulphonamides should not be administered during the third trimester because of the possible development of kernicterus and hyperbilirubinemia. Also, the fluoroquinolones should not be given because of their potential to inhibit cartilage and bone development in the newborn.

CATHETERIZED PATIENTS

- When Bacteriuria occurs in the asymptomatic, short-term catheterized patient (less than 30 days), the use of systemic antibiotic therapy should be withheld and the catheter removed as soon as possible. If the patient becomes symptomatic, the catheter should again be removed, and treatment as described for complicated infections should be started.

- The use of prophylactic systemic antibiotics in patients with short-term catheterization reduces the incidence of infection over the first 4 to 7 days. In long-term catheterized patients, however, antibiotics only postpone the development of bacteriuria and lead to emergence of resistant organisms.

PROSTATITIS

- Prostatitis is an inflammation of the prostate gland and surrounding tissue as a result of infection. It can be either acute or chronic. The acute form is characterized by a severe illness characterized by a sudden onset of fever and urinary and constitutional symptoms. Chronic bacterial prostatitis (CBP) represents a recurring infection with the same organism (relapse). Pathogenic bacteria and Significant inflammatory cells must be present in prostatic secretions and urine to make the diagnosis of bacterial prostatitis.

PATHOGENESIS AND ETIOLOGY

- The exact mechanism of bacterial infection of the prostate is not well understood. The possible routes of infection include ascending infection of the urethra, reflux of infected urine into prostatic ducts, invasion by rectal bacteria through direct extension or lymphatic spread, and by hematogenous spread.
- Gram-negative enteric organisms are the most frequent pathogens in acute bacterial prostatitis. *E. coli* is the predominant organism, occurring in 75% of cases.
- CBP is most commonly caused by *E. coli*, with other gram-negative organisms isolated much less often.

CLINICAL FEATURES AND DIAGNOSIS

- The clinical presentation of bacterial prostatitis is presented in Table 65.3.
- Digital palpation of the prostate via the rectum may reveal a swollen, tender, warm, tense, or indurated prostate. Massage of the prostate will express a purulent discharge, which will readily grow the pathogenic organism. However, prostatic massage is contraindicated in acute bacterial
- Prostatitis because of a risk of inducing bacteremia and associated pain.

Table 65.3

Clinical presentation of bacterial prostatitis

Signs and symptoms
Acute bacterial prostatitis: High fever, chills, malaise, myalgia, localized pain (perineal, rectal, sacrococcygeal), frequency, urgency, dysuria, nocturia, and retention
Chronic bacterial prostatitis: Voiding difficulties (frequency, urgency, dysuria), low back pain, and perineal and suprapubic discomfort
Physical examination
Acute bacterial prostatitis: Swollen, tender, tense, or indurated gland
Chronic bacterial prostatitis: Boggy, indurated (enlarged) prostate in most patients
Laboratory tests
Bacteriuria
Bacteria in expressed prostatic secretions

- CBP is characterized by recurrent UTIs with the same pathogen.
- Urinary tract localization studies are critical to the diagnosis of CBP. Clinical Presentation of Bacterial Prostatitis

TREATMENT

- The majority of patients can be managed with oral antimicrobial agents, such as **trimethoprim–sulphamethoxazole** or the fluoroquinolones (**ciprofloxacin, levofloxacin**). When IV treatment is necessary, IV to oral sequential therapy with **trimethoprim–sulphamethoxazole** or a fluoroquinolone, such as ciprofloxacin or **ofloxacin**, would be appropriate.
- The total course of therapy should be 4 weeks, which may be prolonged to 6 to 12 weeks with chronic prostatitis.
- Parenteral therapy should be maintained until the patient is a febrile and less symptomatic. The conversion to an oral antibiotic can be considered if the patient has been a febrile for 48 hours or after 3 to 5 days of IV therapy.
- The choice of antibiotics in CBP should include those agents that are capable of crossing the prostatic epithelium into the prostatic fluid in therapeutic concentrations and that also possess the spectrum of activity to be effective.
- Currently, the fluoroquinolones (given for 4 to 6 weeks) appear to provide the best therapeutic option in the management of CBP.

REFERENCES

1. Nicolle LE (2008). "Uncomplicated urinary tract infection in adults including uncomplicated pyelonephritis". *Urol Clin North Am* **35** (1): 1–12,
2. Lane, DR; Takhar, SS (2011 Aug). "Diagnosis and management of urinary tract infection and pyelonephritis. "*Emergency medicine clinics of North America* **29** (3): 539–52.
3. Colgan, R; Williams, M (2011-10-01). "Diagnosis and treatment of acute uncomplicated cystitis.". *American family physician* **84** (7): 771–6.
4. Salvatore, S; Salvatore, S, Cattoni, E, Siesto, G, Serati, M, Sorice, P, Torella, M (2011 Jun). "Urinary tract infections in women.". *European journal of obstetrics, gynecology, and reproductive biology* **156** (2): 131–6.
5. Dielubanza, EJ; Schaeffer, AJ (2011 Jan). "Urinary tract infections in women.". *The Medical clinics of North America* **95** (1): 27–41.
6. Gould CV, Umscheid CA, Agarwal RK, Kuntz G, Pegues DA (2010). "Guideline for prevention of catheter-associated urinary tract infections 2009". *Infect Control Hosp Epidemiol* **31** (4): 319–26.
7. Infectious Disease, Chapter Seven, Urinary Tract Infections from *Infectious Disease Section of Microbiology and Immunology On-line*. By Charles Bryan MD. University of South Carolina. This page last changed on Wednesday, April 27, 2011
8. Dai, B; Liu, Y; Jia, J; Mei, C (2010). "Long-term antibiotics for the prevention of recurrent urinary tract infection in children: a systematic review and meta-analysis". *Archives of Disease in Childhood* **95** (7): 499–508.
9. Raynor, MC; Carson CC, 3rd (2011 Jan). "Urinary infections in men.". *The Medical clinics of North America* **95** (1): 43–54.

CHAPTER 66

Infective Meningitis

It is an inflammation of the arachnoid and pia matter associated with presence of bacteria, viruses, fungi or protozoa in CSF.

PREVALENCE

Bacterial meningitis occurs in about 3 people per 100,000 annually in Western countries. Population-wide studies have shown that viral meningitis is more common, at 10.9 per 100,000, and occurs more often in the summer. In Brazil, the rate of bacterial meningitis is higher, at 45.8 per 100,000 annually. Sub-Saharan Africa has been plagued by large epidemics of meningococcal meningitis for over a century, leading to it being labeled the "meningitis belt". Epidemics typically occur in the dry season (December to June), and an epidemic wave can last two to three years, dying out during the intervening rainy seasons. Attack rates of 100–800 cases per 100,000 are encountered in this area, which is poorly served by medical care. These cases are predominantly caused by meningococci. The largest epidemic ever recorded in history swept across the entire region in 1996–1997, causing over 250,000 cases and 25,000 deaths.

ETIOLOGY

- *Neisseria meningitides, Streptococcus pneumonia* account for 75% of cases – occurs in young children.
- In neonatal period – Gp B. streptococci are most common cause of bacterial meningitis, also E.Coli and enterobacteriaceae.
- Also occur as a complication of Neurosurgery, paticnts who have ventriculoatrial shunts.
- May also occur due to multi system bacterial diseases such as syphilis, leptospriosis, lyme disease

PATHOPHYSIOLOGY

Bacterial meningitis is preceded by nasopharyngeal colonization by causative organism.

In colonized individuals → Infection will progress → local invasion occurs

Leads to Bacteremia and Meningeal invasion

Routes by which organism reach Meninges include

(a) Direct spread from nasopharynx
(b) Blood-borne spread from other foci of colonization or injection.

(c) Abnormal communications with skin or mucous membranes
Eg: Skull fractures, anatomical defects.
(d) Spread from an infected adjacent focus.

Mechanism by which microorganisms cause meningitis.
(a) Attachment to host mucosal surfaces.
(b) Evasion of phagocytosis and other host defences
(c) Meningeal invasion
(d) Disruption of B^3 (Blood –Brain-Barrier)
(e) Secondary brain damage.
(f) Induction of pathophysiological changes in CSF space.

CLINICAL FEATURES

- Sudden onset of headache, neck stiffness, photophobia, fever and vomiting.
- Presence of haemorrhagic skin rash. Untreated patients may develop seizures, focal cerebral signs, and cranial nerve palsies.
- In infants with meningitis signs include fever, diarrhea, lethargy, feeding difficulties and respiratory distils

DIAGNOSIS

- Detection of the causative organism, demonstration of biochemical changes and cellular response in CSF.
- In bacterial meningitis, organisms may be visible in Gram stained smears of CSF. Special strains such as Zeihl – Neelsen method to visualize Mycobacteria.
- Polymerase chain reaction is increasingly being used to diagnose pneumococcal meningitis & nuclear acid amplification techniques are used to detect M.tuberculosis and several viruses.

TREATMENT

DRUG TREATMENT (TABLE 66.1)

Table 66.1

Drug treatment of infective meningitis and their dosages

S.No.	Age group	1st choice Antibiotic therapy	Alternative therapies
1.	Neonates < 7 days	Ampicillin, 50mg/kg twice daily or Amoxicillin 25 mg/kg twice daily & Cefotaxime 50 mg/kg twice daily or ceftazidime 50mg/kg twice day.	Benzyl penicillin 50mg twice daily & Ampicillin 50 mg/kg twice daily or amoxicillin 25 mg/kg twice daily & Gentamicin 2.5 mg/kg twice daily
2.	Neonates 8-28 days	Ampicillin 50mg/kg 4 times daily or Amoxicillin25 mg/kg 3 times daily and Cefotaxime 50mg/kg 3 times daily or Ceftazidime 50 mg/1kg 3 times daily	Benzyl penicillin 50 mg 3 or 4 times daily or Ampicillin 50mg/kg 3 or 4 times or Amoxicillin: 25mg/kg & Gentamicin – 2.5mg/kg 3 times daily
3.	Infants 1-3 months	Ampicillin 50mg/kg 4 times daily or amoxicillin 25mg/kg 3 times daily Cefotaxime – 50mg/kg three times. Ceftazidime – 75 -100mg once daily	
4.	Infants, > 3 months	Cefotaxime – 50mg/kg 3 times daily. Ceftriaxone -75 to 100mg/kg once daily	Ampicillin 50mg/kg daily 4 times. Amoxicillin – 25mg/kg 4times 3 times Chloramphenicol 25mg/kg

Table 66.1 *Contd...*

S.No.	Age group	1st choice Antibiotic therapy	Alternative therapies
5.	Adults	Cefotaxime 2g 3 times daily or Ceftriaxone 2-4g once daily.	Benzyl penicillin 2.4 g-4 hours. Ampicillin 2-3 g four times daily or Amoxicillin -2g 3 or 4 times daily & Chloramphenicol 12/.5-25mg/kg 4 times daily.

Table 66.2

Common therapeutic problems in infective meningitis

Sl.No	Infection	Antibiotic	Common problems	Resolution
1	Bacterial Meningitis	Chloramphenicol	Serious toxicity in neonates	Close monitoring of serum levels
2	Neonatal Meningitis	Aminoglycosides	Poor CSF penetration	Substitute With Better CSF Penetration Antibiotic (Cephalosporin)
3	Strep.penumoniae meningitis	Penicillin, Cefotaxime or Ceftriaxone, Vancomycin (I.V)	Resistance is increasing, unreliable CSF penetration	Use Cefotaxime or Ceftriaxone ± Vancomycin
4	Listeria monocytogenes meningitis	Any	Relapse rate up to 10% after short courses of therapy	Give prolonged therapy (3-4 weeks)
5	Cryptococcal meningitis	Amphotericin Flucytosine	Fever, nausea, vomiting, anemia, bone marrow depression	Replace with Fluconazole monitor screen levels.

REFERENCES

1. Warrell DA, Farrar JJ, Crook DWM (2003). "24.14.1 Bacterial meningitis". *Oxford Textbook of Medicine Volume 3* (Fourth ed.). Oxford University Press. pp. 1115–29.
2. WHO (September 2000). "Detecting meningococcal meningitis epidemics in highly-endemic African countries" (PDF). *Weekly Epidemiological Record* 75(38): 306–9.
3. Marc Laforce, F.; Ravenscroft, N.; Djingarey, M.; Viviani, S. (2009). "Epidemic meningitis due to Group a Neisseria meningitidis in the African meningitis belt: A persistent problem with an imminent solution". *Vaccine* 27: B13–B19.
4. Weisfelt M, de Gans J, van der Poll T, van de Beek D (April 2006). "Pneumococcal meningitis in adults: new approaches to management and prevention". *Lancet Neurol* 5 (4): 332–42.
5. Fraser A, Gafter-Gvili A, Paul M, Leibovici L (2006). Fraser, Abigail. ed. "Antibiotics for preventing meningococcal infections". *Cochrane Database of Systematic Reviews* (4): CD004785. .
6. Weichselbaum A (1887). "Ueber die Aetiologie der akuten Meningitis cerebro-spinalis" (in German). *Fortschrift der Medizin* 5: 573–583.

CHAPTER 67

Tuberculosis

DEFINITION

Tuberculosis, **MTB**, or **TB** (short for *tubercle bacillus*) is a common, and in many cases lethal, infectious disease caused by various strains of mycobacterium, usually *Mycobacterium tuberculosis*. Tuberculosis typically attacks the lungs but can also affect other parts of the body. It is spread through the air when people who have an active TB infection cough, sneeze, or otherwise transmit their saliva through the air.

PREVALENCE

Tuberculosis is the second most common cause of death from infectious disease (after those due to HIV/AIDS). The absolute number of tuberculosis cases ("prevalence") has been decreasing since 2005, while new cases ("incidence") have decreased since 2002. China has achieved particularly dramatic progress, with an approximate 80% decline in its TB mortality rate. Tuberculosis is more common in developing countries; about 80% of the population in many Asian and African countries test positive in tuberculin tests, while only 5%–10% of the US population test positive. Hopes of totally controlling the disease have been dramatically dampened because of a number of factors, including the difficulty of developing and making available an effective vaccine, the highly expensive and time-consuming diagnostic process, the necessity to provide many months of treatment, and the emergence of drug-resistant cases in the 1980s.

ETIOLOGY

Pulmonary tuberculosis (TB) is caused by the bacteria *Mycobacterium tuberculosis (M. tuberculosis)*. TB spreads by breathing in air droplets from a cough or sneeze of an infected person. This is called primary TB.

Most people who develop symptoms of a TB infection first became infected in the past. However, in some cases, the disease may become active within weeks after the primary infection.

The following people are at higher risk for active TB:

- Elderly
- Infants
- People with weakened immune systems, for example due to AIDS, chemotherapy, diabetes, or certain medications

Risk of TB increases if person:

- Are in frequent contact with people who have TB
- Have poor nutrition

- Lives in crowded or unsanitary living conditions

The following factors may increase the rate of TB infection in a population:

- Increase in HIV infections
- Increase in number of homeless people (poor environment and nutrition)
- The appearance of drug-resistant strains of TB

PATHOPHYSIOLOGY

- TB infection begins when the Mycobacteria reach the pulmonary alveoli, where they invade and replicate within endosomes of alveolar macrophages. The primary site of infection in the lungs, known as the "Ghon focus", is generally located in either the upper part of the lower lobe, or the lower part of the upper lobe. Tuberculosis of the lungs may also occur via infection from the blood stream. This is known as a Simon focus and is typically found in the top of the lung. This haematogenous transmission can also spread infection to more distant sites such as peripheral lymph nodes, the kidneys, the brain, and the bones. All parts of the body can be affected by the disease, though for unknown reasons it rarely affects the heart, skeletal muscles, pancreas, or thyroid.
- Tuberculosis is classified as one of the granulomatous inflammatory diseases. Macrophages, T lymphocytes, B lymphocytes, and fibroblasts are among the cells that aggregate to form granulomas, with lymphocytes surrounding the infected macrophages. The granuloma prevents dissemination of the Mycobacteria and provides a local environment for interaction of cells of the immune system. Bacteria inside the granuloma can become dormant, resulting in latent infection. Another feature of the granulomas is the development of abnormal cell death (necrosis) in the center of tubercles.
- If TB bacteria gain entry to the bloodstream from an area of damaged tissue, they can spread throughout the body and set up many foci of infection, all appearing as tiny, white tubercles in the tissues. This severe form of TB disease, most common in young children and those with HIV, is called miliary tuberculosis. People with this disseminated TB have a high fatality rate even with treatment (about 30%).

CLINICAL FEATURES

The primary stage of TB usually doesn't cause symptoms. When symptoms of pulmonary TB occur, they may include:

- Cough (usually cough up mucus)
- Coughing up blood
- Excessive sweating, especially at night
- Fatigue
- Fever
- Unintentional weight loss

Other symptoms that may occur with this disease:

- Breathing difficulty
- Chest pain
- Wheezing

DIAGNOSIS

Tests may include:

- Biopsy of the affected tissue (rare)

- Bronchoscopy
- Chest CT scan
- Chest x-ray
- Interferon-gamma blood test such as the QFT-Gold test to test for TB infection
- Sputum examination and cultures; Tuberculin skin test (also called a PPD test)

TREATMENT

GENERAL PRINCIPLES

- Drug treatment is the cornerstone of TB management. A minimum of two drugs, and generally three or four drugs, must be used simultaneously.
- Drug treatment is continued for at least 6 months and up to 2 to 3 years for some cases of multidrug-resistant TB (MDR-TB).
- Measures to assure adherence, such as directly observed therapy, are important.
- Patients with active disease should be isolated to prevent spread of the disease.
- Public health departments are responsible for preventing the spread of TB, finding where TB has already spread using contact investigation.
- Debilitated patients may require therapy for other medical conditions, including substance abuse and HIV infection, and some may need nutritional support.
- Surgery may be needed to remove destroyed lung tissue, space-occupying lesions, and some extra pulmonary lesions.

PHARMACOLOGICAL TREATMENT (TABLE 67.1, 67.2)

LATENT INFECTION

- **Isoniazid** (INH) 300 mg daily in adults is the preferred treatment for latent TB in the United States, generally given for 9 months.
- Individuals likely to be noncompliant may be treated with a regimen of 15 mg/kg (to a maximum of 900 mg) twice weekly with observation.
- Rifampin (RIF) 600 mg daily for 4 months can be used when INH resistance is suspected or when the patient cannot tolerate INH. Rifabutin 300 mg daily may be substituted for RIF for patients at high risk of drug interactions.
- Pregnant women, alcoholics, and patients with poor diets who are treated with INH should receive pyridoxine, 10 to 50 mg daily, to reduce the incidence of CNS effects or peripheral neuropathies.

ACTIVE DISEASE

- The standard TB treatment regimen **INH, RIF, Pyrazinamide, and Ethambutol** for 2 months followed by INH and RIF for 4 months.
- Appropriate samples should be sent for culture and susceptibility testing prior to initiating therapy for all patients with active TB. This data should guide the initial drug selection for the new patient. If susceptibility data are not available, the drug resistance pattern in the area where the patient likely acquired TB should be used.
- If the patient is being evaluated for the retreatment of TB, it is imperative to know what drugs were used previously and for how long.
- Patients must complete 6 months or more of treatment. HIV-positive patients should be treated for an additional 3 months and at least 6 months from the time that they

Table 67.1

Properties of first-line anti-TB agents

Agent	Description	Adverse effects
Isoniazid	Highly active against replicating but not dormant or near-dormant tubercle bacilli. No cross-resistance with other anti-TB agents. Converted to an inactive form by acetylation, the rate of which is genetically determined; people are either rapid or slow acetylators. The rate of acetylation does not affect the efficiency of standard short-course-anti-TB therapy but slow acetylators are more prone to adverse drug reactions and interactions.	Uncommon and mostly involve the nervous system, manifesting as restlessness, insomnia, muscle twitching and psychiatric disorders. Risk is greatly reduced by prescription of pyridoxine) vitamin B_6) at 10 mg/day. Occasionally causes hypersensitivity skin reactions, notably in patients with disease caused by HIV.
Rifampicin (rifampin)	A member of the rifamycin group of antibiotics and the most powerful anti-TB agent currently available; effective concentrations are obtained in all tissues. No cross resistance with other anti-TB agents, except for other rifamycins. Its red colour is imparted to urine, tears and sweat.	Include mild itching and erythema (usually self-limiting), gastrointestinal upsets and impaired liver function in alcoholics and those with liver diseases. A few patients develop the "flu syndrome", with fever, chills, headache, and bone pain and, rarely, a mild thrombocytopenic purpura. The flu syndrome occurs more often into hose on intermittent than on daily treatment. Rate serious complications, also more frequent in those on intermittent therapy, include respiratory collapse, low platelet counts leading to purpura and hemorrhages, hemolytic anemia and renal failure.
Ethambutol	Active during the early, intensive, phase of treatment and may enhance the activity of other anti-TB agents by increasing the permeability of the mycobacterial cell wall.	Include peripheral neuritis, joint pain, low platelet counts, jaundice and optic neuritis. The latter is very uncommon (especially if the maximum recommended dose is not exceeded and the drug is only given in the 2-month intensive phase), but is very serious as it may cause irreversible blindness. National codes of practice for detection and prevention of this adverse effect should therefore be strictly adhered .
Pyrazinamide	Active against tubercle bacilli in acidic inflammatory lesions but not in the neutral or slightly alkaline cavity wall.	Uncommon and include gastro-intestinal upsets and anorexia, photosensitization of the skin, arthralgia and gout. Hepatic toxicity is rare, except in patients with pre-existing liver disease.
Streptomycin	A member of the aminoglyco-side group of antibiotics. In contrast to Pyrazinamide, it is active in neutral or alkaline conditions. It must be given by intramuscular injection, with the risk of transmission of HIV and other viruses	Include renal and inner ear damage the latter leading to vertigo and deafness which may be permanent if treatment is not stopped.

Table 67.2

Properties of second-line anti-TB[a] agents

Agent	Description	Adverse effects
Fluoroquinolones	Include ofloxacin, moxifloxacin, gatifloxacin and levofloxacin, which are being evaluated for the treatment of drug resistant TB.	
Ethionamide and prothionamide	Closely related to each other and also to Isoniazid, although there is no cross-resistance with the latter. They are weak drugs and the bacteriostatic rather than bactericidal agents.	Distressing gastric irritation is common
Other aminoglycoside, e.g. kanamycin and amikacin		Like streptomycin, they are given by intramuscular injection and they have similar adverse effects.
Capreomycin and viomycin	Of restricted availability and rarely used. Although unrelated structurally to the amino-glycoside, partial Cross-resistance occurs.	Must be given by intramuscular injection and their adverse effects are similar to those of the aminoglycoside.
para-Aminosalicylic acid (PAS)	of limited availability and very rarely used nowadays. Has only limited bacteriostatic activity.	Gastrointestinal upsets are common.
Thiacetazone	A weak drug that should be dropped from the list of agents used to treat TB.	A cause of an unacceptably high incidence of severe and life-threatening skin reactions, particularly in those with disease caused by HIV.
Cycloserine	A weak bacteriostatic drug.	Use is limited by the high incidence of neurological and psychiatric adverse effects including headache, dizziness, depression and confusion.
Other agents	Other members of the rifamycin group of antibiotics, notably rifabutin and rifapentine, are used as alternatives to rifampicin under some circum-stances. Rifabutin is used as an alternative to rifampicin in HIV-infected patients receiving antiretroviral therapy, as adverse drug interactions are less frequent. Other agents, with some evidence of efficacy, induce newer Macrolides, (azithromycin, Clarithromycin, the antileprosy drug clofazimine (Lamprene) and β-Lactam/ β-Lactam inhibitors.	

Table 67.3

Dosages of first-line anti-TB agents

Drugs	Daily doses (mg/kg)	Route	Thrice weekly Dosage (mg/kg/dose)
Isoniazid (H)	5 (4-6)	Oral	10 (8-12)
Rifampin (R)	10 (8-12)	Oral	10 (8-12)
Ethambutol (E)	15 (15-20)	Oral	30 (25-35)
Pyrazinamide (Z)	25 (25-30)	Oral	35 (30-40)
Streptomycin (S)	15 (12-18)	Oral	15 (12-18)

Table 67.4

Dosages of second-line anti-TB agents

Drugs	Daily doses (mg/kg)	Route	Maximum daily dose
Kanamycin (K)	15	IM	Up to 1 g
Amikacin (A)	15	IM	Up to 1 g
Ethionamide (Eto)	10-15	Oral	Up to 1 g
Cycloserine (Cs)	10	Oral	Up to 1 g
Para amino salicylic acid (PAS)	250	Oral	Up to 1 g
Ofloxaxin (Ofx)	15-20	Oral	800-10000 mg
Levofloxacin	7.5-10	Oral	750-1000 mg
Moxifloxacin	7.5-10	Oral	400 mg

convert to smear and culture negativity. When INH and RIF cannot be used, treatment duration becomes 2 years or more, regardless of immune status.

- Patients who are slow to respond, those who remain culture positive at 2 months of treatment, those with cavitary lesions on chest radiograph, and HIV-positive patients should be treated for 9 months and for at least 6 months from the time they convert to smear and culture negativity.

DRUG RESISTANCE

- If the organism is drug resistant, the aim is to introduce two or more active agents that the patient has not received previously. With MDR-TB, no standard regimen can be proposed. It is critical to avoid monotherapy or adding only a single drug to a failing regimen.
- Drug resistance should be suspected in the following situations:
  - ✓ Patients who have received prior therapy for TB
  - ✓ Patients from geographic areas with a high prevalence of resistance (New York City, Mexico, Southeast Asia, the Baltic countries, and the former Soviet states
  - ✓ Patients who are homeless, institutionalized, IV drug abusers, and/or infected with HIV

- ✓ Patients who still have acid-fast bacilli–positive sputum smears after 2 months of therapy
- ✓ Patients who still have positive cultures after 2 to 4 months of therapy
- ✓ Patients who fail therapy or relapse after retreatment
- ✓ Patients known to be exposed to MDR-TB cases

SPECIAL POPULATIONS

Tuberculous meningitis and extra pulmonary disease

- In general, **INH, Pyrazinamide, Ethionamide,** and **Cycloserine** penetrate the cerebrospinal fluid readily. Patients with CNS TB are often treated for longer periods (9 to 12 months). Extra pulmonary TB of the soft tissues can be treated with conventional regimens. TB of the bone is typically treated for 9 months, occasionally with surgical debridement.

CHILDREN

- TB in children may be treated with regimens similar to those used in adults, although some physicians still prefer to extend treatment to 9 months. Pediatric doses of drugs should be used.

PREGNANT WOMEN

- The usual treatment of pregnant women is INH, RIF, and Ethambutol for 9 months.
- Women with TB should be cautioned against becoming pregnant, as the disease poses a risk to the fetus as well as to the mother. INH or Ethambutol are relatively safe when used during pregnancy. Supplementation with B vitamins is particularly important during pregnancy. **RIF** has been rarely associated with birth defects, but those seen are occasionally severe, including limb reduction and CNS lesions. **Pyrazinamide** has not been studied in a large number of pregnant women, but anecdotal information suggests that it may be safe. **Ethionamide** may be associated with premature delivery, congenital deformities, and Down's syndrome when used during pregnancy. **Streptomycin** has been associated with hearing impairment in the newborn, including complete deafness. **Cycloserine** is not recommended during pregnancy.

RENAL FAILURE

- In nearly all patients, INH and RIF do not require dose modifications in renal failure. Pyrazinamide and Ethambutol typically require a reduction in dosing frequency from daily to three times weekly.

DOTS THERAPY

DOTS stands for "Directly Observed Treatment, Short-course" and is a major plank in the WHO Global Plan to Stop TB. The DOTS strategy focuses on five main points of action. These include government commitment to control TB, diagnosis based on sputum-smear microscopy tests done on patients who actively report TB symptoms, direct observation short-course chemotherapy treatments, a definite supply of drugs, and standardized reporting and recording of cases and treatment outcomes.

The WHO advises that all TB patients should have at least the first two months of their therapy observed (and preferably the whole of it observed): this means an independent observer watching patients swallow their anti-TB therapy. The independent observer is often not a healthcare worker and may be a shopkeeper or a tribal elder or similar senior person within that society.

The WHO extended the DOTS programme in 1998 to include the treatment of MDR-TB (called "DOTS-Plus"). Implementation of DOTS-Plus requires the capacity to perform drug-susceptibility testing (not routinely available even in developed countries) and the availability of second-line agents, in addition to all the requirements for DOTS. DOTS-Plus is therefore much more resource-expensive than DOTS, and requires much greater commitment from countries wishing to implement it. Resource limitations mean that the implementation of DOTS-Plus may lead inadvertently to the diversion of resources from existing DOTS programmes and a consequent decrease in the overall standard of care.

Bacillus Calmette-Guérin (or **Bacille Calmette-Guérin, BCG**) is a vaccine against tuberculosis that is prepared from a strain of the attenuated (weakened) live bovine tuberculosis bacillus, *Mycobacterium bovis*, that has lost its virulence in humans by being specially sub cultured (230 passages) in an artificial medium for 13 years, and also prepared from *Mycobacterium tuberculosis*. The bacilli have retained enough strong antigenicity to become a somewhat effective vaccine for the prevention of human tuberculosis. At best, the BCG vaccine is 80% effective in preventing tuberculosis for duration of 15 years; however, its protective effect appears to vary according to geography.

Except in neonates, a tuberculin skin test should always be done before administering BCG. A reactive tuberculin skin test is a contraindication to BCG. Someone with a positive tuberculin reaction is not given BCG, because there is a high risk of severe local inflammation and scarring, not because of the common misconception that tuberculin reactors "are already immune" and therefore do not need BCG.

BCG is given as a single intradermal injection at the insertion of the deltoid. If BCG is accidentally given subcutaneously, then a local abscess may form (a BCG-oma) that can sometimes ulcerate, and may require treatment with antibiotics. However, it is important to note an abscess is not always associated with incorrect administration, and it is one of the more common complications that can occur with the vaccination.

REFERENCES

1. Ellner JJ. Tuberculosis. In: Goldman L, Schafer AI, eds.*Cecil Medicine*. 24th ed.Philadelphia,PA: Saunders Elsevier; 2011:chap 332.
2. Fitzgerald DW, Sterling TR, Haas DW. *Mycobacterium tuberculosis*. In: Mandell GL, Bennett JE, Dolan R, eds. *Mandell, Douglas, and Bennett's Principles and Practice of Infectious Diseases*. 7th ed. Orlando, FL: Saunders Elsevier; 2009:chap 250.
3. Konstantinos A (2010). "Testing for tuberculosis". *Australian Prescriber* **33** (1): 12–18.
4. World Health Organization (2009). "Epidemiology". *Global tuberculosis control: epidemiology, strategy, financing*. pp. 6–33. ISBN 9789241563802. Retrieved 12 November 2009.

5. Schiffman G (15 January 2009). "Tuberculosis Symptoms". eMedicine Health.
6. Behera, D. (2010). *Textbook of pulmonary medicine* (2nd ed. ed.). New Delhi: Jaypee Brothers Medical Pub.. pp. 457. ISBN 9788184487497.
7. Jindal, editor-in-chief SK. *Textbook of pulmonary and critical care medicine*. New Delhi: Jaypee Brothers Medical Publishers. pp. 549. ISBN 97893502 50730.
8. American Thoracic Society (1997). "Diagnosis and treatment of disease caused by non tuberculous mycobacteria. This official statement of the American Thoracic Society was approved by the Board of Directors, March 1997. Medical Section of the American Lung Association". *Am J Respir Crit Care Med* **156** (2 Pt 2): S1–25. PMID 9279284.
9. Bonah C (2005). "The 'experimental stable' of the BCG vaccine: safety, efficacy, proof, and standards, 1921–1933". *Stud Hist Philos Biol Biomed Sci* **36** (4): 696–721.

CHAPTER 68

HIV Infection

DEFINITION

Acquired immune deficiency syndrome or **acquired immunodeficiency syndrome** (**AIDS**) is a disease of the human immune system caused by the human immunodeficiency virus (HIV).

PREVALENCE

AIDS is the sixth leading cause of death among people ages 25 - 44 in the United States, down from number one in 1995. The World Health Organization estimates that more than 25 million people worldwide have died from this infection since the start of the epidemic. In 2008, there were approximately 33.4 million people around the world living with HIV/AIDS, including 2.1 million children under age 15.

ETIOLOGY

Human immunodeficiency virus (HIV) causes AIDS. The virus attacks the immune system and leaves the body vulnerable to a variety of life-threatening infections and cancers.

Common bacteria, yeast, parasites, and viruses that usually do not cause serious disease in people with healthy immune systems can cause fatal illnesses in people with AIDS.

HIV has been found in saliva, tears, nervous system tissue and spinal fluid, blood, semen (including pre-seminal fluid, which is the liquid that comes out before ejaculation), vaginal fluid, and breast milk. However, only blood, semen, vaginal secretions, and breast milk have been shown to transmit infection to others.

The virus can be spread (transmitted):

- Through sexual contact including oral, vaginal, and anal sex
- Through blood — via blood transfusions (now extremely rare in the U.S.) or needle sharing
- From mother to child — a pregnant woman can transmit the virus to her fetus through their shared blood circulation, or a nursing mother can transmit it to her baby in her breast milk

Other methods of spreading the virus are rare and include accidental needle injury, artificial insemination with infected donated semen, and organ transplantation with infected organs.

HIV infection is NOT spread by:

- Casual contact such as hugging
- Mosquitoes
- Participation in sports
- Touching items that were touched by a person infected with the virus

AIDS and blood or organ donation:

- AIDS is NOT transmitted to a person who DONATES blood or organs. People who donate organs are never in direct contact with people who receive them. Likewise, a person who donates blood is never in contact with the person receiving it. In all these procedures, sterile needles and instruments are used.
- However, HIV can be transmitted to a person RECEIVING blood or organs from an infected donor. To reduce this risk, blood banks and organ donor programs screen donors, blood, and tissues thoroughly.

People at highest risk for getting HIV include:

- Injection drug users who share needles
- Infants born to mothers with HIV who didn't receive HIV therapy during pregnancy
- People engaging in unprotected sex, especially with people who have other high-risk behaviors, are HIV-positive, or have AIDS
- People who received blood transfusions or clotting products between 1977 and 1985 (before screening for the virus became standard practice)
- Sexual partners of those who participate in high-risk activities (such as injection drug use or anal sex)

CLINICAL FEATURES

AIDS begins with HIV infection. People who are infected with HIV may have no symptoms for 10 years or longer, but they can still transmit the infection to others during this symptom-free period. If the infection is not detected and treated, the immune system gradually weakens and AIDS develops.

Acute HIV infection progresses over time (usually a few weeks to months) to asymptomatic HIV infection (no symptoms) and then to early symptomatic HIV infection. Later, it progresses to AIDS (advanced HIV infection with CD4 T-cell count below 200 cells/mm^3).

Almost all people infected with HIV, if they are not treated, will develop AIDS. There is a small group of patients who develop AIDS very slowly, or never at all. These patients are called nonprogressors, and many seem to have a genetic difference that prevents the virus from significantly damaging their immune system.

The symptoms of AIDS are mainly the result of infections that do not normally develop in people with a healthy immune system. These are called opportunistic infections.

People with AIDS have had their immune system damaged by HIV and are very susceptible to these opportunistic infections. Common symptoms are:

- Chills
- Fever
- Sweats (particularly at night)
- Swollen lymph glands
- Weakness
- Weight loss

DIAGNOSIS

CD4 cells are a type of T cell. T cells are cells of the immune system. They are also called "helper cells."

The following is a list of AIDS-related infections and cancers that people with AIDS may get as their CD4 count decreases. In the past, having AIDS was defined as having HIV infection and getting one of these other diseases. Today, according to the Centers for Disease Control and Prevention, a person may also be diagnosed with AIDS if they are HIV-positive and have a CD4 cell count below 200 cells/mm^3, even if they don't have an opportunistic infection.

AIDS may also be diagnosed if a person develops one of the opportunistic infections and cancers that occur more commonly in people with HIV infection. These infections are unusual in people with a healthy immune system.

Many other illnesses and their symptoms may develop, in addition to those listed here.

The following illnesses are common with a CD4 count below 350 cells/mm^3:

- Herpes simplex virus — causes ulcers/ small blisters in the mouth or genitals, happens more often and usually much more severely in an HIV-infected person than in someone without HIV infection
- Herpes zoster (shingles) — ulcers/small blisters over a patch of skin, caused by reactivation of the varicella zoster virus, the same virus that causes chickenpox
- Kaposi's sarcoma — cancer of the skin, lungs, and bowel due to a herpes virus (HHV-8). It can happen at any CD4 count, but is more likely to happen at lower CD4 counts, and is more common in men than in women.
- Non-Hodgkin's lymphoma — cancer of the lymph nodes
- Oral or vaginal thrush — yeast (typically *Candida albicans*) infection of the mouth or vagina
- Tuberculosis — infection by tuberculosis bacteria mostly affects the lungs, but can also affect Other organs such as the bowel, lining of the heart or lungs, brain, or lining of the central nervous system (brain and spinal cord)

Common with CD4 count below 200 cells/mm^3:

- Bacillary angiomatosis — skin sores caused by a bacteria called *Bartonella,* which may be caused by cat scratches
- Candida esophagitis — painful yeast infection of the esophagus
- *Pneumocystis jiroveci pneumonia*, "PCP pneumonia," previously called *Pneumocystis carinii* pneumonia, caused by a fungus

Common with CD4 count below 100 cells/mm^3:

- AIDS dementia — worsening and slowing of mental function, caused by HIV
- Cryptococcal meningitis — fungal infection of the lining of the brain
- Cryptosporidium diarrhea — Extreme diarrhea caused by a parasite that affects the gastrointestinal tract
- Progressive multifocal leukoencephalopathy — a disease of the brain caused by a virus (called the JC virus) that results in a severe decline in mental and physical functions
- Toxoplasma encephalitis — infection of the brain by a parasite, called *Toxoplasma gondii*, which is often found in cat feces; causes lesions (sores) in the brain
- Wasting syndrome — extreme weight loss and loss of appetite, caused by HIV itself

Common with CD4 count below 50/mm^3:

- Cytomegalovirus infection — a viral infection that can affect almost any organ system, especially the large bowel and the eyes
- Mycobacterium avium — a blood infection by a bacterium related to tuberculosis

In addition to the CD4 count, a test called HIV RNA level (or viral load) may be used to monitor patients. Basic screening lab tests and regular cervical Pap smears are important to monitor in HIV infection, due to the increased risk of cervical cancer in women with a compromised immune system. Anal Pap smears to detect potential cancers may also be important in both HIV-infected men and women.

TREATMENT

GENERAL APPROACH TO TREATMENT OF HUMAN IMMUNODEFICIENCY VIRUS INFECTION

- Regular, periodic measurement of plasma HIV RNA levels and CD4 cell counts is necessary to determine the risk of disease progression in an HIV infected individual and to determine when to initiate or modify antiretroviral treatment regimens.
- Treatment decisions should be individualized by level of risk indicated by plasma HIV RNA levels and CD4 counts.
- The use of potent combination antiretroviral therapy to suppress HIV replication to below the levels of detection of sensitive plasma HIV RNA assays limits the potential for selection of antiretroviral-resistant HIV variants, the major factor limiting the ability of antiretroviral drugs to inhibit virus replication and delay disease progression.
- The most effective means to accomplish durable suppression of HIV replication is the simultaneous initiation of combinations of effective anti- HIV drugs with which the patient has not been previously treated and that are not cross resistant with antiretroviral agents with which the patient has been treated previously.
- Each of the antiretroviral drugs used in combination therapy regimens should always be used according to optimum schedules and dosages.
- Women should receive optimal antiretroviral therapy regardless of pregnancy status.
- The same principles of antiretroviral therapy apply to both HIV infected children and adults, although the treatment of HIV-infected children involves unique pharmacologic, virologic, and immunologic considerations.
- Persons with acute primary HIV infections should be treated with combination antiretroviral therapy to suppress virus replication to levels below the limit of detection of sensitive plasma HIV RNA assays.
- HIV-infected persons, even those with viral loads below detectable limits, should be considered infectious and should be counseled to avoid sexual and drug-use behaviors that are associated with transmission or acquisition of HIV and other infectious pathogens.
- Treatment is recommended for all HIV-infected persons with an AIDS defining event, symptomatic disease, or a CD4 lymphocyte count below 200 cells/mm^3 should be offered therapy. Treatment is generally not recommended in persons with CD4 counts above 350 cells/mm^3.

Those between 201 and 350 cells/mm^3 should be offered therapy

PHARMACOLOGICAL THERAPY

ANTIRETROVIRAL AGENTS

- Inhibiting viral replication with combination of potent antiretroviral therapy has been the most clinically successful strategy in the treatment of HIV infection. There have been three primary groups of drugs used: **Nucleoside and Non-nucleoside reverse transcriptase inhibitors** and **protease inhibitors** (PIs) (Table 68.1).
- Reverse transcriptase inhibitors are of two types: those that are derivatives of purine- and pyrimidine-based nucleosides and nucleotides (NtRTIs) and those that are not nucleoside or nucleotide based (NNRTIs).
- Current recommendations for treating HIV infection advocate a minimum of three antiretroviral agents. The typical regimen consists of two NtRTIs and either a ritonavir-boosted PI or NNRTI. The dual NtRTI backbone should include tenofovir plus emtricitabine (co-formulated as Truvada) or Zidovudine plus Lamivudine (co-formulated as Combivir). Abacavir plus lamivudine is an alternative. Recommended initial NtRTIs include Atazanavir- Ritonavir, Lopinavir-Ritonavir, or Fosamprenavir-Ritonavir. Efavirenz is the recommended NNRTI except for women who plan to become pregnant or who do not have adequate contraception.
- Significant drug interactions can occur with many antiretroviral agents:

✓ The latest information on drug interactions of antiretroviral drugs should be consulted.

✓ **Ritonavir** is a potent inhibitor of cytochrome P450 enzyme 3A and is used to reduce clearance of other PIs.

✓ Two NtRTIs, **Zidovudine** and **Stavudine**, antagonize each other's metabolism and should not be given together.

✓ Rifampin may substantially reduce the concentrations of PIs and is contraindicated with use of most PIs.

✓ Saint John's wort is a potent inducer of metabolism and is contraindicated with PIs and NNRTIs.

TREATMENT DURING PREGNANCY

- Therapy during pregnancy is warranted, particularly in light of the dramatic reduction in transmission seen with **Zidovudine** monotherapy. In general, pregnant women should be treated similar to nonpregnant adults; if possible, Zidovudine should be used for both mother and infant. Efavirenz should not be used, particularly in the first trimester, because of the risk of teratogenicity.

POST EXPOSURE PROPHYLAXIS

- Post exposure prophylaxis with a triple-drug regimen consisting of two NtRTIs and a boosted-PI is recommended for percutaneous blood exposure involving significant risk (i.e., large-bore needle or large volume of blood or blood from patients with advanced AIDS).
- Two NtRTIs may be offered to healthcare workers with lower risk of exposure such as that involving either the mucous membrane or skin. Treatment is not necessary if the source of exposure is urine or saliva.

Table 68.1

Highly active antiretroviral therapy medications, adult dosage and side effects

Medication	Adult dosage	Side effect and toxicities
Lopinavir/ritonavir (Kaletra)	3 tablets twice daily 400mg lopinavir/100mg ritonavir	Diarrhea, nausea, vomiting; asthenia; elevated transaminases; hyperglycemia; fat redistribution; lipid abnormalities; possible increased bleeding in persons with hemophilia; and pancreatitis
Zidovudine/lamivudine (Combivir)	1 tablet twice daily. 300mg Zidovudine/150 mg lamivudine	See following individual medications
Zidovudine/lamivudine (Combivir)/abacavir (Trizivir)	1 tablet twice daily 300mg Zidovudine/150 mg lamivudine/ 300 mg abacavir	See following individual medications
Lamivudine/abacavir (Epzicom)	1 tablet once daily 300 mg lamivudine/600 mg abacavir	See following individual medications
Emtricitabine/tenofovir (Truvada)	1 tablet once daily 200 mg emtricitabine/300 mg tenofovir	See following individual medications
Nucleoside and nucleotide reverse transcriptase inhibitors (side effects as a class: lactic acidosis, severe hepatomegaly with steatosis, including some fatal cases)		
Abacavir (Ziagen, ABC)	300 mg twice daily or 600 mg once daily	Severe hypersensitivity reactions (can be fatal); nausea; and vomiting
Didanosine (Videx, ddl)	>60 kg (132lb) body weight; 200mg twice daily or 400 mg daily; if with tenofovir, 250 mg/daily. <60kg (132lb): 125mg twice daily or 250 mg daily: if with tenofovir, dose not established. Do not use with Stavudine (Zerit) during pregnancy; avoid ddl/d4T combination in general because of increased risk for adverse events (e.g., neuropathy, pancreatitis).	Pancreatitis; nausea, diarrhea; and peripheral neuropathy
Emtricitabine (Emtriva, FTC)	200 mg once daily	Minimal toxicity; lactic acidosis and hepatic steatosis a rare but possible life threatening event
Lamivudine (Epivir, 3TC)	150 mg twice daily or 300 mg once daily	Minimal toxicity; lactic acidosis and hepatic steatosis a rare but possible life threatening event

Table 68.1 *Contd...*

Medication	Adult dosage	Side effect and toxicities
Stavudine (Zerit, d4T)	>60 kg (132 lb) body weight; 40 mg twice daily <60kg (132lb) body weight 30 mg twice daily. Do not use with didanosine (ddl, Videx) during pregnancy; avoid ddl d4T combination in general because of increased risk for adverse events (e.g., neuropathy, pancreatitis, and hyperiactatemia)	Pancreatitis; nausea, diarrhea; and peripheral neuropathy; rapidly progressive ascending neuromuscular weakness (rare)
Tenofovir (Viread)	300 mg daily	Nausea, vomiting, diarrhea; headache; asthenia; flatulence; and renal impairment
Zidovudine (Retrovir, AZT)	200 mg three times daily or 300 mg twice daily	Bone marrow suppression (anemia, neutropenia); gastrointestinal intolerance; headache; insomnia; asthenia; and myopathy
Non-nucleoside reverse transcriptase Inhibitors (Side effects as a class: Stevens-Johnson syndrome)		
Efavirenz (Sustiva)	600 mg daily at bedtime. Do not use during known or possible pregnancy	Rash; central nervous system symptoms (e.g., dizziness, impaired concentration, insomnia, and abnormal dreams); transaminase elevation; and false positive cannabinoid test.
Protease inhibitors (Side effects as a class: gastrointestinal intolerance, hyperlipidemia, hyperglycemia, diabetes, fat redistribution, and possible increased bleeding in hemophiliacs)		
Atazanavir (Reyataz)	400 mg once daily; if administered with tenofovir plus ritonavir, 300 mg once daily	Indirect hyperbilirubinemia; prolonged PR interval (use caution in patients with underlying cardiac conduction defects or on concomitant medications that can cause PR prolongation)
Fosamprenavir (Lexiva)	1,400 mg twice daily	Gastrointestinal intolerance, nausea, vomiting, diarrhea; rash; elevated transaminases; and headache
Indinavir (Crixivan)	800 mg every 8 hours. Without ritonavir (might increase risk for renal adverse events): 800 mg indinavir and 100 mg ritonavir every 12 hours or 800 mg indinavir and 200 mg ritonavir every 12 hours	Gastrointestinal intolerance, nausea; nephrolithiasis; headache; asthenia; blurred vision; metallic taste; thrombocytopenia; hemolytic anemia; and indirect hyperbilirubinemia

Table 68.1 *Contd...*

Medication	Adult dosage	Side effect and toxicities
Nelfinavir (Viracept)	750 mg three times daily or 1,250 mg twice daily	Diarrhea; and elevated transaminases
Ritonavir (Norvir)	See doses used in combination with other specific protease inhibitors	Gastrointestinal intolerance; nausea, vomiting, diarrhea; paresthesias; hepatitis; pancreatitis; asthenia; and taste perversion; many drug interactions
Saquinavir (hard-gel capsule) (Invirase)	With ritonavir: 400mg saquinavir and 400 mg ritonavir twice daily or 1,000 mg saquinavir and 100 mg ritonavir twice daily	Gastrointestinal intolerance; nausea, diarrhea; headache;; and elevated transaminases
Saquinavir (soft-gel capsule) (Fortavase)	With ritonavir: 400mg saquinavir and 400 mg ritonavir twice daily or 1,000 mg saquinavir and 100 mg ritonavir twice daily	Gastrointestinal intolerance; nausea, diarrhea; headache; abdominal pain; dyspepsia; headache; and elevated transaminases.

REFERENCES

1. Del Rio C, Curran JW. Epidemiology and prevention of acquired immunodeficiency syndrome and human immunodeficiency virus infection. In: Mandell GL, Bennett JE, Dolin R, eds. *Principles and Practice of Infectious Diseases*. 7th ed. Philadelphia, Pa: Elsevier Churchill Livingstone; 2009:chap 118.
2. Piot P. Human immunodeficiency virus infection and acquired immunodeficiency syndrome: A global overview. In: Goldman L, Ausiello D, eds. *Cecil Medicine*. 23rd ed. Philadlelphia, Pa: Saunders Elsevier; 2007:chap 407.
3. Sterling TR, Chaisson RE. General clinical manifestations of human immunodeficiency virus infection (including the acute retroviral syndrome and oral, cutaneous, renal, ocular, metabolic, and cardiac diseases). In: Mandell GL, Bennett JE, Dolin R, eds. *Principles and Practice of Infectious Diseases*. 7th ed. Philadelphia, Pa: Elsevier Churchill Livingstone; 2009: chap 121.

CHAPTER 69

GI Infection

INTRODUCTION

GI infections are among the more common causes of morbidity and mortality around the world. Most are caused by viruses, and some are caused by bacteria or other organisms. In underdeveloped and developing countries, acute gastroenteritis involving diarrhea is the leading cause of mortality in infants and children younger than 5 years of age. In the United States, there are approximately 211 million episodes of acute gastroenteritis each year, causing over 900,000 hospitalizations and over 6,000 deaths.

REHYDRATION THERAPY

- Fluid replacement is the cornerstone of therapy for diarrohea regardless of etiology.
- Initial assessment of fluid loss is essential for rehydration. Weight loss is the most reliable means of determining the extent of water loss. Clinical signs such as changes in skin turgor, sunken eyes, dry mucous membranes, decreased tearing, decreased urine output, altered mentation, and changes in vital signs can be helpful in determining approximate deficits (Table 69.1).
- The necessary components of oral rehydration therapy (ORT) solutions include glucose, sodium, potassium, chloride, and water (Table 69.2).
- The maintenance phase should not exceed 100 to 150 mL/kg/day and is generally adjusted to equal stool losses.
- Weight loss of 9% to 10% is considered severe and requires IV fluid replacement with Ringer's lactate or 0.9% sodium chloride. IV therapy is also indicated in patients with uncontrolled vomiting, the presence of paralytic ileus, stool output greater than 10 mL/kg/hour, shock, or loss of consciousness.
- Early refeeding as tolerated is recommended. Age-appropriate diet may be resumed as soon as dehydration is corrected. Early initiation of feeding shortens the course of diarrhea. Initially, easily digested foods, such as bananas, applesauce, and cereal, may be added as tolerated. Foods high in fiber, sodium, and sugar should be avoided.

Table 69.1

Clinical assessment of degree of dehydration in children based on percentage of body weight loss[a]

Variable	Mild, 3–5%	Moderate, 6–9%	Severe, ≥10%
Blood pressure	Normal	Normal	Normal to reduced
Quality of Pulses	Normal	Normal or slightly decreased	Moderately decreased
Heart rate	Normal		
Skin turgor	Normal	Increased	Increased (bradycardia in severe cases)
Fontanelle	Normal		
Mucous membranes	Slightly dry	Decreased	Decreased
Eyes		Sunken	Sunken
Extremities	Normal	Dry	Dry
Mental status	Warm, normal capillary refill	Sunken orbits/ decreased tears	Deeply sunken orbits/decreased tears
Urine output	Normal	Delayed capillary refill	Cool, mottled
Thirst	Slightly decreased	Normal to listless	Normal to lethargic or comatose<1 mL/kg/hour Very thirsty or too lethargic to indicate
Fluid replacement	Slightly increased	<1 mL/kg/hour	Ringer's lactate 40 mL/kg in 15–30 minutes, then 20–40 mL/kg if skin turgor, alertness, and pulse have not returned to normal or Ringer's lactate or normal saline 20 mL/kg, repeat if necessary, and then replace water and electrolyte deficits over 1–2 days
	ORT 50 mL/kg over 2–4 hours Replace ongoing losses with low sodium ORT (40–60 mEq/L Na+) at 10 mL/kg per stool or emesis	Moderately increased ORT 100 mL/kg over 2–4 hours Replace ongoing losses with low sodium ORT (40–60 mEq/L Na+) at 10 mL/kg per stool or emesis	

Table 69.2

Comparison of common solutions used in oral rehydration and maintenance

Product	Na (mEq/L)	K (mEq/L)	Base (mEq/L)	Carbohydrate (mmol/L)	Osmolality (mOsm/L)
Naturalyte (unlimited beverage)	45	20	48	140	265
Pediatric electrolyte	45	20	30	140	250
(NutraMax)	45	20	30	140	250
Pedialyte (Ross)	50	25	30	70	200
Infalyte (formerly Ricelyte; Mead Johnson)	75	20	30	140	310
Rehydralyte (Ross)	90	20	30	111	310
World Health Organization/ United Nations Children's Fund oral rehydration salts	2	0	13	700	750
Cola	5	32	0	690	700
Apple juice	250	8	0	0	500
Chicken broth	20	3	3	255	330
Sports beverage					

BACTERIAL INFECTIONS

- The bacterial species most commonly associated with GI infection and infectious diarrhea in the United States are *Shigella* spp., *Salmonella* spp., *Campylobacter* spp., *Yersinia* spp., *Escherichia* spp., *Clostridium* spp., and *Staphylococcus* spp.
- Antibiotics are not essential in the treatment of most mild diarrheas, and empirical therapy for acute GI infections may result in unnecessary antibiotic courses. Antibiotic choices for bacterial infections are given in Table 69.3.

Table 69.3

Recommendations for antibiotic therapy

Pathogen	First-Line Agents	Alternative Agents
Enterotoxigenic (cholera-like) diarrhea Vibrio cholera O1 or O139	Doxycycline 300 mg oral single dose; tetracycline 500 mg orally four times daily × 3 days; or trimethoprim-sulfamethoxazole DS tablet twice daily × 3 days; norfloxacin 400 mg orally twice daily × 3 days; or ciprofloxacin 500 mg orally twice daily × 3 days or 1 g orally single dose	Chloramphenicol 50 mg/kg IV every 6 hours, erythromycin 250–500 mg orally every 6–8 hours, and furazolidone
Enterotoxigenic Esche-richia col	Norfloxacin 400 mg or ciprofloxacin 500 mg orally twice daily × 3 days	Trimethoprim–sulfamethoxazole DS tablet every 12 hours
Clostridium difficile	Metronidazole 250 mg four times daily to 500 mg three times daily × 10 days	Vancomycin 125 mg orally four times daily × 10 days; bacitracin 20,000–25,000 units four times daily × 7–10 days

Table 69.3 *Contd...*

Pathogen	First-Line Agents	Alternative Agents
Invasive (dysentery-like) diarrhea Shigella species[a]	Trimethoprim–sulfamethoxazole DS twice daily × 3–5 days	Ofloxacin 300 mg, norfloxacin 400 mg, or ciprofloxacin 500 mg twice daily × 3 days, or nalidixic acid 1 g/day 5 days; azithromycin 500 mg orally × 1 day, then 250 mg orally daily × 4 days
Salmonella Nontyphoidal[a]	Trimethoprim–sulfamethoxazole DS twice daily; ofloxacin 300 mg, norfloxacin 400 mg, or	Azithromycin 1,000 mg orally 1 day, followed by 500 mg orally once daily × 6 days
Enteric fever	Ciprofloxacin 500 mg twice daily × 5 days or Ceftriaxone 2 g IV daily or Cefotaxime 2 g IV three times daily × 5 days	Azithromycin 1,000 mg orally × 1 day, followed by 500 mg daily × 5 days; or cefixime, cefotaxime, and cefuroxime; or chloramphenicol 500 mg four times daily orally or IV × 14 days.
Campylobacter[a]	Erythromycin 500 mg orally twice daily 5 days; Azithromycin 1,000 mg orally× 1 day, followed by 500 mg daily or Clarithromycin 500 mg orally twice daily	Ciprofloxacin 500 mg or norfloxacin 400 mg orally twice daily × 5 days
Yersinia species[a]	A combination therapy with Doxycycline, aminoglycosides, trimethoprim sulfame-thoxazole, or fluoroquinolones	
Traveler's diarrhea Prophylaxis[a]	Norfloxacin 400 mg or ciprofloxacin 500 mg orally daily (in Asia, Africa, and South America); trimethoprim–sulfamethoxazole DS tablet orally daily (in Mexico)	Rifaximin 200 mg one to three times daily × 2 weeks
Treatment	Norfloxacin 400 mg or Ciprofloxacin 500 mg orally twice daily × 3 days, or trimethoprim–sulfamethoxazole DS tablet orally twice daily × 3 days (in Mexico), or Azithromycin 500 mg orally once daily × 3 days (only in areas of high prevalence of quinolone-resistant Campylobacter species, such as Thailand)	Rifaximin 200 mg three times a day or 400 mg twice a day × 3 days

ENTEROTOXIGENIC (CHOLERA-LIKE) DIARRHEA

CHOLERA (VIBRIO CHOLERA)

Vibrio cholerae is the serogroup that most often causes human epidemics and pandemics. Four mechanisms for transmission have been proposed: Animal reservoirs, chronic carriers, asymptomatic or mild disease victims,or water reservoirs.

- Most pathology of cholera is thought to result from an enterotoxin that increases cyclic adenosine monophosphate–mediated secretion of chloride ion into the intestinal lumen, which results in isotonic secretion (primarily in the small intestine) exceeding the absorptive capacity of the intestinal tract (primarily the colon).

- The incubation period of *V. cholera* is 1 to 3 days.
- Cholera is characterized by a spectrum from the asymptomatic state to the most severe typical cholera syndrome. Patients may lose up to 1 L of isotonic fluid every hour. The onset of diarrhea is abrupt and is followed rapidly or sometimes preceded by vomiting. Fever occurs in less than 5% of patients. In the most severe state, this disease can progress to death in a matter of 2 to 4 hours if not treated.

TREATMENT

- The mainstay of treatment for cholera consists of fluid and electrolyte replacement with ORT to restore fluid and electrolyte losses. Rice-based rehydration formulations are the preferred ORT for cholera patients. In patients who cannot tolerate ORT, IV therapy with Ringer's lactate can be used.
- Antibiotics shorten the duration of diarrhea, decrease the volume of fluid lost, and shorten the duration of the carrier state (see Table 69.3). A single dose of oral doxycycline is the preferred agent. In children younger than 7 years of age, **trimethoprim–sulfamethoxazole, erythromycin, furazolidone** can be used. In areas of high tetracycline resistance, fluoroquinolones are effective.

ESCHERICHIA COLI

- *Escherichia coli* GI disease may be caused by enterotoxigenic (ETEC), enteroinvasive *E. coli*, enteropathogenic *E. Coli*, enteroadhesive, and enterohemorrhagic *E. Coli* . ETEC is now incriminated as being the most common cause of traveler's diarrhea.
- ETEC is capable of producing two plasmid-mediated enterotoxins: heat-labile toxin and heat-stable toxin. The net effect of either toxin on the mucosa is production of a cholera-like secretory diarrhea.
- Nausea and watery stools, with or without abdominal cramping, are characteristic of the disease caused by ETEC. Most ETEC diarrhea is typically abrupt in onset and resolves within 24 to 48 hours without complication.
- Most cases respond readily to ORT, and although antibiotic therapy is seldom necessary, prophylaxis has been shown to effectively prevent the development of ETEC diarrhea.
- Fluid and electrolyte replacement should be initiated at the onset of diarrhea.
- Antibiotics used for treatment are found in Table 69.3.
- Loperamide should not be used in patients with fever or dysentery.
- Effective prophylaxis of ETEC diarrhea can be accomplished with **doxycycline, trimethoprim–sulfamethoxazole,** or a **fluoroquinolone**, but this approach is not routinely recommended.

PSEUDOMEMBRANOUS COLITIS (*CLOSTRIDIUM DIFFICILE*)

- Pseudomembranous colitis (PMC) results from toxins produced by *Clostridium difficile*. It occurs most often in epidemic fashion and affects high risk groups such as the elderly, debilitated patients, cancer patients, surgical patients, any patient receiving antibiotics, patients with nasogastric tubes, or those who frequently use laxatives.
- PMC has been associated most often with broad-spectrum antimicrobials, including clindamycin, ampicillin, or third-generation cephalosporins.

- PMC may result in a spectrum of disease from mild diarrhea to enterocolitis. In colitis without pseudomembranes, patients present with malaise, abdominal pain, nausea, anorexia, watery diarrhea, low-grade fever, and leukocytosis. With pseudomembranes, there is more severe illness with severe abdominal pain, perfuse diarrhea, high fever, and marked leukocytosis. Symptoms can start a few days after the start of antibiotic therapy to several weeks after antibiotics have been stopped.
- Diagnosis is made by colonoscopic visualization of pseudomembranes, finding cytotoxins A or B in stools, or stool culture for *C. difficile*.
- Initial therapy of PMC should include discontinuation of the offending agent. The patient should be supported with fluid and electrolyte replacement.
- Both vancomycin and metronidazole are effective, but **metronidazole** 250 mg orally four times daily is the drug of choice. Oral **vancomycin**, 125 mg orally four times daily, is second-line therapy. It should be reserved for patients not responding to metronidazole, organisms resistant to metronidazole, patients allergic or intolerant to metronidazole, other treatments that include alcohol-containing solutions, patients who are pregnant or younger than 10 years, critically ill patients, or those with diarrhea that is caused by *Staphylococcus aureus*. Bacitracin is the third-line agent.
- Drugs that inhibit peristalsis, such as **diphenoxylate**, are contraindicated.
- Relapse can occur in 20% to 25% of patients and may be treated with metronidazole or vancomycin for 10 to 14 days.

INVASIVE (DYSENTERY-LIKE) DIARRHEA

BACILLARY DYSENTERY (SHIGELLOSIS)

- Four species of *Shigella* are most often associated with disease: *S. Dysenteriae* type I, *S. flexneri, S. boydii,* and *S. sonnei*.
- Poor sanitation, poor personal hygiene, inadequate water supply, malnutrition, and increased population density are associated with increased risk of *Shigella* gastroenteritis epidemics, even in developed countries. The majority of cases are thought to result from fecal–oral transmission.
- *Shigella* spp. cause dysentery upon penetrating the epithelial cells lining the colon. Microabscesses may eventually coalesce, forming larger abscesses. Some *Shigella* species produce a cytotoxin, or shigatoxin, the pathogenic role of which is unclear, although it is thought to damage endothelial cells of the lamina propria, resulting in microangiopathic changes that can progress to hemolytic uremic syndrome. Watery diarrhea commonly precedes the dysentery and may be a result of these toxins.
- Initial signs and symptoms include abdominal pain, cramping, and fever followed by frequent watery stools. Within a few days, patients experience a decrease in fever, severe abdominal pain, and tenderness prior to the development of bloody diarrhea and other signs of dysentery.
- If untreated, bacillary dysentery usually lasts about 1 week (range 1 to 30 days).
- Shigellosis is usually a self-limiting disease. Most patients recover in 4 to 7 days. Treatment of bacillary dysentery generally includes correction of fluid and electrolyte disturbances and, occasionally, antimicrobials.

- Antimicrobials are indicated in the infirm, those who are immunocompromised, children in daycare centers, the elderly, malnourished children, and healthcare workers. Antimicrobials may shorten the period of fecal shedding and attenuate the clinical illness.
- The agent of choice depends on location. **Trimethoprim–Sulfamethoxazole** is used for infections acquired in the United States. For infections acquired outside the United States, the agents of choice are **Ciprofloxacin, Norfloxacin,** and **Azithromycin**. Fluoroquinolones are generally contraindicated in children and adolescents.
- Fluid and electrolyte losses can generally be replaced with oral therapy, as dysentery is generally not associated with significant fluid loss. IV replacement is necessary only for children or the elderly.
- Antimotility agents such as diphenoxylate are not recommended because they can worsen dysentery.

SALMONELLOSIS

- Human disease caused by *Salmonella* generally falls into four categories: acute gastroenteritis (enterocolitis), bacteremia, extraintestinal localized infection, and enteric fever (typhoid and paratyphoid fever), and a chronic carrier state. *S. typhimurium* is the most common cause of salmonellosis. Salmonellosis is a disease primarily of infants, children, and adolescents.
- Conditions which predispose to infection include those which decrease gastric acidity, antibiotic use, malnutrition, and immunodeficiency states. Contaminated food or water is implicated in most cases.
- With enterocolitis, patients often complain of nausea and vomiting within 72 hours of ingestion followed by crampy abdominal pain, fever, and diarrhea, although the actual presentation is quite variable.
- Stool cultures inevitably yield the causative organism, if obtained early. However, recovery of organisms continues to decrease with time so that by 3 to 4 weeks, only 5% to 15% of adult patients are passing *Salmonella*.
- Some patients may continue to shed *Salmonella* for 1 year or longer. These "chronic-carrier" states are rare for serotypes other than *S. typhi*.
- *Salmonella* can produce bacteremia without classic enterocolitis or enteric fever. The clinical syndrome is characterized by persistent bacteremia and prolonged intermittent fever with chills. Stool cultures are frequently negative.
- Extraluminal infection and/or abscess formation can occur at any site after any of the other syndromes or may be the primary presentation. Metastatic infections have been reported to involve bone, cysts, heart, kidney, liver, lungs, pericardium, spleen, and tumors.
- Enteric fever caused by *S. typhi* is called typhoid fever. If caused by any other serotype, it is referred to as paratyphoid fever. The onset of symptoms is gradual. Nonspecific symptoms of fever, dull headache, malaise, anorexia, and myalgias are most common. Initially, fever tends to be remittent but gradually progresses over the first week to temperatures that are often sustained over 40°C (104°F). Other frequently encountered symptoms include chills, nausea, vomiting, cough, weakness, and sore throat.
- About 80% of patients with enteric fever have positive blood cultures. Bacteremia persists in about one-third of patients for several weeks if not treated. Diagnostic tests other than culture are unreliable.

TREATMENT

- Most patients with enterocolitis require no therapeutic intervention. The most important part of therapy for *Salmonella* enterocolitis is fluid and electrolyte replacement. Antimotility drugs should be avoided because they increase the risk of mucosal invasion and complications.
- Antibiotics have no effect on the duration of fever or diarrhea, and their frequent use increases the likelihood of resistance and the duration of fecal shedding. Antibiotics should be used in neonates or infants younger than 6 months, patients with primary or secondary immunodeficiency, severely symptomatic patients with fever and bloody diarrhea, and patients after splenectomy.
- Recommended antibiotics with adult doses include:

✓ Fluoroquinolones, trimethoprim–sulfamethoxazole, ampicillin, third generation cephalosporins

- For bacteremia, life-threatening treatment should include the combination of a third-generation cephalosporin (ceftriaxone 2 g IV daily) and ciprofloxacin 500 mg orally twice daily. The duration of antibiotic therapy is dictated by the site.
- Fluoroquinolones such as **ciprofloxacin** (500 mg orally twice daily for 10 days in adults) are the drugs of choice for enteric fever, particularly in areas where multidrug resistance is common. A short course of 3 to 5 days is effective but a minimum of 10 days is recommended in severe cases.
- The drug of choice for chronic carriers of *Salmonella* is **norfloxacin**, 400 mg orally twice daily for 28 days.
- Vaccines are recommended for high-risk groups. Live oral attenuated vaccine Ty21a and parenteral polysaccharide vaccine have been shown to confer 42% to 77% efficacy for a duration of 3 to 5 years.

CAMPYLOBACTERIOSIS

- *Campylobacter* species are thought to be a major cause of diarrhea. Transmission of infection occurs primarily by ingestion of contaminated food or water.
- Incubation usually averages 2 to 4 days. The most common symptoms include diarrhea of varying consistency and severity, abdominal pain, and fever. Nausea, vomiting, headache, myalgias, and malaise may also occur. Bowel movements may be numerous, bloody (dysentery-like), foul smelling, and melenic and range from loose to watery (dysentery-like).
- The disease is self-limiting, and signs and symptoms usually resolve in about 1 week but may persist longer in 10% to 20% of patients.
- As with other acute diarrheal illnesses, fluid and electrolyte support is a mainstay of therapy, mainly with ORT.
- Antibiotics are not useful unless started within 4 days of the start of illness, as they do not shorten the duration or severity of diarrhea.
- Antibiotics are warranted in patients who present with high fevers, severe bloody diarrhea, prolonged illness (greater than 1 week), pregnancy, and immunocompromised states, including human immunodeficiency virus infection.
- Erythromycin is considered the drug of choice for treatment. Clarithromycin or azithromycin is equally effective. Antimotility drugs are contraindicated.

YERSINIOSIS

- *Yersinia enterocolitica* and *Y. pseudotuberculosis* are associated with intestinal infection. The organisms have been isolated from a variety of food sources, including raw goat and cow milk.
- These bacteria cause a wide spectrum of clinical syndromes. The majority of

cases present with enterocolitis that is mild and self-limiting. Symptoms, generally lasting 1 to 3 weeks, include vomiting, abdominal pain, diarrhea, and fever. A clinical syndrome seen in older children may resemble appendicitis.

- Many patients develop a reactive arthritis 1 to 2 weeks after recovery from enteritis.
- These diseases are generally self-limiting and are easily managed with oral rehydration solutions.
- Antibiotics should be used in high-risk patients who develop bacteremia (i.e., infants younger than 3 months and patients with cirrhosis or iron overload) or in patients with bone and joint infections.
- Drugs of choice are not yet identified. *Y. enterocolitica* is generally susceptible to **fluoroquinolones**, alone or in combination with **third-generation cephalosporins** or **aminoglycosides**. Alternative agents include **chloramphenicol, tetracycline,** and **trimethoprim–sulfamethoxazole**.
- Suggested antibiotics of choice are given in Table 69.3.

ACUTE VIRAL GASTROENTERITIS

ROTAVIRUSES

- The highest frequency of rotavirus-associated diarrhea appears in children less than 5 years of age. The incubation period is typically 1 to 3 days.
- Clinical manifestations of rotavirus infections vary from asymptomatic (which is common in adults) to severe nausea, vomiting, and diarrhea with dehydration. Symptoms are characterized initially by nausea and vomiting. The symptoms begin abruptly, with vomiting often preceding the onset of diarrhea. Other signs and symptoms include fever, respiratory symptoms, irritability, lethargy, pharyngeal erythema, rhinitis, red tympanic membranes, and palpable cervical lymph nodes. Dehydration and electrolyte disturbances occur more frequently in children.
- Oral fluid and electrolyte replacement is the cornerstone of treatment. Oral Lactobacillus therapy may reduce the duration of diarrhea and or viral excretion. There is no role for antibiotics.
- Antimotility agents are not recommended.

CALICIVIRUSES

- Caliciviruses include Norovirus (including Norwalk virus) and Sapovirus. Calicivirus gastroenteritis is characterized by sudden onset of abdominal cramps with nausea and/or vomiting. Although adults frequently experience nonbloody diarrhea, children experience vomiting more often. Other frequent complaints are myalgias, headache, and malaise, which are accompanied by fever in about 50% of cases. Signs and symptoms generally last only 12 to 48 hours.
- The disease is generally self-limiting and does not require therapy. On occasion, oral rehydration may be required. Rarely is parenteral hydration necessary.

REFERENCES

1. Solomkin JS, Mazuski JE, Bradley JS, Rodvold KA, Goldstein EJ, Baron EJ, O'Neill PJ, Chow AW, Dellinger EP, Eachempati SR, Gorbach S, Hilfiker M, May AK, Nathens AB, Sawyer RG, Bartlett JG. Diagnosis and management of complicated intra-abdominal infection in adults and children: guidelines by the Surgical Infection Society and the Infectious Diseases Society of America. Surg Infect (Larchmt) pp. 79–109.
2. Solomkin JS, Mazuski JE, Baron EJ, Sawyer RG, Nathens AB, DiPiro JT, Buchman T, Dellinger EP, Jernigan J, Gorbach S, Chow AW, Bartlett J. Guidelines for the selection of anti-infective agents for complicated intra-abdominal infections. Clin Infect Dis. 2003;37(8):997–1005.
3. Weigelt JA. Empiric treatment options in the management of complicated intra-abdominal infections. Cleve Clin J Med. 2007;74(Suppl 4):S29–37.

CHAPTER 70

Sexually Transmitted Diseases

DEFINITION

The spectrum of sexually transmitted diseases (STDs) includes the classic venereal diseases—gonorrhea, syphilis, chancroid, lymphogranuloma venereum, and granuloma inguinale—as well as a variety of other pathogens known to be spread by sexual contact Table 70.1. Common clinical syndromes associated with STDs are listed in Table 70.2.

Table 70.1

Sexually transmitted diseases

Disease	Associated Pathogens
Bacterial	
Gonorrhea	*Neisseria gonorrhoeae*
Syphilis	*Treponema pallidum*
Chancroid	*Haemophilus ducreyi*
Granuloma inguinale	*Calymmatobacterium granulomatis*
Enteric disease	*Salmonella* spp., *Shigella,* spp.,*Campylobacter fetus*
Campylobacter infection	*C. jejuni*
Bacterial vaginosis	*Gardnerella vaginalis, Mycoplasma hominis, Bacteriodes* spp. *Mobiluncus* Spp
Group B streptococcal infections	Group B *Streptococcus*
Chlamydial	
Nongonococcal urethritis	*Chlamydia trachomatis*
Lymphogranuloma venereum	*C. trachomatis,*type L
Viral	Human immunodeficiency
Acquired immune deficiency syndrome	Virus Herpes simplex virus, types I and II
Herpes genitalis	Hepatitis A, B, C, and D viruses
Viral hepatitis	Human papillomavirus
Condylomata Acuminate	Poxvirus
Molluscum contagiosum	Cytomegalovirus
Cytomegalovirus infection	
Mycoplasmal	*Ureaplasma urealyticum*
Nongonococcal urethritis	
Protozoal	*Trichomonas vaginalis*
Trichomoniasis	*Entamoeba histolytica*
Amebiasis	*Giardia lamblia*
Giardiasis	

Table 70.1 *Contd...*

Disease	Associated Pathogens
Fungal Vaginal candidiasis	*Candida albicans*
Parasitic Scabies Pediculosis pubis Enterobiasis	*Sarcoptes scabiei* *Phthirus pubis* *Enterobius vermicularis*

Table 70.2

Selected syndromes associated with common sexually transmitted pathogens

Syndrome	Commonly Implicated Pathogens	Common Clinical Manifestations[a]
Urethritis	*Chlamydia trachomatis* herpes simplex virus, *Neisseria gonorrhoeae, Trichomonas vaginalis, Ureaplasma urealyticum*	Urethral discharge, dysuria
Epididymitis Cervicitis/vulvovaginitis	*C. trachomatis, N. Gardnerella* *C. trachomatis, N. Gardnerella* *C. trachomatis, Gardnerella vaginalis, herpes simplex virus, human papillomavirus, N.gonorrhocac, T. vaginalis*	Scrotal pain, inguinal pain, flank pain, urethral discharge normal vaginal discharge, vulvar itching/irritation, dysuria, dyspareunia
Genital ulcers (painful)	*Haemophilus ducreyi, herpes simplex virus*	Usually multiple vesicular/pustular (herpes) or papular/pustular (H. ducreyi) lesions that may coalesce; painful, tender lymphadenopathy coalesce; painful, tender lymphadenopathy[b]
Genital ulcers (painless) Genital/anal warts	*Treponema pallidum* Human papillomavirus	Usually single papular lesion Multiple lesions ranging in size from small papular warts to large exophytic condylomas
Pharyngitis	*C. trachomatis* (?), herpes simplex virus, *N. gonorrhoeae*	Symptoms of acute pharyngitis, cervical lymphadenopathy, fever[c]
Proctitis	*C. trachomatis*, herpes simplex virus, *N. gonorrhoeae, T. pallidum*	Constipation, anorectal discomfort, tenesmus, mucopurulent rectal discharge
Salpingitis	*C. trachomatis, N. gonorrhoeae*	Lower abdominal pain, purulent cervical or vaginal discharge, adnexal swelling, fever[d]

[a]For some syndromes, clinical manifestations may be minimal or absent.
[b]Recurrent herpes infection may manifest as a single lesion.
[c]Most cases of pharyngeal gonococcal infection are asymptomatic.
[d]Salpingitis increases the risk of subsequent ectopic pregnancy and infertility.

GONORRHEA

Gonorrhea (gah-nuh-REE-uh), a bacterial STD, infects at least 700,000 people every year in the United States. Rates were declining until 1998, but they have been rising in recent years. Gonorrhea is on the rise in young people, especially women between the ages of fifteen and nineteen.

Gonorrhea is caused by the bacterium *Neisseria gonorrhoeae*. Because it is a bacterial infection, it is curable with antibiotics. Almost all men who get gonorrhea have symptoms one to fourteen days after exposure, but women may not. Gonorrhea occurs in the genital and anal areas from vaginal and anal intercourse and oral sex.

It can also arise in the throat from oral sex and in the eyes from touching an infected area and then rubbing the eyes. Some typical symptoms of genital gonorrhea in a woman include abdominal pain, bleeding between periods, pain during urination or intercourse, and a yellowish vaginal discharge. Men often have a yellow discharge from the penis, burning during urination, and a feeling of irritation in the penis.

Anal infection can cause itching, pain with bowel movements, bleeding, and discharge. When the throat becomes infected, it may cause soreness or trouble swallowing. Gonorrhea in the eyes can cause redness, a thick yellow discharge, and vision problems. People cannot catch gonorrhea from a toilet seat or towel or through casual contact.

Untreated gonorrhea can lead to serious, permanent health problems. Men can end up with epididymitis, which can cause infertility. Women can get pelvic inflammatory disease (PID) or have ectopic pregnancies. Pregnant women can pass the infection to their babies during delivery, causing infants to become blind or have joint infections or life-threatening blood infections.

DIAGNOSIS

Testing involves taking swabs from the urethra and cervix in women, the urethra in men, and sometimes from the throat and anal area. Bacteria can often be seen under the microscope right away; if not, a culture will need to be done, which takes forty-eight hours to grow. A new test, nucleic acid hybridization, detects DNA in gonorrhea bacterium in urine or in swabs from infected areas. The nucleic acid amplification test (NAAT) is also used to diagnose gonorrhea.

TREATMENT

Antibiotics are also used to treat genital and anal gonorrhea. Cefriaxone is administered as a shot, and ciprofloxacin, levofloxacin, and ofloxacin are given in pill form. Unfortunately, these last three drugs are becoming less effective in treatment ,because the bacteria are becoming resistant.

Antibiotics must be taken for a longer time if gonorrhea has caused PID or epididymitis. Gonorrhea that infects the eyes must be treated by an eye doctor. If the infection has spread to other organs, such as the joints or heart, hospitalization and treatment with intravenous (into a vein) antibiotics is necessary.

SYPHILIS

Syphilis (SIH-fuh-lis) is a common infection caused by the bacterium *Treponema pallidum*. It causes sores in the genital area and the mouth.

PREVALENCE

Syphilis is most prevalent in Africa and Southeast Asia. In the United States, more people have it in the South and in cities along the coasts. Poor people, people who use drugs, and people infected with HIV are especially susceptible to syphilis. In the United States, the number of people with syphilis peaked in the 1940s, but after penicillin was discovered, the numbers declined. In 2000, syphilis cases reached an all-time low, but since then, they have been steadily increasing every year. In 2006, U.S. health officials reported more than 36,000 cases of the disease, mostly in women aged twenty to twenty-four and men aged thirty five to thirty-nine.

PATHOPHYSIOLOGY

This infection is spread through intercourse, oral sex, or touching an infected area, including kissing. It can also be spread from a mother to her unborn baby. It cannot spread from toilet seats, swimming pools or hot tubs, or eating utensils. Syphilis occurs in several stages, and people are contagious during all of them. The primary stage occurs about twenty-one days after contact with an infected person and produces the classic syphilis symptom, the chancre (SHANG-kur). This small, round, painless sore appears at the location where syphilis entered the body. Usually, only one chancre appears, and many people do not even realize they have a sore if it is inside the vagina or the penis. Without treatment, the sore lasts for three to six weeks and goes away on its own. But then the disease progresses to the secondary stage. Secondary stage syphilis occurs as the chancre is healing or several weeks later, when the infection enters the bloodstream.

CLINICAL FEATURES

Symptoms include a red rash that covers the whole body, even the palms of the hands and soles of the feet, but does not itch; wart-like growths in the genital area; hair loss in patches; and fever, headache, tiredness, muscle aches, and swollen glands. However, some people have only a mild rash and may mistake their illness for the flu, especially when the symptoms disappear on their own. But this does not mean the infection has gone away. If people do not get treated, the disease will progress to the latent (hidden) and late phases. The latent stage of syphilis occurs when all the symptoms have disappeared. However, the bacteria are still in the body and the infected person is still contagious. The latent stage can last for years or for the rest of the person's life. About 15 percent of those with untreated syphilis progress to the late stage, which can occur ten to twenty years after exposure. In the late stage, the disease can damage the internal organs, including the brain, eyes, and heart. It can even be fatal. Luckily, late stage syphilis is rare today because of antibiotics. If syphilis is cured during the first two stages, the infected person has no lasting complications. However, mothers can pass syphilis to their unborn children during any stage of the disease. Infants may be born dead or die shortly after birth. If they are born without signs of the disease and do not receive treatment immediately, they can become blind, have seizures, or have other birth defects.

DIAGNOSIS

Two types of tests are used to diagnose syphilis: blood tests to detect antibodies and swabs taken from chancres to detect the syphilis bacterium. Most clinics do not have the special microscope necessary to perform this test, so blood tests are usually used for diagnosis. The most common ones are called the Venereal Disease Research Laboratory test and the Rapid Plasma Reagin test. The bacteria may take up to three months after infection to appear in the blood, although most people test positive within a few weeks.

TREATMENT

The treatment for syphilis is penicillin—one of the first antibiotics invented. It is always given as a shot, and one dose usually gets rid of primary, secondary, and early latent stage syphilis. Because the dose is so high and the bacteria are killed off so quickly, some people get chills, headache, muscle aches, and fever about eight hours after the shot. The rash or chancres may even get worse temporarily. This is called the Jarisch-Herxheimer reaction and usually goes away in twenty-four hours. People with late-stage latent syphilis and those who do not know how long they have been infected need penicillin shots every week for three weeks.

Other antibiotics, such as doxycycline or tetracycline, are used for people with primary or secondary syphilis who have penicillin allergies. However, experts and drug manufacturers advise that it may not be safe to give these drugs to children and teens because they can cause staining of developing teeth. Penicillin is the only safe antibiotic for pregnant women.

Table 70.3

Drug therapy and follow-up of syphilis

Stage/Type of Syphilis	Recommended	Follow-Up Serology
Primary, secondary, or latent syphilis of less than 1-year's duration (early latent syphilis)	Benzathine penicillin G 2.4 million units IM in a single dose [c]	Quantitative nontreponemal tests at 6 and 12 months for primary and secondary syphilis; at 6, 12, and 24 months for early latent syphilis[d]
Latent syphilis of more than 1-year's duration (late latent syphilis) or syphilis of unknown duration	Benzathine penicillin G 2.4 million units IM once a week for 3 successive weeks (7.2 million units total)	Quantitative nontreponemal tests at 6, 12, and 24 months[e]
Neurosyphilis	Aqueous crystalline penicillin G 18–24 million units IV (3–4 million units every 4 hours or by continuous infusion) for 10–14 days[f] *or* Aqueous procaine penicillin G 2.4 million units IM daily plus probenecid 500 mg orally four times daily, both for 10–14 days[e]	Cerebrospinal fluid[f] examination every 6 months until the cell count is normal; if it has not decreased at 6 months or is not normal by 2 years, retreatment should be considered

Table 70.3 *Contd...*

Stage/Type of Syphilis	Recommended	Follow-Up Serology
Congenital syphilis	Aqueous crystalline penicillin G 50,000 units/kg IV every 12 hours during the first 7 days of life and every 8 hours thereafter for a total of 10 days *or* Procaine penicillin G 50,000 units/kg IM daily for 10 days	Serologic follow-up only recommended if antimicrobials other than penicillin are used
Penicillin-allergic patients[g] primary, secondary, or early latent syphilis	Doxycycline 100 mg orally two times daily for 2 weeks[g,h] *or* Tetracycline 500 mg orally four times daily for 2 weeks[h] or Tetracycline 500 mg orally four times daily for 2 weeksh or Ceftriaxone 1 g IM or IV daily for 8–10 days	Same as for non–penicillin-allergic patients
Latent syphilis of more than 1 year's duration (late latent syphilis) or syphilis of unknown duration	Doxycycline 100 mg orally two times a day for 28 days[h,i] or Tetracycline 500 mg orally four times daily for 28 days[h,i]	Same as for non–penicillin-allergic patients

*a*Recommendations are those of the Centers for Disease Control and Prevention.
*b*The Centers for Disease Control and Prevention recommends that all patients diagnosed with syphilis be tested for human
immunodeficiency virus (HIV) infection.
*c*Some experts recommend multiple doses of benzathine penicillin G or other supplemental antibiotics in addition to benzathine
penicillin G in HIV-infected patients with primary or secondary syphilis; HIV-infected patients with early latent syphilis should be treated
with the recommended regimen for latent syphilis of more than 1-year's duration.
*d*More frequent follow-up (i.e., 3, 6, 9, 12, and 24 months) recommended for HIV-infected patients.
*e*More frequent follow-up (i.e., 6, 12, 18, and 24 months) recommended for HIV-infected patients.
*f*Some experts administer benzathine penicillin G 2.4 million units IM once per week for up to 3 weeks after completion of the
neurosyphilis regimens to provide a total duration of therapy comparable to that used for late syphilis in the absence of neurosyphilis.
*g*For nonpregnant patients; pregnant patients should be treated with penicillin after desensitization.
*h*Pregnant patients allergic to penicillin should be desensitized and treated with penicillin.
*i*Limited data suggest that ceftriaxone may be effective, although the optimal dosage and treatment duration are unclear.

CHLAMYDIA

- Infections caused by *C. trachomatis* are believed to be the most common STD in the United States that has more than doubled in the past 10 years. *C. trachomatis* is an obligate intracellular parasite that has some similarities to viruses and bacteria.

Table 70.4

Treatment of chlamydial infections

	Males	Females
General	Incubation period—35 days Symptom onset—7–21 days	Incubation period—7–35 days Usual symptom onset—7–21 days
Site of infection	Most common—urethra Others—rectum (receptive anal intercourse), oropharynx, eye	Most common—endocervical canal Others—urethra, rectum (usually due to perineal contamination), oropharynx, eye
Symptoms	More than 50% of urethral and rectal infections are asymptomatic Urethral infection—mild dysuria, discharge Pharyngeal infection—asymptomatic to mild Pharyngitis	More than 66% of cervical infections are asymptomatic Urethral infection—usually subclinical; dysuria and frequency uncommon Rectal and pharyngeal infection—symptoms same as for men
Signs	Scant to profuse, mucoid to purulent urethral or rectal discharge Rectal infection—pain, discharge, bleeding	Abnormal vaginal discharge or uterine bleeding, purulent urethral, or rectal discharge can be scant to profuse
Complications	Epididymitis, Reiter's syndrome (rare)	Pelvic inflammatory disease and associated complications (i.e., ectopic pregnancy, infertility) Reiter's syndrome (rare)

CLINICAL PRESENTATION

- In comparison with gonorrhea, chlamydial genital infections are more frequently asymptomatic, and when present, symptoms tend to be less noticeable. Table 70-6 summarizes the usual clinical presentation of chlamydial infections.
- Similar to gonorrhea, chlamydia may be transmitted to an infant during contact with infected cervicovaginal secretions. Nearly two-thirds of infants acquire chlamydial infection after endocervical exposure, with the primary morbidity associated with seeding of the infant's eyes, nasopharynx, rectum, or vagina.

DIAGNOSIS

- Culture of endocervical or urethral epithelial cell scrapings is the most specific method (close to 100%) for detection of chlamydia, but sensitivity is as low as 70%. Between 3 and 7 days are required for results.
- Tests that allow rapid identification of chlamydial antigens in genital secretions are the direct fluorescent antibody test, the enzyme immunoassay (requires just 30 minutes for results), the DNA hybridization probe and nucleic acid amplification tests.

TREATMENT

- Recommended regimens for treatment of chlamydial infections are given in Table 74.7. Single-dose **Azithromycin** and 7-day **Doxycycline** are the agents of choice.

- For prophylaxis of ophthalmia neonatorum, various groups have proposed the use of **Erythromycin** (0.5%) or **Tetracycline** (1%) ophthalmic ointment in lieu of silver nitrate. Although silver nitrate and antibiotic ointments are effective against gonococcal ophthalmia neonatorum, silver nitrate is not effective for chlamydial disease and may cause a chemical conjunctivitis.
- Treatment of chlamydial infections with the recommended regimens is highly effective; therefore, post treatment cultures are not routinely recommended.
- Infants with pneumonitis should receive follow-up testing, because erythromycin is only 80% effective.

GENITAL HERPES

- The term *herpes* is used to describe two distinct but antigenically related serotypes of herpes simplex virus (HSV). HSV type 1 (HSV-1) is most commonly associated with oropharyngeal disease; type 2 (HSV-2) is most closely associated with genital disease.

CLINICAL PRESENTATION

- A summary of the clinical presentation of genital herpes is provided in Table 70.5.
- A presumptive diagnosis of genital herpes commonly is made on the basis of the presence of dark-field-negative, vesicular, or ulcerative genital lesions. A history of similar lesions or recent sexual contact with an individual with similar lesions also is useful in making the diagnosis.
- Tissue culture is the most specific (100%) and sensitive method (80% to 90%) of confirming the diagnosis of first-episode genital herpes.

TREATMENT

- The goals of therapy in genital herpes infection are to shorten the clinical course, prevent complications, prevent the development of latency and/or subsequent recurrences, decrease disease transmission, and eliminate established latency.
- Palliative and supportive measures are the cornerstone of therapy for patients with genital herpes. Pain and discomfort usually respond to warm saline baths or the use of analgesics, antipyretics, or antipruritics.
- Specific treatment recommendations are given in Table 70.6.
- Oral acyclovir, valacyclovir, and famciclovir are the treatments of choice for outpatients with first-episode genital herpes. Treatment does not prevent latency or alter the subsequent frequency and severity of recurrences.
- Continuous oral antiviral therapy reduces the frequency and the severity of recurrences in 70% to 90% of patients experiencing frequent recurrences.
- Acyclovir, valacyclovir, and famciclovir have been used to prevent reactivation of infection in patients seropositive for HSV who undergo transplantation procedures or induction chemotherapy for acute leukemia.
- The safety of acyclovir therapy during pregnancy is not established, although there is no evidence of teratogenic effects in humans.

Table 70.5

Presentation of genital herpes infections

General	Incubation period 2–14 days (mean, 4 days) Can be caused by either HSV-1 or HSV-2
Classification of infection First-episode primary	Initial genital infection in individuals lacking antibody to either HSV-1 or HSV-2
First-episode nonprimary	Initial genital infection in individuals with clinical or serologic evidence of prior HSV (usually HSV-1) infection
Recurrent	Appearance of genital lesions at some time following healing of first-episode infection
Signs and symptoms First-episode infections	Most primary infections are asymptomatic or minimally symptomatic Multiple painful pustular or ulcerative lesions on external genitalia developing over a period of 7–10 days; lesions heal in 2–4 weeks (mean, 21 days) Flu-like symptoms (e.g., fever, headache, malaise) during first few days after appearance of lesions Others—local itching, pain or discomfort; vaginal or urethral discharge, tender inguinal adenopathy, paresthesias, urinary retention Severity of symptoms greater in females than in males Symptoms are less severe (e.g., fewer lesions, more rapid lesion healing, fewer or milder systemic symptoms) with nonprimary infections Symptoms more severe and prolonged in the immunocompromised On average viral shedding lasts approximately 11–12 days for primary infections and 7 days for nonprimary infections
Recurrent	Prodrome seen in approximately 50% of patients prior to appearance of recurrent lesions; mild burning, itching, or tingling are typical prodromal symptoms Compared to primary infections, recurrent infections associated with (1) fewer lesions that are more localized, (2) shorter duration of active infection (lesions heal within 7 days), and (3) milder symptoms Severity of symptoms greater in females than in males Symptoms more severe and prolonged in the immunocompromised On average, viral shedding lasts approximately 4 days
Therapeutic implications of HSV-1 versus HSV-2 genital infection Complications	Primary infections due to HSV-1 and HSV-2 virtually indistinguishable Recurrence rate is greater after primary infection with HSV-1 Recurrent infections with HSV-2 tend to be more severe Secondary infection of lesions; extragenital infection due to autoinoculation; disseminated infection (primarily in immunocompromised patients); meningitis or encephalitis; neonatal transmission

Table 70.6

Treatment of genital herpes

Type of Infection	Recommended Regimens[a,b]	Alternative Regimen
First clinical episode of genital herpes[c]	Acyclovir 400 mg po three times daily for 7– 10 days[d], *Or* Acyclovir 200 mg po five times daily for 7–10 days[d], *or* Famciclovir 250 mg po three times daily for 7–10[d] days[d], *or* Valacyclovir 1 g po twice daily for 7–10 days[d]	Acyclovir 5–10 mg/kg IV every 8 hours for 2–7 days or until clinical improvement occurs, followed by oral therapy to complete at least 10 days of total therapy[e]
Recurrent infection Episodic Therapy	Acyclovir 400 mg po three times daily for 5 days, *or* Acyclovir 800 mg po twice daily for 5 days[f] *or* Acyclovir 800 mg po three times daily for 2 days[f] *or* Famciclovir 125 mg po twice daily for 5 days[f] *or* Valacyclovir 500 mg po twice daily for 3–5 days[f] *or* Valacyclovir 1 g po once daily for 5 days[f]	
Suppressive therapy	Acyclovir 400 mg po twice daily, *or* Famciclovir 250 mg po twice daily, *or* Valacyclovir 500 mg or 1,000 mg po once daily[g]	

CDC, Centers for Disease Control and Prevention; HIV, human immunodeficiency virus.
[a]Recommendations are those of the CDC. [b]HIV-infected patients can require more aggressive therapy. [c]Primary or nonprimary first episode. [d]Treatment duration can be extended if healing is incomplete after 10 days. [e]Only for patients with severe symptoms or complications that necessitate hospitalization. [f]Requires initiation of therapy within 24 hours of lesion onset or during the prodrome that precedes some outbreaks. [g]Valacyclovir 500 mg appears less effective than valacyclovir 1,000 mg in patients with approximately 10 recurrences per year.

TRICHOMONIAS

- Trichomoniasis is caused by *Trichomonas vaginalis*, a flagellated, motile protozoan that is responsible for 3 million to 5 million cases per year in the United States.
- Coinfection with other STDs (such as gonorrhea) is common in patients diagnosed with trichomoniasis.

CLINICAL PRESENTATION

- The typical presentation of trichomoniasis in males and females is presented in Table 70.7.
- *T. vaginalis* produces nonspecific symptoms also consistent with bacterial vaginosis, and thus laboratory diagnosis is required.
- The simplest and most reliable means of diagnosis is a wet-mount examination of the vaginal discharge. Trichomoniasis is confirmed if characteristic pear-shaped, flagellating organisms are observed. Newer diagnostic tests such as monoclonal antibody or DNA probe techniques, as well as polymerase chain reaction tests are highly sensitive and specific.

TREATMENT

- **Metronidazole** and **tinidazole** are the only antimicrobial agents available in the United States that are consistently effective in *T. vaginalis* infections.
- Treatment recommendations for *Trichomonas* infections are given in Table 70.8.
- GI complaints (e.g., anorexia, nausea, vomiting, diarrhea) are the most common adverse effects, with the single 2-g dose of metronidazole or tinidazole, occurring in 5% to 10% of treated patients. Some patients complain of a bitter metallic taste in the mouth.
- Patients intolerant of the single 2-g dose because of GI adverse effects usually tolerate the multidose regimen.

Table 70.7

Presentation of *trichomonas* infections

	Males	Females
General	Incubation period 3–28 days Organism may be detectable within 48 hours after exposure to infected partner	Incubation period 3–28 days
Site of infection	Most common—urethra Others—rectum (usually due to rectal intercourse in men who have sex with men), oropharynx, eye	Most common—endocervical canal Others—urethra, rectum (usually due to perineal contamination), oropharynx, eye
Symptoms	May be asymptomatic (more common in males than females) or minimally symptomatic Urethral discharge (clear to mucopurulent) Dysuria, pruritus	May be asymptomatic or minimally symptomatic Scant to copious, typically malodorous vaginal discharge (50–75%) and pruritus (worsen during menses) Dysuria, dyspareunia
Signs	Urethral discharge	Vaginal discharge Vaginal pH 4.5–6 Inflammation/erythema of vulva, vagina, and/or cervix Urethritis
Complications	Epididymitis and chronic prostatitis (uncommon) Male infertility (decreased sperm motility and viability)	Pelvic inflammatory disease and associated complications (i.e., ectopic pregnancy, infertility) Premature labor, premature rupture of membranes, and low-birth-weight infants (risk of neonatal infections is low) Cervical neoplasia

Table 70.8

Treatment of trichomoniasis

Type	Recommended Regimen[a]	Alternative Regimen
Symptomatic and asymptomatic infections	Metronidazole 2 g po in a single dose[d] *or* Tinidazole 2 g po in a single dose[e]	Metronidazole 500 mg po 2 times daily for 7 days[c] *or* Tinidazole 2 g po in a single dose[d]
Treatment in pregnancy	Metronidazole 2 g po in a single dose[e]	

CDC, Centers for Disease Control and Prevention. [a]Recommendations are those of the CDC. [b]Treatment failures should be treated with metronidazole 500 mg po twice daily for 7 days. Persistent failures should be managed in consultation with an expert. Metronidazole or tinidazole 2 g po daily for 5 days has been effective in patients infected with Trichomonas vaginalis strains mildly resistant to metronidazole, but experience is limited; higher doses also have been used. [c]Metronidazole labeling approved by the FDA does not include this regimen. Dosage regimens for treatment of trichomoniasis included in the product labeling are the single 2-g dose; 250 mg three times daily for 7 days; and 375 mg twice daily for 7 days. The 250 mg and 375 mg dosage regimens are currently not included in the CDC recommendations. [d]For treatment failures with metronidazole 2 g as a single dose. [e]Metronidazole is pregnancy category B and tinidazole is pregnancy category C; both drugs are contraindicated in the first trimester of pregnancy. Some clinicians recommend deferring metronidazole treatment in asymptomatic pregnant women until after 37 weeks' gestation.

Table 70.9

Treatment regimens for miscellaneous sexually transmitted diseases

Infection	Recommended Regimen [a]	Alternative Regimen
Chancroid (Haemophilus ducreyi)	Azithromycin 1 g orally in a single dose or Ceftriaxone 250 mg intramuscularly in a single dose or Ciprofloxacin 500 mg orally twice daily for 3 days[b] or Erythromycin base 500 mg orally four times daily for 7 days	—
Lymphogranuloma venereum	Doxycycline 100 mg orally twice daily for 21 days[c]	Erythromycin base 500 mg orally four times daily for 7 days
Human papillomavirus infection External genital warts	Provider-administered therapies: Cryotherapy (e.g., liquid nitrogen or cryoprobe) or Podophyllin 10–25% in compound tinc- ture of benzoin applied to lesions; repeat weekly if necessary[d,e] or Trichloroacetic acid 80–90% or bichlora- cetic acid 80–90% applied to warts; repeat weekly if necessary or Surgical removal (tangential scissor exci- sion, tangential shave excision, curettage, or electrosurgery) Patient-applied therapies: Podofilox 0.5% solution or gel applied twice daily for 3 days, followed by 4 days of no therapy; cycle is repeated as necessary for a total of four cycles[e] or Imiquimod 5% cream applied at bedtime three times weekly for up to 16 weeks[e]	Intralesional interferon or laser surgery
Vaginal, urethral meatus, and anal warts	Cryotherapy with liquid nitrogen, or trichloroacetic acid or bichloracetic acid 80–90% as for external human papillomavirus warts; repeat weekly as necessary[f] Surgical removal (not for vaginal or urethral meatus warts)	
Urethral meatus warts	Cryotherapy with liquid nitrogen, or podophyllin resin 10–25% in compound tincture of benzoin applied at weekly intervals [e,g]	

[a]Recommendations are those of the Centers for Disease Control and Prevention. [b]Ciprofloxacin is contraindicated for pregnant and lactating women and for persons aged <18 years. [c]Azithromycin 1 g orally once weekly for 3 weeks can be effective. [d]Some experts recommended washing podophyllin off after 1–4 hours to minimize local irritation. [e]Safety during pregnancy is not established. [f]Surgical removal of anal warts is also a recommended treatment. [g]Some specialists recommend the use of podofilox and imiquimod for treating distal meatal warts.

- To achieve maximal cure rates and prevent relapse with the single 2-g dose of metronidazole, simultaneous treatment of infected sexual partners is necessary.
- Patients who fail to respond to an initial course usually respond to a second course of metronidazole or tinidazole therapy.
- Patients taking metronidazole should be instructed to avoid alcohol ingestion during therapy and for 1 to 2 days after completion of therapy because of a possible disulfiram-like effect.
- At present, no satisfactory treatment is available for pregnant women with *Trichomonas* infections. Metronidazole and tinidazole are contraindicated during the first trimester of pregnancy.
- Follow-up is considered unnecessary in patients who become asymptomatic after treatment with metronidazole.
- When patients remain symptomatic, it is important to determine if reinfection has occurred. In these cases, a repeat course of therapy, as well as identification and treatment or retreatment of infected sexual partners, is recommended.

PREVENTION OF STDs

Just about everyone knows that having unprotected sex with an infected partner can cause an STD. Then why do so many people get STDs every year? The answer is simple. They are lacking the necessary information about how STDs spread and how they can be prevented. Knowing the kinds of behaviors that will make sex safer can make all the difference.

ABSTINENCE

The only effective way to avoid STDs hundred percent of the time is to say "no" to sex—all sex. Some people abstain forever. Other people say no until they feel they are ready to have sex. Still other people abstain from sex for different reasons and at different times in their lives. Many teens today take "virginity pledges"—pledges to abstain from sex until they are married. What does it mean to abstain from sex? To abstain means to "avoid something by your own choice." So what does "sex" mean? Is it vaginal intercourse? Does it include oral sex? What about mutual masturbation? The last two acts are not sex to some people, but all three of them can transmit STDs.

One five-year study showed that 4.6 percent of teens who were consistent virginity pledgers had chlamydia, trichomoniasis, or gonorrhea at the end of the study. The non-pledgers had a 6.9 percent rate. Also, sixty-one percent of pledgers said they had intercourse by the end of the study or before they married. Abstinence has to be perfect to work. Young people who choose that route need to be informed about other options, too, for their own safety.

CONDOMS

If saying no to sex is not an option, sex with condoms is the only way to go. Condoms cannot give you 100 percent protection from STDs, but they can reduce your risk. It is important to realize that risk reduction is not risk elimination. Condoms must be used the right way, every time you have sex. Studies show that people using latex condoms *correctly and consistently* during vaginal sex can reduce their risk of HIV by 85 percent. The risk for genital herpes and syphilis is reduced only when the infected areas are also covered or protected by a condom. Whether or not condoms can prevent HPV is unknown, but using them has been associated with a lower incidence of cervical cancer, a disease associated with HPV. Talking with a partner about condoms before having sex is a good idea. Some people are uncomfortable with the topic, but a little embarrassment is easier to get over than an STD. If a partner feels that a condom will interfere with sexual pleasure, knowing about condoms will help you explain the need for them.

OTHER WAYS TO REDUCE RISK

The following additional practices can reduce STD risk.

Limiting sexual partners. Choosing one partner who has sex only with you is called mutual monogamy. Both partners still need to get tested though, because either could have been infected by a previous partner and not know it. Some people believe that "serial monogamy"—having sex with one person at a time, even if just for a few weeks—is safe. This practice will not protect someone from STDs.

Avoiding drugs and alcohol. They impair good judgment, something people need to have when considering sex. Drugs and alcohol can make people feel aroused, but watch out. They also can make it difficult for a guy to have an erection! If someone is feeling so anxious about having sex that he or she needs drugs or alcohol to relax, maybe that person should wait. Responsible—and enjoyable—sex requires a clear head.

COMMUNICATING

People need to talk with partners about STDs, past sex partners, condoms, and getting tested. Young people should also communicate with their friends and parents. Being able to discuss sex and ask questions freely results in lower rates of STDs.

GETTING EDUCATED ABOUT STDs

Besides reading this book, look for other information about sexual health, STDs, protection, and prevention. Learn about the different STDs, their symptoms, and how they spread. Check out condom use and other ways to reduce risk. Find out how to be tested and treated for the different STDs. Then educate everyone else—friends, family, and especially partners.

Getting tested for STDs. Chlamydia screening is recommended for all sexually active women from ages fifteen to twenty-four, whether or not they have symptoms. Many young women believe that doctors routinely test for it. In 2003, however, only 30 percent of women under twenty-five with commercial health care plans were screened for chlamydia.

Getting vaccinated against STDs. Newborns and children are now being given a vaccine to prevent hepatitis B as part of their immunization schedule. It is also recommended for sexually active adults. People involved in both oral and anal sex should also consider a vaccine against hepatitis A. Since 2006, a new HPV vaccine called Gardisil has been available. It protects against four HPV types that together cause seventy percent of cervical cancers and 90 percent of genital warts. The vaccine is given in three shots over six months to girls and women from ages nine to twenty-six.

Getting treated for STDs. Someone diagnosed with an STD should take advantage of the treatments available. Many STDs are curable, and others can be managed. Getting treated will help prevent STDs from being passed on to others. People with STDs also have a responsibility to let their partners know so they can be tested, too.

REFERENCES

1. Centers for Disease Control and Prevention, author. Sexually transmitted diseases treatment guidelines, 2010. MMWR Recomm Rep. 2010; 59 (RR-12).
2. Centers for Disease Control and Prevention, author. Sexually transmitted diseases treatment guidelines, 2006. MMWR Recomm Rep. 2006; 55 (RR-11): 42–49.

CHAPTER 71

Sepsis and Septic Shock

DEFINITIONS

Definitions of terms related to sepsis are given in Table 71.1. Physiologically similar systemic inflammatory response syndrome can be seen even in the absence of identifiable infection.

Table 71.1

Definitions of terms related to sepsis

Condition	Definition
Bacteremia (fungemia)	Presence of viable bacteria (fungi) in the bloodstream.
Infection	Inflammatory response to invasion of normally sterile host tissue by the microorganisms.
Systemic inflammatory response syndrome	Systemic inflammatory response to a variety of clinical insults that can be infection, but can be noninfectious etiology. The response is manifested by two or more of the following conditions: Temperature >38°C (100.4°F) or <36°C (96.8°F); heart rate >90 beats/min; respiratory rate >20 breaths/min or Pa <32 torr; white blood cell count >12,000cells/mm3 CO_2, <4,000 cells/mm3, or >10% immature (band) forms.
Sepsis	Systemic inflammatory response syndrome secondary to infection.
Severe sepsis	Sepsis associated with organ dysfunction, hypoperfusion, or hypotension. Hypoperfusion and perfusion abnormalities may include, but are not limited to, lactic acidosis, oliguria, or acute alteration in mental status.
Septic shock	Sepsis with hypotension, despite fluid resuscitation, along with the presence of perfusion abnormalities. Patients who are on inotropic or vasopressor agents may not be hypotensive at the time perfusion abnormalities are measured.
Multiple-organ dysfunction Syndrome	Presence of altered organ function requiring intervention to maintain homeostasis.
Compensatory antiinflammatory response syndrome	Compensatory physiologic response to systemic inflammatory response syndrome that is considered secondary to the actions of anti-inflammatory cytokine mediators.

PATHOPHYSIOLOGY

The word sepsis originates from the Greek words sepsis meaning to decay and sepein meaning to putrefy. Sepsis, in fact, represents the body's systemic response to severe infection, and is the result of a complex interaction between the host and the invading organism resulting in the release of a myriad of inflammatory mediators. Importantly, it is the presence of an infectious organism which elicits this inflammatory response and infection is therefore implicit in the definition and diagnosis of sepsis. The terms 'infection' and 'sepsis' are often used as synonyms, but their meanings are not the same. Infection is a microbiological event caused by bacteria, fungi, viruses, etc. Sepsis is the systemic response to that infection. Thus, while infection can exist without sepsis, the reverse is not true; genuine sepsis can only be present if there is also an infection (Fig. 71.1). Once sepsis has been diagnosed, septic shock is generally accepted as being the association of sepsis with hypotension (systolic arterial pressure < 90 mmHg, mean arterial pressure < 60 mmHg) requiring vasopressor agents, and signs of tissue hypoperfusion such as increased blood lactate levels, oliguria, altered mentation, etc.

Over the last decade, macrophage migration inhibitory factor (MIF) has emerged to be an important mediator of the innate immune system. Originally discovered as áT-cell cytokine, MIF was identified recently to be released by a vast array of cells, including immune(monocytes/ macrophages, T cells, B cells, eosinophils, mast cells), endocrine (pituitary and adrenal cells) and epithelial cells in response to infection and stress. Bacteria, microbial toxins (LPS, TSST-l,SPEA) and cytokines (TNFα. IFNy) were found to be powerful inducers of MIF secretion by monocytes and macrophages. High blood levels of MIF were measured in mice with bacterial peritonitis and in humans with severe sepsis and septic shock. Immunoneutralization of MIF or deletion of the MIF gene protected mice against lethal endotoxemia, staphylococcal

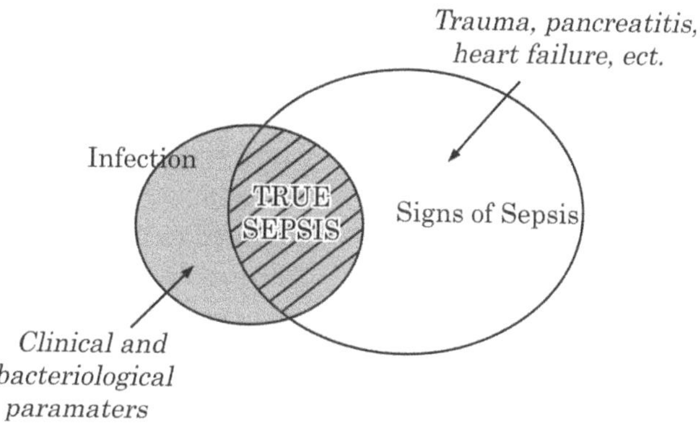

FIGURE 71.1

The interrelation between infection and signs of sepsis.

toxic shock and peritonitis induced by *E. coli* or cecal ligation and puncture. MIF stimulates the expression of pro-inflammatory mediators by immune cells, and thus vigorously promotes inflammatory and immune responses. The surprising observations that MIF release was induced by glucocorticoids and that MIF had the unique feature to override the anti-inflammatory and immunosuppressive effects of glucocorticoids on macrophages and T -cells functions further emphasized the critical regulatory role played by MIF within the immune system.

Primary proinflammatory cytokines like TNF and IL-l induce secondary pro- and antiinflammatory mediators like IL-6 and IL-I0. Both, TNF and IL-l, are capable of inducing the same symptoms in experimental settings as well as in humans . Genetic variations in the TNF and IL-l genes are of major interest given the influences they might have in determining the host's response to endotoxin.

CLINICAL FEATURES

Sepsis is characterized by the presence of a variety of clinical signs, altered biochemical parameters, and typical hemodynamic changes (Table 71.2). However, many of the so-called 'classical' signs of sepsis are also present in patients without infection. For example, fever is a common feature of sepsis, but is also often present in non-infected ICU patients, for example following myocardial infarction or pulmonary embolism, or postoperatively . In addition, some patients with sepsis, may show hypothermia which may, in fact, be associated with a worse outcome . Similarly a raised white cell count is common in sepsis, but again may be caused by other disease processes, and some patients with sepsis will show a reduced white cell count. Thus, none of these signs listed in Table 71.2 is specific for sepsis

Table 71.2

Signs and symptoms associated with sepsis

Early Sepsis	Late Sepsis
Fever or hypothermia Rigors, chills Tachycardia Tachypnea Nausea, vomiting Hyperglycemia Myalgias Lethargy, malaise Proteinuria Hypoxia Leukocytosis Hyperbilirubinemia	Lactic acidosis Oliguria Leukopenia DIC Myocardial depression Pulmonary edema Hypotension (shock) Hypoglycemia Azotemia Thrombocytopenia ARDS Gastrointestinal hemorrhage Coma

DIAGNOSIS (TABLE 71.3)

Inflammatory markers used in the diagnosis of sepsis like C-reactive protein (CRP), are used mostly. CRP has been indicative of infection than the white cell count or fever. CRP levels> 17 mg/dl indicates that separation of patients with sepsis from those with a non-septic inflammatory response due to trauma. Pro calcitonin has also been proposed as a marker of infection . Various other molecules have been suggested as markers of sepsis including neopterin and elastase. However, as with cytokine levels, these are all markers of inflammation rather than infection, and none are specific for sepsis

Table 71.3

Some proposed laboratory markers of sepsis

White blood cell count
C-reactive protein (CRP)
Cytokine levels: INF, IL-6, IL-8, IL- 10, INF receptors,
Procalcitonin
Serum amyloid protein
Neopterin
Elastase
Phospholipase A2
Endothelin-l
Nitrates/nitrites
P-selectinlE-selectin
Prolactin
Lactoferrin
Lipopolysaccharide binding protein

TREATMENT

Beneficial and detrimental actions of Corticosteroids in sepsis Corticosteroids act in many different ways. One of the most critical actions of steroids on the inflammatory process is their inhibitory effect on almost all known cytokines. It is believed that a prolonged and exaggerated release of these inflammatory mediators leads to organ dysfunction and steroids can reverse this process. The major component of the anti-inflammatory action of glucocorticoids may be their inhibition of the nuclear factor kappa B (NF-KB) which activates the cytokine cascade. The inhibition is mediated via the induction of IKBa. Inhibitory protein, which traps activated NF-KB in inactive cytoplasmic complexes . Corticosteroids may also suppress inflammation by increasing the synthesis of anti-inflammatory proteins, such as lipocortin 1, that have inhibitory effects on phospholipase A2, the rate-controlling enzyme governing the release of arachidonic acid from membrane phospholipids. In addition, steroids may inhibit the synthesis of inflammatory mediators through an inhibitory effect on enzyme induction such as the inhibition of the inducible cyc1ooxygenase 2 (COX-2), and by preventing the release of adhesion molecules. There are several mechanisms for the beneficial actions of corticosteroids in sepsis (Table 71.4). The most physiologic benefit of corticosteroids would be replacement of the hormone in adrenal insufficiency. Unfortunately, most patients with severe sepsis and septic shock do not have adrenal insufficiency and many patients have elevated cortisol levels in sepsis. However, septic patients may have relative adrenal insufficiency. Corticosteroids may also act as vasodilators and improve cardiac function. Other metabolic effects of corticosteroids include increased glucagon secretion, liver protein synthesis and gluconeogenesis. Steroids stabilize cell and lysosomal membranes. Steroids have been shown to inhibit complement-induced granulocyte aggregation, disaggregate granulocytes and decrease endothelial cell damage by preventing oxygen-radical production. Corticosteroids also shift the oxyhemoglobin dissociation curve to the right, allowing an increased oxygen availability to the cells. Corticosteroids may also inhibit corticotrophin releasing factor (CRF) which regulates the release of adreno- corticotropic hormone (ACTH) and -endorphin. The latter may depress cardiac function in shock. In fact, adreno-hypothalamo pituitary interactions may be extremely important in the shock response. Corticosteroids restore the receptivity of catecholamine receptors. Glucocorticoids can prevent desensitization of a-adrenergic receptors and decrease the number of down regulated receptors. They may recouple catecholamine induced, desensitized adrenergic receptors and increase adrenergic receptor density in tissues.

Table 71.4

Beneficial actions of corticosteroids in sepsis

Improve decreased adrenal function
Improve myocardial performance
Stimulate gluconeogenesis
Stabilize lysosomal and cell membranes
Inhibit complement-induced granulocyte aggregation and prevent oxygen radical mediated injury
Rightward shift in oxygen-hemoglobin dissociation curve
Interaction with endorphins
Enhance adrenergic receptivity

Despite the potential beneficial actions of corticosteroids, there are also detrimental effects, especially when steroids are given in high doses for long periods of time (Table 71.5). In humans, complications have included superinfections, hyperglycemia, gastrointestinal bleeding, electrolyte disturbances, psychosis and arrhythmias.

Table 71.5

Detrimental actions of corticosteroids in sepsis

Inhibit of neutrophilic bactericidal competency
Interfere with phagocytosis of antigens and subsequent intracellular digestion
Inhibition migration of cells to areas of inflammation
Large doses suppress cell-mediated hypersensitivity
Inhibit antigen processing by macro phages
Inhibit inflammatory response after antigen-antibody union

MEDIATOR- SPECIFIC ANTI-INFLAMMATORY THERAPY IN SEPSIS

The pro inflammatory mediator thought primarily responsible and therefore most implicated was tumor necrosis factor-a (TNF-α). There have been nine published trials of monoclonal antibodies to TNF-α, enrolling over 4000 patients. In addition, three published trials used soluble tumor necrosis factor receptors (sTNFr) to limit the effects of circulating TNF-α.

INTERLEUKIN-L RECEPTOR ANTAGONISTS

Interleukin-l is another pro-inflammatory cytokine that when administered to humans or animals can reproduce many of the manifestations of the sepsis syndrome. Interleukin-l receptor antagonist (ILI ra) is a protein produced by macrophages, which binds to interleukin receptors, thus limiting the biologic activity of interleukin-l. These IL-l inhibitors were given in three clinical trials in patients with sepsis and septic shock.

ANTI-ENDOTOXIN THERAPY IN SEPSIS

Endotoxin, a lipopolysaccaride present on the outer cell wall of gram negative bacteria, has been offered as a key mediator in the development of the sepsis syndrome and septic shock. Endotoxin is composed of two antigens, a highly conserved lipid -A moiety, which appears to cause many of the toxic effects of the molecule, and an 0- side chain. Infusion of endotoxin into experimental animals and normal human volunteers can reproduce many of the hemodynamic manifestations of the sepsis syndrome. Some have hypothesized that endotoxin may be important not only in patients with gram-negative sepsis but in those with gram-positive sepsis also. In such patients, inadequate perfusion of the gut mucosa during grampositive infection could allow endotoxin from gut flora to enter the systemic circulation, and thereby worsen the cardiovascular abnormalities. Thus endotoxin might be a therapeutic target not only in patients with gram negative infections, but possibly in all types of shock associated with inadequate gut perfusion. The first studies of anti-endotoxin agents used antiserum or polyclonal antibodies directed at common epitopes among gram-negative bacteria.

AT THE EARLY PHASE OF SEPSIS

TOLL-LIKE RECEPTORS

Gram-negative bacteria endotoxin binds to a specific plasma acute phase protein (lipopolysaccharide-binding protein, LBP), and this complex binds the macrophage membrane CDI4 receptor. Endotoxin is then presented to another receptor, recently identified as Toll-like receptor (TLR), which promotes transmembrane signaling . Gram-positive organisms can trigger sepsis by superantigens and, more frequently, by cell wall components that bind to another member of the TLR family, TLR2. TLRs and CDI4 represent attractive therapeutic targets, since their blockade may blunt cytokine release in response to both gram-negative and gram-positive bacteria.

FILTRATION OF MEDIATORS

Blood purification via mechanical filtration has also been proposed as a therapy in sepsis. It has been hypothesized that an excessive inflammatory response could be neutralized with hemofiltration, especially using high flow and large-pore hemofilters. However, the evidence for the clinically effective elimination of inflammatory mediators, as well as evidence for a beneficial effect of hemofiltration on outcome remains poor . In contrast, plasma filtration coupled with adsorption techniques may be more efficient for the removal of endotoxin and cytokines.

INHIBITORS OF INDUCIBLE NITRIC OXIDE SYNTHASE (INOS)

Nitric oxide (NO), a free radical gas produced by numerous cell types, isimplicated in a wide range of disease processes, exerting both detrimental and beneficial effects . NO is synthesized intracellularly by the oxidation of L-arginine as catalyzed by nitric oxide synthases (NOS). These enzymes exist in a constitutive and calciumdependent (cNOS) form and in an inducible and calcium independent (iNOS) one. iNOS expression can be induced by specific pro inflammatory agents in many types of cells. Once produced, NO can react with the superoxide anion to form peroxynitrite (ONOO-), a powerful oxidant with toxic effects on many molecules including nucleic acids, lipids and proteins. In different animal models, sepsis has been shown to increase the constitutive release of NO by the endothelium and the activity of the iNOS enzyme . In such conditions, limiting the indirect effects of NO may be a viable therapeutic option .

A viable strategy to modulate the effects of NO should protect its positive effects while eradicating its negative ones. Selective iNOS inhibitors may achieve this better than nonselective agents, but these compounds have not undergone clinical testing yet. It may be that different agents are needed at different times during the septic process. Other approaches include therapies aimed at limiting peroxynitrite generation (e.g. scavengers). Such agents should be efficient in removing excess NO, superoxide anion and peroxynitrite.

OXYGEN FREE RADICAL SCAVENGERS

Excessive production of oxygen free radicals are implicated in endothelial cell damage and multiple organ failure during septic shock. endogenous antioxidant like N acetylcysteine is used. It has been used with promising results in patients with septic shock.

COAGULATION/FIBRINOLYSIS PATHWAY

During sepsis, bacterial components and pro-inflammatory cytokines causes the tissue factor expression.This promotes the activation of the extrinsic coagulation pathway and the consumption of coagulation factors and their endogenous inhibitors, leading to disseminated intravascular coagulation (DIC). Thrombosis of the microvasculature associated with DIC is currently believed to play a significant role in organ dysfunction related to sepsis. Regulatory mechanisms that prevent coagulation from being generalized under normal conditions involve tissue factor pathway inhibitor (TFPI), antithrombin III (AT III), and protein C.

TFPI is an endogenous antagonist of the extrinsic pathway of coagulation that inhibits factor Xa directly and the factor Vlla/TF catalytic complex. Administration of TFPI improved survival and organ function when given to rabbits with septic peritonitis and to baboons infused with E.coli. It was effective even when given several hours after the insult and in doses lacking significant anticoagulant effect. TFPI was found to also exhibit anti-inflammatory activities as reflected by decreases of IL-6 and IL-8 plasma levels in the treated animals. It is well tolerated in human volunteers, although high doses increased thromboplastin time. In contrast to a high dose pilot study, a new phase II study using low doses was not associated with bleeding complications, and showed a trend toward improvement of survival.

COMPLEMENT BLOCKADE

It is generally accepted that the complement network that works through generation of the opsonic factor, C3b, which promotes phagocytosis and intracellular killing of bacteria provides essential protection against bacteria . The low molecular- weight anaphylatoxin C5a is a potent agonist for neutrophils and endothelial cells, and increases vasodilation and vascular permeability.

AT THE LATE PHASE OF SEPSIS

LOW DOSES OF GLUCOCORTICOIDS

Small randomized studies provided the theoretical basis for the use of low-doses of glucocorticoids during the late phase of sepsis.

MACROPHAGE MIGRATION INHIBITORY FACTOR (MIF)

MIF, a pleiotropic cytokine released by macrophages, T cells and the pituitary gland has emerged as a pivotal cytokine in the innate immune system. It is capable of overriding the "anti-inflammatory" effects of glucocorticoids. Once released, MIF induces the expression of pro inflammatory releasers and causes promotion of inflammatory and immune responses.

Neutralization of MIF prevented death. The progressive appearance of MIF in peritoneal fluid and blood may explain the MIF treatment is efficacious when given for post-infection.

HIGH MOBILITY GROUP-L (HMG-L)

High mobility group-1 (HMG-1) protein was found to be released by cultured macrophages more than 8 hours after stimulation with endotoxin, TNF, or IL-1. Delayed administration of antibodies to HMG-1 attenuated endotoxin lethality in mice. Septic patients who succumbed to infection had increased serum HMG-1 levels.

Table 71.6

Empiric antimicrobial regimens in sepsis

Infection (Site or Type)	Antimicrobial Regimen		
	Community-Acquired	Hospital-Acquired	
Urinary tract	Ciprofloxacin or levofloxacin	Ciprofloxacin, levofloxacin or ceftazidime, ceftriaxone	± gentamicin
Respiratory tract	Newer fluoroquinolones ceftriaxone + clarithromycin/ azithromycin	Piperacillin, ceftazidime, or cefepime	+ gentamicin or ciprofloxacin
Intraabdominal	ß-Lactamase inhibitor combo[b] or ciprofloxacin + metronidazole	Piperacillin/tazobactam or carbapenem	
Skin/soft tissue	Vancomycin or linezolid or daptomycin	ß-Lactamase inhibitor combo b or clindamycin plus ciprofloxacin or carbapenem	
Catheter-related Unknown		Vancomycin Piperacillin or ceftazidime/cefepime or imipenem/meropenem	+ gentamicin ± vancomycin

Vancomycin should be added whenever the risk of methicillin-resistant staphylococci is significant.

- The average duration of antimicrobial therapy in the normal host with sepsis is 10 to 14 days.
- Suspected systemic mycotic infection leading to sepsis in neutropenic and critically ill patients should be empirically treated with parenteral Amphotericin B or caspofungin, especially if the patient is clinically unstable.

HEMODYNAMIC SUPPORT

- Maintenance of adequate tissue oxygenation is important in the treatment of sepsis and is dependent on adequate perfusion and adequate oxygenation of the blood.
- Rapid fluid resuscitation is the best initial therapeutic intervention for treatment of hypotension in sepsis. The goal is to maximize cardiac output by increasing the left ventricular preload, which will ultimately restore tissue perfusion.
- Fluid administration should be titrated to clinical endpoints such as heart rate, urine output, blood pressure, and mental status. Isotonic crystalloids, such as 0.9% sodium chloride or lactated Ringer's solution, are commonly used for fluid resuscitation.
- Iso-oncotic colloid solutions (plasma and plasma protein fractions), such as 5% albumin and 6% hetastarch, offer the advantage of more rapid restoration of intravascular volume with less volume infused, but there is no significant clinical outcome differences compared with crystalloids. Clinical outcome differences with the use of crystalloids or colloids have not been demonstrated, so crystalloids are generally recommended.

INOTROPE AND VASOACTIVE DRUG SUPPORT

- When fluid resuscitation is insufficient to maintain tissue perfusion, the use of inotropes and vasoactive drugs is necessary. Selection and dosage are based on the pharmacologic properties of various catecholamines and how they influence hemodynamic parameters .
- **Suggested Protocol for the Use of Inotropes and Vasoactive Agents**
- **Norepinephrine** is a potent-α adrenergic agent (0.01 to 3 mcg/kg/min) that is useful as a vasopressor to restore adequate blood pressure after failure to restore adequate blood pressure and organ perfusion with appropriate fluid resuscitation.
- **Dopamine** in doses greater than 5 mcg/kg/min is used to support blood pressure and to increase cardiac index. Low dose dopamine (1 to 5 mcg/kg/min) is not effective to increase renal and mesenteric perfusion.
- **Dobutamine** (in doses of 2 to 20 mcg/kg/min) is an α-adrenergic inotropic agent that many clinicians prefer for improving cardiac output and oxygen delivery. Dobutamine should be considered in severely septic patients with adequate filling pressures and blood pressure but low cardiac index.
- **Epinephrine**, in doses of 0.1 to 0.5 mcg/kg/min, increases cardiac index and produces peripheral vasoconstriction. It is reserved for patients who fail to respond to traditional therapies.
- Before administering vasoactive agents, aggressive appropriate fluid resuscitation should occur. Vasoactive agents should not be considered an acceptable alternative to volume resuscitation.
- Administration of activated protein C (**drotrecogin**) to promote fibrinolysis and associated antiinflammatory mechanisms may be beneficial in patients with an **APACHE II** (Acute Physiology and Chronic Health Evaluation II) score greater than 25. This agent reduced

mortality in severe sepsis but poses an increased risk of serious bleeding.

REFERENCES

1. Nguyen, H.B., Smith, D. Sepsis in the 21st century: recent definitions and therapeutic advances. Am J Emerg Med. 2007;25:564–571.
2. Cohen, J. et al. Diagnosis of infection in sepsis: an evidence-based review. Crit Care Med. 2004;32:S466–S494.
3. Marshall, J.C. et al. Source control in the management of severe sepsis and septic shock: an evidence-based review. Crit Care Med. 2004;32:S513–S526.

CHAPTER 72

Malaria

It is an acute infectious disease caused by four species of the protozoal genus Plasmodium. The parasite is transmitted to humans through the bite of a female Anopheles mosquito, which thrives in humid, swampy areas. Plasmodium falciparum is the most dangerous species, causing an acute, rapidly fulminating disease that is characterized by persistent high fever, orthostatic hypotension, and massive erythrocytosis (an abnormal elevation in the number of red blood cells accompanied by swollen and reddish condition of the limbs). Plasmodium falciparum infection can lead to capillary obstruction and death if treatment is not instituted promptly. Plasmodium vivax causes a milder form of the disease. Plasmodium malariae is common to many tropical regions, but Plasmodium ovale is rarely encountered. Resistance acquired by the mosquito to insecticides, and by the parasite to drugs, has led to new therapeutic challenges, particularly in the treatment of Plasmodium falciparum.

PREVALENCE

Malaria is presently endemic in a broad band around the equator, in areas of the Americas, many parts of Asia, and much of Africa: however, it is in sub-Saharan Africa where 85%–90% of malaria fatalities occur. The geographic distribution of malaria within large regions is complex, and malaria-afflicted and malaria-free areas are often found close to each other. Malaria is prevalent in tropical regions because of the significant amounts of rainfall, consistent high temperatures and high humidity, along with stagnant waters in which mosquito larvae readily mature, providing them with the environment they need for continuous breeding.

MALARIA TRANSMISSION LIFE CYCLE

When an infected mosquito bites, it injects Plasmodium sporozoites into the bloodstream (Fig. 72.1). The sporozoites migrate through the blood to the liver, where they form cyst-like structures containing thousands of merozoites. [Note: Diagnosis depends on laboratory identification of the parasites in red blood cells of peripheral blood smears]. Upon release, each merozoite invades a red blood cell, becoming a trophozoite and using hemoglobin as a nutrient. The trophozoite multiplies and become merozoites. Eventually, the infected cell ruptures, releasing heme and merozoites that can enter other erythrocytes. [Note: Alternatively, released merozoites can become gametocytes, which are picked up by mosquitoes from the blood they ingest.

The cycle thus begins again, with the gametocytes becoming sporozoites in the insect]. The effectiveness of a drug treatment is related to the particular species of infecting plasmodium and the stage of its

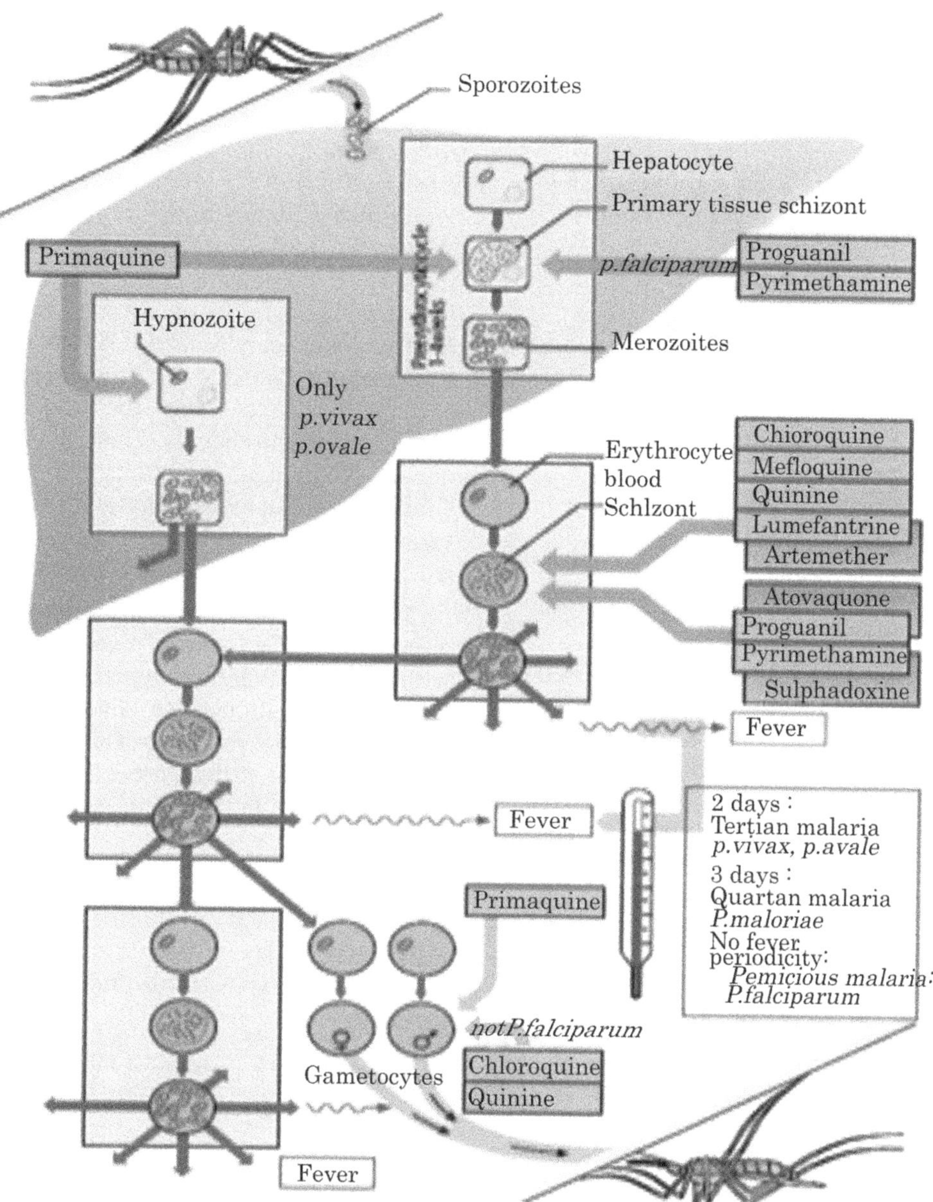

FIGURE 72.1

Life cycle plasmodium falciparum.

Source : Colour Atlas Of Pharmacology ,3rd edition ,Page no.295)

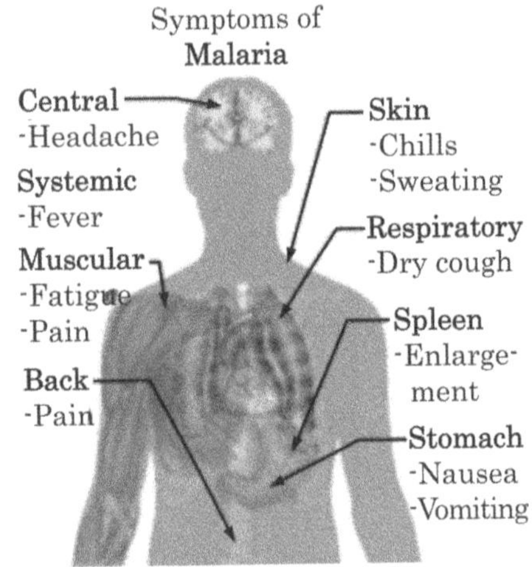

FIGURE 72.2

Symptoms of malaria.

(Source : WebMD > Malaria symptoms Last Updated: May 16, 2007)

life cycle that is targeted.

- Sporozoites → tissue schizonts (in liver) → merozoites infect RBC (blood schizonts) → rupture of RBC (clinical attack) → new crops of merozoites
- Sexual form: some merozoites differentiate into male & female gametocytes α ingested by a mosquito where they form sporozoitesà human

CLINICAL FEATURES

- Malaria infection is generally characterized by recurrent attacks with the following signs and symptoms: (Fig. 72.2)
- Moderate to severe shaking chills, high fever, profuse sweating as body temperature falls, Headache, nausea, vomiting, diarrhea
- Malaria signs and symptoms typically begin within a few weeks after a bite from an infected mosquito. However, some types of malaria parasites can lie dormant in your body for months, or even years.

ETIOLOGY

Malaria parasites are members of thegenus *Plasmodium* (phylum Apicomplexa). In humans malaria is caused by *Plasmodium falciparum*, *Plasmodium malariae*, *Plasmodium ovale*, *Plasmodium vivax* and *Plasmodium knowlesi*. While *Plasmodium vivax* is responsible for the largest number of malaria infections worldwide, infections by *Plasmodium falciparum* account for about 90% of deaths from malaria. Parasitic *Plasmodium* species also infect birds, reptiles, monkeys, chimpanzees and rodents. There have been documented human infections with several simian species of malaria: however, with the exception of *Plasmodium knowlesi*, these are mostly of limited public health importance.

Malaria parasites contain apicoplasts, an organelle usually found in plants, complete with their own functioning genomes. These apicoplast are thought to have originated through the endosymbiosis of algae and play a crucial role in various aspects of parasite metabolism e.g. fatty acid bio-synthesis.

OTHER MODES OF TRANSMISSION

Because the parasites that cause malaria affect red blood cells, people can also catch malaria from exposures to infected blood, including:

From mother to unborn child, through blood transfusions, by sharing needles used to inject drugs

Risk factors: The biggest risk factor for developing malaria is to live in or to visit tropical areas where the disease is common. Many different subtypes of malaria parasites exist. The variety that causes the most lethal complications is most commonly found in:

- African countries south of the Sahara desert, The Indian subcontinent , Solomon islands, Papua New Guinea and Haiti

RISKS OF MORE SEVERE DISEASE

People at increased risk of serious disease include:

- Young children and infants, travelers coming from areas with no malaria, pregnant women and their unborn children

Poverty, lack of knowledge, and little or no access to health care also contribute to malaria deaths worldwide.

IMMUNITY CAN WANE

Residents of a malaria region may be exposed to the disease so frequently that they acquire a partial immunity, which can lessen the severity of malaria symptoms. However, this partial immunity can disappear if we move to a country where you're no longer frequently exposed to the parasite.

COMPLICATIONS

In most cases, malaria deaths are related to one or more of these serious complications:

- **Cerebral malaria.** If parasite filled blood cells block small blood vessels of the brain (cerebral malaria), swelling of the brain or brain damage may occur.
- **Breathing problems.** Accumulated fluid in the lungs (pulmonary edema) can make it difficult to breathe.
- **Organ failure.** Malaria can cause the kidneys or liver to fail, or spleen to rupture. Any of these conditions can be life--- - threatening.

Severe anemia. Malaria damages red blood cells, which can result in severe anemia.

- **Low blood sugar.** Severe forms of malaria itself can cause low blood sugar, as can quinine - one of the most common medications used to combat malaria. Very low blood sugar can result in coma or death.

RECURRENCE MAY OCCUR

Some varieties of the malaria parasite, which typically cause milder forms of the disease, can persist for years and cause relapses.

Diagnosis: Blood tests can help tailor treatment by determining:

- Whether the person have malaria
- Which type of malaria parasite is causing the symptoms
- If the infection is caused by a parasite resistant to certain drugs
- Whether the disease is affecting any of the vital organs

Some blood tests can take several days to complete, while others can produce results in less than 15 minutes.

TREATMENT (TABLE 72.1)

TISSUE SCHIZONTICIDE: PRIMAQUINE

Primaquine [PRIM-a-kwin] is an 8-aminoquinoline that eradicates primary exoerythrocytic forms of *Plasmodium falciparum* and *Plasmodium vivax* and the secondary exoerythrocytic forms of recurring malarias (*Plasmodium vivax* and *Plasmodium ovale*). [Note: Primaquine is the only agent that can lead to radical cures of the *Plasmodium vivax* and *Plasmodium ovale* malarias, which may remain in the liver in the exoerythrocytic form after the erythrocytic form of the disease is eliminated.] The sexual (gametocytic) forms of all four plasmodia are destroyed in the plasma or are prevented from maturing later in the mosquito, thus interrupting the transmission of the disease. [Note: Primaquine is not effective against the erythrocytic stage of malaria and, therefore, is often used in conjunction with a blood schizonticide, such as chloroquine, quinine, mefloquine, or pyrimethamine.]

- ***Mechanism of action***: This is not completely understood. Metabolites of primaquine are believed to act as oxidants that are responsible for the schizonticidal action as well as for the hemolysis and methemoglobinemia encountered as toxicities.
- ***Adverse effects***: Primaquine has a low incidence of adverse effects, except for drug-induced hemolytic anemia in patients with genetically low levels of glucose-6-phosphate dehydrogenase. Other toxic manifestations observed after large doses of the drug include abdominal discomfort, especially when administered in combination with chloroquine (which may affect patient compliance), and occasional methemoglobinemia. Granulocytopenia and agranulocytosis are rarely seen, except in patients with lupus or arthritis (both conditions are aggravated by the drug). Primaquine is contraindicated during pregnancy. All Plasmodium species may develop resistance to primaquine.

BLOOD SCHIZONTICIDE: CHLOROQUINE

Chloroquine [KLOR-oh-kwin] is a synthetic 4-aminoquinoline that has been the mainstay of antimalarial therapy, and it is the drug of choice in the treatment of erythrocytic *Plasmodium falciparum* malaria, except in resistant strains. Chloroquine is less effective against *Plasmodium vivax* malaria. It is highly specific for the asexual form of plasmodia. Chloroquine is also effective in the treatment of extra intestinal amebiasis. [Note: The anti-inflammatory action of chloroquine explains its occasional use in rheumatoid arthritis and discoid lupus erythematosus.]

- ***Mechanism of action:*** Although a detailed explanation of the mechanisms by which chloroquine kills plasmodial parasites is still incomplete, the following processes are essential for the drug's lethal action. After traversing the erythrocytic and plasmodial membranes, chloroquine (a diprotic weak base) is concentrated in the organism's acidic food vacuole, primarily by ion trapping. It is in the food vacuole that the parasite digests the host cell's hemoglobin to obtain essential amino acids. However, this process also releases large amounts of soluble heme (ferriprotoporphyrin IX), which is toxic to the parasite. To protect itself, the parasite ordinarily polymerizes the heme to hemozoin (a pigment), which is sequestered in the parasite's food vacuole. Chloroquine specifically binds to heme, preventing its polymerization to hemozoin. The increased pH and the accumulation of heme result in oxidative damage to the membranes, leading to lysis of both the parasite and the red blood cell. The binding to heme and prevention of its polymerization appear to be a crucial step in the drug's antiplasmodial activity, and this may represent a unifying mechanism for such diverse compounds as chloroquine, quinidine, and mefloquine.

Adverse effects: Side effects are minimal at the low doses used in the chem suppression of malaria. At higher doses, many more toxic effects occur, such as gastrointestinal upset, pruritus, headaches, and blurring of vision. [Note: An ophthalmologic examination should be routinely performed.] Discoloration of the nail beds and mucous membranes may be seen on chronic administration. Chloroquine should be used cautiously in patients with hepatic dysfunction or severe gastrointestinal problems or in patients with neurologic or blood disorders. Chloroquine can cause electrocardiographic changes, because it has a quinidine-like effect. It may also exacerbate dermatitis produced by gold or phenylbutazone therapy. [Note: Patients with psoriasis or porphyria should not be treated with chloroquine, because an acute attack may be provoked.]

- ***Resistance:*** Resistance of plasmodia to available drugs has become a serious medical problem throughout Africa, Asia, and most areas of Central and South America. Chloroquine-resistant *Plasmodium falciparum* exhibit multigenic alterations that confer a high level of resistance. [Note: When a chloroquine-resistant organism is encountered, therapy usually consists of an orally administered combination of quinine, pyrimethamine, and a sulphonamide, such as sulphadoxine.]

BLOOD SCHIZONTICIDE: MEFLOQUINE

Mefloquine [MEF-lo-kween] appears to be promising as an effective single agent for suppressing and curing infections caused by multidrug-resistant forms of *Plasmodium falciparum*. Its exact mechanism of action remains to be determined, but like quinine, it can apparently damage the parasite's membrane. Resistant strains have been identified. Mefloquine is absorbed well after oral administration and concentrates in the liver and lung. It has a long half-life (17 days) because of its concentration in various tissues and its continuous circulation through the enterohepatic and enterogastric systems. The drug undergoes extensive metabolism. Its major excretory route is the feces. Adverse reactions at high doses range from nausea, vomiting, and dizziness to disorientation, hallucinations, and depression. Electrocardiographic abnormalities and cardiac arrest are possible if mefloquine is taken concurrently with quinine or quinidine.

BLOOD SCHIZONTICIDES: QUININE AND QUINIDINE

Quinine [KWYE-nine] and its stereoisomer, quinidine [KWIH-ni-deen], interfere with heme polymerization, resulting in death of the erythrocytic form of the plasmodial parasite. These drugs are reserved for severe infestations and for malarial strains that are resistant to other agents, such as chloroquine. Taken orally, quinine is well distributed throughout the body and can reach the fetus. Alkalinization of the urine decreases its excretion. The major adverse effect of quinine is Cinchonism a syndrome causing nausea, vomiting, tinnitus, and vertigo. These effects are reversible and are not considered to be reasons for suspending therapy. However, quinine treatment should be suspended if a positive Coombs' test for hemolytic anemia occurs. Drug interactions include potentiation of neuromuscular-blocking agents and elevation of digoxin levels if taken concurrently with quinine. Quinine absorption is retarded when the drug is taken with aluminum-containing antacids. Quinine is fetotoxic.

BLOOD SCHIZONTICIDE: ARTEMISININ

Artemisinin [ar-te-MIS-in-in] is derived from the qinghaosu plant, which has been used in Chinese medicine for more than two millennia in the treatment of fevers and malaria. Artemisinin (or one of its derivatives) is available for the treatment of severe, multidrug-resistant *Plasmodium falciparum* malaria. Its antimalarial action involves the production of free radicals within the plasmodium food vacuole, following cleavage of the drug's endoperoxide bridge by heme iron in parasitized erythrocytes. It is also believed to covalently bind to and damage specific malarial proteins. Oral, rectal, and intravenous preparations are available, but the short half-lives preclude their use in chemoprophylaxis. They are metabolized in

Table 72.1

Dosage of antimalarials

Recommend Drug	Adults	Children
Mefloquine	(I tablet = 250 mg mefloquine) 250 mg (1 tablet) every 7 days, starting 1 week before entering the area, once weekly while in the area, and once weekly for 4 weeks after leaving the area. Restrict use to 1 year.	Not recommended for children who are less than 3 months old or who weigh less than 5kg. Weight (kg) Dosage 5 – 20 ¼ tablet 21 – 30 ½ tablet 31 – 45 ¾ : tablet > 45 Adult dose
Doxycycline	(1 tablet = 100 mg doxycycline) (1 capsule = 50mg, 100 mg or 200 mg doxycycline) 100mg once daily starting one day before entering the area, continuing daily while in the area, and daily for 4 weeks after leaving the area. Not to be used for longer than 4-6 months.	Contraindicated in children under 8 years. 2mg/kg of body weight at the same intervals as for adults. Age (years) Weight (kg) Dosage 8 – 15 31 – 45 2 mg/kg > 15 > 45 Adult dose
OR		
Chloroquine	(1 tablet = 150 mg chloroquine base) 300mg base (2 tablets) once every 7 days, starting at least one day before entering the area, but preferable one week before, once wekly while in the area, and once weekly for 4 weeks after leaving the area.	5 mg/kg of body weight taken at the same intervals as for adults. Age (year) Weight (kg) Dosage <1 < 10 ¼ - ½ tab 1 – 4 10 – 19 ½ tablet 5 – 8 20 – 30 1 tablet 9 – 15 31 – 45 1 ½ tablets > 15 > 45 Adult dose Two strengths of chloroquine syrup are available for children (37.5 mg chloroquine base per 5 ml and 50mg chloroquine base per 5 ml). The dose is 5 mg/kg to be taken at the same intervals as for adults. See package insert for dosages.
PLUS Proguanil	(1 tablet = 100mg proguanil) 200mg (2 tablets) daily starting 1 day before entering the area, continuing daily while in the area and daily for 4 weeks after leaving the area.	3mg/kg of body weight at the same intervals as for adults Age (years) weight (kg) Dosage <1 <10 ¼ tablet 1-4 0-19 ½ tablet 5-8 20-30 1 tablet 9-15 31-45 1 ½ tablets > 15 > 45 Adult dose

Table 72.1 *Cont...*

Recommend Drug	Adults	Children
Atovaquone – Proguanil not yet registered in south Africa	1 adult tablet = 250mg atovaquone plus 100mg proguanil. It should be taken 1 day before exposure, continued daily during exposure and for 7 days after the last exposure to malaria.	1 paediatric tablet = 62.5 atovaquone plus 25mg proguanil 11-20kg 1 paediatric tablet daily 21 – 30kg 2 paediatric tablet daily 31 – 40kg 3 paediatric tablet daily > 40kg 1 adult tablet daily
STANDBY THERAPY		
Artemether-lumefantrine 1 tablet contains artemether 20mg plus lumefantrine 120mg.	10- < 15kg : One tablet stat, followed by one after 8 hours and then one twice daily on each of the following two days (total course = 6 tablets) 15 - <25kg : Two tablets stat, followed by two after 8 hours and then two twice daily on each of the following two days (total course = 12 tablets) 25 - <35kg : Three tablets stat, followed by three after 8 hours and then three twice daily on each of the following two days (total course = 18 tablets) 35 - <65 kg : Four tablets stat, followed by four after 8 hours and then four twice daily on each of the following two days (total course = 24 tablets)	

the liver and are excreted primarily in the bile. Adverse effects include nausea, vomiting, and diarrhea, but overall, artemisinin is remarkably safe. Extremely high doses may cause neurotoxicity and prolongation of the QT interval.

BLOOD SCHIZONTICIDE AND SPORONTOCIDE: PYRIMETHAMINE

The antifolate agent pyrimethamine [peer-i-METH-a-meen] is frequently employed to effect a radical cure as a blood schizonticide. It also acts as a strong sporontocide in the mosquito's gut when the mosquito ingests it with the blood of the human host. Pyrimethamine inhibits plasmodial dihydrofolate Reductase at much lower concentrations than those needed to inhibit the mammalian enzyme. The inhibition deprives the protozoan of tetrahydrofolate"a cofactor required in the de novo biosynthesis of purines and pyrimidines and in the interconversions of certain amino acids. Pyrimethamine alone is effective against *Plasmodium falciparum*. In combination with a sulphonamide, it is also used against *Plasmodium malariae* and *Toxoplasma gondii*. If megaloblastic anemia occurs with pyrimethamine treatment, it may be reversed with leucovorin shows some therapeutic options in the treatment of malaria.

PREVENTION

REDUCING EXPOSURE TO MOSQUITOES

In countries where malaria is common, prevention also involves keeping mosquitoes away from humans. Strategies include:

- **Spraying your home.** Treating home's walls with insecticide can help kill adult mosquitoes that come inside.
- **Sleeping under a net.** Bed nets, particularly those treated with insecticide, are especially recommended for pregnant women and young children.
- **Covering skin.** During active mosquito times, usually from dusk to dawn, wear pants and long -sleeved shirts.

Spraying clothing and skin. Sprays containing permethrin are safe to use on clothing, while sprays containing DEET can be used on skin.

REFERENCES

1. Adjuik M et al. Artesunate combinations for treatment of malaria: Meta-analysis. Lancet 2004:363:9.
2. Baird JK: Effectiveness of antimalarial drugs. N Engl J Med 2005:352:1565.
3. Barnes KI et al. Efficacy of rectal artesunate compared with parenteral quinine in initial treatment of moderately severe malaria in African children and adults: A randomized study. Lancet 2004:363:1598.
4. Dorsey G et al. Sulphadoxine/pyrimethamine alone or with amodiaquine or artesunate for treatment of uncomplicated malaria: A longitudinal randomized trial. Lancet 2002:360:2031.
4. Guerin PJ et al. Malaria: Current status of control, diagnosis, treatment, and a proposed agenda for research and development. Lancet Infect Dis 2002:2:564.
5. Lang T, Greenwood B: The development of Lapdap, an affordable new treatment for malaria. Lancet Infect Dis 2003:3:162.

CHAPTER 73

Filaria

DEFINITION

Filariasis (philariasis) is a parasitic disease and is considered an infectious tropical disease, that is caused by thread-like nematodes (roundworms) belonging to the superfamily *Filarioidea*, also known as "filariae". These are transmitted from host to host by blood-feeding arthropods, mainly black flies and mosquitoes.

PREVALENCE

Filariasis is considered endemic in tropical and subtropical regions of Asia, Africa, Central and South America and Pacific Island nations, with more than 120 million people infected and one billion people at risk for infection. In communities where lymphatic Filariasis is endemic, as many as 10% of women can be afflicted with swollen limbs and 50% of men can suffer from mutilating genital symptoms. Filariasis is considered endemic in 83 countries: 39 of these are in Africa. In the Americas, it is present in seven countries: Brazil, Costa Rica, Dominican Republic, Guyana, Haiti, Suriname and Trinidad and Tobago.

In the Middle East, it is present in three countries: Egypt, Sudan and Yemen. In Asia, it is present in Bangladesh, Cambodia, India, South Korea, Indonesia, Laos, Malaysia, Maldives, the Philippines, Sri Lanka, Thailand, Timor-Leste and Vietnam.

ETIOLOGY

Eight known filarial nematodes use humans as their definitive hosts. These are divided into three groups according to the niche within the body they occupy: 'lymphatic Filariasis', 'Subcutaneous Filariasis', and 'Serous Cavity Filariasis'.

- ***Lymphatic Filariasis*** is caused by the worms *Wuchereria bancrofti*, *Brugia malayi*, and *Brugia timori*. These worms occupy the lymphatic system, including the lymph nodes, and in chronic cases these worms lead to the disease elephantiasis.
- ***Subcutaneous Filariasis*** is caused by *Loa loa* (the eye worm), *Mansonella streptocerca*, and *Onchocerca vol-vulus*. These worms occupy the subcutaneous layer of the skin, in the fat layer. *Loa loa*causes *Loa loa* filariasis while *Onchocerca volvulus* causes river blindness.
- ***Serous cavity Filariasis*** is caused by the worms *Mansonella perstans* and *Mansonella ozzardi*, which occupy the serous cavity of the abdomen.

PATHOPHYSIOLOGY

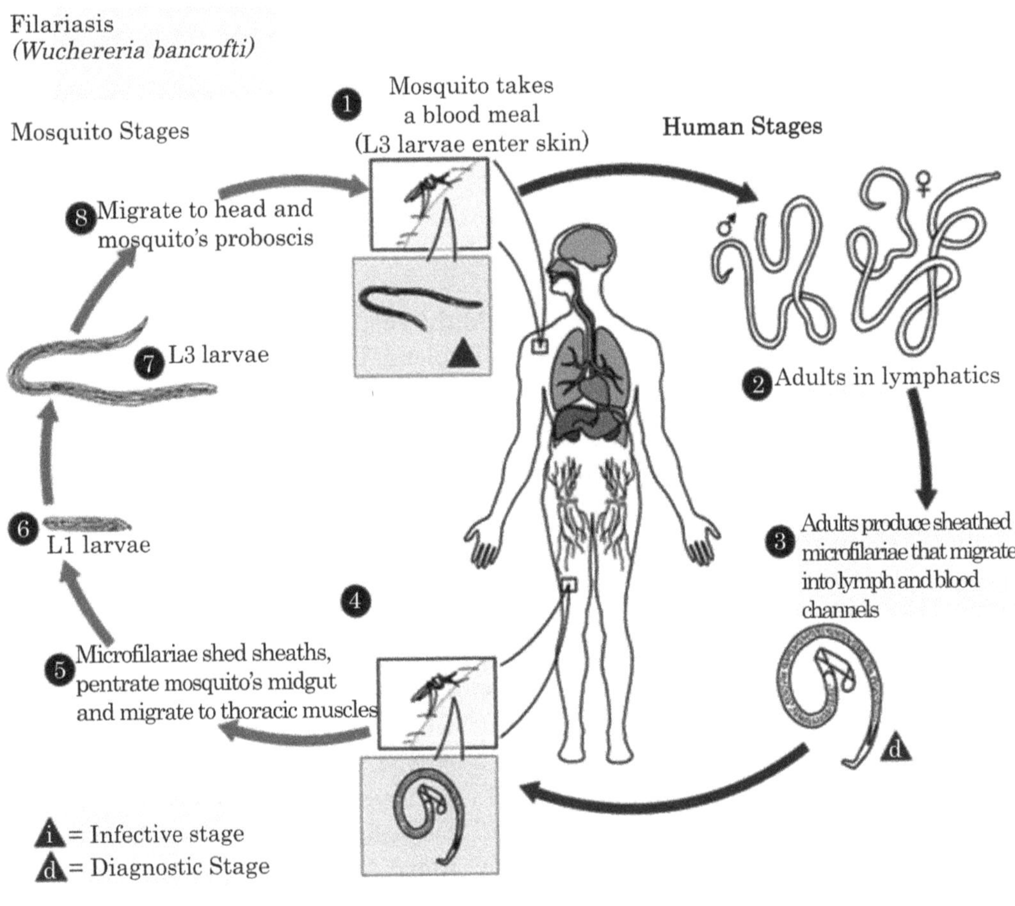

FIGURE 73.1

Wuchereria bancrofti life cycle.

(Source : http://www.parasitesinhumans.org/wuchereria-bancrofti-lymphatic-filariasis.html)

Human filarial nematode worms have complicated life cycles, which primarily consists of five stages. After the male and female worms mate, the female gives birth to live microfilariae by the thousands. The microfilariae are taken up by the vector insect (intermediate host) during a blood meal. In the intermediate host, the microfilariae molt and develop into third-stage (infective) larvae. Upon taking another blood meal, the vector insect injects the infectious larvae into the dermis layer of the skin. After about one year, the larvae molt through two more stages, maturing into the adult worms (Fig. 73.1).

Individuals infected by filarial worms may be described as either "microfilaraemic" or "amicrofilaraemic", depending on whether or not microfilaria can be found in their peripheral blood. Filariasis is diagnosed in microfilaraemic cases primarily through direct observation of microfilaria in the peripheral blood. Occult Filariasis is diagnosed in amicrofilaraemic cases based on clinical observations and, in some cases, by finding a circulating antigen in the blood.

CLINICAL FEATURES

The most spectacular symptom of lymphatic Filariasis is elephantiasis-edema with thickening of the skin and underlying tissues-which was the first disease discovered to be transmitted by mosquito bites. Elephantiasis results when the parasites lodge in the lymphatic system.

Elephantiasis affects mainly the lower extremities, while the ears, mucous membranes, and amputation stumps are affected less frequently. However, different species of filarial worms tend to affect different parts of the body: *Wuchereria bancrofti* can affect the legs, arms, vulva, breasts, and scrotum (causing hydrocele formation), while *Brugia timori* rarely affects the genitals. Interestingly, those who develop the chronic stages of elephantiasis are usually amicrofilaraemic, and often have adverse immunological reactions to the microfilaria, as well as the adult worms.

The subcutaneous worms present with skin rashes, urticarial papules, and arthritis, as well as hyper- and hypo pigmentation macules. *Onchocerca volvulus* manifests itself in the eyes, causing "river blindness" (onchocerciasis), one of the leading causes of blindness in the world. Serous cavity Filariasis presents with symptoms similar to subcutaneous Filariasis, in addition to abdominal pain, because these worms are also deep tissue dwellers.

DIAGNOSIS

Filariasis is usually diagnosed by identifying microfilariae on Giemsa stained, thin and thick blood film smears, using the "gold standard" known as the finger prick test. The finger prick test draws blood from the capillaries of the finger tip; larger veins can be used for blood extraction, but strict windows of the time of day must be observed. Blood must be drawn at appropriate times, which reflect the feeding activities of the vector insects. Examples are *W. bancrofti*, whose vector is a mosquito; night time is the preferred time for blood collection. Loa loa's vector is the deer fly; daytime collection is preferred. This method of diagnosis is only relevant to microfilariae that use the blood as transport from the lungs to the skin. Some filarial worms, such as *M. streptocerca* and *Onchocerca volvulus*, produce microfilarae that do not use the blood; they reside in the skin only. For these worms, diagnosis relies upon skin snips, and can be carried out at any time.

New advances in diagnosis

The recent developments in the diagnosis of Lymphatic Filariasis are given below:

Membrane filtration method for microfilaria detection: Venous blood drawn at night and filtered through millepore membrane filters, enables an easy detection of microfilaria and quantifies the load of infection. They are usually observed in the early stages of the disease before clinical manifestations develop. Once lymphoedema develops microfilaria are generally absent in the peripheral-blood.

Ultrasonography: Recently, ultrasonography has helped to locate and visualise the movements of living adult filarial worms of W. bancrofti in the scrotal lymphatics of asymptomatic males with microfilaraemia. The constant thrashing movement of the adult worms in their 'nests' in the scrotal lymphatic's is described as the 'Filaria dance sign'. The lymphatic vessels lodging the parasite are dilated and this dilation is not seen to revert to normal even after the worms are killed by diethylcarbamazine administration. Ultrasonography is not useful in patients with filarial lymphoedema because living adult worms are generally not present at this stage of the disease. Similarly ultrasonography has not helped in locating the adult worms of *Brugia malayi* in the scrotal lymphatics since they do not involve the genitalia.

Lymphoscintigraphy: After injecting radiolabelled albumin or dextran in the web space of the toes, the structural changes are imaged using a gamma camera. Lymphatic dilatation, dermal back flow and obstruction can be directly demonstrated in the oedematous limbs by this method. Lymphoscintigraphy has shown that even in the early, clinically asymptomatic stage of the disease, lymphatic abnormalities in the affected limbs of people harbouring microfilaria may occur.

Immunochromatographic test (ICT): Highly sensitive and specific filarial antigen detection assays, both as card test and in ELISA based format are now available for the diagnosis of *Wuchereria bancrofti* infection. This test is positive in early stages of the disease when the adult worms are alive and becomes negative once they are dead.

DNA probes using Polymerase Chain Reaction (PCR): These tests are of high specificity and sensitivity, and are able to detect parasite DNA in humans as well as vectors in both bancroftian and Brugian Filariasis.

TREATMENT

Diethylcarbamazine (DEC): This drug is effective against both microfilaria and adult worms. DEC markedly lowers the blood microfilaria levels even in single annual doses of 6 mg/kg, and this effect is sustained even after one year. Even though DEC kills the adult worms, this effect is only observed in 50% of patients. By ultrasonography it is shown that even single doses of DEC kill the adult worms when they are sensitive to the drug. When they are not sensitive even repeated doses do not show any effect on the adult parasite. This drug does not act directly on the parasite but its action is mediated through the immune system of the host. The earlier recommended dose of this drug was 6 mg/kg given daily for 12 days. Recent studies have shown that a single dose of DEC 6mg/kg is as effective as the above standard dose given for 12 days. The sustained destruction of microfilaria by this drug even in annual single doses makes it a good tool to prevent the transmission of this disease.

The adverse effects produced by the drug are mostly observed in patients who have microfilaria in their blood and are due to their rapid destruction which is characterized by fever, headache, myalgia, sore throat or cough lasting for 24 to 48 hours. They are usually mild and self-limiting requiring only symptomatic treatment. Direct adverse effects related to the drug are very rare. Recent trials have clearly shown that DEC has no action either in the treatment or prevention of the acute ADL attacks occurring in lymphoedema. DEC is the drug of choice in the treatment of Tropical Eosinophilia syndrome in which it should be given for longer periods of 3 to 4 weeks.

***Ivermectin**:* This drug acts directly on the microfilaria and in single doses of 200 to 400 ugm/ kg keeps the blood microfilaria counts at very low levels even after one year, such as DEC. The adverse effects noticed in microfilaraemic patients are similar to those produced by DEC but are milder due to the slower clearance of the parasitaemia. Ivermectin has no proven action against the adult parasite or in tropical Eosinophilia. Ivermectin is the drug of choice for the treatment of onchocerciasis because of its safety and efficacy, when compared to DEC. It is also the drug of choice for the prevention of Filariasis in African countries endemic for onchocerca and Loa loa, where DEC cannot be used due to possible severe adverse reactions. Ivermectin is also effective against human ectoparasites such as head and body lice, scabies var hominis and many intestinal helminths. This drug is not licensed for human use in India.

Albendazole: This antihelmintic drug is shown to destroy the adult filarial worms when given in doses of 400 mg twice a day for two weeks. The death of the adult worm induces severe scrotal reactions in bancroftian Filariasis since this is the common site where they are lodged.Albendazole has no direct action against the microfilaria and does not immediately lower the microfilaria counts. When given in single dose of 400 mg in association with DEC or ivermectin, the destruction of microfilaria by these drugs becomes more pronounced. Albendazole combined With DEC or invermectin is recommended in the global Filariasis elimination programme. The strategy that appears most suitable for the elimination of Filariasis in India is the administration of a single annual dose of Albendazole 400 mg along with DEC 6 mg/kg of body weight. This not only prevents transmission of Filariasis in the community by reducing the microfilaria levels, but also has the added benefit of clearing the intestinal helminth.

PREVENTION OF CHRONIC MANIFESTATIONS

Once lymphoedema is established there is no cure and the following treatment offers relief and may prevent further progression of the swelling: using elastocrepe bandage or tailor made stockings while ambulant; keeping the limb elevated at night or while resting, after removing the bandage; regular exercise of the affected limb; regular light massage of the limb to stimulate the lymphatic's and to promote flow of lymph towards larger patent vessels; intermittent pneumatic compression of the affected limb using single or multicell jackets; heat therapy either using wet heat or hot oven; surgical procedures such as lymph filariasis nodo-venous shunts, omentoplasty, excisional surgery, skin grafting; prolonged treatment with oral or topical coumarin or flavonoids is considered to be effective in reducing the lymphoedema.

REFERENCES

1. Hoerauf A, Mand S, Fischer K, Kruppa T, Marfo-Debrekyei Y, Debrah AY, Pfarr KM, Adjei O, Buttner DW (2003), "Doxycycline as a novel strategy against bancroftian

filariasis-depletion of Wolbachia endosymbionts from Wuchereria bancrofti and stop of microfilaria production", *Med Microbiol Immunol (Berl)* **192** (4): 211–6.

2. ^ Taylor MJ, Makunde WH, McGarry HF, Turner JD, Mand S, Hoerauf A (2005), "Macrofilaricidal activity after doxycycline treatment of Wuchereria bancrofti: a double-blind, randomised placebo-controlled trial", *Lancet* **365** (9477): 2116–21,
3. Outland, Katrina (2005 Volume 13), *New Treatment for Elephantitis: Antibiotics*, The Journal of Young Investigators.worms detected by ultrasonography in human bancroftian filariasis. *Am J Trop Med Hyg* 1994; 50: 735-57.
4. Shenoy RK, John A, Hameed S, et al. Apparent failure of ultrasonography to detect adult worms of Brugia malayi. *Ann Trop Med Parasitol* 2000; 94: 77-82.
5. Andrade LA, Medeiros Z, Pires ML, et al. Comparative efficacy of three different diethylcarbamazine regimens in lymphatic filariasis. *Trans Royal Soc Trop Med Hyg* 1995; 89:319-21.

CHAPTER 74

Thyroid Disorders

DEFINITION

Thyroid disorders encompass a variety of disease states affecting thyroid hormone production or secretion that result in alterations in metabolic stability. Hyperthyroidism and hypothyroidism are the clinical and biochemical syndromes resulting from increased and decreased thyroid hormone production, respectively.

THYROID HORMONE PHYSIOLOGY

- The thyroid hormones thyroxine (T_4) and triiodothyronine (T_3) are formed on thyroglobulin, a large glycoprotein synthesized within the thyroid cell. Inorganic iodide enters the thyroid follicular cell and is oxidized by thyroid peroxidase and covalently bound (organified) to tyrosine residues of thyroglobulin.
- The iodinated tyrosine residues monoiodotyrosine (MIT) and diiodotyrosine (DIT) combine (couple) to form iodothyronines in reactions catalyzed by thyroid peroxidase. Thus, two molecules of DIT combine to form T_4, and MIT and DIT join to form T_3.
- Thyroid hormone is liberated into the bloodstream by the process of proteolysis within thyroid cells. T_4 and T_3 are transported in the blood stream by three proteins: thyroid-binding globulin, thyroid-binding prealbumin, and albumin. Only the unbound (free) thyroid hormone is able to diffuse into the cell, elicit a biologic effect, and regulate thyroid-stimulating hormone (TSH) secretion from the pituitary.
- T_4 is secreted solely from the thyroid gland, but less than 20% of T_3 is produced there; the majority of T_3 is formed from the breakdown of T_4 catalyzed by the enzyme 5'-monodeiodinase found in peripheral tissues. T_3 is about five times more active than T_4.
- T_4 may also be acted on by the enzyme 5'-monodeiodinase to form reverse T_3, which has no significant biologic activity.
- Thyroid hormone production is regulated by TSH secreted by the anterior pituitary, which in turn is under negative feedback control by the circulating level of free thyroid hormone and the positive influence of hypothalamic thyrotropin-releasing hormone. Thyroid hormone production is also regulated by extrathyroidal deiodination of T_4 to T_3, which can be affected by nutrition, nonthyroidal hormones, drugs, and illness.

THYROTOXICOSIS (HYPERTHYROIDISM)

PATHOPHYSIOLOGY

- Thyrotoxicosis results when tissues are exposed to excessive levels of T_4, T_3, or both.
- TSH-secreting pituitary tumors release biologically active hormone that is unresponsive to normal feedback control. The tumors may co secrete prolactin or growth hormone; therefore, patients may present with amenorrhea, galactorrhea, or signs of acromegaly.
- In Graves' disease, hyperthyroidism results from the action of thyroid-stimulating antibodies (TSAb) directed against the thyrotropin receptor on the surface of the thyroid cell. These immunoglobulin G antibodies bind to the receptor and activate the enzyme adenylate cyclase in the same manner as TSH.
- An autonomous thyroid nodule (toxic adenoma) is a discrete thyroid mass whose function is independent of pituitary control. Hyperthyroidism usually occurs with larger nodules (i.e., those greater than 3 cm in diameter).
- In multinodular goiters (Plummer's disease), follicles with a high degree of autonomous function coexist with normal or even nonfunctioning follicles. Thyrotoxicosis occurs when the autonomous follicles generate more thyroid hormone than is required.
- Painful sub acute (granulomatous or de Quervain's) thyroiditis is believed to be caused by viral invasion of thyroid parenchyma.

  Painless (silent, lymphocytic, postpartum) thyroiditis is a common cause of thyrotoxicosis; its etiology is not fully understood and may be heterogeneous; autoimmunity may underlie most cases.
- Thyrotoxicosis factitia is hyperthyroidism produced by the ingestion of exogenous thyroid hormone. This may occur when thyroid hormone is used for inappropriate indications, when excessive doses are used for accepted medical indications, or when it is used surreptitiously by patients.
- Amiodarone may induce thyrotoxicosis (2% - 3% of patients) or hypothyroidism. It interferes with type I 5'-deiodinase, leading to reduced conversion of T_4 to T_3, and iodide release from the drug may contribute to iodine excess. Amiodarone also causes a destructive thyroiditis with loss of thyroglobulin and thyroid hormones.

CLINICAL FEATURES

- Symptoms of thyrotoxicosis include nervousness, anxiety, palpitations, emotional liability, easy fatigability, heat intolerance, loss of weight concurrent with an increased appetite, increased frequency of bowel movements, proximal muscle weakness (noted on climbing stairs or arising from a sitting position), and scanty or irregular menses in women.
- Physical signs of thyrotoxicosis may include warm, smooth, moist skin and unusually fine hair; separation of the ends of the fingernails from the nail beds (onycholysis); retraction of the eyelids and lagging of the upper lid behind the globe upon downward gaze (lid lag); tachycardia at rest, a widened pulse pressure, and a

systolic ejection murmur; occasional gynecomastia in men; a fine tremor of the protruded tongue and outstretched hands; and hyperactive deep tendon reflexes.

- Graves' disease is manifested by hyperthyroidism, diffuse thyroid enlargement, and the extrathyroidal findings of exophthalmos, pretibial myxedema, and thyroid acropachy. The thyroid gland is usually diffusely enlarged, with a smooth surface and consistency varying from soft to firm. In severe disease, a thrill may be felt and a systolic bruit may be heard over the gland.
- In subacute thyroiditis, patients complain of severe pain in the thyroid region, which often extends to the ear on the affected side. Low-grade fever is common, and systemic signs and symptoms of thyrotoxicosis are present. The thyroid gland is firm and exquisitely tender on physical examination.
- Painless thyroiditis has a triphasic course that mimics that of painful subacute thyroiditis. Most patients present with mild thyrotoxic symptoms; lid retraction and lid lag are present but exophthalmos is absent. The thyroid gland may be diffusely enlarged, but thyroid tenderness is absent.
- Thyroid storm is a life-threatening medical emergency characterized by severe thyrotoxicosis, high fever (often greater than 39.4°C [103°F], tachycardia, tachypnea, dehydration, delirium, coma, nausea, vomiting, and diarrhea. Precipitating factors include infection, trauma, surgery, radioactive iodine (RAI) treatment, and withdrawal from anti thyroid drugs.

DIAGNOSIS

- An elevated 24-hour radioactive iodine uptake (RAIU) indicates true hyperthyroidism: the patient's thyroid gland is overproducing T_4, T_3, or both (normal RAIU 10%-30%). Conversely, a low RAIU indicates that the excess thyroid hormone is not a consequence of thyroid gland hyperfunction but is likely caused by thyroiditis or hormone ingestion.
- TSH-induced hyperthyroidism is diagnosed by evidence of peripheral hypermetabolism, diffuse thyroid gland enlargement, elevated free thyroid hormone levels, and elevated serum immunoreactive TSH concentrations. Because the pituitary gland is extremely sensitive to even minimal elevations of free T_4, a "normal" or elevated TSH level in any thyrotoxic paticnt indicates inappropriate production of TSH.
- TSH-secreting pituitary adenomas are diagnosed by demonstrating lack of TSH response to thyrotropin-releasing hormone stimulation, inappropriate TSH levels, elevated TSH á-subunit levels, and radiologic imaging.
- In thyrotoxic Graves' disease, there is an increase in the overall hormone production rate with a disproportionate increase in T_3 relative to T_4. Saturation of thyroid-binding globulin is increased due to the elevated levels of serum T_4 and T_3, which is reflected in an elevated T_3 resin uptake. As a result, the concentrations of free T_4, free T_3, and the free T_4 and T_3 indices are increased to an even greater extent than are the measured serum total T_4 and T_3 concentrations. The TSH level is

undetectable due to negative feedback by elevated levels of thyroid hormone at the pituitary. In patients with manifest disease, measurement of the serum free T_4 concentration (or total T_4 and T_3 resin uptake), total T_3, and TSH will confirm the diagnosis of thyrotoxicosis. If the patient is not pregnant, an increased 24-hour RAIU documents that the thyroid gland is inappropriately using the iodine to produce more thyroid hormone when the patient is thyrotoxic.

- Toxic adenomas may result in hyperthyroidism with larger nodules. Because there may be isolated elevation of serum T_3 with autonomously functioning nodules, a T_3 level must be measured to rule out T_3 toxicosis if the T_4 level is normal. After a radioiodine scan demonstrates that the toxic thyroid adenoma collects more radioiodine than the surrounding tissue, independent function is documented by failure of the autonomous nodule to decrease its iodine uptake during exogenous T_3 administration.
- In multinodular goiters, a thyroid scan shows patchy areas of autonomously functioning thyroid tissue.
- A low RAIU indicates the excess thyroid hormone is not a consequence of thyroid gland hyper function. This may be seen in painful subacute thyroiditis, painless thyroiditis, struma ovarii, follicular cancer, and factitious ingestion of exogenous thyroid hormone.
- In subacute thyroiditis, thyroid function tests typically run a triphasic course in this self-limited disease. Initially, serum T_4 levels are elevated due to release of preformed thyroid hormone from disrupted follicles. The 24- hour RAIU during this time is less than 2% because of thyroid inflammation and TSH suppression by the elevated T_4 level. As the disease progresses, intrathyroidal hormone stores are depleted, and the patient may become mildly hypothyroid with an appropriately elevated TSH level. During the recovery phase, thyroid hormone stores are replenished and serum TSH elevation gradually returns to normal.
- During the thyrotoxic phase of painless thyroiditis, the 24-hour RAIU is suppressed to less than 2%. Anti-thyroglobulin and antimicrosomal antibody levels are elevated in more than 50% of patients.

Thyrotoxicosis factitia should be suspected in a thyrotoxic patient without evidence of increased hormone production, thyroidal inflammation, or ectopic thyroid tissue. The RAIU is low because thyroid gland function is suppressed by the exogenous thyroid hormone. Measurement of plasma thyroglobulin reveals the presence of very low levels.

TREATMENT

NONPHARMACOLOGICAL THERAPY

- Surgical removal of the thyroid gland should be considered in patients with a large gland (>80 g), severe ophthalmopathy, or a lack of remission on antithyroid drug treatment. If thyroidectomy is planned, **propylthiouracil** (PTU) or **methimazole** (MMI) is usually given until the patient is biochemically euthyroid (usually 6 to 8 weeks), followed by the addition of **iodides** (500 mg/day) for 10 to 14 days before surgery to decrease the vascularity of the gland. **Levothyroxine** may be added to maintain the euthyroid state while the thionamides are continued.

- **Propranolol** has been used for several weeks preoperatively and 7 to 10 days after surgery to maintain a pulse rate less than 90 beats/min. Combined pre-treatment with propranolol and 10 to 14 days of **Potassium Iodide** also has been advocated.
- Complications of surgery include persistent or recurrent hyperthyroidism (0.6% to 18%), hypothyroidism (up to about 49%), hyperparathyroidism (up to 4%), and vocal cord abnormalities (up to 5%). The frequent occurrence of hypothyroidism requires periodic follow-up for identification and treatment.

ANTITHYROID PHARMACOTHERAPY

THIOUREAS (THIONAMIDES)

- **PTU** and **MMI** block thyroid hormone synthesis by inhibiting the peroxidaze enzyme system of the thyroid gland, thus preventing oxidation of trapped iodide and subsequent incorporation into iodotyrosines and ultimately iodothyronine ("organification"); and by inhibiting coupling of MIT and DIT to form T_4 and T_3. PTU (but not MMI) also inhibits the peripheral conversion of T_4 to T_3.
- Usual initial doses include PTU 300 to 600 mg daily (usually in three or four divided doses) or MMI 30 to 60 mg daily given in three divided doses. Evidence exists that both drugs can be given as a single daily dose.
- Improvement in symptoms and laboratory abnormalities should occur within 4 to 8 weeks, at which time a tapering regimen to maintenance doses can be started. Dosage changes should be made on a monthly basis because the endogenously produced T_4 will reach a new steady-state.
- Concentration in this interval. Typical daily maintenance doses are PTU 50 to 300 mg and MMI 5 to 30 mg.
- Antithyroid drug therapy should continue for 12 to 24 months to induce a long-term remission.
- Patients should be monitored every 6 to 12 months after remission. If a relapse occurs, alternate therapy with RAI is preferred to a second course of anti thyroid drugs, as subsequent courses of therapy are less likely to induce remission.
- Minor adverse reactions include pruritic maculopapular rashes, arthralgias, fever, and a benign transient leucopenia (white blood cell count less than 4,000/mm^3). The alternate thioureas may be tried in these situations, but cross-sensitivity occurs in about 50% of patients.
- Major adverse effects include agranulocytosis (with fever, malaise, gingivitis, oropharyngeal infection, and a granulocyte count less than 250/mm^3), aplastic anemia, a lupus-like syndrome, polymyositis, GI intolerance, and hypoprothrombinemia. If it occurs, agranulocytosis almost always develops in the firehepatotoxicityst 3 months of therapy; routine monitoring is not recommended because of its sudden onset. Patients who have experienced a major adverse reaction to one Thioureas should not be converted to the alternate drug because of cross sensitivity.

IODIDES

- **Iodide** acutely blocks thyroid hormone release, inhibits thyroid hormone biosynthesis by interfering with intrathyroidal iodide use, and decreases the size and vascularity of the gland.
- Symptom improvement occurs within 2 to 7 days of initiating therapy, and serum T_4 and T_3 concentrations may be reduced for a few weeks.
- Iodides are often used as adjunctive therapy to prepare a patient with Graves' disease for surgery, to acutely inhibit thyroid hormone release and quickly attain the euthyroid state in severely thyrotoxic patients with cardiac decompensation, or to inhibit thyroid hormone release after RAI therapy.
- **Potassium iodide** is available as a saturated solution (**SSKI**, 38 mg iodide per drop) or as **Lugol's solution**, containing 6.3 mg of iodide per drop.
- The typical starting dose of SSKI is 3 to 10 drops daily (120 to 400 mg) in water or juice. When used to prepare a patient for surgery, it should be administered 7 to 14 days preoperatively.
- As an adjunct to RAI, SSKI should not be used before but rather 3 to 7 days after RAI treatment so that the RAI can concentrate in the thyroid.
- Adverse effects include hypersensitivity reactions (skin rashes, drug fever, rhinitis, conjunctivitis); salivary gland swelling; "iodism" (metallic taste, burning mouth and throat, sore teeth and gums, symptoms of a head cold, and sometimes stomach upset and diarrhea); and gynecomastia.

ADRENERGIC BLOCKERS

- β-Blockers have been used widely to ameliorate thyrotoxic symptoms such as palpitations, anxiety, tremor, and heat intolerance. They have no effect on peripheral thyrotoxicosis and protein metabolism and do not reduce TSAb or prevent thyroid storm. **Propranolol** and **nadolol** partially block the conversion of T_4 to T_3, but this contribution to the overall therapeutic effect is small.
- β-Blockers are usually used as adjunctive therapy with antithyroid drugs, RAI, or iodides when treating Graves' disease or toxic nodules; in preparation for surgery; or in thyroid storm. β-Blockers are primary therapy only for thyroiditis and iodine-induced hyperthyroidism.
- **Propranolol** doses required to relieve adrenergic symptoms vary, but an initial dose of 20 to 40 mg four times daily is effective for most patients (heart rate less than 90 beats/min). Younger or more severely toxic patients may require as much as 240 to 480 mg/day.
- β-Blockers are contraindicated in patients with decompensated heart failure unless it is caused solely by tachycardia (high output). Other contraindications include sinus bradycardia, concomitant therapy with monoamine oxidaze inhibitors or tricyclic antidepressants, and patients with spontaneous hypoglycemia. Side effects include nausea, vomiting, anxiety, insomnia, lightheadedness, bradycardia, and hematologic disturbances.
- Centrally acting sympatholytics (e.g., **clonidine**) and calcium channel antagonists (e.g., **diltiazem**) may be useful for symptom control when contraindications to β-blockade exist.

RADIOACTIVE IODINE

- **Sodium iodide 131** is an oral liquid that concentrates in the thyroid and initially disrupts hormone synthesis by incorporating into thyroid hormones and thyroglobulin. Over a period of weeks, follicles that have taken up RAI and surrounding follicles develop evidence of cellular necrosis and fibrosis of the interstitial tissue.

- RAI is the agent of choice for Graves' disease, toxic autonomous nodules, and toxic multinodular goiters. Pregnancy is an absolute contraindication to the use of RAI.
- β-Blockers are the primary adjunctive therapy to RAI, since they may be given anytime without compromising RAI therapy.
- Patients with cardiac disease and elderly patients are often treated with thionamides prior to RAI ablation because thyroid hormone levels will transiently increase after RAI treatment due to release of preformed thyroid hormone.
- If iodides are administered, they should be given 3 to 7 days after RAI to prevent interference with the uptake of RAI in the thyroid gland.
- The goal of therapy is to destroy overactive thyroid cells, and a single dose of 4,000 to 8,000 rad results in a euthyroid state in 60% of patients at 6 months or less. A second dose of RAI should be given 6 months after the first RAI treatment if the patient remains hyperthyroid.
- Hypothyroidism commonly occurs months to years after RAI. The acute, short-term side effects include mild thyroidal tenderness and dysphagia. Long-term follow-up has not revealed an increased risk for development of thyroid carcinoma, leukemia, or congenital defects.

TREATMENT OF THYROID STORM

- The following therapeutic measures should be instituted promptly:

1. Suppression of thyroid hormone formation and secretion;
2. Antiadrenergic therapy;
3. Administration of corticosteroids; and
4. Treatment of associated complications or coexisting factors that may have precipitated the storm.

- **PTU** in large doses is the preferred thionamides because it interferes with the production of thyroid hormones and blocks the peripheral conversion of T_4 to T_3.
- **Iodides**, which rapidly block the release of preformed thyroid hormone, should be administered after PTU is initiated to inhibit iodide use by the overactive gland.
- Antiadrenergic therapy with the short-acting agent **esmolol** is preferred because it can be used in patients with pulmonary disease or at risk for cardiac failure and because its effects can be rapidly reversed.
- **Corticosteroids** are generally recommended, but there is no convincing evidence of adrenocortical insufficiency in thyroid storm; their benefits may be attributed to their antipyretic action and stabilization of blood pressure.
- General supportive measures, including **acetaminophen** as an antipyretic (aspirin or other nonsteroidal anti-inflammatory drugs may displace bound thyroid hormone), **fluid and electrolyte replacement, sedatives, digoxin, antiarrhythmics, insulin,** and **antibiotics** should be given as indicated. Plasmapheresis and peritoneal dialysis have been used to remove excess hormone in patients not responding to more conservative measures.

Table 74.1

Thyroid preparations used in the treatment of hypothyroidism

Drug / Dosage form	Content	Relative Dose
Thyroid USP		
Thyroid (T_4:T_3 ratio) 9.5mcg:2.25mcg, 19mcg: 4.5mcg, 19mcg: 4.5mcg, 38mcg: 9mcg, 27 mcg: 13.5 mcg, 76mcg: 18mcg, 114mcg: 27mcg, 152 mcg : 36 mcg, 190 mcg : 45 mcg tablets	Desiccated beef or pork thyroid gland	1 grain (equivalent to 60 mcg of T_4)
Thyroglobulin		
Proloid 32-65, 100-130, 200-mg tablets	Partially purified park thyroglobulin	1 grain
Levothyroxine		
Synthroid, levothroid, levozyl, Unithroid, and other generics 25-, 50-, 75-, 88-, 100-, 112-, 125-, 137-, 150 - 175-, 200-, 300-mcg tablets; 200-and 500-mcg/vial injections	Synthetic T_4	50-60 mcg
Liothyronine		
Cytomel 5-, 25-, and 50-mcg tablets	Synthetic T_3	15-37.5 mcg

HYPOTHYROIDISM

PATHOPHYSIOLOGY

- The vast majority of hypothyroid patients have thyroid gland failure (primary hypothyroidism). The causes include chronic autoimmune thyroiditis (Hashimoto's disease), iatrogenic hypothyroidism, iodine deficiency, enzyme defects, thyroid hypoplasia, and goitrogens.
- Pituitary failure (secondary hypothyroidism) is an uncommon cause resulting from pituitary tumors, surgical therapy, external pituitary radiation, postpartum pituitary necrosis, metastatic tumors, tuberculosis, histiocytosis, and autoimmune mechanisms.

CLINICAL FEATURES

- Adult manifestations of hypothyroidism include dry skin, cold intolerance, weight gain, constipation, weakness, lethargy, fatigue, muscle cramps, myalgia, stiffness, and loss of ambition or energy. In children, thyroid hormone deficiency may manifest as growth retardation. Physical signs include coarse skin and hair, cold or dry skin, periorbital puffiness, bradycardia, and slowed or hoarse speech. Objective weakness (with proximal muscles being affected more than distal muscles) and slow relaxation of deep tendon reflexes are common. Reversible neurologic syndromes such as carpal tunnel syndrome, polyneuropathy, and cerebellar dysfunction may also occur.

- Most patients with pituitary failure (secondary hypothyroidism) have clinical signs of generalized pituitary insufficiency such as abnormal menses and decreased libido, or evidence of a pituitary adenoma such as visual field defects, galactorrhea, or acromegaloid features.
- Myxedema coma is a rare consequence of decompensated hypothyroidism manifested by hypothermia, advanced stages of hypothyroid symptoms, and altered sensorium ranging from delirium to coma. Untreated disease is associated with a high mortality rate.

DIAGNOSIS

- A rise in the TSH level is the first evidence of primary hypothyroidism. Many patients have a free T_4 level within the normal range (compensated hypothyroidism) and few, if any, symptoms of hypothyroidism. As the disease progresses, the free T_4 concentration drops below the normal level. The T_3 concentration is often maintained in the normal range despite a low T_4. Antithyroid peroxidaze antibodies and Antithyroglobulin antibodies are likely to be elevated. The RAIU is not a useful test in the evaluation of hypothyroidism because it can be low, normal, or even elevated.
- Pituitary failure (secondary hypothyroidism) should be suspected in a patient with decreased levels of T_4 and inappropriately normal or low TSH levels.

Treatment of Hypothyroidism (Table 74.1)

- Levothyroxine (L-thyroxine, T_4) is the drug of choice for thyroid hormone replacement and suppressive therapy because it is chemically stable, relatively inexpensive, free of antigenicity, and has uniform potency; however, any of the commercially available thyroid preparations can be used. Once a particular product is selected, therapeutic interchange is discouraged.
- Because T_3 (and not T_4) is the biologically active form, Levothyroxine administration results in a pool of thyroid hormone that is readily and consistently converted to T_3.
- Young patients with long-standing disease and patients older than 45 years without known cardiac disease should be started on 50 mcg daily of Levothyroxine and increased to 100 mcg daily after 1 month. The recommended initial daily dose for older patients or those with known cardiac disease is 25 mcg/day titrated upward in increments of 25 mcg at monthly intervals to prevent stress on the cardiovascular system.
- The average maintenance dose for most adults is about 125 mcg/day, but there is a wide range of replacement doses, necessitating individualized therapy and appropriate monitoring to determine an appropriate dose.
- Patients with subclinical hypothyroidism and marked elevations in TSH (greater than 10 milli-international units per liter [mIU/L]) and high titers of TSAb or prior treatment with sodium iodide 131 may benefit from treatment with levothyroxine.

- Levothyroxine is the drug of choice for pregnant women, and the objective of the treatment is to decrease TSH to 1 mIU/L and to maintain free T_4 concentrations in the normal range.
- Cholestyramine, calcium carbonate, sucralphate, aluminum hydroxide, ferrous sulphate, soybean formula, and dietary fiber supplements may impair the absorption of levothyroxine from the GI tract. Drugs that increase nondeiodinative T_4 clearance include rifampin, carbamazepine, and possibly phenytoin. Amiodarone may block the conversion of T_4 to T_3.
- **Thyroid, USP** (or desiccated thyroid) is derived from hog, beef, or sheep thyroid gland. It may be antigenic in allergic or sensitive patients. Inexpensive generic brands may not be bioequivalent.
- **Thyroglobulin** is a purified hog-gland extract that is standardized biologically to give a T_4:T_3 ratio of 2.5:1. It has no clinical advantages and is not widely used.
- **Liothyronine** (synthetic T_3) has uniform potency but has a higher incidence of cardiac adverse effects, higher cost, and difficulty in monitoring with conventional laboratory tests.
- **Liotrix** (synthetic T_4:T_3 in a 4:1 ratio) is chemically stable, pure, and has a predictable potency but is expensive. It lacks therapeutic rationale because about 35% of T_4 is converted to T_3 peripherally.
- Excessive doses of thyroid hormone may lead to heart failure, anginapectoris, and myocardial infarction. Allergic or idiosyncratic reactions can occur with the natural animal-derived products such as desiccated thyroid and thyroglobulin, but they are extremely rare with the synthetic products used today. Excess exogenous thyroid hormone may reduce bone density and increase the risk of fracture.

TREATMENT OF MYXEDEMA COMA

- Immediate and aggressive therapy with IV bolus **levothyroxine**, 300 to 500 mcg, has traditionally been used. Initial treatment with IV **liothyronine** or a combination of both hormones has also been advocated because of impaired conversion of T_4 to T_3.
- Glucocorticoid therapy with IV **hydrocortisone** 100 mg every 8 hours should be given until coexisting adrenal suppression is ruled out.
- Consciousness, lowered TSH concentrations, and normal vital signs are expected within 24 hours.
- Maintenance levothyroxine doses are typically 75 to 100 mcg IV until the patient stabilizes and oral therapy is begun.

  Supportive therapy must be instituted to maintain adequate ventilation, euglycemia, blood pressure, and body temperature. Underlying disorders such as sepsis and myocardial infarction must be diagnosed and treated.

REFERENCES

1. The thyroid gland in *Endocrinology: An Integrated Approach* by Stephen Nussey and Saffron Whitehead (2001) Published by BIOS Scientific Publishers Ltd.
2. Boron WF, Boulpaep E (2003). "Chapter 48: "synthesis of thyroid hormones" ". *Medical Physiology: A Cellular And Molecular Approaoch.* Elsevier/Saunders. pp. 1300.
3. Kester MH, Martinez de Mena R, Obregon MJ, Marinkovic D, Howatson A, Visser TJ,

Hume R, Morreale de Escobar G (2004). "Iodothyronine levels in the human developing brain: major regulatory roles of iodothyronine deiodinases in different areas".*J Clin Endocrinol Metab* **89** (7): 3117–3128.

4. Treatment for Thyroid disease Retrieved on 2010-02-07.
5. Yamamoto M, Shibuya N, Chen LC, Ogata E (February 1988). "Seasonal recurrence of transient hypothyroidism in a patient with autoimmune thyroiditis". *Endocrinol. Jpn.* **35** (1): 135–42.
6. Patrick L (June 2008). "Iodine: deficiency and therapeutic considerations" (PDF). *Altern Med Rev* **13** (2): 116-27.

CHAPTER 75

Parathyroid Disorders

Many conditions are associated with disorders of the function of the parathyroid gland. **Parathyroid diseases** can be divided into those causing hyperparathyroidism, and those causing hypoparathyroidism.

MOLECULAR AND PATHOLOGIC CORRELATES OF DISEASE

- Calcium metabolism depends upon a complex interplay among dietary calcium, absorption, and excretion; hormonal interactions of parathormone, vitamin D, and calcitonin; immobilization or exercise status; and other diseases and medications.
- An average daily intake of calcium varies with the type of diet and the amount ingested. For example, consumers of large amounts of dairy products have a high calcium intake. Also, consumption of calcium-containing antacids or mineral supplements containing calcium and vitamin D intake influence calcium levels.
- The recommended daily allowance for healthy individuals is 1 g. This is increased under various conditions (e.g., osteoporosis and pregnancy).Calcium is poorly absorbed from the small intestine; the average varies from 10%-30%, with the residual being eliminated in the faeces. Vitamin D directly increases serum calcium by increasing protein synthesis in the intestinal wall, which in turn enhances intestinal calcium transport and absorption.
- Vitamin D also increases renal tubular reabsorption of calcium as well as phosphorus. Vitamin D actually possess hormonal activity, since, through corresponding blood levels, there is a homeostatic interplay mechanism between serum calcium and parathyroid hormone production.

Parathormone, produced in the parathyroid glands, controls calcium levels by influencing bone breakdown or resorption. This hormone is regulated in feedback fashion by the level of serum calcium. Parathormone also influences the hydroxylation of vitamin D as well as the kidney reabsorption of phosphate and calcium.

- Calciferol (vitamin D2) is the most inert form of vitaminD and is obtained from plant sources. This is the active ingredient in most proprietary vitamin D preparations.
- Cholecalciferol (vitamin D3) is obtained through the diet from animal sources or conversion from fat stores in the skin by

ultraviolet light. The most active form of vitamin D is the 1,25-dihydroxy-cholecalciferol.

- The hydroxylation takes place first in the liver (the 25- position) and then sequentially in the kidney (the 1-position). This process takes place in the mitochondria. Obviously then, liver disease decreases the amount of the active form of vitamin D. Therefore, such conditions as Cirrhosis or the ingestion of drugs, such as phenytoin and Phenobarital, influence the levels of vitamin D activity.
- Circulating parathyroid hormone also influences the 1-hydroxylation in the kidney by feedback control. Thus, if there is excess parathyroid hormone and an increase in serum calcium levels, the 1-hydroxylation kidney activity is depressed. This in turn reduces vitamin D activity and lowers intestinal calcium absorption.
- Serum calcium levels have ranges of normal that vary from laboratory to laboratory. However, the limits are rigid, and values slightly above or below normal usually reflect a significant abnormality.
- 50% of serum calcium is usually protein-bound. Up to 200 mg of calcium may be excreted through the urine daily; but the average amount approximates 125 mg. Tubular reabsorption of calcium is efficient, approximating 97%. This process of reabsorption is influenced by serum levels of calcium, vitamin D, and parathormone. When calcium levels exceed normal, the risk for kidney damage increases. The exchange pool between serum calcium and bone usually approximates 350 mg per day, with accretion equaling resorption, under normal conditions.
- Calcitonin is a hormone that tends to preserve the skeleton by controlling calcium and phosphate levels, probably by reducing bone resorption by inhibiting the action of osteoclasts. Its production is primarily from the ultimobranchial cells distributed in thyroid, parathyroid, and thymus glands.

CLINICAL FEATURES

There are innumerable causes of hypercalcemia. Fortunately, the body's homeostatic mechanisms are capable of maintaining serum calcium within normal limits under most circumstances. Following are some of the common causes of hypercalcemia.

1. Cancer that invades bone. Tumours can elaborate parathyroid hormone-like substances leading to release of calcium; this is seen often in advanced head and neck cancers.
2. Milk-alkali syndrome caused by the ingestion of antacids that contain soluble calcium salts.
3. Hyperparathyroidism.
4. Excess vitamin D ingestion.
5. Diuretic therapy using thiazide.
6. Sarcoidosis.
7. Immobilization.

The clinical picture of excessive circulating calcium depends upon the level and duration of hypercalcemia. Primary hyperparathyroidism is caused by the development of benign tumors (adenomas) or hyperplasia of one or more of the parathyroid glands. Early detection and adequate surgical treatment are extremely important, since delay may lead to irreversible kidney damage, hypertension, and death. Tests include the measurement of parathormone as well as biochemical assessment for abnormal calcium, phosphorus, and alkaline phosphatase levels.

Secondary hyperparathyroidism is usually a reflection of renal disease, with sequelae of calcium loss and compensatory parathyroid hyperactivity to maintain adequate serum calcium levels.

The dental findings between primary and secondary disease are indistinguishable. The dental findings of hyperparathyroid disease are usually found as abnormalities on dental radiographs

The changes include one or more of the following:

1. Complete or partial loss of lamina dura;
2. Alveolar bone demineralization (ground-glass appearance); and
3. Fibrous giant-cell bone lesions (brown tumour, osteitis fibrosa cystica), which must be confirmed by biopsy. Bone changes almost always reflect late-stage disease.

Hypoparathyroidism is relatively rare and may be attributable to a genetic disorder (congenital), or induced by parathyroid or thyroid surgery, or radiation to that area. These events can lead to a low serum calcium level (hypocalcaemia), which can lead to muscular spasms and tetany. The dental manifestations only occur in the congenital form, which affects the teeth at the developmental stage, causing mottling (hypoplastia) and discoloration. There are no dental findings in acquired hypoparathyroidism. Vitamin D-resistant rickets is a congenital genetic condition that lowers serum calcium. In one form of the disease, for unknown reasons, spontaneous pulpal death and abscess formation occurs in one or more teeth.

DIAGNOSIS

From the dental point-of-view, the diagnosis of disturbed calcium metabolism is based upon the abnormal radiographic findings of altered lamina dura, demineralised bone, or radiographic cysts. When biopsy specimens from bone show giant cells in the fibrous stroma, hyperparathyroidism must be ruled out. Biochemically, the diagnosis is established by parathyroid hormone levels and, indirectly, by serum levels of high calcium, low phosphate, and high alkaline phosphatase. Confusion in determining the differential diagnosis often arises because of many nonendocrine conditions that may mimic characteristics found in hypercalcemic states.

TREATMENT

Treatment for calcium disorders requires surgery for gland tumours and medications to adjust calcium and phosphorus levels. Abnormalities in bone revert to normal after calcium metabolism is stabilized .Therefore, specific local treatment to the dental structures, other than routine care, is contraindicated.

- It must be remembered that similar radiographic bone alterations may represent several different diseases. Correlations between clinical, radiographic, and microscopic findings are critical to arriving at a definitive diagnosis. For example, giant-cell lesions of bone can be the manifestation of an inflammatory process, neoplasia, or a parathyroid adenoma.

- Fibrous dysplasia is a benign, idiopathic demineralization of one bone or a part of a bone (monotonic) or numerous bones (polyostotic). The clinical appearance may show expansion of the mandible or maxilla with confirmation by a ground-glass or demineralised appearance.
- It is usually painless, has limited growth, and requires no treatment. Surgical trimming is sometimes done for esthetics or interference with prostheses. Polyostotic fibrous dysplasia is rare. The bone expansion is differentiated from an osteoma, which has continued growth and usually a radiographic presentation of radiopacity.
- Paget's disease of bone usually occurs in people over 40 years of age. It is a condition in which osteoclastic activity and compensatory disorganized bone overgrowth occur side by side. Mandibular overgrowth and malocclusion are oral manifestations, and sometimes are the first sign of this idiopathic disease. Long bones may bow, and there is often associated pain. Diagnosis can be confirmed by biopsy, radiographs, and chemistry (normal calcium, high alkaline phosphatase). There might be some clinical confusion with acromegaly, since both conditions may present with the Class III malocclusion. But acromegaly is a reflection of anterior pituitary adenoma with an increase in growth hormone that stimulates condylar cartilagenous reactivation and Mandibular growth.
- Other endocrinopathies, such as diabetes mellitus, occur simultaneously. Osteomalacia is a disease of insufficient bone matrix calcification as a result of intestinal malabsorption of minerals or renal disorders. Osteomalacia commonly follows sprue, a disease of disturbed small intestine function characterized by impaired nutrient absorption.
- Fractures and bone pain are major findings. Osteoporosis is an extremely common condition of aging, particularly in postmenopausal women. Osteoporosis is not a primary disorder of calcium metabolism.
- It may result from inadequate stimulation of osteoblasts (post menopause, disuse) or excess catabolic agents (adrenal cortex over activity). Pain and fractures are common findings. Control is usually on the basis of steroid hormone replacement, nutrient replacement (diet, supplements), and exercise. It has been shown that osteoporosis affects jaw bones; however, the clinical implications are not clear.
- Haemorrhagic pseudo cysts are asymptomatic bone cavities occurring more commonly in the mandible. Although they are often called traumatic cysts, their cause is unknown. These areas will usually remineralize spontaneously. They can resemble the bone lesions of hyperparathyroid disease.

REFERENCES

1. Delmas PD, Meunier PJ. The management of Paget's disease of bone. N Engl J Med 1997;336:558–66.
2. Eastell R. Treatment of postmenopausal osteoporosis. N Engl J Med 1998; 338:736–46.
3. Holick MF, Schnoes THK, DeLuca HF, et al. Isolation and identification of 1,25-dihydroxycholecalciferol. A metabolite of vitamin D active in intestine. J NIH Res 1992;4:88–95.

4. Jeffcoat MK, Chestnut CH. Systemic osteoporosis and oral bone loss: evidence shows increased risk factors. J Am Dent Assoc 1993;124:49–56.
5. Reichel H, Klieffler HP, Norman AW. The role of the vitamin D endocrine system in health and disease. N Engl J Med 1989;320:980–91.
6. Ruggieri P, Sim FH, Bond JR, Unni KK. Malignancies in fibrous dysplasia. Cancer 1994;73:1411–24.
7. Silverberg SJ, Shane E, Jacobs TP, et al. A 10-year prospective study of primary hyperparathyroidism with or without parathyroid surgery. N Engl J Med 1999;341:1249–54.
8. Slavkin HC. Building a better mousetrap: toward an understanding of osteoporosis. J Am Dent Assoc 1999;130: 1632–6.

CHAPTER 76

Diabetes Mellitus

DEFINITION

Diabetes mellitus (DM) is a group of metabolic disorders characterized by hyperglycemia and abnormalities in carbohydrate, fat, and protein metabolism. It results from defects in insulin secretion, insulin sensitivity, or both. Chronic microvascular, macrovascular, and neuropathic complications may ensue.

PREVALENCE

Globally, as of 2010, an estimated 285 million people had diabetes, with type 2 making up about 90% of the cases. Its incidence is increasing rapidly, and by 2030, this number is estimated to almost double. Diabetes mellitus occurs throughout the world, but is more common (especially type 2) in the more developed countries. The greatest increase in prevalence is, however, expected to occur in Asia and Africa, where most patients will probably be found by 2030. The increase in incidence in developing countries follows the trend of urbanization and lifestyle changes, perhaps most importantly a "Western-style" diet. This has suggested an environmental (i.e., dietary) effect, but there is little understanding of the mechanism(s) at present, though there is much speculation, some of it most compellingly presented.

PATHOPHYSIOLOGY

- Type 1 DM accounts for 5% to 10% of all diabetes cases. It generally develops in childhood or early adulthood and results from immune mediated destruction of pancreatic β-cells, resulting in an absolute deficiency of insulin. There is a long preclinical period (up to 9 to 13 years) marked by the presence of immune markers when β-cell destruction is thought to occur. Hyperglycemia occurs when 80% to 90% of β-cells are destroyed. There is a transient remission ("honeymoon" phase) followed by established disease with associated risks for Complications and death. The factors that initiate the autoimmune process are unknown, but the process is mediated by macrophages and T lymphocytes with circulating auto antibodies to various β-cell antigens (e.g., islet cell antibody, insulin antibodies) (Fig. 76.1).
- Type 2 DM accounts for as many as 90% of DM cases and is usually characterized by the presence of both insulin resistance and relative insulin deficiency. Insulin resistance is manifested by increased lipolysis and free fatty acid production, increased hepatic glucose production, and decreased skeletal muscle uptake of

glucose. β-Cell dysfunction is progressive and contributes to worsening blood glucose control over time. Type 2 DM occurs when a diabetogenic lifestyle (excessive calories, inadequate exercise, and obesity) is superimpozed upon a susceptible genotype.

- Uncommon causes of diabetes (1% to 2% of cases) include endocrine disorders (e.g., acromegaly, Cushing's syndrome), gestational diabetes mellitus (GDM), diseases of the exocrine pancreas (e.g., pancreatitis), and medications (e.g., glucocorticoids, pentamidine, niacin, and α-interferon).
- *Impaired fasting glucose* and *impaired glucose tolerance* are terms used to describe patients whose plasma glucose levels are higher than normal but not diagnostic of DM (see Diagnosis). These disorders are risk factors for developing DM and cardiovascular disease and are associated with the insulin-resistance syndrome.
- Microvascular complications include retinopathy, neuropathy, and nephropathy. Macrovascular complications include coronary heart disease, stroke, and peripheral vascular disease.

CLINICAL FEATURES

TYPE 1 DIABETES MELLITUS

Individuals with type 1 DM are often thin and are prone to develop diabetic ketoacidosis if insulin is withheld or under conditions of severe stress with an excess of insulin counter regulatory hormones.

- Between 20% and 40% of patients present with diabetic ketoacidosis after several days of polyuria, polydipsia, polyphagia, and weight loss.

TYPE 2 DIABETES MELLITUS

- Patients with type 2 DM are often asymptomatic and may be diagnosed secondary to unrelated blood testing. However, the presence of complications may indicate that they have had DM for several years.

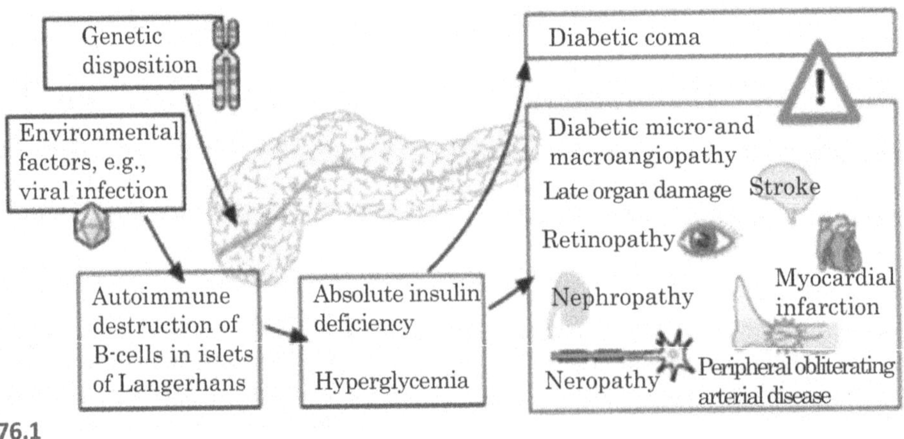

FIGURE 76.1

Type 1 Diabetes mellitus pathogenesis and complications.

(Source : Colour Atlas Of Pharmacology ,3rd edition ,Page no.261)

- Lethargy, polyuria, nocturia, and polydipsia can be present on diagnosis; significant weight loss is less common.

DIAGNOSIS

- Screening for type 2 DM should be performed every 3 years in all adults beginning at the age of 45. Testing should be considered at an earlier age and more frequently in individuals with risk factors (e.g., family history of DM, obesity, signs of insulin resistance).
- The recommended screening test is fasting plasma glucose (FPG). Normal FPG is less than 100 mg/dL (5.6 mmol/L).
- Impaired fasting glucose is defined as FPG of 100 to 125 mg/dl (5.6 to 6.9 mmol/L).
- Impaired glucose tolerance is diagnosed when the 2-hour postload sample of the oral glucose tolerance test is between 140 and 199 mg per dL (7.8 to 11.0 mmol/L).
- The diagnostic criteria for DM are contained in Table 76.1

Pregnant women should undergo risk assessment for GDM at their first prenatal visit and proceed with glucose testing if at high risk (e.g., positive family history, personal history of GDM, marked obesity, or member of a high-risk ethnic group).

TREATMENT

GENERAL APPROACH

- Near-normal glycemia reduces the risk of microvascular disease complications, but aggressive management of traditional cardiovascular risk factors (i.e., smoking cessation, treatment of dyslipidemia, intensive blood pressure control, antiplatelet therapy) is needed to reduce macrovascular disease risk.
- Appropriate care requires goal setting for glycemia, blood pressure, and lipid levels; regular monitoring for complications; dietary and exercise modifications; appropriate self-monitoring of blood glucose (SMBG); and appropriate assessment of laboratory parameters.

NONPHARMACOLOGICAL THERAPY

- Medical nutrition therapy is recommended for all patients. For

Table 76.1

Criteria for the diagnosis of diabetes mellitus
Symptoms of diabetes plus casual[b] plasma glucose concentration e” 200 mg/dl (11.1 mmol/l)
or
Fasting[c] plasma glucose e” 126 mg/dl (7.0 mmol/l)
or
2-Hour post load glucose e” 200 mg/dl (11.1 mmol/l) during an OGTT[d]

(a) In the absence of unequivocal hyperglycemia, these criteria should be confirmed by repeat testing on a different day. The third measure (oral glucose tolerance test; OGTT) is not recommended for routine clinical use.

(b) Casual is defined as any time of day without regard to time since last meal. The classic symptoms of diabetes include polyuria, polydipsia, and unexplained weight loss.

(c) Fasting is defined as no caloric intake for at least 8 hours.

(d) The test should be performed as described by the World Health Organization, using a glucose load containing the equivalent of 75 g anhydrous glucose dissolved in water.

individuals with type 1 DM, the focus is on regulating insulin administration with a balanced diet to achieve and maintain a healthy body weight. A meal plan that is moderate in carbohydrates and low in saturated fat, with a focus on balanced meals is recommended. In addition, patients with type 2 DM often require caloric restriction to promote weight loss. Bedtime and between-meal snacks are not usually needed if pharmacologic management is appropriate.

- Aerobic exercise can improve insulin resistance and glycemic control in most patients and may reduce cardiovascular risk factors, contribute to weight loss or maintenance, and improve well-being. Exercise should be started slowly in previously sedentary patients. Older patients and those with atherosclerotic disease should have a cardiovascular evaluation prior to beginning a substantial exercise program.

PHARMACOLOGICAL THERAPY

Insulin and other injectable preparations (Tables 76.2 and 76.3) (Fig. 76.2)

- **Regular insulin** has a relatively slow onset of action when given subcutaneously; requiring injection 30 minutes prior to meals to achieve optimal postprandial glucose control and to prevent delayed post meal hypoglycemia.
- **Lispro, aspart,** and **glulisine insulins** are analogs that are more rapidly absorbed, peak faster, and have shorter durations of action than regular insulin. This permits more convenient dosing within 10 minutes of meals (rather than 30 minutes prior), produces better efficacy in lowering postprandial blood glucose than regular insulin in type 1 DM, and minimizes delayed post meal hypoglycemia. **Neutral protamine hagedorn (NPH)** is intermediate-acting. Variability in absorption, inconsistent preparation by the patient, and inherent pharmacokinetic differences may contribute to a labile glucose response, nocturnal hypoglycemia, and fasting hyperglycemia.
- **Glargine** and **detemir** are long-acting "peak less" human insulin analogs that result in less nocturnal hypoglycemia than NPH insulin when given at bedtime.
- In type 1 DM, the average daily insulin requirement is 0.5 to 0.6 units/kg. Requirements may fall to 0.1 to 0.4 units/kg in the honeymoon phase. Higher doses (0.5 to 1 unit/kg) are warranted during acute illness or ketosis. In type 2 DM, a dosage range of 0.7 to 2.5 units/kg is often required for patients with significant insulin resistance.
- Hypoglycemia and weight gain are the most common adverse effects of insulin. Treatment of hypoglycemia is as follows:
  - o **Glucose** (10 to 15 g) given orally is the recommended treatment in conscious patients.
  - o **Dextrose** IV may be required in individuals who have lost consciousness.
  - o **Glucagon**, 1 g intramuscular, is the treatment of choice in unconscious patients when IV access cannot be established.
- **Exenatide** is a synthetic analog of exendin-4, a 39-amino acid peptide isolated from the saliva of the Gila monster that enhances glucose dependent insulin secretion and reduces hepatic glucose production. It also decreases appetite and slows gastric emptying,

which may reduce caloric intake and cause weight loss. It significantly decreases postprandial glucose excursions but has only a modest effect on FPG values. The average A1C reduction is approximately 0.9%. The most common adverse effects are nausea, vomiting, and diarrhea. The initial dose is 5 mcg subcutaneously twice daily, titrated to 10 mcg twice daily in 1 month if needed and as tolerated. It should be injected 0 to 60 minutes before the morning and evening meals. Exenatide should be used as adjunctive therapy in patients who have not achieved adequate glycemic control despite treatment with metformin, a sulphonylurea, and/or a thiazolidinedione. **Pramlintide** is a synthetic analog of amylin, a neurohormone co secreted from β-cells with insulin. Pramlintide suppresses inappropriately high postprandial glucagon secretion, reduces food intake (which can cause weight loss), and slows gastric emptying. The average A1C reduction is approximately 0.6%, but optimization of concurrent insulin therapy may result in further A1C decreases. Pramlintide decreases prandial glucose excursions but has little effect on FPG concentrations. Its main advantage is in type 1 DM, where it helps stabilize wide, postprandial glycemic swings. The most common adverse effects are nausea, vomiting, and anorexia. It does not cause hypoglycemia when used alone, but it is indicated only in patients receiving insulin, so hypoglycemia can occur. If a prandial insulin dose is used, it should be reduced by 30% to 50% when pramlintide is started to minimize severe hypoglycemic reactions. In type 2 DM, the starting dose is 60 mcg subcutaneously prior to major meals; the dose is titrated up to 120 mcg per dose as tolerated and as warranted based on postprandial plasma glucose levels. In type 1 DM, dosing starts at 15 mcg prior to each meal, titrated up to a maximum of 60 mcg prior to each meal if tolerated and warranted.

Sulphonylureas (Table 76.4) (Fig. 76.3)

- Sulphonylureas exert a hypoglycemic action by stimulating pancreatic secretion of insulin. All Sulphonylureas are equally effective in lowering blood glucose when administered in equipotent doses. On average, the A1C will fall by 1.5% to 2% with FPG reductions of 60 to 70 mg/dL (3.3 to 3.9 mmol/L).
- The most common side effect is hypoglycemia, which is more problematic with long half-life drugs. Individuals at high risk include the elderly, those with renal insufficiency or advanced liver disease, and those who skip meals, exercise vigorously, or lose a substantial amount of weight. Weight gain is common; less common adverse effects include skin rash, haemolytic anemia, GI upset, and cholestasis. Hyponatremia is most common with chlorpropamide but has also been reported with tolbutamide.
- The recommended starting doses (see Table 76.4) should be reduced in elderly patients who may have compromised renal or hepatic function. Dosage can be titrated every 1 to 2 weeks (longer interval with chlorpropamide) to achieve glycemic goals.

Short-acting insulin secretagogues (meglitinides)

- Similar to Sulphonylureas, meglitinides lower glucose by stimulating pancreatic insulin secretion, but insulin release is glucose dependent and diminishes at low blood glucose concentrations. Hypoglycemic risk appears to be less with meglitinides than with Sulfonylureas. The average reduction in A1C is about 0.8% to 1%. These agents can be used to provide increased insulin secretion during meals (when it is needed) in patients who are close to glycemic goals. They should be administered before each meal (up to 30 minutes prior). If a meal is skipped, the medication should also be skipped.

- **Repaglinide** (Prandin) is initiated at 0.5 to 2 mg with a maximum dose of 4 mg per meal (up to four meals per day or 16 mg/day). **Nateglinide** (Starlix) dosing is 120 mg three times daily before each meal.

Biguanides

- **Metformin** is the only biguanide available in the United States. It enhances insulin sensitivity of both hepatic and peripheral (muscle) tissues. This allows for increased uptake of glucose into these insulin-sensitive tissues. Metformin consistently reduces A1C levels by 1.5% to 2%, FPG levels by 60 to 80 mg/dl, and retains the ability to reduce FPG levels when they are very high (>300 mg/dL). It reduces plasma triglycerides and low-density lipoprotein (LDL) cholesterol by 8% to 15% and modestly increases high-density lipoprotein (HDL) cholesterol (2%). It does not induce hypoglycemia when used alone.
- Metformin should be included in the therapy for all type 2 DM patients (if tolerated and not contraindicated) because it is the only oral antihyperglycemic medication proven to reduce the risk of total mortality and cardiovascular death.
- The most common adverse effects are abdominal discomfort, stomach upset, diarrhoea, anorexia, and a metallic taste. These effects can be minimized by titrating the dose slowly and taking it with food. Extended release Metformin (Glucophage XR) may reduce some of the GI side effects. Lactic acidosis occurs rarely and can be minimized by avoiding its use in patients with renal insufficiency (serum creatinine 1.4 mg/dl or greater in women and 1.5 mg/dl or greater in men), congestive heart failure, or conditions predisposing to hypoxemia or inherent lactic acidosis. Metformin should be discontinued 2 to 3 days prior to IV radiographic dye studies and withheld until normal renal function has been documented post study.
- **Metformin immediate-release** is usually initiated at 500 mg twice daily with the largest meals and increased by 500 mg weekly until glycemic goals or 2,000 mg/day is achieved. Metformin 850 mg can be dosed once daily and then increased every 1 to 2 weeks to a maximum of 850 mg three times daily (2,550 mg/day).
- **Metformin extended-release** (Glucophage XR) can be initiated with 500 mg with the evening meal and increased by 500 mg weekly to a maximum dose of 2,000 mg/day. Administration two to three times a day may help minimize GI side effects and improve glycemic control. The 750-mg tablets can be titrated weekly to the maximum dose of 2,250 mg/day.

Thiazolidinediones (glitazones)

- These agents activate PPAR-γ, a nuclear transcription factor important in fat cell differentiation and fatty acid metabolism. PPAR-γ agonists enhance insulin sensitivity in muscle, liver, and fat tissues indirectly. Insulin must be present in significant quantities for these actions to occur.
- When given for about 6 months, pioglitazone and rosiglitazone reduce A1C values by about 1.5% and FPG levels by about 60 to 70 mg/dL at maximal doses. Maximal glycemic-lowering effects may not be seen until 3 to 4 months of therapy. Monotherapy is often ineffective unless the drugs are given early in the disease course when sufficient β-cell function and hyperinsulinemia are present.
- Pioglitazone decreases plasma triglycerides by 10% to 20%, whereas rosiglitazone tends to have no effect. Pioglitazone does not cause significant increases in LDL cholesterol, whereas LDL cholesterol may increase by 5% to 15% with rosiglitazone.
- Fluid retention may occur, perhaps as a result of peripheral vasodilation and/or improved insulin sensitization with a resultant increase in renal sodium and water retention. Edema is reported in 4% to 5% of patients when Glitazones are used alone or with other oral agents. When used in combination with insulin, the incidence of edema is about 15%. Glitazones are contraindicated in patients with New York Heart Association Class III and IV heart failure and should be used with great caution in patients with Class I or II heart failure or other underlying cardiac disease.
- Weight gain is dose related, and an increase of 1.5 to 4 kg is not uncommon. Rarely, rapid gain of a large amount of weight may necessitate discontinuation of therapy. Weight gain positively predicts a larger A1C reduction but must be balanced with the potential adverse effects of long term weight gain.
- Several case reports of Hepatotoxicity with pioglitazone or rosiglitazone have been reported, but improvement in alanine aminotransferase (ALT) was consistently observed upon drug discontinuation. Baseline ALT should be obtained prior to therapy and then periodically thereafter at the practitioner's discretion. Neither drug should be started if the baseline ALT exceeds 2.5 times the upper limit of normal. The drugs should be discontinued if the ALT is more than 3 times the upper limit of normal.
- Rosiglitazone has been associated with an increased risk of myocardial ischemic events such as angina or myocardial infarction in several studies. Although causality has not been conclusively established, the FDA has required that a "black box" warning be added to the labeling. A new long term study to evaluate potential cardiovascular risks is planned.
- **Pioglitazone** (Actos) is started at 15 mg once daily. The maximum dose is 45 mg/day.
- **Rosiglitazone** (Avandia) is initiated with 2 to 4 mg once daily. The maximum dose is 8 mg/day. A dose of 4 mg twice daily can reduce A1C by 0.2% to 0.3% more than a dose of 8 mg taken once daily.

α-Glucosidase Inhibitors

- These agents prevent the breakdown of sucrose and complex carbohydrates in the small intestine, thereby prolonging the absorption of carbohydrates. The net effect is a reduction in the postprandial glucose concentrations (40 to 50 mg/dl) while fasting glucose levels are relatively unchanged (about 10% reduction). Efficacy on glycemic control is modest, with average reductions in A1C of 0.3% to 1%. Good candidates for these drugs are patients who are near target A1C levels with near-normal FPG levels but high postprandial levels.
- The most common side effects are flatulence, bloating, abdominal discomfort, and diarrhoea, which can be minimized by slow dosage titration. If hypoglycemia occurs when used in combination with a hypoglycemic agent (sulphonylurea or insulin), oral or parenteral glucose (dextrose) products or glucagon must be given because the drug will inhibit the breakdown and absorption of more complex sugar molecules (e.g., sucrose).
- **Acarbose** (Precose) and **Miglitol** (Glyset) are dosed similarly. Therapy is initiated with a very low dose (25 mg with one meal a day) and increased very gradually (over several months) to a maximum of 50 mg three times daily for patients weighing 60 kg or more, or 100 mg three times daily for patients above 60 kg. The drugs should be taken with the first bite of the meal so that the drug is present to inhibit enzyme activity.

Dipeptidyl Peptidase-IV Inhibitors

- Dipeptidyl peptidaze-IV inhibitors prolong the half-life of an endogenously produced glucagon-like peptide-1. These agents partially reduce the inappropriately elevated glucagon post prandially and stimulate glucose dependent insulin secretion. The average reduction in A1C is approximately 0.7% to 1% at a dose of 100 mg/day.
- The drugs are well tolerated, weight neutral, and do not cause GI side effects. Mild hypoglycemia appears to be the only significant adverse effect, but long-term safety data are limited.
- **Sitagliptin** (Januvia) is usually dosed at 100 mg orally once daily. In patients with renal impairment, the daily dose should be reduced to 50 mg (creatinine clearance 30–50 mL/min) or 25 mg (creatinine clearance <30 mL/min).
- **Vildagliptin** was not approved in the United States at the time of this writing (June 2008). The usual dose is expected to be similar to Sitagliptin.

PHARMACOTHERAPY OF TYPE 1 DIABETES MELLITUS

- All patients with type I DM require insulin, but the type and manner of delivery differ considerably among individual patients and clinicians.
- Therapeutic strategies should attempt to match carbohydrate intake with glucose-lowering processes (usually insulin) and exercise. Dietary intervention should allow the patient to live as normal a life as possible.
- Fig. 76.2 depicts the relationship between glucose concentrations and insulin secretion over the course of a day and how various insulin regimens may be given.

- The timing of insulin onset, peak, and duration of effect must match meal patterns and exercise schedules to achieve near-normal blood glucose values throughout the day.
- A regimen of two daily injections that may roughly approximate physiologic insulin secretion is split-mixed injections of a morning dose of NPH insulin and regular insulin before breakfast and again before

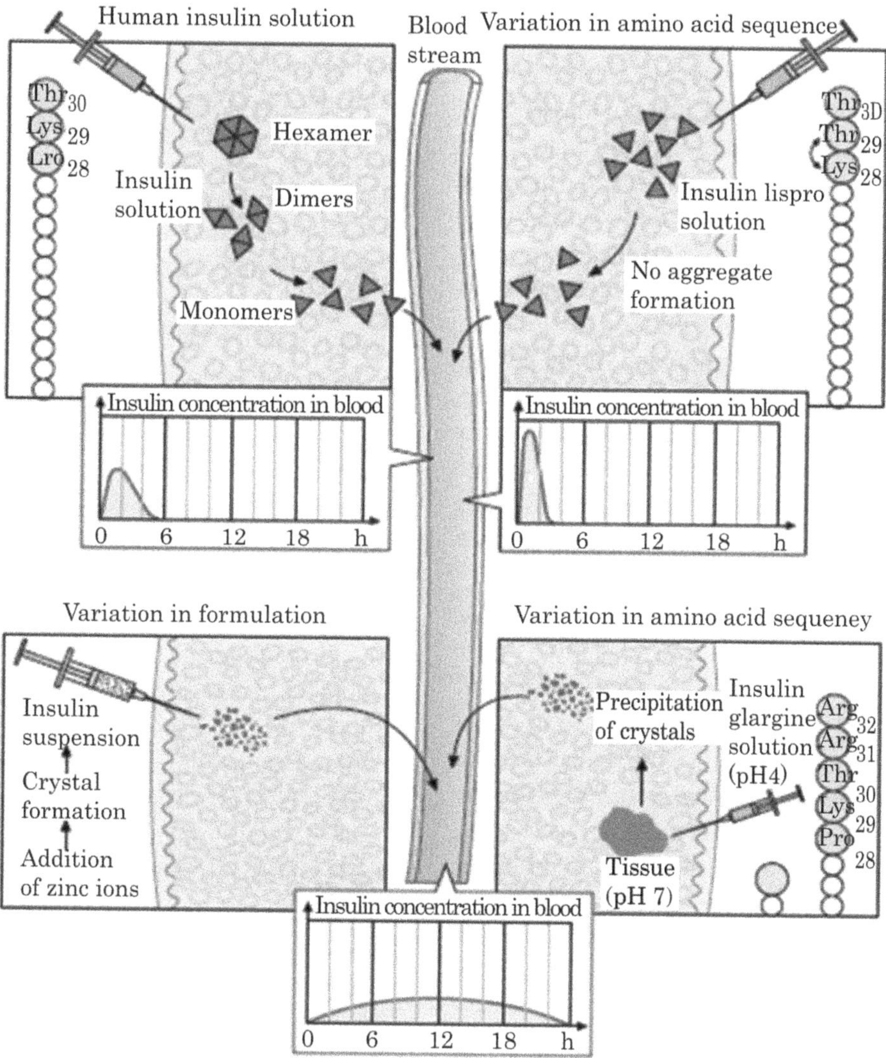

FIGURE 76.2

Human insulin release from injection site.

(Source : Colour Atlas Of Pharmacology ,3rd edition ,Page no.259)

the evening meal. This assumes that the morning NPH insulin provides basal insulin for the day and covers the midday meal, the morning regular insulin covers breakfast, the evening NPH insulin gives basal insulin for the rest of the day, and the evening regular insulin covers the evening meal. Patients may be started on 0.6 units/kg/day, with two-thirds given in the morning and one-third in the evening. Intermediate-acting insulin (e.g., NPH) should comprise two-thirds of the morning dose and one-half of the evening dose. However, most patients are not sufficiently predictable in their schedule and food intake to allow tight glucose control with this approach. If the fasting glucose in the morning is too high, the evening NPH dose may be moved to bedtime (now three total injections per day). This may provide sufficient intensification of therapy for some patients.

- The basal insulin component may be provided by once- or twice-daily **NPH** or **detemir**, or once-daily **insulin glargine**. Most type 1 DM patients require two injections of all insulins except insulin glargine. All of the insulins (with the exception of insulin glargine) have some degree of peak effect that must be considered in planning meals and activity. Insulin glargine or insulin detemir is a feasible basal insulin supplement for most patients.

As an example, patients may begin on about 0.6 units/kg/day of insulin, with basal insulin 50% of the total dose and prandial insulin 20% of the total dose before breakfast, 15% before lunch, and 15% before dinner. Most patients require total daily doses between 0.5 and 1 unit/kg/day.

The bolus insulin component is given before meals with **regular insulin, insulin lispro, insulin aspart,** or **insulin glulisine**. The rapid onset and short duration of rapid-acting insulin analogs more closely replicate normal physiology than regular insulin, allowing the patient to vary the amount of insulin injected based on the pre-prandial SMBG level, upcoming activity level, and anticipated carbohydrate intake. Most patients have a prescribed dose of insulin preprandially that they vary based on an insulin algorithm. Carbohydrate counting is an effective tool for determining the amount of insulin to be injected preprandially.

PHARMACOTHERAPY OF TYPE 2 DIABETES MELLITUS

- Symptomatic patients may initially require insulin or combination oral therapy to reduce glucose toxicity (which may reduce â-cell insulin secretion and worsen insulin resistance).Patients with A1C of about 7% or less are usually treated with therapeutic lifestyle measures with or without an insulin sensitizer. Those with A1C >7% but <8% are initially treated with a single oral agent. Patients with higher initial A1C values may benefit from initial therapy with two oral agents or insulin. Most patients with A1C values >9% to 10% require two or more agents to reach glycemic goals.
- Obese patients (>120% ideal body weight) without contraindications should be started on **metformin** initially, titrated to about 2,000 mg/day. A thiazolidine-diones **(rosiglitazone, piog-litazone)**

Table 76.2

Available insulins and other injectable preparations

Generic Name	Administration Options
Rapid-acting insulins	
Humalog (insulin lispro)	Insulin pen3-mL, vial, and 3-mL pen catridge
NovolLog (Insulin aspart)	Insulin pen3-mL, vial, or 3-mL pen catridge
Adidra (insulin gluisine)	3-mL pen cartridge or OptiClik pen system
Short-acting insulins	
Humulin R (regular)	100units, 10-mL vial; 500 units, 20-mL vial
Novalin R (regular)	Insulin pen, vial, or 3-mL pen catridge, and InnoLet
Intermediate-acting insulins (NPH)	
Humulin N	Vial, prefilled pen
Novolin N	Vial, prefilled pen, and InnoLet
Long-acting insulins	
Lantus (insulin glargine)	Vial, 3mL OptiClik pen system
Levemir (insulin detemir)	Vial, 3 mL pen cartridge and InnoLet
Premixed insulins	
Premixed insulin analogs	
Humalog Mix 75/25 (75% neutral protamine lispro, 25% lispro)	Vial, prefilled pen
Novolog Mix 70/30 (70% aspart protamine suspension, 30% aspart)	Vial, prefilled pen, 3-mL pen catridge
Humalog Mix 50/50 (50% neutral protamine lispro, 50% lispro)	3-mL Pen
NPH-regular combinations	
Humulin 70/30	Vial, prefilled pen
Novolin 70/30	Vial, pen cartridge, InnoLet
Humulin 50/50	Vial
Other injectable preparations	
Exenatide (Byeta)	5-mcg/dose and 10-mcg/dose, 60 doses prefilled pen
Pramlintide (Symlin)	5-mL vial, 1-5mL and 2.7-mL Symlin Pen

may be used in patients intolerant of or having a contraindication to metformin.

- Near-normal-weight patients may be treated with **insulin secretagogues**.
- Failure of initial therapy should result in addition of another class of drug. Substitution of a drug from another class should be reserved for drug intolerance.

Metformin and an insulin secretagogue are often first- and second-line therapy.

- Initial combination therapy should be considered for patients with A1C >9% to 10% and several oral combination products are available.
- If a patient has inadequate control on two drugs, adding a third class can be

Table 76.3

Pharmacokinetics of various insulin administered subcutaneously

Type of Insulin	Onset	Peak (hours)	Duration (hours)	Maximum Duration (hours)	Appearance
Rapid-acting					
Aspart	15-30 minutes	1-2	3-5	5-6	Clear
Lispro	15-30 minutes	1-2	3-4	4-6	Clear
Gluisine	15-30 minutes	1-2	3-4	5-6	Clear
Short-acting					
Regular	30-60 minutes	2-3	3-6	6-8	Clear
Intermediate -acting					
NPH	2-4 hours	4-6	8-12	14-18	Cloudy
Long-acting					
Glargine	4-5 hours	--	22-2	24	Clear
Detemir	2 hours	6-9	14-24	24	Clear

considered (e.g., a glitazone, exenatide, a dipeptidyl peptidase-IV inhibitor, or basal insulin). Therapy should be guided by the A1C, FPG, cost, additional benefits (e.g., weight loss), and avoidance of side effects).

- Virtually all patients ultimately become insulinopenic and require insulin therapy. Patients are often transitioned to insulin by using a bedtime injection of intermediate- or long-acting insulin with oral agents used primarily for glycemic control during the day. This results in less hyperinsulinemia during the day and less weight gain than more traditional insulin strategies. Insulin sensitizers are commonly used with insulin because most patients are insulin resistant.
- When the combination of bedtime insulin plus daytime oral medications fails, a conventional multiple daily dose insulin regimen with an insulin sensitizer can be tried.
- Because of the variability of insulin resistance, insulin doses may range from 0.7 to 2.5 units/kg/day or more.

TREATMENT OF COMPLICATIONS

RETINOPATHY

- Patients with established retinopathy should be examined by an ophthalmologist at least every 6 to 12 months.
- Early background retinopathy may reverse with improved glycemic control. More advanced disease will not regress with improved control and may actually worsen with short-term improvements in glycemia.
- Laser photocoagulation has markedly improved sight preservation in diabetic patients.

Table 76.4

Oral agents for the treatment of type 2 diabetes mellitus

Generic Name (generic version available? Y = yes, N=no)	Non elderly	Elderly	Recommended Starting Dosage (mg/day)			
			Equivalent Therapeutic Dose (mg)	Maximum Dose (mg/day)	Duration of Action	Metabolism or Therapeutic Notes
Sulphonylurea Acetohexamide (Y)	250	125-250	500	1,500	Up to 16 hours	Metabolized n liver; metabolite potency equal to parent compound; renally eliminated
Chlorpropamide	250	100	250	500	Up to 72 hours	Metabolized in liver; also excreted unchanged renally
Tolazamide (Y)	100-250	100	250	1,000.00	Up to 24 hours	Metabolized in liver, metabolite less active than parent compound; renally eliminated.
Tolbutamide (Y)	1,000-2,000	500-1,000	1,000	3,000	Up to 12 hours	Metabolized in liver to inactive metabolites that are renally excreted
Glipizide (Y)	5	2.5-5	5	40	Up to 20 hours	Metabolized in liver to inactive metabolites
Glipizide (Y)	5	2.5-5	5	20	24 hours	slow-release form; do not cut tablet
Glyburide (Y)	5	1.25-2.5	5	20	Up to 24 hours	Metabolized in liver, elimination ½ renal, ½ feces.
Glyburide, micronized (Y)	3	1.5-3	3	12	Up to 24 hours	Equal control, but better absorption from micronized preparation
Glimepiride (Y)	1-2	0.5-1	2	8	24 hours	Metabolized in liver to inactive metabolites
Nateglilnide (N)	120 with meals	120 with meals	N/A	120 mg three times a day	Up to 4 hours	Metabolized by cytochrome P450 (CYP-45002C9 and 3A4 to weakly active metabolites; renally eliminated
Biguanides Metformin (Y)	500mg twice a day	Assess renal function	N/A	2,550	Up to 24 hours	No metabolism; renally secreted and excreted.

Table 76.4 *Contd...*

Generic Name (generic version available? Y = yes, N=no)	Non elderly	Elderly	Recommended Starting Dosage (mg/day)			
			Equivalent Therapeutic Dose (mg)	Maximum Dose (mg/day)	Duration of Action	Metabolism or Therapeutic Notes
Metformin extended release (Y)	500-1,000 mg with evening meal	Assess renal function	N/A	2,550	Up to 24 hours	Take with evening meal or may split dose, may consider trial if intolerant to immediate release.
			N/A	45	24 hours	Metabolized by CYP 2C8 and 3A4' two metabolites have longer half lives than parent compound
			N/A	8mg/day or 4 mg twice a day	24 hours	Metabolized by CYPO 2C8 and 2C9 to inactive metabolites that are renally excreted.
α-glucosidase inhibitors Acarbose (N)	25mg 1-3 times a day	25mg 1-3 times a day	N/A	25-100mg three times a day	1-3 Hours	Eliminated in bile
Miglitol (N)	25mg 1-3 times a day	25mg 1-3 times a day	N/A	25-100mg three times a day	1-3 Hours	Eliminated renally
Dipeptidyl deptidase-IV (DPP-IV) inhibitors Sitagliptin (N)	100mg daily	25-100 mg daily based on renal function	N/A	100 mg daily	24 hours	50 mg daily if creatinine clearance > 30 to <50ml/min; 25mg daily if creatinine clearance <30mL/min
Example combination products Glyburide/ metformin (Y)	2.5-5/500mg twice a day	1.25/250mg twice a day; assess renal function	N/A	20 mg of Glyburide, 2,000 mg of metformin	Combination medication	Used as initial therapy: 1.25/250mg twice a day
Glipizide/ metformin (N)	2.5-5/500mg twice a day	2.5/250mg; assess renal function	N/A	20mg of Glipizide, 2000 mg of metformin	Combination medication	Used as initial therapy: 2.5/250mg twice a day
Rosiglitazone/metformin (N)	1-2/500 mg twice a day	1/500 mg twice a day; assess renal function	N/A	8mg of Rosiglitazone; 2,000 mg of metformin	Combination medication	Can use as initial therapy

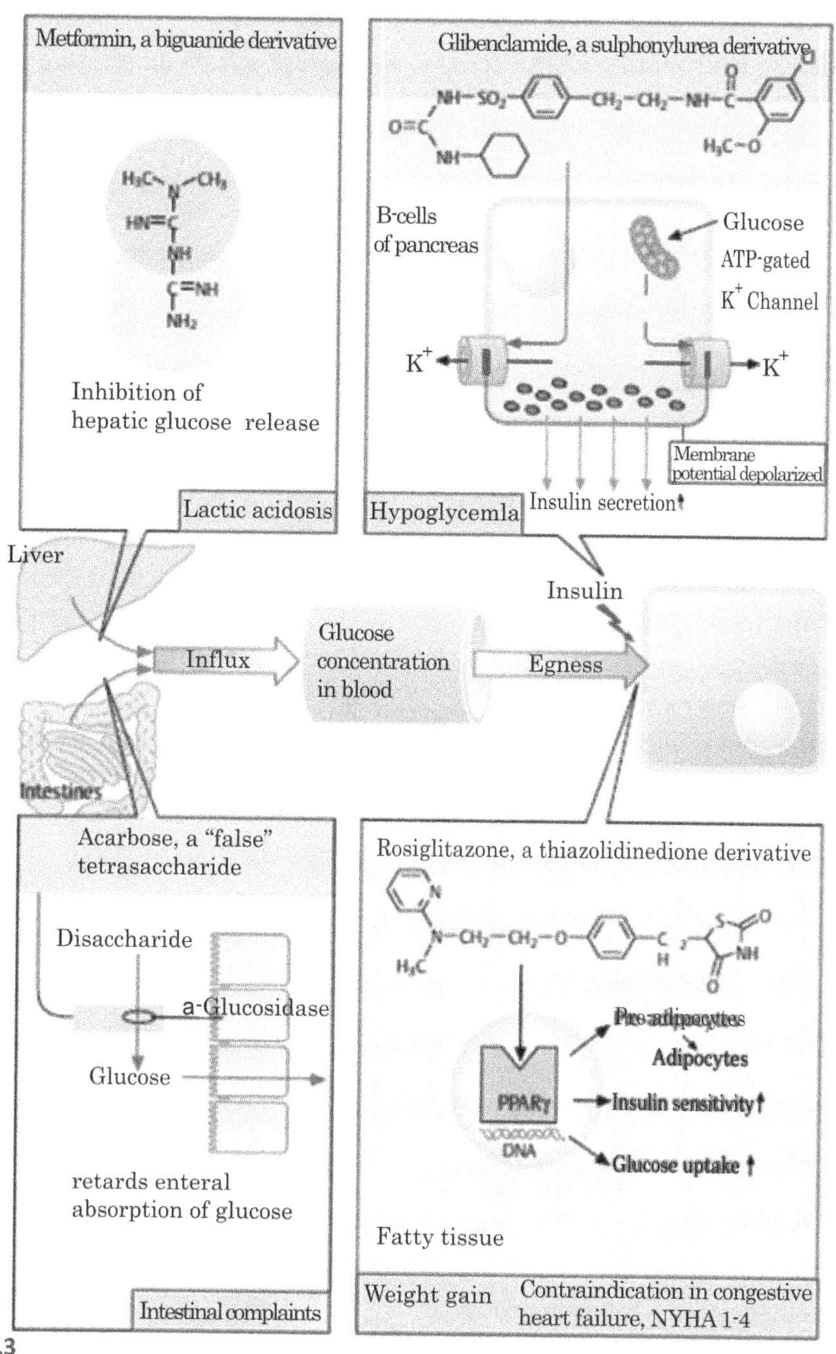

FIGURE 76.3

Oral antidiabetics.

(Source : Colour Atlas Of Pharmacology, 3rd edition, Page no.265)

NEUROPATHY

- Peripheral neuropathy is the most common complication in type 2 DM outpatients. Paresthesias, numbness, or pain may be predominant symptoms. The feet are involved far more often than the hands. Improved glycemic control may alleviate some of the symptoms. Pharmacologic therapy is symptomatic and empiric, including low-dose **tricyclic antidepressants**, anticonvulsants (e.g., **Gabapentin, Pregabalin, carbamazepine**), **Duloxetine, venlafaxine, topical capsaicin,** and various analgesics, including **tramadol** and **nonsteroidal anti-inflammatory drugs**.
- Gastroparesis can be severe and debilitating. Improved glycemic control, discontinuation of medications that slow gastric motility, and use of **metoclopramide** (preferably for only a few days at a time) or **erythromycin** may be helpful.
- Patients with orthostatic hypotension may require mineralocorticoids or adrenergic agonists.
- Diabetic diarrhea is commonly nocturnal and frequently responds to a 10 to 14 day course of an antibiotic such as **doxycycline** or **metronidazole**. **Octreotide** may be useful in unresponsive cases.
- Erectile dysfunction is common, and initial treatment should include one of the oral medications currently available (e.g., **sildenafil, vardenafil, tadalafil**).

NEPHROPATHY

- Glucose and blood pressure control are most important for prevention of nephropathy, and blood pressure control is most important for retarding the progression of established nephropathy.
- Angiotensin-converting enzyme inhibitors and angiotensin receptor blockers have shown efficacy in preventing the clinical progression of renal disease in patients with type 2 DM. Diuretics are frequently necessary due to volume-expanded states and are recommended second-line therapy.

PERIPHERAL VASCULAR DISEASE AND FOOT ULCERS

- Claudication and nonhealing foot ulcers are common in type 2 DM. Smoking cessation, correction of dyslipidemia, and antiplatelet therapy are important treatment strategies.
- **Pentoxifylline** (Trental) or **cilostazol** (Pletal) may be useful in selected patients. Revascularization is successful in selected patients.
- Local debridement and appropriate footwear and foot care are important in the early treatment of foot lesions. Topical treatments may be beneficial in more advanced lesions.

CORONARY HEART DISEASE

- Multiple-risk-factor intervention (treatment of dyslipidemia and hypertension, smoking cessation, antiplatelet therapy) reduces macrovascular events.

- The National Cholesterol Education Program Adult Treatment Panel III guidelines classify the presence of DM as a coronary heart disease risk equivalent, and the goal LDL cholesterol is <100 mg/dl. An optional LDL goal in high-risk DM patients is <70 mg/dl. After the LDL goal is reached (usually with a **statin**), treatment of high triglycerides (e"200 mg/dl) is considered. The non-HDL goal for patients with DM is <130 mg/ dl. **Niacin** or a **Fibrate** can be added to reach that goal if triglycerides are 201 to 499 mg/dl or if the patient has low HDL cholesterol (<40 mg/dl).
- The American Diabetes Association and the National Kidney Foundation recommend a goal blood pressure of <130/80 mm Hg in patients with DM.

Angiotensin-converting enzyme inhibitors and **angiotensin receptor blockers** are generally recommended for initial therapy. Many patients require multiple agents, so diuretics, calcium channel blockers, and â-**blockers** are useful as second and third agents.

REFERENCES

1. Shoback, edited by David G. Gardner, Dolores (2011). *Greenspan's basic & clinical endocrinology* (9th ed. ed.). New York: McGraw-Hill Medical. pp. Chapter 17.
2. *Williams textbook of endocrinology* (12th ed.). Philadelphia: Elsevier/Saunders. pp. 1371–1435.
3. Lambert, P.; Bingley, P. J. (2002). "What is Type 1 Diabetes?". *Medicine* **30**: 5.
4. "Diabetes Mellitus (DM): Diabetes Mellitus and Disorders of Carbohydrate Metabolism: Merck Manual Professional". Merck.com. Retrieved 2010-07-30.
5. "Diabetes mellitus, fasting blood glucose concentration, and risk of vascular disease: a collaborative meta-analysis of 102 prospective studies : The Lancet".
6. Risérus U, Willett WC, Hu FB (January 2009). "Dietary fats and prevention of type 2 diabetes". *Progress in Lipid Research* **48** (1): 44–51.
7. "Definition and Diagnosis of Diabetes Mellitus and Intermediate Hyper-glycemia" (pdf). *World Health Organization*. www.who.int. 2006. Retrieved 2011-02-20.
8. Ripsin, CM; Kang, H, Urban, RJ (2009-01-01). "Management of blood glucose in type 2 diabetes mellitus". *American family physician* **79** (1): 29–36.
9. Wild, S; Roglic, G; Green, A; Sicree, R; King, H (2004). "Global prevalence of diabetes: Estimates for the year 2000 and projections for 2030". *Diabetes Care* **27** (5): 1047–53.
10. American Diabetes Association (2005). "Total Prevalence of Diabetes & Pre-diabetes". Archived fromthe original on 2006-02-08. Retrieved 2006-03-17.
11. Ripoll, Brian C. Leutholtz, Ignacio (2011-04-25). *Exercise and disease management* (2nd ed.). Boca Raton: CRC Press. pp. 25.
12. Greenstone MA, Shaw AB: Alternate day corticosteroid causes alternate day hyperglycemia. *Postgrad Med J* 63:761-64, 1987.
13. Grunfled C, Baird K, Van Obberghen E, Kahn CR: Glucosteroid-induced insulin

resistance in vitro: evidence for both receptor and post-receptor defects. *Endocrinol*109:1723, 1981.

14. Hirsch IB, Paauw DS: Diabetes management in special situations. *Endocrinol Metab Clin North Am* 26:631-43, 1997.
14. Tanaka M, Endo K, Suzuki T, Maruyama Y, Kondo A: Treatment of steroid-induced diabetes with alpha-glucosidase inhibitor voglibose. *Eur J Neurol* 5:315, 1998.

CHAPTER 77

Cushing's Syndrome

INTRODUCTION

Cushing's syndrome is an adrenal gland multisystem disorder that results from sustained exposure to glucocorticoids, that when untreated results in increase in the relative cardiovascular mortality risk.

The various conditions of high prevalence like hypertension, osteoporosis, depression and obesity may present with the anomalism of the hypothalamicpituitary adrenal axis (i.e., elevated levels of cortisol urinary excretion and abnormal responses to dexamethasone suppression) that in general do not reflect the sustained pathologic hypercortisolemia ("pseudo-Cushing's states").

ETIOLOGY AND PATHOGENESIS

Pituitary-Dependent Hypercortisolism

Pituitary tumors are the most important and frequent anatomic etiology for CD. Thus, microadenomas (tumors under 10 mm), noninvasive macroadenomas (tumors larger than 10 mm, but confined to the sella), and invasive macroadenomas are all known to cause CD. Rare cases of CD secondary to hyperplasia of the corticotropes probably represent the early stages in the evolution of the disease. Microadenomas represent the most common etiology, accounting for nearly 80% of CD. While the anatomical etiology of CD is relatively clear, the pathophysiological basis for the development of the disease is far from explicit. It is believed that an abnormality in the hypothalamopituitary-adrenal (HPA) axis sets the stage for the development of this disorder. The characteristic hallmark of a normal HPA axis is prompt recognition by and brisk suppression of ACTH to even minor increases in circulating cortisol levels. This unique sensitivity to suppress in response to negative feedback is blunted in pituitary-dependent CD. Consequently, the hypothalamic pituitary threshold for suppression is raised and the ACTH secretory rate is consistently inappropriate, relative to the circulating cortisol levels at any given time. 'The raised threshold to negative feedback is evidenced by the response of patients with CD to the standard dexamethasone suppression tests (i.e., lack of physiological suppression to low-dose dexamethasone, but preservation of suppression to "higher" doses). The degree of abnormality is variable from patient to patient, some requiring a higher dose than that used in the conventional test. Nevertheless, they do suppress, denoting preservation of physiological cues, albeit operating at a higher threshold. This response pattern is classic for pituitary-dependent CD.

The aforementioned simplistic concept of "reset" hypothalamic pituitary axis has come under rigorous scrutiny in the past decade. The controversy revolves around a very basic issue-is CD a "primary derangement of the pituitary gland" as characterized, or is it a result of an overactive hypothalamic driving mechanism. The proponents of both theories have drawn on histological, biochemical, hormonal, and pharmacological facts to support their respective premise. The ongoing polemic has great significance in terms of its impact on choosing the options for therapy; if the disease is a result of a primary pituitary tumor, a properly performed transsphenoidal microadenectomy should be curative, while if a hypothalamic overdrive was causing the problem, then medical therapy to correct the overdrive would be the logical initial choice.

PRIMARY HYPOTHALAMIC ETIOLOGY

There are several lines of evidence to suggest that CD is a result of corticotrope overactivity secondary to an accentuated hypothalamic drive. *Anatomically* this is supported by the observation that a small, but significant number of patients with CD fail to show any tumor in the pituitary gland despite the most scrutinizing exploration. Indeed, remission of pituitary-dependent CD after removal of nonneoplastic pituitary gland has been reported. The availability of assays for circulating ACTH level in the plasma has greatly facilitated study of ACTH dynamics in pituitary-dependent CD. The pituitary ACTH secretion in CD responds to a variety of seemingly unrelated agents. Thus, thyrotropin-releasing hormone (TRH),5 vasopressin,5,6 and luteinizing-hormone-releasing hormones are all capable of releasing ACTH from pituitary tumors that cause CD, denoting nonautonomy of the tumor and partial preservation of responsiveness.

A major pharmacological link of evidence that points to a central nervous system site as the cause of pituitary-dependent CD comes from studies with cyproheptadine. This drug is a serotonin antagonist which in some patients with CD effectively lowers cortisol and ACTH levels, restores normal suppressibility, and can even induce a sustained remission of CD and Nelson's syndrome.

While the action of this drug is not completely understood, it acts on the central nervous system and is capable of blocking the release of corticotropin-releasing factor (CRF) from the hypothalamus of the rat. More specifically, does cyproheptadine reverse the abnormality in ACTH feedback inherent to patients with CD.

Another pharmacological agent, bromocriptine, can also lower ACTH levels in patients with CD. The characterization and isolation of CRF has provided perhaps the strongest support to the notion that hypothalamic (or even more central) influences underlie the pathophysiology of CD. The demonstration of brisk ACTH response to the intravenous administration of ovine CRF dearly implies that the pituitary adenoma cells are not only nonautonomous, but are possibly hypersensitive to the hypothalamic peptide. Finally, ACTH-dependent Cushing's syndrome can result from ectopic secretion of CRH.

The pituitary demonstrated hyperplasia of the corticotropes, while the extracts from the tumor and the metastases contained CRF (but not ACTH) measurable by both radioimmunoassay and bioassay. This was the first documentation of CRF-induced hypercortisolism. The development of Nelson's syndrome following bilateral adrenalectomy for CD is often cited as evidence to support a hypothalamic etiology for CD. Nelson's syndrome, characterized by markedly increased plasma ACTH levels, despite glucocorticoid replacement, shares several similarities in hormone dynamics with untreated CD. The response to TRH, cyproheptadine, bromocriptine, and CRH administration is strikingly identical in both diseases.

PRIMARY PITUITARY DISORDER

The two major reasons for considering the pituitary gland as the primary seat of the disease are the high percentage of microadenomas found during surgery and the increasing number of "cures" attained following successful microadenomectomy by transsphenoidal surgery (TPS). The ability to study the behavior of corticostrope adenoma cells in tissue culture has provided insight into this phenomenon.

Several recent in vitro studies have also evaluated the effect of various drugs on the isolated tumor cells grown in tissue culture. cyproheptadine and reserpine directly inhibit the release of

ACTH and endorphin in vitro from adenomas removed from patients with pituitary-dependent CD. Similar observations have been extended to bromocriptine. These powerful data have clearly dealt a blow to the hypothalamic theory of origin of CD, since obviously these drugs can directly act on the pituitary gland, circumventing all mediation by the hypothalamus. Additional support to the primary pituitary origin of CD is derived from the observation that transient hypoadrenalism develops after successful extirpation of the ACTH-secreting microadenoma.

While controversy continues regarding the pathophysiology of CD, evidence for the presence of *both* subtypes of CD has been presented . The cortisol pulses, i.e., variations in the circulating cortisol levels in the plasma over a 24-hr period were studied . The "cortisol profile" of normal subjects shows a characteristic jagged pattern with 7-10 pulsatile bursts of secretory activity. The cortisol spikes are due to concomitant ACTH spikes, which in turn are presumed to be due to pulsatile release of CRF by the hypothalamus.

INTERMEDIATE-LOBE PATHOLOGY

While indeed most ACTH-secreting microadenomas arise from the anterior lobe, they can also arise from the intermediate lobe, an area of the pituitary that is anatomically not well delineated in the human. Yet, tumors arising from this region assume special importance in CD. The five characteristics of ACTH-secreting adenomas that arise from the intermediate lobe are:

1. The presence of argyrophilic nerve fibers coursing in and around the tumor, suggesting a neural origin.
2. Resistance to dexamethasone suppression, but response to dopamine agonists such as bromocriptine.
3. Frequent association with hyperprolactinemia.
4. Poor visualization by computed tomography of the pituitary.

5. Frequent failure to respond to transsphenoidal microadenectomy, i.e., persistence or recurrence of tumor despite the apparently complete removal of the tumor.

The relatively unsatisfactory response to surgery contrasts sharply with the highly favorable outcome following TPS for adenomas of the anterior pituitary and has tremendous impact when planning the surgical approach for such patients. The reasons for the unique differences that set apart these tumors of the intermediate lobe from conventional microadenomas of the anterior pituitary are less clear.

It was proposed that depletion of hypothalamic dopaminergic neural input may be the biochemical abnormality that underlies the development of hyperlasia of the corticotropes in the intermediate lobe followed by adenoma formation in some. An identical syndrome occurs in an strikingly parallel animal model in the horse ("equine CD"). A horse and a pony suffering from myopathy, diabetes, and hirsutism were described . The animals manifested hypercortisolism with elevated plasma levels of ACTH, disproportionate elevation of α and β melanophore-stimulating hormones, and poor suppressibility to dexamethasone, with responsiveness to intravenous dopamine, bromocriptine, and pergolide.

CLINICAL FEATURES

The clinical features of CD are a result of prolonged overproduction of cortisol. The classic manifestations are fat deposition in the face, neck, supraclavicular area, and neck resulting in the familiar moon face, buffalo hump, and truncal obesity with relative sparing of extremities are less common these days. For descriptive purposes the clinical features can be viewed from the following vantage points: the "classic" presentation, the early manifestations, the atypical manifestations, and the clinical differences between the various types of hypercortisolism.

THE "CLASSIC" PRESENTATION

The evolution of pituitary-dependent CD is a slow process, gradually evolving into the plethoric features that have become strongly associated with that disease. Several series have analyzed the incidence of the numerous physical findings encountered in patients with hypercortisolism in general. The recurring themes that emerge upon reviewing the literature are that (1) a high index of suspicion is required to make an early diagnosis, and (2) although several features of hypercortisolism can be caused by diverse disorders, when they occur collectively in the same patient CD is more likely to be present.

Hypertension, one of the most common features in patients with pituitary dependent CD, is modest, often responding excellently to therapy. The mechanism(s) that underlie the hypertension of CD are not well delineated.

The oral administration of captopril, an angiotensin I-converting enzyme inhibitor, reduced the blood pressure effectively. The possibility that the blood pressure elevation in patients with Cushing's syndrome might be secondary to suppression of depressor systems, coupled with enhanced pressor response to vasoactive substances, awaits further elucidation.

The *psychopathy* of Cushing's syndrome deserves special emphasis since it often highlights the clinical presentation. Mental changes are reported to occur in 50-60% of patients with Cushing's syndrome. These include marked emotional lability, paranoid ideation, confusion, and disorientation. In severe cases delusions, hallucinations, depression, and delirium may occur. It is interesting to note that euphoria is an uncommon facet of Cushing's psychopathy, whereas patients placed on steroids are often euphoric. It is known that steroids may have a direct effect on neuronal tissue. It has been shown that steroids directly induce electrophysiological changes in the neurons, such as diminished synaptic delay and slowing of axonal conduction. Historically, Harvey Cushing recognized that emotional disturbances were prominent features of the disease; in fact, one of his patients was found in a mental hospital with depression, irritability, and memory loss. The spectrum of psychiatric abnormalities encountered in patients with Cushing's syndrome and the relief of these abnormalities with lowering of cortisol have been amply documented .

The obvious assumption is that ACTH contributes more to the psychopathy of Cushing's syndrome than the cortisol levels. The implication that beta endorphins may be related to the Cushing's psychopathy has generated considerable interest in recent years. Beta endorphin is an opiatelike peptide extracted from the normal pituitary gland. Beta endorphin and ACTH are often secreted concomitantly to various stimuli that normally stimulate ACTH. Therefore, it seems plausible that when excessive ACTH secretion is present (central CD), a concomitant hypersecretion of beta endorphins may also occur. A single report demonstrating high endorphin levels in the cerebrospinal fluid (CSF) of psychotic patients has attempted to link mental disease with endorphins.

The significance of ACTH, endorphins, and the mental illness seen in Cushing's disease awaits elucidation. The *myopathy* associated with hypercortisolism is primarily due to protein catabolism caused by excess glucocorticoids. Like most endocrine myopathies, the proximal group of muscles are involved more commonly than the distal, subjective features are more striking than objective evidence, and the biochemical abnormalities are even less striking. Rarely, overt severe wasting of the muscles may be encountered.

Force measurements, using both the myometer and strain gauge techniques, demonstrated quadriceps weakness in every patient. The histological appearance by light microscopy was consistent with type II fiber atrophy in some, but not all, patients with endogenous hypercortisolism. Electromyographic evidence of myopathy was common to both endogenous and exogenous hypercortisolism.

The skeletal muscle content of sodium was high, but that of creatine was low. Notably, the skeletal muscle content of potassium was normal. Several of these abnormalities were reversible upon restoration of eucortisolemia.

The *thinning* of the skin, in many an experienced endocrinologist's view, is a remarkably good clue to hypercortisolism, which is the only endocrine cause for this phenomenon. The easy *bruisability* is not due to any abnormalities in coagulation, but merely represents increased fragility of the capillaries in the thinned-out skin. The *striae,* which can be quite impressive when classic, assume a violaceous hue, and are due to loss of collagen caused by glucocorticoid excess

Hyperpigmentation, is due to the pigmentary effects of lipotropin. This finding is more frequent in patients with ectopic ACTH secretory syndrome. Hirsutism, glucose intolerance, and hypertension is an impressive triad seen in a high percentage of patients with non-Cushingoid obesity as well. In many obese patients, these features may even be associated with subjective fatigue, mild depression, and menstrual irregularities, all secondary to obesity . Therefore, it is easy to miss CD in a patient with obesity. The occurrence of easy bruisability, puffy facies, significant psychopathy, or edema should increase the index of suspicion to detect hypercortisolism.

EARLY MANIFESTATIONS

As alluded to earlier, a high index of suspicion is required to recognize the disease in its early stages. Since pituitary-dependent CD evolves slowly and progresses gradually, the changes in appearance may be so insidious as to not concern the patient. In this regard pituitary-dependent CD resembles acromegaly, a closely related disorder of the pituitary gland. The following clues may be helpful in suspecting the disease in its early phase.

1. The "puffiness" (plethora) of the face develops in a patient with hypertension of recent onset .
2. The combination of edema of the feet and recent-onset hypertension in an obese patient.
3. Any patient with a history of recent weight gain, easy bruisability, and hypertension.
4. The presence of spontaneous hypokalemia in patients with recent-onset hypertension.
5. The combination of hirsutism and menstrual irregularities in a patient with recent weight gain.
6. Obesity with significant muscle weakness.
7. Unexplained psychiatric distrubances, especially depression, in association with any of the other factors.
8. Growth retardation in an obese child.

Only a small percentage of obese patients turn out to harbor CD, and indeed, Cushing's syndrome seldom if ever causes morbid obesity. Nevertheless, CD, a disorder that can kill if unrecognized, but can be cured if detected, is an important etiology to be kept in mind when evaluating any patient with recent onset of obesity.

ATYPICAL FEATURES

The term *atypical* may not be quite appropriate in discussing certain unusual findings in a disease that is as rare, as unpredictable, and as fascinating as Cushing's syndrome. Unusual deposition of fat in uncommon areas, "lipomatosis," may be seen in this syndrome. The most well-known example of this phenomenonis the mediastinal widening that occurs as a consequence of mediastinal lipomatosis. The location for fat accumulation is the epidural space. Such epidural lipomatosis has been reported to be severe enough to cause compression of the spinal cord. Very rarely the rectum can be displaced anteriorly by the presacral deposition of fat or a fatty mass can be seen in the liver, Although these phenomena occur more often with exogenous steroid administration, they are recognized features of endogenous hypercortisolism of any etiology.

Nephrolithiasis, once considered to be unusual in hypercortisolism, is being noted with increasing frequency. Renal calculi were present in 15% of patients with endogenous hypercortisolism. In the same series *loss* of *scalp hair* was present in a small, but significant percent (13%) of patients.

Since the vast majority of patients with pituitary-dependent CD harbor only small (micro-) adenomas, headaches, visual field cuts, and other parasellar phenomena are highly unusual. These features, when present, strongly point to the presence of invasive macroadenomas. However, headaches are extremely common in patients with hypercortisolism. Other unusual but important features include the occurrence of cyclical edema, increased tendency for developing superficial cutaneous fungal infections, and thromboembolic phenomena.

ETIOLOGICAL DIAGNOSIS OF CUSHING'S SYNDROME

The distinction between the various etiologies for Cushing's syndrome is crucial for proper therapy. The individual features of each variety of Cushing's syndrome is outlined , underscoring the fact that these are broad generalizations.

Pituitary-Dependent Cushing's Disease

The typical patient with pituitary-dependent CD demonstrates preservation of suppression to high-dose dexamethasone and responds to metyrapone with an increase in ll-deoxycortisol; the basal plasma ACTH concentrations are normal to minimally elevated, with further increments with the administration of ovine CRH. The plasma dehydroepiandrosterone (DHEA) sulfate levels are normal to mildly elevated. The CT of the adrenals reveal normal-sized to slightly enlarged glands bilaterally, while the pituitary gland may reveal an abnormality in 35-60% of patients. Some patients with CD may show a paradoxical ACTH response to TRH or LHRH.

Adrenal Adenoma

When Cushing's syndrome is caused by adenomas of the adrenal cortex, the patient fails to suppress with high-dose dexamethasone and fails to respond to metyrapone administration. The plasma ACTH levels are low and show no response to exogenous administration of CRH. The adrenal steroids respond, in a significant number of patients, to exogenous ACTH administration. The level of the adrenal androgen DHEA sulfate is depressed in patients with adrenal adenomas that cause Cushing's syndrome, often remaining low for as long as 2 years following surgical extirpation of the tumor. This feature, a reflection of chronic suppression of endogenous ACTH levels, is characteristic of adrenal adenoma. Computed tomographic examination almost always demonstrates a unilateral mass with a "shrunken" adrenal on the contralateral side.

Macronodular Hyperplasia

Macronodular adrenocortical hyperplasia may be associated with conflicting dynamic data since this entity is characterized by varying degrees of adrenal autonomy coupled with varying degrees of pituitary dependency; suppression tests, basal ACTH levels, and ACTH response to CRF may not always provide clear separation of this entity from CD or from unilateral tumors of the adrenal. Computerized tomography mayor may not reveal the macro nodular disease, but usually bilateral disease.

Adrenal Carcinoma

Adrenal carcinoma should be suspected when virilization occurs in association with hypercortisolism. This rare disease is a devastating disorder affecting younger patients, although it can occur at any age. The most common presentations of adrenal carcinomas are the development of Cushing's syndrome and virilization. In most instances these two syndromes occur together. Adrenal carcinomas causing virilization alone, without a concomitant increase in glucocorticoids, have been described, but the reverse has not; i.e., whenever an adrenal carcinoma causes Cushing's syndrome, there is invariably an elevation of 17-ketosteroids. The hormonal hypersecretion by an adrenal carcinoma is a rather paradoxical phenomenon because when adrenal cells become malignant they lose many enzyme systems needed to produce hormones. Therefore, these tumors are regarded as rather inefficient hormone producers. The implications of this observation are twofold. First, when there is evidence of hormone hypersecretion at the time of diagnosis, it means that the tumors have been present for a long time and have grown large enough to produce hormone hypersecretion. Second, because of the enzyme deletions several precursors are released in the circulation. Thus, DHEA, estrone, estradiol, and ll-deoxycortisol may be detected in the urine before virilization has occurred. The rapid development of Cushing's syndrome, the presence of virilizing signs, and a palpable mass would clearly indicate the clinical diagnosis of adreno-cortical carcinoma. In addition to virilization, adrenal carcinomas can result in precocious puberty in both sexes and feminization of males.

Ectopic ACTH Syndrome

The recognition of *ectopic ACTH syndrome* in its characteristic presentation of weight loss and pigmentation with metabolic phenomena (hypokalemia, alkalois, hyper-glycemia, and so forth) is relatively simple. In most patients the underlying malignancy is apparent and the plethoric features of Cushing's syndrome are absent. The cortisol levels are usually quite high (>,50 f.Lg) as is the plasma ACTH level (>250 pg). These patients are usually nonresponsive to the administration of dexamethasone, metyrapone, and CRF(corticotrophin releasing Factor). The exceptional features of the ectopic secretion of ACTH by carcinoids have already been alluded to. The occurrence of plethoric Cushing's syndrome in the setting of suppressibility to high dose dexamethasone, with only modest increments in plasma ACTH levels closely resembles pituitary-dependent CD. The metyrapone test or the CRF test has not been evaluated in a large series of patients with dexamethasone-suppressible ectopic ACTH syndrome. The only definite method of excluding a pituitary source of ACTH in such patients with an occult primary is by measuring the ACTH gradient by simultaneous bilateral inferior petrosal catheterization, preferably coupled with administration of CRF just prior to sampling.

Periodic Hormonogenesis

It is difficult to establish the diagnosis (much less the etiology) of hypercortisolism when it occurs in the setting of *periodic hormonogenesis.* Apparently these represent examples of a "tumor on a timer." The responses to dexamethasone administration are highly variable, ranging from no response to a "paradoxical" response. The cyclical change in steroid levels in these cases was unaffected by dexamethasone, and the apparent paradoxical response to dexamethasone was fortuitous. The obvious difficulty is that one cannot interpret the steroid levels as an effect of drug administration, and the increase or decrease in steroid levels is totally a reflection of periodic hormogenesis. The phenomenon of periodic hormonogenesis (cyclical Cushing's syndrome) is not restricted to pituitary-dependent CD. Even though pituitary and ACTH-secreting tumors predominate in the display of this astonishing colorful spectable of periodic hormonogenesis, adrenal tumors are not exempt. The importance of recognizing the phenomenon of periodic hormonogenesis is fourfold. First, the results of a high-dose dexamethasone test could be misinterpreted as nonsuppressible when, in fact, they are due to the periodic hormonogenesis; second, between cycles the hormone data may be "normal," and hence even establishing the hormonal diagnosis could be difficult; third, intermittent hypokalemia, periodic mental changes, intermittent loss of diabetic control, and osteopenia can elude diagnosis if this entity is not kept in mind. Finally, intermittent or cyclical hypercortisolism may result in "spontaneous remissions" of the disease.

TREATMENT

The treatment of Cushing's syndrome is based on the etiology of hypercortisolism. Although the adrenal glands are the ultimate target regardless of the etiology, therapy is directed against the primary pathogenic mechanism that stimulated the adrenals in the first place. Thus, pituitary-dependent CD is treated by pituitary surgery, pituitary radiation, and adjunctive drug therapy with neuropharmacotherapeutic agents. Cushing's syndrome caused by ectopic ACTH secretion is managed by therapy directed against the primary neoplasm, coupled with drug therapy that lowers cortisol (metyrapone, ketoconazole) or newer agents that antagonize the peripheral effects of glucocorticoids .

The ideal treatment for pituitary-dependent CD should be one that will completely remove the source of ACTH hypersecretion, restore cortisol secretion to normal, avoid hypopituitarism, and would be associated with negligible morbidity and mortality. These ideals, at least theoretically, are best fulfilled by selective micro-adenectomy by trans sphenoidal pituitary surgery (TPS). Other forms of therapy-bilateral adrenalectomy, radiation of the pituitary gland, and therapy with agents that lower ACTH-cortisol hypersecretion-fall short of these ideal requisites of therapy. The most satisfactory results for a "cure" are obtained when primary treatment is directed at the pituitary gland. Attempts at treating the hypothalamus with chemical therapy are fraught with unpredictable and transitory responses, while therapy aimed at the adrenals is drastic, with the potential for trading off two diseases (Addison's and Nelson's) for one disorder.

The options for treating patients with pituitary-dependent CD are several and include the following:

1. Transsphenoidal pituitary microsurgery,
2. Pituitary radiation.
3. Bilateral total adrenalectomy.
4. Neuropharmacotherapeutic drugs.

TRANSSPHENOIDAL PITUITARY MICROSURGERY

The procedure of trans sphenoidal pituitary surgery has gained immense popularity in the past decade. Several workers have published their experience with this procedure in the treatment of pituitary-dependent CD. It is now generally accepted that the cure rate of TPS far exceeds that of every other available therapeutic modality for CD. The success rate drops significantly when the tumor is no longer confined to the sella (25-48%). It can therefore be emphatically stated that when the tumor is confined to the sella, TPS offers the patient the best chance of a cure. The initial incision is in the midline carried into the neurohypophysis. If an adenoma is not visualized, both the lateral wings should be inspected to detect a resectable adenoma. If no adenoma is seen in either location, a final surgical sweep of the pars intermedia is made to detect a tumor in that region. If the exploration is completely negative, and the surgeon has data from selective inferior petrosal sinus cathetherization that denote a unilateral source, then a hemipituitectomy on the side of the increased gradient is performed. If no catheterization data are available, the choice between a medial wedge resection and a total hypophysectomy is difficult, often resting with the individual neurosurgeon's prior experience.

The success of TPS can be evaluated within a few days after surgery. If the source of the pituitary ACTH was completely removed, the adrenals rapidly become hypo functional. This is because the normal corticotropes have been rendered dormant owing to the suppressive effect of chronic hypercortisolism. It follows, then, that secondary hypoadrenalism (transient as it may be) is an anticipated reflection of successful resection of an ACTH-producing pituitarymicroadenoma. The transient secondary hypoadrenal state caused by prolonged suppression of normal corticotropes lasts for a variable period of time, ranging from weeks to even months. Hypocortisolism (with a low ACTH level) in the postoperative period is the best prognostic parameter for predicting cure.

The adverse effects of TPS are few. The morbidity associated with the procedure is very low. Transient diabetes insipidus is the most frequent complication. Less commonly cerebrospinal fluid leak, meningitis, and optic nerve damage may occur. The mortality, when it occurs, is more likely to be seen in patients with invasive tumors. There are several reasons for the persistence or recurrence of hypercortisolism following TPS. The three major reasons for such failure are when corticotrope hyperplasia underlies the disorder; when the tumor is invasive; and when tumors originate from the intermediate lobe to cause CD. There is a fourth reason-erroneous diagnosis, the most notorious example being ectopic ACTH secretion caused by an occult, relatively benign neoplasm mimicking the dynamics of pituitary-dependent CD. *Corticotrope hyperplasia* can be the cause of pituitary-dependent CD in a minority of patients. Although corticotrope hyperplasia can occur in a diffusely scattered form, clusters of corticotrope nests are especially found in the central posterior area of the adenohypophysis.

BILATERAL ADRENALECTOMY

This surgical method reverses hypercortisolism immediately, and for the most part permanently. The only instances of recurrence are when some adrenal tissue is inadvertently left behind; when the capsule is ruptured and clusters of cells are released into the retroperitoneal bed, where they "germinate" and gradually begin to hyperfunction ("retroperitoneal adrenal remnants"); or when adrenal rest cells in the gonads (usually testes) become functional under the chronic stimulatory influence of ACTH. The objections to bilateral total adrenalectomy as the *first* line of therapy for Cushing's disease are the following:

1. Removing the target organ(s) without removing the obvious seat of primary pathology is scientifically unsound strategy.
2. Permanent adrenal failure, with the need for lifelong replacement therapy, is a high price to pay at an age when selective microadenectomy of the pituitary is an established procedure.
3. The morbidity and mortality of bilateral adrenalectomy are significant. Most centers acknowledge a 5% mortality with this procedure. The postoperative complications include infection, bleeding, thromboembolic phenomena, and pancreatitis.
4. The most important objection to bilateral total adrenalectomy is the possibility of developing Nelson's syndrome. This entity is characterized by the development of generalized hyperpigmentation, progressive enlargement of the sella turcica, and the development of visual-field cuts.

The indications for bilateral adrenalectomy are

1. When the hypercortisolism is life threatening, and a rapid 100% effective modality is imminently required to correct it.
2. When pituitary surgery has failed to cure the patient's disease.
3. When hypercortisolism recurs after a period of remission following pituitary surgery.
4. When macronodular hyperplasia is suspected on the basis of hormonalstudies or CT of the adrenals.

PITUITARY RADIATION

Conventional radiation to the pituitary gland is a time-honored therapeutic modality for CD. About 5000 rads are delivered to the pituitary gland over a 4-5-week period. The main advantage of the procedure is that it is relatively free from major side effects. Conventional radiation has enjoyed the reputation of being an innocuous form of therapy since it is devoid of complications such as hypopituitarism or optic nerve damage. The major drawback of conventional pituitary radiation, particularly in adults, is the relatively low cure rates attained. The low cure rate, and the long delay in attaining a remission have been compelling reasons to minimize the enthusiasm for this therapy. The lack of adverse effects, particularly hypopituitarism, is especially important in this group of patients where preservation of growth and sexual maturation are vital concerns while planning therapy.

Considering this factor, and coupled with its high cure rate, conventional radiation is favored by many as the first option in children and adolescents with CD. Proton beam (or heavy-particle) radiation is a highly effective method to treat pituitary-dependent CD. The major limitation of this modality is the nonavailability of the procedure in most centers and the higher incidence of complications such as hypopituitarism and oculomotor nerve palsies.

NEUROPHARMACOTHERAPY

The role of neuropharmacological agents in the treatment of CD is at best adjunctive. The basis for the use of drugs that modulate ACTH secretion rests on the ability of certain drugs to impair or deplete monoamine concentrations in the hypothalamus. Hypothalamic release of CRH can be affected by neurotransmitter concentration in the hypothalamus. Thus inhibitors of serotonin (and in some instances dopamine agonists) are capable of lowering CRH and indirectly ACTH concentrations. The notion that these drugs exert their action solely on the hypothalamus must be reexamined in view of in vitro data that show a direct inhibitory effect of these drugs on the adenoma cells maintained in culture. In addition to serotonin antagonists and dopaminergic agonists, noreprinephrine depletors as well as agonists to gamma-aminobutyric acid (GABA) have extended the neuropharmacological armamentarium. Several general observationsare pertinent in this regard:

1. Although the basis for drug therapy is solidly based on the abnormal hormone dynamics that characterize pituitary-dependent CD, these data cannot be transposed to all patients with CD. The heterogeneity of this disease precludes predictability of response in an individual case.
2. Even when drug therapy works, as exemplified by cyproheptadine, discontinuation of the drug is usually attended by a return of hypercortisolism.
3. Side effects of the drugs employed should be considered when long-term therapy is contemplated.
4. Definitive therapy should not be deferred while waiting for a drug induced remission that may never come.

Cyproheptadine is the most notable drug used to treat pituitary-dependent CD. Administration of cyproheptadine is attended by lowering of cortisol and ACTH levels, restoration of suppressibility to dexamethasone, and even a clinical remission in some patients with pituitary-dependent CD. The drug has to be administered in large doses (24 mg/day), with the expectation of no more than a 50% chance of remission, which lasts only as long as the drug iscontinued. There are no definite methods of prospectively identifying the patients who are unlikely to respond. The most serious and undesirable effect of cyproheptadine therapy is weight gain.

The use of bromocriptine is likely to benefit patients with CD originating from the intermediate lobe. Although the suppressive effect of dopamine agonists is well established in such patients. Valproate sodium, a GABA agonist, has been shown to be effective in lowering the ACTH level in some patients with CD and Nelson's syndrome. The drug has also been successfully employed to lower ACTH levels in patients with Nelson's syndrome. Adrenolytic agents (e.g., 0 pi DDD, aminoglutethimide, trilostane) are used in the preoperative preparation of the patient when the clinical expression is severe. Most authorities who perform TPS do not employ these agents routinely in the preoperative management. Prolonged use of ketoconazole in the management of CD to correct the hypercortisolism quickly, following unsuccessful TPS.

Table 77.1

Possible treatment plans in cushing's syndrome based on etiology

Treatment			Dosing		
Etiology	Nondrug	Generic (Brand) Drug Name	Initial	Usual	Max
Ectopic ACTH syndrome	irradiation Surgery, chemotherapy,	Metyrapone (Metopirone) 250-mg capsules Aminoglutethimide (Cytadren) 250-mg tabs	0.5–1 g/day, divided every 4–6 hours 0.5–1 g/day, divided two to four times a day for 2 weeks	1–2 g/day, divided every 4–6 hours 1 g/day, divided every 6 hours	6 g/day 2 g/day
Pituitary-dependent		Cyproheptadine (Periactin) 2 mg/5 mL syrup or 4-mg tabs Mitotane (Lysodren) 500-mg tabs Metyrapone	4 mg twice a day 0.5–1 g/day, increased by See above	24–32 mg/day, divided four times a day 1–4 g daily, with food to decrease GI effects See above	32 mg/day 12 g/day See above
Adrenal adenoma	Surgery, irradiation	Ketoconazole (Nizoral) 200-mg tabs	0.5–1 g/day every 1–4 weeks See above 200 mg once or twice a day	200–1,200 mg/day, divided twice a day	1,600 mg/day divided four times a day
Adrenal carcinoma	Surgery, postoperative replacement Surgery	Mitotane	See above	See above	See above

REFERENCES

1. Cushing H: The basophillic adenomas of the pituitary body and their clinical manifestations. *BullJohns Hopkins Hosp* 50:137, 1932.
2. Taylor HC, Velasco ME, Brodkey JS: Remission of pituitary dependent Cushing's disease after removal of nonneoplastic pituitary gland. *Arch Intern Med* 140: 1366, 1980.
3. Liddle GW: Tests of pituitary-adrenal suppressibility in the diagnosis of Cushing's syndrome. *] Clin Endocrinol* 20: 1539, 1960.
4. Schweizer-Cagianut M, Froesch ER, Hedinger C: Familial Cushing's syndrome with primary adrenocortical microadenomatosis (primary adrenocortical nodular dysplasia). *Acta Endocrinol* 94:529, 1980.

5. Meador CK, Bowdoin B, Owen WC, et al. Primary adrenocortical nodular dysplasia: A rare cause of Cushing's syndrome.] *Clin Endocrinol Metab* 27: 1255, 1967.
6. Choi Y, Werk EEJr, Sholiton LJ: Cushing's syndrome with dual pituitary-adrenal control. *Arch Intern Med* 125:1045, 1970.
7. Burke CW, Beardwell CG: Cushing's syndrome. *Q] Med* 42:175,1973.
8. Meador CK, Liddle GW, Island DP, et al. Cause of Cushing's syndrome in patients with tumors arising from "nonendocrine" tissue.] *Clin Endocrinol Metab* 22:693, 1962.
9. Oates TW, McCourt JP, Friedman WA, et al. Cushing's disease with cyclic hormonogenesis and diabetes insipidus. *Neurosurgery* 5:598, 1979.
10. Spark RF, Connolly PB: ACTH secretion from a functioning pheochromocytoma. *N Engl Med* 301:416, 1979.
11. Cook DM, KendallJW: Cushing's syndrome-Current concepts of diagnosis and therapy. *West Med* 132:111, 1980.

CHAPTER 78

Addisons Disease

Primary adrenal insufficiency (Addison's disease) most often involves the destruction of all regions of the adrenal cortex. There are deficiencies of cortisol, aldosterone, and the various androgens. Medications that inhibit cortisol synthesis (e.g., ketoconazole) or accelerate cortisol metabolism (e.g., phenytoin, rifampin, phenobarbital) can also cause primary adrenal insufficiency.

Secondary adrenal insufficiency most commonly results from exogenous corticosteroid use, leading to suppression of the hypothalamic-pituitary adrenal axis and decreased release of ACTH, resulting in impaired androgen and cortisol production. Mirtazapine and progestins (e.g., medroxyprogesterone acetate, megestrol acetate) have also been reported to induce secondary adrenal insufficiency. Secondary disease typically presents with normal mineralocorticoid concentrations.

ETIOLOGY

The main cause of primary adrenal failure is autoimmune disease of the adrenal cortex. Autoimmune adrenalitis occupies the center of the stage in syndromes characterized by polyglandular endocrine failure. Next to autoimmunity, infectious diseases constitute an important etiology. These include tuberculosis and fungal infections such as histoplasmosis and coccidioidomycosis. An emerging cause for adrenal failure is the setting of acquired immune deficiency syndrome (AIDS). The third category of causes for adrenocortical failure is destruction of the adrenal cortex by metastatic spread from diverse malignant diseases. The fourth cause of adrenal failurc is adrenal hemorrhage. The term *Waterhouse-Friderichsen Syndrome* is used to denote acute adrenal hemorrhage that results from septicemic shock. While fulminant meningococcal infection was originally linked with the syndrome of bilateral adrenal hemorrhage. Bilateral adrenal hemorrhage is a well-recognized, but rare complication of anticoagulation. Finally, adrenocortical insufficiency can result from use of drugs that interfere with steroidogenesis. In addition to the five categories mentioned (autoimmune, infectious, metastatic, hemorrhagic, and drug related), rare causes of adrenal insufficiency include sarcoidosis and amyloidosis (Table 78.1). At times, none of the causes mentioned can be identified, and these represent the truly "idiopathic" variety of the disorder.

Table 78.1

Etiology of addison's disease
I. Autoimmune adrenalitis
II. Infectious organisms
Tuberculous
Fungal infections
III. Metastatic disease
Lung
Breasts
Stomach
Non-Hodgkin's lymphoma
IV. Adrenal hemorrhage
"Waterhouse-Fredrichsen syndrome"
Meningococcus
Pneumococcus
E. coil
Hemophilus
DF-2 bacillus
Anticoagulation therapy
Bilateral adrenal vein catheterization
V. Drug-induced or related causes
Withdrawal from steroid therapy
Adrenolytic therapy
op'DDD
Aminoglutethimide
Trilostane
Other agents
Ketoconazole
Etomidate
Rifampin
Cyproterone acetate
Anticoagulation (coumadin, heparin)
VI. Rare causes
Acquired immune deficiency syndrome
Sarcoidosis
Amyloidosis
VII. Neonatal adrenal insufficiency
Enzymatic blocks in cortisol synthesis
Maternal Cushing's svndrome
Adrenal hypoplasia
Adrenal leukodystrophy

AUTOIMMUNE ADRENAL FAILURE

Autoimmune adrenalitis is the most common cause of adrenal failure. The indirect immunofluorescence technique using unfixed human adrenal tissue has become established as a widely used, sensitive method for detecting complement-fixing adrenal antibodies. The ability to accurately measure adrenal antibodies has had a more impact in adrenal endocrinology in three ways: first, it has simplified the etinological approach to adrenal failure; second, it has permitted evaluation of the presence and prevalence of immune markers for the adrenals in patients with other autoimmune disorders; and third, the technique has led to an understanding of the natural history of euadrenal asymptomatic patients with positive antiadrenal antibody titers.

Autoimmune destruction is the most common cause of Addison's disease. The salient clinical aspects are the following:

1. This may occur as an isolated entity or as part of autoimmune alteration in the function of several endocrine glands, notably the ovaries, parathyroids, the thyroid, and the 13 cells of the pancreas.
2. Even in the absence of overt involvement of other endocrine glands, autoimmune adrenalitis is associated with a high prevalence of circulating antibodies against other endocrine glands.
3. Females are more commonly affected by autoimmune Addison's disease than males.
4. The condition can be familial. However, a clear pattern of inheritance or an HLA connection has not been convincingly established.

5. The evolution of adrenal failure is slow in autoimmune adrenalitis, the mean duration of the process being approximately 3 years.
6. Patients with autoimmune adrenal failure often go through a phase of compensated adrenal reserve followed by a limited adrenal reserve before eventually decompensating.
7. The autoimmune destruction is mainly related to the adrenal cortex and does not involve the medulla (in contrast to tuberculous adrenal disease).
8. More than 70% of patients with autoimmune adrenal failure demonstrate autoadrenal antibodies by indirect immunofluorescence.
9. The CT appearance, while of diverse nature, fails to show evidence of calcification, a frequent finding in tuberculous and other diseases that cause adrenal destruction.

INFECTIONS

Several infectious process can lead to Addison's disease by causing progressive destruction of the adrenal glands. Tuberculosis and fungal diseases are the two broad categories of chronic infections that merit consideration.

TUBERCULOSIS

Tuberculosis of the adrenal gland was once considered the most common cause of adrenocortical failure. Tuberculosis in general, and of the adrenal glands in particular, is still a frequent cause of Addison's disease.

Tuberculosis of the adrenals may appear as primary or secondary disease. The adrenal involvement can occur in conjunction with evidence of other tuberculous involvement. Tuberculous Addison's disease can occur in patient's with active tuberculosis elsewhere or can occur years after the initial manifestation of tuberculosis at the primary focus. Thus, it is important to recognize that the absence of overt tuberculosis does not exclude the possibility of adrenal involvement by this disease. Among the usual locations affected by tuberculosis, pulmonary and genitourinary infections predominate.

Clinically, tuberculous adrenal insufficiency evolves more rapidly than the autoimmune variety of the disease. The mean duration of history in tuberculosis of the adrenal gland is approximately 1 year. Also, the destruction by tuberculosis is not limited to the adrenal cortex, since adrenal medullary involvement is often seen at autopsy. Perhaps for this reason, patients with tuberculous adrenalitis suffer more severe symptoms of orthostasis, which may reflect combined loss of mineralocorticoids and catecholamines. Indeed, tests of adrenomedullary reseve are often impaired in tuberculosis of the adrenals.

In summary, the salient features of tuberculosis of the adrenals are

1. Tuberculosis of the adrenal continues to remain as important as an etiology for adrenal failure today as it did in the days of Thomas Addison.
2. A past history of tuberculosis or the presence of contemperaneous active disease elsewhere is usually evident; pulmonary, genitourinary, and even gastrointestinal tuberculosis may be present. The implied importance of a careful search for disease at these sites is obvious.

3. The evolution of adrenal failure is more rapid in comparison to autoimmune adrenal failure.
4. Both sexes are equally affected.
5. The destruction by tuberculosis does not spare the medulla, resulting in impairment of adrenomedullary reserve.
6. Autoantibodies to adrenals are characteristically absent in 98-99% of patients with tuberculosis of the adrenals.
7. The presence of adrenal calcification is a hallmark of tuberculous involvement of the adrenals and can be seen roentgenologically in more than 50% of patients.
8. Enlargement of the adrenals is the most frequent finding seen by CT. In long-standing disease atrophy can be demonstrated.

FUNGAL DISEASES

Adrenal involvement by histoplasmosis, coccidioidomycosis, or blastomycosis can result in the development of Addison's disease. Of these, histoplasmosis is the more frequently encountered fungal disease . Recognition of this group of etiological agents has a threefold importance: First, the administration of antifungal chemotherapy with ketoconazole can cause further deterioration in adrenal function already compromised by the fungal disease. The precipitation of adrenal crisis during antifungal therapy is well recognized. Second, early treatment with antifungal therapy, may restore adrenal reserve. Third, fungal disease can mimic a unilateral mass lesion and resemble an adrenal tumor.

HISTOPLASMOSIS

Adrenal involvement by histoplasmosis is generally encountered in the progressive disseminated form of that disease. The presence of dissemination of histoplasmosis can be diagnosed by demonstration of systemic (hepatic, hematological, renal, gastrointestinal, or cutaneous) involvement by the fungus, or by culturing the fungus from blood, bone marrow, or tissues. The symptoms of disseminated histoplasmosis reflect systemic involvement and are characterized by fever, weight loss, night sweats, malaise, constitutional symptoms, and cough. Dissemination of histoplasmosis is more common in males, those with underlying illnesses, and those with occupational exposure. It is believed that all cases of primary histoplasmosis probably have hematogenous dissemination of the fungus, but in some the organisms continue to progressively disseminate.

Adrenal involvement may be seen during the active phase of dissemination. There exists a correlation between the presence of active or cavitary lung disease and the presence of dissemination. However, most patients with adrenal failure secondary to histoplasmosis demonstrate other evidence of systemic involvement by the fungus.

The range of adrenal involvement by histoplasmosis is also impressive.

1. The mildest form of adrenal involvement characterized by isolated cortical foci of parasitized macrophages.
2. Extensive caseation necrosis with swelling of both adrenals.
3. Extensive infarction.

4. Granulomatous replacement of the adrenals.
5. Calcified mass lesions that can mimic tuberculous or metastatic lesions.

BLASTOMYCOSIS

South American blastomycosis, caused by the fungus *Paracoccidioides brasiliensis,* is known to frequently involve the adrenals. This involvement, which has been noted more frequently postmortem than antemortem, varies between 20 and 80%, with an average of 50%. Like *H. capsulatum* infection, the adrenal involvement by South American blastomycosis is often associated with presence of disease elsewhere, usually from an ulcerated lesion. Adrenal calcification is relatively uncommon. Blastomycosis of the adrenals results in a granulomatous form of Addison's disease, where appropriate antimicrobial therapy has been known to restore adrenal reserve.

METASTATIC DISEASE

Autopsy studies indicate that the adrenal glands are a frequent site of metastases. The relative infrequency of clinical recognition of adrenal failure, despite the high frequency of finding metastatic involvement of the adrenals at autopsy, may be due to several factors.

First, it is commonly held that more than 90% of the adrenal tissue needs to be replaced before adrenal insufficiency results. This concept, of course, implies the development of complete adrenocortical insufficiency and fails to address the development of limited adrenal reserve due to metastatic destruction (a "pre-Addisonian" state).

Second, the symptoms experienced by patients suffering from disseminated malignancy are strikingly similar to those caused by adrenal insufficiency. Thus, weight loss, weakness, fatigue, lassitude, anorexia, vomiting, and orthostatic hypotension are shared by both groups. Consequently, these symptoms are likely to be attributed to malignant disease, resulting in missing or underdiagnosing adrenocortical insufficiency. Further, the increased pigmentation and gastrointestinal symptoms may be mistakenly attributed to the chemotherapy that most such patients receive, when in fact these symptoms may have been caused by adrenocortical insufficiency.

The problem can be further compounded by the fact that hyponatremia, a reflection of adrenocortical failure. Finally, the steroid therapy given to many patients with malignant diseases, as part of the chemotherapy protocols, can lead to masking of partial or complete adrenal insufficiency.

The following observations are pertinent as they relate to metastatic etiology of adrenal failure.

1. The increasing survival rate of patients with cancer and the increasing use of CT are resulting in an increased recognition of adrenal metastastes antemortem.
2. Adrenal insufficiency in patients with malignant disease is probably under diagnosed, perhaps owing to the mistaken attribution of symptoms to the underlying neoplasm.
3. Since CT of the adrenals is a simple, noninvasive procedure, it should be recommended as a part of the workup for patients with disseminated malignancy.

4. The demonstration of enlarged adrenal glands by CT is reason enough to recommend adrenal function testing even in the absence of symptoms of adrenal insufficiency.
5. Compromised adrenal function in metastatic adrenal disease can be partial or complete. The diagnosis of limited adrenal reserve in such a setting would necessitate prophylactic glucocorticoid therapy.
6. While the routine prophylactic administration of maintenance glucocorticoid therapy to all patients with malignancy and enlarged adrenals by CT has been recommended, this practice is not universally accepted.
7. The diagnosis of adrenal insufficiency and the resultant institution of therapy can considerably palliate the suffering of these patients.

ADRENAL HEMORRHAGE

Etiologically, the three classic settings associated with bilateral adrenal hemorrhage are fulminant infections, anticoagulant therapy, and trauma to the abdomen or thorax.

WATERHOUSE-FRIDERICHSEN SYNDROME

The adrenal hemorrhage associated with fulminant septicemia is termed the Waterhouse-Friderichsen syndrome (WF syndrome). The notable feature described in most cases was the enormous size of the adrenal glands, which exhibited a hemorrhagic purplish hue. The shock occurring during the course of endotoxemia seems to be the cause of adrenal hemorrhage, and not vice versa. The role of the meningococcus is believed to be important in causing endothelial damage and subsequent thrombosis in addition to the endotoxin release. The development of WF syndrome in septicemic shock is multifactorial and unresolved. The presentation is characterized by overwhelming sepsis, hypotension progressing to shock, a hemorrhagic diathesis, and often a purpuric rash. The bleeding is, at least in some cases, related to the rapidly developing disseminated intravascular coagulation caused by endotoxins.

ANTICOAGULATION

The sudden development of abdominal or back pain, anorexia, nausea, vomiting, hypotension, and altered sensorium in a patient on anticoagulation therapy should immediately raise the possibility of adrenal hemorrhage. While this complication can occur in any person anticoagulated with both Coumadin and heparin, its occurrence is more common in older patients with increased capillary fragility and in those over anticoagulated. Prompt clinical recognition of acute adrenal hemorrhage in anticoagulated patients can be quite difficult owing to its similarity to other disorders. A high index of suspicion coupled with immediate adrenal reserve testing and CT would readily permit accurate diagnosis.

TRAUMA

Adrenal hemorrhage can occur secondary to thoracic or abdominal trauma, Crushing of one or both adrenals, particularly the right, against the vertebral columns can result in rupture of the central vessels. As a result of the bleeding, the adrenal glands are distended by the blood, with destruction of the cortex and medulla. Thrombosis of the adrenal veins with hemorrhagic infarction can also result in loss of adrenal function.

In addition to overwhelming septicemia, anticoagulation therapy, and trauma, several other causes for adrenal hemorrhage have been reported in the literature. Table 78.2 outlines the common and rare causes of adrenal hemorrhage.

Table 78.2

Causes of adrenal hemorrhage
I. Overwhelming septicemia (Waterhouse-Friderichsen syndrome)
Neisseria meningitidis
Diplococcus pneumoniae
Hemophilus influenzae type b
DF-2 bacillus
II. Anticoagulant therapy
III. Trauma
Abdominal and thoracic surgery
Postadrenal venography
IV. Rare causes
Hemorrhagic diathesis
Neonatal adrenal hemorrhage
Burns
Pregnancy
Hematological diseases (leukemia)
Pancreatitis
V. Metastatic disease

DRUG-INDUCED ADRENOCORTICAL INSUFFICIENCY

Drug-induced adrenocortical insufficiency constitutes a rare, but important cause of hypoadrenalism. Several classes of drugs can contribute to partial or complete adrenal failure.

1. Of course, the classic example of adrenal failure occurs after withdrawal of steroid therapy.
2. The adrenal insufficiency that results from the use of antiadrenal agents is often deliberate and intentional to treat hypercortisolism.
3. The adrenal insufficiency that results from anticoagulation therapy with heparin and coumadin occurs as a consequence of adrenal hemorrhage. In addition to this mechanism, use of heparin can result in hypo-aldosteronism even in the absence of adrenal hemorrhage.
4. Finally drugs administered for other purposes may inadvertently result in the development of adrenal insufficiency. Four such drugs deserve mention- ketoconazole, rifampin, etomidate and cyproterone acetate.

KETOCONAZOLE

Ketoconazole, an imidazole derivative, is a broad-spectrum antifungal drug, widely used in treatment of infections caused by the *Coccidioides, Histoplasma, Candida, Blastomyces,* and *Cryptococcus* species of fungi.

The mechanism of ketoconazole-induced adrenal suppression is believed to be mediated by inhibition of the cytochrome P-450-dependent enzymes. Inhibition of ll-~hydroxylation and inhibition of a more proximal step in the side-chain cleavage that converts cholesterol to pregnenolone. Both ll-13-hydroxylase and the sidechain cleaving enzyme are mitochondrial enzymes that are cytochrome P-450 dependent. Ketoconazole did not inhibit conversion of progesterone to DOC or the other steps in adrenal steroid synthesis mediated by non-PA50-dependent enzymes. Thus, it appears that ketoconazole has a predilection to inhibit mitochondrial enzymes, especially those that are dependent on P-450.

ETOMIDATE

Low plasma cortisol levels in patients receiving etomidate were reported. Since etomidate is an imidazole derivative, structurally analogous to ketoconazole, considerable attention has been focused on the effect of this anesthetic on adrenal steroid synthesis. Etomidate produced a concentration dependent blockade of two mitochondrial enzymes, the cholesterol side chain cleaving enzyme and ll-13-hydroxylase, both dependent on cytochrome P-450. Thus, the antisteroid effects of etomidate bear a striking resemblance to those of ketoconazole, without the peripheral effects of the latter that cause glucocorticoid antagonism at the end-organ level.

RIFAMPIN

Rifampin, is used in the chemotherapy of tuberculosis. While administration of rifampin borderline adrenal disease may result in precipitation of adrenal crisis. In most patients in whom rifampin precipitated acute adrenal crisis, the event occurred within 2 weeks of institution of therapy. Therefore, in patients with tuberculosis placed on rifampin the importance of considering adrenal insufficiency in the first 2 weeks of rifampin therapy is emphasized.

Addison's disease may have near-normal basal plasma cortisol levels, our recommendation is to perform a rapid ACTH stimulation test in all patients with tuberculosis prior to placement on rifampin.

CYPROTERONE ACETATE

Cyproterone acetate possesses antiandrogenic and progestational properties; it has found therapeutic application in Europe in treatment of such diverse disorders as virilization in women, hypersexuality and "deviationism" in males, and precocious puberty in children of both sexes. Cyproterone is known to cause secondary adrenal insufficiency.

RARER CAUSES OF PRIMARY ADRENAL FAILURE

Rare causes of a rare disease need to be considered only rarely. Sarcoidosis can affect the adrenal glands. Most reports of sarcoid involvement of the adrenal glands are based on autopsy findings. Adrenal failure may occur during the granulomatous phase or during the phase of healing when fibrosis supervenes. In general, adrenal failure due to sarcoidosis occurs in the presence of diffuse sarcoid involvement of several organs, such as lung or liver. The ability of sarcoidosis to involve multiple endocrine glands can result in the development of multiple-target-organ failure mimicking the autoimmune pluriglandular failure syndromes.

Adrenocortical failure secondary to disseminated cytomegalovirus (CMV) infection used to be considered a rare event. Patients with AIDS may develop primary adrenal failure. Disseminated infection involving the adrenal glands has occasionally been described in AIDS. Amyloidosis, by virtue of its diffuse infiltration of almost every organ, can also involve the adrenals. Hepatomegaly is invariably present, and the diagnosis of amyloidosis can be established by demonstrating amyloid deposits in the rectal mucosa, liver, kidney, or peripheral nerve.

Hemochromatosis can infiltrate the adrenals and result in adrenal insufficiency. Secondary hemochromatosis is more likely to cause iron deposition in the adrenals than the primary form. Primary hemochromatosis involves the pituitary more frequently than it involves the adrenals. Adrenal failure in the newborn can be due to hypoplasia of the adrenals.

CLINICAL FEATURES

The symptoms can be so nonspecific as to be passed off as insignificant. The presentations of the disease can be so diverse and the recognition so difficult that the patient may have seen several specialists in widely different disciplines before the diagnosis is made. Thus, it is not uncommon for the chronically ill patient to have seen the gastroenterologist (for diarrhea), neurologist (for muscle weakness), hematologist (for anemia), cardiologist (for "dizzy spills"), psychiatrist (for depression),and dermatologist (for skin problems) before the entire picture is put together by the astute generalist and referred to the endocrinologist.

Addison's disease, in its early stages, is insidious in onset and evolves gradually and imperceptibly. The symptoms of weakness and lassitude my persist on such a chronic basis that many patients hopelessly attribute their state of ill being as a basal state. Many such patients, after having sought several medical opinions that disclosed "non-disease," are placed on vitamins. Some turn to bizarre remedies rather than face multiple physicians and a possible diagnosis of hypochondriasis. Most patients give the typical history that their energy level is fair in the morning, but experience rapid tiring as the day progresses. The classic picture described by Addison consisting of "typical pigmentary changes and wasting in a patient with a feeble pulse" should not be allowed to develop if the diagnosis is suspected early.

The three major symptoms of Addison's disease are weight loss, fatigue, and pigmentary changes. Since fatigability and weight loss may occur in the absence of other stigmata of Addison's disease, it is reasonable to screen all patients with unexplained weight loss and fatigue for the presence of adrenocortical failure.

Addison's disease can involve almost all the systems. Therefore, the symptoms and signs are best viewed in terms of individual systems.

CONSTITUTIONAL

These are the most frequent symptoms experienced by patients with adrenocortical failure. Malaise, loss of energy, lassitude, and a general feeling of ill health are important symptoms of adrenal failure, which are, unfortunately, highly nonspecific. These symptoms are mistakenly attibuted to overwork, stress, or psychological factors. As anorexia and weight loss manifest, once again Addison's disease tends to be missed because the focus has often shifted to a malignancy workup. Once again, too many Addisonian patients too often have undergone gastrointestinal investigations and total body imaging before a simple and careful history is put together and an adrenal reserve testing is done. Weight loss, weakness, and fatigability were also universally noted in the patients with Addison's disease .

DERMATOLOGICAL

Increased pigmentation of skin and mucous membrane, a reflection of an increase in circulating 3-lipotropin levels, was encountered. The increased pigmentation is seen in whites as well as in blacks. Patients often are intrigued by the ease with which their skin tans, and by the lingering of suntan for longer periods than usual. The degree of pigmentation can be highly variable.

The three characteristics of the hyperpigmentation of Addison's disease are:

1. Striking involvement of dorsum of the hands, (especially over the joints), elbows, knees, and palmar creases.
2. Mucosal pigmentation involving the lips, buccal mucosa, dental gingival margin, and the tongue.
3. Pigmentation of the scars, especially those acquired after the onset of Addison's disease.

It is generally considered that hyper-pigmentation in Addison's disease indicates chronicity. It was also generally observed that when hyperpigmentation is present in Addison's disease, the other manifestations of the disease are quite apparent. In addition to hyperpigmentation, vitiligo may be evident in patients with autoimmune adrenal failure.

GASTROINTESTINAL

Lower abdominal cramps, anorexia, and nausea are seen often in these patients. In some patients with Addison's disease, the gastrointestinal symptoms can be severe enough to dominate the clinical picture. The stress of an intense gastrointestinal workup, including panendoscopies, can be conducive to the precipitation of decompensation. In Addisonian crises, the gastrointestinal manifestations become severe and are invariably present. Adrenal crisis is often ushered in by nausea, vomiting, lower abdominal cramps, and diarrhea. Indeed, the diarrhea can be severe enough that the initial clinical suspicion may be gastroenteritis. The diarrhea and vomiting seen in Addisonian crisis contribute significantly 10 the dehydration and volume depletion seen with this catastrophe.

CARDIOVASCULAR

Moderate to occasionally severe orthostasis is encountered in nearly all patients with hypotension due to Addison's disease. Infrequently, the supine blood pressure may be entirely normal, but may demonstrate striking changes when the patient assumes erect posture. A history of chronic hypertension that ameliorated spontaneously despite discontinuation of antihypertensive medications is an excellent clue to the presence of Addison's disease. While orthostatic hypotension is a frequently demonstrable sign, less than 20% of patients complain of postural dizziness. In fact, unlike patients with other forms of postural hypotension, Addisonian patients feel well in the morning when they arise from a long period of recumbency.

MUSCULOSKELETAL

Muscle weakness is a subjective symptom that is present in most patients with adrenal failure. The lack of anabolic androgen steroids probably underlies the muscle weakness of adrenal failure. Although the subjective symptoms may be severe, muscle power is often reasonably well preserved. Rarely, flexion contractures have been reported in association with Addison's disease, gradually improving with replacement therapy.

RENAL

Several abnormalities in renal function can be encountered in patients with Addison's disease.

1. A decrease in the glomerular filtration rate and in the renal blood flow is a frequent accompaniment of Addison's discase.
2. An elevated blood urea nitrogen (13 UN) and/or creatinine levels are often seen as a consequence of the decreased glomerular filtration rate (GFR) and the prerenal azotemia.
3. Decreased secretion of ammonia and hydrogen ion results in mild metabolic acidosis. Administration of an acid load is less readily cleared by the kidneys in patients with adrenal insufficiency. The acidifying defect is due to the absence of mineralocorticoids.
4. In addition to the problem with hydrogen ion excretion, patients with Addison's disease demonstrate an inability to normally excrete a water load. It is believed that the abnormalities in urinary dilution seen in Addison's disease are a result of the decreased GFR caused by salt and water depletion. This results in increased reabsorption of water in the proximal tubule (vasopressin independent), reducing the delivery of filtrate to the diluting segments of the nephron. Consequently, the urine is less than maximally dilute. The natriuresis from the mineralocorticoid deficiency further contributes to urinary concentration.

PSYCHIATRIC

The psychiatric symptom seen most often in association with adrenal failure is depression. The lassitude seen in many Addisonian patients may reflect a mild form of endogenous depression.

GONADAL

Oligomenorrhea, even amenorrhea, and impotence are often present in patients with Addison's disease. While these symptoms may occur as a consequence of the chronic illness and debilitation seen in Addison's disease, primary autoimmune gonadal failure may be the underlying mechanism in some cases.

BRONCHOPULMONARY

The possibility that adrenocortical insufficiency may play a role in the natural history of bronchial asthma has been a matter of controversy.The frequency of bronchial asthma and the rarity of its association with Addison's disease diminish the impact of these reports.

In summary, the clinical features of Addison's disease can be striking enough to afford detection at first glance or can be subtle enough to be missed unless a high index of suspicion is entertained. Screening for Addison's disease is justifiable under the following circumstances:

1. Unexplained weight loss
2. Weakness and asthenia
3. Orthostatic hypotension
4. Hyperpigmentation
5. Presence of nonspecific symptoms in patients with pluriglandular failure or vitiligo
6. Electrolyte abnormalities (hyponatremia, hyperkalemia)
7. Dehydration and shock, especially in the presence of hypoglycemia

ASSOCIATIONS OF ADDISON'S DISEASE

Addison's disease, especially the autoimmune variety, can be associated with several syndromes. The most important association of Addison's disease is with the polyglandular autoimmune syndrome. Less commonly, Addison's disease can be part of a neurological syndrome characterized by progressive demyelination of the white matter of the brain. The syndromes of adrenoleuko-dystrophy and adrenomyeloneuropathy belong in this category. Even rarer are the associations of adrenal failure with the beguiling POEMS syndrome, achalasia cardia, and renal microangiopathy.

POLYGLANDULAR DEFICIENCY SYNDROMES

Autoimmune adrenal failure is often associated with deficiency syndromes that involve other endocrine glands. Primary hypoadrenalism, primary hypothyroidism, primary hypogonadism, and diabetes mellitus constitute an important tetrad, the common factor being autoimmunity.

Primary hypoadrenalism and primary hypothyroidism are the two most frequent components of the type II pluriglandular syndrome, being present in 100% and 69% of patients, respectively.

Gonadal failure is especially prevalent in females with autoimmune adrenal disease. Antisteroid cell antibodies were demonstrable in more than 50% of patients with Addison's disease and secondary amenorrhea, whereas very few males had circulating anti-leydig cell antibodies. Thus, gonadal failure is more often encountered in females with autoimmune Addison's disease than in males.

In addition to its association with hypothyroidism, hypogonadism, and diabetes mellitus, autoimmune adrenal failure has been associated with hypoparathyroidism, vitilgo, and pernicious anemia.

Autoimmune Addison's disease is an important constituent of types I and II. Type I polyglandular autoimmune disease (Table 78.3) has its onset in childhood. The most prevalent endocrine dysfunction in type I is hypoparathyroidism (82%), followed by adrenal failure (67%). Less frequent endocrinopathies noted in the type I syndrome include gonadal failure (12- 17%), autoimmune thyroid disease (10%), and diabetes mellitus (2-4%). Type I polyglandular autoimmune syndrome is highlighted by two other facets; mucocutaneous candidiasis is present in 73-78% of patients with this syndrome. The type II polyglandular autoimmune syndrome is characterized by the universal presence of autoimmune failure. Less common associations include gonadal failure, vitiligo, pernicious anemia, and celiac disease (Table 78.4).

Table 78.3

Type I polyglandular autoimmune syndrome
A. Components
1. Endocrine
Hypoparathyroidism (82%)
Addison's disease (67%)
Hypogonadism (12-17%)
Autoimmune thyroid disease (10%)
Diabetes mellitus (2-4%)
2. Nonendocrine
Age
Chronic mucocutaneous candidiasis (73-78%)
Pernicious anemia (13-15%)
Chronic active hepatitis (12%)
Malabsorption syndromes (22-24%)
Vitiligo (8%)
Alopecia (26-32%)
Childhood onset

Absence of Addison's disease, but the presence of IDDM (Insulin Dependent Diabetes Mellitus), pernicious anemia, vitiligo, alopecia, or other organ-specific autoimmune disorders. It is a "catchall" category to include autoimmune disorders other than Addison's disease. Should Addison's disease eventually evolve in this category of patients, this would necessitate reclassification into type I or type II. The list of organ-specific antibodies that can be demonstrated in patients with all three types of polyglandular autoimmune syndromes is bewildering. These antibodies are listed in Table 78.5.

The importance of recognizing the coexistence of multiple endocrinopathies in patients with Addison's disease has several clinical implications. First, the presence of hypogonadism is common to polyglandular syndromes as well as hypopituitarism. .Of course, the measurement of pituitary trophic hormones would clearly differentiate between the two entities. Second, the likelihood of patients with autoimmune Addison's disease developing a second or even third endocrinopathy is as high as 25%. This, obviously, underscores the need for careful search for the presence of other endocrine dysfunction not only at the time at which Addison's disease manifested, but prospectively for the rest of the Patient's life. Third, and from a nonendocrine perspective, the patient with autoimmune adrenal failure needs to be screened for other systemic autoimmune disorders, particularly pernicious anemia. Fourth, the role of HLA *(human leukocyte antigen)* antigens in predisposing patients to the polyglandular autoimmune syndrome is undergoing intense investigation.

Table 78.4

Type II Polyglandular Autoimmune Syndrome
A. Components
1. Endocrine
Addison's disease (100%)
Autoimmune thyroid disease (69%)
Diabetes (usually IDDM) (52%)
Hypogonadism (3.5%)
2. Nonendocrine
Pernicious anemia (less than 1 %)
Vitiligo (4.5%)
Celiac disease
B. Age
Adult onset

Table 78.5

Organ-specific antibodies in polyglandular autoimmune syndrome

Thyroid	Antithyroglobulin; antimicrosomal; antibodies against TSH receptors and thyroid cell surface antigen; antibodies against retroorbital tissues
Pancreas	Antibodies against pancreatic 13 cells, a cells, and 1 cells; antibodies against insulin receptors
Parathyroid	Anti-chief cell antibodies; anti-oxyphil cell antibodies
Gonads	Antibodies against steroid-producing cells; antiova and antisperm antibodies; anti-Leydig cell antibodies
Pituitary	Antibodies against lactotropes and somatotropes
Other organ-specific antibodies	Antiparietal cell gastric antibodies; anti-intrinsic factor antibodies; anti melanocyte antibodies; anti-smooth muscle antihodies; anti-acetylcholine receptor antibodies
Nonorgan-specific antibodies	Antimitochondrial antibodies; anti-DNA and RNA antibodies

ADRENOMYELONEUROPATHY AND ADRENOLEUKODYSTROPHY

Adrenomyeloneuropathy and Adrenoleukodystrophy are progressive degenerative disorders of the brain and spinal cord occurring in association with primary adrenal failure. The classic adrenoleukodystrophy (ALD) is characterized by progressive development of dementia, blindness, quadriparesis, and adrenal insufficiency. Progressive degeneration of the white matter of brain ultimately results in death. Histopathologically, linear cycloplasmic inclusion bodies are found in brain macrophages and adrenocortical cells. The condition is believed to be inherited as an X-linked disorder. Adrenoleukodystrophy resembles other demyelinating disorders of the brain in its tendency to relentlessly progress. The clinical lines that separate adrenoleukodystrophy, Schilder's disease, metachromatic leukodystrophy, and subacute sclerosing panencephalitis are extremely nebulous.

Adrenoleukodystrophy typically affects children during the first decade of life. Behavioral problems, school failure, visual disturbances, and motor deficits with caudal-rostral progression is the usual presentation. Inexorable decline, progressing to death within 6 years of developing neurological symptoms, is the usual course of this disease. The adrenal insufficiency can evolve before, simultaneously, or after the development of the neurological syndrome. In addition to this childhood form, ALD can also afflict adults. Visual deterioration, mental confusion, behavioral changes, and spastic paraplegia eventually supervene.

Adrenomyeloneuropathy (AMN) is a clinical variant of ALD. In addition to the association of primary adrenal failure and neurological deterioration, this entity is characterized by variable degrees of hypogonadism and distal polyneuropathy. The same pathological process that involves the white matter of brain also involves the Leydig cells of the testes. In addition to primary hypogonadism, the spectrum of adrenomyeloneuropathy has extended to involve the hypothalamus and the pituitary.

RARE ASSOCIATIONS

Rarely, Addison's disease can be part of the POEMS syndrome, may be associated with achalasia cardia with alacrimation, or can occur with renal microangiopathy.

The term *POEMS syndrome* refers to a constellation characterized by polyneuropathy, organomegaly, endocrinopathy, M proteins, and skin changes (POEMS). The mechanism for the development of this multisystem disorder is not known. The disease is predominantly seen in middle- aged men, particularly in Japanese, and is characterized by the universal occurrence of polyneuropathy, which is both sensory and motor, and is usually progressive. Biopsy of the nerves reveals varying degrees of axonal degeneration. Hepatomegaly, splenomegaly, and lymphadenopathy are present in 68%, 39%, and 65% of patients, respectively. The endocrinopathies encountered in the syndrome include gynecomastia (69%), impotence (68%), amenorrhea (100%), glucose intolerance (50%), primary hypothyroidism (12%), and Addison's disease (9%).

ACHALASIA, ALACHRYMIA SYNDROME

The rare syndrome of isolated adrenal glucocorticoid failure with normal aldosterone production associated with achalasia cardia and defective tear production (alacrimation) has recently been described. There has been no satisfactory explanation for this rare syndrome. Postulated mechanisms include ACTH insensitivity, degenerative processes that affect the adrenal glands and the autonomic nerve structure, and a loss of parasympathetic input to the adrenal gland.

LABORATORY DIAGNOSIS

The laboratory diagnosis of Addison's disease can be viewed in terms of several perspectives. First, the nonspecific clues derived from the routine tests will be outlined. Second, the screening tests for adrenocortical insufficiency will be discussed. Third, the confirmatory tests to establish the diagnosis will be discussed. Fourth, the steps taken to identify the cause of adrenal insufficiency will be outlined.

NONSPECIFIC ROUTINE TESTS

Nonspecific, but important, information from routine tests might often raise the first suspicion of adrenal insufficiency. Particularly relevant are the changes in serum electrolytes, glucose, BUN/creatinine, and calcium.

The typical electrolyte abnormality in Addison's disease is the combination of hyponatremia and hyperkalemia. The two reasons for these changes are the loss of mineralocorticoid effect on the renal handling of these ions and the loss of glucocorticoid action on the sodium-potassium pump that maintains a normal gradient between the intracellular and extracellular sodium and potassium.

Hyperkalemia can be masked in Addisonian patients with potassium loss from vomiting, diarrhea, or diuretic abuse. Hyperkalemia is nearly always present during adrenal crises. Treatment with glucocorticoids alone can lower the serum potassium level, ascribing an important role to the effect of glucocorticoids on the sodium-potassium pump. In the absence of cortisol, there is loss of the normal Na+ – K + gradient across the cell, with resultant movement of potassium out of the cell, and sodium into it. With glucocorticoid administration, he gradient is reestablished, and the hyperkalemia promptly resolves. The BUN and creatinine are mildly elevated in patients with adrenocortical failure due to a decrease in the GFR and renal flow. In patients with acute adrenal crises, the presence of dehydration magnifies these effects, often resulting in impressive prerenal azotemia.

Hypoglycemia in Addison's disease is due to inadequate hepatic gluconeogenesis. The decreased food intake due to anorexia usually compounds the problems. Patients with adrenocortical failure poorly tolerate fasting. Profound, symptomatic hypoglycemia may develop when Addisonian patients are fasted for diagnostic procedures. Also, hypoglycemia with hypotension may be seen in patients with Addisonian crisis. The counterregulatory mechanisms to combat hypoglycemia are extremely impaired in these patients owing to loss of glucocorticoids and often catecholamines. The presence of hypoglycemia in a patient with "shock" must immediately bring Addisonian crisis to mind, since in most other situations characterized by shock, the blood sugar is not low, because the "stress hormones" are present in adequate amounts.

The degree of hypercalcemia is generally mild to modest, although occasionally hypercalcemic crisis has been reported. The mechanism of hypercalcemia is unclear, but seems to be related to cortisol deficiency, since it completely normalizes after cortisol replacement. Glucocorticoids increase urinary excretion of calcium, probably as a consequence of expansion of extracellular fluid volume which suppresses reabsorption of sodium and calcium by the proximal nephron. It is, therefore, possible that mineralocorticoid deficiency with resultant contraction of extracellular fluid volume could lead to enhanced proximal tubular reabsorption of calcium.

SCREENING TESTS

The three screening tests utilized for detecting adrenal insufficiency are measurement of basal steroid levels in plasma; evaluation of the cortisol and aldosterone response to an intravenous bolus of cosyntropin; and evaluation of plasma II-deoxycortisollevel following an overnight metyrapone test. Of these, the cosyntropin test is the most sensitive.

BASAL STEROID MEASUREMENT

Measurement of 8 A.M. (or 4 P.M.) cortisol levels in the plasma is used for screening. When the 8 A.M. plasma cortisol level is below 5 JLg/dl, the diagnosis of adrenal insufficiency is strongly suspect, while a level in excess of 25 JLg/dl excludes it. Plasma cortisol levels in the range of 10-20 JLg/dl can still be associated with adrenal insufficiency, when the disease is partial and the adrenals are functioning at maximal capacity. Thus, in such instances, screening with only basal cortisol levels in plasma carries the dangerous risk of missing the diagnosis of a potentially fatal disease. When the disease is suspected, the presence of normal basal cortisol levels should not deter one from pursuing further diagnostic tests.

For the same reasons, measurement of basal 24-hr urinary free cortisol and 17-hydroxycorticosteroids fails to achieve a desirable sensitivity in screening for Addison's disease. The inconvenience of urine collection, and the low sensitivity of these tests have been major reasons for discarding these determinations for screening purposes.

THE RAPID ACTH STIMULATION TEST

This dynamic procedure evaluates the immediate response of the adrenal cortex to the exogenous administration of synthetic ACTH ("cosyntropin"). Cosyntropin contains the first 24 amino acids of ACTH and has all the biological activity of the intact hormone. This is a simple test to detect adrenal insufficiency. The test involves, in its simplest form, measuring the serum cortisol at the basal state and 30, 60, and 90 min following the intravenous administration of 2.5 flg of cosyntropin. The "normal" response varies according to different workers, but a widely accepted criterion is a peak level that doubles and increases by at least 10 flg/dl above the baseline, following ACTH. An absolute peak level of 25 flg/ dl of cortisol has also been considered as a normal response .

Three important statements need to be emphasized regarding the rapid ACTH test.

First, the test is, at best, only a screening procedure and separates the normal responder from the nonresponder. The demonstration of a clearly normal response precludes the possibility of primary adrenal failure.

Second, a blunted or flat cortisol response to rapid ACTH administration can be seen in both primary and secondary (pituitary) hyponadrenalism.

Finally, and most important, the response patterns of patients with partial adrenal insufficiency and those under stress can be quite variable and can often defy interpretation. For instance, some patients with partial adrenal insufficiency may show a near-normal response on the rapid challenge, while decompensating under continuous stimulation. In contrast, normal subjects under stress may show no appreciable rise following ACTH since they are functioning at full capacity.

THE METYRAPONE TEST

Metyrapone is an inhibitor of the 11-I3-hydroxylase enzyme that converts ll-deoxycortisol (compound S) to cortisol. The "short" version of the test is performed by administering 30 mg/kg of metyrapone orally at midnight and measuring the levels of cortisol, compound S, and ACTH at 8 A.M. the next morning. The danger of precipitating acute adrenal insufficiency by further lowering the cortisol due to administration of metyrapone is not a significant problem with the overnight test.

The screening for adrenal insufficiency in a patient receiving no steroid coverage consists of the following steps:

1. The basal plasma cortisol at 8 A.M. is first measured. If the 8 A.M. cortisol is greater than 25-30 fJ.g/dl, the diagnosis of adrenal insufficiency is no longer considered, and no further investigations are pursued in that direction.
2. If the cortisol level is below normal, a rapid ACTH test, using cosyntropin, is

performed. A basal sample for plasma ACTH is collected and saved for future assay if necessary. Similarly, the samples for aldosterone are also saved for future assay, if deemed appropriate. Thus, for cost effectiveness, only the cortisol determinations are performed in the samples before and after ACTH. If the cortisol response is unequivocally normal, the diagnosis of primary adrenal insufficiency has been excluded with reasonable certainty. The other stored samples are discarded.

3. If the cortisol response to ACTH is subnormal, or absent, the diagnosis of hypoadrenalism is entertained. Now, the plasma aldosterone levels are determined in the sample that was saved. An absent or impaired aldosterone response, in the presence of an absent or impaired cortisol response to ACTH, would suggest primary adrenal disease. If the aldosterone response is normal, pituitary disease needs to be excluded. The plasma ACTH level in the stored sample can now be assayed to provide additional help.
4. If the cortisol response to cosyntropin is borderline (i.e., neither completely normal nor completely abnormal), an overnight metyrapone test is performed. This test has the advantage of screening the entire hypothalamic- pituitary-adrenal axis.

CONFIRMATORY TESTS

The confirmation of primary adrenal failure rests on demonstrating impaired or absent adrenal responsiveness to protracted exogenous ACTH administration, coupled with elevated basal ACTH levels. The concept that theophylline may be used to evaluate adrenocortical function is interesting. Theophylline presumably stimulates intracellular steroidogenesis by circumvention of ACTH-receptor interaction.

ETIOLOGICAL DIAGNOSIS OF ADDISON'S DISEASE

Once the diagnosis of Addison's disease has been established, it is important to find the etiology of the primary adrenal failure for several reasons. First, if autoimmune disease of the adrenal, the most common cause today, is established, the physician should screen for endocrine dysfunction involving other endocrine glands. Second, if an infectious cause is identified [tuberculosis (TB), fungal disease], appropriate therapy for the offending pathogen needs to be instituted. Rarely, the institution of such therapy can result in "reversing" adrenal insufficiency. Third, if metastatic disease is established as the cause of adrenal disease, appropriate therapy for the primary neoplasm may become necessary. Rarely, the adrenal manifestation may indeed be the first clue to the presence of neoplastic disease.

With this reasoning in mind, several lines of approach can be utilized for the etiological evaluation of primary adrenocortical failure. These include the use of CT, measurement of antibodies against the adrenal cortex, and reviewing routine biochemical data to detect evidence of infectious disease.

COMPUTERIZED TOMOGRAPHY OF THE ADRENALS

CT of the adrenals can provide extremely valuable information regarding the etiology of primary adrenal failure. The size, the density, the contours, and the presence of calicification can provide clues to the underlying cause.

Size of the Adrenals: The adrenal size can be variable even in normal subjects. The normal left adrenal gland is 21.5 ± 4.6 mm in greatest diameter (length), and 6.7 ± 1.7 mm in thickness; the normal right adrenal measures 22.8 ± 6.3 mm in greatest diameter, and 5.1 ± 1.1 mm in thickness. 291 Demonstration of enlarged ad rena Is in a patient with Addison's disease is compatible with tuberculosis, metastatic disease, and fungal infections. Decreased size of the adrenals, on the other hand, is indicative of autoimmune disease, idiopathic atrophy, and late sequelae of TB.

Density: Acute tuberculous involvement of the adrenals may cause multiple lucent areas seen by CT, representing necrosis. Bilaterally enlarged, nonhomogenous adrenals can also be seen with histoplasmosis. Secondary hemochromatosis presents as bilaterally hyperdense glands with normal or reduced size, the hyperdensity being caused by iron deposition within the adrenals. Malignant disease generally appears as bilaterally enlarged glands of homogenous density, except in the case of metastases from malignant melanoma, which tend to bleed and necrose. Adrenal hemorrhage also causes irregular enlargement with nonhomogenous densities due to the blood within.

Contours: Metastatic disease typically causes round or oval intraadrenal masses, altering the normal adrenal contours. Inflammatory causes generally are associated with preservation of normal adrenal contours.

***Calcification*:** Historically, radiographic demonstration of intraadrenal calcification has been regarded as a classic sign for tuberculous origin of adrenal failure. The incidence of detecting calcification by plain films of the abdomen in tuberculosis of the adrenals ranges from 30 to 50%. Computed tomography of the adrenals is the most sensitive method for detecting calcification. Adrenal calcification is extremely unusual when autoimmune atrophy underlies the etiology of Addison's disease. Whilc tuberculosis is associated with calcification in more than half the cases, rarely other diseases processes can cause calcification; thus, fungal infections, metastatic disease, and adrenal hemorrhage may produce calcific changes detectable by CT. In summary, CT has been suggested as an important tool to determine the etiology of Addison's disease.

MEASUREMENT OF ADRENAL ANTIBODIES

The titers of antiadrenal antibodies are elevated in more than 80% of patients with autoimmune disease while being undetectable in tuberculous adrenalitis is of enormous help in distinguishing these two forms of Addison's disease.

TESTS FOR INFECTIOUS DISEASE

The presence of TB elsewhere, the background of endemicity for fungal disease, positive skin tests or serology (ELISA test for TB or fungal serology), and nonspecific biochemical clues, such as elevated globulins or alkaline phosphatase, would help in marshalling evidence for the presence of underlying infections.

CT -guided biopsy of the adrenal masses can establish the diagnosis of metastasis or fungal disease.

The etiological separation between tuberculous and autoimmune adrenal disease can present difficulties. The four most important clues to assist in making the separation are duration of symptoms, size of adrenal glands, presence of calcification, and presence of extraadrenal tuberculosis or other autoimmune diseases .

The fact that medullary function is spared in autoimmune adrenal failure may assist in separating the two, but this has not found wide application in the literature.

EXTRA-ADRENAL ENDOCRINE DYSFUNCTION IN ADDISON'S DISEASE

In patients diagnosed as having autoimmune adrenal failure, it is mandatory to evaluate other endocrine glandular function. Thus, screening for primary hypothyroidism, hypoparathyroidism, diabetes mellitus, and gonadal failure (particularly in females) constitutes part of the workup. The other part includes evaluation of pituitary hormones, since several of these demonstrate perturbations which are reversible with glucocorticoid treatment.

SCREENING FOR POLYGLANDULAR FAILURE SYNDROME

Evaluation of gonadal function, hypoparathyroidism, and diabetes mellitus in patients with Addison's disease is relatively simple and straightforward. Measurement of testosterone, 17 -13-estradiol, LH, and FSH and the determination of antibodies that react with steroid-secreting cells would disclose the presence of autoimmune gonadal failure. The simple measurement of serum calcium level with simultaneous assay of parathyroid hormone would disclose the presence of parathyroid failure. Hyperglycemia or an abnormal glucose tolerance test, often in conjunction with the presence of circulating, anti-islet cell antibodies, would establish the autoimmune diabetes syndrome.

Primary hypothyroidism clearly occurs with greater frequency in primary autoimmune adrenal failure than can be attributed to chance alone. Measurement of basal TSH level in plasma is considered one of the hallmarks of diminished thyroid reserve. However, in patients with Addison's disease, regardless of etiology, an elevated basal TSH need not always imply the presence of underlying thyroid failure.

EVALUATION OF PITUITARY HORMONES

While an elevated ACTH is the hallmark of primary adrenal failure, [3 lipotropin, TSH, and prolactin can undergo significant alterations. The reversible elevation in TSH secondary to glucocorticoid lack has already been alluded to; the perturbations in ACTH, [3-lipotropin, and prolactin in patients with Addison's disease deserve brief mention.

ACTH

Basal ACTH levels are variably elevated in almost all patients with Addison's disease, ranging between 200 and 1000 pg. In general, the degree of elevation bears little correlation to the severity of adrenal failure or the duration of the disease. The spontaneous fluctuation in plasma ACTH level can cause difficulties in interpretation. The availability of sensitive and standardized assays for ACTH has permitted evaluation of plasma levels of ACTH in patients with Addison's disease who are on long-term, conventional glucocorticoid replacement. While most patients demonstrate suppression of the raised ACTH following glucocorticoid therapy, some Addisonian patients demonstrate only partial suppression.

The clinical correlation of these observations is that ACTH measurements be obtained in all patients with Addison's disease, and if ACTH is found to be extraordinarily elevated, a CT scan of the pituitary is indicated. Also, the reappearance or intensification of pigmentation in Addisonian patients on replacement therapy would warrant a similar approach.

β-LIPOTROPIN

β-Lipotropin and ACTH share "similar dynamics but different kinetics." Thus, 13-lipotropin is more stable in the plasma and has a longer half-life. The correlation between the magnitude of elevation in plasma levels of ACTH and 13- lipotropin is an assumed one and has not been demonstrated in any large series of Addisonian patients. Similarly, the correlation between the degree of hyperpigmentation and the magnitude of elevation of these pituitary hormones has not been conclusively established. Unless measurement of 13-lipotropins in the plasma is routinely performed in all Addisonians before and during treatment, questions regarding these correlations cannot be resolved.

TSH

The elevated TSH levels seen in co~unction with untreated adrenal failure might lead to mistakenly conferring a diagnosis of concomitant primary hypothyroidism. The nature of the relationship between glucocorticoids and TSH has already been alluded to in this chapter in the section, "Extraadrenal Endocrine Dysfunction in Addison's Disease."

PROLACTIN

Prolactin dynamics can also undergo significant alteration as a consequence vof primary adrenal failure. These changes parallel the changes in TSH. For instance, glucocorticoid administration suppresses prolactin secretion in humans, while adrenalectomy can result in elevations of serum prolactin. Adrenalectomy has also been shown to increase the prolactin response to ether stress in rats. Development of the amenorrhea galactorrhea syndrome in a patient with primary adrenal failure, which reversed on glucocorticoid replacement, has been reported

COMPLICATIONS (ACUTE ADDISONIAN CRISIS)

The most important complication of hypoadrenalism is the development of Addisonian crisis that is potentially fatal. Adrenal crisis develops when the marginally adequate adrenal reserve becomes suddenly inadequate to combat the rising needs for cortisol during stress. Addisonian crisis is almost always precipitated by some form of stress. Physical, emotional, anesthetic, or traumatic stress can all be responsible for triggering a crisis. But the most notable factor that precipitates adrenal crisis is infection. Even a seemingly simple viral cold can trigger adrenal crisis. At times adrenal crisis can be triggered by the use of medications. Initiating thyroxine therapy in a patient with marginal adrenal insufficiency is a classic setting where the sudden increase in metabolic demands cannot be met by the compromised adrenals. Similarly, the use of rifampin, which accelerates the turnover of cortisol, can be conducive for precipitating decompensation in a marginally compromised situation. Of course, the sudden withdrawal of steroid therapy is another classic setting where the chronically suppressed hypothalamic pituitary adrenal axis cannot muster a response to stress.

The clinical presentation of acute adrenal crisis is easy to recognize if the background of adrenocortical failure is known. For instance, the development of crisis in the Addisonian patient on steroid replacement is often detected even at the very early stages of its evolution. In contrast, the diagnosis is often missed when the adrenal crisis is the presenting manifestation of Addison's disease. The syndrome is ushered in by anorexia, nausea, vomiting, and diarrhea with vague abdominal cramps. Fever, chills, and diaphoresis may accompany the gastrointestinal manifestations of acute adrenal crisis. As the untreated syndrome evolves, patients develop volume depletion and dehydration, often severe enough to culminate in shock. Hyponatremia and hyperkalemia are usually apparent, often associated with mild to moderate metabolic acidosis, hypoglycemia, and occasionally hypercalcemia. Unfortunately, when the hyperkalemia is masked by severe vomiting and diarrhea, the diagnosis of adrenal crisis can be missed by even experienced clinicians. The list of initial diagnoses that are often made in patients who were subsequently documented as being in Addisonian crisis includes acute gastroenteritis, salmonellosis, ruptured ectopic pregnancy, toxic shock syndrome, septic shock, acute myocardial failure with shock, and others.

Acute adrenal crisis should be a diagnostic concern under the following conditions.

1. Dehydration and electrolyte abnormalities in patients with a chronic history of ill health characterized by weight loss and weakness.
2. Shock in the background of tuberculosis, or carcinomatosis.
3. Diarrhea and dehydration in the presence of normal or elevated potassium and low sodium concentrations in the plasma.
4. The unusual combination of hypoglycemia in association with hypotension; most conditions characterized by hypotension are associated with a brisk release of several counterinsulin hormones that usually increase the blood glucose levels.
5. The presence of hyperpigmentation or absence of axillary hair in females in the setting of hypotension should strongly point to underlying adrenal disease as the cause of illness.

The recognition of Addisonian crisis is crucial since early administration of glucocorticoids can make the difference between life and death. The beneficial effects of therapy are often dramatically evident within 24 hr of steroid therapy. Little time should be wasted on performing tests when acute adrenal crisis is considered. A pretreatment cortisol, often coupled with a rapid ACTH stimulation test, is all that is required. When the patient's condition is deemed too dangerous to allow even a I-hr delay in therapy, the rapid ACTH test can be still performed while covering the patient with a bolus of 20 mg of methylprednisolone and 10 mg of desoxycorticosterone acetate. Vigorous normal saline coupled with stress doses of hydrocortisone (100 mg intravenously three times a day) rapidly corrects the dehydration, electrolyte disturbances, and cortisol deficiency of acute adrenal crisis.

TREATMENT

Addison's disease is indeed one of the most gratifying diseases to treat. The transformation of a listless, withdrawn, helpless person into a normal being, capturing the lost vigor and vitality with a vengeance, is an unforgettable experience. The replacement therapy for Addison's disease consists of glucocorticoids and mineralocorticoid administration, which, in physiological doses, is remarkably devoid of adverse effects. The treatment of Addison's disease can be viewed from four perspectives-glucocorticoid replacement, mineralocorticoid replacement, treatment of acute adrenal crisis, and therapy for the disease that is responsible for the adrenal failure.

GLUCOCORTICOID THERAPY

Replacement glucocorticoid therapy consists of administering cortisone acetate or hydrocortisone hemisuccinate. To simulate the physiological diurnal rhythm, cortisone acetate is administered orally as 25 mg in the morning and 12.5 mg in the evening, while hydrocortisone hemisuccinate is given in the dosage of 20 mg in the morning and 10 mg in the evening. Administration of these two glucocorticoids, although well tolerated, entails some inherent problems. First, since these steroids are short acting, it is inevitable that such therapy be associated with intermittent periods of unsuppressed ACTH levels in the plasma.

The patterns of plasma cortisol and ACTH concentrations in patients with Addison's disease treated with conventional corticosteroid replacement and showed that some patients failed to show adequate suppression of ACTH with the use of conventional doses of either drug. Second, therapy with cortisone acetate may be hampered by inadequate absorption of steroid acetate by the gastrointestinal tract and impaired *in vivo* conversion of cortisone to cortisol. Obviously, these phenomenona may be conducive to reducing the bioavailability of the drug. Third, unlike replacement therapy of primary hypothyroidism, where the dosage of thyroxine can be finely adjusted, there are no scientific tools to provide fine titration of glucocorticoid therapy. Thus, adequacy of replacement is often judged on the basis of clinical response, and on the subjective symptoms of the patient.

The efficacy of four different glucocorticoids (cortisone, hydrocortisone, dexamethasone, and prednisolone) as replacement therapy for Addison's disease. Dexamethasone was strikingly potent in suppressing ACTH levels at the lowest total glucocorticoid dose. However, the same potency of dexamethasone may also play an important role in predisposing patients to adverse effects of long-term glucocorticoid activity. Besides, dexamethasone possesses little mineralocorticoid activity. These two factors limit the usefulness of dexamethasone in treatment of Addison's disease, despite its longer-acting effects and its ability to suppress ACTH more effectively than cortisone or hydrocortisone. In addition, it is unclear whether complete suppression of ACTH is necessary in treatment of Addison's disease, in contrast to adrenogenital syndrome where total suppression of ACTH has great therapeutic benefit.

The parameters to follow in Addisonian patients on glucocorticoid replacement are mostly clinical. Thus, if fatigue, malaise, weight loss, and hyperpigmentation persist, the dose of cortisone or hydrocortisone is increased, while the presence of signs indicative of steroid excess necessitates reduction of glucocorticoid dosage. In general, measurement of serum cortisol is not a good parameter for dose titration in patients receiving cortisone or hydrocortisone. The measurement of serum cortisol might prove valuable in studying the absorption characteristics of these medications when a question of bioavailability arises. Of course, serum cortisol measurements are of absolutely no value in patients receiving dexamethasone. As for measurement of serum ACTH level to titrate the dose of glucocorticoid, this marker has not assumed the status or sophistication of measurement of TSH for adjustment of thyroxine dosage in patients with primary hypothyroidism. The relatively short half-life of cortisone (or hydrocortisone), the pulsatile nture of ACTH secretion, the heterogeneity of ACTH levels in treated Addisonians, and the limited availability of ACTH determinations have all limited the use of serum ACTH level as a parameter for titrating the glucocorticoid dosage.

The measurement of urine free cortisol might be a useful tool for detecting undertreatment or excess dose of the orally administered cortisone or hydrocortisone. Notably, the 24-hr urine free cortisol showed little day-to-day variation, and in the nine patients with Addison's disease on oral replacement regimens with cortisone or hydrocortisone, the urine free cortisol is correlated well . Again, this measurement is meaningless in patients receiving dexamethasone or prednisolone, steroids that do not get converted into hydrocortisone in the body. Individual variations in the absorption of the cortisone acetate or hydrocortisone hemisuccinate which are orally administered are the most frequent reasons for undertreatment despite administration of a conventional replacement dose. The development of diarrhea, vomiting, and other side effects would mandate an increment (usually doubling) in the dose of oral cortisone. If the problem is severe, as with gastroenteritis, parenteral hydrocortisone becomes necessary. Patients with Addison's disease should be repeatedly reinforced as to the need for increasing their glucocorticoid dose during periods of stress. Also, it is mandatory that such patients wear on their person some form of identification as to their disease, with instructions to use intravenous hydrocortisone in the event the patient is found unconscious.

MINERALOCORTICOID REPLACEMENT

Mineralocorticoid replacement for patients with Addison's disease is provided by oral administration of 9-a-fludrocortisone, 0.05-0.1 mg/day. Initially, nearly all patients with Addison's disease require both gluco- and mineralocorticoids. However, after several months to years, many patients continue to do well despite exclusion of mineralocorticoids. Adjustment of the dose of mineralocorticoid is also empirical and is based on clinical and biochemical data. Thus, the persistence of orthostatic hypotension, dizziness, hyperkalemia, or hyponatremia is an indication to start, or increase the preexisting dose of, mineralocorticoid. Similarly, the development of hypertension, edema, or cardiac failure is an indication to decrease the dose or discontinue the mineralocorticoid altogether. During the initial stages of therapy with florinef, some patients with Addison's disease may demonstrate exquisite mineralocorticoid sensitivity and may rapidly develop edema. In such cases withdrawal of the drug with very careful reinstitution becomes necessary. While clinical judgment and electrolyte monitoring continue to remain the parameters to evaluate dosage of mineralocorticoid replacement, measurement of plasma renin activity (PRA) has been advocated as a sensitive tool to assess the need and dose of mineralocorticoid replacement. A raised PRA indicates the presence of sodium depletion and hence the need for more mineralocorticoid, even when the serum potassium concentrations are still within the normal range. However, PRA determinations cannot clearly distinguish between adequate dosage and overdosage.

Patients with Addison's disease generally learn to include a high salt intake in their diet. This, coupled with adequate glucocorticoid replacement, may allow elimination of all mineralocorticoid. However, a careful assessment of blood pressure, pulse, cardiac status, electrolytes, and perhaps plasma renin is indicated before oral mineralocorticoid replacement is discontinued. Occasionally, mimetic action can provide mineralocorticoid converge. This, however, is not to be recommended since sooner or later these effects are lost andacute mineralocorticoid deficiency is likely to manifest.

ADRENAL CRISIS

This represents an emergency situation where early therapeutic intervention can be lifesaving. The four-pronged approach to treatment of Addisonian crisis is administration of hydrocortisone, 100 mg three times a day, intravenously; use of mineralocorticoid, 10 mg DOC intramuscularly once or twice a day, or 9-0: fludrocortisone, 0.1 mg orally; liberal administration of normal saline until the patient has been adequately hydrated and volume-repleted; and treatment of precipitating causes, if identified. Glucose-containing solutions should be incorporated in the fluid regimen to provide adequate caloric support. With timely intervention, patients with Addisonian crisis improve with dramatic and startling rapidity. The key here is early intervention. Once the patient has developed hypoperfusion and shock, the prognosis is gloomy. The electrolyte abnormalities and metabolic acidosis rapidly improve with hydration andsteroid therapy. Within 24-48 hr, the patient can be switched to oral replacement therapy.

TREATMENT OF UNDERLYING CAUSE

This aspect of therapy assumes importance when infectious etiologies underlie the adrenal failure. Two in particular merit attention-TB and fungal disease.

Although the scourge of TB has declined over the past two decades, it still continues to be an important cause of Addison's disease. Several important statements are relevant in terms of specific therapy.

I. The mere presence of a reactive tuberculin test should not deter the physician from searching for another cause for Addison's disease. The coexistence of idiopathic adrenal atrophy in patients exposed to tuberculosishas been emphasized.
2. The presence of "active" tuberculosis elsewhere (e.g., lung, genitourinary tract) in a patient with Addison's disease clearly indicates the need for conventional antituberculous therapy with three drugs-isoniazid, rifampin, and ethambutal-along with replacement therapy.
3. When active tuberculosis cannot be demonstrated in extraadrenallocations, the combination of a reactive tuberculin test, exclusion of other causes of Addison's disease, and demonstration of bilaterally enlarged adrenal glands by CT constitutes an adequate basis for the diagnosis oftuberculous Addison's disease. In these cases, institution of a full course of antituberculous treatment is justified, along with, of course, full hormonal replacement.
4. When active tuberculosis cannot be demonstrated in extraadrenallocations, but the patient demonstrates a reactive tuberculin test with bilaterally atrophied adrenals by CT and without evidence of other causes for Addison's disease, the diagnosis can be presumed. In such cases, institution of a full course of antituberculous therapy is of dubious value.
5. When antituberculous therapy is administered to patients with Addison's disease on replacement, the effect of rifampin on the catabolism of cortisol should be borne in mind. An increase in the glucocorticoid dosage should be anticipated, since rifampin increases the hepatic catabolism of glucocorticoids. Failure to realize this fact may result in the development of acute adrenal crisis due to inadequate bioavailability of the glucocorticoid administered.
6. Finally, there are reports of improvement in adrenal function after treatment of tuberculous adrenalitis. However, these cases were reported in the early 1960s, without complete documentation by present standards.

Fungal infections, when documented as a cause of adrenal failure, demand antifungal chemotherapy with either ketoconazole or amphotericin B.

REFERENCES

1. Goudie RB, AndersonJR, Gray KK, et al. Autoantibodies in Addison's disease. *Lancet* **1**: 1173, 1966.
2. Irvine Wj, Barnes EW: Adrenocortical insufficiency. *Clin Endocr Metab* 1:549, 1972.
3. Crispell KR, Parson W, Hamlin J, et al. Addisons disease associated with histoplasmusis. *Am J Med* 20:23, 1956.
4. Abrams, HL, Spiro R, Golstein N: Metastases in carcinoma. *Cancer* 3:74,1950.
5. Guenthner EE, Rabinowe SL, Van Niel A, et al: Primary Addison's disease in a patient with the acquired immuno-deficiency syndrome. *Ann Intern Med* 100:847, 1984.
7. Farid NR, Larsen B, Payne R, et al. Polyglandular autoimmune disease and HLA. *Tissue*

8. *Antigenl* 16:23, 1980.
9. Fettes I, Killinger D. Volpe R: Adrenoleukodystrophv: Report of a familial case. *Clin Enliorrinol*11:151, 1979.
10. Walker DA, Davies M: Addison's disease presenting as a hypercalcaemic crisis in a patient with idiopathic hypoparathyroidism. *Clin Endocrinol* 14:419, 1978.
11. Vita JA, Silverberg SJ, Goland RS, et al. Clinical clues to the cause of Addison's disease. *Am]Med* 78:461, 1985.
12. Leiba S, Landau B, Ber A: Target gland insufficiency and pituitary tumours. *Acta Endocrinol (Kbh)* 60: 112, 1969.
13. Nelson DH: Diagnosis and treatment of Addison's disease. In DeGroot **LI** (ed): *Endocrinology,* vol. 2. Grune & Stratton, New York, 1979, p. 1199.
14. Burch WM: Urine free-cortisol determination: A useful tool in the management of chronic hypoadrenal states. *]AMA* 247: 2002, 1982.

CHAPTER 79

Pheochromocytoma

Pheochromocytoma is the neoplasm of the neural crest derived chromaffin cells. Synthesis and secretion of catecholamines in an uncontrolled and oftentimes life threatening manner is the characteristic feature of this rare tumor. Chromaffin cells are most frequently found in the adrenal medulla, where they normally function to secrete catecholamines, which modulate stress response, metabolism, and blood pressure. When catecholamine producing chromaffin cell tumors arise in an extra-adrenal location they are referred to as paragangliomas, or extra-adrenal pheochromocytomas. Although there is similarity in ontogeny, minor differences exist in the biology of disease between adrenal and extra-adrenal pheochromocytomas, which impact clinical decision making. A thorough understanding of the natural history of the various manifestations of chromaffin cell tumors guides the clinician in the most appropriate and efficacious treatment.

EPIDEMIOLOGY

Pheochromocytomas can occur sporadically or in association with a number of syndromes. Familial syndromes that are associated with the development of pheochromocytomas includes mainly multiple endocrine neoplasia (MEN) types 2A and 2B, von Recklinghausen's neurofibromatosis (NF1) and von Hippel-Lindau disease (VHL).

Pheochromocytomas may also be associated with other un-familiarly syndromes such as tuberous sclerosis , Sturge-Weber syndrome, , and Carney's triad. Pheochromocytomas in patients with suffering with familial syndromes are unlikely to be malignant.

MEN 2A and 2B are autosomal dominant syndromes caused by mutations in the RET proto-oncogene. Common to MEN2 syndromes are medullary thyroid cancer (MTC; nearly 100% penetrance) and pheochromocytoma (approximately 40%). Pheochromocytomas in MEN 2 are bilateral in approximately 70% and are usually multicentric. Bilateral medullary hyperplasia is almost always present in these patients.

Pheochromocytomas are rarely cancerous or extra-adrenal in MEN2. von Recklinghausen's neurofibromatosis (NF1) is an autosomal dominant disorder associated with widespread neurofibromatosis, and the rare (1%) development of pheochromocytomas. Inheritance of VHL is autosomal dominant, and is characterized by cerebellar hemangioblastoma, retinal hemangiomatosis, pancreatic cysts & tumors, kidney cysts or tumors, epididymal cystadenoma, and pheochromocytoma. Other neuroectodermal disorders that are associated with pheochromocytoma include tuberous sclerosis, Sturge-Weber syndrome, and Carney's triad. Carney's triad is a syndrome of pulmonary chondroma, gastric leiomyosarcoma, and functional extra-adrenal pheochromocytoma.

UNTREATED PHEOCHROMOCYTOMA

Untreated and undiagnosed pheochromocytoma may lead to heavy morbidity due to the uncontrolled oversecretion of catecholamines. Most of the complications are cardiovascular related. Increase or decrease in blood pressure, myocardial infarction, dysrhythmias, cardiac failure, and cerebral vascular accidents account for 75% of mortalities in undiagnosed or untreated pheochromocytomas. Patients may present with convulsions, elevated glucose levels, hypercalcemia, retinopathy, cardiomegaly, shock, and lactic acidosis. Symptoms are commonly misdiagnosed as anxiety or panic attacks . Other rare manifestations reported includes mainly renal infarction, rhabdomyolysis, acute pancreatitis, vasculitis, retroperitoneal tumor hemorrhage, kidney failure, and disseminated intravascular coagulopathy.

HISTOPATHOLOGY

SITE OF TUMOR

Pheochromocytomas originate from the chromaffin cells of the sympathoadrenal system. Nearly 85-90% of the time the tumor originates from the adrenal medulla. In 10-15% of cases, the tumor is extraadrenal. These sites include the paraganglia cells of the sympathetic chain (particularly from the lumbar and paraaortic sympathetic ganglia); the organ of Zuckerkandl, a structure composed of chromaffin-staining cells situated near the mesenteric artery and extending along the aorta as far down as its bifurcation 7-9; the chest «2%), particularly from the sympathetic chain in the posterior mediastinum; the neck «0.1%); and the urinary bladder. Rarely, the pheochromocytoma can be intrapericardial.

The familial variety of pheochromocytoma is regarded as a distinct entity, owing to the fact that tumors are commonly bilateral in this group of pheochromocytoma. Even when unilateral, the familial pheochromocytoma tends to demonstrate multicentricity within the gland. It is generally held that the incidence of extraadrenal pheochromocytoma is the same in familial as well as sporadic pheochromocytomas.

MACROSCOPIC APPEARANCE

Morphologically, adrenal pheochromocytomas average 100 g in weight and less than 10 cm in diameter. Extraadrenal pheochromocytomas weigh less and are usually less than 5 cm in diameter. Adrenal pheochromocytomas are highly vascular and often display a tendency to be supplied by all three suprarenal arteries-middle, superior, and inferior. Hemorrhage, necrosis, and cyst formation (from infarction and liquefaction) are often encountered in adrenal pheochromocytomas.

MICROSCOPIC APPEARANCE

Microscopically, pheochromoctytomas are composed of large pleomorphic chromaffin cells. As with other endocrine tumors, it is difficult to determine whether the tumor is benign or malignant on the basis of the microscopic appearance alone. Less than 10% of adrenal pheochromocytomas are malignant, based on the presence of local invasion or distant spread. It is generally believed that the incidence of malignant pheochromocytomas is higher in three types of pheochromocytomas: the familial variant, the extraadrenal pheochromocytomas, and those in children. Ultrastructural studies of tumor tissue show that the tumor contains large amounts of chromaffin granules, which are subcellular particles that store catecholamines. These chromaffin granules, for the most part, appear no different than the granules seen within normal adrenal medullary cells. There are no consistent data to suggest differences in the mechanisms of intragranular binding, storage, and release of catecholamines between normal and tumorous adrenal medullary tissue. Considerable variability exists in the biosynthesis, storage, turnover, and release of catecholamine in pheochromocytomas. This precludes any assumptions in postulating differences in the manner in which tumor tissue synthesizes catecholamine in comparison to normal tissue. It is not clear whether a change in the rate-limiting step involving tyrosine hydroxylase leads to an uncontrolled rate of catecholamine synthesis by the tumor cells. There seems to be a correlation between the size of the tumor and the turnover rate of catecholamines within the tumor. Thus, small pheochromocytomas tend to show relatively lower concentrations of catecholamines within the tumor, with a high turnover rate of catecholamines and lower urinary ratios of vanillyl mandelic acid (VMA) to catecholamines. In contrast, the larger tumors contain higher concentrations of catecholamines within the tumor, with a lower turnover rate, resulting in a higher urinary ratio of VMA to catecholamine. It is possible that smaller tumors cause symptoms earlier, since more catecholamines are secreted into the system.

ASSOCIATIONS OF PHEOCHROMOCYTOMA

Although rare, several associations of pheochromocytomas need to be kept in mind and the disease sought in the presence of these "background disorders." The four most important associations are, von Hippel-Lindau disease, von Recklinghausen's disease (neurofibromatosis), the multiple endocrine neoplasia syndromes type II and III (MEN II and III), and acromegaly. A fifth, cholelithiasis, is frequently mentioned as an association of pheochromocytoma.

VON RECKLINGHAUSEN'S DISEASE

The classic concept has been that the prevalence of pheochromocytoma in patients with multiple cutaneous neurofibromatosis is approximately 1-2%,13-15. About 5% of patients with pheochromocytoma may have neurofibromatosis. One of the clinical hallmarks of von Recklinghausen's disease is the presence of more than two cafe-au-lait spots greater than 2 cm in diameter with the presence of freckles in the axilla. Since von Recklinghausen's disease may be transmitted as an incomplete form, minor manifestations such as pigmentary or vertebral anomalies, may suggest the presence of the von Recklinghausen trait. The conventionally ascribed low rate of association (1-2%) of pheochromocytoma with von Recklinghausen's disease should be reevaluated in light of recent data. The pheochromocytomas were detected within or adjacent to the adrenal gland and secreted both epinephrine as well as norepinephrine.

VON HIPPEL-LINDAU DISEASE

von Hippel-Lindau disease refers to a familial syndrome characterized by the variable occurrence of retinal, cerebellar, and cerebral hemangioblastomas. Pheochromocytoma is regarded as an unusual but notable association with von Hippel-Lindau disease, approximately 61 cases having been reported. In a collected series of 50 patients with von Hippel-Lindau disease from nine families, the prevalence of pheochromocytoma was noted to be 10%. 20 In contrast to this low incidence, in another series, pheochromocytomas were found in 12 of 13 affected members with von Hippel-Lindau's disease. Thus, it seems that the prevalence of pheochromocytomas in this syndrome is highly variable. The usual site of the tumor is adrenal, but rarely extraadrenal pheochromocytoma has been reported in patients with von Hippel-Lindau disease.

MEN II AND MEN III

The association of pheochromocytoma with MEN II and III is well recognized. Type II MEN consists of medullary carcinoma of the thyroid, pheochromocytoma, and hyperparathyroidism. Type III MEN, which is believed to represent an entity distinct from type II MEN, consists of medullary thyroid carcinoma, pheochromocytoma, and a unique constellation of somatic stigmata. These stigmata include a Marfanoid habitus, mucosal neuromas (particularly of the tongue, lips, and eyelids), thickening of corneal nerves, and ganglioneuromatosis of the alimentary tract. Type III MEN is also characterized by the lack of hyperparathyroidism, the heightened frequency of bilateral pheochromocytomas, the often aggressive nature of the medullary thyroid carcinoma, and the onset at a relatively younger age in comparison to MEN II. The pheochromocytomas that occur in association with familial syndromes, particularly the MEN types, are unique for the following reasons:

1. These tumors are often extremely small, increasing the likelihood of being missed by conventional localizational and imaging procedures.
2. Familial pheochromocytomas may remain clinically silent, with very few symptoms until a crisis supervenes. In some instances, the first manifestation of the pheochromocytoma, for instance during anesthesia, may well be the last.
3. The small size of these tumors, when combined with the rapid turnover within the tumor, may result in unimpressive biochemical data, which may result in missing the condition when conventional screening tests are employed.
4. The pheochromocytomas of familial variety are usually bilateral. Very often, even when the tumor is demonstrably unilateral, the contralateral adrenal medulla may show changes of "medullary hyperplasia." Whether the bilateral nature of such tumors is universal is rather controversial.
5. Familial pheochromocytomas tend to demonstrate a proclivity toward

malignancy more often than the sporadic variants.

6. Familial pheochromocytomas often demonstrate a tendency to selectively or predominantly secrete epinephrine, a phenomenon that is relatively uncommon in the sporadic variety of pheochromocytoma.
7. Finally, the familial variety of pheochromocytoma does not often lend itself to successful diagnostic testing by employing provocative maneuvers such as intravenous glucagon.

The frequent occurrence of familial pheochromocytoma with such diverse conditions as von Hippel-Lindau's disease, neurofibromatosis, the MEN syndromes, and carcinoid tumors has led to the concept that all these conditions may be ultimately related to an aberration in the migration, growth, and differentiation of the neural crest cells.

ACROMEGALY

The association between acromegaly and pheochromocytoma is less well recognized. Pheochromocytomas with acromegaly suggests that the combination may represent a nonfamilial variety of multiple endocrine neoplasia syndrome. These patients tend to have sustained hypertension rather than the episodic hypertension characteristic of pheochromocytoma. Symptoms of pheochromocytoma had persisted for an average of 7 years before the diagnosis was established. Even more important was the fact that 4 of the 10 patients died from causes directly related to pheochromocytoma. This emphasizes the importance of a careful search for pheochromocytoma in acromegalics with hypertension. Hyperparathyroidism has been variably associated with the syndrome. As with MEN I, aberrant neural crest development may underlie the development of both the pituitary tumor and the pheochromocytoma.

CHOLELITHIASIS

The increased incidence (up to 30%) of cholelithiasis in association with pheochromocytoma is well recognized but unexplained. The possibility that such a combination, at least in some instances, may represent gallstones caused by a somatostinoma is speculative.

CLINICAL FEATURES

The clinical features of pheochromocytoma can be viewed from several perspectives: the acute paroxysms, which can be so characteristic as to permit instant recognition; the sustained manifestations, which may render the disease as unremarkable as any garden-variety essential hypertension; unusual manifestations, and finally, the features that result from complications of chronic catecholamine excess, the brunt of which are shouldered by the cardiovascular system.

Table 79.1

Precipitating factors for a paroxysm
1. **Increase in intraabdominal pressure**
Massage, or steady pressure on the tumor
Valsalva maneuver
Straining at stool
Coughing, sneezing, laughing, tight clothing
Sexual intercourse
Parturition
Abdominal trauma

Table 79.1 *Contd...*

2. **Anxiety**
   - Pain
   - Nervousness
   - Hyperventilation
3. **Administration of certain drugs**
   - Histamine
   - Glucagon
   - ACTH
   - Nicotine
   - Phenothiazine
   - Saralasin
   - Epinephrine
   - Tyramine
4. **Procedures**
   - Anesthesia
   - Surgery
   - Endoscopy

ACUTE PAROXYSMS

Patients with pheochromocytoma often experience sudden "attacks," which are due to intermittent release of catecholamines from the tumor into the circulation. Paradoxically, smaller tumors are more often associated with more dramatic and explosive paroxysms than larger-sized tumors. These episodes of paroxysms are highlighted by the occurrence of moderate to severe hypertension. At times, the paroxysm can be so explosive as to result in stroke, myocardial infarction, or death. The precipitating factors for the development of an attack can be several. Numerous "trigger factors" have been recognized (Table 79.1). Three factors seem to be the most commonly associated precipitating factors-increase in the intraabdominal pressure, anxiety, and use of certain drugs or procedures. Of particular interest is the precipitation of paroxysms from the use of drugs. There are primarily three mechanisms whereby drugs can precipitate a paroxysm, even a crisis. First, certain drugs may result in direct release of catecholamines from the tumor. The precipitation of crisis by the use of histamine, glucagon, ACTH, saralasin, and opiates belongs in this category. More important, fentanyl, a potent opiate agonist, can provoke catecholamine release. The second mechanism involves release of catecholamines stored in the sympathetic nerve endings.

Methyldopa and decongestants containing sympathomimetic amines belong in this category. The third mechanism involves the use of drugs that inhibit reuptake of catecholamines by the sympathetic neurons; guanethidine and tricyclic antidepressants belong to this category.

The frequency of attacks can be highly variable in individual patients, ranging from occurring once in few months to occurring 25 times daily. The attacks, which evolve so dramatically and rapidly, resolve more slowly than they started. The symptoms that accompany the paroxysm of hypertension are headaches, excessive perspiration, and palpitations.

Paroxysmal hypertension is encountered in more than 50% of patients with pheochromocytoma. The degree of hypertension during some of these attacks can be dangerously high, exceeding a diastolic greater than 130 mm Hg ("hypertensive crisis"). Headaches, which generally accompany the paroxysmal hypertension, are severe, are located in the frontal or occipital regions, and are described as throbbing or pounding. The increased diaphoresis can be severe enough to drench the patient in sweat.

Palpitations, tachycardia, or both are present in more than 70% of patients who experience paroxysms of pheochromocytoma. In addition, patients may experience nervousness, panic, or a sense of impending doom, dizziness, weakness, and tremulousness during an attack. The classic attack of catecholamine excess is typical enough to be diagnosed by the history.

SUSTAINED HYPERTENSION

In approximately 49% of patients with pheochromocytoma the blood pressure elevation may be sustained without discernible evidence of the presence of paroxysms. 40 In such patients, the presentation and behavior of the hypertensive condition bear a close resemblance to those of patients with essential hypertension. Unremarkable as the hypertension may seem, an underlying pheochromocytoma should be suspected under the following conditions:

1. Alterations of the blood pressure, often spontaneously.
2. Little or no response to conventional antihypertensive medications.
3. The presence of orthostatic hypotension; spontaneous orthostatic hypotension can be a prominent feature of pheochromocytoma. Such a finding in an untreated hypertensive patient should raise the suspicion of pheochromocytoma. The pathogenesis of orthostatic hypotension in pheochromocytoma is ill understood. The proposed mechanisms include increased venous tone with resultant decrease in plasma volume; an adverse effect of catecholamines on the sympathetic reflexes that normally maintain the cybernetic response; and tachyphylaxis to the catecholamines.
4. Adverse or paradoxical increases in blood pressure in response to betablockade or ganglion-blocking agents.
5. Presence of hypermetabolic features such as weight loss, heat intolerance, or glucose intolerance.
6. A marked presser response during induction with any anesthetic agent.

While all hypertensive patients with the 4 Hs (headache, hyperhidrosis, hypermetabolism, and hyperglycemia) should be mandatorily screened for the presence of a pheochromocytoma, the reported rarity of the disease in the hypertensive population at large should be kept in mind. On the other hand, pheochromocytoma is a curable cause of hypertension, and therefore, the cost of prolonged antihypertensive therapy must be weighed against the cost of screening, as well as the price extracted by missed diagnosis. There is no unanimity of opinion in the matter of screening the entire hypertensive population for pheochromocytoma. Some degree of selectivity is of course desirable, and patients with even the most subtle clues in the history should be screened for the presence of this disease.

UNUSUAL MANIFESTATIONS (TABLE 79.2)

Pheochromocytoma, as indicated earlier, can be the proverbial "great masquerader." The diversity of manifestations is illustrated by the fact that no less than 80 manifestations have been reported. Several unusual manifestations are listed in the Table 79.2.

Table 79.2

Unusual manifestations of pheochromocytomas
1. Shock or circulatory collapse
2. "Normotensive" pheochromocytoma
3. Fever ("FUO")
4. Gastrointestinal manifestations
5. Vasomotor phenomena
6. Neuropsychiatric manifestations
7. Cardiovascular disease
8. "Paraneoplastic" disease
Hypercalcemia
Rarer syndromes
9. Hypermetabolic phenomena
10. Asymptomatic ("nonfunctional")

COMPLICATIONS

Occasionally patients with pheochromocytoma come to attention for the first time owing to manifestations from the complications of the disease. As can be seen from Table 79.3, cardiovascular complications lead the list.

Table 79.3

Complications of pheochromocytoma
1. Cardiac
Cardiomyopathy
Congestive failure
Myocarditis
Myocardial infarction
Dissecting aneurysm
2. Central nervous system
Cerebrovascular accident
Encephalopathy
3. Gastrointestinal
Pseudoobstruction
Ischemic enterocolitis
Hemorrhage within tumor
4. Shock

LABORATORY DIAGNOSIS

The laboratory diagnosis of pheochromocytoma can be viewed from three perspectives: establishing the biochemical diagnosis, the use of dynamic studies, and localization of the tumor. It is unacceptable to "explore" a patient for the possible presence of a pheochromocytoma in the absence of documented biochemical or radiological proof of the tumor.

BIOCHEMICAL DIAGNOSIS

With the currently available hormonal tests to document catecholamine hypersecretion, the diagnosis of pheochromocytoma can be established with certainty in more than 90-95% of cases. When combined with dynamic testing (such as glucagon stimulation or clonidine suppression), the diagnostic accuracy approaches virtually 100%. The three major screening tests for pheochromocytoma involve determining the urinary excretion of catecholamine metabolites, measurement of free catecholamines in the urine, and determination of plasma catecholamines.

CATECHOLAMINE METABOLITES

Measurement of 24-hr urinary metanephrine, normetanephrine, and VMA (Vanillyl-mandelic acid) have stood the test of time as simple, reasonably accurate, and inexpensive firstline screening tests for detection of a pheochromocytoma.

Metanephrine, Normetanephrine: The metanephrine and normetanephrine levels in the 24-hr urine measure the methylated metabolites of epinephrine and norepinephrine; of the urinary indices of catecholamine production, measurement of metanephrine and normetanephrine provides the most reliable clues for the presence of an underlying pheochromocytoma. The normal range of these metabolites is from 0.02 to 1.7 mg/24 hr in a well-collected specimen. Collection of urine for catecholamines or their metabolites is done in an acidified bottle, preferably on ice. When the 24-hr meta- and normetanephrines exceed 1.8 mg/24 hr, the diagnosis of pheochromocytoma is highly suspect. It is essential to avoid the use of drugs that interfere with the assay; particular attention should be paid to the use of antihypertensive agents (methyldopa), catecholamine-containing drugs, benzodiazepines, MAO inhibitors, and alcohol, all of which can give an apparent increase in urinary metanephrine and normetanephrine. On the other end of the spectrum, spurious lowering of values might be seen in patients who have received radiographic dyes containing methyglucamine (renografin, renovist), and in those taking large doses of fenfluramine. Of course, in the hospital setting, the main reason for encountering elevated levels of urinary metanephrine, normetanephrine values is stress. Thus, patients with severe illness, burns, myocardial infarction, and stroke tend to show elevation of these metabolites. The impact of chronic renal failure on the urinary metabolites of catecholamines is also another factor to be kept in mind while interpreting these values.

***VMA* (Vanillylmandelic acid):** The 24-hr urinary VMA excretion is seldom recommended as the sole screening test for detection of pheochromocytoma. The normal range for VMA excretion in 24 hr in adults is 1-14 mg/24 hr. In children, the VMA excretion correlates with weight as well as creatinine excretion. VMA excretion is affected by diet (especially foods rich in vanillin) as well as the same drugs that affect metanephrine and normetanephrine values in the 24-hr urine. In addition, nalidexic acid, L-dopa, and rapid clonidine withdrawal may also spuriously increase VMA levels. In contrast, MAO inhibitors, clofibrate, disulfiram, and large doses of fenfluramine tend to decrease the apparent value of VMA measurements. Despite these disadvantages, when the VMA levels are greater than 13 mg/24 hr, the diagnosis of pheochromocytoma is strongly supported.

URINARY CATECHOLAMINES

Measurement of urinary excretion of free catecholamines, when collected and performed properly, provides 95% accuracy in detecting pheochromocytoma. However, free catecholamines are metabolized too rapidly to provide an accurate index of catecholamine production. It has been suggested that samples of urine obtained after sleep and analyzed for norepinephrine excretion, expressed as f.Lg/hr, may provide accurate discrimination in detecting a pheochromocytoma.

The major limitations of using 24-hr free catecholamine levels to diagnose pheochromocytoma are the methodological problems associated with the assay, as well as the interference from physiological and chemical factors. Urinary catecholamines can increase with stress, as well as with the use of bronchodilators, sympathomimetic drugs, and in rare diseases such as certain posterior fossa tumors and acute intermittent porphyria. Despite these obvious limitations, several laboratories combine measurement of urinary total catecholamines [norepinephrine (NE) and epinephrine (E)] with metanephrines, normetanephrines, and VMA. When all three are completely normal, the diagnosis of pheochromocytoma can be excluded with 90% certainty. This is especially true when the urine collections have been performed during or shortly after a paroxysm. Fractionation of free catecholamines and measuring E and NE in the urine may reveal important diagnostic information. If the patient secretes predominantly E or secretes both E and NE, the tumor is likely to be in adrenals. The conversion of NE to E takes place only in the adrenal medulla (and perhaps to a smaller extent in the organ of Zuckerkandl) and requires the permissive effect of adrenocortical hormones. However, rarely E-secreting tumors have been reported in the bladder, and even in the lungs. In addition to providing insight into the possible site of the tumors, selective measurement of urinary E has been found to be extremely useful and sensitive in detection of the small-sized pheochromocytomas, particularly those associated with medullary thyroid carcinoma.

PLASMA CATECHOLAMINES

The two most important factors that determine the usefulness of this test are the method of collection (and handling) of the sample, as well as the expertise in performing the assay. The patient should be supine, and rested for at least 20 to 30 min, and should have blood drawn through an indwelling needle to avoid the stress of venipuncture. The blood should be collected in special tubes, on ice, and immediately centrifuged to separate the red blood cells (RBC). This is because the RBCs quickly and avidly consume the catecholamines. It has been emphasized that approximately half the amount of catecholamines disappear from the plasma within 20 min, if the RBC are present in the sample. In addition, a highly specialized laboratory is needed to perform and interpret catecholamine levels in the plasma.

The difficulties with methodology aside, elevation of plasma catecholamines can be encountered in several settings. Stress, hypoglycemia, acute myocardial infarction, and congestive failure are a few conditions where plasma catecholamines are elevated. More important, a small but significant number of patients with essential hypertension may show elevations in the supine resting plasma catecholamine concentrations. While as a group the levels in patients with essential hypertension may not overlap the levels seen in association with pheochromocytoma, in individual patients the differentiation can be difficult. It is in such a setting that the clonidine suppression test can be employed to differentiate patients with essential hypertension and high basal plasma catecholamine levels from those with pheochromocytoma.

Nevertheless, the measurement of basal plasma concentrations is exceedingly valuable during a paroxysm. Impressive elevations in plasma levels of catecholamines (ranging from 2000 to 20,000 *pg/mL)* can be seen in patients with hypertensive crisis caused by pheochromocytoma. The plasma catecholamine levels are also invaluable while studying the response to glucagon or clonidine administration.

DYNAMIC STUDIES

The advent of sophisticated methodology to measure catecholamines and their metabolites has led to near abandonment of several provocative tests used in the not-so-distant past. Of many tests, only the phentolamine test may still have a diagnostic role in patients who present in hypertensive crisis. The failure to lower the diastolic pressure in a patient presenting in hypertensive crisis excludes pheo-chromocytoma as a cause of the hypertension. The presence of a response, however, does not establish the diagnosis of pheo-chromocytoma, since a small number of patients with severe essential hypertension my respond to phentolamine. Even in the setting of a hypertensive crisis, measurement of plasma catecholamines and initiation of urine collection (even a 4-hr collection) for metanephrines, normetanephrines, VMA, and free catecholamines has more diagnostic value than the response to phentolamine. The two dynamic studies that still may have a role in the diagnosis of pheochromocytoma are the glucagon response study and the clonidine suppression test.

CLONIDINE SUPPRESSION TEST

The clonidine suppression test is based on the principle that oral administration of this drug, which is a centrally acting alpha-adrenergic agonist, suppresses the release of neurogenically mediated catecholamine output, but not the release of catecholamines from a pheochromocytoma.

Thus, it was anticipated that patients with essential hypertension and elevated plasma catecholamines could be distinguished from those with catecholamine excess from a pheochromocytoma by the plasma catecholamine response to oral administration of 0.3 mg of clonidine. Several important observations regarding the clonidine suppression test are observed. First, the blood pressure response to clonidine does not differentiate patients with pheo-chromocytoma from those with essential hypertension. This is owing to the inhibition of central sympathetic outflow by clonidine in both groups of patients. Second, in their experience, significant or symptomatic hypotension was not a commonly encountered adverse side effect from clonidine. Such a complication is more likely to occur in patients with pheochromocytoma in whom clonidine is administered in the presence of other antihypertensive drugs. In particular, patients with pheochromocytoma receiving beta blockers are more likely to develop hypotension with clonidine, which has potent vagotonic effects. It is advisable to avoid beta blockers and marked volume depletion for at least 48 hr prior to testing. Third, a false positive response, i.e., failure to suppress below 500 *pg/ml* in the absence of pheochromocytoma, is more likely to occur when radioimunoassays that measure both free and conjugated catecholamines are employed. It is believed that measurement of free catecholamines by radioenzymatic assays that employ catecholamine- o-methyltransferase are superior and preferred for the proper interpretation of the clonidine suppression test. False positive responses to the clonidine suppression test can be also encountered when propranolol and other beta blockers are used.

GLUCAGON PROVOCATIVE TEST

The administration of 1 mg of glucagon intravenously to patients harboring a pheochromocytoma leads to a prompt increase in the blood pressure, as well as in the circulating catecholamine levels. The test is considered positive if the pressor response to glucagon exceeded by *20/10* mm Hg the response caused by the nonspecific cold pressor stimulation. The sensitivity of the glucagon stimulation test improves when plasma catecholamines are measured before and after glucagon administration. The mechanisms that underlie the catecholamine release following glucagon in patients with pheochromocytoma are dual. Glucagon may directly enhance the release of catecholamines from the tumor, or alternatively the drug may cause vasodilatation with subsequent release of catecholamines from extratumor storage sites. Administration of glucagon to an already hypertensive patient with pheochromocytoma may potentially result in severe hypertension. Therefore, parenteral phentolamine must be readily available in case of this adverse effect of the test. The incidence of false negative responses to the glucagon stimulation test in patients with pheochromocytoma is probably quite low. When pheochromocytoma occurs as part of the spectrum of MEN II, the glucagon challenge test may be normal. The test is probably most useful when quiescent tumor is suspected and provocative maneuvers are called upon to diagnose its presence. In comparison to the histamine or tyramine stimulation tests, the glucagon provocative test provides far superior diagnostic yield.

LOCALIZATION

Localization of a pheochromocytoma can be as simple as a single-step procedure utilizing computed tomography (CT) of the adrenals (and the abdomen) or can involve the use of arteriography, venography, or venous effluent studies. The development of [131 I]meta-iodobenzylguanidine ([131 I]MIBG) scintigraphy has added a new and exciting dimension in the localization of pheochromocytoma.

COMPUTERIZED TOMOGRAPHY

Current experience suggests that a properly performed CT study of the adrenals and abdomen should virtually eliminate the need for invasive and potentially hazardous angiographic procedures. Several reports have repeatedly confirmed the high diagnostic yield by CT in locating the adrenal pheochromocytoma. The procedure accurately localizes tumors larger than 1 cm, with a precision of approximately 90-95%. The tumors that are most likely to be missed are those originating from the periaortic sympathetic chain and the organ of Zuckerkandl. If these areas are included in the scanning area, the likelihood of missing extraadrenal, intraabdominal pheochromocytomas would be minimized. Clearly, CT represents the first line of investigation for localization of pheochromocytoma. When the CT study provides no help, additional procedures such as arteriography or venous effluent studies may have to be performed.

[^{131}I]META-IODOBENZYL GUANIDINE SCAN

[^{131}I] MIBG is a radiopharmaceutical with a striking affinity for the adrenal medulla. This

analog of guanethedine resembles NE in its molecular structure and enters adrenergic tissues by a mechanism similar to the neurotransmitter. Thus, the radioisotope is concentrated in the catecholamine storage vesicles such as the adrenal medulla, or within adrenergic tumors such as pheochromocytoma or paraganglioma. The scintigraphic localization of pheochromocytoma is based on the principle that tissues that contain numerous adrenergic vesicles retain the radio nuclide for a protracted period of time, usually days. First, small tumors that are not visualized adequately by CT can be visualized by *[^{131}I]* MIBG; second, MIBG scintigraphy is probably unparalleled in its ability to detect extraadrenal and malignant pheochromocytomas; third, MIBG scintigraphy is uniquely applicable for anatomical localization of recurrent or residual disease; and finally, abnormal scintigraphy may provide a clue for the presence of medullary hyperplasia, a situation that is particularly likely to be encountered in familial pheochromocytomas, especially those in association with the spectrum of MEN II or MEN III.

The advantage of *[^{131}I]* MIBG scintigraphy is its ability to screen the whole body with remarkable specificity and precision for locating extraadrenal sites of the tumor, as well as metastatic lesions. The limitations of the procedure are the lack of widespread availability and the possibility of false positive results. While CT visualized nearly 95% of tumors, scintigraphy had the potential of false negative results in about 10% of patients. Superiority of scintigraphy in (1) detecting lesions that were negative by CT, (2) detecting recurrent pheochromocytoma, and (3) detecting malignant, less differentiated catecholamine-secreting tumors such as paragangliomas.

INVASIVE STUDIES

When both CT and scintigraphy have failed, and the hormonal evidence of pheochromocytoma is indisputable, invasive studies are indicated for localization of the tumor. Arteriography, combined with and guided by the stepup in NE concentrations in the venous effluents, can be diagnostic for localization. Blood samples from sequential points in the vena cava demonstrate an abrupt rise in NE concentrations, permitting identification of the anatomical site of tumor. Arteriography may also be helpful in identifying the presence of "cryptic" tumors. Patients with pheochromocytoma undergoing invasive studies should be adequately alpha-blocked to prevent the occurrence of a crisis.

TREATMENT

The treatment of the disease pheochromocytoma mainly includes surgical, after adequate preparation of the patient.

MEDICAL THERAPY

The preparation of the patient with pheochromocytoma consists of medical therapy with alpha-adrenergic blocking agents, the prototype of which is the alpha blocker phenoxybenzamine. The triple purposes that underlie such preparation are to control blood pressure, to prevent paroxysms, and to promote intravascular volume expansion.

PHENOXYBENZAMINE

Phenoxybenzamine is an noncompetitive adrenergic blocking agent. In contrast to phenotolamine, which has equal affinity for both αl and α2 receptors, phenoxybenzamine is 100 times more potent in blocking α1 than α2 receptors. The pharmacological importance of this property of phenoxybenzamine is readily apparent if one views the physiology of blocking both versus á1receptors alone: α1 receptors are postsynaptic, while α2 receptors are presynaptic.

Stimulation of α1 receptors leads to vasoconstriction and increase in peripheral resistance and in blood pressure. In contrast, the stimulation of α2 receptors (which serve the function of providing "feedback" regulation for NE release from the nerve) leads to inhibition of NE release from the nerve terminal with an attendant diminution in constriction of the vascular bed. Thus, if á1 receptors are blocked, the blood pressure declines, while with α2 blockade the blood pressure can rise owing to increased release of NE from the nerve terminal. When these phenomena are applied to a blocker therapy, important differences may rise in the actions exerted by phenotolamine and phenoxybenzamine. Phentolamine, because of its ability to block both α1 and α2 receptors to an equal degree, would result in dual effects-the α1 blockade leads to a drop in the blood pressure immediately; however, with progressive α2 blockade, more NE is released from the presynaptic terminal, leading to eventual displacement of phentolamine from the α1 terminal. The net result would be an eventual rise in the blood pressure and loss of alpha blocking effects of the drug. Phenoxybenzamine, on the other hand, has a much more potent blocking effect on the α1 receptors in comparison to the α2 receptors; as a result, there is negligible effect in causing. NE release from the nerve terminal. Thus, chronic therapy is less likely to result in loss of α1-blocking effect.

In addition to its predominant α1 -blocking effect, the advantages of phenoxybenzamine includes ease of administration (oral), few side effects, and a long half-life, which permits a twice-a-day regimen. The initial dose is 10 mg twice daily, with gradual increments to 20-40 mg twice (or even thrice) daily until the blood pressure is perfectly normalized. The track record of phenoxybenzamine for long-term control of pheochromocytic hypertension is excellent;

OTHER DRUGS

The role for other drugs in the medical management of pheochromocytoma is limited. Three, however, deserve comment-prazosin, beta blockers, and drugs that inhibit catecholamine synthesis.

Prazosin: Prazosin hydrochloride has been used in isolated cases of pheochromocytoma for effective control of blood pressure, either alone or in combination with beta blockers. Prazosin is a specific cell postsynaptic antagonist and has seemingly impressive advantages over pheoxybenzamine therapy. First, the hypotensive action of prazosin is not associated with an increase in the heart rate, in contrast to nonselective alpha-adrenergic antagonists. Second, the adverse effects of complete alpha blockade are seldom seen with chronic prazosin therapy. Third, patients with pheochromocytoma are quite sensitive to the drug and respond with minimum dosage of the drug, a factor that may promote compliance. Finally, in atleast one study long-term dosage requirements could be predicted based on the blood pressure response to a single1-mg oral dose. Despite these superficial advantages, prazosin has not been scrutinized in large numbers of patients with pheochromocytoma. Further, it has been noted that surgical management of the tumor, i.e., intra- and perioperative management, was less than optimal with prazosin alone, requiring the use of intravenous phentolamine to suppress the pressor surges during manipulation.

Beta Blockers: Treatment with propranolol is indicated only in the presence of persistent tachycardia, angina, or hazardous arrythmias. Propranolol should never be administered alone, owing to the unopposed alpha effects, which may result in severe hypertension. Even in the presence of alpha-blocker therapy, use of propranolol can elevate the blood pressure in patients with pheochromocytoma. If beta-blocker therapy is deemed necessary, it should be initiated cautiously by starting at a low dose (10 mg orally twice a day), with gradual increments of 10 mg every day or 2 until the tachycardia or arrythmia is brought under control. Labetalol, a drug that has both alpha- and beta-adrenergic blocking properties, has been effectively used in some patients with pheochromocytoma.

Drugs That Inhibit Catecholamine Synthesis: The drug alpha-methyl paratyrosine (metyrosine) blocks the synthesis of norepinephrine by inhibiting the enzyme tyrosine hydroxylase. In a dosage of 2-2.5 g/day, metyrosine therapy can result in acceptable reductions in catecholamine synthesis. The effectiveness of the drug can be monitored by following the reduction in the excretion of catecholamine metabolites in the urine. Treatment with metyrosine is often initiated with 250 mg, twice daily, and gradually increased to 2 g/day. The drug is relatively long-acting, and therefore, dosage increments should be made slowly, with the guide of urinary metabolite excretion. The side effects of metyrosine include drowsiness, diarrhea, and crystalluria. The latter can be minimized by liberalizing fluid intake. The majority of patients can be kept relatively asymptomatic with the use of metyrosine.

Other drugs that inhibit catecholamine synthesis are currently under investigation. One such drug, fusaric acid (a dopamine hydroxylase inhibitor), has been found to be useful by some investigators. Finally, there is at least one report of pheochromocytoma associated with a profound decline in urinary NE levels following calcium channel blockade. Medical therapy with adrenergic blockade and or me tyrosine is the mainstay of therapy for surgical preparation of the patient with pheochromocytoma. While there is no controversy as to the need for adrenergic blockade prior to surgical exploration of the tumor, some controversy exists as to the time frame of discontinuing adrenergic blockade before the surgery. There are two schools of thought in this regard. One subscribes to continuation of adrenergic blockade up to the time of surgery. The arguments in favor of this opinion include prevention of catecholamine surges during the operation, reversal of hypovolemia, promotion of smooth anesthetic induction, and prevention of severe postoperative manifestations of hyper-catecholism. The other school of thought argues against continuation of alpha blockade up to the time of surgery based on the fact that complete alpha blockade removes the surgical advantage of locating the tumor by observing blood pressure responses to manipulation. The controversy remains unsettled, with individual preferences prevailing. One approach is to continue metyrosine until the day of surgery in the partially alpha-blocked patient, especially if tumor location is uncertain or if multiple tumors are anticipated.

SURGICAL TREATMENT

Surgical excision of the tumor provides the best and possibly the only cure for unilateral benign pheochromocytoma. The mortality and morbidity from surgery, in experienced hands, is acceptably low, particularly when preoperative preparation is excellent. The incision usually employed is an anterior, transperitoneal approach that permits adequate exposure of both adrenal glands, the urinary bladder, and the entire paraaortic sympathetic chain. When one tumor is found, all areas of sympathetic tissue must be carefully examined to exclude the presence of a second tumor. Greater scrutiny is required in the familial pheochromocytomas. Should a hypertensive crisis occur during the period of anesthesia or tumor manipulation, this should be treated with IV sodium nitroprusside or phenotolamine or Cardiac arrythmias may be treated by the use of lidocaine. Postoperative hypotension can complicate the course of the patient recovering from surgery. Volume expansion, normalization of the blood pressure, and liberal replacement of blood lost during surgery would minimize the frequency and severity of the postoperative hypotension. Postoperative hypotension is best managed by vigorous fluid expansion rather than by pressor agents, since considerable difficulty exists in withdrawal of these agents. The success rate of surgical excision of pheochromocytoma is excellent, approaching 95%. Failure to restore the normal blood pressure by surgical excision indicates the presence of a second (or multiple) tumor(s) missed during exploration or the concomitant presence of nephrosclerosis as result of the chronic hypertensive process. Rarely the persistence of hypertension following surgery may be the clue to the presence of malignant pheochromocytoma with metastases.

REFERENCES

1. van Heerden JA, Sheps SG, Hamberger B, et al. Pheochromocytoma: Current status and changing trends. *Surgery* 91:367, 1979.
2. Manger WM, Gifford RW Jr: *Pheochromocytoma.* Springer-Verlag, New York, 1977.
3. Sheps SG: Pheochromocytoma. In SpittellJAJr (ed): *Clinical Medicine,* vol. 7. Harper & Row, Philadelphia, 1981, pp. 1-22.
4. Jones DH, Reid JL, Hamilton CA, et al. The biochemical diagnosis, localization and follow up of phaeochromocytoma: The role of plasma and urinary catecholamine measurements. *QJ Med* 49:341, 1980.
5. Remine WH, Chong GC, van Heerden JA, et al. Current management of pheochromocytoma. *Ann Surg* 182:740, 1974.
6. Sjoerdsma A: Sympatho-adrenal system: Pheochromocytoma. In Beeson PB, McDermott W(eds): *Cecil Loeb Textbook of Medicine.* 13th ed. Saunders, Philadelphia, 1971, pp. 1832-1836.
7. Bravo EL, Gifford RW Jr: Phaeochromocytoma: Diagnosis, localization and management. *N Engl] Med* 311:1298, 1984
8. SissonJC, Frager MS, Valk TW, et al: Scintigraphic localization of pheochromocytoma. *N Engl] Med* 305:12, 1981.

CHAPTER 80

Menstrual Cycle Disorders

INTRODUCTION

There are a number of different menstrual disorders. Problems can range from heavy, painful periods to no period at all. There are many variations in menstrual patterns, but in general women should be concerned when periods come fewer than 21 days or more than 3 months apart, or if they last more than 10 days. Such events may indicate ovulation problems or other medical conditions.

DYSMENORRHEA (PAINFUL CRAMPS)

Dysmenorrhea is severe, frequent cramping during menstruation. Pain occurs in the lower abdomen but can spread to the lower back and thighs. Dysmenorrhea is usually referred to as primary or secondary.

PRIMARY DYSMENORRHEA

Cramps occur from contractions in the uterus. These contractions are a normal part of the menstrual process. With primary dysmenorrhea, cramping pain is directly related to and caused by menstruation. About half of menstruating women have primary dysmenorrhea. It usually begins 2 - 3 years after a woman begins to menstruate. The pain typically develops when the bleeding starts and continues for 32 - 48 hours. Cramps are generally most severe during heavy bleeding.

SECONDARY DYSMENORRHEA

Secondary dysmenorrhea is menstrual-related pain that accompanies another medical or physical condition, such as endometriosis or uterine fibroids.

HEAVY BLEEDING

During a normal menstrual cycle, the average woman loses about 1 ounce (30 mL) of blood. Most women change their tampons or pads around 3 - 6 times per day. Menorrhagia is the medical term for significantly heavier bleeding. Menorrhagia can be caused by a number of factors.

Women often overestimate the amount of blood lost during their periods. Clot formation is fairly common during heavy bleeding and is not a cause for concern. However, women should consult their doctor if any of the following occurs:

- Soaking through at least one pad or tampon every 1-2 hours for several hours
- Heavy periods that regularly last 10 or more days
- Bleeding between periods or during pregnancy. Spotting or light bleeding

between periods is common in girls just starting menstruation and sometimes during ovulation in young adult women, but it is still a good idea to speak with a doctor.

Several terms are often used to describe different patterns of heavy bleeding:

- ***Menorrhagia*** refers to long (greater than 7 days) or excessive (more than 80 mL) bleeding that occurs at regular intervals
- ***Metrorrhagia*** refers to bleeding which occurs at frequent but irregular intervals, and with variable amounts
- ***Menometrorrhagia*** refers to prolonged episodes of bleeding that occur at irregular intervals.

AMENORRHEA (ABSENCE OF MENSTRUATION)

Amenorrhea is the absence of menstruation. There are two categories: **primary amenorrhea and secondary amenorrhea**. These terms refer to the time when menstruation stops:

- Primary amenorrhea occurs when a girl does not begin to menstruate by age 16. Girls who show no signs of sexual development (breast development and pubic hair) by age 13 should be evaluated by a doctor. Any girl who does not have her period by age 15 should be evaluated for primary amenorrhea.
- Secondary amenorrhea occurs when periods that were previously regular stop for at least three months.

OLIGOMENORRHEA (LIGHT OR INFREQUENT MENSTRUATION)

Oligomenorrhea is a condition in which menstrual cycles are infrequent, greater than 35 days apart. It is very common in early adolescence and does not usually indicate a medical problem.

When girls first menstruate they often do not have regular cycles for a couple of years. Even healthy cycles in adult women can vary by a few days from month to month. Periods may occur every 3 weeks in some women, and every 5 weeks in others. Flow also varies and can be heavy or light. Skipping a period and then having a heavy flow may occur; this is most likely due to missed ovulation rather than a miscarriage.

PREMENSTRUAL SYNDROME (PMS)

Premenstrual syndrome (PMS) is a set of physical, emotional, and behavioral symptoms that occur during the last week of the luteal phase (a week before menstruation) in most cycles. The symptoms typically do not start until at least day 13 in the cycle, and resolve within 4 days after bleeding begins. Women may begin to have premenstrual syndrome symptoms at any time during their reproductive years. Once established, the symptoms tend to remain fairly constant until menopause, although they can vary from cycle to cycle.

CAUSES

Many different factors can trigger menstrual disorders, such as hormone imbalances, genetic factors, clotting disorders, and pelvic diseases.

DYSMENORRHEA

- ***Contraction-Causing Chemicals:*** Powerful chemicals known as *prostaglandins* and *arachidonic acid* can induce uterine muscle contractions. Prostaglandins also play a large role in the heavy bleeding that causes dysmenorrhea.

- ***Abnormal Nervous System Response:*** Some women with primary dysmenorrhea may have autonomic nervous systems that are overly sensitive to menstrual cycle changes. The autonomic nervous system regulates heart rate and blood pressure, and it contains the pain receptors in nerve fibers in the uterus and pelvic area. As a result, women with autonomic nervous system abnormalities may have a more intense response to pain.
- ***Abnormalities in the Arteries in the Uterus:*** Impaired blood flow through the arteries in the uterus may cause severe dysmenorrhea for some women.
- ***Genetic Factors:*** Genetic factors may play a role in primary dysmenorrhea cases.
- ***Endometriosis:*** Endometriosis is a chronic and often progressive disease that develops when the tissue that lines the uterus (endometrium) grows onto other areas, such as the ovaries, bowels, or bladder (Fig. 80.1).

  Endometriosis is the condition in which the tissue that normally lines the uterus (endometrium) grows on other areas of the body, causing pain and irregular bleeding.
- ***Uterine Fibroids:*** Fibroids are noncancerous growths that grow on the walls of the uterus. They can cause heavy bleeding during menstruation and cramping pain.
- ***Other Causes*:** Pelvic inflammatory disease, ovarian cysts, and ectopic pregnancy. The intrauterine device (IUD) contraceptive can also cause dysmenorrhea.

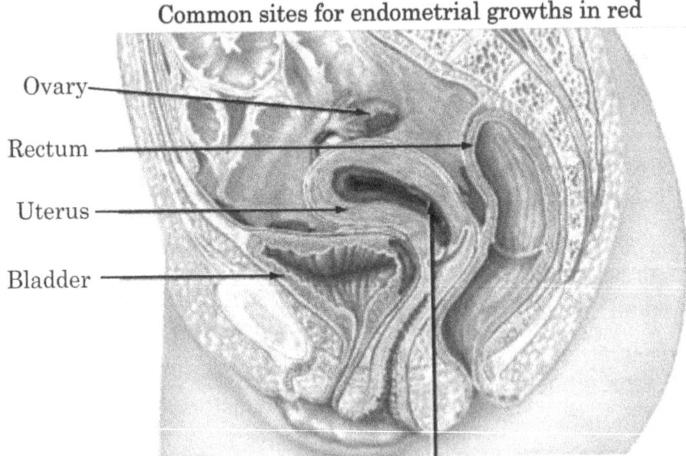

FIGURE 80.1

Common sites for endometrial growths
(Source: http://www.nytimes.com/health/guides/disease/endometriosis/print.html)

ABNORMAL UTERINE BLEEDING

Abnormal uterine bleeding may occur as infrequent episodes, excessive flow, prolonged duration of menses, or bleeding between menses.

Examples of abnormal bleeding include:

- Bleeding or spotting between periods
- Bleeding after sex
- Bleeding heavier or for more days than normal
- Bleeding after menopause

DYSFUNCTIONAL UTERINE BLEEDING (DUB)

DUB is a general term for abnormal uterine bleeding that usually refers to extra or excessive bleeding caused by hormonal problems. DUB usually occurs either when girls begin to menstruate or when women approach menopause, but it can occur at any time during a woman's reproductive life.

About 90% of DUB events happen when ovulation is not occurring (anovulatory DUB). In such cases, women do not properly develop and release a mature egg. As a result, estrogen is produced continuously, causing an overgrowth of the uterus lining. The period is delayed in such cases, and when it occurs menstruation can be very heavy and prolonged.

The other 10% of DUB cases occur in women who are ovulating (ovulatory DUB), but progesterone secretion is prolonged because estrogen levels are low. This causes irregular shedding of the uterine lining and break-through bleeding.

Other Causes of Abnormal Uterine Bleeding: Abnormal uterine bleeding may also be related to other causes unrelated to the natural cycle or ovulation:

- ***Uterine Fibroids.***
- ***Von Willebrand Disease and Other Bleeding Disorders:*** Bleeding disorders that stop blood from clotting can cause heavy menstrual bleeding. Most of these disorders have a genetic basis. Von Willebrand disease is the most common of these bleeding disorders and may be under diagnosed in many women with unexplained menorrhagia.
- ***Abnormalities in the Uterus:*** Structural problems or other abnormalities in the uterus may cause bleeding. They include uterine polyps (small benign growths in the uterus), uterine fibroids (Fig. 80.2), endometriosis, adenomyosis, and miscarriage. Infections or inflammation in the vagina or pelvic area can also cause heavy bleeding.
- ***Medications and Contraceptives:*** Certain drugs, including anticoagulants and anti-inflammatory medications, can cause heavy bleeding. Problems linked to some birth control methods, such as birth control pills or intrauterine devices (IUDs) can cause bleeding.
- ***Cancer:*** Rarely, uterine, ovarian, and cervical cancer can cause excessive bleeding
- ***Infection:*** Infection of the uterus or cervix can cause bleeding.
- ***Pregnancy or Miscarriage.***

Other Medical Conditions: Systemic lupus erythematosus, diabetes, pelvic inflammatory disorder, cirrhosis, and thyroid disorders can cause heavy bleeding. Women who have migraine headaches may be more likely to have menorrhagia and endometriosis.

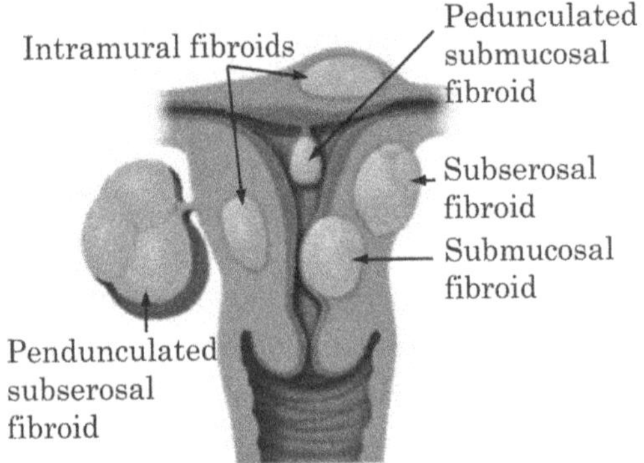

FIGURE 80.2

Fibroid tumors.
(source : http://www.gynaecologistauckland.co.nz/womens-health/what-are-fibroid-tumors/)

Fibroid tumors may not need to be removed if they are not causing pain, bleeding excessively, or growing rapidly.

AMENORRHEA AND OLIGOMENORRHEA

Normal causes of skipped or irregular periods include pregnancy, breast-feeding, hormonal contraception, and perimenopause. Skipped periods are also common during adolescence, when it may take a while before ovulation occurs regularly. Consistently absent periods may be due to the following factors:

- ***Delayed Puberty:*** A common cause of primary amenorrhea is delayed puberty due to some genetic factor that delays physical development. Failure of ovarian development is the most common cause of primary amenorrhea.
- ***Hormonal Changes and Puberty:*** Oligomenorrhea is a frequent complaint during puberty who are just beginning to have their periods
- ***Weight Loss and Eating Disorders:*** Another common cause of amenorrhea in adolescent girls is eating disorders. Extreme weight loss and reduced fat stores lead to hormonal changes that include low thyroid levels (hypothyroidism) and elevated stress hormone levels (hypercortisolism). These changes produce a reduction in reproductive hormones. A syndrome known as the female athlete triad is associated with hormonal changes that occur with the combination of eating disorders, amenorrhea, and osteopenia (loss of bone density that can lead to osteoporosis) in young women who excessively exercise.
- ***Polycystic Ovarian Syndrome (PCOS):*** PCOS is a condition in which the ovaries produce high amounts of androgens (male hormones), particularly testosterone. PCOS occurs in about 10% of women of childbearing age, and amenorrhea or oligomenorrhea (infrequent menses) is quite common (Fig. 80.3).
- ***Elevated Prolactin Levels (Hyperprolactinemia):*** Prolactin is a hormone produced in the pituitary gland that stimulates breast development and milk production in association with pregnancy. High levels of prolactin (hyperprolactinemia) in women who are not pregnant or nursing can reduce gonadotropin hormones and inhibit ovulation, thus causing amenorrhea.
- ***Premature Ovarian Failure (POF):*** POF is the early depletion of follicles before age 40. In most cases, it leads to premature menopause. POF is a significant cause of infertility.
- ***Structural Problems:*** In some cases, structural problems or scarring in the uterus may prevent menstrual flow. Inborn

genital tract abnormalities may also cause primary amenorrhea.

- *Stress*. Physical and emotional stress may block the release of luteinizing hormone, causing temporary amenorrhea.
- ***Athletic Training***. Amenorrhea or oligomenorrhea associated with vigorous activity is related to stress and not weight loss. Female athletes who use anabolic steroids will often have amenorrhea or oligomenorrhea.

Other Medical Conditions. Epilepsy, thyroid problems,metabolic syndrome, and Cushing's disease are associated with amenorrhea.

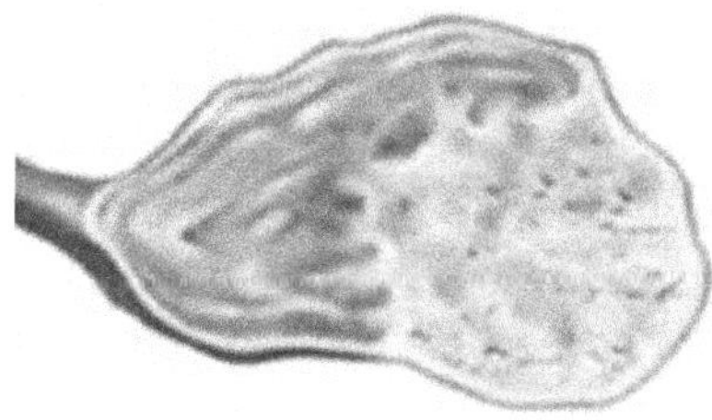

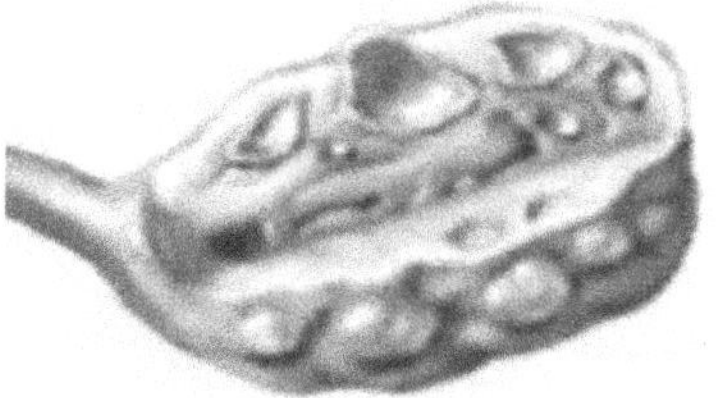

FIGURE 80.3

Ovarian tumor and polycystic ovary.

(Source : https://hubpages.com/health/PCOS-and-tips-on-dealing-with-it)

If the ovaries produce too much androgen (hormones such as testosterone) a woman may develop male characteristics. This ovarian imbalance can be caused by tumors in the ovaries or adrenal glands, or polycystic ovarian disease. Virilization may include growth of excess body and facial hair, amenorrhea (loss of menstrual period) and changes in body contour.

RISK FACTORS

Age plays a key role in menstrual disorders. Girls who start menstruating at age 11 or younger are at higher risk for severe pain, longer periods, and longer menstrual cycles. Between 20 - 90% of teenage girls report menstrual pain, and about 15% report that it is severe. Adolescents may develop amenorrhea before their ovulating cycles become regular.

Women who are approaching menopause (perimenopause) may also skip periods. Occasional episodes of heavy bleeding are also common as women approach menopause.

Other risk factors include:

- ***Weight***: Being either excessively overweight or underweight can increase the risk for dysmenorrhea and amenorrhea.
- ***Smoking and Alcohol Use***: Smokers have a 50% higher risk than nonsmokers for menstrual pain. Alcohol does not cause menstrual pain, but in women with dysmenorrhea, alcohol consumption may prolong the pain.
- ***Stress***: Physical and emotional stress may block the release of luteinizing hormone, causing temporary amenorrhea. Emotional problems, including history of sexual abuse, may predispose to dysmenorrhea.
- ***Menstrual Cycles and Flow***: Longer and heavier menstrual cycles can cause dysmenorrhea.

- ***Pregnancy History*:** Women who have had a higher number of pregnancies are at increased risk for menorrhagia. Women who have never given have a higher risk of dysmenorrhea, while women who first gave birth at a young age are at lower risk.
- ***Chronic Pelvic Pain*:** Many women feel chronic pain in the pelvic area. This pain can be due to gynecologic reasons (such as fibroids, endometriosis, or pelvic inflammatory disease) or non-gynecologic causes (such as irritable bowel syndrome, interstitial cystitis, or diverticulitis).

Exercise and oral contraceptive use may help protect against dysmenorrhea.

POSSIBLE COMPLICATIONS

ANEMIA

Menorrhagia is the most common cause of anemia (reduction in red blood cells) in premenopausal women. A blood loss of more than 80mL (around three tablespoons) per menstrual cycle can eventually lead to anemia. Most cases of anemia are mild. Nevertheless, even mild anemia can reduce oxygen transport in the blood, causing fatigue and a diminished physical capacity. Moderate-to-severe anemia can cause shortness of breath, rapid heart rate, lightheadedness, headaches, ringing in the ears (tinnitus), irritability, pale skin, restless legs syndrome, and mental confusion. Heart problems can occur in prolonged and severe anemia that is not treated.

OSTEOPOROSIS (FIG. 80.4)

Amenorrhea caused by reduced estrogen levels increases the risk for osteopenia (loss of bone density) and osteoporosis (more severe bone loss that increases fracture risk). Conditions that are associated with low estrogen levels include eating disorders, pituitary tumors, and premature ovarian failure. Because bone growth is at its peak in adolescence and young adulthood, losing bone density at that time is very dangerous, and early diagnosis and treatment is essential for long-term health.

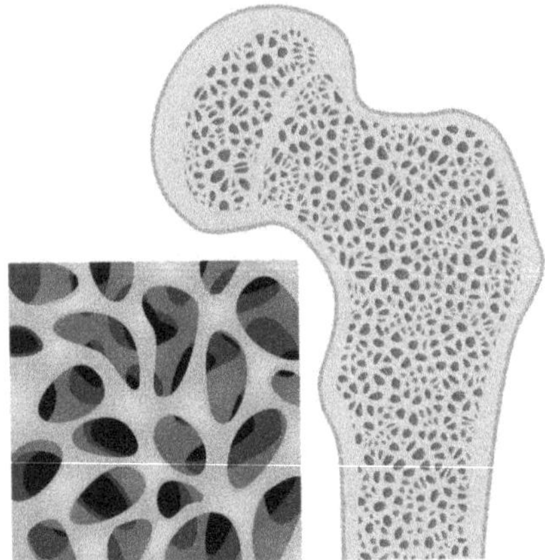
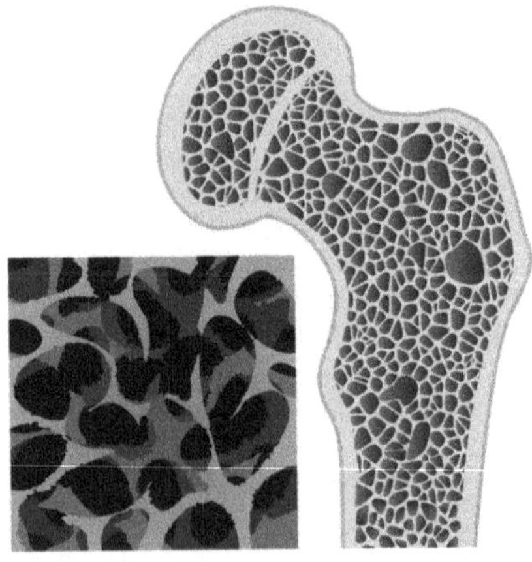

FIGURE 80.4

Bone osteoporosis.
(source : http://rehabilitaciontacna.com/osteoporosis-y-osteopenia/)

Osteoporosis is a condition characterized by progressive loss of bone density, thinning of bone tissue, and increased vulnerability to fractures. Osteoporosis may result from disease, dietary or hormonal deficiency, or advanced age. Regular exercise and vitamin and mineral supplements can reduce and even reverse loss of bone density.

INFERTILITY

Some conditions associated with heavy bleeding, such as ovulation abnormalities, fibroids, or endometriosis, are important contributors to infertility. Many conditions that cause amenorrhea, such as ovulation abnormalities and polycystic ovary syndrome, can also cause infertility. Irregular periods from any cause may make it more difficult to conceive. Sometimes treating the underlying condition can restore fertility. In other cases, specific fertility treatments that use assisted reproductive technologies may be beneficial.

QUALITY OF LIFE

Menstrual disorders, particularly pain and heavy bleeding, can affect school and work productivity and social activities.

DIAGNOSIS

The doctor will ask for the patient's complete medical history. This information can help determine whether a menstrual problem is caused by another medical condition. For example, non-menstrual conditions that may cause abdominal pain include appendicitis, urinary tract infections, ectopic pregnancy, and irritable bowel syndrome. Endometriosis and fibroids may cause heavy bleeding and pain. Doctors may ask questions concerning:

- Menstrual cycle patterns — length of time between periods, number of days that periods last, number of days of heavy or light bleeding
- The presence or history of any medical conditions that might be causing menstrual problems
- Any family history of menstrual problems
- History of pelvic pain
- Regular use of any medications (including vitamins and over-the-counter drugs)
- Diet history, including caffeine and alcohol intake
- Past or present contraceptive use
- Any recent stressful events
- Sexual history

Menstrual Diary: A menstrual diary is a helpful way to keep track of changes in menstrual cycles. Patients can record when their period starts, how long it lasts, and the amount of bleeding and pain that occurs during the course of menstruation.

Pelvic Examination: A pelvic exam is a standard part of diagnosis. A Pap test may be done during this exam.

BLOOD AND HORMONAL TESTS

Blood tests can help rule out other conditions that cause menstrual disorders. For example, a doctor may test thyroid function to make sure that low thyroid (hypothyroidism) is not present. Blood tests can also check follicle-stimulating hormone, estrogen, and prolactin levels. Patients who have menorrhagia may get tests for bleeding disorders. If patients are losing a lot of blood, they should also get tested for anemia.

Patients who have amenorrhea may need to receive special hormonal tests. The progestational challenge test uses oral or injected progesterone to test for a functional uterine lining (endometrium):

- Bleeding that occurs up to 3 weeks after the progesterone dose suggests that the woman has normal estrogen levels but is not ovulating, particularly if thyroid and prolactin levels are normal. In such cases, the doctor will check for stress, recent weight loss, and any medications. Such results could also suggest polycystic ovaries or stress.
- A failure to bleed could indicate an abnormal uterus that prevents outflow or insufficient estrogen. In such cases, the next step may be to administer estrogen followed by progestin. If bleeding occurs after that, the cause of amenorrhea is related to low estrogen levels. The doctor will then check for ovarian failure, anorexia, or other causes of low estrogen. If bleeding does not occur, the doctor would check for obstructions that are preventing outflow of menstruation.

ULTRASOUND

Imaging techniques are often used to detect certain conditions that may be causing menstrual disorders. Imaging can help diagnose fibroids, endometriosis, or structural abnormalities of the reproductive organs.

Ultrasound and Sono-hysterography: Ultrasound is the standard imaging technique for evaluating the uterus and ovaries, detecting fibroids, ovarian cysts and tumors, and finding obstructions in the urinary tract. It uses sound waves to produce an image of the organs. Ultrasound carries no risk and causes very little discomfort.

Transvaginal sonohysterography uses ultrasound along with saline injected into the uterus to enhance the visualization of the uterus.

OTHER DIAGNOSTIC PROCEDURES

Hysteroscopy: Hysteroscopy is a procedure that can detect the presence of fibroids, polyps, or other causes of bleeding. It may miss cases of uterine cancer, however, and is not a substitute for more invasive procedures, such as dilation and curettage (D&C) or endometrial biopsy, if cancer is suspected.

It is done in the office setting and requires no incisions. The procedure uses a long flexible or rigid tube called a *hysteroscope*, which is inserted into the vagina and through the cervix to reach the uterus. A fiber optic light source and a tiny camera in the tube allow the doctor to view the cavity. The uterus is filled with saline or carbon dioxide to inflate the cavity and provide better viewing. This can cause cramping.

Hysteroscopy is non-invasive, but many women find the procedure painful. The use of an anesthetic spray such as lidocaine may help in preventing pain from this procedure. Other complications include excessive fluid absorption, infection, and uterine perforation. Hysteroscopy is also performed as part of surgical procedures.

Laparoscopy: Diagnostic laparoscopy, an invasive surgical procedure, is currently the only definitive method for diagnosing endometriosis, a common cause of dysmenorrhea. It may also be used to treat endometriosis. Laparoscopy normally requires a general anesthetic, although the patient can go home the same day. The procedure involves inflating the abdomen with gas through a small abdominal incision. A fiber optic tube equipped with small camera lenses (the laparoscope) is then inserted. The doctor uses the laparoscope to view the uterus, ovaries, tubes, and peritoneum (lining of the pelvis).

Endometrial Biopsy: When heavy or abnormal bleeding occurs, an endometrial (uterine) biopsy can be performed in the office. This procedure can help identify abnormal cells, which suggest that cancer may be present. It may also help the doctor decide on the best hormonal treatment to use. This procedure may often be done without anesthesia, or local anesthetic is injected.

- The patient lies on her back with her feet in stirrups. An instrument (speculum) is inserted into the vagina to hold it open and allow the cervix to be viewed.
- The cervix is cleaned with an antiseptic liquid and then grasped with an instrument (tenaculum) that holds the uterus steady. A device called a cervical dilator may be needed to stretch the cervical canal if there is tightness (stenosis). A small, hollow plastic tube is then gently passed into the uterine cavity.
- Gentle suction removes a sample of the lining. The tissue sample and instruments are removed. A specialist called a pathologist examines the sample under a microscope.

Dilation and Curettage (D&C): Dilation and curettage (D&C) is a more invasive procedure:

- A D&C is usually done in an outpatient setting so that the patient can return home the same day, but it sometimes requires a general anesthetic. It may need to be performed in the operating room to rule out serious conditions or treat some minor ones that may be causing the bleeding.
- The cervix (the neck of the uterus) is dilated (opened).
- The surgeon scrapes the inside lining of the uterus and cervix.

The procedure is used to take samples of the tissue and to relieve heavy bleeding in some instances. D&C can also be effective in scraping off small endometrial polyps, but it is not very useful for most fibroids, which tend to be larger and more firmly attached.

LIFESTYLE CHANGES

DIETARY FACTORS

Making dietary adjustments starting about 14 days before a period may help some women with certain mild menstrual disorders, such as cramping. The general guidelines for a healthy diet apply to everyone; they include eating plenty of whole grains, fresh fruits and vegetables, and avoiding saturated fats and commercial junk foods.

Limiting salt may help bloating. Reducing caffeine, sugar, and alcohol intake may also be beneficial.

PREVENTING AND TREATING ANEMIA

Dietary Forms of Iron: Women who have heavy menstrual bleeding can sometimes become anemic. Eating iron-rich foods can help prevent anemia. Iron found in foods is either in the form of heme or non-heme iron. Heme iron is better absorbed than non-heme iron.

- Foods containing heme iron are the best for increasing or maintaining healthy iron levels. Such foods include (in order of iron-richness) clams, oysters, organ meats, beef, pork, poultry, and fish.
- Non-heme iron is less well absorbed. About 60% of iron in meat in non-heme (although meat itself helps absorb non-heme iron). Eggs, dairy products, and iron-containing vegetables have only the non-heme form. Such vegetable products include dried beans and peas, iron-fortified cereals, bread, and pasta products, dark green leafy vegetables (chard, spinach, mustard greens, kale), dried fruits, nuts, and seeds.

Increasing intake of vitamin C rich foods can enhance absorption of non-heme iron.

Iron Supplements: There are two forms of supplemental iron: ferrous and ferric. Ferrous iron is better absorbed and is the preferred form of iron tablets. Ferrous iron is available in three forms: ferrous fumarate, ferrous sulfate, and ferrous gluconate. Depending on the severity of the anemia, as well as your age and weight, the doctor will recommend a dosage of 60 - 200 mg of elemental iron per day. This means taking one iron pill 2 - 3 times each day.

OTHER LIFESTYLE MEASURES

Exercise: Exercise may help reduce menstrual pain .

Sexual Activity: There have been reports that orgasm reduces the severity of menstrual cramps.

Applying Heat: Applying a heating pad to the abdominal area, or soaking in a hot bath, can help relieve the pain of menstrual cramps.

Menstrual Hygiene: Change tampons every 4 - 6 hours. Avoid scented pads and tampons; feminine deodorants can irritate the genital area. Women should not douche during or between periods. Women who douche on a weekly basis are more likely to contract cervical cancer than those who do not. Douching may destroy the natural bacteria normally present in the vagina. Bathing regularly is sufficient. than those who do not.

ALTERNATIVE REMEDIES

Acupuncture and Acupressure: Some studies have reported relief from pelvic pain after acupuncture or acupressure, a technique that applies small pins or pressure to specific points on the body.

Yoga and Meditative Techniques: Yoga and meditative techniques that promote relaxation may help relieve menstrual cramps.

Herbs and Supplements: Generally, manufacturers of herbal remedies and dietary supplements do not need approval from the Food and Drug Administration to sell their products. Just like with drugs, herbs and supplements can affect the body's chemistry, and therefore have the potential to produce side effects that may be harmful. There have been a number of reported cases of serious and even lethal side effects from herbal products. Patients should check with their doctor before using any herbal remedies or dietary supplements.

Studies have not generally found herbal or natural remedies to be any more effective than placebos for reducing menstrual disorders. Natural remedies promoted for menstrual symptoms include:

- Black cohosh (also known as *Cimicifuga racemosa* or squawroot) contains a plant estrogen and is the most studied herbal remedy for treating menopausal symptoms, including dysmenorrhea, although most studies have indicated it is ineffective. Headaches and gastro-intestinal problems are common side effects. At this time, doctors do not recommend taking it for more than 6 months.
- Ginger tea or capsules may help to relieve nausea and bloating.
- Aromatherapy with topically-applied lavender, sage, and rose oils may help ease menstrual cramps, according to some small studies.
- Pycnogenol, an extract from the bark of the French maritime pine tree, may help reduce menstrual pain and discomfort, according to some small studies.

MEDICATIONS

There are a number of different medicines prescribed for menstrual disorders.

COMMON PAIN RELIEVERS FOR CRAMPS

Nonsteroidal Anti-inflammatory Drugs (NSAIDs). Nonsteroidal anti-inflammatory drugs (NSAIDs) block prostaglandins, the substances that increase uterine contractions. They are effective painkillers that also help control the inflammatory factors that may be responsible for heavy menstrual bleeding. Aspirin is the most common NSAID, but there are dozens of others available over the counter or by prescription.

Among the most effective NSAIDs for menstrual disorders are ibuprofen (such as Advil, Motrin, and Midol PMS), naproxen (such as Aleve), and mefenamic acid (Ponstel). Long-term daily use of any NSAID can increase the risk for GI bleeding and ulcers, as well as heart attack and stroke (Fig. 80.5).

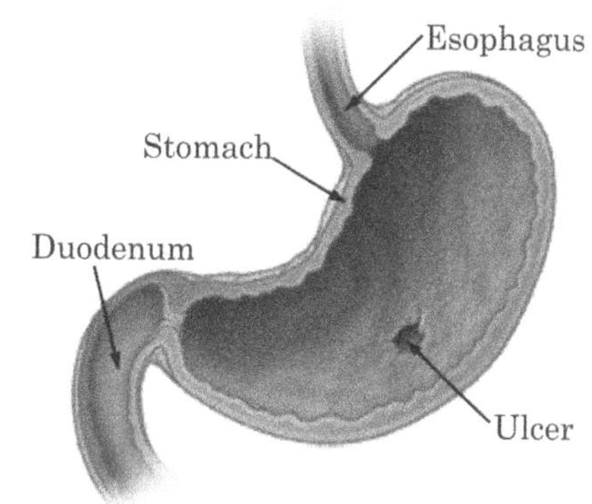

FIGURE 80.5

Stomach ulcers.

(source : http://www.fairview.org/healthlibrary/Article/116655EN)

An ulcer is a crater-like lesion on the skin or mucous membrane caused by an inflammatory, infectious, or malignant condition. To avoid irritating an ulcer a person can try eliminating certain substances from their diet such as caffeine, alcohol, aspirin, and avoid smoking. Patients can take certain medicines to suppress the acid in the stomach causing the erosion of the stomach lining. Endoscopic therapy can be used to stop bleeding from the ulcer.

Acetaminophen: Acetaminophen (Tylenol) is a good alternative to NSAIDs, especially when stomach problems, ulcers, or allergic reactions prohibit their use. Some products (Pamprin, Premsyn) combine acetaminophen with other drugs, such as a diuretic, to reduce bloating. Little evidence exists to indicate whether they are more or less effective than NSAIDs or other mild pain relievers.

ORAL CONTRACEPTIVES

Oral contraceptives (OCs), commonly called "the Pill" collectively, contain combinations of an estrogen and a progestin (either natural progesterone or the synthetic form called progestogen). The estrogen compound used in most combination OCs is estradiol. There are many different progestins, but common types include **Levonorgestrol, Dros-pirenone, Norgestrol, Nore-thindrone, and Desogestrel**. (Combination contra-ceptives are also available in other forms, including patches and vaginal rings, but they may increase the risk for menstrual cramping and bleeding.)

OCs are often used to regulate periods in women with menstrual disorders, including menorrhagia (heavy bleeding), dysme-norrhea (severe pain), and amenorrhea (absence of periods). Oral contraceptives are as effective for treating pain from endometriosis as the more potent gonadotropin releasing hormone agonists. They also protect against ovarian and endometrial cancers.

High-dose OCs has been specifically helpful for adolescents with severe dysmenorrhea. Studies with low-dose OCs have also shown they can reduce menstrual pain for adolescents and adults.

OCs may be taken in cycles that include pills of the same or different strengths. These are categorized as monophasic (one-phase), biphasic (two-phase), or triphasic (three-phase). Monophasic pills contain the same amount of hormones in each dose. Biphasic and triphasic pills contain different dosages of hormones with the pill packs. The monophasic regimen is the most studied regimen and is usually recommended for dysmenorrhea as well as premenstrual symptoms.

***Continuous-Dosing OCs*:** Standard OCs usually come in a 28-pill pack with 21 days of "active" (hormone) pills and 7 days of "inactive" (placebo) pills. Newer "continuous-dosing" (also called "continuous-use") oral contraceptives aim to reduce — or even eliminate — monthly menstrual periods. These OCs contain a combination of estradiol and the progesterone levonorgestrel, but they use extending dosing of active pills.

Continues-dosing oral contraceptives include:

- Seasonale, with an average period every 3 months
- Seasonique, with about 4 periods a year
- Lybrel, which completely eliminates monthly menstrual periods in many women

***Side effects*:** Common side effects of combination OCs include headache, nausea, bloating, breast tenderness, and bleeding between periods. The estrogen component in combination OCs is usually responsible for these side effects. In general, today's OCs are much safer than OCs of the past because they contain much lower dosages of estrogen.

However, all OCs can increase the risk for migraine, stroke, heart attack, and blood clots. The risk is highest for women who smoke or who have a history of heart disease risk factors (such as high blood pressure or diabetes) or past cardiac events. Women who have certain metabolic disorders, such as polycystic ovary syndrome (PCOS), are also at higher risk for the heart-related complications associated with these pills.

PROGESTINS

Progestins (either natural progesterone or synthetic progestogen) are used by women with irregular or skipped periods to restore regular cycles. Because of this, they may also help menstrual pain. They also reduce heavy bleeding and may protect against uterine and ovarian cancers. Progestin-only contraceptives may be a good option for women who are not candidates for estrogen-containing OCs, such as women smokers over the age of 35.

Progestins can be delivered in various forms.

Oral Progesterone: Short-term treatment of anovulatory bleeding may involve a 21-day course of oral progesterone on days 5 - 26. Oral medroxypro-gesterone (Provera) has shown benefit in treating patients with chronic pelvic pain (but not those with pain due to endometriosis, primary dysmenorrheal or chronic active pelvic inflammatory disease).

Levonorgestrel-Releasing Intrauterine System (LNG-IUS): An intrauterine device (IUD) that releases progestin can be very beneficial for menstrual disorders, regardless of its contraceptive effects. In the United States, a levonorgestrel-releasing intrauterine system, also called an LNG-IUS, is sold under the brand name Mirena. The LNG-IUS has been proven to reduce heavy bleeding and pain in many women who suffer from menorrhagia and dysmenorrhea.

Many doctors now recommend the LNG-IUS as a first-line treatment for severe heavy menstrual bleeding, particularly for women who may face hysterectomy (removal of uterus) or conservative surgery such as endometrial ablation (destruction of the endometrial lining). This device is considered a good long-term option, particularly for women who may desire future pregnancies. Research also indicates that women who choose the LNG-IUS are as satisfied with their quality of life as those who choose surgery.

The LNG-IUS remains in place in the uterus and releases the progestin levonorgestrel for up to 5 years. Progestin released by an IUD mainly affects the uterus and cervix, and so it causes fewer widespread side effects than progestin pills do. (However, the other major IUD — the Copper T — may increase bleeding.)

After the LNG-IUS is inserted, heaver periods may occur during the first 3 - 6 months as the lining of the uterus is shed. This shedding may also cause irregular periods and light bleeding ("spotting") between menstrual cycles. Eventually, the LNG-IUS results in a shorter period, with little or no blood flow. For many women, the LNG-IUS completely stops menstrual periods.

Common side effects include cramping, acne, back pain, breast tenderness, headache, mood changes, and nausea. The LNG-IUS may increase the risk for ovarian cysts, but such cysts usually cause no symptoms and resolve on their own. Women who have a history of pelvic inflammatory disease or who have had a serious pelvic infection should not use the LNG-IUS. Because of the risks associated with pelvic infection, doctors recommend that women who use the LNG-IUS be in a stable monogamous relationship. The LNG-IUS does not protect against sexually transmitted diseases.

Injections (Depo-Provera): Depo-Provera uses a progestin called medroxyprogesterone. Most women who use Depo-Provera stop menstruating altogether after a year. Depo-Provera may be beneficial for women with heavy bleeding, or pain due to endometriosis. Women who eventually want to have children should be aware that Depo-Provera can cause persistent infertility for up to 22 months after the last injection, although the average is 10 months.

Weight gain can be a problem, particularly in women who are already overweight. Women should not use Depo-Provera if they have a history of liver disease, blood clots, stroke, or cancer of the reproductive organs. Long-term (more than 2 years) use of Depo-Provera can cause loss of bone density. Because of this, Depo-Provera should not be used for longer than 2 years.

GnRH AGONISTS

Gonadotropin releasing hormone (GnRH) agonists are used on occasion to treat severe menorrhagia for women who desire future pregnancy. GnRH agonists block the release of the reproductive hormones LH (luteinizing hormone) and FSH (follicular-stimulating hormone). As a result, the ovaries stop ovulating and no longer produce estrogen. GnRH agonists include goserelin (Zoladex), buserelin, a monthly injection of leuprolide (depot Lupron), and a nasal spray, Nafarelin (Synarel). Such drugs may be used alone or in preparation for procedures used to destroy the uterine lining. They are not generally suitable for long-term use.

Commonly reported side effects, which can be severe in some women, include menopausal-like symptoms. These symptoms include hot flashes, night sweats, changes in the vagina, weight change, and depression. The side effects vary in intensity depending on the GnRH agonist. They may be more intense with leuprolide and persist after the drug has been stopped.

The most important concern is possible osteoporosis from estrogen loss. Women ordinarily should not take these drugs for more than 6 months. Add-back therapy, which provides doses of estrogen and progestin that are high enough to maintain bone density but are too low to offset the beneficial effects of the GnRH agonist, may be used.

GnRH treatments used alone do not prevent pregnancy. Furthermore, if a woman becomes pregnant during their use, there is some risk for birth defects. Women who are taking GnRH agonists should use non-hormonal birth control methods, such as the diaphragm, cervical cap, or condoms while on the treatments.

DANAZOL

Danazol (Danocrine) is a synthetic substance that resembles a male hormone. It suppresses estrogen, and therefore menstruation, and is occasionally used (sometimes in combination with an oral contraceptive) to help prevent heavy bleeding. It is not suitable for long-term use, and due to its masculinizing side effects it is only used in rare cases. GnRH agonists have largely replaced the use of Danazol.

Adverse side effects include facial hair, deepening of the voice, weight gain, acne, and reduced breast size. Danazol may also increase the risk for unhealthy cholesterol levels and it may cause birth defects.

SURGERY

Women with heavy menstrual bleeding, dysmenorrhea, or both have medical and surgical options available to them. Most procedures eliminate or significantly affect the possibility for childbearing, however. Hysterectomy removes the entire uterus while endometrial ablation destroys the uterine lining.

For some women, an intrauterine device (IUD) that releases hormones is proving to be a good medical alternative to surgery. The levonorgestrel-releasing intrauterine system, or LNG-IUS (Mirena), is increasingly being used instead of surgery to treat heavy menstrual bleeding. Studies have found the LNG-IUS to work just as well as ablation. Women should be sure to ask their doctors about all medical options before undergoing surgical procedures.

ENDOMETRIAL ABLATION

In endometrial ablation, the entire lining of the uterus (the endometrium) is removed or destroyed. For most women, this procedure stops the monthly menstrual flow. In some women, menstrual flow is not stopped but is significantly reduced.

Candidates: Endometrial ablation is not appropriate for women who:

- Have gone through menopause
- Have recently been pregnant
- Would like to have children in the future
- Have certain gynecologic conditions such as cancer of the uterus, endometrial hyperplasia, uterine infection, or an endometrium that is too thin

Considerations: Endometrial ablation significantly decreases the likelihood a woman will become pregnant. However, pregnancy can still occur and this procedure increases the risks of complications, including miscarriage. Women who have this procedure must be committed to not becoming pregnant and to using birth control. Sterilization after ablation is another option.

A main concern of endometrial ablation is that it may delay or make it more difficult to diagnose uterine cancer in the future. (Postmenopausal bleeding or irregular vaginal bleeding can be warning signs of uterine cancer.) Women who have endometrial ablation still have a uterus and cervix, and should continue to have regular Pap smears and pelvic exams.

Types of Endometrial Ablation: Endometrial ablation used to be performed in an operating room using electrosurgery with a resectoscope (a hysteroscope with a heated wire loop or roller ball.) Laser ablation was another older procedure. These types of endometrial ablation have largely been replaced by newer types of procedure that do not use a resectoscope.

The newer procedures can be performed either in an operating room or a doctor's office. They include:

- **Radiofrequency:** The NovaSure system uses a mesh electrode probe that emits electromagnetic energy to destroy the lining.

- **Heated fluid:** In the HydroThermAblator system, a saline solution is inserted into the uterus with a hysteroscope and heated until the lining is destroyed. In the thermal balloon method, a balloon inserted into the uterus with hysteroscope is filled with heated fluid and expanded until it touches and destroys the endometrium.
- **Freezing:** Cryoablation uses liquid nitrogen to freeze the uterine lining.
- **Microwave:** Microwave endometrial ablation applies very low-power microwaves to the uterus.

Before the Procedure: In preparing for the ablation procedure, the doctor will perform an endometrial biopsy to make sure that cancer is not present. If the woman has an intrauterine device (IUD), it must be removed before the procedure. In some cases, hormonal drugs, such as GnRH analogs, may be given a few weeks before ablation to help thin the endometrial lining.

During the Procedure: Endometrial ablation is an outpatient procedure. The doctor usually applies a local anesthetic around the cervix. (The patient also receives medication for pain and to help her relax.) The doctor will dilate the cervix before starting the procedure. Patients may feel some mild cramping or discomfort, but many of the newer types of endometrial procedures can be performed in under 10 minutes.

After the Procedure: Patients may experience menstrual-like cramping for several days and frequent urination during the first 24 hours. The main side effect is watery or bloody discharge that can last for several weeks. This discharge is especially heavy in the first few days following ablation. (Patients need to wear pads, not tampons during this time, and to wait to have sex until the discharge has stopped.) Patients are generally able to return to work or normal activities within a few days after the procedure.

Complications: Complications of endometrial ablation may include perforation of the uterus, injury to the intestine, hemorrhage, or infection. If heated fluid is used in the procedure, it may leak and cause burns. However, in general, the risk of complications is very low.

Nearly all women have reduced menstrual flow after endometrial ablation, and nearly half of women have their periods stop. Some women, however, may continue to have bleeding problems and ultimately decide to have a hysterectomy.

HYSTERECTOMY

Hysterectomy is the surgical removal of the uterus.

Heavy bleeding, often from fibroids, and pelvic pain are the reasons for many hysterectomies. However, with newer medical and surgical treatments available, hysterectomies are performed less often than in the past. In its support, hysterectomy, unlike drug treatments and less invasive procedures, cures menorrhagia completely, and most women are satisfied with the procedure. Less invasive hysterectomy procedures are also improving recovery rates and increasing satisfaction afterward.

Still, any woman who is uncertain about a recommendation for a hysterectomy to treat fibroids or heavy bleeding should certainly seek a second opinion.

NERVE DESTRUCTION TECHNIQUES FOR TREATING DYSMENORRHEA

Some evidence suggests that surgically cutting the pain-conducting nerve fibers leading from the uterus diminishes the pain from dysmenorrhea. Two procedures, uterine nerve ablation and laparoscopic presacral neurectomy, can block such nerves. Small studies have shown benefits from these procedures, but stronger evidence is needed before they can be recommended for women with severe primary dysmenorrhea.

REFERENCES

1. American Academy of Pediatrics Committee on Adolescence; American College of Obstetricians and Gynecologists Committee on Adolescent Health Care; Diaz A, Laufer MR, Breech LL. Menstruation in girls and adolescents: using the menstrual cycle as a vital sign. *Pediatrics* . 2006 Nov;118(5): 2245-50.
2. Apgar BS, Kaufman AH, George-Nwogu U, Kittendorf A. Treatment of menorrhagia. *Am Fam Physician* . 2007 Jun 15; 75(12): 1813-9.
3. Beaumont H, Augood C, Duckitt K, Lethaby A. Danazol for heavy menstrual bleeding. *Cochrane Database Syst Rev.* 2007 Jul 18; (3): CD001017.
4. Casablanca Y. Management of dysfunctional uterine bleeding.*Obstet Gynecol Clin North Am* . 2008 Jun; 35(2): 219-34.
5. Chen EC, Danis PG, Tweed E. Clinical inquiries. Menstrual disturbances in perimenopausal women: what's best? *J Fam Pract* . 2009 Jun; 58(6): E3.
6. Damlo S. ACOG guidelines on endometrial ablation. Am Fam Physician. 2008 Feb 15; 77(4): 545-549.
7. Dietrich JE. Von Willebrand's disease. *J Pediatr Adolesc Gynecol* . 2007 Jun; 20(3): 153-5.
8. Kaunitz AM, Meredith S, Inki P, Kubba A, Sanchez-Ramos L. Levonorgestrel-releasing intrauterine system and endometrial ablation in heavy menstrual bleeding: a systematic review and meta-analysis. *Obstet Gynecol* . 2009 May; 113(5): 1104-16.
9. Lethaby A, Irvine G, Cameron I. Cyclical progestogens for heavy menstrual bleeding. *Cochrane Database Syst Rev* . 2008 Jan 23; (1): CD001016.

CHAPTER 81

Menopause

DEFINITION

Menopause is time in a woman's life when her periods (menstruation) eventually stop and the body goes through changes that no longer allow her to get pregnant. It is a natural event that normally occurs in women age 45 - 55.

ETIOLOGY

During menopause, a woman's ovaries stop making eggs and they produce less estrogen and progesterone. Changes in these hormones cause menopause symptoms. Periods occur less often and eventually stop. Sometimes this happens suddenly. But most of the time, periods slowly stop over time.

Menopause is complete when woman have not had a period for 1 year. This is called postmenopause. Women who are post-menopausal can no longer get pregnant.

Surgical menopause is when medical treatments cause a drop in estrogn. This can happen if your ovaries are removed, or if woman receive chemotherapy or hormone therapy for breast cancer.

CLINICAL FEATURES

Symptoms vary from woman to woman. They may last 5 or more years. Some women may have worse symptoms than others. Symptoms of surgical menopause can be more severe and start more suddenly.

The first thing to notice is that your periods start to change. They might occur more often or less often. Some women might get their period every 3 weeks. This might last for 1-3 years before the periods completely stop.

Common symptoms of menopause include (Fig. 81.1):

- Menstrual periods that occur less often and eventually stop.
- Heart pounding or racing
- Hot flashes, usually worst during the first 1-2 years
- Night sweats
- Skin flushing
- Sleeping problems (insomnia)

Other symptoms of menopause may include:

- Decreased interest in sex, possibly decreased response to sexual stimulation
- Forgetfulness (in some women)
- Headaches
- Mood swings including irritability, depression, and anxiety
- Urine leakage
- Vaginal dryness and painful sexual intercourse
- Vaginal infections
- Joint aches and pains
- Irregular heartbeat (palpitations)

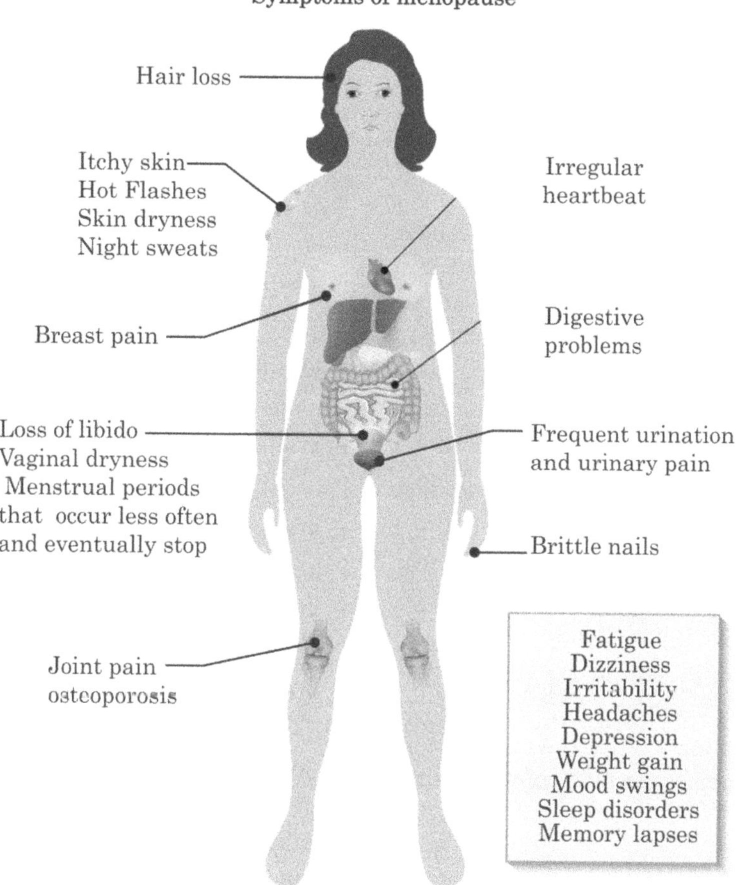

FIGURE 81.1

Clinical features of menopause.

(source : https://www.shutterstock.com/image-vector/menopause-sign-symptoms-woman-silhouette-highlighted-316559192)

DIAGNOSIS

Blood and urine tests can be used to look for changes in hormone levels. Test results can help to determine if woman is close to menopause or have already gone through menopause.

Tests that may be done include:

- Estradiol
- FSH
- LH

Bone loss increases during the first few years after your last period. Your doctor may order a bone density test to look for bone loss related to osteoporosis.

TREATMENT

Treatment for menopause depends on many things, including how bad symptoms are, overall health, and preference. It may include lifestyle changes or hormone therapy.

HORMONE THERAPY

Hormone therapy may help if women have severe hot flashes, night sweats, mood issues, or vaginal dryness. Hormone therapy is treatment with estrogen and, sometimes, progesterone.

Several major studies have questioned the health benefits and risks of hormone therapy, including the risk of developing breast cancer, heart attacks, strokes, and blood clots.

Current guidelines support the use of HT for the treatment of hot flashes. Specific recommendations:

- HT may be started in women who have recently entered menopause.
- HT should not be used in women who started menopause many years ago, except for estrogen vaginal creams.
- The medicine should not be used for longer than 5 years.
- Women taking HT have a low risk for stroke, heart disease, blood clots, or breast cancer.

To reduce the risks of estrogen therapy, the doctor may recommend:

- A lower dose of estrogen or a different estrogen preparation (for instance, a vaginal cream or skin patch rather than a pill)
- Frequent and regular pelvic exams and Pap smears to detect problems as early as possible
- Frequent and regular physical exams, including breast exams and mammograms

ALTERNATIVES TO HORMONE THERAPY

There are other medicines available to help with mood swings, hot flashes, and other symptoms. These include:

- Antidepressants, including **paroxetine** (Paxil), **venlafaxine** (Effexor), **bupropion** (Wellbutrin), and **fluoxetine** (Prozac)
- A blood pressure medicine called **Clonidine**
- **Gabapentin**, a seizure drug that also helps reduce hot flashes

DIET AND LIFESTYLE CHANGES

Hormones are not always needed to reduce symptoms of menopause. There are many steps to reduce symptoms.

Diet changes:

- Avoid caffeine, alcohol, and spicy foods
- Eat soy foods. Soy contains estrogen
- Get plenty of calcium and vitamin D in food or supplements

Exercise and relaxation techniques:

- Get plenty of exercise.
- Do exercises every day. They strengthen the muscles of vagina and pelvis.
- Practice slow, deep breathing whenever a hot flash starts to come on. Try taking six breaths a minute.
- Try yoga, tai chi, or meditation.

Other tips:

- Dress lightly and in layers.
- Keep having sex.
- Use water-based lubricants or a vaginal moisturizer during sex.

COMPLICATIONS

Some women have vaginal bleeding after menopause. This is often nothing to worry about. However, women should tell your health care provider if this occurs. It may be an early sign of other health problems, including cancer.

Decreased estrogen levels have been linked with some long-term effects, including:

- Bone loss and osteoporosis in some women
- Changes in cholesterol levels and greater risk of heart disease

PREVENTION

Menopause is a natural and expected part of a woman's development and does not need to be prevented. Woman can reduce your risk of long-term problems such as osteoporosis and heart disease by taking the following steps:

- Control blood pressure, cholesterol, and other risk factors for heart disease.
- Do NOT smoke. Cigarette use can cause early menopause.
- Eat a low-fat diet.
- Get regular exercise. Resistance exercises help strengthen bones and improve balance.
- If you show early signs of bone loss or have a strong family history of osteoporosis are observed, talk to doctor about medications that can help stop further weakening.
- Take calcium and vitamin D.

REFERENCES

1. American College of Obstetricians and Gynecologists Committee on Gynecologic Practice. ACOG Committee Opinion No. 420, November 2008: hormone therapy and heart disease. *Obstet Gynecol.* 2008 Nov;112(5):1189-92.
2. Management of osteoporosis in postmenopausal women: 2010 position statement of The North American Menopause Society.*Menopause.* 2010 Jan-Feb;17(1):25-54; quiz 55-6.
3. North American Menopause Society. Estrogen and progestogen use in postmenopausal women: 2010 position statement of The North American Menopause Society. *Menopause.* 2010 Mar;17(2):242-55.
4. Col NF, Fairfield KM, Ewan-Whyte C, Miller H. In the clinic. Menopause. *Ann Intern Med.* 2009 Apr 7;150(7):ITC4-1-15.
5. Brunner RL, Aragaki A, Barnabei V, et al. Menopausal symptom experience before and after stopping estrogen therapy in the Women's Health Initiative randomized, placebo-controlled trial. *Menopause.* 2010 Sep-Oct;17(5):946-54.
6. Freeman EW, et al. Efficacy of Escitalopram for Hot Flashes in Healthy Postmenopausal Women. *JAMA.* 2011; 305(3): 267-274.

CHAPTER 82

Drug Therapy in Pregnancy

PHARMACOKINETICS

Most drugs taken by pregnant women can cross the placenta and expose the developing embryo and fetus to their pharmacologic and teratogenic effects. Critical factors affecting placental drug transfer and drug effects on the fetus include the following: (1) The physicochemical properties of the drug; (2) the rate at which the drug crosses the placenta and the amount of drug reaching the fetus; (3) The duration of exposure to the drug; (4) Distribution characteristics in different fetal tissues; (5) The stage of placental and fetal development at the time of exposure to the drug; and (6) The effects of drugs used in combination.

LIPID SOLUBILITY

As is true also of other biologic membranes, drug passage across the placenta is dependent on lipid solubility and the degree of drug ionization. Lipophilic drugs tend to diffuse readily across the placenta and enter the fetal circulation. For example, thiopental, a drug commonly used for cesarean sections, crosses the placenta almost immediately and can produce sedation or apnea in the newborn infant. Highly ionized drugs such as succinylcholine and tubocurarine, also used for cesarean sections, cross the placenta slowly and achieve very low concentrations in the fetus. Impermeability of the placenta to polar compounds is relative rather than absolute. If high enough maternal-fetal concentration gradients are achieved, polar compounds cross the placenta in measurable amounts. Salicylate, which is almost completely ionized at physiologic pH, crosses the placenta rapidly. This occurs because the small amount of salicylate that is not ionized is highly lipid-soluble.

MOLECULAR SIZE

The molecular weight of the drug also influences the rate of transfer and the amount of drug transferred across the placenta. Drugs with molecular weights of 250–500 can cross the placenta easily, depending upon their lipid solubility and degree of ionization; those with molecular weights of 500–1000 cross the placenta with more difficulty; and those with molecular weights greater than 1000 cross very poorly. An important clinical application of this property is the choice of heparin as an anticoagulant in pregnant women. Because it is a very large (and polar) molecule, heparin is unable to cross the placenta. Unlike warfarin, which is teratogenic and should be avoided during the first trimester and even beyond (as the brain continues to develop), heparin may be safely given to pregnant women who need anticoagulation. Yet the placenta contains drug transporters, which can carry larger molecules to the fetus. For example, a variety of maternal antibodies cross the placenta and may cause fetal morbidity, as in Rh incompatibility.

PLACENTAL TRANSPORTERS

During the last decade, many drug transporters have been identified in the placenta, with increasing recognition of their effects on drug transfer to the fetus. For example, the P-glycoprotein transporter encoded by the *MDR1* gene pumps back into the maternal circulation a variety of drugs, including cancer drugs (e.g., vinblastine, doxorubicin) and other agents. Similarly, viral protease inhibitors, which are substrates to P-glycoprotein, achieve only low fetal concentrations—an effect that may increase the risk of vertical HIV infection from the mother to the fetus. The hypoglycemic drug glyburide cannot be measured in umbilical blood despite therapeutic maternal concentrations. Recent work has documented that this agent is effluxed from the fetal circulation by the BCRP transporter as well as by the MRP3 transporter located in the placental brush border membrane.

PROTEIN BINDING

The degree to which a drug is bound to plasma proteins (particularly albumin) may also affect the rate of transfer and the amount transferred. However, if a compound is very lipid-soluble (e.g., some anesthetic gases), it will not be affected greatly by protein binding. Transfer of these more lipid-soluble drugs and their overall rates of equilibration are more dependent on (and proportionate to) placental blood flow. This is because very lipid-soluble drugs diffuse across placental membranes so rapidly that their overall rates of equilibration do not depend on the free drug concentrations becoming equal on both sides. If a drug is poorly lipid-soluble and is ionized, its transfer is slow and will probably be impeded by its binding to maternal plasma proteins. Differential protein binding is also important since some drugs exhibit greater protein binding in maternal plasma than in fetal plasma because of a lower binding affinity of fetal proteins. This has been shown for sulphonamides, barbiturates, phenytoin, and local anesthetic agents.

PLACENTAL AND FETAL DRUG METABOLISM

Two mechanisms help protect the fetus from drugs in the maternal circulation: (1) The placenta itself plays a role both as a semi-permeable barrier and as a site of metabolism of some drugs passing through it. Several different types of aromatic oxidation reactions (e.g., hydroxylation, N-dealkylation, demethylation) have been shown to occur in placental tissue. Pentobarbital is oxidized in this way. Conversely, it is possible that the metabolic capacity of the placenta may lead to creation of toxic metabolites, and the placenta may therefore augment toxicity (e.g., ethanol, benzpyrenes). (2) Drugs that have crossed the placenta enter the fetal circulation via the umbilical vein. About 40%–60% of umbilical venous blood flow enters the fetal liver; the remainder bypasses the liver and enters the general fetal circulation. A drug that enters the liver may be partially metabolized there before it enters the fetal circulation. In addition, a large proportion of drug present in the umbilical artery (returning to the placenta) may be shunted through the placenta back to the umbilical vein and into the liver again. It should be noted that metabolites of some drugs may be more active than the parent compound and may affect the fetus adversely.

PHARMACODYNAMICS

MATERNAL DRUG ACTIONS

The effects of drugs on the reproductive tissues (breast, uterus, etc) of the pregnant woman are sometimes altered by the endocrine environment appropriate for the stage of pregnancy. Drug effects on other maternal tissues (heart, lungs, kidneys, central nervous system, etc) are not changed significantly by pregnancy, although the physiologic context (cardiac output, renal blood flow, etc) may be altered, requiring the use of drugs that are not needed by the same woman when she is not pregnant. For example, cardiac glycosides and diuretics may be needed for heart failure precipitated by the increased cardiac workload of pregnancy, or insulin may be required for control of blood glucose in pregnancy-induced diabetes.

THERAPEUTIC DRUG ACTIONS IN THE FETUS

Fetal therapeutics is an emerging area in perinatal pharmacology. This involves drug administration to the pregnant woman with the fetus as the target of the drug. At present, corticosteroids are used to stimulate fetal lung maturation when preterm birth is expected. Phenobarbital, when given to pregnant women near term, can induce fetal hepatic enzymes responsible for the glucuronidation of bilirubin, and the incidence of jaundice is lower in newborns when mothers are given Phenobarbital than when Phenobarbital is not used. Before phototherapy became the preferred mode of therapy for neonatal indirect hyperbilirubinemia, Phenobarbital was used for this indication. Administration of Phenobarbital to the mother was suggested recently as a means of decreasing the risk of intracranial bleeding in preterm infants. However, large randomized studies failed to confirm this effect. Antiarrhythmic drugs have also been given to mothers for treatment of fetal cardiac arrhythmias. Although their efficacy has not yet been established by controlled studies, digoxin, flecainide, procainamide, verapamil, and other antiarrhythmic agents have been shown to be effective in case series. During the last decade it has been shown that maternal use of zidovudine decreases by two thirds transmission of HIV from the mother to the fetus, and use of combinations of three antiretroviral agents can eliminate fetal infection almost entirely .

PREDICTABLE TOXIC DRUG ACTIONS IN THE FETUS

Chronic use of opioid by the mother may produce dependence in the fetus and newborn. This dependence may be manifested after delivery as a neonatal withdrawal syndrome. A less well understood fetal drug toxicity is caused by the use of angiotensin-converting enzyme inhibitors during pregnancy. These drugs can result in significant and irreversible renal damage in the fetus and are therefore contraindicated in pregnant women. Adverse effects may also be delayed, as in the case of female fetuses exposed to diethylstilbestrol, who may be at increased risk for adenocarcinoma of the vagina after puberty.

TERATOGENIC DRUG ACTIONS

A single intrauterine exposure to a drug can affect the fetal structures undergoing rapid development at the time of exposure. Thalidomide is an example of a drug that may profoundly affect the development of the limbs after only brief exposure. This exposure, however, must be at a critical time in the development of the limbs. The thalidomide phocomelia risk occurs during the fourth through the seventh weeks of gestation because it is during this time that the arms and legs develop Listed in Following Fig. 82.1.

TERATOGENIC MECHANISMS

The mechanisms by which different drugs produce teratogenic effects are poorly understood and are probably multifactorial. For example, drugs may have a direct effect on maternal tissues with secondary or indirect effects on fetal tissues. Drugs may interfere with the passage of oxygen or nutrients through the placenta and therefore have effects on the most rapidly metabolizing tissues of the fetus. Finally, drugs may have important direct actions on the processes of differentiation in developing tissues. For example, vitamin A (retinol) has been shown to have important differentiation-directing actions in normal tissues. Several vitamin A analogs (isotretinoin, etretinate) are powerful teratogen, suggesting that they alter the

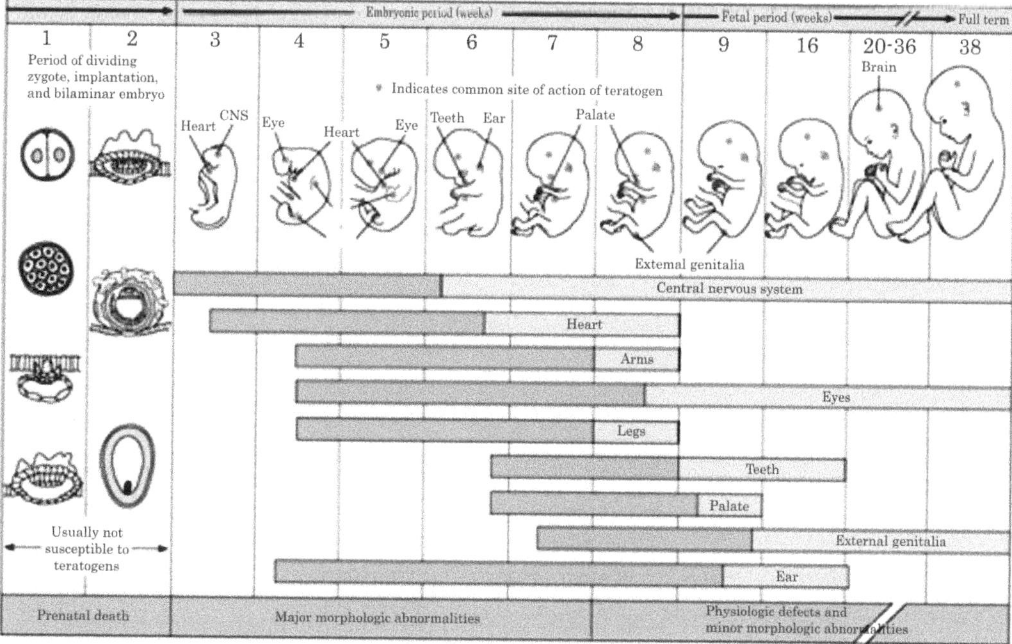

FIGURE 82.1

Schematic diagram of critical periods of human development.

normal processes of differentiation. Finally, deficiency of a critical substance appears to play a role in some types of abnormalities. For example, folic acid supplementation during pregnancy appears to reduce the incidence of neural tube defects (e.g., spina bifida).

Continued exposure to a teratogen may produce cumulative effects or may affect several organs going through varying stages of development. Chronic consumption of high doses of ethanol during pregnancy, particularly during the first and second trimesters, may result in the fetal alcohol syndrome. In this syndrome, the central nervous system, growth, and facial development may be affected.

DEFINING A TERATOGEN

To be considered teratogenic, a candidate substance or process should (1) Result in a characteristic set of malformations, indicating selectivity for certain target organs; (2) Exert its effects at a particular stage of fetal development, i.e., during the limited time period of organogenesis of the target organs and (3) Show a dose-dependent incidence. Some drugs with known teratogenic or other adverse effects in pregnancy are listed in Following Table 82.1.

Table 82.1

Drugs with known teratogenic or other adverse effects

Drug	Trimester	Effect
ACE inhibitors	All, especially second and third	Renal damage
Aminopterin	First	Multiple gross anomalies
Amphetamines	All	Suspected abnormal developmental patterns, decreased school performance
Androgens	Second and third	Masculinization of female fetus
Antidepressants, tricyclic	Third	Neonatal withdrawal symptoms have been reported in a few cases with clomipramine, desipramine, and imipramine
Barbiturates	All	Chronic use can lead to neonatal dependence.
Busulfan	All	Various congenital malformations; low birth weight
Carbamazepine	First	Neural tube defects
Chlorpropamide	All	Prolonged symptomatic neonatal hypoglycemia
Clomipramine	Third	Neonatal lethargy, hypotonia, cyanosis, hypothermia
Cocaine	All	Increased risk of spontaneous abortion, abruption placenta, and premature labor; neonatal cerebral infarction, abnormal development, and decreased school performance
Cyclophosphamide	First	Various congenital malformations
Cytarabine	First, second	Various congenital malformations
Diazepam	All	Chronic use may lead to neonatal dependence
Diethylstilbestrol	All	Vaginal adenosis, clear cell vaginal adenocarcinoma

Table 82.1 *contd...*

Drug	Trimester	Effect
Ethanol	All	Risk of fetal alcohol syndrome and alcohol-related neurodevelopment defects
Etretinate	All	High risk of multiple congenital malformations
Heroin	All	Chronic use leads to neonatal dependence
Iodide	All	Congenital goiter, hypothyroidism
Isotretinoin	All	Extremely high risk of CNS, face, ear, and other malformations
Lithium	First	Ebstein's anomaly
Methadone	All	Chronic use leads to neonatal dependence
Methotrexate	First	Multiple congenital malformations
Methylthiouracil	All	Hypothyroidism
Metronidazole	First	May be mutagenic (from animal studies; there is no evidence for mutagenic or teratogenic effects in humans)
Organic solvents	First	Multiple malformations
Misoprostol	First	Möbius sequence
Penicillamine	First	Cutis laxa, other congenital malformations
Phencyclidine	All	Abnormal neurologic examination, poor suck reflex and feeding
Phenytoin	All	Fetal hydantoin syndrome
Propylthiouracil	All	Congenital goiter
Streptomycin	All	Eighth nerve toxicity
Smoking (constituents of tobacco smoke)	All	Intrauterine growth retardation; prematurity; sudden infant death syndrome; perinatal complications
Tamoxifen	All	Increased risk of spontaneous abortion or fetal damage
Tetracycline	All	Discoloration and defects of teeth and altered bone growth
Thalidomide	First	Phocomelia (shortened or absent long bones of the limbs) and many internal malformations
Trimethadione	All	Multiple congenital anomalies
Valproic acid	All	Neural tube defects, cardiac and limb malformations
Warfarin	First	Hypoplastic nasal bridge, chondrodysplasia
	Second	CNS malformations
	Third	Risk of bleeding. Discontinue use 1 month before delivery.

FDA PREGNANCY CATEGORIES (TABLE 82.2)

A – Studies in pregnant woman, no risk.

B – Animal studies no risk, but human not adequate or animal toxicity but human studies no risk.

C – Animal studies show toxicity, human studies inadequate but benefit of use may exceed risk.

D – Evidence of human risk, but benefit may outweigh.

X – Fetal abnormalities in humans, risk > benefit: contraindicate in pregnant women.

*Category with a subscript M (e.g., CM) refers to the risk factor that the manufacturer rated its product in its professional literature.

Table 82.3

Effect of drugs during pregnancy analgesics and anti-inflammatory drugs

Drugs	FDA Pregnancy Categories	Nature of Effect
Acetaminophen	B	Acetaminophen is analgesic-antipyretic of choice for use near Term.
Aspirin	C (D if full-dose aspirin in 3rd trimester)	Maternal – aspirin use late in gestation can cause increased bleeding at delivery and delay the onset of labor. Neonatal – prolong constriction of ductus arteriosus, pulmonary hyper-tension, platelet function, and bleeding, intracranial hemorrhage.
Indomethacin	B (D if use long term than 48 hrs or after 34-week gestation)	Premature closure of ductus arteriosus, neonatal pulmonary hypertension.
Ibuprofen	B (D if use in the 3rd trimester)	Similar to aspirin and indomethacin.
Diclofenac	B_M (D if use in the 3rd trimester)*	Inhibition of labor, prolongation of pregnancy and suppression of fetal renal function. If use in the 3rd trimester close to delivery, persistant pulmonary hypertension of the newborn may occur.
Piroxicam	B (D if use in the 3rd trimester)	Inhibition of labor, prolongation of pregnancy. If use in the 3rd trimester close to delivery, persistent pulmonary hypertension of the newborn may occur.
	Anticoagulants	
Heparin	C	Heparin is usually the drug of choice for anticoagulation during
Warfarin	D	Warfarin may produce the "Fetal Warfarin Syndrome" or "Warfarin Embryopathy" include nasal hypoplasia, neonatal respiratory distress, axial skeleton and proximal femur are affected, spontaneous abortion, stillbirths, CNS defects.
	Anticonvulsants	
Phenytoin	D	Mild-to-moderate growth deficiency, wide anterior fontanelle,hypertelorism, depressed nasal bridge, short nose with bowed upper lip, cleft lip and palate, hypoplasia of distal phalanges with

Table 82.2 *Contd...*

Drugs	FDA Pregnancy Categories	Nature of Effect
Sodium valproate	D	High forehead, epicanthal folds, broad nasal bridge, long philtrum, small mouth, cleft lip, neural tube defect, hypospadias.
Carbamazepine	C	Craniofacial defect, neural tube defects.
Phenobarbital	D	Cleft lip and palate, cardiac defects.
		Antimicrobial Drugs
Penicillins	B	Penicillins are without teratogenic risk.
Cephalosporins	B	Cephalosporins are thought to be without teratogenic risk.
Erythromycin	B	Pregnant women are at increased risk for hepatotoxicity caused
Aminoglycosides	C	Congenital hearing loss, deafness.
Chloramphenicol	C	Risk for development of blood dyscrasias and aplastic anemia.Particular caution should be exercised near term because the "Gray Baby" syndrome is resulted.
Tetracycline's	D; B (topical)	Tetracycline's have been reported to cause congenital Abnormalities, particularly staining of the teeth and retardation of the developing skeletal system.
Fluoroquinolones (e.g. Ciprofloxacin, Norfloxacin, Ofloxacin)	C	Fluoroquinolones were shown to cause erosion of the cartilage and other arthropathies in fetuses. These drugs should not be used in pregnancy.
Sulphonamides (e.g. Sulphadiazine)	B (D at term)	Evidence associating sulfonamide use near term with hyperbilirubinemia, hemolytic anemia (in G-6-PD deficiency), competition of albumin site-neonatal kernicterus.
Co-Trimoxazole	C	Do not use at term to avoid kernicterus in the new born and use during pregnancy only if risk outweigh the benefits since folic acid metabolism may be effected.
Metronidazole	BM*	The manufacturer and the Centers for Disease Control (CDC) consider Metronidazole to be contraindicated during 1st trimester in patients with trichomoniasis. Use for trichomoniasis during the 2nd and 3rd trimester may be acceptable if alternate therapies have failed.
		Cardiovascular Drugs
Antiarrhythmics -Amiodarone	D	Neonatal hypothyroidism with or without goiter, as well as Hyperthyroidism.
-Digoxin	C	Digoxin is not a teratogen. It may be given to pregnant women to treat fetal CHF and supra-ventricular tachycardia. Maternal digitalis toxicity has been associated with fetal toxicity.
β-Adrenergic blocking agents -Atenolol -Pindolol -Metoprolol -Propranolol	 C B B C	These agents are thought to be generally safe in pregnancy but these have also been associated with intrauterine growth Retardation and neonatal hypoglycemia and hypotension.

Table 82.2 *Contd...*

Drugs	FDA Pregnancy Categories	Nature of Effect
Angiotensin-converting enzyme (ACE) inhibitors (e.g. Captopril, enalapril, lisinopril, fosinopril)	C	Fetal abnormalities, including death can be caused and these drugs should not be used in pregnancy.
Calcium – channel blocking agents (e.g. Nifedipine, Diltiazem, verapamil)	C	A small, transient decrease in uterine activity occurred with all doses.
Diuretics Hydrochlorothiazide (HCTZ) -Furosemide -Amiloride 5 mg.+ HCTZ 50 mg. (Moduretic®)	 B C BM*	 Neonatal hypoglycemia, hyponatremia, hypokalemia and thrombocytopenia. Crosses the placenta. Increases fetal urine production, electrolyte disturbances reported. Animal studies using amiloride alone had not shown adverse effects in the fetus but in human studies some newborns had hypospadias, renovascular hypertension.
Isosorbide dinitrate	CM*	No reports on the use in human pregnancy. If produces embryo toxicity in rabbits.
Hydralazine	B (oral); C (IV)	Hydralazine is the Parentral drug of choice used in pregnancy.
Methyldopa	C	Antihypertensive of choice used in pregnancy.
Reserpine	C	Produces edema of the nasal mucosa in the neonate, hypothermia and bradycardia.
Gastrointestinal Drugs		
Antacid -Magnesium hydroxide -Aluminum hydroxide -Sucralphate	 B C B	 The safety of antacid use during the 1st trimester of pregnancy has not been established. 2nd and 3rd trimester use appears to be without adverse effects. Sucralfate is poorly absorbed and no adverse effects to the fetus have been reported.
-Antiulcer **H2-blocker** -Cimetidine -Famotidine -Ranitidine -Nizatidine Proton-Pump Inhibitor -Omeprazole	 B B B C C_M*	 Crosses the placenta. Available evidence suggests safe use during pregnancy and breast-feeding. Severe congenital anomalies; anencephaly, severe talipes inhuman. Long term high dose consumption was carcinogenic in rats, producing gastrointestinal tumors.
Laxative -Bulk laxatives (Psyllium) - Mineral oil - Castor oil	 B C X	 These are agent of choice. Mineral oil should be avoided. Castor oil may cause pelvic congestion.

Table 82.2 *Contd...*

Drugs	FDA Pregnancy Categories	Nature of Effect
Metoclopramide	B	Crosses the placenta. Available evidence suggests safe use during pregnancy and breastfeeding.
Sedative and Hypnotics		
Benzodiazepines (e.g. Clorazepate, Diazepam, Lorazepam)	D	Neonatal depression, apnoeic spells, "floppy baby syndrome" (muscular relaxation, poor sucking, disturbances in thermoregulation and regurgitation), withdrawal symptom.
Phenobarbital	D	Neonatal depression, neonatal feeding difficulties, neonatal bleeding, withdrawal symptom.
Antidiabetic Agents		
Sulphonylurea's (e.g. Chlorpropamide, glyburide, glipizide) Biguanides (e.g. Metformin)	C B	May cause prolonged hypoglycemia or hyperinsulinism in the newborn.
Insulin	B	Does not cross the placenta. Insulin is the drug of choice for the control of diabetes mellitus during pregnancy.
Sex Hormone		
Diethyl Stilbestrol (DES)	X	DES causes a number of reproductive tract abnormalities in both female and male offspring exposed in utero.
Estradiol	X	Vaginal adenosis Feminization of male fetus hypotrophic testis, abnormal spermatogenesis, epididymal cyst.
Progesterone	X ; B (oral capsules per manufac-turer)	It may produces the "VACTERL syndrome" (vertebral, anal, cardiovascular, tracheal, esophageal, renal and limb defects)
Respiratory Drugs		
Antitussives -Codeine	C (D if used for prolonged periods or in high dose at term)	Typical symptoms of narcotic withdrawal were noted in the infants shortly after birth but not in the mother.
-Dextromethorphan	C	Toxicity in the fetus and newborn after the use of dextromethorphan.
Bronchodilators -Aminophylline -Theophylline	C C	Theophylline is the bronchodilator of choice for asthma and COPD in the pregnant patient but should have theophylline concentration monitored frequently for dosage adjustments.
-Terbutaline	BM*	Only rare reports of serious toxicity in the fetus or newborn have Appeared.

Table 82.2 *Contd...*

Drugs	FDA Pregnancy Categories	Nature of Effect
Antihistamines and Nasal Decongestants		
Chlorpheniramine Cetirizine Loratadine Diphenhydramine Dimenhydrinate	B B B B B	These agents use during pregnancy has not been associated with an increase risk of fetal malformation.
Pseudoephedrine	C	Some study shown about six major birth defect categories: cardiovascular defects, oral clefts, spina bifida, polydactyly, limb reduction defects and hypospadias.
Tripolidine	CM*	Cardiovascular, spina bifida, polydactyly and limb reduction defects.
Miscellaneous		
Smoking	X	Increased Perinatal Risk: Spontaneous abortion, Preterm birth, Intrauterine growth restriction/small for gestation age –100 to 320g. reduction in expected birthweight.Increased Postnatal Risk: Small head circumference; decreased Auditory, language and cognitive performance; low IQ; increased incidence of asthma, bronchitis, pneumonia; increased risk of sudden infant death syndrome.
Caffeine	Should be avoided	High dose (>7 cups/day); low birth weight (<2500 g.) neurological impairment, growth retardation.
Alcohol	X	Fetal Alcohol Syndrome includes Intrauterine Growth Retardation (IUGR), microcephaly, postnatal growth deficiency, developmental delay, mental retardation and craniofacial anomalies.
Isotretinoin	X	Isotretionin is potent teratogen (e.g. CNS, cardiac anomalies, facial abnormalities, deafness and blindness)
Lithium	D	Neonatal hypotonia, poor sucking power, diminished reflexes for days.
Corticosteroids	C	When appropriate, corticosteroids can be administered by aerosol inhalation or intrasynovial injection to minimize systemic availability. Corticosteroids use during pregnancy may cause an Increased risk for maternal gestation diabetes, hypertension, and excessive weight gain.

REFERENCES

1. Barbara GW, Joseph TD, Terry LS, Cynthia WH. Pharmacotherapy Handbook. 2nd ed.Stamford (CT): Appleton & Lange; 2000.
2. Charles FL, Lora LA, Morton PG, Leonard LL. Drug Information Handbook. 8th ed. Hudson (OH):Lexi-Comp; 2000-2001.
3. Gerald GB, Roger KF, Sumner JY. Drugs in Pregnancy and Lactation. 5th ed. Baltimore (MD): Lippincott Williams & Wilkins; 1998.
4. Philip OA, James EK. Handbook of Clinical Drug Data. 8th ed. Stamford (CT): Appleton & Lange; 1997-1998.
5. Robert JB. Effects of Certain Prenatal Drugs on the Fetus and Newborn. Pediatrics in Review 2002 Jan; 23(1):17-23.
6. van Lingen RA et al. The effects of analgesia in the vulnerable infant during the perinatal period. Clin Perinatol 2002;29:511.
7. Nottarianni LJ: Plasma protein binding of drugs in pregnancy and in neonates. Clin Pharmacokinet 1990;18:20.
8. Koren G, Pastuszak A: Prevention of unnecessary pregnancy terminations by counseling women on drug, chemical, and radiation exposure during the first trimester. Teratology 1990;41:657.

CHAPTER 83

Drug Therapy in Lactation

LACTATION

Drugs present in the maternal organism can be secreted in breast milk and thus be ingested by the infant. Evaluation of risks should be done. In case of doubt, potential danger to the infant can be averted only by weaning.

Most drugs are transferred to breast milk only in small amounts and the dose to which the infant is exposed is very low and well below the therapeutic dose for an infant Fig. 83.1. **However, all infants exposed to drugs via breast milk should be observed for drug-related side effects.**

As the number of nursing mothers continues to increase, so does the use of drugs, both legal and recreational. As a nursing mother, should be aware that there are four things to know for sure about drugs and breast milk.

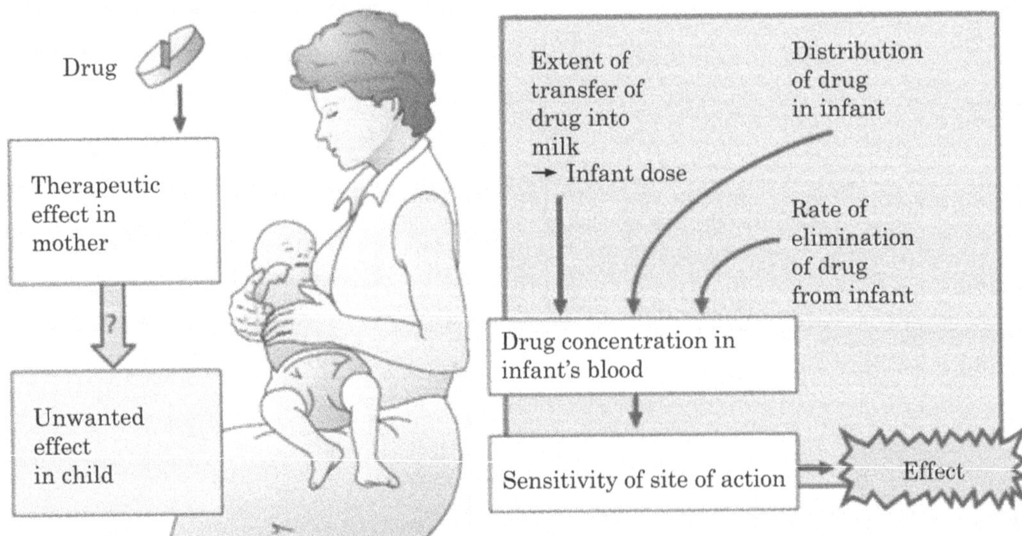

FIGURE 83.1

Drug action during breast feeding.

Drugs must pass into the bloodstream before they can appear in the milk. Most drugs pass into human milk.

Almost all medication appears in very small amounts, usually less than 1% of the maternal dose.

Very few drugs are contraindicated for nursing mothers (Table 83.1).

The list of drugs which are unsafe for breastfeeding moms is very small. The vast majority of medications can be taken without harm to the baby. The issue of which drugs are safe to take during lactation is quite complicated.

Many factors must be taken into consideration, such as:

- **The route of administration** (The baby is always exposed through the GI tract, but drugs can enter the system several different ways: orally, intravenously, intramuscularly, topically, or through inhalation – topical medications (skin creams) and medications inhaled or applied to the eyes or nose reach the milk in lesser amounts and more slowly than other routes and are almost always safe for nursing mothers: oral medications take longer to get into the milk than IV and IM routes (the drug must first go through the mother's GI tract before it enters the bloodstream, and the milk supply)-with IV drugs, the medications bypasses the barriers in the GI tract to enter the milk quickly and at higher levels, and with IM injections, drugs transfer quickly into the milk because the muscles have so many blood vessels, so the drug enters the bloodstream quickly.
- **The amount taken** (The higher the dosage, the more the drug transfers into milk).
- **How often you take the drug** (medications taken 30 to 60 minutes before feed are likely to be a peak blood levels when your baby nurses).
- **Baby's age and maturity level** (premature infants have immature kidney and liver functions and may have trouble processing and eliminating even small quantities of drugs that might not cause problems for larger, full-term infants: however, even full-term baby's protective metabolic systems are not fully developed for the first week of life, so they may not be able to handle chemicals in the milk as well as a baby who is several months old).
- **The frequency and volume of feedings** (the baby who is nursing once or twice a day, and is supplemented the rest of the time, will receive less of a drug than the baby who is totally breastfed and may nurse 10-12 times a day). Duration of drug therapy (a medication taken for weeks or months may have a greater impact on nursing than one taken for just a few days).
- **The type of medication** (characteristics such as the molecular weight, how fat soluble the drug is, and how long it takes for it to be eliminated from the system, or it's half-life, all affect how much of the drug is transferred into the milk).

GENERAL GUIDELINES FOR TAKING DRUGS WHILE NURSING

- Only take a medication if it is really needed. Consider alternative, non drug therapies if possible.
- If have a choice, delay starting the drug until the baby is older. A drug which might cause problems for a newborn may be

fine for an older, larger, more mature infant.

- Take the lowest possible dose for the shortest possible time.
- Avoid drugs with long-half lives, sustained-release preparations, or high M/P (milk to blood) ratio. If the M/P ratio is one or higher, that means that more of it is transferred into the milk.
- Schedule the doses so that the lowest amount gets into the milk (take it soon after a feeding, preferably a night feeding, rather than right before nursing).
- Watch for reactions such as sleepiness, rashes, diarrhea, colic, etc. Although reactions are rare, it is important to keep the doctor informed of any changes.
- If have to take a drug that is contraindicated, and no alternatives are available, get a good electric pump to maintain the milk supply if need to wean for more than a day or two. The supply will build up when the baby starts nursing again.

Table 83.1

Drugs often used during lactation and possible effects on the nursing infant

Drug	Effect on Infant	Comments
Ampicillin	Minimal	No significant adverse effects: possible occurrence of diarrhea or allergic sensitization.
Aspirin	Minimal	Occasional doses probably safe: high doses may produce significant concentration in breast milk.
Caffeine	Minimal	Caffeine intake in moderation is safe: concentration in breast milk is about 1% of total dose taken by mother.
Chloral hydrate	Significant	May cause drowsiness if infant is fed at peak concentration in milk.
Chloramphenicol	Significant	Concentrations too low to cause grey baby syndrome: possibility of bone marrow suppression does exist: recommend not taking chlorampheni-col while breast-feeding.
Chlorothiazide	Minimal	No adverse effects reported.
Chlorpromazine	Minimal	Appears insignificant.
Codeine	Minimal	Safe in most cases. Neonatal toxicity described when the mother is ultra rapid 2D6 metabolizer, producing substantially more morphine from codeine.
Diazepam	Significant	Will cause sedation in breast-fed infants: accumulation can occur in newborns.
Dicumarol	Minimal	No adverse side effects reported: may wish to follow infant's prothrombin time.
Digoxin	Minimal	Insignificant quantities enter breast milk.
Ethanol	Moderate	Moderate ingestion by mother unlikely to produce effects in infant: large amounts consumed by mother can produce alcohol effects in infant.
Heroin	Significant	Enters breast milk and can prolong neonatal narcotic dependence.

Table 83.1 ***Contd...***

Drug	Effect on Infant	Comments
Iodine (radioactive)	Significant	Enters milk in quantities sufficient to cause thyroid suppression in infant.
Isoniazid (INH)	Minimal	Milk concentrations equal maternal plasma concentrations. Possibility of pyridoxine deficiency developing in the infant.
Kanamycin	Minimal	No adverse effects reported.
Lithium	Significant	Mother should avoid breast-feeding unless levels can be measured.
Methadone	Significant	(See heroin.) Under close physician super-vision, breast-feeding can be continued. Signs of opioid withdrawal in the infant may occur if mother stops taking methadone or stops breast-feeding abruptly.
Oral contraceptives	Minimal	May suppress lactation in high doses.
Penicillin	Minimal	Very low concentrations in breast milk.
Phenobarbital	Moderate	Hypnotic doses can cause sedation in the infant.
Phenytoin	Moderate	Amounts entering breast milk are not sufficient to cause adverse effects in infant.
Prednisone	Moderate	Low maternal doses (5 mg/d) probably safe. Doses 2 or more times physiologic amounts (> 15 mg/d) should probably be avoided.
Propranolol	Minimal	Very small amounts enter breast milk.
Propylthiouracil	Significant	Can suppress thyroid function in infant.
Spironolactone	Minimal	Very small amounts enter breast milk.
Tetracycline	Moderate	Possibility of permanent staining of developing teeth in the infant. Should be avoided during lactation.
Theophylline	Moderate	Can enter breast milk in moderate quantities but not likely to produce significant effects.
Thyroxine	Minimal	No adverse effects in therapeutic doses.
Tolbutamide	Minimal	Low concentrations in breast milk.
Warfarin	Minimal	Very small quantities found in breast milk.

- Most antibiotics taken by nursing mothers can be detected in breast milk. Tetracycline concentrations in breast milk are approximately 70% of maternal serum concentrations and present a risk of permanent tooth staining in the infant. Isoniazid rapidly reaches equilibrium between breast milk and maternal blood. The concentrations achieved in breast milk are high enough so that signs of pyridoxine deficiency may occur in the infant if the mother is not given pyridoxine supplements.
- Most sedatives and hypnotics achieve concentrations in breast milk sufficient to produce a pharmacologic effect in some infants. Barbiturates taken in hypnotic doses by the mother can produce lethargy, sedation, and poor suck reflexes in the infant. Chloral hydrate can produce sedation if the infant is fed at peak milk concentrations. Diazepam can have a sedative effect on the nursing infant, but, most importantly, its long half-life can result in significant drug accumulation.

- Opioids such as heroin, methadone, and morphine enter breast milk in quantities potentially sufficient to prolong the state of neonatal narcotic dependence if the drug was taken chronically by the mother during pregnancy. If conditions are well controlled and there is a good relationship between the mother and the physician, an infant could be breast-fed while the mother is taking methadone. She should not, however, stop taking the drug abruptly: the infant can be tapered off the methadone as the mother's dose is tapered. The infant should be watched for signs of narcotic withdrawal. Although codeine has been believed to be safe, a recent case of neonatal death from opioid toxicity revealed that the mother was an ultra rapid metabolizer of cytochrome 2D6 substrates, producing substantially higher amounts of morphine. Hence, polymorphism in maternal drug metabolism may affect neonatal exposure and safety.
- Minimal use of alcohol by the mother has not been reported to harm nursing infants. Excessive amounts of alcohol, however, can produce alcohol effects in the infant. Nicotine concentrations in the breast milk of smoking mothers are low and do not produce effects in the infant. Very small amounts of caffeine are excreted in the breast milk of coffee-drinking mothers.
- Lithium enters breast milk in concentrations equal to those in maternal serum. Clearance of this drug is almost completely dependent upon renal elimination, and women who are receiving lithium may expose the infant to relatively large amounts of the drug.
- Radioactive substances such as iodinated ^{125}I albumin and radioiodine can cause thyroid suppression in infants and may increase the risk of subsequent thyroid cancer as much as tenfold. Breast-feeding is contraindicated after large doses and should be withheld for days to weeks after small doses. Similarly, breast-feeding should be avoided in mothers receiving cancer chemotherapy or being treated with cytotoxic or immune-modulating agents for collagen diseases such as lupus erythematous or after organ transplantation.

REFERENCES

1. Benitz WE, Tatro DS: *The Pediatric Drug Handbook,* 3rd ed. Year Book, 1995.
2. Bennett PN: *Drugs and Human Lactation,* 2nd ed. Elsevier, 1996.
3. Briggs GG, Freeman RK, Yaffe SJ: *Drugs in Pregnancy and Lactation. A Reference Guide to Fetal and Neonatal Risk,* 6th ed. Williams & Wilkins, 2002.
4. Koren G: *Medication Safety during Pregnancy and Breastfeeding: A Clinician's Guide,* 4th ed. McGraw Hill, 2006.

CHAPTER 84

Leukemia

DEFINITION

The word Leukemia comes from the Greek *leukos* which means "white" and *aima* which means "blood". It is cancer of the blood or bone marrow (which produces blood cells). A person who has leukemia suffers from an abnormal production of blood cells, generally leukocytes (white blood cells).

PREVALENCE

According to the Leukemia and Lymphoma Society, there were approximately 13,410 new cases of AML (2007), 5,200 new cases of ACL (2007), 4,570 cases of CML (2007), and 15,110 new cases of CLL (2008) diagnosed in the USA.

ETIOLOGY

Experts say that different leukemia's have different causes. The following are either known causes, or strongly suspected causes:

- Artificial ionizing radiation
- Viruses-HTLV-1 (human T-lymphotropic virus) and HIV (human immunodeficiency virus)
- Benzene and some petrochemicals
- Alkylating chemotherapy agents used in previous cancers
- Maternal fetal transmission (rare)
- Hair dyes
- Genetic predisposition - Some studies researching family history and looking at twins have indicated that some people have a higher risk of developing leukemia because of a single gene or multiple genes.
- Down syndrome - People with Down syndrome have a significantly higher risk of developing leukemia, compared to people who do not have Down syndrome. Experts say that because of this, people with certain chromosomal abnormalities may have a higher risk.
- Electromagnetic energy - Studies indicate there is not enough evidence to show that ELF magnetic (not electric) fields that exist currently might cause leukemia. The International Agency for Research on Cancer (IARC) says that studies which indicate there is a risk tend to be biased and unreliable.

PATHOPHYSIOLOGY

The DNA of immature blood cells, mainly white cells, becomes damaged in some way. This abnormality causes the blood cells to grow and divide chaotically. Normal blood cells die after a while and are replaced by new cells which are produced in the bone marrow. The abnormal blood cells do not die so easily, and accumulate, occupying more and more space. As more and more space is occupied by these faulty blood cells there is less and less space for the normal cells - and the sufferer becomes ill. Quite simply, the bad cells crowd out the good cells in the blood.

CLASSIFICATION

Chronic and Acute: Experts divide leukemia into four large groups, each of which can be *Acute*, which is a rapidly progressing disease that results in the accumulation of immature, useless cells in the marrow and blood, or *Chronic*, which progresses more slowly and allows more mature, useful cells to be made. In other words, *acute* leukemia crowds out the good cells more quickly than *chronic* leukemia.

Lymphocytic and Myelogenous: Leukemia's are also subdivided into the type of affected blood cell. If the cancerous transformation occurs in the type of marrow that makes lymphocytes, the disease is called *lymphocytic leukemia*. A lymphocyte is a kind of white blood cell inside your vertebrae immune system. If the cancerous change occurs in the type of marrow cells that go on to produce red blood cells, other types of white cells, and platelets, the disease is called *myelogenous leukemia*. To recap, there are two groups of two groups - four main types of leukemia, as you can see in the illustration below:

Acute Lymphocytic Leukemia (ALL) also known as Acute Lymphoblastic Leukemia - This is the most common type of leukemia among young children, although adults can get it as well, especially those over the age of 65. Survival rates of at least five years range from 85% among children and 50% among adults. The following are all subtypes of this leukemia: precursor B acute lymphoblastic leukemia, precursor T acute lymphoblastic leukemia, Burkitt's leukemia, and acute biphenotypic leukemia.

Chronic Lymphocytic Leukemia (CLL): This is most common among adults over 55, although younger adults can get it as well. CLL hardly ever affects children. The majority of patients with CLL are men, over 60%. 75% of treated CLL patients survive for over five years. Experts say CLL is incurable. A more aggressive form of CLL is B-cell prolymphocytic leukemia.

Acute Myelogenous Leukemia (AML)

ML is more common among adults than children, and affects males significantly more often than females. Patients are treated with chemotherapy. 40% of treated patients survive for over 5 years. The following are subtypes of AMS - acute promyelocytic leukemia, acute myeloblastic leukemia, and acute megakaryoblastic leukemia.

Chronic Myelogenous Leukemia (CML)

The vast majority of patients are adults. 90% of treated patients survive for over 5 years. Gleevec (imatinib) is commonly used to treat CML, as well as some other drugs. Chronic monocytic leukemia is a subtype of CML.

CLINICAL FEATURES (FIG. 84.1)

- Blood clotting is poor - As immature white blood cells crowd out blood platelets, which are crucial for blood clotting, the patient may bruise or bleed easily and heal slowly - he may also develop petechiae (a small red to purple spot on the body, caused by a minor hemorrhage).
- Affected immune system - The patient's white blood cells, which are crucial for fighting off infection, may be suppressed or not working properly. The patient may experience frequent infections, or his immune system may attack other good body cells.
- Anemia - As the shortage of good red blood cells grows the patient may suffer from anemia - this may lead to difficult or labored respiration (dyspnea) and pallor (skin has a pale color caused by illness).
- Other symptoms - Patients may also experience nausea, fever, chills, night sweats, flu-like symptoms, and tiredness. If the liver or spleen becomes enlarged the patient may feel full and will eat less, resulting in weight loss. Headache is more common among patients whose cancerous cells have invaded the CNS (central nervous system).

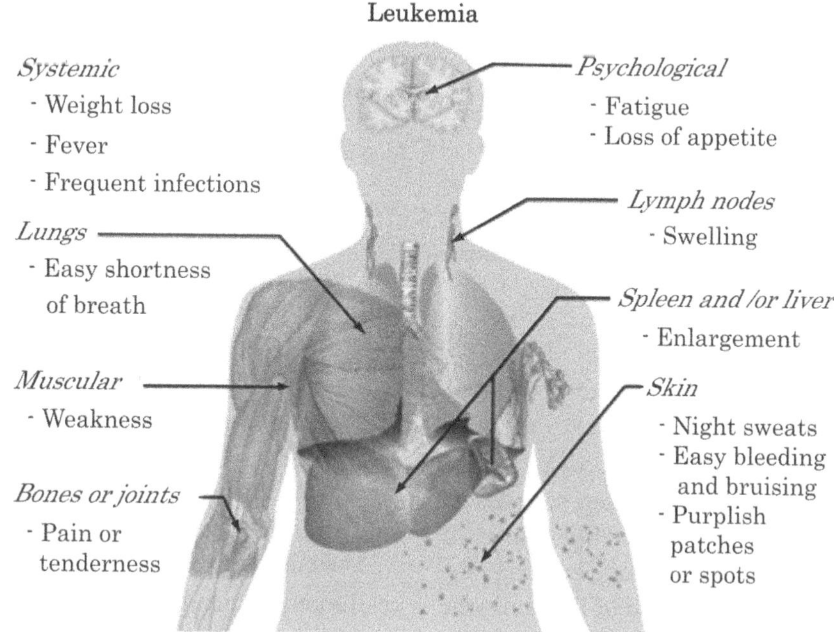

FIGURE 84.1

Clinical features of leukemia.

(source : MedicineNet.com Leukemia (cont.), Symptoms Retrieved on November 3, 2009)

DIAGNOSIS

- **Physical exam:** Check for swollen lymph nodes, spleen, or liver.
- **Blood tests:** Complete blood count was performed to check the number of white blood cells, red blood cells, and platelets. Leukemia causes a very high level of white blood cells. It may also cause low levels of platelets and hemoglobin, which is found inside red blood cells.
  - **Biopsy**: A tissue was removed to observe for cancer cells. A biopsy is the only sure way to know whether leukemia cells are in the bone marrow. Before the sample is taken, local anesthesia is used to numb the area. This helps reduce the pain A pathologist uses a microscope to check the tissue for leukemia cells. There are two ways to obtain bone marrow.
  - **Bone marrow aspiration**: The doctor uses a thick, hollow needle to remove samples of bone marrow.
  - **Bone marrow biopsy**: The doctor uses a very thick, hollow needle to remove a small piece of bone and bone marrow.

OTHER TESTS

The tests depend on your symptoms and type of leukemia.

- **Cytogenetics:** The lab looks at the chromosomes of cells from samples of blood, bone marrow, or lymph nodes. If abnormal chromosomes are found, the test can show what type of leukemia the person have. For example, people with CML have an abnormal chromosome called the Philadelphia chromosome.
- **Spinal tap:** Some of the cerebrospinal fluid (the fluid that fills the spaces in and around the brain and spinal cord) will be removed using a long, thin needle to remove fluid from the lower spine. The procedure takes about 30 minutes and is performed with local anesthesia. Person must lie flat for several hours afterward to keep from getting a headache. The lab checks the fluid for leukemia cells or other signs of problems.
- **Chest X-ray:** An X-ray can show swollen lymph nodes or other signs of disease in the chest.

TREATMENT FOR LEUKEMIA

Leukemia is not a single disease. Instead, the term leukemia refers to a number of related cancers that start in the blood-forming cells of the bone marrow. There are both acute and chronic forms of leukemia, each with many subtypes that vary in their response to treatment. In addition, children with leukemia have special needs that are best met by care in pediatric cancer centers.

Leukemia treatment plans often are personalized and geared toward each individual patient. In general, there are five major approaches to the treatment of leukemia:

1. Chemotherapy to kill leukemia cells using strong anti-cancer drugs;
2. Interferon therapy to slow the reproduction of leukemia cells and promote the immune system's anti-leukemia activity;
3. Radiation therapy to kill cancer cells by exposure to high-energy radiation;
4. Stem cell transplantation (SCT) to enable treatment with high doses of chemotherapy and radiation therapy; and

5. Surgery to remove an enlarged spleen or to install a venous access device (large plastic tube) to give medications and withdraw blood samples.

ACUTE LYMPHOBLASTIC

Management of ALL focuses on control of bone marrow and systemic (whole-body) disease. Additionally, treatment must prevent leukemic cells from spreading to other sites, particularly the central nervous system (CNS) e.g. monthly lumbar punctures. In general, ALL treatment is divided into several phases:

- *Induction chemotherapy* to bring about bone marrow remission. For adults, standard induction plans include prednisone, vincristine, and an anthracycline drug; other drug plans may include L-asparaginaze or cyclophosphamide. For children with low-risk ALL, standard therapy usually consists of three drugs (prednisone, L-asparaginaze, and vincristine) for the first month of treatment.
- *Consolidation therapy* or *intensification therapy* to eliminate any remaining leukemia cells. There are many different approaches to consolidation, but it is typically a high-dose, multi-drug treatment that is undertaken for a few months. Patients with low to average risk ALL receive therapy with antimetabolite drugs such as methotrexate and 6-mercaptopurine (6-MP). High-risk patients receive higher drug doses of these drugs, plus additional drugs.
- *CNS prophylaxis* (preventive therapy) to stop the cancer from spreading to the brain and nervous system in high-risk patients. Standard prophylaxis may include radiation of the head and/or drugs delivered directly into the spine.
- *Maintenance treatments* with chemotherapeutic drugs to prevent disease recurrence once remission has been achieved. Maintenance therapy usually involves lower drug doses, and may continue for up to three years.
- Alternatively, *allogeneic bone marrow transplantation* may be appropriate for high-risk or relapsed patients.

CHRONIC LYMPHOCYTIC

Hematologists base CLL treatment on both the stage and symptoms of the individual patient. A large group of CLL patients have low-grade disease, which does not benefit from treatment. Individuals with CLL-related complications or more advanced disease often benefit from treatment. In general, the indications for treatment are:

- Falling hemoglobin or platelet count
- Progression to a later stage of disease
- Painful, disease-related overgrowth of lymph nodes or spleen
- An increase in the rate of lymphocyte production

TYPICAL TREATMENT APPROACH

CLL is probably incurable by present treatments. The primary chemotherapeutic plan is combination chemotherapy with **chlorambucil or cyclophosphamide**, plus a corticosteroid such as prednisone or **prednisolone**. The use of a corticosteroid has the additional benefit of suppressing some related autoimmune diseases, such as immunohemolytic anemia or immune-mediated thrombocytopenia. In resistant cases, single-agent treatments with nucleoside drugs such as **Fludarabine, Pentostatin, or Cladribine** may be successful. Younger patients may consider allogeneic or autologous bone marrow transplantation.

ACUTE MYELOGENOUS

Many different anti-cancer drugs are effective for the treatment of AML. Treatments vary somewhat according to the age of the patient and according to the specific subtype of AML. Overall, the strategy is to control bone marrow and systemic (whole-body) disease, while offering specific treatment for the central nervous system (CNS), if involved.

In general, most oncologists rely on combinations of drugs for the initial, *induction phase* of chemotherapy. Such combination chemotherapy usually offers the benefits of early remission and a lower risk of disease resistance. *Consolidation* and *maintenance* treatments are intended to prevent disease recurrence. Consolidation treatment often entails a repetition of induction chemotherapy or the intensification chemotherapy with additional drugs. By contrast, maintenance treatment involves drug doses that are lower than those administered during the induction phase.

CHRONIC MYELOGENOUS

There are many possible treatments for CML, but the standard of care for newly diagnosed patients is **Imatinib** (Gleevec) therapy. Compared to most anti-cancer drugs, it has relatively few side effects and can be taken orally at home. With this drug, more than 90% of patients will be able to keep the disease in check for at least five years, so that CML becomes a chronic, manageable condition.

In a more advanced, uncontrolled state, when the patient cannot tolerate imatinib, or if the patient wishes to attempt a permanent cure, then an allogeneic bone marrow transplantation may be performed. This procedure involves high-dose chemotherapy and radiation followed by infusion of bone marrow from a compatible donor. Approximately 30% of patients die from this procedure.

T-CELL PROLYMPHOCYTIC

Most patients with T-cell prolymphocytic leukemia, a rare and aggressive leukemia with a median survival of less than one year, require immediate treatment.

T-cell prolymphocytic leukemia is difficult to treat, and it does not respond to most available chemotherapeutic drugs. Many different treatments have been attempted, with limited success in certain patients: purine analogues (**pentostatin, fludarabine, cladribine**, **chlorambucil**), and various forms of combination chemotherapy (**cyclophosphamide, doxorubicin, vincristine, prednisone CHOP, Cyclophosphamide, vincristine, prednisone [COP], vincristine, doxorubicin, prednisone, etoposide, Cyclophosphamide, bleomycin VAPEC-B**). **Alemtuzumab** (Campath), a monoclonal antibody that attacks white blood cells, has been used in treatment with greater success than previous options.

Some patients who successfully respond to treatment also undergo stem cell transplantation to consolidate the response.

JUVENILE MYELOMONOCYTIC

Treatment for juvenile myelomonocytic leukemia can include splenectomy, chemotherapy, and bone marrow transplantation.

INTERFERON THERAPY TO TREAT LEUKEMIA

Interferons are a class of proteins that are released by virus-infected cells. They help normal cells to make antiviral proteins. Interferon's also help the body to reduce leukemia cell proliferation (growth and reproduction), while strengthening the body's immune response.

Interferon-alpha (INFα) is a type of interferon that frequently is used to treat leukemia. In addition, based on an patient's response to INFα, a physician can better predict the anticipated length of survival.

Interferon-alpha can be given by a number of methods—that is, by injection into a vein, into a muscle, or under the skin—although subcutaneous (under the skin) injection is the customary route. INF-α usually is offered to all newly diagnosed patients who are not candidates for stem cell transplantation. Often IFN-α is started at a low dose (e.g., 3 MIU daily), with gradual increases over time. Unfortunately, though, this drug is not without side effects. Possible IFN-related complaints include fevers, chills, muscle aches, bone pain, headaches, concentration difficulties, fatigue, nausea, vomiting, and general flu-like symptoms when starting the drug. Such symptoms usually last for 1 to 2 weeks, but may be lessened by drugs such as acetaminophen. Side effects recur if the INF-α dosage is increased, but they are temporary and usually improve after INF-α therapy is completed.

REFERENCES

1. Leukemia, in Mosby's Medical, Nursing &Allied Health Dictionary, Fourth Edition, Mosby-Yearbook, Inc.,1994, p. 903
2. Colvin GA, Elfenbein GJ (2003). "The latest treatment advances for acute myelogenous leukemia". *Med Health R I* **86** (8): 243–6.
3. American Cancer Society (2010). "How is Leukemia Diagnosed?". *Detailed Guide: Leukemia - Adult Chronic*. American Cancer Society. Retrieved 4 May 2010.
4. "Do We Know What Causes Leukemia". *Detailed Guide: Leukemia*. American Cancer Society. 2010. Retrieved 18 May 2010.[dead link]
5. Stass, Sanford A.; Schumacher, Harold R.; Rock, William R. (2000). *Handbook of hematologic pathology*. New York, N.Y: Marcel Dekker. pp. 193–194.
6. Leonard, Barry (1998). *Leukemia: A Research Report*. DIANE Publishing. p. 14.
7. Eichhorst BF, Busch R, Hopfinger G, Pasold R, Hensel M, Steinbrecher C, Siehl S, Jäger U, Bergmann M, Stilgenbauer S, Schweighofer C, Wendtner CM, Döhner H, Brittinger G, Emmerich B, Hallek M, German CLL Study Group. (2006). "Fludarabine plus cyclophosphamide versus fludarabine alone in first-line therapy of younger patients with chronic lymphocytic leukemia". *Blood* **107** (3): 885–91.
8. Gribben JG (January 2008). "Stem cell transplantation in chronic lymphocytic leukemia". *Biol. Blood Marrow Transplant.* **15** (1 Suppl): 53–8.
9. American Cancer Society (6 July 2009). "Typical Treatment of Acute Myeloid Leukemia". *Detailed Guide: Leukemia - Acute Myeloid (AML)*. American Cancer Society. Retrieved 4 May 2010.
10. Fausel C (October 2007). "Targeted chronic myeloid leukemia therapy: seeking a cure". *J Manag Care Pharm* **13** (8 Suppl A): 8–12.

CHAPTER 85

Lymphoma

DEFINITION

Lymphomas are a heterogenous group of malignancies that arise from immune cells residing predominantly in lymphoid tissues. Differences in histology have led to classification as Hodgkin's and non-Hodgkin's lymphoma (HL and NHL, respectively).

PREVALENCE

Lymphoma is the most common form of haematological malignancy, or "blood cancer", in the developed world. Taken together, lymphomas represent 5.3% of all cancers (excluding simple basal cell and squamous cell skin cancers) in the United States and 55.6% of all blood cancers. According to the U.S. National Institutes of Health, lymphomas account for about 5% of all cases of cancer in the United States, and Hodgkin's lymphoma in particular accounts for less than 1% of all cases of cancer in the United States. Because the whole system is part of the body's immune system, patients with a weakened immune system such as from HIV infection or from certain drugs or medication also have a higher incidence of lymphoma.

HODGKIN'S LYMPHOMA

ETIOLOGY

The first sign of Hodgkin's lymphoma is often a swollen lymph node, which appears without a known cause. The disease can spread to nearby lymph nodes. Later it may spread to the spleen, liver, bone marrow, or other organs.

The cause is not known. Hodgkin's lymphoma is most common among people ages 15 - 35 and 50 - 70. Past infection with the Epstein-Barr virus (EBV) is thought to contribute to some cases. Patients with HIV infection are more at risk than the general population.

PATHOPHYSIOLOGY

- Current hypotheses indicate that B-cell transcriptional processes are disrupted, which prevent expression of B-cell surface markers and production of immunoglobulin messenger RNA. Alterations in the normal apoptotic pathways favour cell survival and proliferation.
- Malignant Reed-Sternberg cells over express nuclear factor-κ B, which is associated with cell proliferation and anti-

apoptotic signals. Infections with viral and bacterial pathogens up regulate nuclear factor-κ B. Epstein- Barr virus is found in many, but not all, HL tumours.

CLINICAL FEATURES

- Most patients with HL present with a painless, rubbery lymph node. Adenopathy is usually localized to the cervical region but can also occur in the mediastinal, hilar, and retroperitoneal regions.
- Constitutional, or "B," symptoms (e.g., fever, night sweats, weight loss, and pruritus) are present at diagnosis in approximately 25% of patients with HL.

DIAGNOSIS

- Diagnosis requires the presence of Reed-Sternberg cells in the lymph node biopsy.
- Staging is performed to provide prognostic information and to guide therapy. Clinical staging is based on non-invasive procedures such as history, physical examination, laboratory tests, and radiography. Pathologic staging is based on biopsy findings of strategic sites (e.g., muscle, bone, skin, spleen, abdominal nodes) using an invasive procedure (e.g., laparoscopy).
- Approximately half of the patients have localized disease (stages I, II, and IIE). The other half has advanced disease at diagnosis, of which 10% to 15% is stage IV.
- Prognosis predominantly depends on age and stage; patients older than 65 to 70 years are 50% as likely to be cured as younger patients. Patients with limited stage disease (stages I to II) have a 90% to 95% cure rate, whereas those with advanced disease (stages III to IV) have a 65% to 75% cure rate.

TREATMENT SUMMARY

- The treatment goal for HL is to maximize curability while minimizing treatment-related complications.
- Treatment options include radiation therapy, chemotherapy, or both (combined- modality therapy). The therapeutic role of surgery is limited, regardless of stage.
- Combination chemotherapy is the primary treatment modality for most HL patients.
- Radiation therapy is an integral part of treatment and can be used alone for selected patients with early-stage disease, although most patients will receive chemotherapy and radiation. Involved-field radiation therapy targets a single field of HL. Extended-field or subtotal nodal radiation targets the involved field and an uninvolved area. Total nodal radiation therapy targets all areas.
- Long-term complications of radiotherapy, chemotherapy, and chemoradiotherapy include gonadal dysfunction, secondary malignancies, and cardiac disease. Patients treated for HL are at increased risk of developing leukemia, GI tumours, lung cancer, and breast cancer.

INITIAL CHEMOTHERAPY

- Two to eight cycles of chemotherapy should be administered, depending on the stage of disease and presence of risk factors.

SALVAGE CHEMOTHERAPY

- Response to salvage therapy depends on the extent and site of recurrence, previous therapy, and duration of first remission. Choice of salvage therapy should be guided by response to initial therapy and a patient's ability to tolerate therapy.
- Patients who relapse after an initial complete response can be treated with the same regimen, a non–cross-resistant regimen, radiation therapy, or high dose chemotherapy and autologous hematopoietic stem cell transplantation (HSCT).
- Lack of complete remission after initial therapy or relapse within one year after completing initial therapy is associated with poor prognosis. Patients with these prognostic factors are candidates for high-dose chemotherapy and HSCT.

NON-HODGKIN'S LYMPHOMA

PATHOPHYSIOLOGY

- Chromosomal translocations have become a hallmark of many lymphomas and are helpful in the diagnosis and classification of lymphoid malignancies. NHL often involves extranodal sites and does not spread through contiguous lymph nodes.
- NHLs are derived from monoclonal proliferation of B or, less commonly lymphocytes and their precursors. Two categories of B- and T-cell neoplasm's are "precursor" neoplasm's corresponding to the earliest stages of differentiation, and "peripheral" neoplasm's corresponding to the more differentiated cell stages.

CLINICAL FEATURES

- Patients present with a variety of symptoms, which depend on the site of involvement and whether it is nodal or extranodal.
- Adenopathy can be localized or generalized. Involved nodes are painless, rubbery, and discrete and are usually located in the cervical and supraclavicular regions. Mesenteric or GI involvement can cause nausea, vomiting, obstruction, abdominal pain, palpable abdominal mass, or GI bleeding. Bone marrow involvement can cause symptoms related to anemia, neutropenia, or thrombocytopenia.
- 40% of patients with NHL present with B symptoms—fever, night sweats, and weight loss.

DIAGNOSIS AND STAGING

- Diagnosis is established by biopsy of an involved lymph node.
- Diagnostic workup of NHL is generally similar to that of HL.
- Systems for classifying NHLs continue to evolve. Lymphomas can be classified by degree of aggressiveness. Slow-growing or indolent lymphomas are favourable (untreated survival measured in years), whereas rapid growing or aggressive lymphomas are unfavourable (untreated survival measured in weeks to months).
- Prognosis depends on histologic subtype and clinical risk factors (e.g., age more than 60 years, performance status of 2 or more, elevated lactic dehydrogenaze, extranodal involvement, and stage III or

IV disease). These risk factors are used to calculate the International Prognostic Index.

- A newer prognostic index uses similar risk factors except that poor performance status is replaced with low haemoglobin (less than 12 g/dl). Current research is focused on the prognostic importance of phenotypic and molecular characteristics of NHL.

TREATMENT

GENERAL PRINCIPLES

- Appropriate therapy for NHL depends on many factors including patient age, histologic type, stage and site of disease, presence of adverse prognostic factors, and patient preference.
- Treatment is divided into two categories: limited disease (e.g., localized disease; Ann Arbor stages I and II) and advanced disease (e.g., Ann Arbor stage III or IV and stage II patients with poor prognostic features).
- Treatment options include radiation therapy, chemotherapy, and biologic agents.
- Radiation therapy is rarely suitable for remission induction because NHL is rarely localized at diagnosis. Radiation therapy is used more commonly in advanced disease, mainly as a palliative measure.
- Effective chemotherapy ranges from single-agent therapy for indolent lymphomas to aggressive, complex combination regimens for aggressive lymphomas. Paradoxically, indolent or favourable lymphomas are rarely curable, whereas aggressive or unfavourable lymphomas are potentially curable.
- Treatment strategies are summarized for the most common NHLs as examples of how to treat indolent (i.e., follicular) and aggressive (i.e., diffuse large B-cell) lymphomas. Strategies are also summarized for acquired immune deficiency syndrome (AIDS)–related lymphoma.

INDOLENT LYMPHOMAS

- Follicular lymphomas occur in older adults with a majority having advanced disease at diagnosis. The clinical course is generally indolent, with median survival of 8 to 10 years. The natural history of follicular lymphoma is unpredictable with spontaneous regression of objective disease seen in 20 % to 30 % of patients.

LOCALIZED FOLLICULAR LYMPHOMA

- Options for stage I and II follicular lymphoma include locoregional radiation therapy, chemotherapy followed by radiation therapy, and extended-field radiation therapy.
- Radiation therapy is the standard treatment and is usually curative. Chemotherapy is not recommended, unless the patient has high-risk, stage II disease.

ADVANCED FOLLICULAR LYMPHOMA

- Management of stages III and IV indolent lymphoma is controversial because standard approaches are not curative. Time to relapse is only 18 to 36 months. After relapse, response can be reinduced; however, response rates and durations decrease with each retreatment.

- Therapeutic options are diverse and include watchful waiting, single-agent therapy, combination chemotherapy, biologic therapy, radio immunotherapy, and combined-modality therapy. Immediate aggressive therapy does not improve survival compared with conservative therapy (i.e., watchful waiting followed by single-agent chemotherapy, rituximab or radiation therapy, only when needed).
- Oral alkylating agents, chlorambucil, 0.1 to 0.2 mg/kg, or cyclophosphamide, 1.5 to 2.5 mg/kg (adjusted to white blood cell and platelet counts), are the mainstay of treatment. These single agents are as effective as combination regimens and produce minimal toxicity, but secondary acute myelogenous leukemia (AML) is a concern. Fludarabine and cladribine produce high response rates without secondary AML, but they are more myelosuppressive.
- Rituximab, a chimeric monoclonal antibody directed at the CD20 molecule on B cells, has become one of the most widely used therapies for follicular lymphoma. Rituximab is approved for first-line therapy either alone or combined with chemotherapy and as maintenance therapy for patients with stable disease or with partial or complete response following induction chemotherapy.
- The rituximab dosage is 375 mg/m^2 weekly for 4 weeks. Maintenance schedules include 375 mg/m2 weekly for 4 weeks every 6 months for 2 years or 375 mg/m2 every 2 to 3 months for 1 to 2 years.
- Adverse effects are usually infusion related, especially after the first infusion of rituximab. Adverse effects include fever, chills, respiratory symptoms, fatigue, headache, pruritus, and angioedema. Patients should receive acetaminophen, 650 mg, and diphenhydramine, 50 mg, 30 minutes before the infusion.
- Anti-CD20 radioimmunoconjugates are mouse antibodies linked to radioisotopes (e.g., 131 I-tositumomab and 90 Y-ibritumomab tiuxetan). They have the advantage of delivering radiation to tumour cells expressing the CD20 antigen and to adjacent tumour cells that do not express it. They have the disadvantage of damaging adjacent normal tissue (e.g., bone marrow).
- Radioimmunotherapy was initially used as salvage therapy and is being evaluated as first-line therapy in combination with CHOP (cyclophosphamids, doxorubicin, vincristine, and prednisone).
- Radioimmunotherapy is generally well tolerated. Toxicities include infusion-related reactions, myelosuppression, and possibly myelodysplastic syndrome or AML.131_I-tositumomab can cause thyroid dysfunction.
- The decision to use radioimmunotherapy requires consideration of the complexity, risks, and cost. The ideal candidate has limited bone marrow involvement and adequate blood cell counts.
- High-dose chemotherapy followed by HSCT is an option for relapsed follicular lymphoma. The recurrence rate is lower after allogeneic than after autologous HSCT, but the benefit is offset by increased treatment related mortality. The ideal candidate is young and does not have serious co morbidities.

AGGRESSIVE LYMPHOMAS

- Diffuse large B-cell lymphomas are the most common lymphoma in patients of all ages but most commonly seen in the seventh decade. Extranodal disease is present at diagnosis in 30% to 40% of patients.

EARLY-STAGE DIFFUSE LARGE B-CELL LYMPHOMA

- Stage I and nonbulky stage II should be treated with three to four cycles of Rituximab and CHOP (R-CHOP) followed by locoregional radiation therapy.
- Patients with at least one adverse risk factor should receive six to eight cycles of R-CHOP followed by locoregional radiation therapy.

LYMPHOMA DISEASE

- Bulky stage II and stages III and IV lymphoma should be treated with RCHOP or rituximab and CHOP-like chemotherapy until achieving complete response (usually four cycles). Two or more additional cycles should be given following complete response for a total of six to eight cycles. Maintenance therapy following a complete response does not improve survival.
- High-dose chemotherapy with autologous HSCT should be considered in high-risk patients who respond to standard chemotherapy and are candidates for autologous HSCT.

SALVAGE THERAPY FOR AGGRESSIVE LYMPHOMA

- Approximately one-third of patients with aggressive lymphoma will require salvage therapy at some point. Salvage therapy is more likely to induce response if the response to initial chemotherapy was complete (chemosensitivity) than if it was primarily or partially resistant to chemotherapy.
- High-dose chemotherapy with autologous HSCT is the therapy of choice for younger patients with chemosensitive relapse.
- Salvage regimens incorporate drugs not used as initial therapy. Commonly used regimens include DHAP (dexamethasone, high-dose cytarabine, and cisplatin), ESHAP (etoposide, methylprednisolone, high-dose cytarabine, and cisplatin), and MINE (mesna, ifosfamide, mitoxantrone, and etoposide). None is clearly superior to the others.
- ICE (ifosfamide, carboplatin, and etoposide) appears to be better tolerated than cisplatin-containing regimens, especially in elderly adults.
- Rituximab is being evaluated in combination with many salvage regimens.

REFERENCES

1. Horning SJ. Hodgkin's lymphoma. In: Abeloff MD, Armitage JO, Niederhuber JE, Kastan MB, Mckena WG, eds. *Clinical Oncology*. 4th ed. Philadelphia, Pa: Elsevier Churchill Livingstone; 2008:chap 111.
2. Armitage JO. Early-stage Hodgkin's lymphoma. *N Engl J Med*. 2010 Aug 12;363(7):653-62.
3. Ziegler JL, et al. Non-Hodgkin's lymphoma in 90 homosexual men. Relation to generalized lymphadenopathy and the acquired immunodeficiency syndrome. N Engl J Med 1984;9:565-70.

CHAPTER 86

Breast Cancer

DEFINITION

Breast cancer is a malignancy originating from breast tissue.

EPIDEMIOLOGY

The strongest risk factors for breast cancer are female gender and increasing age. Additional risk factors include endocrine factors (e.g., early menarche, nulliparity, late age at first birth, hormone replacement therapy), genetic factors (e.g., personal and family history, mutations of tumor suppresser genes [*BRCA1*and *BRCA2*]), and environmental and lifestyle factors (e.g., radiation exposure).

Breast cancer cells often spread undetected by contiguity, lymph channels, and through the blood early in the course of the disease, resulting in metastatic disease after local therapy. The most common metastatic sites are lymph nodes, skin, bone, liver, lungs, and brain.

CLINICAL PRESENTATION

- Cysts may be developed which are the epithelial lined, fluid filled that occurs in glandular part of the breast as a part of breast involution.
- There may be musculoskeletal chest wall pain and cyclical breast pain in the persons suffering with breast cancer.
- The nipple discharge is present in few patients and various factors like the type of discharge, whether the discharge is spontaneous or not or is it troublesome.
- The other features includes the Benign nipple retraction which has a characteristic symmetrical appearance with a central horizontal slit.
- Alteration in breast size may be associated with malignancy due to tumor involvement of breast connective tissue. This may cause lumps and skin dimpling. It should be carefully monitored.
- Due to this there will be development of hard pink lump or ulceration in nipple . breast edema develops due to blockade of skin lymphatics by the breast cancer cells.

DIAGNOSIS

Breast cancer is mainly assessed by the combination of clinical, radiological, and pathological evaluation of a breast lesion.

CLINICAL EXAMINATION

Breast examination should be done in good light and examined by observing symmetry, inversion of nipple, skin changes and alteration in the contour of the breast. The chest wall muscles tensed and changes in the dynamic setting should be noted by raising the both arms. Tenderness of the chest should be examined, the patient is asked to be in sitting position the hand is pushed up behind the breast and the patient is asked to roll on other side so that edge of the pectoral muscle for palpitation is examined. The patient is asked for any discomfortness or any tenderness on chest wall palpitation.

IMAGING

MAMMOGRAPHY

In this study the breast is compressed between the two plates, oblique and craniocaudal view of the each breast are taken. Mass lesions, parenchymal distortions and micro-calcifications can be detected. It is not performed in the persons below 35yrs age because in younger women Breasts are relatively radiodense. Prior to surgery this test should be carried out for in assessing extent of disease. The introduction of digital technology offers opportunities in image manipulation, storage, and transmission.

ULTRASOUND

In this breast is exposed to high-frequency sound waves and those reflections detected are converted into images. It mainly depends upon the operator skill, equipment quality, but is having several advantages like safety, painless, and suitable for use in all ages. It is used for detecting only specific sites of breast but not the entire breast. It is not useful in all patients with an mammographic or palpable abnormality. In those with cancer, it is useful to guide core biopsy and assess size.

MAGNETIC RESONANCE IMAGING

In this study usage of powerful magnets to affect the hydrogen atoms behavior . It is expensive equipment and need specialist for operating. Invasive malignant breast lesions can be detected.

PATHOLOGICAL ASSESSMENT

FINE NEEDLE ASPIRATION CYTOLOGY

It involves usage of 21 or 23 gauge needle to obtain cells from suspected area and these are spread onto a microscope slide and observed for the changes. The result will be obtained in 45 min.

STAGING

The UICC (Union Internationale Contre le Cancre) TNM (Tumour/Node/Metastasis) classification is commonly used but is not ideally suited to breast cancer. (Table 86.1)

PATHOLOGICAL EVALUATION

- The development of malignancy is a multistep process with preinvasive (or noninvasive) and invasive phases. The goal of treatment for noninvasive carcinomas is to prevent the development of invasive disease.
- The pathologic evaluation of breast lesions establishes the histologic diagnosis and presence or absence of prognostic factors.
- Most breast carcinomas are adenocarcinomas and are classified as ductal or lobular.

Table 86.1

TNM staging

T – Primary tumour
TX-Primary tumour cannot be assessed
T0-No evidence of primary tumour
Tis Carcinoma *in situ*: intraductal carcinoma, or lobular carcinoma *in situ*, or Paget's disease of the nipple with no tumour
T1-Tumour 2 cm or less in greatest dimension
T1mic-Microinvasion 0.1 cm or less in greatest dimension
T1a-More than 0.1 cm but not more than 0.5 cm in greatest dimension
T1b-More than 0.5 cm but not more than 1 cm in greatest dimension
T1c-More than 1 cm but not more than 2 cm in greatest dimension
T2-Tumour more than 2 cm but not more than 5 cm in greatest dimension
T3-Tumour more than 5 cm in greatest dimension
T4-Tumour of any size with direct extension to chest wall or skin
T4a-Extension to chest wall wall (not including pectoralis muscle)
T4b-Oedema (including *peau d'orange*), or ulceration of the skin of the breast, or satellite skin nodules confined to the same breast
T4c-Both 4a and 4b, above
T4d-Inflammatory carcinoma

N – Regional lymph nodes
NX-Regional lymph nodes cannot be assessed (e.g. previously removed)
N0-No regional lymph node metastasis
N1-Metastasis to movable ipsilateral axillary node(s)
N2-Metastasis to ipsilateral axillary node(s) fixed to one another or to other structures, or clinically apparent ipsilateral internal mammary nodes in absence of axillary node metastasis
N2a Metastasis to ipsilateral axillary node(s) fixed to one another or to other structures
N2b Metastasis only in clinically apparent internal mammary nodes in absence of clinically evident axillary node metastasis
N3-Metastasis to ipsilateral infraclavicular node(s), or ipsilateral internal mammary lymph node(s) with axillary lymph node metastasis, or metastasis in ipsilateral supraclavicular node(s)
N3a-Metastasis in ipsilateral infraclavicular node(s)
N3b-Metastasis in ipsilateral internal mammary lymph node(s) and axillary lymph node(s)
N3c-Metastasis in ipsilateral supraclavicular node(s)

M – Distant metastasis
MX-Distant metastasis cannot be assessed
M0-No distant metastasis
M1-Distant metastasis

Summary of stages:

Stage 0	Carcinoma *in situ*
Stage I	Tumor (T) does not involve axillary lymph nodes (N)
Stage IIA	T 2–5 cm, N negative, or T <2 cm and N positive
Stage IIB	T >5 cm, N negative, or T 2–5 cm and N positive (<4 axillary nodes)
Stage IIIA	T >5 cm, N positive, or T 2–5 cm with 4 or more axillary nodes
Stage IIIB	T has penetrated chest wall or skin, and may have spread to <10 axillary nodes
Stage IIIC	T has >10 axillary nodes, 1 or more supraclavicular or infraclavicular nodes, or internal mammary nodes
Stage IV	Distant metastasis (M)

PROGNOSTIC FACTORS

- The ability to predict prognosis is used to design treatment recommendations to maximize quantity and quality of life.
- Tumor size and the presence and number of involved axillary lymph nodes are primary factors in assessing the risk for breast cancer recurrence and subsequent metastatic disease. Other disease characteristics that provide prognostic information include histologic subtype, nuclear or histologic grade, lymphatic and vascular invasion, and proliferation indices.
- Hormone receptors are used as indicators of prognosis and to predict response to hormone therapy.
- HER2/*neu* (HER2) overexpression is associated with transmission of growth signals that control aspects of normal cell growth and division. Overexpression of HER2 may be associated with a poor prognosis. HER2 status should be obtained for all invasive breast cancers.
- Genetic profiling tools provide additional prognostic information to aid in treatment decisions for subgroups of patients with otherwise favourable prognostic features.

TREATMENT

EARLY BREAST CANCER

Local-Regional Therapy

- Most of the patients suffering with breast cancer can be cured by surgery alone if it is diagnosed immediately.
- For most of the women suffering with stage I and stage II disease the Breast Conservation therapy is the appropriate one. To prevent local recurrence lumpectomy (i.e., excision of the primary tumor and adjacent breast tissue) followed by radiation therapy is a part of Breast-conserving therapy.
- To eradicate residual disease after BCT RT is administered over entire breast for 4 to 6 weeks. It results in minor complications like Reddening, erythema and shrinkage of total breast mass.
- The procedure of simple or total mastectomy includes the removal of the entire breast without disturbing underlying muscle or axillary nodes and is used mainly for carcinoma where axillary node involvement is only 1%.

SYSTEMIC ADJUVANT THERAPY

- It involves administration of systemic therapy followed by local therapy (surgery, radiation, or both) when there is no metastatic disease but there is a chance disease recurrence
- Disease-free survival and/or overall survival (OS) for all treated patients includes mainly chemotherapy, hormonal therapy, or both .
- Genetic tests are used as a support tools in decision making for Systemic Adjuvant Therapy in patients to identify primary tumour characteristics that may indicate the likelihood of metastases and death.

Adjuvant Chemotherapy

- Early administration of effective combination chemotherapy at a time of low tumor burden should increase the likelihood of cure and minimize emergence of drug-resistant tumor cell clones. Combination regimens have historically been more effective than single agent chemotherapy (Table 86.2).

Table 86.2

Common chemotherapy regimens for breast cancer

Adjuvant Chemotherapy Regimens	
AC Doxorubicin 60 mg/m^2 IV, day 1 Cyclophosphamide 600 mg/m^2 IV, day 1 Repeat cycles every 21 days for four cycles	**AC → Paclitaxel** Doxorubicin 60 mg/m^2 IV, day 1 Cyclophosphamide 600 mg/m IV, day 1 Repeat cycles every 21 days for four cycles Followed by: Paclitaxel 175 mg/m^2 IV over 3 hours Repeat cycles every 21 days for four cycles
FAC Fluorouracil 500 mg/m2 IV, days 1 and 4 Doxorubicin 50 mg/m2 IV continuous infusion over 72 hours ^{v} Cyclophosphamide 500 mg/m2 IV, day 1 Repeat cycles every 21–28 days for six cycles	**TAC** Docetaxel 75 mg/m^2 IV, day 1 Doxorubicin 50 mg/m^2 IV bolus, day 1 Cyclophosphamide 500 mg/m^2 IV, day 1 (Doxorubicin should be given first) Repeat cycles every 21 days for six cycles (must be given with growth factor support)
CAF Cyclophosphamide 600 mg/m2 IV, day 1 Doxorubicin 60 mg/m2 IV bolus, day 1 Fluorouracil 600 mg/m2 IV, day 1 Repeat cycles every 21–28 days for six cycles	**Paclitaxel → FAC** Paclitaxel 80 mg/m^2 per week IV over 1 hour every week for 12 weeks Followed by: Fluorouracil 500 mg/m^2 IV, days 1 and 4 Doxorubicin 50 mg/m^2 IV continuous infusion over 72 hours Cyclophosphamide 500 mg/m^2 IV, day 1 Repeat cycles every 21–28 days for four cycles
FEC Fluorouracil 500 mg/m^2 IV, day 1 Epirubicin 100 mg/m^2, IV bolus, day 1 Cyclophosphamide 500 mg/m^2 IV, day 1 Repeat cycle every 21 days for six cycles	**CMF** Cyclophosphamide 100 mg/m^2 per day orally, days 1–14 Methotrexate 40 mg/m^2 IV, days 1 and 8 Fluorouracil 600 mg/m^2 IV, days 1 and 8 Repeat cycles every 28 days for six cycles or Cyclophosphamide 600 mg/m^2 IV, day 1 Methotrexate 40 mg/m^2 IV, day 1 Fluorouracil 600 mg/m^2 IV, days 1 and 8 Repeat cycles every 21 days for six cycles
CEF Cyclophosphamide 75 mg/m^2 per day orally on days 1–14 Epirubicin 60 mg/m^2 IV, days 1 and 8 Fluorouracil 600 mg/m^2 IV, days 1 and 8 Repeat cycles every 21 days for six cycles (requires prophylactic antibiotics or growth factor support)	**Dose-Dense AC → Paclitaxel** Doxorubicin 60 mg/m^2 IV bolus, day 1 Cyclophosphamide 600 mg/m^2 IV, day 1 Repeat cycles every 14 days for four cycles (must be given with growth factor support) Followed by: Paclitaxel 175 mg/m^2 IV over 3 hours Repeat cycles every 14 days for four cycles (must be given with growth factor support)w

Table 86.2 *Contd...*

Adjuvant Chemotherapy Regimens	
Metastatic Single-Agent Chemotherapy **Paclitaxel** Paclitaxel 175 mg/m^2 IV over 3 hours Repeat cycles every 21 days or Paclitaxel 80 mg/m^2 per week IV over 1 hour Repeat dose every 7 days	**Vinorelbine** Vinorelbine 30 mg/m^2 IV, days 1 and 8 Repeat cycles every 21 days or Vinorelbine 25–30 mg/m^2 per week IV Repeat cycles every 7 days (adjust dose based on absolute neutrophil count; see product information)
Docetaxel Docetaxel 60–100 mg/m^2 IV over 1 hour Repeat cycles every 21 days or Docetaxel 30–35 mg/m^2 per week IV over 30 minutes Repeat dose every 7 days	**Gemcitabine** Gemcitabine 600–1,000 mg/m^2 per week IV, days 1, 8, and 15 Repeat cycles every 28 days (may need to hold day 15 dose based on blood counts)[q]
Capecitabine Capecitabine 2,000–2,500 mg/m per day orally divided twice daily for 14 days Repeat cycles every 21 days	**Liposomal doxorubicin** Liposomal doxorubicin 30–50 mg/m^2 IV over 90 minutes Repeat cycles every 28 days
Metastatic Combination Chemotherapy Regimens Docetaxel + capecitabine[t] Docetaxel 75 mg/m^2 IV over 1 hour, day 1 Capecitabine 2,000–2,500 mg/m^2 per day orally divided twice daily for 14 days Repeat cycles every 21 days	**Metastatic Combination Chemotherapy Regimens** Paclitaxel + Gemcitabine[u] Paclitaxel 175 mg/m^2 IV over 3 hours, day 1 Gemcitabine 1,250 mg/m^2 IV days 1 and 8 Repeat cycles every 21 days

AC, Adriamycin (doxorubicin), Cytoxan (cyclophosphamide); CAF, Cytoxan (cyclophosphamide), Adriamycin (doxorubicin), 5fluorouracil; CEF, cyclophosphamide, epirubicin, 5-fluorouracil; CMF, cyclophosphamide, methotrexate, 5-flourouracil; FAC, 5fluorouracil, Adriamycin (doxorubicin), cyclophosphamide; FEC, 5-fluorouracil, epirubicin, cyclophosphamide; TAC, Taxol (paclitaxel), Adriamycin (doxorubicin), cyclophosphamide.

- Anthracycline-containing regimens (e.g., **doxorubicin** and **epirubicin**) significantly reduce the rate of recurrence and improve OS 5 and 10 years after treatment as compared with regimens that contain **cyclophosphamide, methotrexate,** and **fluorouracil**. Both node-negative and node positive patients benefit from anthracycline-containing regimens.
- The addition of taxanes, **docetaxel** and **paclitaxel**, a newer class of agents, to adjuvant regimens comprised of the drugs listed above resulted in consistently and significantly improved disease-free survival and OS in node-positive breast cancer patients.
- Primary tumour removal is followed immediately by 3 weeks of Chemotherapy and continued for a duration of about 12 to 24 weeks.
- The amount of drug administered per unit of time *is the Dose intensity* and where

as by decreasing time between treatment cycles *Dose density* is achieves dose intensity.

- For node-positive breast cancer adjuvant therapy includes dose dense regimens.
- Standard regimens increasing doses may not be beneficial and sometimes harmful.
- Serotonin-antagonist, substance P / neurokinin 1-antagonist antiemetics and colony-stimulating factors, short-term toxicities of adjuvant chemotherapy are well tolerated.

ADJUVANT BIOLOGIC THERAPY

- Trastuzumab in combination with adjuvant chemotherapy is indicated in patients with early stage, HER2-positive breast cancer. The risk of recurrence was reduced up to 50% in clinical trials.
- Unanswered questions with the use of adjuvant trastuzumab include optimal concurrent chemotherapy, optimal dose, schedule and duration of therapy, and use of other concurrent therapeutic modalities.

Adjuvant Endocrine Therapy

- **Tamoxifen** has been the gold standard for adjuvant endocrine therapy. It has both estrogenic and antiestrogenic properties, depending on the tissue and gene in question.
- Tamoxifen 20 mg daily, beginning soon after completing chemotherapy and continuing for 5 years, reduces the risk of recurrence and mortality. Tamoxifen is usually well tolerated. Symptoms of estrogen withdrawal (hot flashes and vaginal bleeding) may occur but decrease in frequency and intensity over time. Tamoxifen increases the risks of stroke, pulmonary embolism, deep vein thrombosis, and endometrial cancer, particularly in women age 50 years or older.
- Premenopausal women benefit from ovarian ablation with luteinizing hormone-releasing hormone (LHRH) agonists (e.g., **goserelin**) in the adjuvant setting, either with or without concurrent tamoxifen.
- Options for adjuvant hormonal therapy in postmenopausal women include aromatase inhibitors (e.g. **anastrozole, letrozole,** or **exemestane**) either in place of or after tamoxifen. Adverse effects with aromatase inhibitors include hot flashes, myalgia/arthralgia, vaginal dryness/atrophy, mild headaches, and diarrhea.
- The optimal drug, dose, sequence, and duration of administration of aromatase inhibitors in the adjuvant setting are not known.

LOCALLY ADVANCED BREAST CANCER (STAGE III)

- The initial treatment of choice is Neoadjuvant or primary chemotherapy . Rendering inoperable tumors resectable and increasing the rate of BCT are the benefits associated with this therapy.
- An anthracycline- or taxane-containing regimen is Primary chemotherapy recommended. For patients with HER2-positive tumors the use of trastuzumab with chemotherapy is appropriate
- To minimize local recurrence Surgery is followed by chemotherapy and adjuvant RT.

METASTATIC BREAST CANCER (STAGE IV)

- Based on the site of disease involvement and presence or absence of certain characteristics, the choice of therapy for MBC is described below.

ENDOCRINE THERAPY

- For the patients who have hormone receptor-positive metastases in soft tissue, bone, pleura, or, if asymptomatic, viscera Endocrine therapy is the primary treatment of choice. Endocrine therapy has an equal probability of response and a better safety profile compared with chemotherapy.
- Endocrine therapy is given to the patients until their tumors cease to respond, at which time chemotherapy can be given.
- Historically, the choice of an endocrine therapy was based primarily on toxicity and patient preference but study results have led to changes in MBC treatment (Table 86.3).

Table 86.3

Endocrine therapies used for metastatic breast cancer

Class	Drug	Dose	Side Effects
Aromatase inhibitors			
Nonsteroidal	Anastrozole	1 mg orally daily	Hot flashes, arthralgias, myalgias, headaches, diarrhea, mild nausea
	Letrozole	2.5 mg orally daily	
Steroidal	Exemestane	25 mg orally daily	
Antiestrogens			
SERMs	Tamoxifen	20 mg orally daily	Hot flashes, vaginal dis charge, mild nausea, thromboembolism, endometrial cancer
	Toremifene	60 mg orally daily	
SERDs	Fulvestrant	250 mg IM every 28 days	Hot flashes, injection site reactions, possibly thromboembolism
LHRH analogs	Goserelin	3.6 mg SC every 28 days	Hot flashes, amenorrhea, menopausal symptoms, injection site reactions (extended formulations are not recommended for the treatment of breast cancer).
	Leuprolide	3.75 mg IM every 28 days	
	Triptorelin	3.75 mg IM every 28 days	
Progestins	Megestrol acetate	40 mg orally four times a day	Weight gain, hot flashes, vaginal bleeding, edema, thromboembolism.
	Medroxyprogesterone	400–1,000 mg IM every week	
Androgens	Fluoxymesterone	10 mg orally twice a day	Deepening voice, alopecia, hirsutism, facial/truncal acne, fluid retention, menstrual irregularities, cholestatic jaundice

Table 86.3 *Contd...*

Class	Drug	Dose	Side Effects
Estrogens	Diethylstilbestrol	5 mg orally three times a day	Nausea/vomiting, fluid retention, anorexia, thromboembolism, hepatic dysfunction
	Ethinyl estradiol	1 mg orally three times a day	
	Conjugated estrogens	2.5 mg orally three times a day	

- Aromatase inhibitors reduce circulating and target organ estrogens by blocking peripheral conversion from an androgenic precursor, the primary source of estrogens in postmenopausal women. Newer agents are more selective and better tolerated than the prototype, **aminoglutethimide**. **Anastrozole, letrozole,** and **exemestane** are approved as second-line therapy; anastrozole and exemestane have been shown to improve OS and time to progression compared with progestins. As first-line therapy, anastrozole and letrozole increase time to progression and are better tolerated compared with tamoxifen.
- **Tamoxifen** is the antiestrogen of choice in premenopausal women whose tumors are hormone-receptor positive, unless metastases occur within 1 year of adjuvant tamoxifen. Maximal beneficial effects do not occur for at least 2 months. In addition to the side effects described for adjuvant therapy, tumor flare or hypercalcemia occurs in approximately 5% of patients with MBC.
- **Toremifene** has similar efficacy and tolerability as tamoxifen and is an alternative to tamoxifen in postmenopausal patients. **Fulvestrant** is a second-line intramuscular agent with similar efficacy and safety when compared to anastrozole in patients who progressed on tamoxifen.
- Medical castration with an LHRH analogue, **goserelin, leuprolide,** or **triptorelin**, is a reversible alternative to surgery. In premenopausal women , Ovarian ablation (oophorectomy) is the endocrine therapy of choice and produces same response as tamoxifen.
- For third-line therapy progestins are generally reserved and they may cause weight gain, fluid retention, and thromboembolic events.

CHEMOTHERAPY

- For women suffering with rapidly progressive lung, liver, or bone marrow involvement; or failure of endocrine therapy or hormone receptor-negative tumors chemotherapy is preferred than endocrine therapy
- Based on the individual the choice of treatment depends and the previously used agents as adjuvant therapy can be repeated unless the cancer recurred within 1 year. Lower response rates occurs with usage of single agents than combination therapy. Single agents are better tolerated.
- **Anthracyclines** and **taxanes** produce response rates of 50% to 60% when used as first-line therapy for MBC. Single agent **capecitabine, vinorelbine,** or **gemcitabine** have response rates of 20% to 25% when used after an anthracycline and a taxane.

- **Ixabepilone**, a microtubule stabilizing agent, is indicated as monotherapy or in combination with capecitabine in MBC patients who have previously received an anthracycline and a taxane. Response rates and time to progression were increased with combination therapy as compared with capecitabine alone. Adverse effects include myelo-suppression, peripheral neuropathy, and myalgias/arthralgias.

BIOLOGIC THERAPY

- **Trastuzumab**, a monoclonal antibody that binds to HER2, produces response rates of 15% to 20% when used as a single agent and increases response rates, time to progression, and OS when combined with chemotherapy. It has been studied in doublet (taxane-trastuzumab; Vinorelbine trastuzumab) and triplet (trastuzumab-taxane-platinum) combinations but the optimum regimen is unknown.
- Trastuzumab is well tolerated, but the risk of cardiotoxicity is 5% with single-agent trastuzumab and unacceptably high in combination with an anthracycline.
- **Lapatinib**, a tyrosine kinase inhibitor that targets both HER2 and the epidermal growth factor receptor, improved response rates and time to progression in combination with capecitabine, as compared to capecitabine alone, in patients previously treated with an anthracycline, taxane, and trastuzumab. The most common adverse events were rash and diarrhea.
- The role of **bevacizumab**, a monoclonal antibody targeted against vascular endothelial growth factor, in MBC is currently not clearly defined.

RADIATION THERAPY

- Radiation is commonly used to treat painful bone metastases or other localized sites of disease including brain and spinal cord lesions. Pain relief is seen in approximately 90% of patients who receive RT.

PREVENTION OF BREAST CANCER

- **Tamoxifen** and **raloxifene** reduce the rates of invasive breast cancer in women at high risk for developing the disease. Rates of endometrial cancer and deep vein thromboses are higher in patients receiving tamoxifen but overall quality of life is similar between the two agents.

REFERENCES

1. Rosen, P. P., Groshen, S., Saigo, P. E., Kinne, D. W. & Hellman, S. Pathological prognostic factors in stage I (T1N0M0) and stage II (T1N1M0) breast carcinoma: a study of 644 patients with median follow-up of 18 years. J. Clin. Oncol. 7, 1239–1251 (1989).
2. Hellman, S. Karnofsky Memorial Lecture. Natural history of small breast cancers. J. Clin. Oncol. 12, 2229–2234 (1994).
3. Ma, X. J. *et al.* Gene expression profiles of human breast cancer progression. Proc. Natl Acad. Sci. USA 100, 5974–5979 (2003).
4. Colditz GA, Colditz GA. Epidemiology and prevention of breast cancer. Cancer Epidemiology, Biomarkers & Prevention 2005 Apr;14(4):768-72.
5. MacMahon B, MacMahon B. Epidemiology and the causes of breast cancer. International Journal of Cancer 2006 May 15;118(10):2373 -8.
6. Morrow M SEBLea. Standard for breast conservation therapy in the management of invasive breast carcinoma. CA Cancer J Clin 52, 277-300. 2002.

CHAPTER 87

Prostate Cancer

DEFINITION

It is a malignant neoplasm that mainly occurs from the prostate gland. Prostate cancer has an indolent course; localized prostate cancer is mainly curable by surgery or radiation therapy but advanced prostate cancer is not yet curable.

PREVALENCE

It is one of the frequently diagnosed non dermatological malignancy and it is the second leading cause for the death. In 2009, just over 40 000 patients were diagnosed with prostate cancer in the United Kingdom, with approximately 10 000 deaths occurring each year. Global rates for prostate cancer generally mirror those found in the United Kingdom, with the highest primarily in the developed countries of Europe, North and South America, and the Oceanic nations.

Most of the prostate tumors remain confined to the organ and will never exhibit clinically during the patient's lifetime, as they may be indolent or because death occurs from competing causes before clinical manifestation of the malignancy.

The causes of prostate cancer most likely reflect a complex interplay between environmental and hereditary genetic factors, most of which remain to be identified, that interact and lead to a critical acquisition of DNA. As the growth these cells depends on the circulating levels of the testosterone metabolites, hormonal factors are likely to have an important role in the natural history of the disease. A slight increase in incidence of prostate cancer has been predicted with high consumption of meat, dairy products, and fats . Although the evidence reveals at best, weak associations are incredibly difficult to interpret in the face of multiple confounding factors.

PATHOPHYSIOLOGY

Most prostate cancers are acinar adenocarcinomas. Unusual histologic variants or types of prostatic carcinoma account for about 5% to 10% of carcinomas that originate in the prostate gland.

DUCTAL ADENOCARCINOMA

The ductal subtype of adenocarcinoma is composed of larger glands that are lined by tall pseudostratified columnar cells. *Endometrial carcinoma* originally described this entity because of its morphologic similarity to endometrium. In pure form, ductal adenocarcinoma accounts for 0.2% to 0.8% of prostate cancers. More commonly, it is seen with an acinar component. Ductal adenocarcinoma on biopsy warrants definitive therapy. Although these cancers are less hormonally responsive than acinar adenocarcinoma, androgen deprivation therapy may provide palliative relief. Serum PSA levels in patients with ductal adenocarcinoma may be normal, especially in patients with only centrally located tumors. Ductal adenocarcinoma may be located near the prostatic urethra and admixed with typical acinar adenocarcinoma. Ductal adenocarcinoma located centrally is associated with a peripherally situated acinar adenocarcinoma. Centrally occurring tumors generally appear as papillary masses protruding into the urethra. Peripherally occurring tumors typically show a white-gray firm appearance similar to that of acinar adenocarcinoma. Periurethral or centrally located ductal adenocarcinoma may cause hematuria, urgency in urine, and urinary retention. In these cases, there may be no abnormalities on rectal examination.

ONCOCYTIC ADENOCARCINOMA

Oncocytic prostatic adenocarcinomas are composed of large cells with granular, eosinophilic cytoplasm. Tumor cells are ovoid hyperchromatic nuclei and are strongly immunoreactive for PSA. Numerous mitochondria are seen on ultrastructural examination. High Gleason grade, elevated serum PSA, and metastasis of similar morphology have been reported with this variant.

LYMPHOEPITHELIOMA-LIKE CARCINOMA

Lymphoepithelioma-like carcinoma is an undifferentiated carcinoma characterized by malignant cells arranged in a syncytial pattern. Malignant cells are PSA-positive. An associated acinar adenocarcinoma has been noted. In situ hybridization has been negative for Epstein-Barr virus.

ATROPHIC ADENOCARCINOMA

Ordinary prostate cancers develops atrophic cytoplasm as a result of treatment , atrophic prostate cancers are usually not associated with a treatment history. The diagnosis of carcinoma in atrophic adenocarcinoma may be based on several features. Atrophic prostate cancer exhibit a truly infiltrative pattern of growth with individual. The glands of benign atrophy may appear to be infiltrative on needle biopsy, because individual benign atrophic glands do not infiltrate between the larger benign glands. Some forms of atrophy are associated with fibrosis, atrophic prostate cancers lack such a desmoplastic stromal response. Atrophy may show enlarged nuclei and prominent nucleoli. Presence of a component of conventional acinar carcinoma can help in recognizing the malignant nature of the adjacent atrophic cancer glands.

SYMPTOMS

The diagnosis of prostate cancer can be made in a number of stages. Symptoms due to prostate cancer are rarely the cause for patient presentation and investigation. If symptomatic, localized prostate cancer can result in urinary symptoms including hematospermia, although the presence of voiding lower urinary tract symptoms (LUTS), hematuria, and/or perineal/ voiding discomfort is likely to result from coexisting BPH/prostatitis. Advanced disease may present with rectal obstruction, bone pain, and more systemic features of malignancy

DIAGNOSIS

FIRST LINE INVESTIGATIONS

First line tests include completion of the physical examination with a digital rectal examination (DRE), and measurement of serum PSA; suspicious findings on either of these tests is followed by more sophisticated diagnostic techniques, beginning with transrectal ultrasound (TRUS) and guided systematic biopsy. Prostate cancer was typically diagnosed as a result of symptomatic metastases or when found during DRE in a patient presenting with urinary complaints. In addition, the biomarker "prostatic acid phosphatase" would often be elevated with the presence of bone metastases. However, the advent of the PSA blood test assay, transformed the diagnostic landscape for prostate cancer, as the antigen became one of the most commonly used tumor markers in modern medicine.

PROSTATE-SPECIFIC ANTIGEN

Prostate-specific antigen (PSA) 240 amino acids glycoprotein. It is secreted by prostate into semen where it causes lysis of seminal coagulum. It exists mainly in three forms: free Prostate-specific antigen (PSA), Prostate-specific antigen (PSA) complexed with alpha-1 antichymotrypsin, and Prostate-specific antigen (PSA) complexed with β1-antichymotrypsin. PSA with DRE, has become a widely used clinical tool , as well as its subsequent staging and monitoring post-diagnosis. The routine use of the PSA blood test as a diagnostic/screening tool has resulted in a substantial increase in the incidence of prostate cancer recorded worldwide. Although the PSA test allows for earlier detection of prostate cancer with the potential for widespread use of relatively aggressive curative treatments by radical surgical, chemotherapeutic and radiation. The abnormal PSA level has been 4.0 ng/ml. When reviewing the performance of a diagnostic test, several parameters need to be assessed. These include sensitivity (probability of identifying true positives with the disease), specificity (probability of identifying the true negatives), and positive/negative predictive values (probability that a test positive/negative individual (actually has/does not have the disease).

TRANS RECTAL ULTRASOUND (TRUS)

TRUS is the most commonly used imaging technique for evaluating prostate cancer. In addition to its role in diagnosing prostate cancer, it also allows estimation of prostate size, guides needle biopsies, provides local staging information, and monitors disease prior to and after treatment. TRUS is not normally used as a primary screening measure but to confirm the diagnosis of prostate cancer in combination with prostate biopsy for those with raised PSA or lesions suspicious on DRE. Technical advances, selection biases, observer differences in TRUS scanning, and the lack of UK studies mean that the evidence concerning the accuracy and effectiveness of TRUS for the detection and diagnosis of prostate cancer remains variable. It is however generally accepted that when used in conjunction with DRE and PSA measurement, TRUS can add to the detection rate of localized prostate cancer.

TRANSRECTAL ULTRASOUND-GUIDED BIOPSY

Needle biopsy is used to confirm the diagnosis of prostate cancer and to provide histological grading information. In the context of the increasing use of the PSA assay, the number of biopsies undertaken in urological practice has increased considerably in recent years. Core biopsy involves the use of a spring-loaded automatic biopsy gun, equipped with an 18- gauge needle. The needle is reliably placed into suspicious lesions in the gland using TRUS which helps to ensure accurate targeting . Foci of cancerous cells within the prostate can appear as hypo- (or even hyper-) echoic lesions on TRUS, although are frequently isoechoic, warranting a standard protocol biopsy (e.g., 12-core). Biopsy does not have a role in first line screening, although it is considered the gold standard diagnostic investigation for histological confirmation of prostate cancer. Biopsy specimens are graded histologically based on the architectural differentiation of the tumor cells. The predominant histological system is the Gleason grading system in which sections of tumor are graded from 1 (least aggressive) to 5 (most aggressive). The two highest grades from each tumor are added to give a score ranging from 2 to 10. In addition to using the Gleason score as a predictor of the biological aggressiveness of prostate cancer, other parameters can also be combined with the Gleason score to estimate disease severity. It was suggested that a stratification of patients into low, intermediate, and high-risk groups by combining the Gleason score, the PSA measurement, and the clinical stage . Although physical examination and the DRE provide the basis for clinical staging, imaging in the form of TRUS, MRI, CT, radionuclide bone scans, and pelvic lymph node evaluation are used to further evaluate the stage of prostate cancer.

TREATMENT

SYSTEMIC THERAPY

There are two main methods of achieving control of prostate cancer by hormonal manipulation:

(i) Withdrawal of androgen (using luteinising hormone-releasing hormone agonists (LHRHa) or bilateral orchidectomy), which removes the supply of endogenous hormone; or (ii) Receptor blockade of androgen (anti-androgens), which reduces the effect of endogenous hormones.

Androgen withdrawal commonly causes hot flushes, loss of sexual drive and weight gain. In addition men may become lethargic and describe loss of drive and energy. In the long term, bone mineral density may decrease with an increase risk of pathological fractures. Anti-androgen therapy is less likely to result in sexual dysfunction and/or lethargy. These agents cause enlargement of breast (gynaecomastia) and breast pain (mastalgia). For many men with locally advanced prostate cancer, hormonal therapy will be the primary therapy. Bicalutamide monotherapy is sometimes used as an alternative to LHRHa's for men with locally advanced disease.

NEOADJUVANT THERAPY

Hormonal therapy is sometimes given for longer duration before radical treatment. It can be used before radical radiotherapy to reduce the size of the prostate. This may reduce the side effects of radiotherapy by allowing smaller radiotherapy fields to be used. Hormonal therapy may also increase the cell killing effect of radiotherapy. Hormonal therapy has also been given before surgery in order to downstage the tumour . Neoadjuvant androgen withdrawal has made the patients disease-free and increased survival of the patients receiving radical radiotherapy for high-risk localised and locally advanced prostate cancer. The role of neoadjuvant androgen withdrawal for low and intermediate-risk disease treated with modern escalated dose radiotherapy has not been well studied.

ADJUVANT THERAPY

Hormonal therapy has been used following both surgery and radiotherapy with the intention of improving survival. The duration of hormonal therapy has ranged from 6 months to indefinite.

Robotic and Laparoscopic Radical Prostatectomy

- A steadily increasing proportion of radical prostatectomies are being performed using laparoscopic techniques.
- Laparoscopic radical prostatectomy (LRP) can be performed with or without the assistance of the da Vinci surgical robot.
- Potential advantages of the da Vinci robot for prostatectomy include the magnified vision, tremor filtering, and motion scaling and instruments with 7 degrees of freedom that more accurately replicate human wrist movements.
- Relative disadvantages of LRP include increased cost, lack of universal availability at all centers, and a steep learning curve for experienced urologic oncologic surgeons trained only in open surgical techniques. As LRP becomes more widely disseminated and integrated fully into residency training throughout urology, these disadvantages will likely become less significant.
- Cancer control using LRP appears to be equivalent to radical prostatectomy using either the traditional open retropubic or the perineal approach.
- LRP, and particularly its robotic variant, is an excellent technique for radical prostatectomy in obese patients, who may be more challenging candidates for open radical prostatectomy.
- Advantages of LRP over open retropubic radical prostatectomy include less blood loss and postoperative pain, as well as an earlier return to full activity.
- Health-related quality of life after LRP appears to be excellent. Reported outcomes are at least equivalent and perhaps superior to outcomes from open retropubic radical prostatectomy, particularly with respect to early return of urinary continence.

PERINEAL PROSTATECTOMY

- Radical perineal prostatectomy (RPP) represents the oldest form of radical prostatectomy and offers the most direct approach to the prostate.
- Appropriate candidates for RPP are patients with clinically organ-confined prostate cancer and an estimated life expectancy of more than 10 years.
- RPP is an excellent approach for many patients but offers distinct advantages over other approaches in patients who have undergone previous extensive

abdominal surgery, those who have had renal transplants, and those who are morbidly obese.

- Advantages of the perineal approach include decreased blood loss, low transfusion requirements, infrequent postoperative ileus, and short hospital stay.
- RPP results in favorable long-term disease control comparable to other surgical techniques with 15-year cancer-associated survival rates approaching 86%.
- RPP demonstrates favorable urinary and sexual health-related quality-of-life outcomes, which appear comparable to those of other approaches such as radical retropubic

HIGH-INTENSITY FOCUSED ULTRASOUND FOR PROSTATE CANCER

The basic principle of transrectal high-intensity focused ultrasound (HIFU) is the destruction of tissue of the prostate gland by depositing large amounts of energy into it. The two principal mechanisms of action are based on mechanical and thermal effects. The thermal effect of HIFU is related to the absorption of ultrasound energy into the tissue, which is converted into heat. Mechanically, damage to cells is due to acoustic cavitation. Both lead to a reduction in prostate volume to 5 mL.

- The use of HIFU in organ-confined prostate cancer was first examined in 1993 and two commercially available devices for HIFU are currently in use: the Ablatherm and the Sonablate. The main differences between the two systems are patient positioning, treatment and planning, ultrasound frequencies, shoot and delay time, intraprostatic treatment mode, and rectal wall control.
- HIFU is generally indicated for patients with prostate cancer who are not candidates for surgery because of their age, general health status or a prohibiting comorbidity, or who would prefer not to undergo a radical prostatectomy.
- The indication for HIFU has been expanded based on clinical experience to include advanced prostate cancer as a debulking process.
- Unlike other local treatment options for prostate cancer, such as surgery, radiation therapy, cryotherapy, and brachytherapy, HIFU treatment can be repeated easily in cases of local recurrence and can be used as a salvage therapy.
- In current practice, a pre-HIFU transurethral resection of the prostate (TURP) allows for the removal of any calcifications, abscesses, middle lobe, and large adenomas because it optimizes the prostate shape for HIFU application.
- A number of studies have reported the outcome with HIFU, including single-center and multicenter European studies.
- Data from one study combining TURP with HIFU in 30 patients with localized prostate cancer with a median follow-up of 20 months report a 83.3% negative biopsy rate at 1 year and an overall negative biopsy rate of 86.6% in patients undergoing one or two HIFU sessions.
- HIFU can be considered a treatment option in patients with high-risk prostate cancer, although long-term studies are still needed. In one study involving 30 patients with locally advanced and advanced

disease at 6 months follow-up, positive biopsies were reported in 23% of patients. At 1 year, only three (10%) patients had a PSA level higher than 0.3 ng/mL and less than 1.0 ng/mL.

- As salvage treatment, HIFU treatment results in a good outcome in locally recurrent prostate cancer. A 30-month actuarial negative biopsy rate of 73% has been reported in one study involving 71 patients.
- Patients treated with HIFU as a primary local therapy combined with TURP generally have low morbidity. Grade 1 (4%–6%) or grade 2 (0%–2%) urinary stress incontinence and secondary intravesical obstruction (5%–10%) are the most commonly reported adverse events. Urinary tract infections are common (5%–13%), but the incidence has been shown to be significantly reduced in patients undergoing the combined TURP/HIFU procedure compared with HIFU alone.

PROSTATE CRYOABLATION

Prostate cryoablation represents an effective image guided percutaneous treatment for clinically localized prostate cancer.

- Metal cryoprobes were first developed in the 1960s for delivering liquid nitrogen and have evolved to 1.4 mm needles that carry argon gas as the cryogen.
- Modern prostate cryoablation was developed with the application of transrectal ultrasound guidance in the 1980s.
- Tissue temperatures below “40ÚC cause cell death through vascular injury, stimulation of apoptosis, and creation of intracellular ice crystals.
- Salvage prostate cryoablation for persistent prostate cancer following radiation therapy eradicates the cancer in 86% to 95% of cases.
- Primary prostatic cryoablation is associated with a positive post procedure biopsy rate of 1% to 5% with a low risk of incontinence.
- Primary prostatic cryoablation is the least costly treatment alternative for clinically localized prostate cancer.
- The technique of prostate cryoablation provides flexibility in treatment planning that allows for a whole gland or subtotal gland destruction.
- A significant minority of men diagnosed with localized prostate cancer harbor small-volume and unilateral cancers that can be destroyed with an individualized subtotal cryoablation, further reducing treatment intensity and cost.

Alternative Medicine for Prostate Cancer: Diet, Vitamins, Minerals, and Supplements

Prostate cancer is an excellent candidate for chemoprevention with nutrition .

- The highest likelihood of chemoprevention of prostate cancer is in the stage called prostatic intraepithelial neoplasia (PIN).
- Current evidence supports a chemopreventive approach that incorporates reduction of inflammation and protection against oxidation.
- Research into nutritional chemoprevention of prostate cancer is ongoing and highly promising, and administered to the patients who are in early stages of prostate cancer.
- Nutritional chemopreventive agents have no negative impact on potency or continence.

NEW THERAPIES IN HORMONE RELAPSED DISEASE

INTRODUCTION

Men with relapsed or metastatic prostate cancer are treated with androgen deprivation therapy (ADT) to achieve surgical or medical castration. However, while metastatic prostate cancer is incurable, progression on ADT therapy no longer signals the end of therapeutic options. Five novel treatments proven to prolong survival in castration-resistant prostate cancer (CRPC) have been reported in the past 2 years. These novel therapies comprise abiraterone acetate and enzalutamide, which act to inhibit androgen receptor (AR) signaling, sipuleucel-T immunotherapy, the bone targeting radionuclide radium223, and second-line cabazitaxel chemotherapy. These new CRPC treatments and other promising agents will be reviewed, including practical management issues. The therapeutic landscape of CRPC is changing rapidly, and this chapter will outline the current options and discuss emerging strategies.

TARGETING ANDROGEN RECEPTOR SIGNALING

Medical or surgical castration causes interruption of AR signaling. Unfortunately, the response to ADT is not durable and is followed by disease progression, with rising prostate-specific antigen (PSA) despite castrate levels of testosterone, indicating a "castration-resistant" state. Several mechanisms are involved, including intratumoral androgen synthesis from peripheral adrenal androgens and *de novo* synthesis directly from cholesterol. Additionally, androstenediol (a progesterone derivative) can be converted to dehydrotestosterone (DHT) via the "backdoor pathway." Novel therapies have been designed recognizing AR activation as a key target in advanced prostate cancer. Successful strategies to overcome AR activation include novel androgen biosynthesis inhibitors and potent AR inhibitors.

CYP17 INHIBITION

The enzyme CYP17, which has dual functions as a 17α-hydroxylase and 17,20 lyase, has an essential role in androgen biosynthesis. ketoconazole and aminoglutethimide, which are nonspecific inhibitors of CYP17, had modest antitumor activity in advanced prostate cancer.

ABIRATERONE ACETATE

The molecular structure of pregnenolone was modified to identify a potent, irreversible, and selective inhibitor of CYP17A1 . Early-phase testing of abiraterone was encouraging, with a favorable toxicity profile at doses up to 2000 mg daily and evidence of PSA and radiological activity. Androgen biosynthesis inhibition with abiraterone results in accumulation of androgen precursor molecules and a positive feedback loop, causing high ACTH levels and increased mineralocorticoid activity. Although concomitant prednisone can cover most of the mineralocorticoid excess, the most common side effects in patients receiving abiraterone were fluid retention and edema (seen in 31% of patients receiving abiraterone, compared with 22% placebo patients), hypokalemia (seen in 17% and 8% patients, respectively), and hypertension (10% and 8%, respectively). These toxicities were generally easily managed with increased glucocorticoid doses or by adding the specific mineralocorticoid antagonist eplerenone.

NEXT-GENERATION ANTIANDROGENS

Antiandrogens are agents that compete with endogenous androgen ligand for the ligand-binding pocket of the AR. Mutations in the AR can cause older "first-generation" antiandrogens to become agonistic, which can contribute to cancer progression. Second-generation oral antiandrogens have been rationally designed as potent AR antagonists with currently no evidence of agonistic activity.

ENZALUTAMIDE

Enzalutamide binds the AR with approximately fivefold greater avidity compared with bicalutamide. In preclinical studies, enzalutamide showed activity in bicalutamide-resistant models, preventing AR nuclear translocation, DNA binding, and AR co-activator recruitment.

Immune targeting in advanced prostate cancer

Harnessing the immune system against cancer cells has proven difficult, but immunotherapies have met with some success in metastatic CRPC. Promising strategies include specific vaccines and more general immune system modulation to decrease cancer immune tolerance by blocking immune checkpoints.

SIPULEUCEL-T

Sipuleucel-T is a vaccine therapy developed for the treatment of CRPC. It is prepared using a sample of a patients' own dendritic cells, which are pulsed *ex vivo* with a recombinant fusion protein of granulocyte macrophage colony stimulating factor (GM-CSF) and prostatic acid phosphatase (PAP). Collection of dendritic cells by apheresis usually requires insertion of a venous catheter. A series of three treatments is administered over 1 month.

IPILIMUMAB

Cytotoxic T-lymphocyte antigen-4 (CTLA-4) is a protein expressed by cytotoxic T cells. T cell activation requires binding of CD28, but CTLA-4 competes for binding with a higher efficiency, and thus acts as an immune inhibitor. Ipilimumab is a humanized monoclonal antibody used as a nonspecific immunotherapy and is approved for use in advanced melanoma.

BONE-TARGETING AGENTS IN ADVANCED PROSTATE CANCER

Bone metastases are the most common metastatic site in prostate cancer, occurring in up to 90% of patients with advanced disease The main cancer-related serious reportable events are spinal cord compressions, and painful bone metastases requiring radiotherapy or surgery.

Bisphosphonates are bone-seeking agents that bind to hydroxyapatite crystals in the bone and inhibit osteoclast activity. The bisphosphonate zoledronic acid is used for the prevention of serious reportable events in patients with prostate cancer and bone metastases.

ALPHARADIN

Several beta-emitting radionuclides are bone-seeking agents that have been investigated in men with prostate cancer and bone metastases. Two drugs have been approved by the FDA: 89Sr (Strontium-89) and 153Sm (Samarium-153), based on trial results showing improved pain control when compared with placebo. Radium 223 chloride is a novel agent that acts as a calcium mimetic and is preferentially integrated into areas of new bone formation such as bone growth around metastases . Radium 223 emits alpha particles.

CABOZANTINIB

Cabozantinib is a novel oral small molecule targeting multiple-key receptor tyrosine kinases, including the receptor of the hepatocyte growth factor and the vascular endothelial growth factor receptor 2 (VEGFR2), but also inhibits KIT, FLT3, and AXL .

SECOND-LINE CHEMOTHERAPY

A number of agents have been tested in men following first-line docetaxel chemotherapy. There is Phase II trial evidence to support docetaxel retreatment as a second-line strategy in selected men who responded well to initial docetaxel. Other agents have been tested second line, but have met with limited success.

CABAZITAXEL

Cabazitaxel (Jevtana, Sanofi, Paris, France) is a partially synthesized taxane compound. Preclinical studies suggested activity in docetaxel-resistant cell lines.

REFERENCES

1. Godley PA. Prostate cancer screening: promise and peril—a review. *Cancer Detect Prev* 1999; 23: 316–324.
2. Ghann PH, Hennekens CH, Stampfer MJ. A prospective evaluation of plasma prostate-specific antigen for detection of prostatic cancer. *J Am Med Assoc* 1995; 273(4): 289.
3. Stamey TA, Yang N, Hay AR, et al. Prostate-specific antigen as a serum marker for adenocarcinoma of the prostate. *N Engl J Med* 1987; 317(15): 909–916.
4. Catalona WJ. Radical surgery for advanced prostate cancer and for radiation failures. *J Urol* 1993; 147: 916.
5. D'Amico AV, Whittington R, Malkowicz SB. Biochemical outcome after radical prostatectomy, external beam radiation therapy or interstitial radiation therapy for clinically localized prostate cancer. *J Am Med Assoc* 1998; 280: 969–974.
6. 24 Wilson JMG, Jungner G. *Principles and Practice of Screening for Disease*. Geneva: WHO;1968.
7. Scardino PT, Weaver R, Hudson MA: Early detection of prostate cancer. Hum Pathol 23: 211, 1992.
8. Sundar S, Dickinson PD. Spironolactone, a possible selective androgen receptor modulator,should be used with caution in patients with metastatic carcinoma of the prostate. *BMJ Case Rep* 2012; 2012.
9. Kawata H, Ishikura N, Watanabe M, et al. Prolonged treatment with bicalutamide induces androgen receptor over-expression and androgen hyper-sensitivity. *Prostate* 2010; 70(7): 745–754.
10. Urbanucci A, Sahu B, Seppala J, et al. Overexpression of androgen receptor enhances the binding of the receptor to the chromatin in prostate cancer. *Oncogene* 2012; 31(17): 2153–2163.
11. Guo Z, Yang X, Sun F, et al. A novel androgen receptor splice variant is upregulated during prostate cancer progression and promotes androgen depletionresistant growth. *Cancer Res* 2009; 69(6): 2305–2313.
12. Hornberg E, Ylitalo EB, Crnalic S, et al. Expression of androgen receptor splice variants in prostate cancer bone metastases is associated with castration-resistance and short survival. *PLoS One* 2011; 6(4): e19059.

CHAPTER 88

Colorectal Cancer

DEFINITION

It is a malignant neoplasm involving the colon, rectum, and anal canal. Colon and rectal cancers develop by the accumu-lation of changes that occur in certain genes within the cells of the mucosal lining of the bowel.

AETIOLOGY OF COLON AND RECTAL CANCER

GENES AND COLORECTAL CANCER

Colon and rectal cancers develop by the accumulation of changes that occur in certain genes within the cells of the mucosal lining of the bowel. The genes that are mainly affected appear to have important roles in the control of the cell cycle, differentiation, contact inhibition, angiogenesis and many other regulatory mechanisms of cellular growth. The alterations that occur in these genes are mainly due to exposure to the carcinogens (e.g. irradiation ,chemicals, dietary, or viral), spontaneous sporadic mutation, or an inherited gene defect . There is also some evidence that environmental factors such as diet may affect certain gene mechanisms. The changes may also arise on the background of chronic diseases such as ulcerative colitis.

There would appear to be two molecular pathways that may result in the development of colorectal cancers. The first pathway is adenomatous cancer sequence or mutation of multisteps. This theory states that there is a progressive mutation of oncogenes and also loss of the functioning of tumour suppressor genes. The gradual accumulation of these genetic events will usually require several years (often 10–20) and is therefore consistent with the epidemiological data regarding the polyp–cancer sequence. Genes responsible for DNA-mismatch repair mediate this pathway. There are several classes of genes are involved in the transformation of normal colonic mucosa to malignant. They include:

- Tumour suppressor genes
- DNA-repair genes
- Oncogenes

Genetic instability is the basis for the development of colorectal cancer. This process may occur in two broad and possibly overlapping ways. The instability may affect the whole chromosome or short segments of repetitive DNA termed ‘microsatellites’.

MICROSATELLITE INSTABILITY AND DNA-REPAIR GENES

Microsatellites are unique repeated segments of DNA. These base segments usually consist of cytosine (C) and adenine (A) nucleotides, or dinucleotides (CA repeats). These segments are found scattered throughout the genome.

In tumours it has been found that these repeated segments are often altered. Typically new alleles may appear, indicating a failure of DNA replication. This failure of DNA replication was termed 'microsatellite instability' or MSI .The failure of the normal replication is thought to result from loss of normal function in the DNA polymerase during replication. The cell subsequently fails to recognize the mismatch. It was the detection of MSI in hereditary non-polyposis coli (HNPC) cancers that led to the discovery of DNA-mismatch repair (MMR) genes.

Studies have suggested that DNA MMR gene deficiency (caused by mutation of *hMSH2*, *hMLH1*, *hPMS1* or *hPMS2* genes) contributes to the development of HPNC (Lynch syndrome). Most tumours in these patients display MSI. DNA-repair genes play an important role in the tumour development by the loss of protein function. After such a loss some oncogenes and tumour suppressor genes may undergo mutation with progression to neoplastic change.

The failure of the cell to recognize and repair the mismatch or defect probably promotes carcinogenesis through the loss of a caretaker function in certain genes. The loss of such a self-regulatory mechanism may result in the accumulation of other genetic errors or mutations.The areas of DNA that appear to be particularly prone to the loss of MMR are segments of DNA that contain repeated short segments. The progressive accumulation of defects occurs in the cancer cells.

ONCOGENES

Oncogenes were originally detected in certain tumour-forming viruses. Oncogenes are in fact normal genes but when they become inappropriately activated or expressed they may result in the development of disease. The products of the oncogenes tend to have vital roles in the control of the cell cycle, growth and differentiation. The activation or expression in an abnormal manner of these genes, and hence in their protein products, can result in a neoplastic transformation. The loss of normal growth control, contact inhibition and other functions gives the cell thc ability to invade surrounding tissues and even metastasis : the cell has become malignant .A number of oncogenes have been identified and are thought to play a role in the development of colorectal cancers. These, then, are some of the building blocks involved in the development of neoplasia .The classic polyp–cancer sequence and the role of MSI theories probably have areas of overlap depending on a given situation. There still remain significant gaps in our knowledge about the pathways and specific triggers that initiate the process.

TUMOUR SUPPRESSOR GENES

Oncogenes often tend to function in a dominant fashion. There is, however, another class of genes that function in a recessive manner. These are termed 'tumour suppressor genes'.

Tumour suppressor genes are those with normal function that appear to be related to the control or suppression of cell proliferation. The inactivation of these genes results in the loss of normal cell growth control. It has been proposed that a mutation of one copy of this type of gene was inherited in such conditions as FAP and that neoplasms resulted from the subsequent somatic mutation of the normal allele. Later on it was proposed that the same germline genes would be altered somatically in the development of both the familial and the non-familial type of bowel cancers.

The tumour suppressor genes are inactivated during the development of tumours is often associated with the loss of the few tumour suppressor DNA. This loss may be detected using sophisticated molecular biological techniques. One such technique is to identify the loss of restriction fragment length polymorphism alleles in the tumour DNA which are present in normal DNA from the same person. The loss of such constitutional heterozygosity in tumours may be used to identify the tumour suppressor genes sites.

DNA METHYLATION

DNA methylation plays a complex role in the development of tumours. Hypomethylation is associated with increase in gene expression and may play a role in the activation of oncogenes such as *k-ras*. Similarly, DNA hypermethylation can coexist with hypomethylation in different areas of the genome in a variety of tumours.

The multistep, polyp–cancer theory of colorectal carcinogenesis

Based on the available epidemiological and molecular evidence, it is now apparent that a multistep pathway is involved in the development of colorectal cancers. In 1976 Nowell proposed the clonal theory of carcinogenesis. Colorectal cancers arise from a single cell that develops by clonal expansion. Genetic events gradually accumulate in clones of cells. These events may be acquired by mutations or be inherited. Some changes would be deleterious to the cell, others would give it a growth advantage. Those cells that developed a growth advantage would gradually produce a subclone of cells that would continue to grow. Gradually further clones would develop and, with successive mutations accumulating within the cells, a polyp; then, gradually with time and further gene changes, a malignant cancer would develop. This theory explained the time lag from patients developing polyps and subsequently tumours in later life. Histological analysis of tumours helps to confirm the theory because analysis often reveals the presence of adenomatous tissue adjacent to the tumour. The tumour has arisen as a clone from the polyp cells.

The pattern of change that occurred in certain genes in colorectal cancers might be reflected in the different stages of development of tumours during the transition from normal mucosa to polyp and subsequent cancer. The altered genes number that occur in oncogenes or tumour suppressor genes appear to be more critical than the exact order in which they occur. There are several genes that have been identified as playing a role in this multistep pathway (Fig. 88.1).

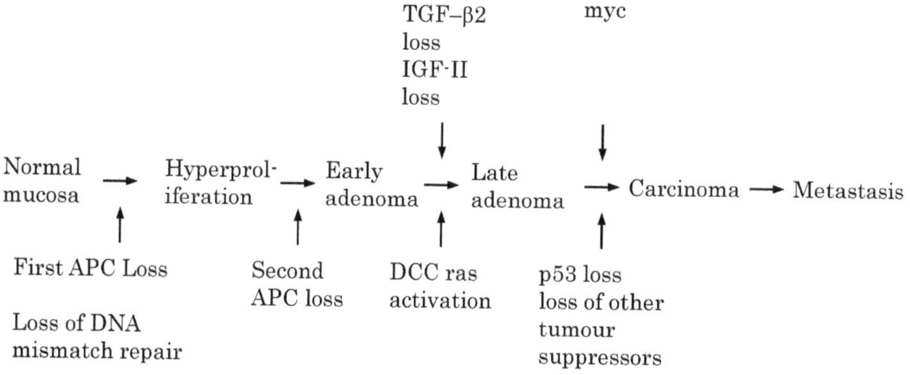

FIGURE 88.1

The multistep model for colorectal carcinogenesis.

THE APC GENE

The investigation for the genetic cause of FAP resulted in the discovery of the adenomatous polyposis gene (*APC*). The *APC* gene is expressed in most tissues and is composed of 19 exons, 16 of which are alternatively expressed.

The *APC* gene has been termed a 'gatekeeper gene'. It would appear that it is probably involved in the initiation of adenomatous polyps. In the development of sporadic polyps, both copies of the *APC* gene must probably be inactive. This permits the initiating trigger for the development of a polyp. As the function of the *APC* gene is lost, a polyp with the potential for malignant transformation (depending on which other gene mechanisms are affected) forms. From the studies to date it would appear that the *APC* gene aids in the control of cell growth by several mechanisms. These include regulation of cell adhesion, processing of signalling pathways, maintaining the cytoskeleton, and cell cycle progression and apoptosis . The loss or inactivation of the *APC* gene results in the disruption of the normal balance between cell division and death. The result is disordered growth.

Familial adenomatous polyposis There are several rare inherited syndromes that predispose to the development of colorectal cancers. One of the best studied is familial adenomatous polyposis or FAP. Studies of this disease have resulted in insights into the development of non-inherited colorectal cancers. FAP is an autosomal dominant condition in which multiple polyps develop throughout the colon and rectum. The patients will usually develop a colorectal cancer in their 20s to 40s unless they undergo a prophylactic panproctocolectomy either with a pouch anal reconstruction or a permanent ileostomy.

Several other genes have now been demonstrated to play a role in the development of colorectal cancers (Table 88.1).

Table 88.1

Some genes involved in the development of colorectal cancers

Gene	Chromosomal site	Syndrome	Protein
APC control c-myc, apoptosis	5q21	FAP	Cell adhesion,
hMSH$_2$ repair	2p16	HNPCC	DNA-mismatch
HMLH1 repair	3p21	HNPCC	DNA-mismatch
p53	17p13	Tumour suppressor repair DNA damage, apoptosis	Cell cycle control,
DCC	18q21	Tumour suppressor	Cell adhesion
MCC	5q21	Tumour suppressor	Not known
K-ras	12p	Oncogene	GTP binding
c-myc	8q24	Oncogene	DNA synthesis
R11 gene		Tumour suppressor	TGF-β2 receptor
IGF-IIR	6q26	Tumour suppressor	Activation of TGF-β

FAP, familial adenomatous polyposis; HNPCC, hereditary non-polyposis coli cancer; TGF, transforming growth factor.

THE MCC GENE

The *MCC* (mutated in colorectal cancer) gene is located on chromosome 5q21, close to the FAP gene. The gene codes for a protein of 829 amino acids, which is similar in structure to that of the *APC* gene product. It is possible that they interact in some way, although at present their exact function remains unknown.

THE P53 GENE

Protein P53 is produced by a gene located on the short arm of chromosome 17 (17p13), and this gene codes for a 53-kDa nuclear phosphoprotein that contains 393 amino acids. It appears to act as a tumour suppressor-type gene. Not only do a high proportion (70 per cent) of colorectal cancers indicates the loss of the allele responsible for the production of the oncoprotein *p53*, but also the abnormality is detected in nearly half of all tumours . The inactivation of *p53* appears to be associated with the transition mechanism from a benign to a malignant polyp. In the development of colorectal neoplasms, *p53* function can be lost by a combination of chromosomal mutation and deletion by the loss of heterozygosity. The *p53* can also lose its function when only one allele is mutated because the mutant *p53* can bind to the wild-type *p53* inactivating it (a dominant negative effect). The *p53* gene seems to possess three main functions in response to DNA damage: cell cycle (G1) arrest, stimulation of DNA repair and promotion of cell death (apoptosis). When *p53* is mutated, these mechanisms are lost and the cell can progress as a neoplastic clone.

THE DCC GENE

The DCC (deleted in colon cancer) gene was identified on chromosome 18q21. Both mutations on chromosomes 17 and 18 are found uncommonly in small adenomas but, as the adenomas develop, carcinoma *in situ* changes the incidence rises. The loss of heterozygosity on the long arm of chromosome 18 (18q) may be a molecular predictor of a poor prognosis. The gene appears to function as a tumour suppressor. This gene has a similarity to a variety of cell-surface glycoproteins including neural cell adhesion molecules.

THE RAS ONCOGENE

There are a variety of *ras* oncogenes (H-*ras*, K-*ras*, N-*ras*), which encode for a 21-kDa protein. Activation of *ras* appears, in most cases, to be caused by point mutations usually occurring at codons .These *ras* oncogenes appear to be present in about 50 per cent of colon and rectal tumours. The *ras* mutations by themselves appear, however, to be insufficient to initiate neoplastic change. The k-*ras* gene is often found mutated in polyps and the incidence appears to rise as the polyp increases in size and dysplastic changes occur.

DIAGNOSIS AND INVESTIGATIONS

Patients with a high probability of having cancer can be identified statistically by the combination and persistence of their symptoms. Diagnostic services would be overwhelmed if all patients with bowel symptoms were referred for hospital assessment. As a large proportion of the population experience bowel symptoms every year, it is important that those who develop new symptoms are observed in general practice. Only those with persistent, progressive or sinister symptoms should be referred for rapid diagnosis.

SYMPTOMS

The site of the tumour in the colon often determines clinical presentation. Right-sided or caecal lesions often present with iron deficiency anaemia, diarrhoea or a palpable mass in the right iliac fossa, but are less likely to present with intestinal obstruction unless the ileocaecal valve itself is involved. Alteration of bowel habit, spurious diarrhoea and intestinal obstruction are more typical of lesions on the left side of the colon. Rectal carcinoma presents with bleeding, tenesmus and change in bowel habit.

Table 88.2

Differential diagnosis for different symptoms

Rectal bleeding	Diarrhoea	Constipation
Haemorrhoids	Diverticular disease	Crohn's disease
Perianal fissure	Infective colitis	Benign stricture
Infective colitis	Inflammatory bowel disease	Benign stricture
Inflammatory bowel disease	Coeliac disease	Poor dietary intake
Diverticular disease		
Angiodysplasia		
Meckel's diverticulum		

RECTAL BLEEDING

The colour of blood and its relationship to stool may give an indication of the site of the bleeding. Bright-red blood on the toilet paper or dripping after defecation is more commonly associated with an anal cause, e.g. haemorrhoids or fissures. Dark-red blood or blood mixed with the stool is more likely to be associated with colorectal cancer, especially when associated with change in bowel habit and/or abdominal pain. Rectal bleeding in cancer patients occurs without anal symptoms in over 60 per cent of patients.

ALTERATION IN BOWEL HABIT

Consistency of stool varies with age, older patients having on average more formed stool, and also with gender, men on average having looser stools. It is important to ascertain exactly what patients mean by a change in bowel habit. Constipation is usually defined as the infrequent passage of hard stool with straining, whereas diarrhoea is the frequent passage of liquid or semi-liquid stool. Not only is consistency of stool important but also the frequency of defecation because change in frequency may be significant without a change in consistency.

PAIN

Abdominal pain is of surprisingly little help in assessing the likelihood of colorectal cancer because it is both very common in the population and large bowel obstruction tends to occur without warning. Abdominal pain is characterized by severity, timing and association with eating. With obstruction of the ileocaecal valve, intestinal colic may be experienced about an hour after eating when the bowel contents reach the caecum.

IRON DEFICIENCY ANAEMIA

A relatively small amount of ingested iron is absorbed in the upper intestinal tract. Occult gastrointestinal blood loss from colorectal cancer, particularly right-sided lesions, is an important cause of iron deficiency in men and postmenopausal women. In the age group where colorectal cancer is most prevalent, i.e. over 70 years, haemorrhoids or non-steroidal anti-inflammatory drugs should initially not be assumed to be the cause of iron deficiency anaemia and a full investigation should be undertaken.

OTHER PRESENTATIONS

Uncommon presentations occur in colorectal cancer as a result of advanced disease. Gastrocolic fistulae may cause faecal vomiting or severe diarrhea and weight loss. Occasionally sigmoid cancers present as an external fistula or a psoas abscess. Internal fistulae can present with passage of faeces vaginally or recurrent urinary tract infections and pneumaturia. Local invasion of disease in rectal cancers produces localized pain and dysfunction. Secondary dissemination of the disease may produce anorexia and weight loss. Occasionally patients present with distant metastases in the lung, brain or bone. These symptoms may be the only presenting features.

EMERGENCY PRESENTATION

Symptoms may have been present for only a short period of time and the patient usually presents with obstruction and/or perforation. Large bowel obstruction is characterized by lower abdominal pain, usually intermittent and colicky in nature, and absolute constipation. Increased bowel sounds (borborygmi), nausea, vomiting and distension usually accompany these. A plain abdominal radiograph achieves confirmation of the diagnosis.

OUTPATIENT ASSESSMENT

A complete history should be taken to include presenting symptoms, past medical history, drug history and family history. Blood tests should include full blood count, liver function tests and carcinoembryonic antigen (CEA). This is a tumour marker for colorectal cancer, but can be raised in other conditions, e.g. smokers.

PHYSICAL EXAMINATION

General examination of the patient should look for evidence of weight loss, signs of general disease, jaundice, etc. Abdominal examination should be conducted with the patient supine and comfortable.

The examination should include:

1. Inspection: abdominal distension, visible peristalsis and scars indicating previous surgery.
2. Palpation: should include all four quadrants of the abdomen and inguinal regions, to elicit tenderness and detect abdominal masses. (May be able to feel palpable sigmoid colon; can be a normal finding in constipated patients.)
3. Percussion: dullness may suggest ascites or fluid-filled loops of bowel. Rebound tenderness indicates the presence of peritonitis.
4. Auscultation: listen for bowel sounds – high-pitched suggests partial obstruction; hypoactive bowel sounds may be present in late obstruction

ANORECTAL EXAMINATION

The anal area should be inspected, in good lighting, for rashes, lesions or skin tags. A digital examination should be performed first. A gloved lubricated finger is placed flat on the anus, gentle pressure applied and when the sphincter yields the finger is passed into the anus. The suggested order of examination is to feel the rectum first, then extrarectal pelvic structures, the pelvic floor and finally the anal canal. The feel of mucosa and the anal canal should be smooth, so any masses are abnormal. An assessment of the pelvic floor relaxed and contracted should be made. The prostate in men and the cervix in women can be felt.

Tenderness can indicate fissures or abscesses. The withdrawn finger should be inspected for stool, pus, mucus or blood.

SIGMOIDOSCOPY

This is usually carried out after the digital examination. Many physicians prefer an unprepared bowel, as enemas can cause irritation that can mimic proctitis. It can also remove important physical signs such as mucus and blood and prevents inspection of stool. However, glycerine suppositories or a small-volume enema can be given if required. It is usually performed in the left lateral position and can be with a rigid or flexible endoscope; the main advantage of the latter is the ability to insert beyond 20 cm. The rigid scope is inserted with the obturator in place, initially in the direction of the umbilicus. When there is a fall in resistance (indicating that the rectum is entered) the obturator is removed and the instrument then angled along the sacrum. The instrument is advanced under direct vision with minimal insufflation, as far as possible or until the patient has discomfort. Inspection is performed during withdrawal, undertaking a circular motion so that all walls of the bowel are visualized.

FLEXIBLE SIGMOIDOSCOPY

This allows examination up to 60 cm and can usually be performed without sedation. Bowel preparation with a phosphate enema is usually sufficient, 1–2 hours before the test. Antibiotic prophylaxis is recommended for those patients at risk of developing endocarditis, e.g. those with prosthetic heart valves. The scope is usually inserted with the right hand and the controls manoeuvred in the left hand. The bowel is insufflated with air.

Examination of the mucosa is made on withdrawal of the instrument, the tip of the sigmoidoscope being rotated to cover all walls of the bowel. The yield of pathological abnormalities is greater than with rigid sigmoidoscopy; about 50 per cent of colorectal carcinomas are within reach of a flexible sigmoidoscope . It provides a clearer visualization of the mucosa of the bowel and also tends to be more comfortable for the patient. Both biopsies and polypectomies can be performed using electrocautery.

FURTHER INVESTIGATIONS

FAECAL OCCULT BLOOD TEST

This test is often used in patients with unexplained iron deficiency anaemia. It is sensitive but not highly specific for colorectal cancer because it identifies any bleeding in the gastrointestinal tract, e.g. from gum disease or gastritis.

COLONOSCOPY

Colonoscopy allows complete examination of the colon, and has a sensitivity and specificity of >95 per cent for all lesions. The major advantage of colonoscopy is greater sensitivity for small polyps and also that it allows tissue diagnosis and treatment when appropriate.

RADIOLOGY

Lower gastrointestinal tract radiological investigation should be considered only after full rectal examination including sigmoidoscopy.

SINGLE CONTRAST BARIUM ENEMA

This is a rarely performed procedure that does not involve insufflation of gas; it is less sensitive and specific than a double-contrast barium enema.

DOUBLE-CONTRAST BARIUM ENEMA

This is the current radiological gold standard for examining the colon. Excellent bowel preparation is essential. This is usually achieved with a low residue diet and sodium picosulphate 24 hours before the procedure.

It is important to maintain an intake of at least 2 litres of clear fluids to avoid dehydration. During the procedure barium liquid is introduced through a balloon catheter placed in the rectum, the patient or table is rotated to coat all walls of the bowel, and most of the barium is removed. Insufflation of air or carbon dioxide through the catheter then enables an outline of the mucosa to be achieved. An antispasmodic may be given during the procedure because instillation of air may cause some discomfort. Using carbon dioxide instead of air as an insufflation gas reduces pain .Patients continue to pass barium for 1–2 days after the test and may need laxatives to prevent constipation.

COLONOGRAPHY/VIRTUAL COLONOSCOPY

This is a relatively new procedure using spiral computed tomography (CT). This involves an X-ray tube that rotates continuously around the patient as he or she moves forwards on a table. This can produce three dimensional images of the abdomen. Scan data are computed to produce images of the colon in three dimensions, similar to those obtained during a real colonoscopy.

ENDOANAL ULTRASONOGRAPHY

Patient preparation is two glycerine suppositories or an enema 1 hour before the test. Usually the patient is placed in jack-knife or left lateral position. The endorectal ultrasound probe is surrounded by a balloon filled with water and inserted into the rectum. It is advanced proximal to the tumour, the examination being performed during withdrawal. The difference in tissue density of the rectal wall produces a five-layer image that can be used to determine tumour invasion. Tumours are hypoechoic and, when invaded by tumour, the separate layers are distorted. It is particularly useful in assessing the depth of penetration in early rectal tumours. Lymph nodes are visible when enlarged, their size being directly proportional to the risk of their containing metastatic disease; those smaller than 5 mm in diameter have a 20 per cent risk, whereas those larger than 9 mm have a 70 per cent risk. The accuracy of determination of mesorectal node involvement is only 50–60 per cent; this may be because many nodes lie outside the field of the probe. The limitations of endoanal ultrasonography are its small field of view and inability to stage high or stenosing tumours.

COMPUTED TOMOGRAPHY

Pelvic CT can be used to detect local spread of rectal cancer. CT scans cannot distinguish the different layers of the rectal wall, and so are not able to distinguish between T1 and T2 tumours. Lymph nodes that appear enlarged are assumed to contain tumour deposits and CT can also identify extension beyond the bowel wall. However, as with endoanal ultrasonography it cannot be determined whether this is caused by invasion or inflammatory reaction.

MAGNETIC RESONANCE IMAGING

This investigation uses the waveform of magnetic resonance of hydrogen nuclei in the body. This is picked up by a scanner and translated into visual images. Hydrogen nuclei are present in large numbers in fat and water, and so show up white. Organs show up in shades of grey. Movement produces blurring or motion artifact so it is vital that the patient stays still during the procedure. The tunnel action and the noise of the machine may cause claustrophobia so patients need to be well informed. There is a need to remove all clothing containing metal objects because they can cause artefacts. For the same reason, this examination cannot be used on patients with implanted metal objects, e.g. hip prostheses. MRI is used in the assessment of spread of rectal cancer, with most studies finding sensitivity equal to that of enlarged nodes can be identified but there is difficulty distinguishing between inflammatory and neoplastic changes. The use of an endorectal coil can enhance the image produced. This is kept in the left lateral position of the patient and held there by use of a clamp to reduce motion artefact. This method provides detailed definition of primary tumour depth. However, they may be difficult to use in stenosing tumours and are more invasive. They are also less accurate in providing information about the circumferential resection margin because of the limited field of view . The most accurate current method is to use an external phased-array coil that provides images with high spatial resolution and also a wide field of view, allowing visualization of the entire mesorectum and surrounding pelvic organs .

CHEST RADIOGRAPH

Up to 25 per cent of patients with distant spread will have pulmonary metastases. A plain chest radiograph will identify most pulmonary metastases, but a CT scan is more sensitive.

ULTRASONOGRAPHY

Ultrasound waves are produced by applying a short burst of electricity to a piezoelectric crystal in the transducer; several of these together comprise a probe. Diagnosis is made by measuring the echoes produced by the scattering of sound waves by the tissue interfaces. To scan a patient the probe is placed on the skin, gel being used to produce an air-free interface. To scan the liver a patient usually has to be nil by mouth for the day of the test because food can obstruct the scan preventing a clear view.

INTRAOPERATIVE ULTRASONOGRAPHY

Intraoperative ultrasonography can be performed either directly or laparoscopically and can obviate the need for preoperative CT as a staging procedure for distant metastases.

POSITRON EMISSION TOMOGRAPHY

PET with 2-fluoro-2-deoxy-D-glucose (FDG) exploits the increased rate of glycolysis in tumour cells to detect disease. Patients are fasted for four hours before the test, FDG is administered IV and a wholebody scan is undertaken. It is used principally to determine local or distant recurrence, especially when there is doubt about appearances on other imaging modalities. It is particularly useful in distinguishing cancer from inflammatory or scar tissue in postoperative patients.

RADIOIMMUNODETECTION

Colorectal tumours express carcino-embryonic antigen (CEA). Arcitumomab is given to the patient by intravenous infusion; imaging can then be carried out externally using a total body scan (radio-immunodetection or RAID). Alternatively a gamma probe can be used intraoperatively to identify any areas of tumour, e.g. in lymph nodes or locally invading other tissues .

TREATMENTS

When the colorectal cancer survival rate is merely 40 per cent, for a potentially curable disease it is essential that any treatments offer optimum prognosis. Surgery is the mainstay treatment for colorectal cancer and therefore should be at the forefront for improving outcomes, using nationally agreed guidelines based on valid research.

PRINCIPLES OF SURGERY

A colorectal surgeon should achieve 'curative resection', i.e. histological confirmation of complete excision and no residual tumour for about 40 per cent of cases. New surgical techniques may now be recommended for selective procedures to effect optimum prognosis; however, there are still traditional principles for cancer surgery:

- Wide resection of the cancer-bearing bowel segment
- Widest feasible excision of the lymphatics draining the cancer-bearing bowel segment
- 'No touch' technique
- Minimum of cancer cell contamination and embolization
- Segmental resection of the colon, removing all possible gross disease with adequate margins and adequate lymph node basin excision to remove regional nodal metastases.

COLON CANCER: SURGICAL PROCEDURES

Colon cancer surgery is predominantly concerned with segmental colonic resection, excision of all gross disease with adequate margins and adequate removal of corresponding lymphatic drainage.

RIGHT HEMICOLECTOMY

Carcinoma of the caecum or right side of the colon is usually managed by right hemicolectomy. The operation, via a right transverse or midline incision, consists of resection from the terminal ileum, past the hepatic flexure along to the mid-transverse colon, preserving the middle colic vessels with end-to-end or stapled side-to-side anastomosis and removal of its regional lymphatic drainage.

In this surgical procedure, as with all other colonic resections, the abdomen is explored to determine respectability and to search for synchronous tumours, distant metastases and associated abdominal disease. The small intestinal mesentery and the transverse mesocolon are divided on a line parallel to the superior mesenteric and middle colic arteries.

The blood vessels are divided and ligated early in the operation, again to avoid dissemination of tumour cells into the portal circulation or the lymphatics.

When the carcinoma is near the ileocaecal valve a substantial segment of the terminal ileum (10–12 cm) with its mesentery should be removed because of the lymphatics along the ileocolic vessels. When the lesion is in the hepatic flexure or mid-transverse colon, less ileum is removed, although careful dissection of the mesentery to the root of the mid-colic from the superior mesenteric is necessary.

A primary tumour on the right side of the colon is usually resected even if distant metastases have occurred, because prevention of obstruction or anaemia may offer best palliation.

If a patient has an unresectable carcinoma, the obstruction may be bypassed by carrying out a palliative side-to-side anastomosis between the ileum and the transverse colon.

LEFT HEMICOLECTOMY

When no intestinal obstruction is present, the treatment of choice for carcinoma of the descending colon is usually managed by left hemicolectomy. The resection extends from the middle of the transverse colon to below the sigmoid colon near the origin of the left branch of the middle colic artery. The resection also incorporates excision of a large proportion of the greater omentum and all of the colic mesentery, the left colic artery, the sigmoid vessels and the superior haemorrhoidal artery that supplies the resected bowel. Primary anastomosis is usually performed.

SIGMOID COLECTOMY

Carcinoma of the sigmoid colon is occasionally managed by sigmoid colectomy with primary anastomosis of the descending colon to the rectum, although more frequently anterior resection or left hemicolectomy is the surgical option of choice.

EMERGENCY SURGERY

Elective surgery is always preferable to help minimize surgical complications and promote optimum prognosis. Patients with malignant obstruction of the colon are known to have a poorer prognosis stage for stage than those with non-obstructing lesions.

Over the past two decades we have seen a major change in the method of surgical intervention. Previously, when intestinal obstruction was present, the traditional surgical intervention was a three-stage procedure: (1) Stoma formation proximal to the obstruction and bowel decompression; (2) Resection of the obstructing lesion; and (3) Reversal of the stoma.

PALLIATION IN COLONIC CANCER

If it is possible to remove the tumour with only a reasonable risk, it is preferable to death from pain, bleeding and faecal discharge of an uncontrolled primary. Obliviously wide clearance of lymphatic drainage is not necessary.

Bypass surgery is indicated when it is not possible or advisable to excise the tumour and the colonic flow is altered, i.e. ileotransverse bypass for unresectable caecal tumour.

At times stoma formation may be indicated to bypass an obstruction but this should be considered only if all other options are not advisable. Trephine or laproscopic stoma formation would be performed to minimize the morbidity risk to the patient and reduce hospitalization.

STENTING

In selected patients with obstructed left colon cancer, non-surgical treatment may be preferred. Deflation of the obstructed colon (often caused by a rectosigmoid lesion) may be achieved by the introduction of a colonic stent to the affected site, using a sigmoidoscope which is highly flexible.

In the patient with a non-resectable tumour and poor prognosis and health status, it improves symptoms without the need (and therefore increased morbidity) for general anaesthesia and probable stoma surgery.

RECTAL CANCER: SURGICAL PROCEDURES

TOTAL MESORECTAL

Traditionally, anterior resection and abdominoperineal excision of the rectum (APER) have produced disappointing results with regard to local recurrence and overall survival for rectal cancer. It may be argued that the use of adjuvant therapies of radiotherapy and chemotherapy has beenpromoted in an effort to improve these outcomes. Heald questioned the value of traditional rectal surgery and, considering the area of spread in rectal cancer, found that this was usually limited to a field that is encompassed by the integral visceral mesentery of the hindgut, i.e. the mesorectum. When disease is not widely disseminated, resection including the mesorectum offers removal of virtally every tumour satellite and minimizes local recurrence. This procedure described by Heald is now known as total mesorectal excision (TME). Excision of the mesorectum, 'the perfect tumour package' as described by Heald, is where the surgical resection technique, under direct vision, recreates the tissue planes around the intact tumour specimen, preventing tearing and compromising of the clearance margins.

ABDOMINOPERINEAL EXCISION OF RECTUM

This is excision of the whole rectum and anal canal via abdominal and perineal approaches, with the formation of a permanent end-colostomy.

At the turn of the twentieth century, surgery performed for rectal cancer affected a high mortality with almost certain future recurrence.

HARTMANN'S PROCEDURE

It is defined as a resection of the sigmoid colon, possibly including a length of rectum being excised, with formation of a terminal colostomy and closure of the rectal stump.

Traditionally this procedure was indicated for carcinoma of the upper and mid-rectum but this has now largely been superseded by anterior resection. A Hartmann's procedure is generally now performed in the emergency setting, when a patient presents with colonic obstruction or perforation secondary to a carcinoma. Primary anastomosis is often not advisable in these situations. A laparotomy is performed to explore the peritoneal cavity and to identify the primary lesion and any associated disease. The proximal dissection is usually at the last part of the descending colon or sigmoid colon. The diseased segment is, where possible, resected by dividing the distal end with suturing of the remaining rectal stump.

A left iliac colostomy is constructed through a separate incision, which preferably has been predetermined by the colorectal or stoma care nurse specialist in conjunction with the patient, and is clearly marked on the patient's skin.

If the disease is advanced, complete resection with suturing of the rectal stump may not be possible and the tumour may be left in situ, draining through the distal rectum. This form of palliative surgery is not recommended because it results in an immeasurably poor quality of life for patients as a result of the physical disruption caused by per rectum tumour drainage.

COMPLICATIONS

- Rectal stump leakage can occur in approximately 10 per cent of cases.
- Stoma complications are uncommon but necrosis may occur perioperatively.
- Wound sepsis, anastomotic leakage and urinary problems are the main complications.
- Anastomotic stenosis can be a late complication.

LOCAL EXCISION

Transanal local excision does play a significant part in the management of rectal carcinoma, albeit a limited one.

The possibility of cure of selected rectal cancers with minimal morbidity, negligible mortality, and maintenance of normal gastrointestinal and genitourinary function has caused a lot of controversy over the past two decades. Does local excision with curative intent and its current techniques compromise the potential for cure, even for a highly selected group? Selection is critical because the tumour must be anatomically accessible and technically amenable to complete excision with free margins, and have pathology of good or moderate differentiation and be < 3 cm in diameter. If poorly differentiated, lymphatic or vascular invasion is present, or histopathology confirms mucinous or signet ring tumours, local excision will be inadequate and more invasive surgery will be warranted.

The advent of endorectal ultrasonography offers improved accuracy in predicting tumour staging with regard to depth of mural invasion and lymph node involvement. Unfortunately, research indicates that, even with improved scan ing techniques, it is still not possible to predict with absolute precision and local excision; certainly, when T2 tumours were treated by this technique, it often resulted in higher than acceptable localrecurrence. Salvage surgery is possible, but overall survival is unknown compared with traditional surgical intervention. Tumours involving the muscle coat of the bowel wall have 10–20 per cent of involved nodes in the mesorectum and therefore, at present, curative intent local excision of rectal carcinoma in good-risk patients should probably be limited to those few, highly favourable T1 tumours.

LAPAROSCOPIC SURGERY

Controversy continues regarding this form of colorectal cancer management; in some research, short-term benefits have been indicated whereas others have indicated that the advantages remain unclear. Advantages to elderly people are reduced complication rate and favourable short-term outcome. Port site recurrence appears to be associated with poor laparoscopic technique (Nduka et al., 1994). In younger patients this form of surgical management of colorectal cancer is not advocated, because longterm benefits/complications are, as yet, unknown.

RECTAL CANCER: FIRST-LINE ADJUVANT TREATMENT

Although surgery remains the mainstay intervention for colorectal cancer, radiotherapy and chemotherapy are now seen as an integral part of the overall treatment package for selective patients, particularly rectal tumours.

Individuals performing surgery without preoperative radiotherapy have demonstrated lower local recurrence rates than those in the Swedish trial, and therefore this posed the question of whether preoperative radiotherapy actually was a benefit in the light of this new accepted surgical procedure.

Side effects experienced by patients are generally minimal, but may include tiredness, diarrhoea and occasionally sore skin. Surgical complications include delayed healing to the perineum and increased risk of wound dehiscence in abdominoperineal excision and higher rates of impotency in both abdominoperineal excision and anterior resection (up to 0 per cent). Long-term complications include fibrosis, small bowel obstruction and, possibly, radiological cancer formation.

Up to 30 per cent of patients with rectal cancer will have locally advanced disease at presentation, which is unresectable or borderline as a result of fixation to adjacent structures, e.g. the prostate and/or the bony pelvis. These fixed or tethered tumours are associated with poor prognosis when compared with mobile tumours, and palliative or incomplete resection has a reported median of 10-month survival. Adjuvant therapy in these cases aims to effect tumour shrinkage and this long-course treatment using synchronous chemotherapy and radiation, known as chemoradiotherapy, is believed to improve the efficacy of radiotherapy by impairing the ability of tumour cells to repair DNA damage.

Treatment consists of 25 fractions of radiotherapy over 33 days in a three-field plan and a chemotherapy regimen of folinic acid and 5-fluorouracil (5FU) on days 1–5 and 29–33.

After this first-line treatment there is a delay of 6–12 weeks before surgical resection, to allow toxicity and subsequent side effects to reduce and possible downstaging of the tumour to occur.

SYNCHRONOUS TUMOURS: SURGICAL MANAGEMENT

About 25 per cent of all colorectal cancer patients will present with coexisting polyps in the colon and 3–8 per cent will have synchronous tumours. At present, there are no strict guidelines regarding surgical management, and surgery performed varies greatly, dependent on tumour locations, possible consultant preference, multidisciplinary team agreement and patient considerations of age, health status and preference.

The following are examples of the range of surgery being performed.

TRADITIONAL COLORECTAL SURGERY

An anterior resection may still be the surgery of choice for synchronous tumours of the sigmoid and mid- or upper rectum.

SUBTOTAL COLECTOMY

For possible synchronous tumours of the descending colon, excision of the descending and sigmoid colon with colorectal anastomosis can be used.

TOTAL COLECTOMY

- Colectomy and anastomosis of ileum to rectum
- Total colectomy and ileostomy and creation of rectal fistula

- Total colectomy and ileostomy with rectal stump.

All are examples of surgery for caecal and sigmoid synchronous tumours.

PANPROCTOCOLECTOMY

- Total excision of the colon with formation of a permanent end-ileostomy
- Possible very low rectal tumour with synchronous tumours elsewhere in the colon

STOMA FORMATION

Traditionally an end stoma is created for diversion or palliation. At present, loop ileostomy tends to be the procedure of choice for diversion and it is estimated that about 20–30 per cent of anterior resections performed will involve formation of a temporary loop ileostomy. This may be the result of anastomotic difficulties at operation or the surgeon's preference for routine protection of the anastomotic site (although the ACPGB&I recommend judicious use of stoma diversion in this instance). Many surgeons will take the following into consideration:

- Low anastomosis is technically more difficult, with greater risk of anastomotic leak.
- Obstructing lesion with inadequate bowel cleansing causes an increased risk of sepsis, leakage, etc.
- Poor colonic vascularity increases anastomotic leak potential.
- When hysterectomy is also performed, closure of the vaginal stump at the same level as the bowel anastomosis increases the risk of rectovaginal fistula.
- Stoma formation, whether temporary or permanent, has an immense impact on a patient's rehabilitation. It is also important to note that there are an appreciable number of supposed temporary stomas where reversal is not performed. Quality of life can deteriorate quite markedly and at times this may lead to incapacitation because of the patient's inability to manage the stoma, and even to institutionalization.

ANAL CANCER

Anal carcinoma is still relatively rare in Western society; Northover (1993) states that there are 100 cases of colorectal cancer for each new anal tumour. Most cases are of epidermoid origin, with 80 per cent being squamous cell carcinoma.

Anal tumours can be categorized into those in the anal canal, at or above the dentate line, or those at the anal margin, below the dentate line. Invasion into the anal sphincters may occur, in the case of a tumour above the dentate line, or to the inguinal lymph nodes for those tumours below the dentate line.

Anal tumours manifest as ulcers or proliferate growths with ulceration present; as they advance they become hard and fixed. Histologically they vary from being well-differentiated, keratinizing, large-cell tumours to poorly differentiated, non-keratinizing, small-cell tumours in the upper anal canal. One major difference between anal and colorectal cancer is that anal tumours spread mainly only within the pelvis and rarely have distant spread.

Traditionally, treatment of anal cancer has been surgical intervention by radical APER. However, in the 1970s an American report suggested chemotherapy treatment as a possible cure. At the same time, Papillon in France reported on the benefits of radiotherapy with early rectal tumours and, following this, others suggested similar benefits to anal tumours. Now radiation therapy, or combined chemoradiation in particular, has become the more optimal treatment of choice. A British study in 1988 (Geh, 1988) reported where combination radiation and chemotherapy resulted in a response rate of 80-90 per cent and a 5-year survival rate of about 83 percent. This combination therapy of about six weeks is arduous for the patient but is now considered the most appropriate first-line treatment. Therefore, most patients undergoing chemoradiation should not require any surgical intervention after biopsy confirmation. A temporary trephine loop stoma may be necessary in isolated cases, if the risk of obstruction is high before the treatment, which becomes unmanageable. If the tumour was initially treated by local excision, chemoradiation should be considered before radical surgery.

Surgical intervention of abdominoperineal excision should be reserved for residual or recurrent disease, permanent anal sphincter damage or the complications of chemo-radiation therapy.

FURTHER TREATMENT: CHEMOTHERAPY AND RADIOTHERAPY

The management of colorectal cancer usually involves one of more of the following treatment modalities:

- Surgery
- Radiotherapy (predominately rectal cancer)
- Chemotherapy.

To achieve the best possible chance of cure, early diagnosis and appropriate surgical therapy are essential. Unfortunately, diagnosis is often delayed as a result of the vagueness of symptoms and a delayed realization of the significance of these symptoms .Many of the Patients have potentially good recovery rate.

RADIOTHERAPY

Radiotherapy is the use of ionizing radiation in the treatment of primarily malignant disease exerting local control over tumour tissue. Ionizing radiation destroys cells in the body by physical, chemical and biological methods. Radiation cannot distinguish between cancer and normal cells, so all cells within the treatment field are damaged, although cancer cells cannot repair radiation damage as effectively as normal cells. The aim of treatment is that the required dose of radiation to the target area must be delivered while minimizing the dose to the surrounding normal tissue. This is achieved by careful treatment planning to produce the best possible outcome in terms of survival, symptom relief and side effects. The treatment area must be accurately imaged so that the radiation beam can be accurately targeted; computed tomography (CT) facilitates precise delivery of radiotherapy to the treatment site, avoiding radiation of normal tissue. A multiple radiotherapy field technique is often used, bombarding the treatment area with multiple beams set to converge at a point deep within the treatment area, ensuring that the normal tissue receives minimal radiation. Different types of energy are required to treat different parts of the body; treatment fields close to the skin require less energy than treatment areas deep inside the body.

Radiation is measured in units called 'grays' (Gy) and the frequency in which it is given is referred to as 'fractionation'.

Dosages are calculated to maintain a balance between killing any cancer cells without causing irreversible side effects to normal cells and tissue. Treatment is also dependent on whether the intent is to cure cancer at an early stage or at symptom relief in more advanced cancer. Radiotherapy can be delivered by various methods.

EXTERNAL BEAM RADIOTHERAPY

This is the most commonly used method of radiation treatment. The radiation beam is administered on to and into the patient from a source external to the patient's body. Treatment is delivered by high-energy Xray machines known as linear accelerators. A course of treatment is prescribed, which can be anything from a single session to treatment lasting up to six weeks, depending on the site and stage performance status of the individual; it lasts about 2–3 minutes a day. The X-ray beam is accurately targeted by markings on the individual's skin or by the use of individually prepared Perspex shells.

BRACHYTHERAPY

Otherwise known as sealed source therapy, brachytherapy is a radioactive source placed within a body cavity or tissue or supported close to the skin surface. It was developed from the use of radium, but has largely been replaced by other radioisotopes, the properties of which make them less of a potential radiation hazard; it allows the radioactive sources to be remotely after-loaded into the tumour site, thus reducing the radiation hazard to individuals.

LIQUID RADIOACTIVE SOURCES

Also known as unsealed source therapy, this is a radioactive substance delivered via injection or taken orally, the most common being radioactive iodine in the treatment of thyroid cancer.

ADJUVANT RADIOTHERAPY FOR RECTAL CANCER

In colon cancer there is no established role for adjuvant radiotherapy. Its goal in rectal cancer is to reduce the incidence of local recurrence, a potentially morbid complication. Local recurrence after complete resection of rectal cancer is more frequent than with colon cancer because the rectum lies below the peritoneal reflection. Of recurrences, 50 percent are in the pelvis rather than at distant sites, and tumour invasion into the surrounding tissue and organs occurs more frequently because the growth of rectal tumours is not limited by a serosa. Adjuvant radiotherapy has been evaluated for rectal cancer both before and after surgical resection.

PREOPERATIVE RADIOTHERAPY

A large number of randomized controlled trials (RCTs) have produced consistent evidence demonstrating that preoperative radiotherapy for rectal cancer reduces local recurrence rates .

MOBILE/TETHERED/OPERABLE TUMOURS

Tumours that have not infiltrated surrounding structures are generally referred to as 'mobile/tethered tumours'. The objective of preoperative radiotherapy is to destroy micrometastatic disease and reduce the incidence of local recurrence. The Swedish rectal trial, which was the largest study of preoperative radiotherapy, demonstrated a reduction in local recurrence compared with surgery alone.

Recent improvements in the surgical excision of rectal cancers, e.g. total mesorectal excision (TME), has in some cases produced local recurrence rates as low as those seen in individuals treated with preoperative radiotherapy. However, preliminary results from a recent Dutch study have shown local recurrence rates of preoperative radiotherapy and TME surgery being further improved.

POSTOPERATIVE RADIOTHERAPY

Postoperative, long-course, adjuvant radiotherapy minimizes the incidence of local recurrence but it is less than that of preoperative radiotherapy. As with preoperative treatment, no benefit in overall survival has been demonstrated, although postoperative radiotherapy combined with 5-fluorouracil (5FU)-based chemotherapy demonstrates a significant survival advantage compared with surgery alone. The chemoradiation is more commonly used in the USA; in European countries the tendency is to opt for preoperative short- or long-course radiotherapy, as previously described in operable tumours.

Individuals who have not had preoperative radiotherapy and shown postoperatively a high risk of tumour recurrence, with tumour involvement of the circumferential resection margin (CRM) or radial margins of < 1 mm clearance, should be considered for longer-course postoperative chemoradiation. Local recurrence rates are slightly improved when chemotherapy is combined with radiotherapy in the postoperative setting (Pahlman, 1998).

RADIOTHERAPY FOR LOCALLY ADVANCED RECTAL CANCER

Large numbers of individuals present with fixed rectal tumours, which have invaded surrounding structures and organs. To increase the respectability rate of fixed rectal tumours, preoperative radiotherapy is administered , at a dose of 45–50 Gy over 5 weeks, with the aim of producing tumour shrinkage. If possible, surgical resection takes place about 4–6 weeks later to allow for maximum tumour regression. The addition of chemotherapy is currently being evaluated in established trials.

PALLIATIVE RADIOTHERAPY FOR ADVANCED COLORECTAL CANCER

Palliative radiotherapy is usually given for the relief of symptoms of advanced disease. The treatment of distant metastases, such as lung, brain and bone as well as the pelvic recurrences, with either single fraction or short courses of radiotherapy can lead to a symptomatic benefit. The aim of palliative radiotherapy is to obtain a balance between symptom management and treatment toxicities.

CHEMOTHERAPY

Chemotherapy drugs used in the treatment of cancer are referred to as cytotoxic agents: 'cyto' means 'cell', and 'toxic' means 'poison'. Cytotoxic drugs can broadly be grouped into classes relating to their anti-tumour action at cell level. Mode of action depends on the individual drug, but most drugs in current use inhibit cellular proliferation, by inhibiting DNA or RNA synthesis. The primary classification of cytotoxic drugs is according to their action on the cell life cycle, those that are cell cycle specific (CCPS) or active in all phases of the cell cycle, and those that are cell cycle phase non-specific (CCPNS) or active in specific phases.

ALKYLATING AGENTS

These exert their main toxicity by forming cross-linkages between DNA chains, which result in the inhibition of DNA replication and subsequent cell division; also by interacting with a number of enzymes involved in protein synthesis, they prevent DNA synthesis and cell division, e.g. cyclophosphamide or oxaliplatin.

ANTIMETABOLITES

These interfere with the production of purine and pyrimidine and thus prevent protein synthesis. They inhibit enzymes, or become incorporated in new nuclear material altering function, e.g. methotrexate, 5-fluorouracil, capecitabine, UFT.

CYTOTOXIC ANTIBIOTICS

These are divided into anthracyclines or non-anthracyclines. Anthracyclines intercalate between DNA base-pairs, inhibiting DNA and RNA synthesis, and also producing free radicals that can break the DNA chain. Both have an alkylating activity and affect permeability of the cell membrane, e.g. doxorubicin.

MITOTIC SPINDLE INHIBITORS

These bind to the protein of cellular microtubles known as tubulin, inhibiting spindle formation and causing metaphase arrest, which leads to the disruption of cell division, e.g. vincristine.

TOPOISOMERASE I INHIBITORS

These are S phase specific, inhibiting the action of topoisomerase I, an enzyme that releases the torsional strain in the supercoiled DNA by catalysing a transient break in one of its strands, allowing replication to take place. They act by stabilizing the complex between the enzyme and DNA strand and, as a result, the cleavable complex does not dissociate and the repair of the strand is prevented, resulting in cessation of the advancement of the replication fork, e.g. irinotecan.

TAXOIDS/TAXANES

These work by arresting cell division during the metaphase of the cell cycle. As the spindle forms during mitosis, the taxoids/taxanes promote the assembly of the microtubules but then stop their disassembly by inhibiting the depolymerization of the contractile protein tubulin. As a result, the microtubular network becomes abnormally rigid and unable to perform vital mitotic and interphase cellular functions, which eventually leads to cell death, e.g. paclitaxel (Taxol).

MISCELLANEOUS AGENTS

These work by various ways of inhibiting cell proliferation. Cytotoxic drugs can be administered by a variety of routes: oral, intramuscular, intravenous, intra-arterial and intravesicular. All are blood borne and have the potential to treat both primary and metastatic disease. As cytotoxic drugs cannot differentiate between cancer and normal cells, they affect all cells. The cells most affected are the rapidly proliferating cells of the mouth, gastrointestinal tract, bone marrow and hair follicles. This is why side effects in these areas are generally more severe.

Adjuvant Chemotherapy for Colorectal Cancer

Adjuvant is derived from the Latin 'ad' meaning 'to' and 'juvare' meaning 'help'.

The aim of adjuvant treatment is to target rapidly cycling foci of cancer cells and destroy them before they become established detectable metastasis.

5-Fluorouracil is a cell-cycle-specific agent, active during one short phase of the cell life. It is a thymidylate synthetase (TS) inhibitor that prevents formation of thymidine, inhibiting DNA and RNA synthesis. The addition of folinic acid (FA) stabilizes the 5FU–TS complex, promoting and maximizing TS inhibition.

Palliative Chemotherapy for Advanced Colorectal Cancer

For individuals with advanced colorectal cancer, chemotherapy is administered with palliative rather than curative intent.

Palliative chemotherapy is now offered to an increasing proportion of patients with advanced colorectal cancer.

The individuals are selected for palliative chemotherapy requires the opinion of an oncologist experienced in the treatment of colorectal cancer. Poor performance status (3 or 4), low serum albumin, high alkaline phosphatase and liver involvement are independent predictors of progression, and low serum albumin, high glutamyl transferase and high carcinoembryonic antigen (CEA) are predictors for poor survival (Fontzilas et al., 1996).

The potential benefits of chemotherapy in the palliative setting must be weighed against any treatment adverse effects and effect on quality of life. The continuing assessment of treatment-related side effects and correct management is essential in determining the acceptability of chemotherapy in the palliative setting.

Irinotecan

It represents a novel class of cytotoxic drug, the camptothecins. The active component of irinotecan causes inhibition of topoisomerase I, an enzyme that plays a pivotal role in DNA transcription, replication and repair, leading to multiple single-strand DNA breaks, which eventually block the replication fork, leading to cell death. Colorectal cancer cells have high levels of the enzyme topoisomerase I; irinotecan's, inhibition of this enzyme explains its activity in colorectal cancer. Multiple RCTs with irinotecan have shown a survival benefit in individuals with advanced colorectal cancer. First-line combination treatment is administered for 48 hours via a centrally placed line a peripherally inserted central catheter (PICC), every 14 days for a total of six cycles before assessment of tumour response. Second-line treatment with irinotecan is given as a single agent. Treatment is administered via an intravenous infusion lasting between 30 and 60 minutes, every 21 days for four cycles before assessment of tumour response.The side effects of irinotecan are generally manageable and non-cumulative.

Acute Cholinergic Syndrome

This usually occurs within 24 hours of treatment administration; it is short lasting, but never life threatening, and is very unpleasant for the patient, treatable and preventable, and should never lead to treatment discontinuation. Treatment is by a subcutaneous injection of atropine sulphate 0.25 mg and is then given prophy-lactically before each administration.

Early Diarrhea

This is diarrhoea that occurs in the first 24 hours of treatment administration; treatment should be with atropine, because this is related to the acute cholinergic syndrome.

Nausea and Vomiting

These can occur concurrently after each administration of treatment. It is usually controllable with effective antiemetic therapy, which is commonly administered intravenously before each cycle, with oral treatment being given to take home as required

Delayed Diarrhoea

This is diarrhoea that usually occurs more than 24 hours after treatment administration. It is predictable at around 5 days and is usually shortlived, lasting about 12–72 hours. Delayed diarrhoea is the most common dose-limiting toxicity of irinotecan therapy.

Neutropenia

This is the second most dose-limiting toxicity; it rarely develops into febrile neutropenia and is non-cumulative. The median day to nadir is 8 days. Once again, the incidence of the grade of neutropenia is different between first-line combination treatment and second-line single-agent treatment. The severity in combination treatment is less.

Alopecia

This is more common when irinotecan is administered as a single agent; incidence and grade are reduced when given with 5FU/FA. Although all patients should be prepared for some hair loss, it occurs gradually as the cycles continue and hair loss is reversed when treatment is discontinued.

Oxaliplatin

Oxaliplatin is a new platinum derivative analogue and is a potent inhibitor of DNA synthesis. It is thought to act as an alkylating agent, making DNA lesions that the cell cannot repair and leading to cell death. It shows synergism with 5FU.

Several RCTs have demonstrated that oxaliplatin added to the 5FU/FA regimen shows an improved response rate and time to progression, but there is no difference in overall survival. One study demonstrated an increased number of individuals undergoing potential curative surgical resection of liver metastasis. The side effects of oxaliplatin are generally manageable and, apart from neurotoxicity, they are non-cumulative.

Sensory Peripheral Neurotoxicity

This is the most distinguishable side effect of oxaliplatin treatment. If symptoms have not resolved between each cycle and there is a loss of function (fine finger control), oxaliplatin should be stopped until the sensoryneuropathy has resolved.

Pharyngeal Dysaesthesia

Otherwise known as 'funny throat syndrome', this is precipitated by cold and can cause considerable distress to an individual if not he or she is reassured about it.

Renal Function

Oxaliplatin is not nephrotoxic but is renally cleared. Renal function should be monitored before treatment administration.

Hair thinning

Alopecia is uncommon but as treatment cycles continue individuals might notice a thinning of hair.

Nausea and vomiting

These can occur concurrently after each administration of treatment. It is usually controllable with effective antiemetic therapy, which is usually administered intravenously before each cycle, and oral treatment is given to take home as required.

Raltitrexed

Raltitrexed is a selective TS inhibitor. It is used for the palliative treatment of colorectal cancer for patients in whom 5FU is not tolerated or is inappropriate. It is a convenient 15-min infusion every three weeks and, although evidence suggests survival data comparable with 5FU. Common toxicities associated with raltitrexed are diarrhoea, nausea and vomiting, myelosuppression and increased liver transaminases.

Capecitabine

Capecitabine is a new class of oral fluoropyrimidines, was designed to mimic continuous infusion 5FU and to generate 5FU preferentially in tumour tissue. The tumour-selective activity of capecitabine is achieved through the exploitation of the high-concentrations of thymidine phosphorylase (TP) present in colorectal cancer cells compared with normal cells. Two RCTs have demonstrated that, in advanced colorectal cancer, capecitabine shows a significantly better response rate, equivalent time to progression, and overall survival when compared with a bolus regimen of 5FU/FA (Hoff, 2000).Capecitabine was also less toxic in most respects and more convenient to administer. It is licensed for use in advanced colorectal cancer. Capecitabine is taken twice daily in equally divided doses for 14 days followed by a rest period for seven days. The most common side effects of capecitabine are similar to those of 5FU; incidence and grade of toxicity vary between individuals and 5FU regimen.

Hand and foot syndrome

This is one of the most commonly reported toxicities and, depending on the grade, can lead to dose reduction.

Diarrhoea, Stomatitis, Nausea and Vomiting, and Alopecia

These are also common toxicities and are managed continuously as per local guidelines. As always, the grade of toxicity has to be effectively monitored to gain maximum benefits from treatment and defer or dose reduce as appropriate.**UFT**Ftorafur is another oral pro-drug of 5FU that has been around since the 1960s. Uracil is added to ftorafur to form UFT, which acts as a competitor for the rate-limiting enzyme in the catabolic inactivation of 5FU, which extends the plasma half-life of 5FU. UFT is licensed for use in advanced colorectal cancer.

Hand and foot syndrome diarrhoea, stomatitis, nausea and vomiting, and alopecia

FATIGUE

Table 88.3

Chemotherapy Regimens for the Adjuvant Treatment of Colorectal Cancer

Regimen	Agents	Comment
FOLFOX4[a]	Oxaliplatin 85 mg/m^2 IV day 1 Folinic acid 200 mg/m^2 per day IV over 2 hours days 1 and 2 Fluorouracil 400 mg/m^2 IV bolus, after folinic acid then 600 mg/m^2 CIV over 22 hours days 1 and 2 • Repeat every 14 days	Improved DFS as compared to infusional fluorouracil-leucovorin–based regimens.
FLOX[b]	Oxaliplatin 85 mg/m^2 IV administered on weeks 1, 3, and 5 Fluorouracil 500 mg/m^2 IV bolus weekly × 6 Folinic acid 500 mg/m^2× IV weekly 6 • Each cycle lasts 8 weeks and is repeated for three cycles	Improved DFS as compared to bolus fluorouracil-leucovorin–based regimens.
Capecitabine	Capecitabine 1,250 mg/m^2 po twice daily on days 1 through 14 every 21 days	Equivalent DFS as compared to the Mayo Clinic regimen with improved tolerability.
Fluorouracil-based regimens Roswell Park regimen[c]	Fluorouracil 600 mg/m^2 per day IV, day 1 Folinic acid 500 mg/m^2 per day IV over 2 hours • Repeat weekly for 6 of 8 weeks	
Mayo Clinic regimen[d]	Fluorouracil 425 mg/m^2 per day IV, days 1–5 Folinic acid 20 mg/m^2 per day IV, days 1–5 • Repeat every 4 to 5 weeks	
De Gramont regimen[e]	Fluorouracil 400 mg/m^2 per day IV bolus, followed by 600 mg/m^2 CIV over 22 hours, days 1 and 2 for 2 consecutive days Folinic acid 200 mg/m^2 per day IV over 2 hours days 1 and 2 • Repeat every 2 weeks	Improved safety as compared to the Mayo Clinic regimen.

REFERENCES

1. Association of Coloproctology of Great Britain and Ireland (2001) Guidelines for the Management of Colorectal Cancer. London: Royal College of Surgeons.
2. Cvikovic E, Betradda M (1999) Oxaliplatin: A new therapeutic option in colorectal cancer. Seminars in Oncology 26: 647–662.
3. Effective Health Care (1997). The Management of Colorectal Cancer. NHS Centre for Reviews and Dissemination, University of York.
4. Association of Coloproctology of Great Britain and Ireland (2001) Guidelines for the Management of Colorectal Cancer. London: ACPGB&I.
5. Boulos PB, Wexner SD (2000) Colorectal Surgery. Philadelphia: WB Saunders.
6. Burkitt HG, Quick CRG, Gatt D (1996) Essential Surgery. Edinburgh: Churchill Livingstone.
7. Cushieri A, Hennessy TPJ, Greenhalgh RA, Rowley DI, Grace PA (1996) Clinical Surgery.Oxford: Blackwell Science.
8. Deans GT, Spence RAJ, Love AHG (1998) Colorectal Disease for Physicians and Surgeons.Oxford: Oxford University Press.
9. Department of Health (2000) The NHS National Cancer Plan. London: HMSO.
10. Forest APM, Carter DC, Macleod IB (1995) Principles and Practice of Surgery. Edinburgh:
11. Goligher J (1984) Surgery of the Anus, Rectum, and Colon. London: Baillière Tindall.
12. Heald RJ (1988) The 'holy plane' of rectal surgery. Journal of the Royal Society of Medicine81: 503–508.
13. Heald RJ, Husband EM, Ryall RDH (1982) The mesorectum in rectal cancer surgery – the clue to pelvic recurrence? British Journal of Surgery 69: 613–616.
14. Adam IJ, Ali Z, Shorthouse AJ (2000) How accurate is the endoscopist's assessment of visualisation of the left colon seen at flexible sigmoidoscopy? Colorectal Disease 2: 41–44.
15. Angelelli G, Scopinaro G, Claudiani F, Davini D, Mallarini G, Saitta S (1990) Rectal carcinoma: CT staging with water as a contrast medium. Radiology 177: 511–514.
16. Association of Coloproctology of Great Britain and Ireland (2001) Guidelines for the Management of Colorectal Cancer. London: Royal College of Surgeons.
17. Association of Coloproctology of Great Britain and Ireland (2002) Referral Guidelines for Bowel Cancer. London: Royal College of Surgeons.
18. Armitage, N (1998) Colorectal cancer: clinical features and investigations. Medicine 26: 975–976.
19. Balthazar EJ, Megibow AJ, Hulnick D, Naidich DP (1988) Carcinoma of the colon: detection and preoperative staging by CT. Radiology 150: 301–306.
20. Bat L, Pines A, Shemesh E et al. (1992) Colonoscopy in patients aged 80 years or older and its contribution to the evaluation of rectal bleeding. Postgraduate Medical Journal 68: 355–358.
21. Aaltonen LA, Peltomaki P, Leach FS, Sistonen P, Pylkkanen L, Mecl JP, Jarvinen H, Powell SM, Jen J, Hamilton SR, et al. (1993) Clues to the pathogenesis of familial colorectal cancer. Science 260: 812–816.
22. Bishop JM (1981) Oncogenes. Scientific American 140: 69.
23. Bishop JM (1985) Trends in oncogenes. Trends in Genetics 245–249.
24. Bishop JM (1987) The molecular genetics of cancer. Science 235: 305–311.
25. R, Smits AM, Bos JL (1988) Genetic alterations during colorectal-tumor development.
26. New England Journal of Medicine 319: 525–532.
27. Weiss RA (1982) RNA Tumour Viruses. Cold Spring Harbor Laboratory, USA .

CHAPTER 89

Rheumatoid Arthritis

DEFINITION

Rheumatoid arthritis (RA) is a chronic and usually progressive inflammatory disorder of unknown etiology characterized by polyarticular symmetric joint involvement and systemic manifestations.

PREVALENCE

The incidence of RA is in the region of 3 cases per 10,000 population per annum. Onset is uncommon under the age of 15 and from then on the incidence rises with age until the age of 80. The prevalence rate is 1%, with women affected three to five times as often as men. It is up to three times more common in smokers than non-smokers, particularly in men, heavy smokers, and those who are rheumatoid factor positive. A study in 2010 found that those who drank modest amounts of alcohol regularly were four times less likely to get rheumatoid arthritis than those who never drank. Some Native American groups have higher prevalence rates (5% – 6%) and people from the Caribbean region have lower prevalence rates. First-degree relative's prevalence rate is 2% – 3% and disease genetic concordance in monozygotic twins is approximately 15% – 20%.

ETIOLOGY

The cause of RA is unknown. It is an autoimmune disease, which means the body's immune system mistakenly attacks healthy tissue.

RA can occur at any age, but is more common in middle age. Women get RA more often than men.

Infection, genes, and hormone changes may be linked to the disease.

PATHOPHYSIOLOGY

- RA results from a dysregulation of the humoral and cell-mediated components of the immune system. Most patients produce antibodies called rheumatoid factors; these seropositive patients tend to have a more aggressive course than patients who are seronegative.
- Immunoglobulins (Igs) can activate the complement system, which amplifies the immune response by enhancing chemotaxis, phagocytosis, and release of lymphokines by mononuclear cells that are then presented to T lymphocytes. The processed antigen is recognized by the major histocompatibility complex proteins on the lymphocyte surface, resulting in activation of T and B cells.

- Tumor necrosis factor (TNF), interleukin-1 (IL-1), and IL-6 are proinflammatory cytokines important in the initiation and continuance of inflammation.
- Activated T cells produce cytotoxins, which are directly toxic to tissues, and cytokines, which stimulate further activation of inflammatory processes and attract cells to areas of inflammation. Macrophages are stimulated to release prostaglandins and cytotoxins.
- Activated B cells produce plasma cells, which form antibodies that, in combination with complement, result in accumulation of polymorphonuclear leukocytes. Polymorphonuclear leukocytes release cytotoxins, oxygen free radicals, and hydroxyl radicals that promote cellular damage to synovium and bone.
- Vasoactive substances (histamine, kinins and prostaglandins) are released at sites of inflammation, increasing blood flow and vascular permeability. This causes edema, warmth, erythema, and pain and makes it easier for granulocytes to pass from blood vessels to sites of inflammation.

CLINICAL FEATURES

- Nonspecific prodromal symptoms that develop insidiously over weeks to months may include fatigue, weakness, low-grade fever, loss of appetite, and joint pain. Stiffness and myalgias may precede development of synovitis
- Joint involvement tends to be symmetric and affect the small joints of the hands, wrists, and feet; the elbows, shoulders, hips, knees, and ankles may also be affected.
- Joint stiffness typically is worse in the morning, usually exceeds 30minutes, and may persist all day.
- On examination, joint swelling may be visible or may be apparent only by palpation. The tissue feels soft and spongy and may appear erythematous and warm, especially early in the course of the disease. Chronic joint deformities commonly involve of the wrists, metacarpophalangeal joints, and proximal interphalangeal joints.

DIAGNOSIS

LABORATORY ABNORMALITIES THAT MAY BE SEEN INCLUDE

- Normocytic, normochromic anemia;
- Thrombocytosis or thrombocytopenia;
- Leukopenia;
- Elevated erythrocyte sedimentation rate and C-reactive protein; positive rheumatoid factor (60% to 70% of patients);
- Positive anticyclic citrullinated peptide antibody (50% to 85% of patients), and positive antinuclear
- Antibodies (25% of patients).
- Examination of aspirated synovial fluid may reveal turbidity, leukocytosis, reduced viscosity, and normal or low glucose relative to serum concentrations.
- Radiologic findings early in the disease course may include soft tissue swelling and osteoporosis near the joint (periarticular osteoporosis).

- Erosions occurring later in the disease course are usually seen first in the metacarpophalangeal and proximal interphalangeal joints of the hands and metatarsophalangeal joints of the feet.

TREATMENT

NONPHARMACOLOGICAL THERAPY

- Adequate rest, weight reduction if obese, occupational therapy, physical therapy, and use of assistive devices may improve symptoms and help maintain joint function.
- Patients with severe disease may benefit from surgical procedures such as tenosynovectomy, tendon repair, and joint replacements.
- Patient education about the disease and the benefits and limitations of drug therapy is important.

PHARMACOLOGICAL THERAPY (TABLE 89.1) (FIG. 89.1)

GENERAL APPROACH

- A disease-modifying antirheumatic drug (DMARD) should be started within the first 3 months of symptom onset. DMARDs should be used in all patients except those with limited disease. Early use of DMARDs results in a more favorable outcome and can reduce mortality.
- First-line DMARDs include methotrexate (MTX), hydroxychloroquine, Sulphasalazine, and leflunomide. The order of agent selection is not clearly defined, but MTX is often chosen initially because long-term data suggest superior outcomes compared with other DMARDs and lower cost than biologic agents. Leflunomide appears to have long-term efficacy similar to MTX.
- Biologic agents with disease-modifying activity include the anti-TNF agents (etanercept, infliximab and adalimumab), the IL-1 receptor antagonist anakinra, and Rituximab, which depletes peripheral B cells. Biologic agents are effective for patients who fail treatment with other DMARDs.
- DMARDs that are less frequently used include azathioprine, penicillamine, gold salts (including auranofin), minocycline, cyclosporine, and cyclophosphamide. These agents have either less efficacy or higher toxicity, or both.
- Combination therapy with two or more DMARDs may be effective when single-DMARD treatment is unsuccessful. Combinations that are particularly effective include (1) MTX plus cyclosporine, and (2) MTX plus sulphasalazine and hydroxychloroquine.
- Non-steroidal anti-inflammatory drugs (NSAIDs) and/or corticosteroids may be used for symptomatic relief if needed. They provide relatively rapid improvement compared with DMARDs, which may take weeks to months before benefit is seen. However, NSAIDs have no impact on disease progression, and corticosteroids have the potential for long-term complications.

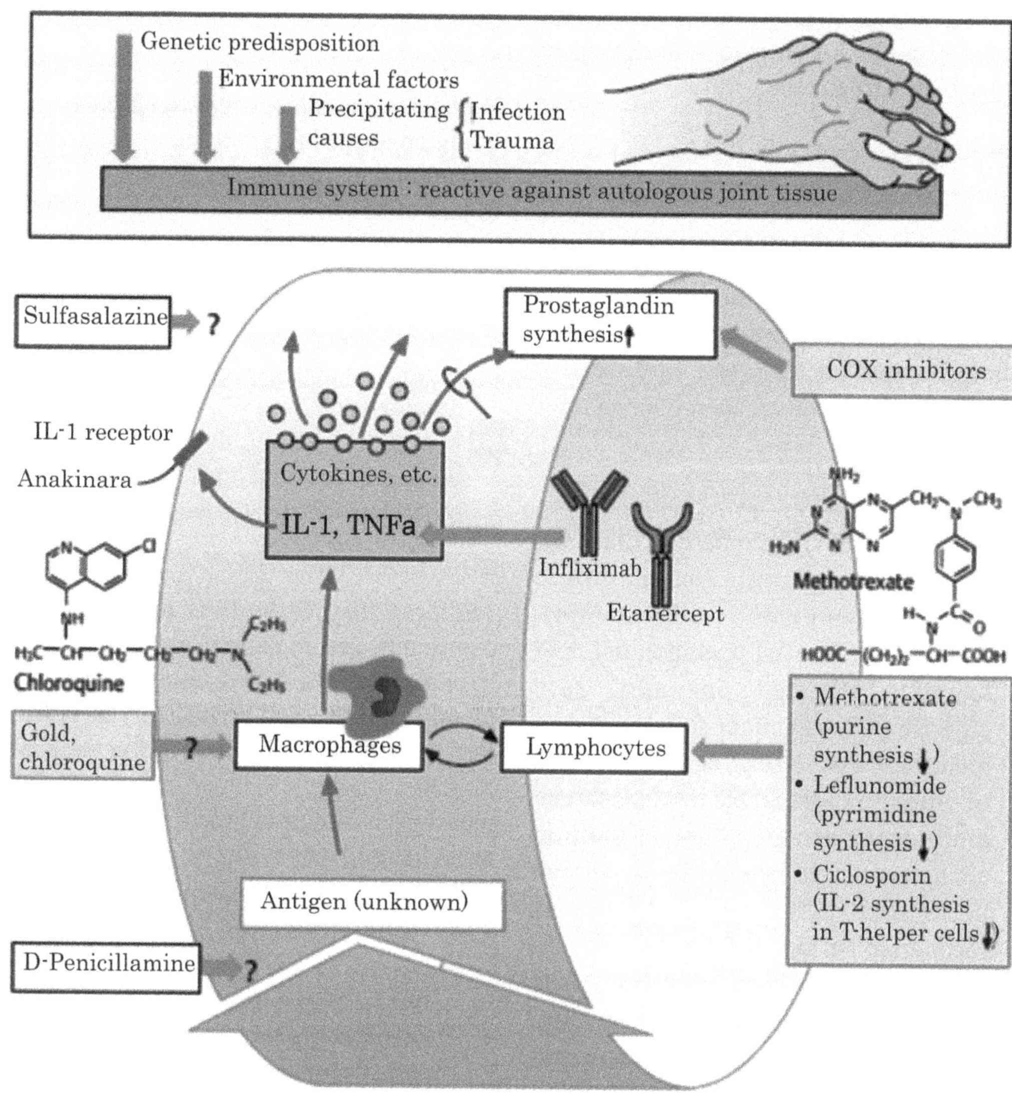

FIGURE 89.1

Anti rheumatoid drugs.

(Source : Colour Atlas of Pharmacology , 3rd edition ,Page no.333)

NON-STEROIDAL ANTI-INFLAMMATORY DRUGS

- NSAIDs act primarily by inhibiting prostaglandin synthesis, which is only a small portion of the inflammatory cascade. They possess both analgesic and anti -inflammatory properties and reduce stiffness but do not slow disease progression or prevent bony erosions or joint deformity. They should seldom be used as monotherapy for RA; instead, they should be viewed as adjuncts to DMARD treatment.

METHOTREXATE

M.O.A.

MTX inhibits cytokine production and purine biosynthesis, which may be responsible for its anti-inflammatory properties. Its onset is relatively rapid (as early as 2 to 3 weeks), and 45% to 67% of patients remained on it in studies ranging from 5 to 7 years.

ADVERSE EFFECTS

- Toxicities are GI (stomatitis, diarrhea, nausea, vomiting), hematologic (thrombocytopenia, leukopenia), pulmonary (fibrosis, pneumonitis), and hepatic (elevated enzymes, rare cirrhosis). Concomitant folic acid may reduce some adverse effects without loss of efficacy. Liver injury tests (aspartate aminotransferase or alanine aminotransferase) should be monitored periodically, but a liver biopsy is recommended during therapy only in patients with persistently elevated hepatic enzymes. MTX is teratogenic, and patients should use contraception and discontinue the drug if conception is planned.

CONTRAINDICATIONS

- MTX is contraindicated in pregnant and nursing women, chronic liver disease, immunodeficiency, pleural or peritoneal effusions, leukopenia, thrombocytopenia, preexisting blood disorders, and creatinine clearance <40 mL/min.

LEFLUNOMIDE (ARAVA)

M.O.A.

It inhibits pyrimidine synthesis, which reduces lymphocyte proliferation and modulation of inflammation. Its efficacy for RA is similar to that of MTX.

DOSE

- A loading dose of 100 mg/day for the first 3 days may result in a therapeutic response within the first month. The usual maintenance dose of 20 mg/day may be lowered to 10 mg/day in cases of GI intolerance, complaints of hair loss, or other dose-related toxicity.

ADVERSE EFFECTS

The drug may cause liver toxicity and is contraindicated in patients with preexisting liver disease. The ALT should be monitored monthly initially and periodically thereafter. Leflunomide may cause bone marrow toxicity; a complete blood cell count with platelets is recommended monthly for 6 months and then every 6 to 8 weeks thereafter. It is teratogenic and should be avoided during pregnancy.

HYDROXYCHLOROQUINE

- Hydroxychloroquine lacks the myelosuppressive, hepatic, and renal toxicities seen with some other DMARDs, which simplifies monitoring. Its onset may be delayed for up to 6 weeks, but the drug should not be considered a therapeutic failure until after 6 months of therapy with no response.

ADVERSE EFFECTS

- Short-term toxicities include GI (nausea, vomiting, diarrhea), ocular (accommodation defects, benign corneal deposits, blurred vision, scotomas, night blindness, preretinopathy), dermatologic (rash, alopecia, skin pigmentation), and neurologic (headache, vertigo, insomnia) effects. Periodic ophthalmologic examinations are necessary for early detection of reversible retinal toxicity.

SULPHASALAZINE

- **Sulphasalazine** use is often limited by adverse effects. Antirheumatic effects should be seen in 2 months.

ADVERSE EFFECTS

- Adverse effects include GI (anorexia, nausea, vomiting, diarrhea), dermatologic (rash, urticaria), hematologic (leukopenia, rare agranulocytosis), and hepatic (elevated enzymes) effects. GI symptoms may be minimized by starting with low doses, dividing the dose more evenly throughout the day, and taking the drug with food.

OTHER DISEASE-MODIFYING ANTIRHEU ANTIRHEUMATIC DRUGS

- The drugs in this section can be effective and may be of value in certain clinical settings. However, they are used less frequently today because of toxicity, lack of long-term benefits, or both.
- Aurothioglucose (solganol) (suspension in oil) and gold sodium thiomalate (myochrysine, aurolate) (aqueous solution) are intramuscular (IM) gold preparations with an onset that may be delayed for 3 to 6 months. They require weekly injections for about 22 weeks before a less frequent maintenance regimen may be initiated. **Auranofin** (ridaura) is an oral gold preparation that is more convenient but less effective than IM gold.

ADVERSE EFFECTS

Include GI (nausea, vomiting, diarrhea), dermatologic (rash, stomatitis), renal (proteinuria, hematuria), and hematologic (anemia, leukopenia, thrombocytopenia) effects. Gold sodium thiomalate is associated with nitritoid reactions (flushing, palpitations, hypotension, tachycardia, headache, blurred vision). Patients receiving IM gold may experience a post injection disease flare for 1 to 2 days after an injection.

AZATHIOPRINE

M.O.A.

It is a purine analog that is converted to 6-mercaptopurine and is thought to interfere with DNA and RNA synthesis. Antirheumatic effects may be seen in 3 to 4 weeks. It should be discontinued if no response is observed after 12 weeks at maximal doses.

ADVERSE EFFECTS

Bone marrow suppression (leukopenia, macrocytic anemia, thrombocytopenia, pancytopenia), stomatitis, GI intolerance, infections, drug fever, hepatotoxicity, and oncogenic potential.

PENICILLAMINE

Onset may be seen in 1 to 3 months, and most responses occur within 6 months.

ADVERSE EFFECTS

Early adverse effects include skin rash, metallic taste, hypogeusia, stomatitis, anorexia, nausea, vomiting, and dyspepsia. Glomerulonephritis may occur, which manifests as proteinuria and hematuria.

Penicillamine is usually reserved for patients who are resistant to other therapies because of the rare but potentially serious induction of autoimmune diseases (e.g., Good pasture's syndrome, myasthenia gravis).

CYCLOSPORINE

M.O.A.

It reduces production of cytokines involved in T-cell activation and has direct effects on B cells, macrophages, bone, and cartilage cells. Its onset appears to be 1 to 3 months.

ADVERSE EFFECTS

Important toxicities at doses of 1 to 10 mg/kg/day include hypertension, hyperglycemia, nephrotoxicity, tremor, GI intolerance, hirsutism, and gingival hyperplasia. Cyclosporine should be reserved for patients refractory to or intolerant of other DMARDs. It should be avoided in patients with current or past malignancy, uncontrolled hypertension, renal dysfunction, immunodeficiency, low white blood cell or platelet counts, or elevated liver function tests.

BIOLOGIC AGENTS

ETANERCEPT (ENBREL)

M.O.A.

It is a fusion protein consisting of two p75-soluble TNF receptors linked to an Fc fragment of human IgG1. It binds to and inactivates TNF, preventing it from interacting with the cell-surface TNF receptors and thereby activating cells. Most clinical trials used etanercept in patients who failed DMARDs, and responses were seen in 60% to 75% of patients. It has been shown to slow erosive disease progression to a greater degree than oral MTX in patients with inadequate response to MTX monotherapy.

ADVERSE EFFECTS

Local injection-site reactions, and there have been case reports of pancytopenia and neurologic demyelinating syndromes. No laboratory monitoring is required. The drug should be avoided in patients with preexisting infection and in those at high risk for developing infection. Treatment should be discontinued temporarily if infections develop during therapy.

INFLIXIMAB (REMICADE)

M.O.A.

It is a chimeric anti-TNF antibody fused to a human constant-region immunoglobulin G1 (IgG1). It binds to TNF and prevents its interaction with TNF receptors on inflammatory cells. To prevent Formation of antibodies to this foreign protein, MTX should be given orally in doses used to treat RA for as long as the patient continues on Infliximab. In clinical trials, the combination of infliximab and MTX halted progression of joint damage and was superior to MTX monotherapy.

ADVERSE EFFECTS

Infliximab may increase the risk of infection, especially upper respiratory infections. An acute infusion reaction with fever, chills, pruritus, and rash may occur within 1 to 2 hours after administration. Auto antibodies and lupus-like syndrome have also been reported.

- **Adalimumab** (Humira) is a human IgG1 antibody to TNF that is less antigenic than Infliximab. It has response rates similar to other TNF inhibitors

ANAKINRA (KINERET)

M.O.A.

It is an IL-1 receptor antagonist (IL-1ra) that binds to IL-1 receptors on target cells, preventing the interaction between IL-1 and the cells. IL-1 normally stimulates release of chemotactic factors and adhesion molecules that promote migration of inflammatory leukocytes to tissues.

ADVERSE EFFECTS

Injection-site reactions were the most common adverse effect (e.g., redness, swelling, pain). Infection risk and precautions are similar to those for the TNF inhibitors.

ABATACEPT (ORENCIA)

M.O.A.

It binds to CD80/CD86 receptors on antigen-presenting cells; abatacept inhibits interactions between the antigen- presenting cells and T cells, preventing T cells from activating to promote the inflammatory process.

ADVERSE EFFECTS

Infusion reactions, headache, nasopharyngitis, dizziness, cough, back pain, hypertension, dyspepsia, urinary tract infection, rash, and extremity pain.

RITUXIMAB (RITUXAN)

Is a monoclonal chimeric antibody consisting of mostly human protein with the antigen-binding region derived from a mouse antibody to CD20 protein found on the cell surface of mature B lymphocytes.

M.O.A.

Binding of rituximab to B cells results in nearly complete depletion of peripheral B cells, with a gradual recovery over several months. Rituximab is useful in patients failing MTX or TNF inhibitors. Methylprednisolone 100 mg should be given 30 minutes prior to rituximab to reduce the incidence and severity of infusion reactions.

CORTICOSTEROIDS

M.O.A.

- **Corticosteroids** have anti-inflammatory and immunosuppressive properties. They interfere with antigen presentation to T lymphocytes, inhibit prostaglandin and leukotrienes synthesis, and inhibit neutrophil and monocyte superoxide radical generation.
- Oral corticosteroids (e.g., **prednisone, methylprednisolone**) can be used to control pain and synovitis while DMARDs are taking effect ("bridging therapy"). This is often used in patients with debilitating symptoms when DMARD therapy is initiated.
- Low-dose, long-term corticosteroid therapy may be used to control symptoms in patients with difficult-to-control disease. Prednisone doses below 7.5 mg/day (or equivalent) are well tolerated but are not devoid of the long-term corticosteroid adverse effects.
- The IM route is preferable in nonadherent patients. Depot forms (**triamcinolone acetonide, triamcinolone hexacetonide, methylprednisolone acetate**) provide 2 to 6 weeks of symptomatic control.

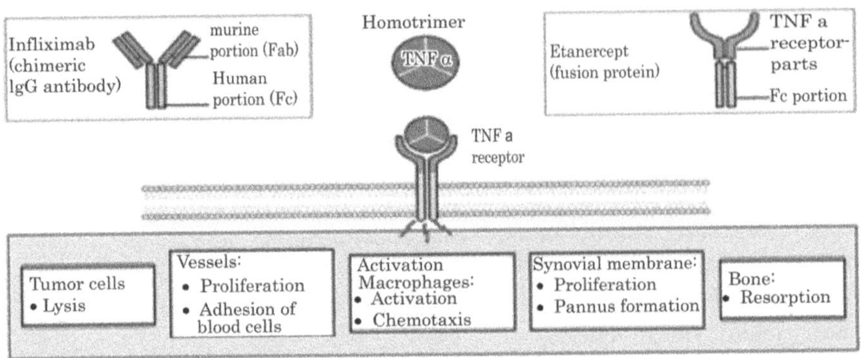

FIGURE 89.2

Tumor necrosis factor α and inhibitors.

(Source : Colour Atlas of Pharmacology, 3rd edition ,page no.333)

Table 89.1

Clinical monitoring of drug therapy in rheumatoid arthritis

Drug	Toxicities Requiring Monitoring	Symptoms to Inquire About
NSAIDs and salicylates	GI ulceration and bleeding renal damage	Blood in stool, dyspepsia, nausea/vomiting weakness, dizziness, abdominal pain, edema, weight gain, shortness of breath
Corticosteroids	Hypertension, hyperglycemia, osteoporosis	Blood pressure if available, polyuria, polydipsia, edema, shortness of breath, visual changes, weight gain, headaches, broken bones or bone pain
Azathioprine	Myelosuppression, hepatotoxicity, lymphoproliferative disorders	Symptoms of myelosuppression (extreme fatigue, easy bleeding or bruising, infection), jaundice
Gold (intramuscular or oral)	Myelosuppression, proteinuria, rash, stomatitis	Symptoms of myelosuppression, edema, rash, oral ulcers, diarrhea
Hydroxchloroquine	Macular damage, rash, diarrhea	Visual changes, including a decrease in night or peripheral vision, rash, diarrhea
Methotrexate	Myelosuppression, hepatic fibrosis, cirrhoiss, pulmonary infiltrates or fibrosis, stomatitis, rash	Symptoms of myelosuppression, shortness of breath, nausea/vomiting lymph node swelling coughing mouth sores, diarrhea, jaundice
Leflunomide	Hepatitis, GI distress, alopecia	Nausea/vomiting, gastritis, diarrhea, hair loss, jaundice
Penicillamine	Myelosuppression, proteinuria, stomatitis, rash, dysgeusia	Symptoms of myelosuppression, edema, rash, diarrhea, altered taste perception, oral ulcers
Sulfasalazine	Myelosuppression, rash	Symptoms of myelosuppression, photo-sensitivity. cash, nausea/vomiting
Etanercept, adali-mumab, anakinra	Local injection-site reactions, infection	Symptoms of infection

REFERENCES

1. Catrina, AI., Trollmo, C., Klint, E., Engstrom, M., Lampa, J., Hermansson, Y., Klareskog, L. & Ulfgren, E.K. Evidence that Anti Tumor Necrosis Factor Therapy with both Etanercept and Infliximab induces apoptosis in macrophages, but not lymphocytes, in Rheumatoid Arthritis joints. *Extended Report Arthritis and Rheumatism.*, 2005, **52**, 61–7.
2. OíDell, JR. Therapeutic strategies for rheumatoid arthritis. *N Engl J Med*, 2004, **350**, 2591–602.
3. Maddison, PJ. Is it SLE? *Best Practice and Research Clinical Rheumatology*, 2002, **16**, 167–18.

CHAPTER 90

Osteoarthritis

DEFINITION

Osteoarthritis (OA) is a common, slowly progressive disorder affecting primarily the weight-bearing diarthrodial joints of the peripheral and axial skeleton. It is characterized by progressive deterioration and loss of articular cartilage, resulting in osteophyte formation, pain and limitation of motion, deformity, and progressive disability. Inflammation may or may not be present in the affected joints .

PREVALENCE

Osteoarthritis affects nearly 27 million people in the United States, accounting for 25% of visits to primary care physicians, and half of all NSAID prescriptions. It is estimated that 80% of the population have radiographic evidence of OA by age 65, although only 60% of those will have symptoms. In the United States, hospitalizations for osteoarthritis increased from 322,000 in 1993 to 735,000 in 2006.

ETIOLOGY

Osteoarthritis is a normal result of aging. It is also caused by 'wear and tear' on a joint.

- Cartilage is the firm, rubbery tissue that cushions the bones at the joints, and allows bones to glide over one another.
- If the cartilage breaks down and wears away, the bones rub together. This causes pain, swelling, and stiffness.
- Bony spurs or extra bone may form around the joint. The ligaments and muscles around the joint become weaker and stiffer.

The symptoms of OA usually appear in middle age. Almost everyone has some symptoms by age 70. However, these symptoms may be minor. Before age 55, OA occurs equally in men and women. After age 55, it is more common in women.

Other factors can also lead to OA.

- OA tends to run in families.
- Being overweight increases the risk of OA in the hip, knee, ankle, and foot joints because extra weight causes more wear and tear.
- Fractures or other joint injuries can lead to OA later in life. This includes injuries to the cartilage and ligaments in your joints.
- Jobs that involve kneeling or squatting for more than an hour a day put you at the highest risk. Jobs that involve lifting, climbing stairs, or walking also put you at risk.
- Playing sports that involve direct impact on the joint (such as football), twisting (such as basketball or soccer), or throwing also increase the risk of arthritis.

Medical conditions that can lead to OA include:

- Bleeding disorders that cause bleeding in the joint, such as haemophilia
- Disorders that block the blood supply near a joint and lead to avascular necrosis
- Other types of arthritis, such as chronic gout, pseudogout, or rheumatoid arthritis

PATHOPHYSIOLOGY (FIG. 90.1)

- Primary (idiopathic) OA, the most common type, has no known cause. Subclasses of primary OA are localized OA (involving one or two sites) and generalized OA (affecting three or more sites). The term erosive OA indicates the presence of erosion and marked proliferation in the proximal and distal interphalangeal (PIP and DIP) hand joints.
- Secondary OA is associated with a known cause such as rheumatoid arthritis or another inflammatory arthritis, trauma, metabolic or endocrine disorders, and congenital factors.
- OA usually begins with damage to articular cartilage through injury, excess joint loading from obesity or other reasons, or joint instability or injury that causes abnormal loading. Damage to cartilage increases the metabolic activity of chondrocytes, leading to increased synthesis of matrix constituents with cartilage swelling. This hypertrophic reparative response to damage does not restore cartilage to normal but instead is the first step in the process leading to further cartilage loss.
- After the hypertrophic phase, there is increased synthesis of matrix metalloproteinase's (MMPs) 1, 3, 13, and 28, which causes collagen destruction to occur faster than synthesis, with a net loss of cartilage. Chondrocytes contribute to collagen loss by secreting MMPs in response to inflammatory mediators present in OA (interleukin-1 and tumour necrosis factor-α). Chondrocytes also undergo apoptosis, probably as a result of induction of nitric oxide synthase and production of toxic metabolites. This leaves fewer chondrocytes to synthesize matrix components. OA chondrocytes are also less responsive to the anabolic stimulus of transforming growth factor-β. The net result of these processes is a progressive cycle of cartilage destruction and chondrocyte loss.
- Subchondral bone adjacent to articular cartilage also undergoes pathologic changes that allow progression of damage to articular cartilage. In OA, subchondral bone releases vasoactive peptides and MMPs. Neovascularization and subsequent increased permeability of the adjacent cartilage occur, which contribute further to cartilage loss.
- Substantial loss of cartilage causes joint space narrowing and leads to painful, deformed joints. The remaining cartilage softens and develops fibrillations, and there is splitting, further cartilage loss, and exposure of underlying bone. Cartilage is eventually eroded completely, leaving denuded subchondral bone that becomes dense, smooth, and glistening (eburnation). A more brittle, stiffer bone results, with decreased weight-bearing ability and development of sclerosis and microfractures. New bone formations (osteophytes) that arise from local and humoral factors appear at joint margins distant from cartilage destruction; evidence indicates that Osteophytes help to stabilize OA joints.

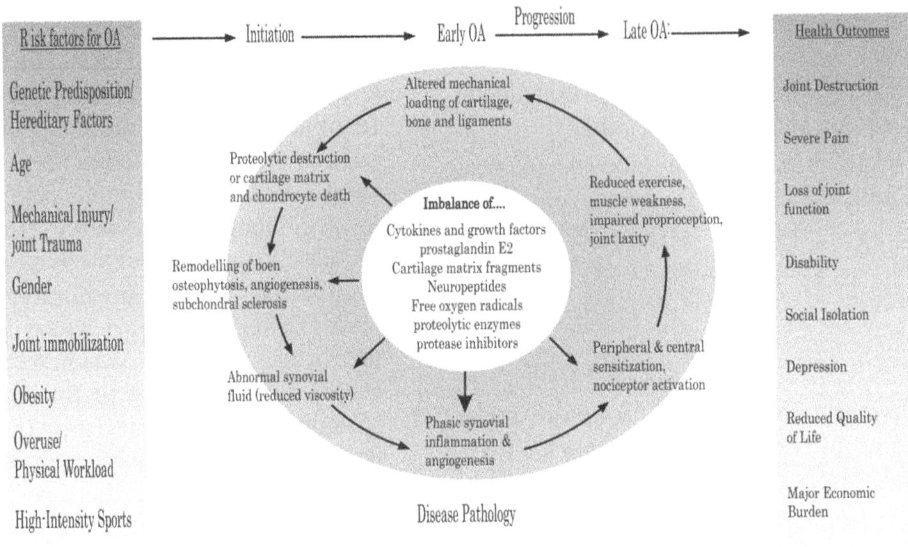

FIGURE 90.1

Vicious cycle of osteoarthritis.

(Source : Chris D. Meletis, ND. Osteoarthritis: New Solutions for a Crippling Concern. Sunday, 01 July 2012; http://www.vrp.co.za/Public/ViewArticle.aspx?ArticleID=314)

- Local inflammatory changes occur in the joint capsule and synovium. The synovium becomes infiltrated with T cells, and immune complexes appear. Crystals or cartilage shards in synovial fluid may contribute to inflammation. There are also increased levels of interleukin-1, prostaglandin E2, tumor necrosis factor-α and nitric oxide in synovial fluid. Inflammatory changes result in effusions and synovial thickening.
- The pain of OA arises from activation of nociceptive nerve endings within joints by mechanical and chemical irritants. OA pain may result from distension of the synovial capsule by increased joint fluid; microfracture; periosteal irritation; or damage to ligaments, synovium, or the meniscus.

CLINICAL FEATURES

Pain and stiffness in the joints are the most common symptoms. The pain is often worse after exercise and when you put weight or pressure on the joint.

If the person osteoarthritis, the joints probably become stiffer and harder to move over time. The person may notice a rubbing, grating, or crackling sound when the person move the joint.

The phrase "morning stiffness" refers to the pain and stiffness you may feel when you first wake up in the morning. Stiffness usually lasts for 30 minutes or less. It is improved by mild activity that "warms up" the joint.

During the day, the pain may get worse when the person is active and feel better when at rest. After a while, the pain may be present during resting. It may even wake the person up at night.

Some people might not have symptoms, even though x-rays show the changes of OA.

DIAGNOSIS

A physical exam can show:

- Joint movement may cause a cracking (grating) sound, called crepitation
- Joint swelling (bones around the joints may feel larger than normal)
- Limited range of motion
- Tenderness when the joint is pressed
- Normal movement is often painful

An x-ray of affected joints will show a loss of the joint space. In advanced cases, there will be a Wearing down of the Ends of the Bone and Bone Spurs.

TREATMENT

NON-PHARMACOLOGICAL THERAPY

- The first step is to educate the patient about the extent of the disease, prognosis, and maximum weight-loss program are recommended for overweight OA patients.
- Physical therapy—with heat or cold treatments and an exercise program—helps to maintain and restore joint range of motion and reduce pain and muscle spasms. Exercise programs using isometric techniques are designed to strengthen muscles, improve joint function and motion, and decrease disability, pain, and the need for analgesic use.
- Assistive and orthotic devices such as canes, walkers, braces, heel cups, and insoles can be used during exercise or daily activities.
- Surgical procedures (e.g., osteotomy, partial or total arthroplasty, joint fusion) are indicated for patients with functional disability and/or severe pain unresponsive to conservative therapy.

PHARMACOLOGICAL THERAPY

GENERAL APPROACH

- For mild or moderate pain, topical analgesics or acetaminophen can be used. If these measures fail or if there is inflammation, non-steroidal anti-inflammatory drugs (NSAIDs) may be useful. Appropriate nondrug therapies should be continued when drug therapy is initiated.

ACETAMINOPHEN

- Acetaminophen is recommended by the ACR as first-line drug therapy for pain management of OA. The dose is 325 to 650 mg every 4 to 6 hours on a scheduled basis (maximum dose 4 g/day; maximum 2 g/day if chronic alcohol intake or underlying liver disease). Comparable relief of mild to moderate OA pain has been demonstrated for acetaminophen (2.6 to 4 g/ day) compared with aspirin (650 mg four times daily), ibuprofen (1,200 or 2,400 mg daily), and naproxen (750 mg daily). However, some patients respond better to NSAIDs.
- Acetaminophen is usually well tolerated, but potentially fatal hepatotoxicity with overdose is well documented. It should be used with caution in patients with liver disease and those who chronically abuse alcohol. Chronic alcohol users (three or more drinks daily) should be warned about an increased risk of liver damage or GI

bleeding with acetaminophen. Other individuals do not appear to be at increased risk for GI bleeding. Renal toxicity occurs less frequently than with NSAIDs.

NON -STEROIDAL ANTI-INFLAMMATORY DRUGS

- NSAIDs at prescription strength are often prescribed for OA patients after treatment with acetaminophen proves ineffective, or for patients with inflammatory OA. Analgesic effects begin within 1 to 2 hours, whereas anti-inflammatory benefits may require 2 to 3 weeks of continuous therapy.
- All NSAIDs have similar efficacy in reducing pain and inflammation in OA although individual patient response differs among NSAIDs.
- Selection of an NSAID depends on prescriber experience, medication cost, patient preference, toxicities, and adherence issues. An individual patient should be given a trial of one drug that is adequate in time (2 to 3 weeks) and dose. If the first NSAID fails, another agent in the same or another chemical class can be tried; this process may be repeated until an effective drug is found. Combining two NSAIDs increases adverse effects without providing additional benefit.
- Cyclooxygenase-2 (COX-2) selective inhibitors (e.g., celecoxib) demonstrate analgesic benefits that are similar to traditional non-selective NSAIDs. Although COX-2 selective inhibition was designed to reduce NSAID induced gastropathy (e.g., ulcers, bleeding, perforation), concerns about adverse cardiovascular events (e.g., myocardial infarction, stroke) have led authorities to recommend their use only in selected patients who are at high risk for NSAID-related GI effects and low risk for cardiovascular toxicity.
- GI complaints are the most common adverse effects of NSAIDs. Minor complaints such as nausea, dyspepsia, anorexia, abdominal pain, flatulence, and diarrhoea occur in 10% to 60% of patients. NSAIDs should be taken with food or milk, except for enteric-coated products (milk or antacids may destroy the enteric coating and cause increased GI symptoms in some patients). All NSAIDs have the potential to cause gastric and duodenal ulcers and bleeding through direct (topical) or indirect (systemic) mechanisms. Risk factors for NSAID-associated ulcers and ulcer complications (perforation, gastric outlet obstruction, GI bleeding) include increased age, comorbid medical conditions (e.g., cardiovascular disease), concomitant corticosteroid or anticoagulant therapy, and history of peptic ulcer disease or upper GI bleeding.
- For OA patients who need an NSAID but are at high risk for GI complications, the ACR recommendations include either a COX-2 selective inhibitor or a non-selective NSAID in combination with either a proton pump inhibitor or misoprostol.
- NSAIDs may also cause kidney diseases, hepatitis, hypersensitivity reactions, rash, and CNS complaints of drowsiness, dizziness, headaches, depression, confusion, and tinnitus. All non-selective NSAIDs inhibit COX-1-dependent thromboxane production in platelets,

thereby increasing bleeding risk. NSAIDs should be avoided in late pregnancy because of the risk of premature closure of the ductus arteriosus.

- The most potentially serious drug interactions include the concomitant use of NSAIDs with lithium, warfarin, oral hypoglycemics, high-dose methotrexate, antihypertensives, angiotensin-converting enzyme inhibitors, β-blockers, and diuretics.

TOPICAL THERAPIES

- Capsaicin, an extract of red peppers that causes release and ultimately depletion of substance P from nerve fibres, has been beneficial in providing pain relief in OA when applied topically over affected joints. It may be used alone or in combination with oral analgesics or NSAIDs.
- Topical diclofenac in a dimethyl sulphoxide carrier (pennsaid) is a safe and effective treatment for OA pain. It is thought to act primarily by local inhibition of COX-2 enzymes.
- Topical rubefacients containing Methyl Salicylate, Trolamine Salicylate, and other salicylates may have modest, short-term efficacy for treating acute pain associated with OA.

GLUCOSAMINE AND CHONDROITIN

- Glucosamine and chondroitin are dietary supplements that were shown to stimulate proteoglycan synthesis from articular cartilage *in vitro*. Although their excellent safety profile makes them appealing for patients at high risk of adverse drug events, enthusiasm waned after results of a large, well-controlled, National Institutes of Health-sponsored clinical trial demonstrated no significant clinical response to glucosamine alone, chondroitin alone, or combination therapy when compared to placebo across all patients. In subgroup analyses, patients with moderate to severe knee pain showed a response to combination glucosamine–chondroitin therapy superior to placebo, but this finding did not reach the predetermined threshold for pain reduction.
- Because of their relative safety, a trial of glucosamine–chondroitin may be reasonable in patients considering alternatives to traditional OA treatment. Dosing should be at least glucosamine sulphate 1,500 mg/day and chondroitin sulphate 1,200 mg/day in divided doses.
- Glucosamine adverse effects are mild and include GI gas, bloating, and cramps; it should not be used in patients with shellfish allergies. The most common adverse effect of chondroitin is nausea.

CORTICOSTEROIDS

- Systemic corticosteroid therapy is not recommended in OA, given the lack of proven benefit and the well-known adverse effects with long-term use.
- Intraarticular corticosteroid injections can provide relief, particularly when a joint effusion is present. Average doses for injection of large joints in adults are Methylprednisolone acetate 20 to 40 mg or triamcinolone hexacetonide 10 to 20 mg. After aseptic aspiration of the effusion and corticosteroid injection, initial pain relief may occur within 24 to 72 hours, with peak relief occurring in

about 1 week and lasting for 4 to 8 weeks. The patient should minimize joint activity and stress on the joint for several days after the injection. Therapy is generally limited to three or Four injections per year because of the potential systemic effects of the drugs and because the need for more frequent injections indicates poor response to therapy.

HYALURONATE INJECTIONS

- High-molecular-weight hyaluronic acid is a constituent of normal cartilage that provides lubrication with motion and shock absorbency during rapid movements. Because the concentration and molecular size of endogenous hyaluronic acid decrease in OA, exogenous administration has been studied in an attempt to reconstitute synovial fluid and reduce symptoms.
- Hyaluronic acid injections temporarily and modestly increase synovial fluid viscosity and were reported to decrease pain, but many studies were short term and poorly controlled with high placebo response rates.
- Four Intraarticular hyaluronic acid preparations are available for treating pain associated with OA of the knee: sodium hyaluronate (Hyalgan 20 mg/2 mL; supartz 25 mg/2.5 mL), hylan polymers (Synvisc 16 mg/2 mL), and hyaluronan (orthovisc 30 mg/2 mL). Hyalgan and supartz are administered once weekly for five injections, whereas synvisc and orthovisc are administered once weekly for three injections.
- Injections are well tolerated, but acute joint swelling and local skin reactions (e.g., rash, ecchymoses, or pruritus) have been reported.
- These products may be beneficial for OA of the knee that is unresponsive to other therapy, but they are expensive because treatment includes both drug and administration costs.

OPIOID ANALGESICS

- Low-dose opioid analgesics (e.g., **oxycodone**) may be useful for patients who experience no relief with acetaminophen, NSAIDs, Intraarticular injections, or topical therapy.
- They are particularly useful in patients who cannot take NSAIDs because of renal failure or for patients in whom all other treatment options have failed and who are at high surgical risk, precluding joint arthroplasty.
- Low-dose opioids should be used initially, usually in combination with acetaminophen. Sustained-release compounds usually offer better pain control throughout the day and are used when simple opioids are ineffective.

TRAMADOL

- Tramadol with or without acetaminophen has modest analgesic effects in patients with OA. It may also be effective as add-on therapy in patients taking concomitant NSAIDs or COX-2 selective inhibitors. As with opioids, Tramadol may be helpful for patients who cannot take NSAIDs or COX-2 selective inhibitors.
- Tramadol should be initiated at a lower dose (100 mg/day in divided doses) and may be titrated as needed for pain control to a dose of 200 mg/ day. Opioid-like adverse effects such as nausea, vomiting, dizziness, constipation, headache, and somnolence are common.

REFERENCES

1. Gregory PJ, Sperry M, Wilson AF. Dietary supplements for osteoarthritis. *Am Fam Physician*. 2008;77:177-184.
2. Hunter DJ. In the clinic: Osteoarthritis. *Ann Intern Med*. 2007;147(3):ITC8-1-ITC8-16.
3. Hunter DJ, Lo GH. The management of osteoarthritis: an overview and call to appropriate conservative treatment. *Med Clin North Am*. 2009;93:127-43, xi.
4. Richmond J, Hunter D, Irrgang J, et al. Treatment of osteoarthritis of the knee (nonarthroplasty). *J Am Acad Orthop Surg*. 2009;17:591-6000.
5. Bijlsma JW, Berenbaum F, Lafeber FP. Osteoarthritis: an update with relevance for clinical practice. *Lancet*. 2011; 377:2115-2126.

CHAPTER 91

Gout and Hyperuricemia

DEFINITION

The term *gout* describes a disease spectrum including hyperuricemia, recurrent attacks of acute arthritis associated with monosodium urate crystals in leukocytes found in synovial fluid, deposits of monosodium urate crystals in tissues (tophi), interstitial renal disease, and uric acid nephrolithiasis.

- Hyperuricemia may be an asymptomatic condition, with an increased serum uric acid concentration as the only apparent abnormality. A urate concentration greater than 7.0 mg/dl is abnormal and associated with an increased risk for gout.

PATHOPHYSIOLOGY

Gouty arthritis is due to the crystallization and deposition of poorly soluble urate. Uric acid arises from the metabolism of endogenous purines, either from excess nucleic acids or increased cell death as in certain disease states (cancer) (Fig. 91.1).

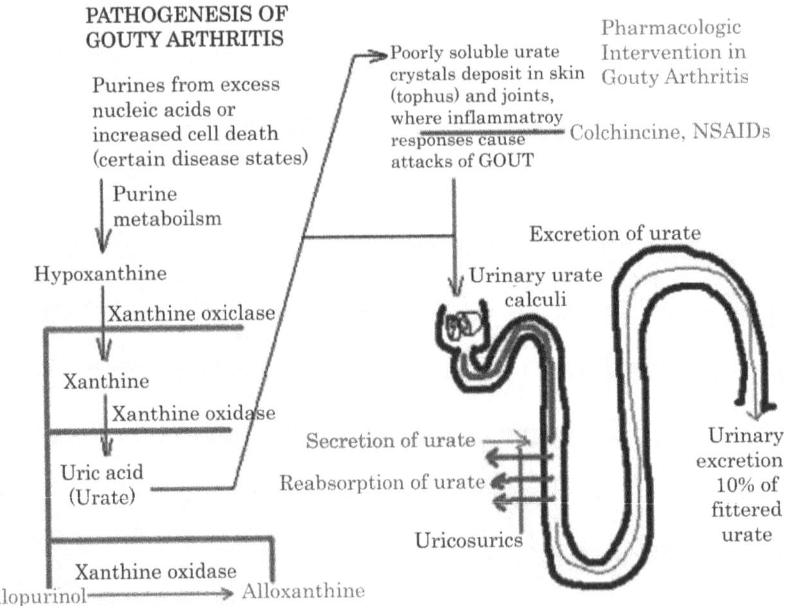

FIGURE 91.1

Pathogenesis of gouty arthritis.

- The purines are metabolized to hypoxanthine which then undergoes further metabolism by the enzyme xanthine oxidaze to xanthine, which is again oxidized by xanthine oxidase to uric acid. The urate may then deposit in soft tissues, such as the skin, as a urate tophus, or in joints.
- Crystals of urate in the joint undergo phagocytosis by local synoviocytes. This releases prostaglandins, interleukin 1, and other inflammatory mediators. These substances then cause the chemotaxis of leukocytes and macrophages to the joint, magnifying the inflammatory response. Alternately, the urate may be excreted.
- Urate is highly filtered through the glomerulus. Additionally, it is actively secreted in the tubules. However, massive tubular reabsorption of urate also occurs so that only about 10% of filtered urate is actually excreted. If urinary conditions are conducive, the urate may crystallize in the urine, forming urinary urate calculi.

CLINICAL FEATURES

- Acute attacks of gouty arthritis are characterized by rapid onset of excruciating pain, swelling, and inflammation. The attack is typically monoarticular at first, most often affecting the first metatarsophalangeal joint (podagra), and then, in order of frequency, the insteps, ankles, heels, knees, wrists, fingers, and elbows. Attacks commonly begin at night, with the patient awakening from sleep with excruciating pain. The affected joints are erythematous, warm, and swollen. Fever and leukocytosis are common. Untreated attacks may last from 3 to 14 days before spontaneous recovery.
- Although acute attacks of gouty arthritis may occur without apparent provocation, attacks may be precipitated by stress, trauma, alcohol ingestion, infection, surgery, rapid lowering of serum uric acid by ingestion of uric acid–lowering agents, and ingestion of certain drugs known to elevate serum uric acid concentrations.

DIAGNOSIS

- The definitive diagnosis is accomplished by aspiration of synovial fluid from the affected joint and identification of intracellular crystals of monosodium urate monohydrate in synovial fluid lcukocytes.
- When joint aspiration is not a viable option, a presumptive diagnosis of acute gouty arthritis may be made on the basis of the presence of the characteristic signs and symptoms, as well as the response to treatment.

ACUTE GOUTY ARTHRITIS (FIG. 91.2)

NON PHARMACOLOGICAL THERAPY

- Patients may be advised to reduce their intake of foods high in purines (e.g., organ meats), avoid alcohol, increase fluid intake, and lose weight if obese.
- Joint rest for 1 to 2 days should be encouraged and local application of ice May be beneficial.

NON-STEROIDAL ANTI-INFLAMMATORY DRUGS

- Non-steroidal anti-inflammatory drugs (NSAIDs) are the mainstay of therapy because of their excellent efficacy and minimal toxicity with short term use. There is little evidence to support one NSAID as more efficacious than another and three drugs (indomethacin, naproxen, and sulindac) have FDA approval for this indication
- Therapy should be initiated with maximum recommended doses for gout at the onset of symptoms and continued for 24 hours after complete resolution of an acute attack, then tapered quickly over 2 to 3 days. Acute attacks generally resolve within 5 to 8 days after initiating therapy.

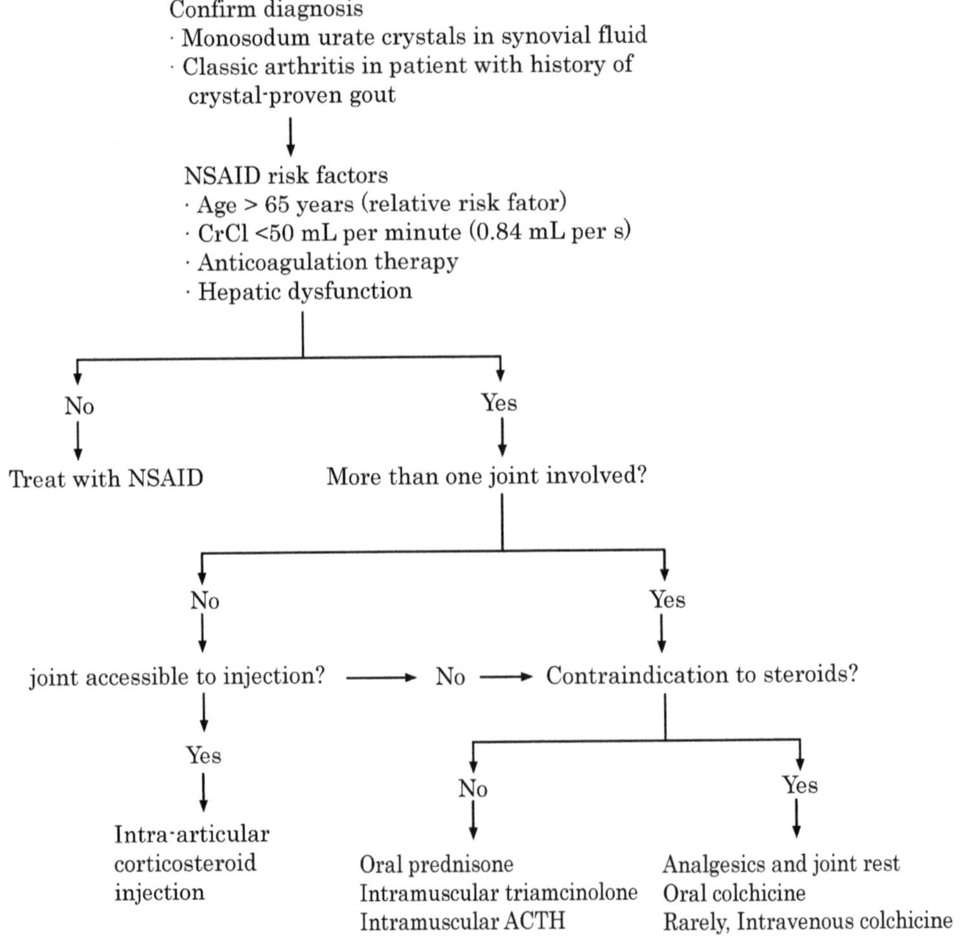

FIGURE 91.2

Treatment algorithm for acute gouty arthritis.

The most common adverse effects involve the GI system (gastritis, bleeding, and perforation), kidneys (renal papillary necrosis, reduced creatinine clearance, cardiovascular system (sodium and fluid retention, increased blood pressure), and CNS (impaired cognitive function, headache, dizziness).

- Although the risk of GI complications is relatively small with short-term therapy, co administration with a proton pump inhibitor should be considered in elderly patients and others at increased GI risk. NSAIDs should be used with caution in individuals with a history of peptic ulcer disease, heart failure, uncontrolled hypertension, renal insufficiency, coronary artery disease, or if they are receiving anticoagulants concurrently.
- The efficacy and safety of cyclooxygenase-2 (COX-2) selective inhibitors (e.g., celecoxib) have not been fully assessed in gouty arthritis, but they are more costly than conventional NSAIDs and are unlikely to result in fewer GI complications because of the short duration of therapy.

COLCHICINE

Colchicine is an alkaloid isolated from the autumn crocus, *Colchicum autumnale*. Pharmacologically, it is classified as an anti-mitotic. This is due to its mechanism of action, which is to inhibit tubulin formation and/or polymerization. Since tubulin is required in the formation of spindles, it prevents mitosis or cell division. This action is responsible for many of the side effects of colchicine. Additionally, tubulin formation and polymerization are the steps necessary for the migration of inflammatory cells. Since this is inhibited, the cells cannot undergo chemotaxis to the insulted area, thus inhibiting subsequent inflammation.

Colchicine is indicated for the treatment of acute attacks of gouty arthritis at a dose of 0.5 to 1 mg stat, followed by 0.5 mg q2h until the pain has subsided or until side effects (nausea, vomiting) occur. Colchicine is also used in the prophylaxis of gouty attacks at a dose of 0.5 mg q.d. to t.i.d. Note that colchicine has a very narrow therapeutic index with as little as 8 mg in a 24h period resulting in fatality. For this reason, the use of colchicine in acute attacks should be limited to not more than once per week.

Side effects of colchicine most commonly encountered are diarrhea, nausea, vomiting, and abdominal cramping. Less often are alopecia and bone marrow depression. Acute toxicity of colchicine may include the above plus a burning pain in the throat, bloody diarrhea, shock, hematuria, oliguria, and CNS depression. The diarrhea, bone marrow depression, and alopecia reflect the ability of colchicine to inhibit the replication of these relatively rapidly dividing cells.

Note: That colchicine therapy inhibits the inflammatory response but does not alter either plasma or urine urate levels.

URICOSURICS

These agents increase the urinary excretion of urate by inhibiting its active reabsorption. Note that the urinary excretion of urates is complicated and varies greatly across species. In humans, it is filtered, secreted, and reabsorbed in great quantities. Furthermore, a single drug may act to either increase or decrease its excretion by affecting either its secretion or reabsorption, often in a dose dependent manner. To further complicate the issue, drugs may interact to offset each other's effect or produce a synergistic effect. However, for the purposes of this course, only those agents that act as Uricosurics will be covered. These agents will decrease plasma urate levels and increase urinary urate levels (thus increasing the risk of renal stones caused by urate crystallization).

Mechanistically, these drugs compete with and inhibit the active reabsorption of urate from the renal tubules, thus lowering the plasma urate levels, increasing its urinary excretion, and decreasing total body load of urate.

SPECIFIC URICOSURICS

Probenecid — May cause allergic dermatitis, GI upset, nephrotic syndrome, aplastic anemia

Sulphinpyrazone — Higher incidence of GI upset, may also cause rash, kidney damage, aplastic anemia

Phenylbutazone — High incidence of GI effects, blood dyscrasia, and kidney damage, no longer used

Azapropazone — A PBZ derivative that produces less agranulocytosis

Benzbromarone — A product currently available in Europe that has fewer side effects.

Uricosurics are most often used when gouty attacks are frequent, there are numerous tophi present, and/or plasma urate levels are high.

ALLOPURINOL

Allopurinol competitively inhibits the enzyme xanthine oxidase. In addition to inhibiting xanthine oxidase it is metabolized by XO to the active metabolite alloxanthine, which also inhibits XO. This mechanism reduces the formation of urate, whose precursors are more water soluble and therefore, excretable. Allopurinol will lower both plasma and urinary concentration of urate. Note that since allopurinol does not eliminate urate it is NOT effective in an acute attack. In fact, the decreased formation of urate will shift the plasma concentration such that the concentration gradient favors the movement of urate from deposited tophi to the plasma which may actually precipitate an acute attack early in therapy. For this reason, Uricosurics are often co-administered, at least initially, with allopurinol.

Side effects observed with allopurinol include GI upset (nausea, vomiting, diarrhea) which are most common, and bone marrow depression, aplastic anemia, neuritis, vasculitis, nephrotoxicity, hepatotoxicity, and cataracts (due to deposition of Allopurinol on the lens).

Allopurinol will interact with the mercaptopurine class of anti-metabolites (azathioprine), inhibiting their metabolism. Therefore the dose of the drugs may have to be reduced.

COMBINATION PRODUCTS

ColBenemid® — Colchicine and Probenecid — for prophylaxis of gouty attacks. This product provides the anti-inflammatory effect of colchicine and the uricosuric effect or probenecid. Allopurinol is often added to reduce urate synthesis. This combination is generally reserved for patients with severe gout.

DIETARY INTERVENTION IN GOUTY ARTHRITIS

A diet that is rich in purines may precipitate an attack of gout. Therefore, as well as drinking copious amount of water to prevent renal calculi, a low-purine diet is desirable in these patients (95% of whom are men). Food that should be limited or avoided includes the following:

Foods that may be eaten sparingly: Dried beans, peas, lentils, oatmeal, whole wheat bread, unprocessed grains and cereals, asparagus, mushrooms, cauliflower, and spinach. Other vegetables that have been associated with gouty attacks include collard, turnip, and mustard greens, broccoli, and Brussels sprouts. In general meats, seafood, and poultry should be limited to once daily.

Foods that should be avoided (higher in purines and incidence of attack) include: shrimp, scallops, sardines, anchovies, herring, mackerel, cured pork (ham, bacon, luncheon meats — both pork and beef based), game meats, and organ meats (liver, kidney, sweetbreads, brains).Alcohol intake should be limited since it may also precipitate an attack.

The overall diet should be relatively rich in carbohydrates and low in fat, avoiding the above foods and replacing meat with milk, cheese, and other sources of dietary protein.

REFERENCES

1. Wortmann RL, Kelley WN. Gout and hyperuricemia. In: Harris ED, Budd RC, Genovese MC, et al., eds. *Kelley's Textbook of Rheumatology.* Philadelphia: WB Saunders, 2005:1402-1429.
2. Rott KT, Agudelo CA. Gout. *JAMA.* 2003;289:2857-2860.
3. Johnson RJ, Rideout BA. Uric acid and diet-Insights into the epidemic of cardiovascular disease. *N Engl J Med.* 2004;350:1071-1073.
4. Choi HK, Atkinson K, Karlson EW, et al. Purine-rich foods, dairy and protein intake, and the risk of gout in men. *N Engl J Med.* 2004;350:1093-1103.
5. Kim KY, Schumacher HR, Hunsche E, et al. A literature review of the epidemiology and treatment of acute gout. *Clin Ther.* 2003;25:1593-1617.
6. Harris MD, Siegel LB, Alloway JA. Gout and hyperuricemia. *Am Fam Physician.* 1999;59:925-934.
7. Clinical Pharmacology. www.clinicalpharmacology.com. Accessed 7/23/2010 Schlesinger N, Schumacher HR. Gout: Can management be improved? *Curr Opin Rheumatol.* 2001;13:240-246.
8. Schlesinger N. Management of acute and chronic gouty arthritis: present state-of-the-art.*Drugs.* 2004; 64:2399-2416.

CHAPTER 92

Glaucoma

DEFINITION

Glaucoma's are ocular disorders characterized by changes in the optic nerve head (optic disk) and by loss of visual sensitivity and field.

ETIOLOGY

Glaucoma is the second most common cause of blindness in the United States. There are four major types of glaucoma:

- Open-angle (chronic) glaucoma
- Angle-closure (acute) glaucoma
- Congenital glaucoma
- Secondary glaucoma

The front part of the eye is filled with a clear fluid called aqueous humor. This fluid is always being made behind the colored part of the eye (the iris). It leaves the eye through channels in the front of the eye in an area called the anterior chamber angle, or simply the angle.

Anything that slows or blocks the flow of this fluid out of the eye will cause pressure to build up in the eye. This pressure is called intraocular pressure (IOP). In most cases of glaucoma, this pressure is high and causes damage to the optic nerve.

Open-angle (chronic) glaucoma is the most common type of glaucoma.

- The cause is unknown. An increase in eye pressure occurs slowly over time. The pressure pushes on the optic nerve.
- Open-angle glaucoma tends to run in families. The risk is higher if the person have a parent or grandparent with open-angle glaucoma. People of African descent are at particularly high risk for this disease.

Angle-closure (acute) glaucoma occurs when the exit of the aqueous humor fluid is suddenly blocked. This causes a quick, severe, and painful rise in the pressure in the eye.

- Angle-closure glaucoma is an emergency. This is very different from open-angle glaucoma, which painlessly and slowly damages vision.
- If the person had acute glaucoma in one eye, is at risk for an attack in the second eye, and the doctor is likely to recommend preventive treatment.
- Dilating eye drops and certain medications may trigger an acute glaucoma attack.

Congenital glaucoma is seen in babies. It often runs in families (is inherited).

- It is present at birth.
- It is caused by abnormal eye development.

Secondary glaucoma is caused by:

- Drugs such as corticosteroids
- Systemic diseases
- Trauma

PATHOPHYSIOLOGY

- There are two major types of glaucoma: **open-angle glaucoma**, which accounts for most cases and is therefore the focus of this chapter, and **closed-angle glaucoma.**
- In open-angle glaucoma, the specific cause of optic neuropathy is unknown. Increased intraocular pressure (IOP) was historically considered to be the sole cause. Additional contributing factors include increased susceptibility of the optic nerve to ischemia, reduced or dysregulated blood flow, excitotoxicity, autoimmune reactions, and other abnormal physiologic processes.
- Although IOP is a poor predictor of which patients will have visual field loss, the risk of visual field loss increases with increasing IOP. IOP is not constant; it changes with pulse, blood pressure, forced expiration or coughing, neck compression, and posture.
- The balance between the inflow and outflow of aqueous humor determines IOP. Inflow is increased by β-adrenergic agents and decreased by α2-, α1-, and β-adrenergic blockers; dopamine blockers; carbonic anhydrase inhibitors (CAIs); and adenylate cyclase stimulators. Outflow is increased by cholinergic agents, which contract the ciliary muscle and open the trabecular meshwork, and by prostaglandin analogs and β - and α2-adrenergic agonists, which affect uveoscleral outflow.
- Secondary open-angle glaucoma has many causes including exfoliation syndrome, pigmentary glaucoma, systemic diseases, trauma, surgery, lens changes, ocular inflammatory diseases, and drugs. Secondary glaucoma can be classified as pretrabecular (normal meshwork is covered and prevents outflow of aqueous humor), trabecular (meshwork is altered or material accumulates in the intertrabecular spaces), or post trabecular (episcleral venous blood pressure is increased).
- Closed-angle glaucoma occurs when there is a physical blockage of the trabecular meshwork, resulting in increased IOP.
- For *closed-angle glaucoma*, the presence of a narrow angle is usually visualized by gonioscopy. IOP is generally markedly elevated (e.g., 40 to 90mm Hg) when symptoms are present. Additional signs include hyperemic conjunctiva, cloudy cornea, shallow anterior chamber, and occasionally edematous and hyperemic optic disk.

CLINICAL FEATURES

OPEN-ANGLE GLAUCOMA

- Most people have no symptoms
- Once vision loss occurs, the damage is already severe

- There is a slow loss of side (peripheral) vision (also called tunnel vision)
- Advanced glaucoma can lead to blindness

ANGLE-CLOSURE GLAUCOMA

- Symptoms may come and go at first, or steadily become worse
- Sudden, severe pain in one eye
- Decreased or cloudy vision, often called "steamy" vision
- Nausea and vomiting
- Rainbow-like halos around lights
- Red eye
- Eye feels swollen

CONGENITAL GLAUCOMA

- Symptoms are usually noticed when the child is a few months old
- Cloudiness of the front of the eye
- Enlargement of one eye or both eyes Red eye
- Sensitivity to light
- Tearing

DIAGNOSIS

A complete eye exam is needed to diagnose glaucoma. The person may be given eye drop to widen (dilate) the pupil. The eye doctor can look at the inside of the eye when the pupil is dilated.

A test called (tonometry) is done to check eye pressure. However, eye pressure always changes. Eye pressure can be normal in some people with glaucoma. This is called normal-tension glaucoma. The doctor need to run other tests to confirm glaucoma.

Some of the tests include:

- Using a special lens to look at the eye (gonioscopy)
- Photographs or laser scanning images of the inside of the eye (optic nerve imaging)
- Examination of the retina in the back of the eye
- Slit lamp examination
- Visual acuity
- Visual field measurement

TREATMENT OF OCULAR HYPERTENSION AND OPEN-ANGLE GLAUCOMA (TABLE 92.1, FIG. 92.1)

- Treatment is indicated for ocular hypertension if the patient has a significant risk factor such as IOP greater than 25 mm Hg, vertical cup-disk ratio greater than 0.5, or central corneal thickness less than 555 micrometers. Additional risk factors to be considered include family history of glaucoma, black race, severe myopia, and presence of only one eye.
- Treatment is indicated for all patients with elevated IOP and characteristic optic disk changes or visual field defects.
- Drug therapy is the most common initial treatment and is initiated in a stepwise manner, starting with a single well tolerated topical agent. Historically, β-blockers (e.g., timolol) were the treatment of choice and continue to be used if there are no contraindications to potential β-blockade caused by systemic absorption. β-Blockers have the advantage of low cost owing to generic formulations.

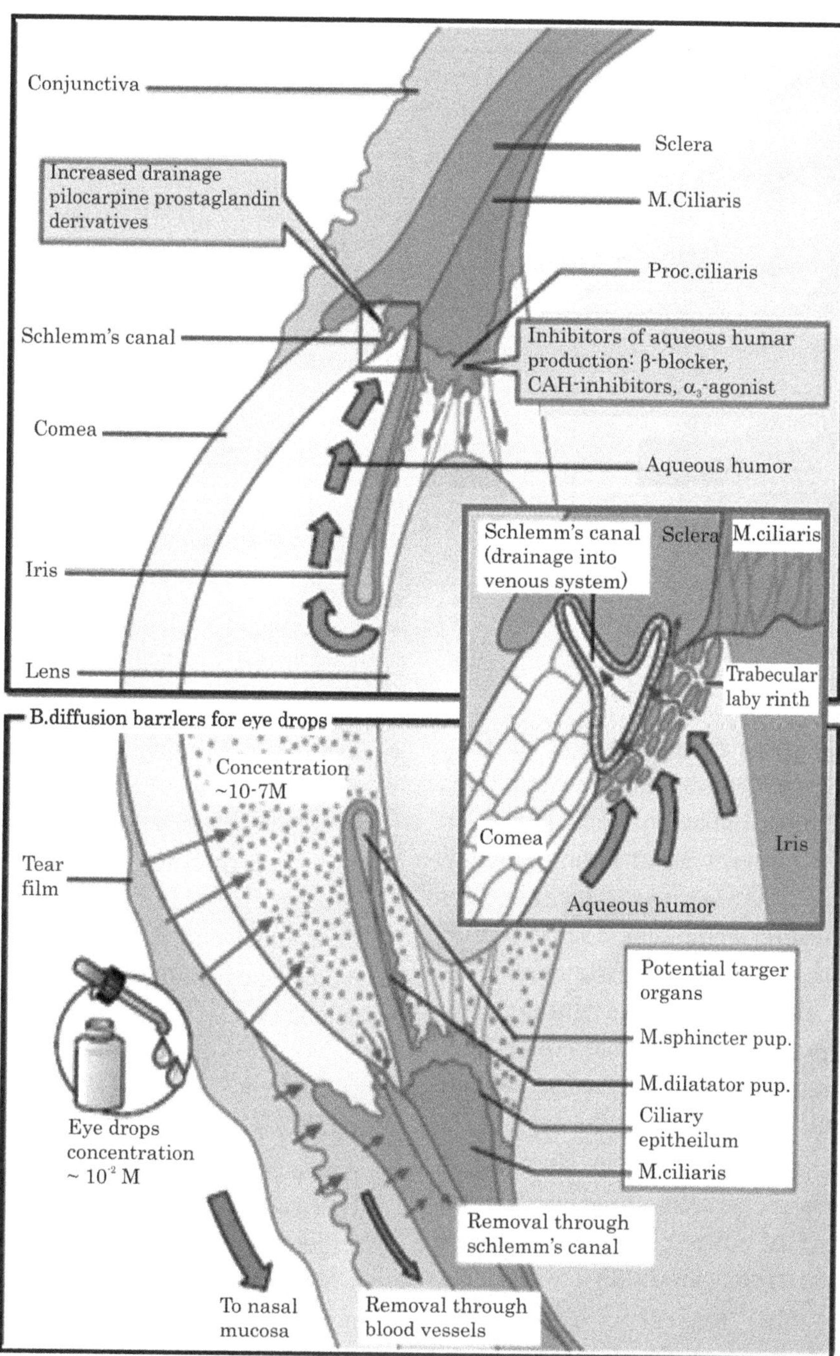

FIGURE 92.1

Local pharmacotherapy of glaucoma.

Table 92.1

Medical treatment of glaucoma

Therapy	Indication	Purpose	Method	Side Effects/ Drawbacks
Beta Blockers	1st line therapy	Reduce IOP	Reduce aqueous humor production	Exacerbate asthma, bradycardia, hypotension
Carbonic Anhydrase Inhibitors	1st line therapy	Reduce IOP	Reduce aqueous humor production	Headache, ocular discomfort, pruritus, keratitis
Alpha 2 agonists	2nd line agents	Reduce IOP	Reduce aqueous humor production, epinephrine prevents PAS formation through mydriatic effect	Palpitations, tachycardia, pallor, sweating
Prostaglandins	3nd line therapy	Reduce IOP	Increase outflow through uveal pathway and ciliary muscle	May worsen inflammation and increase risk of cystoid macular edema in uveitis
Hyperosmotic agents	3rd line therapy	Reduce IOP	Dehydrade the vitreous and reduce vitreous volume	Risk of intravascular fluid overload in patients with suppressed CV function

- Newer agents are also suitable for first-line therapy. Prostaglandin analogs (e.g., Latanoprost, bimatoprost and travoprost) have the advantage of strong potency, unique mechanism suitable for combination therapy, good safety profile, and once-a-day dosing. Brimonidine has the theoretical advantage of neuroprotection, which has not yet been demonstrated in humans. Topical CAIs are also suitable for first-line therapy.
- Pilocarpine and dipivefrin, a prodrug of epinephrine, are used as third line therapies because of adverse events or reduced efficacy as compared with newer agents.
- Carbachol, topical cholinesterase inhibitors, and oral CAIs (e.g., Acetazolamide) are used as last-resort options after failure of less toxic options.
- The optimal timing of laser or surgical trabeculectomy is controversial, ranging from initial therapy to after failure of third- or fourth-line drug therapy. Antiproliferative agents such as fluorouracil and mitomycin C are used to modify the healing process and maintain patency.

TREATMENT OF CLOSED-ANGLE GLAUCOMA

- Acute closed-angle glaucoma with high IOP requires rapid reduction of IOP. Iridectomy is the definitive treatment, which produces a hole in their is that permits aqueous flow to move directly from the posterior to the anterior chamber.
- Drug therapy of an acute attack typically consists of an osmotic agent and secretory

inhibitor (e.g. β-blocker, α2 agonist, latanoprost, or CAI), with or without pilocarpine.

- Osmotic agents are used because they rapidly decrease IOP. Examples include glycerin, 1 to 2 g/kg orally, and mannitol, 1 to 2 g/kg IV.
- Although traditionally the drug of choice, pilocarpine use is controversial as initial therapy. Once IOP is controlled, pilocarpine should be given every 6 hours until Iridectomy is performed.
- Epinephrine should be used with caution because it can precipitate acute closed-angle glaucoma, especially when used with a β-blocker.

REFERENCES

1. Anderson DR. The Optic Nerve in Glaucoma. In: Tasman W, Jaeger EA, eds. *Duane's Ophthalmology*. 15th ed. Philadelphia, Pa: Lippincott Williams & Wilkins; 2009:chap 48.
2. Kwon YK, Caprioli J. Primary Open-Angle Glaucoma. In: Tasman W, Jaeger EA, eds. *Duane's Ophthalmology*. 15th ed. Philadelphia, Pa: Lippincott Williams & Wilkins; 2009:chap 52.
3. Giaconi JA, Law SK, Caprioli J. Primary Angle-Closure Glaucoma. In: Tasman W, Jaeger EA, eds. *Duane's Ophthalmology*. 15th ed. Philadelphia, Pa: Lippincott Williams & Wilkins; 2009:chap 53.
4. Mandelcorn E, Gupta N. Lens-Related Glaucomas. In: Tasman W, Jaeger EA, eds. *Duane's Ophthalmology*. 15th ed. Philadelphia, Pa: Lippincott Williams & Wilkins; 2009:chap 54A.

CHAPTER 93

Diabetic Retinopathy

Diabetic retinopathy is an one of the microvascular complication of diabetes mellitus and 28 million were affected by vision-threatening diabetic retinopathy VTDR. The disease is mainly associated with a decline in best-corrected visual acuity.

INCIDENCE OF DIABETIC RETINOPATHY

The incidence of Diabetic retinopathy prevalence is higher in patients suffering with type I diabetes compared to type II , with sight-threatening retinopathy 2.5 times more common in type I.

Onset of diabetes before age 30 years

- The incidence of any retinopathy developing for the first time over a 4-year and 10-year period is 59% and 90%, respectively.
- The incidence of proliferative retinopathy over a 4-year and 10-year period is 11% and 30%, respectively.

Onset of diabetes after age 30 years

- The incidence of any retinopathy developing for the first time over a 4-year and 10 year period is 34–47% and 67–80%, respectively.
- The incidence of proliferative retinopathy over a 4-year and 10-year period is 2–7% and 10–23%, respectively.

DIABETIC RETINOPATHY RISK FACTORS

HYPERGLYCAEMIA

Chronic hyperglycaemia is the major risk factor in the development of diabetic retinopathy. The US Diabetes Control and Complications Trial (DCCT) evaluated the rates of development of microvascular complications of diabetes mellitus in two groups of type 1 diabetics assigned either to strict or standard glycaemic control over a mean follow-up period of 6.5 years. Those who had no retinopathy at entry into the study and who were assigned to tight control showed a 76% reduction in the mean risk of developing retinopathy. In addition, among those subjects with mild retinopathy at baseline, tight control slowed the progression of retinopathy by 54% and reduced the survival of persons suffering with proliferative retinopathy by 47%. Duration of diabetes is a reliable predictor of the presence of retinopathy, but the severity of the retinopathy is primarily influenced by other risk factors, especially glycaemic control.

HYPERTENSION

Hypertension is an major risk factor in the development of retinopathy in both type 1 and type 2 diabetes. Even among relatively normotensive individuals (BP <140/90 mmHg), those with BP levels above the 90th percentile show a higher prevalence of retinopathy and higher rate of progression. Hypertension is roughly twice as common in diabetic compared with non-diabetic patients. For example, 17–24% of patients with type 1 diabetes and 38% of patients with type 2 diabetes have BP >160/90 mmHg. Because of the link between BP and diabetic renal complications, it has been difficult to establish from epidemiological work that hypertension is an independent risk factor for retinopathy, but several intervention studies have been conclusive.

AGE

Puberty, with its attendant hormonal changes, brings about accelerated changes in retinopathy status; the highest 4-year incidence was among the patients aged ten to twelve years. In those with onset of diabetes below 21 years, females developed retinopathy approximately two years ahead of males, once again suggesting a pubertal influence.

NEPHROPATHY

Patients with diabetic nephropathy are much more likely to have associated microvascular disease in the eye; up to 96% of those with nephropathy also have retinopathy. This indicates similar pathogenic mechanisms, but a significant proportion of patients with advanced retinopathy show no clinical evidence of nephropathy. Similarly, although unusual, advanced renal disease has been described in the absence of retinopathy. It therefore seems likely that each form of microvascular disease has overlapping but not identical pathogenic mechanisms. Beyond its predictive value, nephropathy may also signify the presence of a more severe form of retinopathy, one that is more resistant to the effects of laser therapy.

PLASMA LIPIDS

The role of plasma lipids in the development of diabetic retinopathy is unclear. An association between higher levels of total serum cholesterol, declining ratios of high density lipoproteins (HDL), total cholesterol and more severe retinopathy. In type 1 diabetes, total serum cholesterol was found to have a marginal effect on the rate of progression of retinopathy. Patients with maculopathy were followed-up over seven years and compared with a matched group of patients who are without maculopathy. The group suffering with maculopathy was found to have higher serum cholesterol levels (6.6 vs. 5.9 mmol/L), higher levels of the HDL2 subfraction (0.46 vs. 0.32 mmol/L) and a higher prevalence of hyperlipidaemia (54% vs. 35%).

GENETIC FACTORS

It seems likely that there is a component of inherited susceptibility to the various microvascular complications of diabetes, because some individuals appear not to develop retinopathy despite poor glycaemic control. Familial clustering of diabetic retinopathy was investigated among 372 subjects with type 1 diabetes in the DCCT. The presence and severity of retinopathy was assessed in first-degree diabetic relatives of subjects in the trial. The severity of retinopathy in parents of children probands was found to be linked with the severity of retinopathy in their children, with the link strongest between mother and child. However, no relationship could be established between siblings. Although this observation suggests that the severity of diabetic retinopathy may be influenced by familial factors, the difficulty remains in differentiating environmental from genetic influences.

PREGNANCY

Diabetic retinopathy often gets worse during pregnancy, but it has been difficult to demonstrate that the progression of retinopathy is related to the pregnancy and would not otherwise have occurred. The progression of retinopathy prospectively in two groups of diabetic women who were matched apart from pregnancy status. The pregnant group demonstrated both increased prevalence and severity of retinopathy status compared to the control group. This finding is further supported by a larger study where the rate of progression of retinopathy was also found to be greater in the pregnant group after accounting for the influence of duration of diabetes, glycaemic control and hypertension. It was found that women with the highest glycosylated haemoglobin levels at the start of pregnancy, and those who experienced the greatest improvement in glycaemic control during pregnancy, had the highest risk of progression of retinopathy status. Although current pregnancy may adversely affect retinopathy status, it has been reported that in the long-term parous women have a lower prevalence of any retinopathy and of severe retinopathy. This may be the consequence of the institution of better control during pregnancy continuing into the post-partum period.

Ophthalmic supervision is therefore important during pregnancy particularly when retinopathy status at the start of pregnancy is moderately advanced. Those women with poor glycaemic control at the start of pregnancy also require close supervision.

OCULAR FACTORS

It has been observed that patients with asymmetrical diabetic retinopathy have a higher ophthalmic arterial perfusion pressure in the more severely affected eye. Ocular perfusion pressure is associated with the incidence of retinopathy. Higher intraocular pressure (therefore lower perfusion pressure) may offer some protection against retinopathy. Other factors found to be associated with a reduced risk of retinopathy include myopia, extensive chorioretinal scarring (perhaps simulating the effects of panretinal laser treatment) and amblyopia.

CLINICAL FEATURES

The clinical features of diabetic retinopathy result from pathological changes within the retinal vasculature which are classified into two principal stages, that includes proliferative retinopathy and background retinopathy. Background retinopathy has also been referred to as non-proliferative retinopathy to differentiate it from proliferative retinopathy although the proliferative changes occur amongst the 'background' of non-proliferative features. The terms most commonly used to denote the various stages of diabetic retinopathy are: background retinopathy, preproliferative retinopathy (a subclassification within background retinopathy) and proliferative retinopathy.

BACKGROUND DIABETIC RETINOPATHY

This is common and ranges from the very earliest signs of retinopathy to the severe changes seen just before the development of proliferative retinopathy. Background retinopathy can be subclassified into two subgroups of patients: those with sight-threatening disease and those without. The patterns of retinopathy most likely to reduce vision are those with macular involvement (maculopathy) and preproliferative disease. Maculopathy denotes the lesions of background disease within the macular area, whereas preproliferative retinopathy has additional features which differentiate it from the lesions of less severe background retinopathy. The three basic lesions which make up background retinopathy are microaneurysms, retinal haemorrhages and exudates. Haemorrhages and exudates have a limited lifespan, and, to a lesser extent, this also applies to microaneurysms.

MICROANEURYSMS

These are the very earliest clinically detectable lesions of diabetic retinopathy. They appear as small, round, red dots and may be found in any part of the retina although they predominate in the posterior pole of the eye. They are not associated with any visible blood vessels and represent localized dilatations of retinal capillaries. The number of microaneurysms increases with increasing severity of retinopathy. A microaneurysm indicates a localized area in the microvascular circulation where the blood-retinal barrier is deficient and may therefore be associated with abnormal vascular leakage.

The pathogenesis of microaneurysms is unclear but they may represent outpouchings of capillaries at areas of relative weakness where there is pericyte loss. Pericytes are cells which partly enclose retinal capillaries and may be considered the smooth muscle equivalent of the microvasculature; pericyte numbers diminish early in the development of diabetic retinopathy. Microaneurysms may also represent a localized response to surrounding hypoxia, i.e a limited proliferative process, as they tend to predominate in areas where there is closure of surrounding capillary beds.

HAEMORRHAGES

Haemorrhages co-exist with microaneurysms but are more variable in their appearance. At their smallest, they may be difficult to differentiate from microaneurysms. A haemorrhage, unlike a microaneurysm, is not necessarily round and may take on a variety of outlines; the phrase 'dot and blot' is an apt description. Haemorrhages can occur within the retina, where they remain confined by the retina, or flameshaped haemorrhage where they spread out over the superficial nerve fibre layer taking on a characteristic flame appearance. This latter form of haemorrhage is less obviously a feature of diabetic retinopathy and may suggest the co-existence of hypertensive vessel damage.

Haemorrhages probably occur from rupture of microaneurysms or other weak-walled vascular abnormalities. Small intraretinal haemorrhages occur early in diabetic retinopathy and their numbers increase with increasing severity. In more advanced disease, large dark blot intraretinal haemorrhages suggest severe retinal ischaemia with arteriolar occlusion, a feature of preproliferative disease.

EXUDATES

These are usually small collections of lipoprotein which have accumulated within the retina from abnormal vascular leakage, and are therefore found in the vicinity of microaneurysms. They are usually reflective and may appear to have a rigid, multifaceted contour, ranging in colour from white to yellow. They were previously referred to as 'hard' exudates to differentiate them from soft exudates (now called cotton wool spots); however, this separation is now redundant since it is well established that cotton-wool spots are not the products of exudation.

Like microaneurysms, exudates are most frequently detected in the posterior pole and may be distributed in the form of a whole or partial ring appearance. Such 'circinate' ring arrangements usually have microaneurysms in the centre, which are responsible for the vascular leakage that gives rise to the exudates at the margins. The number of exudates may paradoxically increase as the degree of extravascular fluid diminishes due to precipitation of lipids and proteins, analogous to a saline solution depositing salt upon drying. There may, therefore, be a transient increase in the number of exudates following laser treatment as the macula becomes drier.

DIABETIC MACULOPATHY

The term macula refers to the important centre of the retina. It measures approximately 5 mm in diameter and is the area centred upon the fovea with a radius that extends to the temporal margin of the optic disc.The fovea itself is about the same size as the optic disc (1.5–1.7 mm in diameter), with its centre (foveola) recognizable in normal eyes by the foveolar reflex. More practically, the macula can be considered as the area within the major temporal vascular arcades.

Diabetic maculopathy can be defined as any retinopathy lesion located within the macula. However, the term maculopathy is usually reserved for sight-threatening lesions close to the centre of the macula. The Early Treatment Diabetic Retinopathy Study (ETDRS) group produced the following list of criteria, any one of which is sufficient to diagnose clinically significant macular oedema (CSMO) requiring laser treatment:

- Thickening of the retina located less than 0.5 mm from the centre of the macula.
- Exudates (with thickening of adjacent retina) located less than 0.5 mm from the centre of the macula.
- An area of retinal thickening 1 disc diameter in size located less than 1 disc diameter from the centre of the macula.

PREPROLIFERATIVE DIABETIC RETINOPATHY

Preproliferative retinopathy is a sight-threatening condition that is usually considered separately from background disease. It also differs from background retinopathy in having four new features, i.e. cotton wool spots, retinal venous abnormalities, large blot intraretinal haemorrhages and intraretinal microvascular abnormalities.

COTTON WOOL SPOTS

Cotton wool spots appear as pale cream patches of variable sizes . They do not have clearly defined outlines and are most frequently seen in the posterior pole. A cotton wool spot is an area of infarction in the nerve fibre layer. It therefore represents an area of localized retinal ischaemia and suggests the presence of arteriolar occlusion. Cotton wool spots persist for a long time, ranging from 8–17 months.

INTRARETINAL MICROVASCULAR ABNORMALITIES (IRMA)

These usually appear as irregular loops of vessels within the retina which may straddle normal vessels. IRMA occur adjacent to areas of capillary bed closure and their origin is unclear. Unlike 'new vessels', IRMA do not always leak fluorescein, although some leakage may occur at their growing tips. At least two different theories exist as to what abnormal vasculature are presently classified as IRMA: shunt vessels and intraretinal new vessels.

VENOUS ABNORMALITIES

Various abnormalities occur in the retinal veins in response to the hypoxic environment. These take the form of:

- Beading, e.g. the 'string-of-sausages' appearance;
- Reduplication of veins, whereby the vein appears to divide into two parallel channels over a short segment; and
- Venous loops, where the vein makes a sudden deviation in the form of a loop. Venous abnormalities, particularly those of beading and reduplication, are strong indicators of hypoxia and suggest that new vessel development is imminent.

DEEP RETINAL HAEMORRHAGES

These are large dark haemorrhages within the retina representing haemorrhagic infarction secondary to retinal arteriolar occlusion.

PROLIFERATIVE DIABETIC RETINOPATHY

Ischaemia within the retina due to widespread closure of capillary beds leads to newly formed blood vessels appearing on the retinal surface, or overlying the optic disc. These vessels extend in the plane between the retina and the vitreous and are accompanied by a supporting network of fibroglial proliferation. New vessels developing from the vasculature of the optic disc are called 'disc new vessels' (NVD) whilst those developing on the surface of the retina are called 'new vessels elsewhere' (NVE) . It is thought that NVD represents severe generalized ischaemia of the retina, whereas NVE are a response to local ischaemia in the quadrant of the retina where they occur.

New vessels usually arise from a vein and have a haphazard growth pattern. As they grow, the combination of new vessels and supporting fibroglial tissue becomes adherent to both the retinal and posterior vitreous surfaces, inducing the vitreous to detach from the retina. The subsequent traction may cause haemorrhage either because the fragile new vessels break or because they are avulsed from their point of origin on the main retinal vessel. If bleeding is confined to the space between the retina and the vitreous, a preretinal or retrohyaloid haemorrhage is clearly visible on ophthalmoscopy (the so-called 'boat shaped' haemorrhage with a fluid level appearance). Depending on whether the haemorrhage obscures the macula, vision may be severely affected or minimally compromised. If the haemorrhage is to break through into the main body of the vitreous, the view of the retina may be variably obscured, likewise the patient's vision. The second outcome of neovascular traction is a retinal detachment. A tractional retinal detachment usually occurs slowly, and may remain stable for years assuming laser treatment has been applied to control the neovascular process. A tractional retinal detachment affects vision in two ways. Firstly, if it directly affects the fovea, vision will be reduced; if extrafoveal traction exists, tension induced retinal folds may secondarily affect the fovea, producing visual distortion. Secondly, a stable tractional detachment may suddenly become unstable if a full thickness hole occurs in the retina, leading to a rhegmatogenous retinal detachment which may spread to involve the fovea.

The proliferative process may not be confined to the posterior segment of the eye. Iris neovascularization is a feared complication because of the risk of neovascular or thrombotic glaucoma; a form of glaucoma which is difficult to manage once established. As with retinal neovascularization, fibrous tissue eventually develops which can occlude the trabecular meshwork and the anterior chamber angle leading to uncontrolled neovascular glaucoma or secondary angle closure glaucoma, resulting in a painful, red blind eye.

PATHOGENESIS

Exudative maculopathy or macular oedema is the consequence of a breakdown of the blood-retinal barrier (BRB), more specifically the inner BRB, i.e. the retinal capillary endothelium. This is usually at sites of microaneurysms although other retinopathy lesions also signify breaches in the BRB such as dilated capillaries, IRMA and retinal neovascularization. There is however, also some evidence suggesting a breakdown in the outer BRB may be due to the retinal pigment epithelium . The retinal pigment epithelium forms a barrier between the neural retina and the choriocapillaris, the capillary network of the choroid, which is highly permeable to macromolecules (unlike retinal capillaries). The normally tight junctions of the RPE, therefore, maintain a diffusion gradient for water from retina to choroid because of the higher oncotic pressure within the choroid. It has also recently been demonstrated that a taut, thickened posterior hyaloid (vitreous), which is still attached to the retina, can give rise to traction upon the macula producing intraretinal cystic spaces, and possibly a tractional detachment. These changes in the posterior hyaloid usually occur in response to ischemia and this form of macular oedema occurs very frequently in severe forms of retinopathy. Retinal hypoxia occurs mainly due to closure of the capillaries and arterioles is the major pathophysiological stimulus inducing new vessel formation. Hypoxia induces the local production of diffusible growth factors, e.g. vascular permeability factor (VPF), which initiate formation of new endothelial cellsfrom existing blood vessels.

DIAGNOSIS

Ophthalmoscopic evaluation with the direct or indirect ophthalmoscope is widely used for the diagnosis of diabetic retinopathy. Fluorescein angiography, introduced in 1961, has been the one laboratory test that has dramatically increased our knowledge of the diabetic retinal process and our ability to implement rational treatment procedures. Ultrasonography has permitted the ophthalmologist to document the structural relationship of various parts of the eye even though direct visualization is clouded by blood, debris, or membranes. Electrophysiologic aids, such as electroretinography, permit one to assess the functional capabilities of the retina in order to determine whether surgical intervention, such as cataract extraction or vitrectomy, would prove useful in a particular eye.

FLUORESCEIN ANGIOGRAPHIC EVALUATION

Intravenous fluorescein angiography has been available for the study of posterior segment diseases, like macular degeneration, diabetic retinopathy, and various vasculopathies. With this technique it has been possible to study various chorioretinal diseases.

The technique involves the administration of injection of 5 ml of a 10% solution of sodium fluorescein into the antecubital vein and then taking the results photographically on black and white film at intervals of 0.6-0.8 sec. In this manner the entire transit of the fluorescein-blood mixture can be documented as it enters the retinal and choroidal circulation. All abnormalities of the retinal circulation present in diabetic retinopathy can be visualized and identified with precision, and the appropriate therapeutic steps taken.

In nonproliferative phase of diabetic retinopathy, multiple microaneurysms, areas of patchy retinal edema, hemorrhages, zones of capillary closure, and intraretinal microvascular abnormalities can be visualized by the fluorescein antiography. Usually exudates fail to appear on a fluorescein angiogram, and hemorrhages can be identified by the areas of blocked transmittance of the fluorescent dye from the choroidal circulation. Perhaps the most important use of this technique in nonproliferative diabetic retinopathy is the assessment of the leakage of the retinal vessels in the macular area with the subsequent pooling of fluorescein in the perifoveal space, the disruption of the circumfoveolar capillary network, and the presence of large areas of microinfarction and capillary closure. With the correct evaluation of fluorescein angiograms, the proper treatment technique can be selected and the various photocoagulation parameters adjusted for the degree ofretinopathy.

In case of the proliferative diabetic retinopathy, fluorescein angiography has been shown to be indispensable in identifying not only all of the factors but also the presence of small areas of retinal or optic nerve neovascularization. The extent of the neovascular complexes and their leakage capabilities are important to analyze in conjunction with the degree of capillary closure and other hemodynamic and vascular pathology in the posterior pole of the eye. The various types of neovascularization can be documented, and the amount of background retinopathy and pathologic alterations can be assessed in order to implement the panretinal photocoagulation or focal photocoagulation approach in the proper manner.

ULTRASONOGRAPHY AND ELECTRORETINOGRAPHY

Ultrasonography and bright-flash electroretinography (ERG) should be used as complementary tests when evaluating a patient being considered for vitrectomy. Ultrasonography can provide excellent information regarding the anatomy of theeye with an opaque vitreous or severely opacified lens. The presence and distribution of membranes in the vitreous or traction retinal detachments can be detected by ultrasonography, and these factors can be used to determine the feasibility of vitrectomy intervention. The bright-flash ERG can indicate if the retina is attached and capable of some visual function. When there is a poor response to bright-flash ERG, ultrasonography can be of assistance in clarifying whether the decreased ERG is due to a retinal detachment or to a poorly functioning attached retina. In eyes with a retinal detachment, the visual potential depends on the technical possibility of surgical reattachment of the retina and the potential of the retina to function once it is reattached.

MANAGEMENT

The increasing incidence of diabetic retinopathy in recent decades is a sober reminder that medical therapy for diabetic retinopathy has not proven very successful. For centuries prior to insulin, dietary restriction, often severely imposed, was the only means of coping with diabetes. Such strict measures painfully improved the life expectancy of diabetics.

Insulin lessened the necessity for harsh diets in the treatment of diabetes. Diabetics now enjoy a more normal life, but microvascular complications have only increased as patients live longer. Today there remains significant controversy as to whether or not strict control of blood sugar alleviates complications such as retinopathy.

Until this is achieved, weight reduction and low-fat diets, although seemingly old-fashioned, probably do not receive adequate emphasis in the medical treatment of diabetes and diabetic retinopathy. Numerous drugs have been used to treat diabetic retinopathy, a fact that only emphasizes how ineffective such treatment has proven. However, better understanding of the pathogenesis of diabetic retinopathy will hopefully create new opportunities for successful drug therapy. The need for careful and controlled clinical trials, so often overlooked in the past, is now recognized. This, in itself, is an important step in the search for more effective drugs to treat retinopathy.

PHOTOCOAGULATION

During the last decade, diabetic retinopathy has been proven to be treated effectively in controlled clinical trials by photocoagulation intervention. Photocoagulation therapy involves the channeling of an incandescent or laser light beam to the retina of the eye through a dilated pupil. As the light energy strikes the retina, it is absorbed by melanin, xanthophyll, or oxy- and reduced-hemoglobin. These treatments convert the light energy to heat with varying efficiency but with sufficient heat production to raise the temperature of the retina from 37° C to 65-70° C, thereby producing a coagulum. This coagulum can be produced in strategic areas of the retina in order to destroy microaneurysms, leaky retinal vessels, patches of retinal or vitreal neovascularization, and areas of retinal edema or capillary microinfarction. In this way, the incidence of hemorrhage as well as glial proliferation can be markedly reduced, and, in some cases, can be nearly normalized.

Practical photocoagulation was introduced by Meyer-Schwickerath in 1959 utilizing an incandescent xenon-arc high-pressure bulb source. Although not a laser source, the intense white light produced by this instrument contains all the wavelengths of the visible and near-infrared spectrum. It is still being used effectively as a photocoagulation device in certain circumstances. Argon laser photocoagulation introduced in 1968 has gained wide acceptance in ophthalmic practice because the absorption characteristics of the argon laser beam can be readily determined, an extremely small coagulation spot can be produced, the blue-green beam is highly absorbed by the abnormal red retinal vasculature, and the procedure can be performed without anesthesia other than topically applied drops. Krypton laser photocoagulation introduced in 1972 has also been utilized by ophthalmologists to photocoagulate extremely hemorrhagic areas of diabetic retinopathy, to coagulate abnormal vasculature through a hazy blood-filled vitreous, and to produce pan-retinal photocoagulation ablative retinal procedures in areas where the fragile diabetic neovascularization might be ruptured by the more highly absorbed argon laser beam. Very recently, photocoagulation by the frequency-doubled neodymiumYAG green beam and the organic liquid dye red or yellow laser beam, both introduced in 1971 and 1983, respectively, have been shown to be highly absorbed by critical elements of the retina so that each individual case of diabetic retinopathy can be treated precisely with respect to the particular underlying vascular, hemodynamic, or metabolic defect.

RATIONALE

The basic rationale of photocoagulation is to destroy neovascular complexes, to obliterate areas of microinfarction or capillary closure, to destroy leaking vessels in the macular and paramacular region.

It would seem obvious that these blood vessels are proliferating in a response to some biochemical stimulus, and neovascularization seems to be an appropriate defense for the reparative mechanism of the body. However, the in-growth of neovascularization with the support of glial tissue, as well as the attendant leakage of damaged vessels into the surrounding retinal spaces, the transport of high molecular weight lipoproteinaceous material throughout the neovascular walls into the retina, the resulting hemorrhages, and the dynamic changes occurring from the interposition of the fibrovascular membranes, can irreparably damage the retina. Panretinal photocoagulation appears to obliterate successfully or cause the regression of neovascularization by one of four mechanisms: (1) The reduction or destruction of areas of hypoxic retina that are producing the vasoformative factor that is calling forth neovascularization from more healthy areas of the retina; (2) The creation of a closer apposition of the inner layers of the retina to the choriocapillaris by the multiple scattered photocoagulation scarring around the entire posterior polar region, thereby allowing greater oxygen perfusion from the choroidal layers to the inner retinal layers that have undergone a relatively high degree of microinfarction; (3) The destruction of unhealthy microinfarcted areas of retina and sluggishly perfused capillaries, thereby allowing the available retinal blood to increase nourishment to the remaining retina; and (4) The destruction of leaking blood vessels and other abnormal vascular complexes that are creating an abnormal hemodynamic situation in the diabetic retina, thereby more nearly normalizing the vascular supply of the macular region of the eye. The entire concept of the vasoformative factor being elaborated by hypoxic retina, secondary to microinfarction and capillary closure, is a most inviting explanation for the beneficial effect of panretinal photocoagulation. If the vasoformative factor emanating from the hypoxic areas of retina can be reduced in the posterior vitreous, the neovascular stimulus is thereby decreased, and the new vessels tend to regress or become obliterated. Certainly the better nutrition of the inner portions of the retina by the closer apposition of the inner layers to the choriocapillaris and the choroidal blood supply would also appear to be a beneficial result of the panretinal photocoagulation technique.

PHOTOCOAGULATION RESULTS

The application of photocoagulation is divided either into the focal type of treatment or panretinal photocoagulation. Focal argon laser or xenon-arc photocoagulation of isolated patches of neovascularization involves the coagulation of zones of retinal vessels, leakage, or herniation. The photocoagulation is not extensive, but serves to contain the retinopathy and to destroy those more localized regions of retinal vascular abnormalities. Panretinal photocoagulation involves the systematic photocoagulation of the retina from the region several disc diameters outside the macula to the equator of the eye in six to eight photocoagulation sessions, spaced at weekly intervals. By coagulating approximately 20-30% of the retina in these areas, the demand for oxygen and nutrition is decreased along with the areas of hypoxic retina, thereby theoretically decreasing the vasoformative factor which calls forth and supports neovascular growth and perhaps the glial proliferation process in diabetic retinopathy. This indirect application of photocoagulation, usually away from the neovascularization, by panretinal photocoagulation leads to the partial ablation of the peripheral retina and to the regression or obliteration of the neovascularization in the central retina in more than 80% of cases.

It was recommended that photocoagulation treatment should be considered in eyes with anyone of the following criteria: (1) Moderate or severe new vessels on or within one-disc diameter on the optic disc; (2) Mild new vessels on or within one-disc diameter of the optic disc if a hemorrhage is present; and (3) Moderate or severe new vessels elsewhere if a fresh hemorrhage is present .

It was emphasized that: (1) The presence of vitreous or preretinal hemorrhage, (2) The presence of new vessels, (3) The location of new vessels on or near the optic disc, and (4) The severity of the new vessels has increased the severe visual loss; and photocoagulation was indicated earlier if these particular factors were present. The occurrence of visual acuity less than V200 for two consecutive, completed four-month followup visits, when determined over a four-year period, was reduced approximately 50% in all treated eyes in the study .

VITRECTOMY AND VITREOLYSIS

A promising new therapy for eyes previously blinded from vitreous hemorrhage is pars plana vitrectomy. Vitrectomy involves a technique whereby a needle-like cutting and aspiration device is introduced into the central cavity of vitreous in the eye, and blood, membranes, and fibrin are delicately removed from that region and replaced with clear Ringer's solution. Vitrectomy has been proven to be useful in cases in which blindness is due primarily to vitreous opacification from fibrin or vitreous membranes, and it has not been as useful if the retina has been previously severely damaged by advanced retinopathy, fibrosis, and degeneration. Many blind diabetics are not candidates for this operation because of concurrent retinal deterioration as noted by electrophysiologic tests, advanced traction retinal detachments as documented by ultrasonography, or the development ofdiabetic neovascular glaucoma.

INDICATIONS

The following conditions have been considered as the optimal requirements in order for an eye to be selected for pars plana vitrectomy. Rarely are all of the *ideal* conditions present at the time of vitrectomy. Repeated vitreous hemorrhages, a progressively enlarging retinal detachment, known zones of neovascularization that could be photocoagulated, rapid visual and electrophysiologic deterioration of the eye, or marked debilitation of the fellow eye may all be indications for earlier vitrectomy intervention. These conditions and the following more ideal indications should be integrated with the Diabetic Retinopathy Vitrectomy Study (DRVS) criteria as soon as they have been firmly established:

1. Absence of recurrent hemorrhage or new red blood in the vitreous during the preceding six-month period.
2. No evidence of clearing of the opacified vitreous during the preceding six month period.
3. Presence of light perception and, ideally, the presence of an accurate light projection in two or more fields.
4. No definite ultrasonographic evidence of retinal detachment in eyes with questionable light projection.
5. No previously documented evidence of long-standing retinal gliosis or detachment.
6. Ideally, an ERG response that is present, although possibly diminished in intensity.
7. Complete understanding of the purpose of the procedure by the patient with totally informed patient consent.

Traction retinal detachments often complicate proliferative diabetic retinopathy. In these cases the posterior vitreous is attached to sites of epiretinal proliferation, and they result in a traction detachment of the underlying retina. Characteristically, a retinal detachment occurs along the course of the superotemporal vascular arcade, but other areas may be involved. Although extensive detachment along the vascular arcades often spares the macular region and because of the operative risks associated with these eyes, vitreous surgery is usually not recommended before the macular region has been threatened. However, vitreous surgery should be considered if the macula is partially detached, particularly if the detachment is of recent onset .

PITUITARY ABLATION

Pituitary ablation has been shown to be most effective in the treatment of rapidly progressive, severe, proliferative (florid) retinopathy. Recent controlled clinical trials of pituitary ablation versus no treatment and versus photocoagulation have both shown significantly better retention of vision in the hypophysectomized patients. However, in view of the acknowledged occasional severe side effects of hypophysectomy, it has been recommended that this procedure should be reserved for florid retinopathy.

GENERAL PATIENT MANAGEMENT

The most frequently asked questions, by both physicians and patients, will be answered as simply as possible. The answers to these questions should provide an overall pattern that has been discussed more completely .

1. When should the diabetic patient be seen or referred to an ophthalmologist?

Every patient should be seen by an ophthalmologist when diabetes mellitus has been first diagnosed. Particularly type II diabetic patients who may have some degree of diabetic retinopathy requiring immediate treatment.

2. How frequently should the diabetic patient be seen by an ophthalmologist?

If the patient is newly diabetic and has no obvious retinopathy ophthalmoscopically, the patient is usually observed at yearly intervals. If retinopathy is progressing or is far advanced, patients may be seen as frequently as every two to three months.

3. When are fluorescein angiographic or ultrasonographic evaluations performed on the diabetic patient?

Fluorescein angiography is usually not performed until ophthalmoscopic evidence of the early stages of diabetic retinopathy can be detected. Thereafter, fluorescein angiographic evaluations can be performed at 6- to 12-month intervals, or more frequently, in order to document closely any retinal vascular changes. *Ultrasonography* should be done in some cases in order to produce a baseline study and also is used during later stages of diabetic retinopathy when vitreous hemorrhage, cataract, or corneal changes obstruct the view of the retina which can only be evaluated, at that point in time, by ultrasonographic examination.

4. What restrictions does the diabetic patient have after photocoagulation?

All of these directions should be followed for at least two weeks after photocoagulation unless advised otherwise.

1. Keep head up and move slowly. Do not bend over or move suddenly.
2. Remain calm. Do not worry about the treatment or anything else, if possible. Contact the physician if the person is overly anxious or overly disturbed about your condition or other problems.
3. Do not strain at anything. Do not lift any object heavier than 20 pounds or hold your breath for any reason. Do not strain

during bowel movements and try not to get constipated. Try not to engage in any strenuous or "surge" type activities (athletics, sex, heavy housework, furniture moving, etc.).

4. Vision may be blurry and blotchy for two to three weeks, or longer, after treatment. Nearly always, but not invariably, vision will return to the pretreatment level.
5. The patient may have some discomfort around your treated eye. Aspirin is sufficient to relieve the pain in most cases. Also, the eye may be bloodshot, a common occurrence following photocoagulation.

The following directions should be followed indefinitely.

1. Sleep with the head of your bed raised 15-20 degrees. This is best accomplished by placing a foam rubber wedge seven inches high and one-third the length of the mattress under the mattress. If this wedge is not available, use several pillows to elevate your head. This will decrease the blood pressure in the tiny blood vessels in your eyes.
2. Control coughing and sneezing by cough syrup or other medications. However, do not stifle a sneeze since this raises the blood pressure in your eyes.
3. Continue to avoid bending, straining, and heavy lifting.
4. Do not rub eyes since this may disrupt blood vessels inside the eyes.
5. Try not to use those nose drops, sprays, or inhalators which contain ephedrine or adrenalin. These may raise your blood pressure and predispose to hemorrhage.
6. Use a stool softener, one or two capsules of Colace each bedtime, if constipated.
7. Avoid altitudes over 8,000 feet; e.g., mountain passes, private plane flying. Scheduled commercial aircraft are pressurized to this altitude and are permissible.

5. What exercise can a diabetic patient with nonproliferative diabetic retinopathy do?

Excessive exercise can result in severe retinal, preretinal, or vitreal hemorrhages due to a momentary or sustained increase in systemic hypertension or an extended Valsalva maneuver. A combination of vitreoretinal adhesions, vitreo-retinal traction, and vitreous movement during exercise may cause a *stress* hemorrhage or retinal tear. The combination of hypertension, hypoglycemia, and the Valsalva maneuver will, in many cases, cause a *hypertensive* or "blow-out" hemorrhage. It is recommended that the patient with nonproliferative diabetic retinopathy engage in non-Valsalva maneuver exercises such as swimming, jogging, bicycling, and racket sports.

6. The diabetic person suffering with nonproliferative diabetic retinopathy should *not* do which exercises ?

It is imperative that the patient with any phase of retinopathy refrain from excessive Valsalva maneuvers, such as holding one's breath while lifting or exercising, particularly if the diabetic individual has mild or moderate systemic hypertension. The exercises to be avoided are bowling, yoga, weight-lifting and advanced Nautilus or similar type exercises.

7. What exercises can a diabetic patient with proliferative diabetic retinopathy do?

The patient with proliferative diabetic retinopathy has developed new diabetic retinal blood vessels which may extend from the retina into the vitreous body. These areas of neovascularization do not have sufficient muscular or other reinforcement to withstand increases in blood pressure much above normal day-to-day activity. Therefore, it is recommended that exercise and muscular toning, important to all diabetic patients, be limited to swimming, light jogging or bicycling, passive exercise machines, walking briskly, and mild nonisometric toning.

8. What exercises should a diabetic patient with proliferative diabetic retinopathy not do?

The patient with proliferative diabetic retinopathy runs the risk of producing a disabling intraocular hemorrhage with one or a combination of: (1) An increase in systemic blood pressure; (2) A decrease in the blood sugar level; or (3) A modified Valsalva maneuver. The exercises that should not be attempted by a patient with proliferative diabetic retinopathy include diving, bowling, yoga, Nautilus and similar type workouts, pushups, situps, head-below-the-waist exercises, strenuous jogging, bicycling, strenuous racket sports, or any advanced isometric exercises.

9. What can internists do to help stabilize diabetic retinopathy?

The most important factors appear to be to stabilize, as much as possible, the patient's blood pressure and blood glucose level; closely monitor the renal and retinal condition; and to be certain that the patient is being seen at regular intervalsby his ophthalmologist. Patients with late nonproliferative or proliferative diabetic retinopathy should be controlled in such a way that hypoglycemic shocks should be minimized or eliminated due to the devastating effect that they can have on retinal vessels.

10. What happen to be the most detrimental to diabetic patients with diabetic retinopathy?

The Valsalva maneuver, where external muscles contract against a lungful of air in order to lift or cough, etc., raises the pressure in the vessels of the head and the retina causing hypertensive or blow-out hemorrhages into the vitreous cavity. Therefore, as documented previously, constipation should be avoided, lifting ofany object over 20-30 pounds should be avoided, as well as bending at the waist with the back held horizontally. Vomiting, excessive coughing, frequent bouts of hypoglycemia with or without frank "shocking" all can lead to severe retinal problems. In addition, extreme surge exercises, as noted previously, can be disastrous. Any combination of the multitude of physical states that can dilate or increase the pressure within the retinal vessels can lead to immediate hemorrhaging from the tiny retinal vessels.

11. Do diabetic patients have an increased problem in cataract extraction?

Although a few special precautions should be taken with diabetic patients during a cataract extraction, the actual operation, postoperative healing, and eventual recovery (providing retinal damage is not present) is similar to the nondiabetic population.

12. Can diabetic patients have intraocular lenses as a replacement for the cataractous lens after its removal?

An intraocular lens implant should not be placed in a diabetic eye with advanced retinopathy or in a younger person with less retinopathy but with a greater lifespan in which to develop advanced retinopathy. However, intraocular lens implants can be considered for most diabetic patients without significant retinopathy.

13. Do diabetic patients have an increased incidence of glaucoma?

The incidence of glaucoma in diabetic patients without retinopathy or with early retinopathy is not essentially different from the nondiabetic population. However, the incidence of glaucoma, especially diabetic neovascular glaucoma, increases with the duration of diabetes and, therefore, with the duration and severity of the diabetic retinopathy process. Ophthalmologists and internists should be constantly aware of the potential for their patients to develop an elevation in intraocular pressure.

14. Can diabetic neovascular glaucoma be treated?

Until recently it was difficult to treat diabetic neovascular glaucoma successfully with any assortment of medications and, in many cases, destructive surgery was finally recommended.

However, various types of laser therapy to the anterior portion of the eye have proved successful in a number of patients, and this therapy appears to be promising.

15. Can diabetic patients expect to retain usable visual function during their lifetimes?

The diabetic individual can expect to retain usable visual acuity during his or her lifetime provided he or she is willing to follow the lifestyle and regulations recommended by their internist, nephrologist, neurologist, and other medical care personnel. On the other hand, it is imperative that the internist, nephrologist, and ophthalmologist work closely together to integrate their treatment, so that individual recommendations coordinate with other physicians' recommendations to maximally benefit the patient with regard to their vision and to other organs attacked by the diabetic process.

REFERENCES

1. Brown JK, Jones AT. Retinopathy and diabetic control. Br J Ophthalmol, 48:148-153, 1964.
2. Colwell JA. Effect of diabetic control on retinopathy. Diabetes 15:497-499, 1966.
3. Hardin RC, Jackson RL, Johnston TL, Kelly HG. The development of diabetic retinopathy: effects of duration and control of diabetes. Diabetes 5:397-405, 1956.
4. L'Esperance FA Jr. Ocular photocoagulation. St. Louis: C.V. Mosby Co., 1975.
5. Little HP. In: Diabetic Retinopathy, LynnJR, Snyder WB, Vaiser A (eds). New York: Grune and Stratton, 1974, pp. 133-144.
6. L'Esperance FA Jr. (ed). Current diagnosis and management of chorioretinal diseases. St. Louis: C.V. Mosby Co., 1977.
7. Bachmann MO, Nelson SJ. Impact of diabetic retinopathy screening on a British district population: case detection and blindness prevention in an evidence-based model. *J Epidemiol Community Health* 1998; 52: 45–52.
8. Early Treatment Diabetic Retinopathy Study Research Group: Photocoagulation for diabetic macular oedema: Early Treatment Diabetic Retinopathy Study report number 1. *Arch Ophthalmol* 1985; 103: 1796–1806.

CHAPTER 94

Psoriasis

DEFINITION

Psoriasis is a common chronic inflammatory disease characterized by recurrent exacerbations and remissions of thickened, erythematous, and scaling plaques.

PREVALENCE

Psoriasis affects both sexes equally, and can occur at any age, although it most commonly appears for the first time between the ages of 15 and 25 years.

The prevalence of psoriasis in Western populations is estimated to be around 2% - 3%. The prevalence of psoriasis among 7.5 million patients who were registered with a general practitioner in the United Kingdom was 1.5%. A survey conducted by the National Psoriasis Foundation (a US-based psoriasis education and advocacy group) found a prevalence of 2.1% among adult Americans. The study found 35% of people with psoriasis could be classified as having moderate to severe psoriasis.

ETIOLOGY

Psoriasis is very common. Anyone can get it, but it most commonly begins between ages 15 and 35.

It is not contagious and cannot be spread to others.

Psoriasis seems to be passed down through families. Doctors think it probably occurs when the body's immune system mistakes healthy cells for dangerous substances.

Usually, skin cells grow deep in the skin and rise to the surface about once a month. In persons with psoriasis, this process is too fast. Dead skin cells build up on the skin's surface.

The following may trigger an attack of psoriasis or make the condition more difficult to treat:

- Bacteria or viral infections, including strep throat and upper respiratory infections
- Dry air or dry skin
- Injury to the skin, including cuts, burns, and insect bites
- Some medicines, including antimalarial drugs, β-blockers, and lithium
- Stress
- Too little sunlight
- Too much sunlight (sunburn)
- Too much alcohol

In general, psoriasis may be severe in people who have a weakened immune system. This may include persons who have:

- AIDS
- Autoimmune disorders (such as rheumatoid arthritis)
- Cancer chemotherapy

PATHOPHYSIOLOGY

- Cell-mediated immune mechanisms play a central role in psoriasis. Cutaneous inflammatory T-cell–mediated immune activation requires two T-cell signals mediated via cell–cell interactions by surface proteins and antigen-presenting cells such as dendritic cells or macrophages. The first signal is the interaction of the T-cell receptor with antigen presented by antigen-presenting cells. The second signal (called co-stimulation) is mediated through various surface interactions.
- Once T-cells are activated, they migrate from lymph nodes and the bloodstream into skin and secrete various cytokines (e.g., interferon γ, interleukin 2 [IL-2]) that induce the pathologic changes of psoriasis. Local keratinocytes and neutrophils are induced to produce other cytokines, such as tumor necrosis factor-α (TNF- α), IL-8, and others.
- As a result of pathogenic T-cell production and activation, psoriatic epidermal cells proliferate at a rate sevenfold faster than normal epidermal cells. Epidermal proliferation is also elevated in apparently normal skin of psoriatic patients.
- There is a significant genetic component in psoriasis. Studies of histocompatibility antigens in psoriatic patients indicate a number of significant associations, especially with HLA-Cw6, where the relative likelihood for developing psoriasis is 9 to 15 times normal.
- Climate, stress, alcohol, smoking, infection, trauma, and drugs may aggravate psoriasis. Warm seasons and sunlight improve psoriasis in 80% of patients, whereas 90% of patients worsen in cold weather. Psoriatic lesions may develop at the site of injury (e.g., rubbing, venipuncture, bites and surgery) on normal-appearing skin (Koebner response). Lithium carbonate, β-adrenergic blockers, some antimalarials, nonsteroidal anti-inflammatory drugs, and tetracyclines have been reported to exacerbate psoriasis.

CLINICAL FEATURES

Psoriasis can appear suddenly or slowly. Many times, it goes away and then comes back again and again.

Symptoms include:

- Irritated, red, flaky patches of skin
- Most often seen on the elbows, knees, and middle of the body
- Red patches may appear anywhere on the body, including the scalp

  The skin may be:
- Itchy
- Dry and covered with silver, flaky skin (scales)
- Pink-red in color (like the color of salmon)
- Raised and thick

Other symptoms may include:

- Genital lesions in males
- Joint pain or aching
- Nail changes, including thick nails, yellow-brown nails, dents in the nail, and nail lifts off from the skin underneath

- Severe dandruff on the scalp

Psoriasis may affect any or all parts of the skin. There are five main types of psoriasis:

- Erythrodermic — The skin redness is very intense and covers a large area.
- Guttate — Small, pink-red spots appear on the skin.
- Inverse — Skin redness and irritation occurs in the armpits, groin, and in between overlapping skin.
- Plaque — Thick, red patches of skin are covered by flaky, silver-white scales. This is the most common type of psoriasis.
- Pustular — White blisters are surrounded by red, irritated skin.

DIAGNOSIS

The diagnosis is based on physical examination findings of the characteristic lesions of psoriasis.

- The medical history of a patient with psoriasis should include information about the onset and duration of lesions, family history of psoriasis, presence of exacerbating factors, previous history of antipsoriatic treatment (if any) along with efficacy and adverse effect data, exposure to chemicals and toxins, and allergies (food, drugs, and environmental).
- Skin biopsy of lesional skin is useful in confirming the diagnosis.

TREATMENT

NONPHARMACOLOGICAL THERAPY (FIG. 94.1)

- **Emollients (moisturizers)** hydrate the stratum corneum and minimize water evaporation. They may enhance desquamation, eliminate scaling, and decrease pruritus. The lotions, creams, or ointments often need to be applied up to four times a day to achieve a beneficial response. Adverse effects include folliculitis and allergic or irritant contact dermatitis.
- Balneotherapy (and climatotherapy) involves bathing in waters containing certain salts, often combined with natural sun exposure. The salts in certain waters (e.g., the Dead Sea) reduce activated T cells in skin and may be remittive for psoriasis.

FIRST-LINE TOPICAL PHARMACOTHERAPY

KERATOLYTICS

Salicylic acid is one of the most commonly used keratolytics. It causes a disruption in corneocyte-to-corneocyte cohesion in the abnormal horny layer of psoriatic skin. This serves to remove scales, smooth the skin, and decrease hyperkeratosis. The keratolytic effect enhances penetration and efficacy of some other topical agents such as corticosteroids. It is applied as a 2% to 10% gel or lotion two or three times a day. Salicylic acid produces local irritation. Application to large, inflamed areas may induce salicylism with symptoms of nausea, vomiting, tinnitus, or hyperventilation.

CORTICOSTEROIDS

- **Topical corticosteroids** may halt synthesis and mitosis of DNA in epidermal cells and appear to inhibit phospholipase A, lowering the amounts of arachidonic acid, prostaglandins, and leukotrienes in the skin. These effects, coupled with local vasoconstriction, reduce erythema, pruritus, and scaling. As antipsoriatic agents, they are best used adjunctively with a product that specifically functions to normalize epidermal hyperproliferation.

- Low-potency products (e.g., hydrocortisone 1%) have a weak anti-inflammatory effect and are safest for long-term application, for use on the face and intertriginous areas, for use with occlusion, and for use in infants and young children.
- Medium-potency products are used in moderate inflammatory dermatoses. They may be used on the face and intertriginous areas for a limited time.
- High-potency preparations are used primarily as alternatives to systemic corticosteroids when local therapy is feasible.
- Very high potency products may be used for thick, chronic psoriatic lesions but for only short periods of time and on relatively small surface areas.
- Ointments are the most effective formulations for psoriasis because they have an occlusive oily phase that conveys a hydrating effect and enhances penetration of the corticosteroid into the dermis. They are not suited for use in the axilla, groin, or other intertriginous areas where maceration and folliculitis may develop secondary to the occlusive effect.
- Creams are more cosmetically desirable for some patients. They may be used in intertriginous areas even though their lower oil content makes them more drying than ointments.
- Topical corticosteroids are applied two to four times daily during long-term therapy.
- Adverse effects include local tissue atrophy, skin degeneration, and striae. If detected early, these effects may be reversible with discontinuation. Thinning of the epidermis may result in visibly distended capillaries (telangiectasias) and purpura. Acne form eruptions and masking of symptoms of bacterial or fungal skin infections have been reported. Systemic consequences include risk of suppression of the hypothalamic-pituitary-adrenal axis, hyperglycemia, and development of cushingoid features. Tachyphylaxis and rebound flare of psoriasis after abrupt cessation of therapy can also occur.

VITAMIN D ANALOGS

Vitamin D and its analogs inhibit keratinocyte differentiation and proliferation and have antiinflammatory effects by reducing IL-8, IL-2, and other cytokines. Use of vitamin D itself is limited by its propensity to cause hypercalcemia.

CALCIPOTRIENE

(Dovonex) is a synthetic vitamin D analog used for mild to moderate plaque psoriasis. Improvement is usually seen within 2 weeks of treatment, and approximately 70% of patients demonstrate marked improvement after 8 weeks. Adverse effects occur in about 10% of patients and include lesional and perilesional burning and stinging. Calcipotriene 0.005% cream, ointment, or solution is applied one or two times a day (no more than 100 g/wk).

- Calcitriol and tacalcitol are other vitamin D derivatives that have been studied for treatment of psoriasis.

TAZAROTENE

Tazarotene (Tazorac) is a synthetic retinoid that is hydrolyzed to its active metabolite, tazarotenic acid, which modulates keratinocyte proliferation and differentiation. It is available as a 0.05% or 0.1% gel and cream and is applied once daily (usually in the evening) for mild to moderate plaque psoriasis. Adverse effects are dose- and frequency related and includes mild to moderate pruritus, burning, stinging, and erythema. Application of the gel to eczematous skin or to more than 20% of body surface area is not recommended because this may lead to extensive systemic absorption. Tazarotene is often used with topical corticosteroids to decrease local adverse effects and increase efficacy.

SECOND-LINE TOPICAL PHARMACOTHERAPY

COAL TAR

- **Coal tar** contains numerous hydrocarbon compounds formed from distillation of bituminous coal. Ultraviolet B (UVB) light–activated coal tar photo adducts with epidermal DNA and inhibits DNA synthesis. This normalized epidermal replication rate reduces plaque elevation.
- Coal tar preparations of 2% to 5% tar are available in lotions, creams, shampoos, ointments, gels, and solutions. It is usually applied directly to lesions in the evening and allowed to remain in skin contact through the night. It may also be used in bathwater.
- The risk of carcinogenicity is low, but there may be a higher rate of non-myeloma skin cancers in patients chronically exposed to coal tar and UV light.

ANTHRALIN

- Anthralin possesses antiproliferative activity on keratinocytes, inhibiting DNA synthesis by intercalation between DNA strands.
- Because anthralin exerts its clinical effects at low cellular concentrations, therapy usually starts with low concentrations (0.1% to 0.25%) with gradual increases to higher concentrations (0.5% to 1%). Cream and ointment formulations are usually applied in the evening and allowed to remain overnight.
- Alternatively, short-contact Anthralin therapy (SCAT) with application for 10 to 20 minutes of higher concentrations (1% to 5%) in water-soluble vehicles is effective with decreased local adverse effects.
- Anthralin products must be applied only to affected areas because contact with uninvolved skin may result in excessive irritation and staining, which usually disappear within 1 to 2 weeks of discontinuation. Staining of affected plaques indicates a positive response because cell turnover has been slowed enough to take up the stain.
- Inflammation, irritation, and staining of skin and clothing are often therapy limiting effects.

FIRST-LINE SYSTEMIC PHARMACOTHERAPY

- Biologic therapies—primarily immunomodulating agents designed to alter immune responses—comprise first-line systemic therapy.

- Infliximab (Remicade) is a chimeric monoclonal antibody directed against TNF-α. recently; its indications have been expanded to include psoriatic arthritis and treatment of adults with chronic severe plaque psoriasis. An advantage over other systemic psoriasis treatments is that Infliximab does not adversely affect blood counts, hepatic enzyme levels, or kidney function.
- The recommended dose is 5 mg/kg as an IV infusion at weeks 0, 2, and 6, then every 8 weeks thereafter. For psoriatic arthritis, it may be used with or without methotrexate. Adverse effects include headaches, fever, chills, fatigue, diarrhea, pharyngitis, upper respiratory and urinary tract infections. Hypersensitivity reactions (urticaria, dyspnea, hypotension) and lymphoproliferative disorders have been reported.
- **Etanercept** (Enbrel) is a fusion protein that binds TNF-α, competitively interfering with its interaction with cell-bound receptors. Unlike the chimeric infliximab, Etanercept is fully humanized, thereby minimizing the risk of immunogenicity. It is also indicated for adult patients with chronic moderate to severe plaque psoriasis who are candidates for systemic therapy or phototherapy. The recommended dose for psoriatic arthritis is 50 mg subcutaneously once per week. For plaque psoriasis, the dose is 50 mg subcutaneously twice weekly (administered 3 or 4 days apart) for 3 months followed by a maintenance dose of 50 mg per week. Adverse effects include local reactions at the injection site (20% of patients), respiratory tract and GI infections, abdominal pain, nausea and vomiting, headaches, and rash. Serious infections (including tuberculosis) and malignancies are rare.
- **Adalimumab** (Humira) is a human immunoglobulin G1 monoclonal TNF-α antibody. The binding of Adalimumab results in inactivation of the proinflammatory cytokine TNF-α. It is indicated for psoriatic arthritis and treatment of adults with moderate to severe chronic plaque psoriasis who are candidates for systemic therapy or phototherapy. The recommended dose for psoriatic arthritis is 40 mg subcutaneously every other week. The recommended dose for adults with plaque psoriasis is an initial dose of 80 mg, followed by 40 mg every other week starting 1 week after the initial dose. The most common adverse reactions are infections (e.g., upper respiratory, sinusitis), injection site reactions, headache, and rash.
- **Alefacept** (Amevive) is a dimeric fusion protein that binds to CD2 on T cells to inhibit cutaneous T-cell activation and proliferation. It also produces a dose-dependent decrease in circulating total lymphocytes. Alefacept is approved for treatment of moderate to severe plaque psoriasis and is also effective for treatment of psoriatic arthritis. Significant response is usually achieved after about 3 months of therapy. The recommended dose is 15 mg intramuscularly once weekly for 12 weeks. Adverse effects are mild and

include pharyngitis, flu-like symptoms, chills, dizziness, nausea, headache, injection site pain and inflammation, and nonspecific infection.

- **Efalizumab** (Raptiva) is a humanized monoclonal antibody that inhibits CD11-α integrin, which is involved in T-cell activation, migration into skin, and cytotoxic function. It is approved for adults with chronic, moderate to severe plaque psoriasis who are candidates for systemic therapy or phototherapy. The recommended dose is a single 0.7 mg/kg subcutaneous conditioning dose followed by weekly subcutaneous doses of 1 mg/kg (200 mg maximum single dose). The most frequent adverse effects are mild to moderate flu-like complaints such as headache, nausea, chills, nonspecific infection, pain, fever, and asthenia. Cases of exacerbation of psoriasis on discontinuation have been reported, leading to the suggestion that continuous treatment may be required to maintain disease suppression.

SECOND-LINE SYSTEMIC PHARMACOTHERAPY

- **Acitretin** (Soriatane) is a retinoic acid derivative and the active metabolite of etretinate. It is indicated for severe psoriasis, including erythrodermic and generalized pustular types. However, it is more useful as an adjunct in the treatment of plaque psoriasis. It has shown good results when combined with other therapies, including UVA combined with oral methoxsalen (PUVA) and UVB and topical calcipotriol. The initial recommended dose is 25 or 50 mg; therapy is continued until lesions have resolved. It is better tolerated when taken with meals. Adverse effects include hypervitaminosis A (dry lips/cheilitis, dry mouth, dry nose, dry eyes/conjunctivitis, dry skin, pruritus, scaling, and hair loss), hepatotoxicity, skeletal changes, hypercholesterolemia, and hypertriglyceridemia. Acitretin is a teratogen and is contraindicated in females who are pregnant or who plan pregnancy within 3 years after drug discontinuation.
- **Cyclosporine** demonstrates immunosuppressive activity by inhibiting the first phase of T-cell activation. It also inhibits release of inflammatory mediators from mast cells, basophils, and polymorphonuclear cells. It is used in the treatment of both cutaneous and arthritis manifestations of severe psoriasis. The usual dose is between 2.5 and 5 mg/kg/day given in two divided doses. Adverse effects include nephrotoxicity, hypertension, hypomagnesemia and hyperkalemia, alterations in liver function tests, elevations of serum lipids, GI intolerance, paresthesias, hypertrichosis, and gingival hyperplasia. Cumulative treatment for more than 2 years may increase the risk of malignancy, including skin cancers and lymphoproliferative disorders.
- **Tacrolimus**, an immunosuppressant that inhibits T-cell activation, is a useful alternative in severe recalcitrant psoriasis. Although it is not FDA approved for this indication, patients have received oral doses of 0.05 mg/kg daily, with increases up to 0.15 mg/kg daily, depending on

results. Adverse effects include diarrhea, nausea, paresthesias, hypertension, tremor, and insomnia.

- **Methotrexate**, an antimetabolite, is indicated for moderate to severe psoriasis. It is particularly beneficial for psoriatic arthritis. It is also indicated for patients refractory to topical or UV therapy. Methotrexate can be administered orally, subcutaneously, or intramuscularly. The starting dose is 7.5 to 15 mg per week, increased incrementally by 2.5 mg every 2 to 4 weeks until response; maximal doses are approximately 25 mg/wk. Adverse effects include nausea, vomiting, mucosal ulceration, stomatitis, malaise, headache, macrocytic anemia, and hepatic and pulmonary toxicity. Nausea and macrocytic anemia can be ameliorated by giving oral folic acid 1 to 5 mg/day. Methotrexate should be avoided in patients with active infections and in those with liver disease. It is contraindicated in pregnancy because it is teratogenic.
- **Mycophenolate mofetil** (CellCept) inhibits DNA and RNA synthesis and has been shown to have a specific lymphocyte antiproliferative effect. Although not FDA approved for this indication, oral mycophenolate mofetil appears effective in the treatment of moderate to severe plaque psoriasis. The usual dose is 500 mg orally four times a day, up to a maximum of 4 g/day. Common adverse effects include GI toxicity (diarrhea, nausea, vomiting), hematologic effects (anemia, neutropenia, thrombocytopenia), and viral and bacterial infections. Lymphoproliferative disease or lymphoma has been reported. Sulphasalazine is an antiinflammatory agent that inhibits 5-lipoxygenase. It is used selectively as an alternative treatment, particularly in patients with concurrent psoriatic arthritis. When used alone, it is not as effective as methotrexate, PUVA, or acitretin. However, it has a relatively high margin of safety. The usual oral dose is 3 to 4 g/day for 8 weeks. Its adverse effects are similar to other sulfonamide antibiotics.
- **6-Thioguanine** is a purine analog that has been used as an alternative treatment for psoriasis when conventional therapies have failed. The typical dose is 80 mg twice weekly, increased by 20 mg every 2 to 4 weeks; the maximum dose is 160 mg three times a week. Adverse effects include
- Bone marrow suppression, GI complications (e.g., nausea, diarrhea), and elevation of liver function tests. 6-Thioguanine may be less hepatotoxic and therefore more useful than methotrexate in hepatically compromised patients with severe psoriasis.
- **Hydroxyurea** inhibits cell synthesis in the S phase of the DNA cycle. It is used selectively in the treatment of psoriasis, especially in those with liver disease who would be at risk of adverse effects with other agents. However, it is less effective than methotrexate. The typical dose is 1 g/day, with a gradual increase to 2 g/day as needed and as tolerated. Adverse effects include bone marrow toxicity with leukopenia or thrombocytopenia, cutaneous reactions, leg ulcers, and megaloblastic anemia.

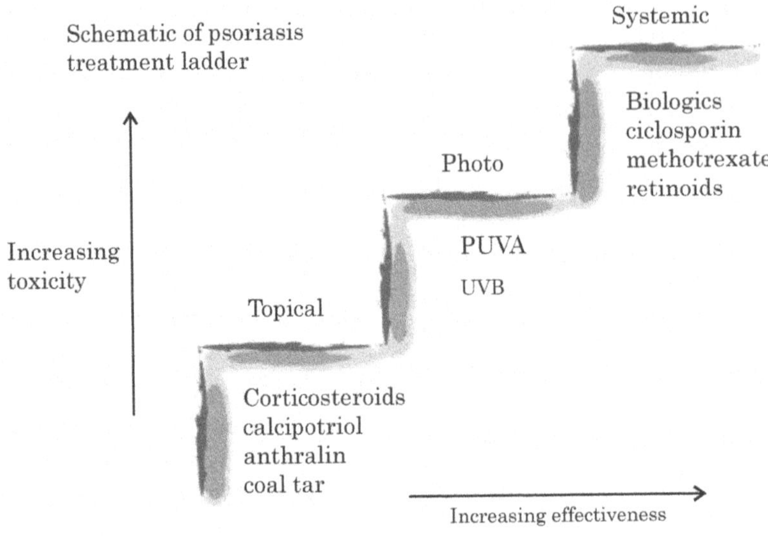

FIGURE 94.1

Psoriasis treatment.

PHOTOTHERAPY AND PHOTOCHEMOTHERAPY

UVB light (290 to 320 nm) therapy is an important phototherapeutic intervention for psoriasis. The most effective wavelength is 310 to 315 nm, which led to development of a UVB narrowband light source, in which 83% of the UVB emission is at 310 to 313 nm. Topical and systemic psoriatic therapies are used adjunctively to hasten and improve the response to UVB phototherapy. Emollients enhance efficacy of UVB and can be applied just before treatments. Combining short-contact Anthralin, Calcipotriene, or topical retinoids to UVB may also improve results. However, topical application should be done after or at least 2 hours before UVB therapy because phototherapy can inactivate the topical product. UVB phototherapy may also be more effective when added to systemic treatments such as methotrexate and oral retinoids.

- **PUVA** is a photo chemotherapeutic approach for selected patients. Candidates for PUVA therapy usually have moderate to severe, incapacitating psoriasis unresponsive to conventional topical and systemic therapies. Systemic PUVA consists of oral ingestion of a potent photosensitizer such as methoxsalen (8-methoxypsoralen) at a constant dose (0.6 to 0.8 mg/kg) and variable doses of UVA depending on patient skin phototype and history of previous response to UV radiation. Two hours after ingesting psoralen, the patient is exposed to UVA light. Photochemotherapy is performed two or three times a week. Partial clearing occurs in most patients by the 25 treatment.
- Another method that may have less carcinogenic potential is to topically deliver the photosensitizer (methoxsalen) to the skin by adding it to bath water **(bath**

PUVA) or as a topical cream (**PUVA cream**) instead of through systemic administration. Advantages of this approach include minimal risk of systemic effects, overall reduction of PUVA dose to one fourth of that required with conventional PUVA, and reduction in the risk of non-melanoma skin cancer.

REFERENCES

1. Gottlieb A, Korman NJ, Gordon KB, Feldman SR, Lebwohl M, Koo JY, et al. Guidelines for the management of psoriasis and psoriatic arthritis. Section 2. Psoriatic arthritis: overview and guidelines of care for treatment with an emphasis on biologics. *J Am Acad Dermatol.* 2008;58:851-864.
2. Menter A, Korman NJ, Elmets Ca, Feldman SR, Gelfand JM, Gordon KB, et al. American Academy of Dermatology guidelines of care for the management of psoriasis and psoriatic arthritis. Section 3. Guidelines of care for the management and treatment of psoriasis with topical therapies. *J Am Acad Dermatol.* 2009;60:643-659.
3. Menter A, Gottlieb A, Feldman SR, Voorhees ASV, Leonardi CL, Gordon KB, et al. Guidelines for the management of psoriasis and psoriatic arthritis. Section 1. Overview of psoriasis and guidelines of care for the treatment of psoriasis with biologics. *J Am Acad Dermatol.* 2008;5:826-850.
4. Stern RS. Psoralen and ultraviolet a light therapy for psoriasis. *N Engl J Med.* 2007;357(7):682-690.

CHAPTER 95

Skin Disorders and Cutaneous Drug Reactions

DEFINITION

The word *dermatitis* denotes an inflammatory erythematous rash. The disorders discussed in this chapter include contact dermatitis, seborrheic dermatitis, diaper dermatitis, and atopic dermatitis. Drug-induced skin disorders have been associated with most commonly used medications and may present as maculopapular eruptions, fixed-drug eruptions, and photosensitivity reactions.

PATHOPHYSIOLOGY

- ***Contact dermatitis*** is an acute or chronic inflammatory skin condition resulting from contact of an inciting factor with the skin. In *allergic contact dermatitis*, an antigenic substance triggers Langerhans cells, and their immunologic responses produce the allergic skin reaction, sometimes several days later. *Irritant contact dermatitis* is caused by an organic substance that usually results in a reaction within a few hours of exposure.
- ***Diaper dermatitis*** (diaper rash) is an acute, inflammatory dermatitis of the buttocks, genitalia, and perineal region. The reaction is a type of contact dermatitis, as it results from direct fecal and moisture contact with the skin in an occlusive environment.
- ***Atopic dermatitis*** is an inflammatory condition with genetic, environmental, and immunologic mechanisms. Many immune cells have demonstrated abnormalities, including Langerhans cells, monocytes, macrophages, lymphocytes, mast cells, and keratinocytes.
- ***Drug-induced cutaneous reactions*** tend to be immunologic in origin and relate to hypersensitivity, but some reactions are nonallergic. The pathogenesis of fixed-drug reactions is not well understood.
- ***Drug-induced photosensitivity reactions*** are divided into *phototoxicity* (a nonimmunologic reaction) and *Photoallergic reactions* (an immunologic reaction). The latter form is far less common. Medications associated with photosensitivity reactions include fluoroquinolones, nonsteroidal anti-inflammatory drugs, phenothiazines, antihistamines, estrogens, progestins, sulphonamides, sulphonylureas, thiazide diuretics, and tricyclic antidepressants.

CLINICAL FEATURES

- The skin lesions of dermatitis may or may not be painful or pruritic. Typically, lesions are described as being less than or greater than 0.5 cm in diameter.

- *Macules* are circumscribed, flat lesions of any shape or size that differ from surrounding skin because of their color. They may result from hyperpigmentation, hypopigmentation, vascular abnormalities, capillary dilatation (erythema), or purpura.
- *Papules* are small, solid, elevated lesions that are usually less than 1 cm in diameter. They may result from metabolic deposits in the dermis, from localized dermal cellular infiltrates, or from localized hyperplasia of cellular elements in the dermis and epidermis.
- *Plaques* are mesa-like elevations that occupy a relatively large surface area in comparison with their height above the skin surface.
- *Seborrheic dermatitis* typically occurs around the areas of skin rich in sebaceous follicles (e.g., the face, ears, scalp, and upper trunk). In infants with involvement of the scalp, the condition is commonly referred to as cradle cap.
- *Diaper dermatitis* results in erythematous patches, skin erosions, vesicles, and ulcerations. Although commonly seen in infants, it can occur in adults who wear diapers for incontinence.
- *Atopic dermatitis* in its acute phase is associated with intensely pruritic, erythematous papules and vesicles over erythematous skin. Scratching may result in excoriations and exudates. Subacute lesions are thicker, paler, scaly, erythematous and excoriated plaques. Chronic lesions are characterized by thickened plaques, accentuated skin markings (lichenification), and fibrotic papules. In all phases, the atopic skin has a dry luster.
- *Drug-induced cutaneous reactions* are unpredictable, ranging from mild, self-limiting episodes to more severe, life-threatening conditions.
- A *fixed-drug reaction* usually presents as an erythematous or hyperpigmented round or oval lesion usually between a few millimeters to 20 cm in diameter. The oral mucosa and genitalia are the most common sites involved, but lesions can appear anywhere on the body. If the patient takes the drug again, the reaction tends to recur within 30 minutes to 8 hours in the same location. Although this is highly indicative of a fixed-drug reaction, rechallenge should be avoided when possible.
- *Sun-induced drug eruptions* appear similar to sunburn and present with erythema, papules, edema, and sometimes vesicles. They appear in areas exposed to sunlight (e.g., the ears, nose, cheeks, forearms, and hands).

DIAGNOSIS

- Patient age and hormonal status in women should be considered in the initial evaluation of patients with skin disorders. Older patients are predisposed to developing psoriasis, seborrhea, and other skin conditions. Atopic dermatitis is most likely to occur in children. Menopausal women tend to develop brown hyperpigmentation, or melasma. Pregnant women may develop hyperpigmentation of the areola and genitalia as well as melasma.
- Patients presenting with a rash or skin lesion should be evaluated for potential anaphylaxis or angioedema (e.g., symptoms of difficulty in breathing, fever, nausea, vomiting).

- The area involved and the number of lesions present is important considerations. A rash involving only the arms and legs suggests a nonsystemic cause, whereas involvement of the trunk as well as the arms and legs indicates a systemic cause.
- Lesions should be inspected for color, texture, size, and temperature. Areas that are oozing, erythematous, and warm to the touch may be infected.
- The duration of the skin condition should be determined, and the temporal relationship with any new medications should be established.
- Assessment for potential drug-induced skin disorders begins with a comprehensive medication history, including episodes of previous drug allergies.
- Diagnostic criteria for atopic dermatitis include the presence of pruritus with three or more of the following: (1) history of flexural dermatitis of the face in children younger than 10 years of age; (2) history of asthma or allergic rhinitis in the child or a first-degree relative; (3) history of generalized xerosis (dry skin) within the past year; (4) visible flexural eczema; (5) onset of rash before 2 years of age.

TREATMENT

CONTACT DERMATITIS

- Initial treatment should focus on identification and removal of the offending agent.
- Products that relieve itching, rehydrate the skin, and decrease the weeping of lesions provide some immediate relief.
- In the acute inflammatory stage, wet dressings are preferred because ointments and creams further irritate the tissue.
- Astringents such as Aluminum acetate or witch hazel decrease weeping from lesions, dry out the skin, and relieve itching. They are applied as a wet dressing for no longer than 7 days.
- For chronic dermatitis, lubricants, emollients, or moisturizers should be applied after bathing. Soap-free cleansers and colloidal oatmeal products also alleviate itching and soothe the skin.
- If the reaction does not subside within a few days, topical or oral corticosteroids may be needed.

SEBORRHEIC DERMATITIS

- Depending on the area of the body that is affected, topical solutions or scalp shampoos may be used.
- Scalp involvement can be treated with twice-daily topical corticosteroids in conjunction with a shampoo containing selenium sulphide, coal tar, or salicylic acid to help soften and remove scales.
- Topical calcineurin inhibitors (e.g., tacrolimus ointment, pimecrolimus cream) have fungicidal and anti-inflammatory properties and can be used for the scalp or face.

DIAPER DERMATITIS

- Effective treatment involves frequent diaper changes and keeping the area dry.
- Lukewarm water and mild soap can be used to clean the area thoroughly, which should then be allowed to dry.
- Occlusive agents (e.g., zinc oxide, titanium dioxide and petrolatum) should be generously applied to the area before the clean diaper is put on the child.

ATOPIC DERMATITIS

- Possible aggravating factors that may trigger a flare-up should be identified and avoided. Moisturizers, including emollients, occlusive's, and humectants should be recommended based on the needs of individual patients.
- Most corticosteroids are applied once or twice daily. High-potency agents are used for less than 3 weeks for flare-ups or for lichenified (thickened) lesions. Moderate potency steroids may be used for more chronic conditions, and low-potency steroids are usually used in children. When used in combination with other topical agents such as moisturizers, the corticosteroid should be applied first, rubbed in well, and followed by the other product.
- Antihistamines are frequently used, but few clinical studies support their efficacy. A sedating antihistamine (e.g., hydroxyzine, diphenhydramine) can offer an advantage by facilitating sleep because pruritus is often worse at night.
- Doxepin is a tricyclic antidepressant that inhibits histamine receptors. It may be helpful in atopic patients who have a component of depression. Doses of 10 to 75 mg at night and up to 75 mg twice daily in adults have been used.
- The topical immunomodulators tacrolimus (Protopic) and pimecrolimus (Elidel) inhibit calcineurin, which normally initiatives T-cell activation. These agents can be used on all parts of the body for prolonged periods without producing corticosteroid-induced adverse effects. Tacrolimus ointment 0.03% and 0.1% is applied twice daily; the lower strength is preferred in children with moderate to severe atopic dermatitis. The most common adverse effect is transient itching and burning at the site of application. Pimecrolimus cream 1% is applied twice daily for mild to moderate atopic dermatitis in adults and children older than age 2.
- Coal tar preparations reduce itching and skin inflammation and are available as crude coal tar (1% to 3%) or liquor carbonis detergens (5% to 20%). They have been used in combination with topical corticosteroids, as adjuncts to permit effective use of lower corticosteroid strengths, and in conjunction with ultraviolet light therapies. Patients can apply the product at bedtime and wash it off in the morning. Factors limiting coal tar use include its strong odor and staining of clothing. Coal tar preparations should not be used on acute oozing lesions, which would result in stinging and irritation.

CUTANEOUS DRUG REACTIONS

- Most maculopapular reactions disappear within a few days after discontinuing the agent, so symptomatic control of the affected area is the primary intervention. Topical corticosteroids and oral antihistamines can relieve pruritus. In severe cases, a short course of systemic corticosteroids may be warranted.
- Treatment of fixed drug reactions involves removal of the offending agent. Other therapeutic measures include corticosteroids, antihistamines to relieve itching, and perhaps cool water compresses on the affected area.

- Photosensitivity reactions typically resolve with drug discontinuation. Some patients benefit from topical corticosteroids and oral antihistamines, but these are relatively ineffective. Systemic corticosteroid (e.g., oral prednisone 1 mg/kg/day tapered over 3 weeks) is more effective for these patients.

REFERENCES

1. American Academy of Dermatology. Guidelines of care for cutaneous adverse drug reactions. *J Am Acad Dermatol.* 1996;35:458-461.
2. Balch JF, Balch PA. *Prescription for Nutritional Healing.* 2nd ed. Garden City Park, NY: Avery Publishing Group; 1997.
3. Fauci AS, Braunwald E, Isselbacher KJ, et al., eds. *Harrison's Principles of Internal Medicine.* 14th ed. New York, NY: McGraw-Hill; 1998.
4. Habif. *Clinical Dermatology.* 5th ed. Philadelphia, PA: Mosby, An Imprint of Elsevier; 2009.
5. Jonas WB, Jacobs J. *Healing with Homeopathy: The Doctors' Guide.* New York, NY: Warner Books; 1996: 255-265.
6. Koh KJ, Pearce AL, Marshman G, et al. Tea tree oil reduces histamine-induced skin inflammation. *Br J Dermatol* 2002;147:1212-7.
7. Shin YW, Bae EA, Lee B, Lee SH, Kim JA, Kim YS, Kim DH. In vitro and in vivo antiallergic effects of *Glycyrrhiza glabra* and its components. *Planta Med.* 2007 Mar;73(3):257-61.

CHAPTER 96

Acne Vulgaris

INTRODUCTION

Acne vulgaris (acne) is the most common type of skin disease encountered, affecting over 80% of the population at some point in their lifetime. Acne not only creates relatively short-term physical and psychological effects for the sufferer, but if recalcitrant to normal treatment or left unchecked, it can also cause more permanent physical effects such as facial scarring that may produce profound psychological consequences.

PATHOPHYSIOLOGY

Acne is caused by follicular hyperkeratosis (plugging) and sebum production abnormal within pilosebaceous units (composed of a hair follicle, sebaceous glands, and a follicular canal) in the skin. Normally, sebum is secreted from the follicular canal to aid in the removal of desquamated follicular epithelial cells via the infundibulum at the top of the follicle.

In acne, the dilated orifice of affected follicles can be blocked with excess amount of sebum and/or keratin from the desquamated cells, promoting the proliferation of bacteria that normally resides in the pilosebaceous unit. This combination of events can result in immune reactions, inflammation, and comedone formation in the pilosebaceous unit lasting for days or weeks. Excess sebum is caused by an increase in the level of androgens, and excess keratin results from an increase in ductal keratinocytes (e.g., from hyperplasia that may also result from high androgen levels), an inadequate separation of the ductal corneocytes, or a combination of the both .

Although one species of normal skin flora, the anaerobic diphtheroid *Propionibacterium acnes*, has been shown as the principal cause of the inflamed comedones in acne vulgaris, other dermal bacterial flora such as *Staphylococcus aureus and Staphylococcus epidermidis* may play a role in the etiology of this condition, particularly as secondary infections. *Propionibacterium acnes* has also mainly associated with various number of other conditions such as sarcoidosis and synovitis, pustulosis, hyperostosis, and osteitis, although its precise role as a causative agent in these skin disorders remains to be determined. *Propionibacterium acnes* will produce a number of virulence factors and it is very well known for its immunomodulatory and inflammatory properties . The organism metabolizes excess sebaceous triglycerides, leading to expanded bacterial growth and the production of chemoattractants that includes the various inflammatory cells (i.e., macrophages and neutrophils) to the infected area. The inflammatory cascade in these host cells includes stimulation of protein kinases , phospholipases, and cyclooxygenases, leading to the production of degradative enzymes and reactive chemicals intended to control or eliminate the infection.

Destructive mechanisms that cause this condition involve the chronic, uncontrolled activation of proteolytic, glycolytic, and lipolytic enzymes, as well as the production of mediators of the inflammation like interleukins 1α and 8 and tumor necrosis factor α, IL-8, TNF-α, and other cytokines that causes incorporation of more cells into the infected area, ultimately resulting in the breakdown of tissue and, if unattended, scarring.

TYPES OF ACNE

Acne is typically categorized into three types: comedonal, papulopustular, and nodular resulting in degrees of severity ranging from noninflammatory comedones (i.e., blackheads and whiteheads) to deep dermal inflammatory papules that appear as erythematous, raised solid lesions that can eventually coalesce and dissect under the skin producing inflamed sinus tracts which can result in scarring, sometimes severe, upon resolution.

TREATMENT TO FIT THE TYPE AND SEVERITY OF ACNE

Once acne is diagnosed, the doctor evaluates the type and severity of a patient's lesions in order to determine what treatment is best. Acne treatment is individualized. It depends on the type of acne a person has as well as how severely acne lesions are inflamed. For example, treatment for whiteheads and blackheads focuses mainly on removing the cells of dead skin that clog the follicles, while treatment for pustules is aimed at destroying infection and reducing inflammation. In an effort to achieve these different goals, different medications are needed.

THE ACNE SCALE

To ensure that each patient receives the most effective treatment for his or her individual problems, doctors employ a special scale known as the acne grading scale. The acne grading scale rates the severity of acne on a scale from zero to eight, with zero indicating very mild acne and eight indicating very severe acne. For example, if a patient has a few comedones, he or she is given a zero rating. The rating increases with the number, size, and severity of a person's lesions. Therefore, a patient with half of his or her face covered with papules, comedones, and a few pustules receives a four rating, which denotes moderate acne. A rating of eight indicates very severe acne, with the patient having acne lesions of all types, including numerous cysts, covering almost all of his or her face. Once a person's acne has been rated, doctors match the rating to specific treatment plans recommended by the American Academy of Dermatology, an organization that studies skin diseases. At the same time, the doctor makes adjustments in the recommended treatment for individual differences. For example, these differences may include such factors as how dry or oily the patient's skin may be, the patient's gender, whether the patient is allergic to any medications, and whether the patient is pregnant or planning to become pregnant soon.

A COMMON GOAL

Because there are many differences in the severity and types of acne lesions, there are a wide variety of acne treatment options. These include over-the-counter medication people can purchase without a doctor's prescription as well as more powerful, doctor-prescribedmedications. Acne medication may be taken orally or applied directly onto the skin in the form of a topical treatment. Often, oral and topical treatments are combined. Once acne outbreaks are eliminated, a special type of surgery known as skin dermabrasion can lessen acne scars.

No matter what form of treatment is used, all acne treatments share a common goal: to control the sequence of events that cause acne outbreaks in order to prevent new outbreaks from occurring. Experts agree that since there are so many different acne treatment options available, most cases of acne outbreaks can be controlled (Fig 96.1).

Degrees of Acne Severity

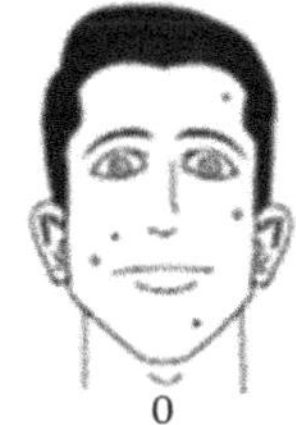
0
Few scattered comedones (blackheads and whiteheads).

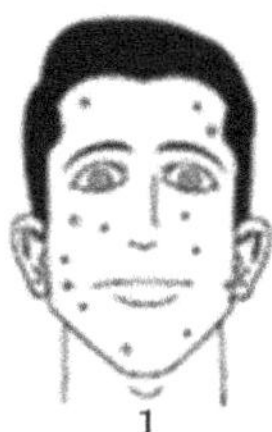
1
Thirty to forty papules and comedones over one-fourth of the face

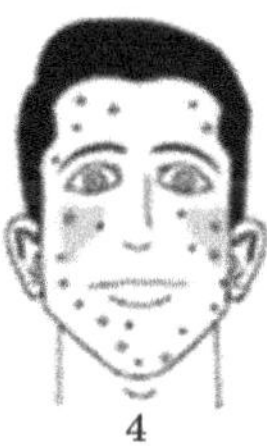
4
about half of the face has papules, comedones, and a few pustules. Some lesions are red and inflamed.

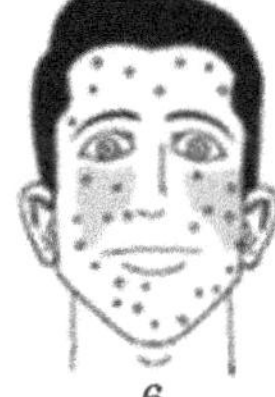
6

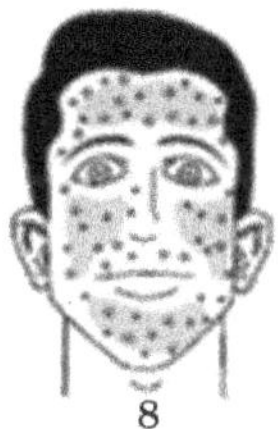
8
All or most of the face is involved. Large, prominent pustules, much inflammation. Healed lesions leave scars.

FIGURE 96.1

Degrees of severity of acne.

TOPICAL TREATMENTS

Some of the most popular and effective treatment options available for acne are topical treatments. Most commonly used to treat cases of mild to moderate acne, topical treatments come in cream, lotion, or gel form and on specially prepared pads. Those used to treat the mildest cases of acne can be purchased without a doctor's prescription.

SALICYLIC ACID

Salicylic acid is a popular topical treatment that is easily available. Salicylic acid does not treat infection or inflammation. Therefore, it is mainly used to treat comedones. When salicylic acid is rubbed onto the skin, it penetrates the pores and gets inside clogged hair follicles. Salicylic acid causes the dead skin cells inside the follicles to dissolve. This allows oil trapped in the follicles to reach the skin. Many patients report that treatment with salicylic acid helps eliminate acne outbreaks.

BENZOYL PEROXIDE

Benzoyl peroxide is another topical treatment. In fact, it is the main ingredient in most over-the-counter acne preparations. Used to treat mild inflammatory acne, benzoyl peroxide is available in different strengths. It is often used with products that contain salicylic acid by patients who have both comedones and mildly inflamed pustules. Benzoyl peroxide is an oxidizing agent, meaning it releases oxygen. The bacteria that cause acne can only exist in an oxygen-free environment, such as a clogged hair follicle. When benzoyl peroxide gets penetrated into the hair follicles and releases oxygen, acne-causing bacteria are killed. This not only relieves existing infection but also stops new pustules from forming.

OTHER ANTIBACTERIAL OINTMENTS AND VITAMIN A

In addition to benzoyl peroxide, there are a number of other antibacterial ointments used to in the treatment of the inflammatory acne. These contain chemicals such as sulfur that kill bacteria. In addition, there are a number of stronger antibiotic creams, gels, and lotions that contain powerful bacteria-killing drugs such as tetracycline and erythromycin, which are used to treat moderately inflamed acne. Although these products do control infection, they have no effect on clogged hair follicles. Therefore, these products are often combined with salicylic acid or a more powerful prescription strength ointment such as Retin A, a popular retinoid.

Retinoids are derived from vitamin A, which has a potent effect on the skin. It was found that when vitamin A is applied to the skin, it slows the growth of skin cells. This is important in preventing acne because when new skin cells form, old skin cells are shed. Slowing the growth of skin cells keeps away the building up of the dead skin cells from inside the hair follicles. This stops new comedones from forming. In addition, for reasons that scientists cannot explain, vitamin A slows down oil production and stimulates the production of collagen. This gives the skin a smoother appearance. Therefore, vitamin A is often used to help smooth out acne scars.

ORAL MEDICATION

In addition to topical treatments, many people with moderate to severe inflammatory acne take oral medication, either alone or in combination with topical ointments. There are three main types of oral medications used to treat acne. They are antibiotics, hormones, and isotretinoin.

ANTIBIOTICS

Bacteria-fighting oral antibiotics such as tetracycline, erythromycin, clindamycin, and doxycycline are often prescribed for people whose acne does not respond well to the topical antibiotic treatment. Oral antibiotics are absorbed into the bloodstream, and then into the skin and hair follicles. Here they kill acne-causing bacteria and reduce inflammation. This helps stop new acne lesions from forming and gives the skin a healthier appearance by lessening redness. However, most oral antibiotics are absorbed into the bloodstream quickly. Consequently, they are eliminated from the body rapidly. Therefore, in order to maintain a constant level of bacteria-fighting medication in the bloodstream, oral antibiotics must be taken frequently for an extended period of time. Indeed, some people with acne take antibiotics two or three times each day for six months to a year. Moreover, once treatment with oral antibiotics is stopped, unchecked bacteria often cause new acne outbreaks. In an effort to prevent this from occurring, when the skin begins to clear, treatment with oral antibiotics is gradually tapered off, rather than stopped abruptly, and replaced with topical antibiotic treatment. This helps restrain the growth of acne-causing bacteria. Despite these drawbacks, treatment with oral antibiotics can be quite successful.

HORMONES

For many teenage girls as well as women with adult-onset acne, treatment with female sex hormones such as estrogen offers another treatment option. Usually taken in the form of low-dose birth control pills, hormonal therapy increases the level of female hormones in a woman's bloodstream. This reduces or blocks the production of androgen. Once androgen is reduced, sebum production also gets decreased simultaeneously. The result is decreased acne outbreaks.

ISOTRETINOIN

For patients with severe cystic acne or for patients with moderate inflammatory acne that has proven to be resistant to oral antibiotics, isotretinoin is the most effective acne treatment available. In fact, it is the only medication that effectively controls severe cystic acne. Commonly sold under the brand name Accutane, isotretinoin is a vitamin A derivative that is administered in pill form. Isotretinoin is an extremely powerful drug that stops all the changes in the skin that cause acne. It kills bacteria and reduces inflammation. At the same time, it shrinks the sebaceous oil glands, reducing sebum production by up to 90 percent. It also slows up the growth of skin cells, which helps in unblocking of the hair follicles and allows pustules and cysts trapped below the surface of the skin to work their way to the surface of the skin, where they burst and heal. Consequently, many patients find that their acne actually worsens in the first month of Accutane treatment but starts improving thereafter. Taken for a period of four to nine months, isotretinoin is effective in 98 percent of all cases. However, in some cases acne symptoms return after isotretinoin treatment ends. In these cases, patients may begin a second cycle of isotretinoin treatment.

TREATMENT OF ACNE SCARS

Eventhough acne medication can lessen and even eliminate acne outbreaks, many patients are left with permanent scars. For these patients, treatment with a form of surgery known as skin dermabrasion can help give the skin a smoother appearance. In this procedure, patients are given a local anesthetic to eliminate pain. Then, a high speed instrument that resembles a wire brush is used to scrape away the top layer of skin and alter the contour of acne scars. Small scars may be completely removed, while the depth of large scars is reduced considerably. Because the top layer of skin is removed, after the procedure the patient's skin often appears red and may remain red for a month or more.

RISKS AND SIDE EFFECTS OF ACNE TREATMENTS

Despite the benefits of acne treatments, like all surgery and medication, those used for acne can cause side effects and health risks. For example, as in all surgical procedures, people who undergo skin dermabrasion can develop an infection or have an allergic reaction to the anesthetic. Acne medicines too, present health risks. Topical ointments, for instance, can dry out and irritate the skin, causing it to become red and scaly. Retin A, in particular, makes the skin extremely sensitive to sunlight. If it is left on the skin when an individual goes out in direct sunlight, he or she is likely to experience a severe sunburn. Oral antibiotics can also present problems for some patients by causing nausea, dizziness, stomachaches, and sensitivity to the sun. Furthermore, because oral antibiotics kill bacteria, they alter the level of normal bacteria present throughout the body. In women, lack of normal bacteria can lead to the growth of yeast in the vagina. This often causes the development of a yeast infection. More troubling is the fact that long-term use of antibiotics can cause people to develop a resistance to these drugs. This can be devastating if a person develops a serious bacterial infection, such as bacterial pneumonia or strep throat, that requires antibiotics to be cured. Hormones, too, can cause side effects such as mood swings, depression, and weight gain.

ISOTRETINOIN AND SERIOUS HEALTH PROBLEMS

Even more disturbing are the health problems that isotretinoin can cause. Like Retin A, isotretinoin dries out the skin. However, because of its potency, its drying effect can cause the skin on the lips, fingers, toes, feet, and palms of the hands to swell, peel off, and bleed. Isotretinoin can also cause frequent nosebleeds, dry tear ducts, and muscular pain. In most cases, these problems disappear when treatment with isotretinoin ends, but in a few cases these problems persist indefinitely.

ISOTRETINOIN AND PSYCHIATRIC PROBLEMS

Isotretinoin has also been linked to psychiatric problems such as depression, violent behavior, and suicide attempts. Scientists do not know why a drug that targets the skin affects the brain. They theorize that isotretinoin may lower serotonin levels in the brain. Low levels of this brain chemical have been linked to depression, violence, and suicide. However, this link is controversial. It is unclear whether isotretinoin actually causes these problems or if the emotional impact of acne itself, combined with normal mood swings common to adolescents, is the cause.

Although the drug has not been banned, due to these and other cases it is illegal for doctors to administer the drug until patients read a detailed medical guide, which describes the possible health risks that isotretinoin presents. The patient must then sign a consent form stating he or she is aware of the risks.

ISOTRETINOIN AND BIRTH DEFECTS

Another health risk that female patients are warned about in the medical guide is the risk of damage to unborn babies. Because everything that enters an expectant mother's bloodstream also enters the fetus's bloodstream, when expectant mothers take isotretinoin, the drug's powerful effect can harm the developing fetus. According to the FDA, 35 percent of babies born to mothers treated with the drug during their pregnancies are born with birth defects. These defects include physical deformities, undeveloped organs, blindness, and mental retardation. Isotretinoin can also cause the death of the fetus before birth, premature births, or the death of the newborn baby. For this reason, the FDA prohibits the dispensation of isotretinoin to pregnant women. In addition, female patients must take two pregnancy tests before the drug can be prescribed, and women are warned not to become pregnant while taking the drug.

Therefore, birth control is mandatory for sexually active women taking isotretinoin, as are monthly pregnancy tests. In addition, women are warned not to become pregnant for at least one month after stopping use of isotretinoin, since it takes at least one month for the drug to clear a person's system.

THREE TYPES OF ALTERNATIVE TREATMENTS FOR ACNE

The most widely used alternative treatments for acne fall into three categories—those that are taken internally, those that are applied on the skin, and those that eliminate stress. Dietary supplements such as herbs, vitamins, and minerals are among the most popular internal treatments. In fact, herbal remedies have been used to treat many diseases, including acne, for thousands of years, and herbs still remain the primary treatment for acne. Herbal remedies use the leaves, roots, and stems of plants that are known to have healing properties. Usually taken ground up in capsule form or as a tea, herbal remedies for acne consist of herbs that balance hormone levels, boost the immune system, and reduce inflammation. Because herbs are natural, many people feel that they are gentler and safer than conventional medicines.

HERBS THAT BALANCE HORMONE LEVELS

Herbs that balance hormone levels are the most commonly prescribed herbs for acne. They mainly includes red clover, black cohosh, wild yam, evening primrose, chaste berry, and dong quai, all of which are prescribed for women. These herbs contain phytoestrogen, a plant-based female hormone-like compound. Therefore, although they are useful for women, they are inappropriate for males due to chemical differences in the male and female body. Herbalists believe phytoestrol increases the effect of the female sex hormone, estrogen, on the body while counterbalancing the the action of androgen.

HERBS TO COMBAT INFECTION AND INFLAMMATION

The various other herbs used in the treatment of the acne are echinacea, burdock, licorice, and dandelion root, are thought to contain compounds that attack bacteria, thus reducing infection and inflammation. Herbs like salvia and red peony, on the other hand, are thought to improve circulation and tissue growth, which increases the skin's ability to heal. The effect of these herbs on acne patients has been studied in China. There they are commonly prescribed for acne in individually formulated combinations based on each patient's particular skin problems.

VITAMINS AND MINERALS

Treatment with vitamin B5, is another widely used alternative treatment for acne. Also known as pantothenic acid, vitamin B5 is believed by some experts to be as effective in reducing the production of sebum as isotretinoin. When there is a shortage of vitamin B5, fat that is normally burned for fuel or stored in cells for future use cannot be processed properly. Instead, it accumulates in the bloodstream. The excess fat in the form of sebum is eliminated through the skin. Thus the presence of excess fat in the bloodstream causes the body to increase sebum production for the removal of the excess fat. Therefore, when acne patients increase the level of vitamin B5 in their bodies, they improve the processing of fat.

REFERENCES

1. Bobbi Brown and Sally Wadyka, *Beauty Evolution.* New York: Harper-Resource, 2002. Beauty experts team up to give skin care tips for women of all ages.
2. Anthony C. Chu and Anne Lovell, *The Good Skin Doctor.* London: HarperCollins, 1999. A dermatologist and an advice columnist team up to discuss the different types of acne, why it occurs, and different conventional and alternative treatments. Gale Maleskey, *Nature's Medicines.* Emmaus, PA: Rodale Press, 1999.
3. Different herbs, what they do, and what illnesses they treat are discussed in detail. Linda Papadopoulous and Carl Walker, *Understanding Skin Problems.* West Sussex, England: Wiley, 2003. Provides information and advice on living with different skin conditions, including acne

CHAPTER 97

Male Sexual Dysfunction

SEXUAL DYSFUNCTION

Sexual dysfunction refers to a problem during any phase of the sexual response cycle that prevents the individual or couple from experiencing satisfaction from the sexual activity. The sexual response cycle has four phases: excitement, plateau, orgasm and resolution.

ETIOLOGY

Causes of sexual dysfunction include:

- **Physical causes** — Many physical and/or medical conditions can cause problems with sexual function. These conditions include diabetes, heart and vascular (blood vessel) disease, neurological disorders, hormonal imbalances, chronic diseases such as kidney or liver failure, and alcoholism and drug abuse. In addition, the side effects of certain medications, including some antidepressants drugs, can affect sexual desire and function.
- **Psychological causes** — These include work-related stress and anxiety, concern about Sexual performance, marital or relationship problems, depression, feelings of guilt, and the effects of a past sexual trauma.

SEXUAL DYSFUNCTION IN MEN

The most common problems related to sexual dysfunction in men include ejaculation disorders, erectile dysfunction and inhibited sexual desire.

EJACULATION DISORDERS

There are different types of ejaculation disorders, including:

- Premature ejaculation — Refers to ejaculation that occurs before or soon after penetration.
- Inhibited or retarded ejaculation — when ejaculation does not occur.
- Retrograde ejaculation — occurs when, at orgasm, the ejaculate is forced back into the bladder rather than through the urethra and out the end of the penis.

In some cases, premature and inhibited ejaculation are caused by psychological factors, including a strict religious background that causes the person to view sex as sinful, a lack of attraction for a partner and past traumatic events (such as being discovered in masturbation or illicit sex, or learning one's partner is having an affair). Premature ejaculation, the most common form of sexual dysfunction in men, often is due to performance anxiety during sex. However, organic causes are sometimes present. Certain drugs, including some anti-depressants, may impair ejaculation, as can nerve damage to the spinal cord or back.

Retrograde ejaculation is most common in males with diabetes who suffer from diabetic neuropathy (nerve damage). This is due to problems with the nerves in the bladder and the bladder neck that allow the ejaculate to flow backward. In other men, retrograde ejaculation occurs after operations on the bladder neck or prostate, or after certain abdominal operations. In addition, certain medications, particularly those used to treat mood disorders, may cause problems with ejaculation.

ERECTILE DYSFUNCTION

Also known as impotence, erectile dysfunction is defined as the inability to attain and/or maintain an erection suitable for intercourse. Causes of erectile dysfunction include diseases affecting blood flow, such as atherosclerosis (hardening of the arteries); nerve disorders; psychological factors such as stress, depression and performance anxiety; and injury to the penis. Chronic illness, certain medications and a condition called Peyronie's disease (scar tissue in the penis) also can cause erectile dysfunction.

INHIBITED SEXUAL DESIRE (REDUCED LIBIDO)

Inhibited desire, or loss of libido, refers to a decrease in desire for or interest in sexual activity. Reduced libido can result from physical or psychological factors. It has been associated with low levels of the hormone testosterone. It also may be caused by psychological problems, such as anxiety and depression; medical illnesses such as diabetes and high blood pressure; certain medications, including some anti-depressants; and relationship difficulties.

DIAGNOSIS

The doctor likely will begin with a physical exam and a thorough history of symptoms. He or she may order other diagnostic tests to rule out any medical problems that may be contributing to the dysfunction. The doctor may refer the patient for consultations with other health care professionals, including an urologist (a doctor specializing in the urinary tract and male reproductive system), an endocrinologist (a doctor specializing in glandular disorders), a neurologist (a doctor specializing in disorders of the nervous system), sex therapists and other counselors.

Tests to evaluate sexual dysfunction include:

- Blood tests — These tests are done to evaluate hormone levels.
- Vascular assessment — This involves an evaluation of the blood flow to the penis. A blockage in a blood vessel supplying blood to the penis may be contributing to erectile dysfunction.
- Sensory testing — Particularly useful in evaluating the effects of diabetic neuropathy, sensory testing measures the strength of nerve impulses in a particular area of the body.
- Nocturnal penile tumescence and rigidity testing — This test is used to monitor erections that occur naturally during sleep. This test can help determine if a man's erectile problems are due to physical or psychological causes.

TREATMENT

Many cases of sexual dysfunction can be corrected by treating the underlying physical or psychological problems. Treatment strategies may include the following:

- Medical treatment — This involves treatment of any physical problem that may be contributing to a man's sexual dysfunction.

Medications — new medications, such as sildenafil (viagra), varderafil (levitra), or Tadalafil (Cialis) may help improve sexual function in men by increasing blood flow to the penis.

PHOSPHODIESTERASE TYPE 5 INHIBITORS

The cyclic nucleotide phosphodiesterases constitute a group of enzymes that catalyze the hydrolysis of the cyclic nucleotides cyclic AMP and cyclic GMP. They exist in different molecular forms and are unevenly distributed throughout the body.

One of the forms of phosphodiesterase is termed PDE5. The prescription PDE5 inhibitors Sildenafil (viagra), vardenafil (levitra) and tadalafil (cialis) are prescription drugs which are taken orally. They work by blocking the action of PDE5, which causes cGMP to degrade.

ALPROSTADIL

Alprostadil in combination with the permeation enhancer DDAIP has been approved in Canada under the brand name Vitaros as a topical cream first line treatment for erectile dysfunction.

Another treatment regimen is injection therapy. One of the following drugs is injected into the penis: papaverine, phentolamine, and Prostaglandin E1.

- Hormones — Men with low levels of testosterone may benefit from hormone injections. The use of a testosterone patch applied to the scrotum or other parts of the body has been approved by the Food and Drug Administration to help increase testosterone levels to a normal range. Testosterone replacement by pills and implantable pellets also is being evaluated.
- Psychological therapy — Therapy with a trained counselor can help a person address feelings of anxiety, fear or guilt that may have an impact on sexual function.
- Mechanical aids — Aids such as vacuum devices and penile implants may help men with erectile dysfunction.
- Education and communication — Education about sex, and sexual behaviors and responses may help a man overcome his anxieties about sexual function. Open dialogue with your partner about your needs and concerns also helps to overcome many barriers to a healthy sex life.

CURING

The success of treatment for sexual problems depends on the underlying cause. The outlook is good for dysfunction that is related to a treatable or reversible physical condition. Mild dysfunction that is related to stress, fear, or anxiety often can be successfully treated with counseling, education, and improved communication between partners.

PREVENTION

While sexual problems cannot be prevented, dealing with the underlying causes of the dysfunction can help to better understand and cope with the problem when it occurs. There are some things help to maintain good sexual function:

- Follow the doctor's treatment plan for any health conditions. Limit alcohol intake, Quit smoking. Deal with any emotional or psychological issues such as stress, depression, and anxiety. Get treatment as needed.

REFERENCES

1. Diaz V.A. & Close J.D. *Male Sexual Dysfunction* Primary Care 2010;37(3): 473 - 489.'
2. Michetti, P M; Rossi, R; Bonanno, D; Tiesi, A; Simonelli, C (2005). "Male sexuality and regulation of emotions: a study on the association between alexithymia and erectile dysfunction (ED)". *International Journal of Impotence Research* **18** (2): 170–4.
3. Merck Sharpe & Dohme. "Male genital and sexual disorders" 2010-02-18.
4. Rodríguez Vela, L; Moncada Iribarren, I; Gonzalvo Ibarra, A; Sáenz de Tejada y Gorman I (1998). "Treatment of erectile dysfunction using intracavernous pharmacotherapy". *Actas urologicas espanolas* **22** (4): 291–319.

CHAPTER 98

Drug Dependence and Drug Abuse

Drug Dependence - State when drug-taking becomes compulsive, taking precedence over other needs. Syn. substance dependence

Drug Addiction - Is not clearly defined but implies a physical dependence, however, sometimes it is used as a synonymn to drug (substance) dependence

Drug Abuse - More general term, includes recurrent use of any illegal/harmful substance, e.g., in sport

Tolerance - The decrease in a pharmacological effect on repeated administration of the drug imply the need to increase the dose to reach the pharmacological effect of the same intensity on repeated administration of the drug often accompanies the state of dependence

Withdrawal (Syn. Abstinence) Syndrome - Adverse effects, both psychological and physical, of stopping taking a drug. Distinguish commonly observed rebound phenomenon from the true dependence.

Rewarding Effect – Important and common feature of psychoactive addictive substances.

The phrases substance abuse and drug abuse are often applied to the use of an illegal or illicit chemical substance (e.g., LSD, heroin). However, these terms may be applied when a legally obtainable medication is used excessively and for unintended purposes or is diverted to someone else's use. Also, some legal substances (e.g., nicotine, alcohol) are used to the detriment of the individual. Inappropriate use, or abuse, is the excessive self-administration of any substance for nonmedical purposes. An additional aspect of drug abuse is the production of hazardous or harmful effects to the individual and/or to society. The etiology of substance abuse is a complicated phenomenon that is sometimes a function of genetics, socioeconomic status, education, peer pressure, thrill seeking, or experimenting behavior and sometimes an inappropriate attempt at self-medication to treat a real or perceived disease state. It is also clear that drug abuse is a function of the pharmacology of each drug. Almost all abused substances produce an effect on the brain that is perceived as desirable and will initiate drug-seeking behavior.

The professionals in the drug abuse field have such diverse backgrounds that adopting a common terminology for terms such as addiction and dependence has been difficult. These terms are best defined in the context of the pattern and consequences of drug use. Regardless of the characteristics of the drug-induced intoxication, the properties of the drug that are responsible for drug-seeking behavior are often referred to as the reinforcing properties. These drugs produce effects that are so desirable that the user is compelled to obtain more of the drug. Recurrent abuse of a drug may properly be termed an addiction when the individual becomes so obsessed with constantly obtaining and using a drug that it becomes a primary goal and disrupts the ability to function in family, social, or career settings. Typically, especially during the initial stages of drug addiction, the primary reinforcing property is the production of euphoria, a term indicating anything from happiness or pleasantness to an excitement resembling sexual orgasm. Euphoria is considered to be a positive reinforcing property, one that the individual would desire or seek.The evaluation of drugs for their reinforcing properties is an assessment of their abuse potential.The craving or desire to obtain additional drug, especially when it is not available, was at one time termed psychological addiction or psychological dependence, though today these terms are not necessarily descriptive or specific. The term addiction should be used to describe recurrent drug abuse, while the term dependence (discussed later) refers to another state, a function of drug use, not drug craving per se. Addiction has also been used to describe recurrent substance abuse by individuals who realize it is harmful to their health but cannot fulfill their desire to stop, such as with tobacco.

Chronic use of a drug over a long period sometimes produces a state of tolerance that may be classified as pharmacokinetic, pharmacodynamic, or behavioral. The degree of tolerance is generally proportional to the drug dose and the duration of use. In some cases, partial or complete tolerance to the euphoric effect of the drug develops. However, tolerance to many of the other acute effects also generally develops. Termination of drug abuse may create a condition of drug abstinence, which coincides with the emergence of a measurable physical syndrome. This abstinence syndrome is an indication of dependence, is often referred to as drug withdrawal, and was once termed physical dependence to distinguish it from psychological dependence. It is assumed that adaptation, or tolerance, to repeated administration of drug is responsible for physical dependence. Generally, the severity of the abstinence syndrome or level of dependence is proportional to the degree of tolerance attained. However, the relationship between tolerance and dependence has not been fully resolved; tolerance and dependence can occur separately. Epidemiological studies indicate that most individuals who abuse any one drug often also abuse, or coabuse, other drugs during the same period. Polydrug abuse complicates conclusions drawn from epidemiological and clinical studies. One reason for coabuse of drugs relates to similarities in pharmacological effects.In these cases, once tolerance to the primary drug develops, the individual also has cross-tolerance to related classes of drugs. For example, the development of tolerance to one CNS depressant, such as barbiturates, anxiolytic agents, or alcohol, simultaneously produces some degree of tolerance to the other depressants. Users may attempt to ameliorate selected drug effects by coabuse of drugs with opposite pharmacological profiles.

Drugs of abuse are derived from numerous chemical classes, and therefore, it is not surprising that they produce distinctive pharmacological effects

OPIOIDS

For centuries opium was used for both medicinal and recreational purposes. Derived from the poppy *Papaver somniferum*, it contains numerous opiates, the primary one of which is morphine. The term opiate has largely been replaced by opioid, which represents all compounds with morphine like activity and includes morphine, morphine derivatives, and peptides. Opiate is used to refer to morphine like drugs derived from the plant and structurally similar analogues. These drugs are frequently referred to as narcotics, a Greek term for stupor, which is scientifically obsolete. Even in its early history, opium presented a problem when it was smoked or taken orally. The introduction of the hypodermic needle and syringe, however, drastically enhanced the euphoric properties of opioids and thereby altered their abuse liability. In addition, the synthesis of heroin resulted in an opioid that was more potent than morphine and ideally suited for intravenous administration.

Extent and Pattern of Abuse

The abuse of opioids falls into two distinct categories of users, those who initiate use solely for recreational purposes and those who become physically dependent as a result of being treated medically with opioids. The primary use of opioids is for the control of moderate to severe pain. However, few patients receiving opioids for pain management become dependent. Furthermore, dependence is less likely if opioids are used judiciously. Acute pain can be controlled with opioids such as hydromorphone or oxycodone, which have a rapid onset and short duration of action. In contrast, chronic pain is better treated with opioids such as methadone or morphine (e.g., Duramorph, MS Contin), which are less likely to produce euphoria because of their slow onset of action. Dependence in patients is most likely to occur in those with pain of unexplained or poorly defined etiology. Avoiding long-term use of opioids in this population reduces the risk of developing dependence. Development of dependence should not be a consideration in the management of terminal cancer pain. The primary illicit opioid is heroin (diacetylmorphine),which was once used almost exclusively by the intravenous route. In recent years, the purity of street heroin has risen to levels that allow it to be smoked or snorted.

Pharmacological Aspects

First-time users frequently experience unpleasant, or dysphoric, effects that may include nausea and vomiting. The frequent user experiences a rush, or warm flushing feeling, in the skin and lower extremities that is often equated with sexual orgasm. This intense euphoria lasts for one to several minutes and is followed by sedation, relaxation, and tranquility lasting up to an hour. This latter period is sometimes called being on the nod. All effects have largely dissipated within 3 to 5 hours, which requires the user to inject at frequent intervals. Pharmacokinetics plays a very important role in the manner in which opioids are abused. Morphine and many of its derivatives are slowly and erratically absorbed after oral administration, which makes this route suitable for long-term management of pain but not for producing euphoria. In addition, opioids undergo considerable first-pass metabolism, which accounts for their low potency after oral administration. Heroin is more potent than morphine, although its effects arise primarily from metabolism to morphine. The potency difference is attributed to heroin's greater membrane permeability and resultant increased absorption into the brain.

Tolerance and Dependence

Tolerance to the unpleasant effects experienced by some individuals at the initiation of opioid use develops readily. Significant tolerance also occurs to the analgesic, respiratory depressant, emetic, and euphoric effects, although it develops somewhat more slowly to respiratory depression. Little tolerance to the GI effects and miosis develops. Cross-tolerance occurs with all known opioid analgesics. Opioid tolerance develops more quickly and to a greater extent than it does for most other drugs of abuse. The lethal opioid dose can be 20-fold higher in a tolerant individual than in a neophyte. Tolerance develops within a few days if potent opioids are given at frequent intervals, such as every 4 to 6 hours. Development of tolerance requires several weeks if the opioid is given only twice a day. The continued use of opioids results in the development of physical dependence, as demonstrated by the appearance of a characteristic abstinence syndrome upon interruption or cessation of use. The symptoms of withdrawal include hyperactivity, anxiety, restlessness, yawning, diarrhea, vomiting, chills, fever, lacrimation, and runny nose. Piloerection (gooseflesh or cold turkey), mydriasis, increased blood pressure and heart rate, and hyperpyrexia may be observed. Tremors, abdominal cramps, and muscle and joint pain may be present. Drug craving is an important feature of opioid withdrawal. In contrast to some other drugs of abuse, withdrawal is not life threatening.

Treatment of Opioid Dependence

Although the ultimate goal of treatment programs is to achieve drug-free status as quickly as possible, it is rarely achieved without pharmacotherapy. The most commonly used strategy is to switch the patient from a short-acting opioid, such as heroin, to a long-acting agonist , such as methadone. It is easier to withdraw patients from methadone because it produces a protracted withdrawal syndrome that is less intense than that produced by heroin. Opioid antagonists, such as naltrexone, provide another treatment option in that addicts who are completely withdrawn from an opioid can be maintained on antagonists that will block the pleasurable effects of subsequent injections of heroin. Mixed opioid agonist–antagonists show promise in that they have sufficient agonist effects to reduce craving while at the same time exhibiting antagonist properties.

STIMULANTS

A variety of drugs in distinct pharmacological and chemical classes can be considered under the broad classification as stimulants. Xanthines and methylxanthines constitute a weak class of stimulants that includes caffeine, theophylline (aminophylline), and theobromine. Caffeine is freely available in coffee, colas, and certain over-the-counter pills. A low degree of tolerance develops to some of their effects and a mild withdrawal syndrome is observed following immediate cessation of their repeated use. The primary class of stimulants for which there is a tremendous addiction problem is the sympathomimetic stimulants, which include cocaine, amphetamine, methamphetamine (Desoxyn), methylphenidate (Ritalin), and phenmetrazine.

Extent and Pattern of Abuse

Sympathomimetic stimulant drugs have very high abuse potential. They are typically used repeatedly for a short period during which time the user escalates the dose to greater and greater levels to attain the desired degree of euphoria. Extended uninterrupted use of stimulants for 24 to 72 hours is often referred to as a run and usually ends in a crash (24–36 hours of sleep) once the individual is exhausted physically. Besides illicit sources of stimulants, approximately 5 billion doses of these drugs are prescribed per year, and there appears to be a significant degree of abuse via prescription diversion. While some stimulants, such as amphetamine and methylphenidate, are taken orally, others are either volatilized for inhalation or snorted as the solid (nasal insufflation). It is necessary to convert cocaine and methamphetamine to their free base so that they can be volatilized. Methamphetamine and cocaine are also abused via the intravenous route.

Pharmacological Aspects

Most of the sympathomimetic stimulants exhibit similar pharmacological properties, differing primarily in the magnitude of their effects. Acute drug administration produces feelings of euphoria, elation, and alertness. Intravenous injections of cocaine and amphetamine can produce a very intense rush of sensations that resemble sexual orgasm. At small doses cognition increases and mood is elevated. As the dose of drug escalates during a run, the overall activity of the individual changes from task performance to one generally characterized by stereotypical movements. The person starts performing certain behaviors repeatedly. Some grind or gnash their teeth. Many continuously touch or pick at their face or extremities. At this stage the individual becomes suspicious and may develop anxiety or paranoia. Acute toxic paranoid psychosis can develop, but it usually requires a longer period of abuse than a single acute session. Besides stimulating the CNS, these drugs activate the autonomic nervous system. Individuals have tachycardia, hypertension, and possibly arrhythmias. Autonomic hyperactivity is also expressed as hyperthermia and mydriasis.More serious effects include the possibility of myocardial infarction, cerebrovascular hemorrhage, seizure and death.

Tolerance and Dependence

Tolerance to stimulants develops fairly rapidly, even in the therapeutic dose range. It is the rapid development of tolerance that leads to the escalation of dose during drug abuse runs.

Other Adverse Effects of Chronic Abuse

Chronic stimulant abuse alters the personality of the abuser. These and related changes are the result of neurotoxicity and are not characterized as either acute drug effects or withdrawal signs. Individuals have delusions of being pursued or persecuted and therefore become suspicious and paranoid. They become self-occupied and hostile toward others. Long-term abuse can produce toxic psychosis that closely resembles schizophrenia and must be treated with neuroleptic drugs (haloperidol, chlorpromazine). This psychosis can develop even within 1 to 2 weeks if the person is on a run of very high doses of stimulants.

NICOTINE

Pharmacological Actions

The behavioral effects of nicotine have been defined as both stimulant and depressant, effects that are influenced by the present mental status and expectations of the smoker. Smokers may feel alert and relaxed. Nicotine produces myriad effects on the central nervous system (CNS), almost all of which appear to be mediated through nicotinic receptors. Additionally, nicotine influences multiple neuronal systems. One of its most prominent effects is stimulated release of dopamine, particularly in the nucleus accumbens, which is a major component of the reward system. Nicotine also stimulates the release of endogenous opioids and glucocorticoids.

Tolerance and Dependence

Tolerance to nicotine's effects develops rapidly and most likely involves multiple processes, although the pattern and extent of tolerance development is not identical for all of nicotine's effects. It has been proposed that rapid tolerance or desensitization occurs to the behavioral or reinforcing effects of nicotine. These effects are of such a short duration that a smoker continually cycles between a sensitized and desensitized state. This notion is consistent with the fact that drugs with high abuse liability have a rapid onset and short duration of action. Regardless of the mechanism of tolerance, nicotine is a highly addicting drug. Even though most individuals are unaware of nicotine's reinforcing properties when smoking, many individuals feel intense, long-lasting craving when attempting to stop.Although most smokers wish to quit, only about one-third attempt to do so each year.

SEDATIVE–HYPNOTICS

The CNS depressants include barbiturates, nonbarbiturate sedatives, and the benzodiazepines. As the medical use of barbiturates decreased, primarily because of their high addiction liability and the danger of acute lethality, the use of the benzodiazepine anxiolytics increased. The most commonly abused barbiturates are secobarbital, pentobarbital, and amobarbital. Phenobarbital is not generally abused, because of its slow onset of action. The most commonly abused anxiolytics include diazepam, chlordiazepoxide, midazolam, lorazepam, and flurazepam. These drugs are readily attainable from illicit sources. Abused nonbarbiturate sedatives include glutethimide and meprobamate.

Pharmacological Aspects

CNS depressants, including barbiturate, benzodiazepine, and ethanol, produce a similar intoxication.These drugs are abused for their euphoric effects and as a means to reduce anxiety and limit insomnia. As the dose of depressant increases, along with the degree of intoxication, the effects progress from anxiety reduction and muscle relaxation to motor impairment and unconsciousness.The difference between the classes of drugs is primarily dose responsiveness. Intoxication progresses from mild to severe over a relatively narrow dose range in the case of the barbiturates. The benzodiazepine dose–response curve is such that great increases in dose are necessary to make such a transition.Thus, the benzodiazepines are a safer class of depressant drugs.The acute effects of depressants can include euphoria, anxiety reduction, anticonvulsant activity, sedation, ataxia, motor incoordination, impaired judgment, anesthesia, coma, and respiratory depression resulting in death. The benzodiazepines are rarely involved in lethality, but all CNS depressants enhance the effects of other depressant drugs. The physiological effects of high-dose depressants include miosis, shallow respiration, and reduction in reflex responses.

Tolerance and Dependence

Tolerance to many of the effects of the depressants develops. Unlike opioids, barbiturate and benzodiazepine tolerance develops slowly. Also, tolerance is incomplete in some instances or does not influence some pharmacological effects. One such exception is the lack of tolerance to barbiturate lethality. The lethal dose in a tolerant individual is not much different from that of the general population. Cross-tolerance develops to some degree between the depressant classes of drugs. Dependence on benzodiazepines, as evidenced by a withdrawal syndrome, can develop to large doses of drugs. Mild dependence is produced at therapeutic doses. Individuals report some craving for drug during withdrawal from benzodiazepines, but the level is not as great as among those who abuse alcohol. Once the withdrawal syndrome has dissipated, the abusers of benzodiazepines are not as likely to resume drug consumption as are alcoholics. Withdrawal signs appear to be more likely following chronic exposure to short acting benzodiazepines, such as alprazolam (half-life of less than 15 hours) or lorazepam than long-acting drugs. Despite gradual dose reduction, individuals may have anxiety attacks, confusion, agitation, restlessness, sweating, clouded sensorium, heightened sensory perception, perceptual disturbances, sleep disruption, muscle cramps, muscle twitches, and tremors; 2% of addicts may have a seizure during withdrawal. Withdrawal signs peak the second day after abrupt withdrawal and last for at least 5 to 7 days. Withdrawal symptoms following long-acting benzodiazepines (diazepam, clorazepate) peak during the second week of abstinence. In contrast to alcohol and the barbiturate sedatives, withdrawal from benzodiazepines is not life threatening.

ETHANOL

Ethanol is the most widely abused drug in the world. There are more than 10 million alcoholics in the United States alone. Excessive consumption of alcoholic beverages has been linked to as many as half of all traffic accidents, two-thirds of homicides, and three-fourths of suicides, and it is a significant factor in other crimes, in family problems, and in personal and industrial accidents. The annual cost to the American economy has been estimated to exceed $100 billion in lost productivity, medical care, and property damage. Alcoholism has been difficult to define because of its complex nature. A person is generally considered an alcoholic, however, when his or her lifestyle is dominated by the procurement and consumption of alcoholic beverages and when this behavior interferes with personal, professional, social, or family relations. A light drinker generally is defined as one who consumes an average of one drink or less per day, usually with the evening meal; a moderate drinker is one who has approximately three drinks per day; and a heavy drinker is one who has five or more drinks per day (or in the case of binge drinkers, at least once per week with five or more drinks on each occasion).

Chemistry

Ethanol (ethyl alcohol, alcohol) is a simple organic molecule composed of a single hydroxyl group and a short two-carbon aliphatic chain, CH_3CH_2OH.The hydroxyl and ethyl moieties confer both hydrophilic and lipophilic properties on the molecule. Therefore, ethanol is an amphophile, a property important to its pharmacological activity.

Absorption, Distribution, Metabolism, and Excretion

After oral administration, ethanol is almost completely absorbed throughout the gastrointestinal tract.The rate of absorption is largely determined by the quantity consumed, the concentration in the beverage, the rate of consumption, and the composition of the gastric contents. Eating food before or during drinking retards absorption, especially if the food has a high lipid content. After absorption, ethanol is distributed throughout body water. In organs with high blood flow, such as the brain, liver, lungs, and kidney, equilibrium occurs rapidly. Conversely, in organs with low blood flow, such as muscle, equilibrium occurs more slowly. Ethanol readily passes through the blood–placenta barrier into the fetal circulation. Although the concentration of ethanol in the blood can be quite predictable, measurements of blood ethanol, especially when the concentrations are rising, may lead to erroneous conclusions, since the values obtained can underestimate the concentration of ethanol in the brain. This fact can confound legal proceedings in drunk-driving cases where blood ethanol concentrations are considered an accurate and legally acceptable determinant of the amount of ethanol consumed. Ethanol is metabolized primarily in the liver by at least two enzyme systems. The best-studied and most important enzyme is zinc dependent: alcohol dehydrogenase. The rate of metabolism catalyzed by alcohol dehydrogenase is generally linear with time except at low ethanol concentrations and is relatively independent of the ethanol concentration (i.e., zero-order kinetics).In adults, ethanol is metabolized at about 10 to 15 mL/hour. Since metabolism of ethanol is slow, ingestion must be controlled to prevent accumulation and intoxication. There is little evidence that chronic ingestion of ethanol leads to a significant induction of alcohol dehydrogenase, even in heavy drinkers.Some populations, most notably East Asians, exhibit an unusual response after drinking ethanol. The symptoms include facial flushing, vasodilation, and tachycardia. These individuals apparently have a genetic deficiency of the enzyme aldehyde dehydrogenase, which leads to an accumulation of acetaldehyde even after they drink relatively small amounts of ethanol. If drugs such as metronidazole, griseofulvin, quinacrine, the hypoglycemic sulfonylureas, phenothiazines, and phenylbutazone are coadministered with ethanol, a similar accumulation of acetaldehyde may occur. In addition to alcohol dehydrogenase, ethanol can be oxidized to acetaldehyde by the microsomal mixedfunction oxidase system (cytochrome P450 2 EI). Although this microsomal ethanol-oxidizing system probably has minor importance in the metabolism of ethanol in humans, it may be involved in some of the reported interactions between ethanol and other drugs that are also metabolized by this system. Microsomal mixed-function oxidases may be induced by chronic ethanol ingestion. Because ethanol is metabolized in the liver, it can interfere with the metabolism of other drugs by blocking microsomal hydroxylation and demethylation. Drug classes whose metabolism is most affected include the barbiturates, coumarins, and anticonvulsants, such as phenytoin. Liver damage resulting from chronic abuse of ethanol can impair metabolism of a variety of drugs. Normally, 90 to 98% of an ingested dose of ethanol is metabolized by the liver. Most of the remaining 2 to 10% is excreted unchanged in the urine and expired air. The ethanol content in the urine is normally about 130% of the blood concentration and is quite constant; the expired air contains about 0.05% of the blood ethanol level, a concentration that also is remarkably consistent.

PHARMACOLOGICAL ACTIONS

CENTRAL NERVOUS SYSTEM

Alcohol is primarily a CNS depressant, and the degree of depression is directly proportional to the quantity of ethanol consumed. However, behavioral stimulation can be found after ingestion of small amounts of ethanol.This stimulation is expressed as decreased social and psychological inhibition and is most likely the result of a depression of inhibitory pathways in the brain with release of cortical activity. The behavioral and physiological effects are associated with different blood ethanol concentrations. As the blood ethanol concentration begins to increase, behavioral activation, characterized by euphoria, talkativeness, aggressiveness, and loss of behavioral control, generally precedes the overt CNS depression induced by ethanol. At progressively higher blood ethanol concentrations, the stage of relaxation is transformed into decreased social inhibitions, slurred speech, ataxia, decreased mental acuity, decreased reflexive responses, coma, and, finally, death resulting from respiratory arrest. In moderation, however, there is no evidence that the judicious use of small amounts of alcoholic beverages (e.g., a glass of wine with meals) is permanently harmful.

Other Body Systems

In general, ethanol in low to moderate amounts, is relatively benign to most body systems.A moderate amount of ethanol causes peripheral vasodilation, especially of cutaneous vessels, and stimulates the secretion of salivary and gastric fluids; the latter action may aid digestion. On the other hand, ethanol consumption in high concentrations, as found in undiluted spirits, can induce hemorrhagic lesions in the duodenum, inhibit intestinal brush border enzymes, inhibit the uptake of amino acids, and limit the absorption of vitamins and minerals. In addition, ethanol can reduce blood testosterone levels, resulting in sexual dysfunction. Ethanol is a diuretic.This effect may be caused by its ability to inhibit secretion of antidiuretic hormone from the posterior pituitary, which leads to a reduction in renal tubular water reabsorption. The large amount of fluid normally consumed with ethanol also contributes to increased urine production.

ADVERSE EFFECTS

ACUTE ETHANOL INTOXICATION AND HANGOVER

Ethanol intoxication is probably the best-known form of drug toxicity. Intoxicated individuals are a threat to themselves and others, particularly if they attempt to drive or operate machinery. Although death can result from ethanol overdose, usually the patient lapses into a coma before ingesting lethal quantities. Ethanol intoxication is sometimes mistakenly diagnosed as diabetic coma, schizophrenia, overdosage of other CNS depressant drugs, or skull fracture. An additional feature commonly associated with excessive ethanol consumption is difficulty in regulating body temperature. Hypothermia frequently results, with body temperature falling toward that of the ambient environment. This problem can be particularly severe in the elderly, who normally have difficulty regulating their body temperature. One of the consequences of ethanol intoxication is the hangover, a condition characterized by headache, nausea, sweating, and tremor. Although unpleasant, a hangover is not dangerous, even though the person having one may feel otherwise.

TREATMENT FOR ACUTE INTOXICATION

Generally, no treatment is required for acute ethanol intoxication. Allowing the individual to sleep off the effects of ethanol ingestion is the usual procedure. Hangovers are treated similarly; that is, no effective remedy exists for a hangover, except for controlling the amount of ethanol consumed. Sometimes ethanol overdose is a medical emergency. For example, prompt treatment is required if the patient is in danger of dying of respiratory arrest, is comatose, has dilated pupils, is hypothermic, or displays tachycardia Treatment for severe ethanol overdose is generally supportive. Increased intracranial pressure can be relieved by intravenous administration of hypertonic mannitol. Hemodialysis can accelerate the removal of ethanol from the body. Stimulants of ethanol metabolism, such as fructose, are not sufficiently effective, and use of analeptics is not recommended because of the possibility of precipitating convulsions.

ALCOHOLISM

Alcoholism is among the major health problems in most countries. Dependence on ethanol, as with other addictive drugs, is expressed as drug-seeking behavior and is abrupt cessation of drinking. The ethanol withdrawal syndrome is characterized by tremors, seizures, hyperthermia, hallucinations, and autonomic hyperactivity. A number of organs are affected adversely by chronic ethanol use, the result of a direct cytotoxic action. Hepatic fatty infiltration and cirrhosis are common in alcoholics; cancer may develop in advanced stages of hepatic disease. Ethanol produces a number of depressant effects on the myocardium. Atrial arrhythmias and ventricular tachycardia may arise from chronic ethanol use. A serious clinical entity, alcoholic cardiomyopathy, has also been described. A high rate of ethanol consumption can lead to inhibition of gastric secretion and irritation of the gastric mucosa. Ethanol irritates the entire gastrointestinal tract, which may lead to constipation and diminished absorption of nutrients. Other pathological effects include pancreatitis and peripheral neuropathy. Severe gonadal failure is often found in both men and women, accompanied by low blood levels of sex hormones.

A variety of pathological problems involving the CNS have been described in chronic alcoholics, the main ones being Wernicke's encephalopathy and Korsakoff's psychosis. Brain damage from chronic ethanol consumption can be especially severe in the elderly and may accelerate aging. Ethanol readily passes across the placenta and into the fetal circulation. The fetal alcohol syndrome has three primary features: microcephaly, prenatal growth deficiency, and short palpebral fissures. Other characteristics include postnatal growth deficiency, fine motor dysfunction, cardiac defects, and anomalies of the external genitalia and inner ear. A definite risk of producing fetal abnormalities occurs when ethanol consumption by the mother exceeds 3 oz daily, the equivalent of about six drinks.

Treatment for Alcoholism

The immediate concern in the treatment of alcoholics is detoxification and management of the ethanol withdrawal syndrome. Once the patient is detoxified, long term treatment requires complete abstinence, psychiatric treatment, family involvement, and frequently support from lay organizations such as Alcoholics Anonymous. One pharmacological approach is aversion therapy using drugs such as disulfiram to associate drinking ethanol with unpleasant consequences. If ethanol is taken after disulfiram administration, blood acetaldehyde concentrations increase 5 to 10 times, resulting in vasodilation, pulsating headache, nausea, vomiting, severe thirst, respiratory difficulties chest pains, orthostatic hypotension, syncope, and blurred vision. In certain cases, marked respiratory depression, cardiac arrhythmias, cardiovascular collapse, myocardial infarction, acute congestive heart failure, unconsciousness, convulsions, and sudden death have been reported. Despite these potentially severe consequences, disulfiram is prescribed for some alcoholic patients. Another pharmacological approach is the use of anticraving drugs, for example serotonin uptake inhibitors, dopaminergic agonists, and opioid antagonists. The only treatment that has shown considerable promise is one that uses the opioid antagonist naltrexone.

MARIJUANA

The hemp plant, or cannabis (Cannabis sativa), continues to be the most frequently abused illicit substance in America. The dried leaves and flowering tops of the plant are referred to as marijuana, and it is typically smoked in pipes or rolled as cigarettes. It also may be consumed in baked goods. Hashish is a solid black resinous material obtained from the leaves of the plant and is usually smoked in a pipe.

Chemistry

The major psychoactive constituent in marijuana use is tetrahydrocannabinol (THC), the prototypical cannabinoid. Although marijuana contains a large number of cannabinoids, they lack behavioral activity with the exception of cannabinol, which is approximately onetenth as potent as THC. The THC content in hashish is more than double that in marijuana.

Pharmacokinetic Aspects

THC is readily absorbed when marijuana is smoked. Pharmacological effects are produced rapidly and generally peak within 30 minutes of the onset of smoking. The dynamics of smoking (number of puffs, spacing, hold time, and lung capacity) substantially influence how much drug is absorbed. Although oral ingestion of marijuana produces similar pharmacological effects, 9-THC is absorbed more slowly than by smoking. Impairment on various performance measures related to driving skills has been demonstrated immediately following marijuana smoking and up to 24 hours thereafter. Generally, behavioral and physiological effects return to baseline levels 4 to 6 hours after usage. Blood concentrations of 9-THC peak prior to drug-induced effects.This time discordance between blood concentrations of 9-THC and effects has made it difficult to establish a meaningful relationship between blood concentrations and effects. 9-THC is rapidly distributed to all tissues despite being tightly bound by plasma proteins. 9-THC is a highly lipophilic substance and so accumulates in tissue high in lipid content.Traces of 9-THC have been found in adipose tissue more than 30 days after the subject smoked a single joint. The terminal half-life of 9-THC in plasma ranges from 18 hours to 4 days.

Pharmacological Actions on Central Nervous System

Marijuana produces a distinctive behavioral syndrome that is easily distinguished from that of most other drugs. The most prominent feature is the initial period of euphoria, or high, which has been described as a sense of well-being and happiness. Euphoria is frequently followed by a period of drowsiness or sedation. Perception of time is altered, along with distortions in both hearing and vision. However, illusions and hallucinations occur infrequently. The subjective effects also include dissociation of ideas. The subjective effects of marijuana vary from individual to individual as a function of dose, route of administration, the experience and expectation of the subjects, and individual vulnerability to certain psychoactive substances.Motor coordination also may decrease, especially in situations requiring highly complex motor skills, such as flying an airplane and driving an automobile. Increased appetite is frequently attributed to smoking marijuana. Cannabinoids are effective antiemetics, particularly in treating emesis arising during chemotherapy. 9-THC has been reported to be as effective as codeine as an analgesic, although pronounced behavioral effects occur with analgesic doses.

Other Organ Systems

The most consistent pharmacological effect produced by marijuana is tachycardia, which is closely associated with the blood levels of 9-THC. There is relatively little effect on blood pressure unless large quantities of marijuana are smoked, in which case there can be marked orthostatic hypotension. Cannabinoids are also vasodilatory, which results in the characteristic conjunctival reddening following marijuana smoking.They also reduce intraocular pressure and are capable of producing bronchodilation.

Adverse Effects

Marijuana is unique among drugs of abuse in that there have been no credible reports of fatal overdose. The most prominent effect of acute marijuana use is intoxication, which can impair the cognitive and motor skills needed to complete complex tasks. Anxiety and panic reactions are occasionally reported in inexperienced users or following use of large quantities of marijuana. 9-THC causes its greatest effects on short-term memory, as measured in free-recall tasks. Marijuana does not affect the retrieval of previously learned facts. In contrast to alcohol, there is no residual hangover from a single use of high quantities of marijuana. Heavy marijuana smoking produces bronchitis, and some individuals have evidence of precancerous lung conditions. However, definitive evidence of the relationship between marijuana smoking and the incidence of lung cancer is lacking. Tolerance develops to many of 9-THC's effects in heavy marijuana users. Although chronic cannabis use does not result in severe withdrawal symptoms, numerous reports attest to development of dependence in subjects taking high doses of THC for several weeks. The most prominent symptoms were irritability and restlessness; others included insomnia, anorexia, increased sweating, and mild nausea. Cessation of mild or moderate use of marijuana, however, does not produce a withdrawal syndrome.

Hallucinogens

The term hallucinogen is often used to describe a drug that produces a change in sensory perception, usually either visual or auditory. Drugs commonly assigned to this class include lysergic acid diethylamide (LSD), mescaline (derived from the peyote cactus), and psilocybin (derived from a mushroom). However, this rather limited definition fails to include the other prominent property of this class of drugs, which is a change in thought and mood. For this reason the term is sometimes used interchangeably with psychedelic or psychotomimetic, the latter term representing the CNS effects beyond the hallucination itself. Most literal definitions of the term hallucinogen are inadequate, but it should be used to signify substances that consistently produce changes in sensory perception, thought, and mood. An hallucinogen is a drug that reliably produces alterations in perceptions as a primary effect. Drugs that should not be included are those that produce alterations in sensory perception only at toxic doses (e.g., antimuscarinic agents, antimalarials, and opioids) and fail to produce these effects in all individuals. This does not preclude a drug's being classified as an hallucinogen if it has other properties as well. Several drugs that reliably alter mood at low doses and produce altered sensory perceptions at slightly higher doses are close chemical analogues to the CNS stimulant class of drugs. These drugs that also reliably produce differing degrees of CNS stimulation in a dose responsive dose responsive fashion include phencyclidine (PCP), methylenedioxymethamphetamine (MDMA), and methylenedioxyaphetamine (MDA).The hallucinogens generally fall into two chemicalclasses.The indole alkylamines include LSD, psilocybin, psilocin, dimethyltryptamine (DMT), and diethyltryptamine (DET), all of which are structurally similar to serotonin. The other chemical subclass of hallucinogens contains phenylethylamine derivatives such as mescaline, MDMA, MDA, and DOM (dimethoxymethyl amphetamine). A related stimulatory hallucinogen, PCP, is a piperidine analogue that produces unique effects.

EXTENT AND PATTERN OF ABUSE

LSD is very potent and produces both CNS and peripheral effects. Because of the rapid tolerance produced with these drugs, the typical abuser does not use the drug on a daily basis. Generally, an hallucinogen is abused approximately once per month. Illicit PCP abuse began in the 1960s, primarily by oral ingestion. However, its use was limited because PCP frequently produced dysphoria, which was unpredictable.

PHARMACOLOGICAL ASPECTS

The effects of LSD may be observed for 8 hours. The specific acute effects of a drug like LSD include euphoria, depersonalization, enhanced awareness of sensory input, alterations in the perception of time or space or body image, and to some extent, minor stimulant effects. Sometimes the dreamlike quality of the experience produces relaxation, good humor, and a sense of wonder or euphoria. Often the effect is a function of expectation and environmental conditions. Someone who is anxious about the use of the hallucinogen may have drug-induced anxiety, panic, or even paranoid ideation. The loss of individuality can be perceived as a disintegration of the person and can lead to a panic attack. Even if the drug experience initially is euphoric, tremendous mood swings can occur and suddenly plunge the abuser into emotions of great anxiety or terror. These negative phenomena are not always precipitated by an unexpected or sudden frightful event but can be a function of the labile mood induced by the drug. The visual hallucinations are often composed of extremely vivid colors of geometric patterns, such as cones, spirals, or cobweb-like structures. Other types of hallucinations are possible. A true hallucination involves the belief by the individual that the (altered) sensations and perceptions actually represent reality. However, generally the person abusing LSD and related drugs retains the ability to test reality versus illusion and knows that the experience is not real. Thus, the typical drug-induced hallucinatory state would be more appropriately termed a pseudohallucination, though real hallucinations are possible. The subjective or psychotomimetic changes are those considered to be changes in mood. These effects are somewhat more and variable than the hallucinatory effects or changes in sensory perception. Though these effects can occur with LSD, they seem to be more common with other specific hallucinogens, such as MDMA and MDA. MDMA (XTC, or ecstasy) possesses hallucinogenic activity similar to that of mescaline but also produces stimulant activity similar to that of amphetamine. Initially MDMA produces euphoria, increases the ability to communicate with others, increases the degree of intimacy one feels toward others in the surroundings, increases self-esteem and mood, and generally appears reduce perceived intensity of psychological problems. Hallucinatory activity occurs at higher doses. One residual effect of abuse is the MDMA hangover, which is the occurrence on the second day after abuse of drowsiness and sore jaw muscles along with other possible side effects due to the stimulant properties of the drug. MDA, which is similar to MDMA, has been termed the love drug because it produces a feeling of closeness to others. Typically, a dose of 75 mg produces the primary psychotomimetic effects, while a dose of 150 mg produces LSD-like effects, and a dose of 300 mg produces amphetamine like CNS stimulation. The amphetamine like stimulation of the CNS and periphery is prominent with both MDA and MDMA. To a lesser degree this stimulation also occurs with LSD. The effects that can be produced by stimulatory doses of hallucinogens include tachycardia, hypertension, and arrhythmias. PCP is unique in terms of its hallucinogenic properties and its other pharmacological effects. It possesses CNS stimulatory actions, but it is also a dissociative anesthetic. It induces a wide variety of psychotomimetic and hallucinatory effects during emergence from anesthesia. Because it possesses CNS stimulant properties comparable with those of amphetamine, it does not produce depression of the cardiovascular system like other anesthetics, though it does depress the respiratory system. At a low dose, individuals believe they are thinking and acting rapidly and efficiently. The general mood is happiness, though (especially at higher doses) the individual can vacillate between euphoria and depression. It primarily produces auditory hallucinations. At higher doses the stimulatory effects are more pronounced and the likelihood of tremendous mood swings more likely. At near anesthetic doses, it produces more typical depressant effects, including motor incoordination, catalepsy, vacant stare, or even amnesia. Coma is produced subsequent to respiratory depression.

Tolerance and Dependence

Tolerance to the effects of hallucinogens develops rapidly. A high degree of tolerance can be produced after as few as three to four daily doses of drug. Generally, the abuser self-imposes the requirement for a 2- to 3-day drug-free period before another drug session. Additionally, there is a tremendous degree of cross-tolerance between the hallucinogens, so other LSD-like hallucinogens cannot be abused during the drug-free period either. One danger with the stimulant subclass of hallucinogens is rapid development of tolerance to some of their effects while the stimulatory properties remain and produce various side effects. Despite the apparent overlap of effects with stimulant drugs, however, there is no cross-tolerance with the CNS stimulants such as amphetamine. There are no observable physical withdrawal signs during drug abstinence, nor is there a tremendous craving for drug during the drug-free period. Therefore,clearly no dependence is attributed to the hallucinogens.Though there is an abuse potential with this class of drug, and individuals express drug-seeking behavior, there does not seem to be the magnitude of craving found with other drug classes, such as the CNS stimulants.

Treatment Strategies

The difference between the abused and the lethal dose of LSD is very large, so little pharmacological intervention is necessary. Treatment involves limiting external stimuli and placing the individual in a safe environment. Treatment of PCP intoxication also involves limiting external stimuli, minimizing lighting, noise, and unnecessary physical contact.The life-threatening nature of PCP overdose, however, may require symptomatic treatment of respiratory depression by artificial respiration or use of neuroleptics to control violent rage or panic anxiety.

INHALANTS

Volatile chemicals and gases that produce behavioral effects are subject to abuse. These agents represent a broad range of chemical classes but in general can be classified as gases, volatile organic solvents, and aliphatic nitrites. Inhalant abuse differs from that of many other drugs in that it is confined primarily to juveniles and young adults. The use of gases is primarily confined to nitrous oxide by young medical professionals who have ready access to this agent. It produces short-lived mild intoxication that typifies the early stages of anesthesia. Deaths occur occasionally by individuals inhaling nitrous oxide alone. Volatile organic solvents are usually aliphatic and aromatic hydrocarbons. They include substances such as gasoline, paint and lacquer thinners, lighter fluid, degreasers (methyl chloride and methylene chloride), and the solvents in airplane glue, typewriter correction fluid, and bathroom deodorizers. These agents produce a sense of exhilaration and light-headedness. Judgment and perception of reality are impaired, and hallucinations may be produced. The mechanism by which inhalants produce their behavioral effects are poorly understood, but there are some indications that their actions are similar to those of other centrally acting depressants, including alcohol. Toxicity depends on the properties of the individual solvents. The consequences of inhaling these substances can be severe, for they have been implicated in producing cancer, cardiotoxicity, neuropathies, and hepatotoxicity.

DESIGNER DRUGS

In an effort to avoid federal regulations, chemists in clandestine laboratories adopted the strategy of synthesizing analogues of controlled substances. Although these drugs are technically not illegal until scheduled, the consequences of their abuse are unpredictable and in some instances lethal. Efforts to make synthetic heroin led to the synthesis of at least six chemicals that are structurally similar to fentanyl.These agents gained considerable attention because their increased potency over fentanyl and heroin led to a rash of overdoses and numerous deaths. The two derivatives are referred to as China White and are 900 and 1,100 times as potent as morphine. Meperidine has also been used as a template for preparing synthetic heroin, the end product being 1-methyl-4-propionoxy-4-phenyl pi-peridine (MPPP). However, MPPP is sometimes contaminated with the side reaction product 1-methyl,4-phenyl-1,2,3,6-tetrahydropyridine (MPTP), which produces a parkinsonian syndrome through nigrostriatal lesions. Several substituted derivatives of amphetamine have also been called designer drugs. The most widely known of this group is the hallucinogen MDMA (ecstasy).

ANABOLIC STEROIDS

Historically, drugs used to increase the ability of an athlete to perform in a given sport included the use of stimulants to diminish the onset of fatigue or opiates to diminish the pain of exertion. Recently, abuse of anabolic–steroids (derivatives of testosterone) has increased. They are used to increase muscle size and definition (in the case of body-building competitors) and are sometimes coabused with other growth enhancers, such as human growth hormone. In sports in which mass, physical size, or even total strength (a function of total muscle mass) is important, the abuse of anabolic steroids provides a shortcut to attainment of the physical stature that might otherwise require much more extensive training and exercise. However, it is a misconception to believe that anabolic steroid abuse is limited to professional athletes and body builders. There is clear evidence that these drugs are abused by adult men and women who are not athletes, who are blue-collar and white-collar workers, and by male and female athletes at the college, high school, and junior high school levels.

REFERENCES

1. Maskos U et al. Nicotine reinforcement and cognition restored by targeted expression of nicotinic receptors. Nature 2005;436:103.
2. Morton J: Ecstasy: Pharmacology and neurotoxicity. Curr Opin Pharmacol 2005;5:79.
3. Nichols DE: Hallucinogens. Pharmacol Ther 2004;101:131.
4. Snead OC 3rd, Gibson KM: Gamma-hydroxybutyric acid. N Engl J Med 2005;352:2721.
5. Sulzer D et al. Mechanisms of neurotransmitter release by amphetamines: A review. Prog Neurobiol 2005;75:406.

CHAPTER 99

Nutraceuticals

OVERVIEW

The term "Nutraceutical" was coined from "Nutrition" and "Pharmaceutical" in 1989 by Stephen DeFelico,

OTHER WORDS USED IN THE CONTEXT

Dietary supplementation, Functional, Multifunctional Foods, etc.

DEFINITION

Nutraceutical can be defined as "A food or part of food or nutrient that provides health benefits including the prevention and treatment of a disease."

INTRODUCTION

Drug and food from natural origin play a significant role in public health care system of any nation. The search for specific constituents of plant, animals, minerals and microbial origin which are beneficial to our mental and physical health has caused coining of terminology such as Nutraceutical, cosma-ceuticals, dermaceuticals, phytochemicals, phytonutrients, phytofoods, pharmafoods, designer foods or functional foods. The term Nutraceutical and functional foods are broad terms describing foods, food ingredients or dietary supplements that demonstrate specific health or medical benefits including the prevention and treatment of disease beyond basic nutritional functions.

A number of Nutraceuticals are available that includes

- Antioxidants,
- Probiotics,
- Prebiotics,
- Omega-3 Fatty Acids and
- Dietary Fibers.

INTEREST IN NUTRACEUTICALS

Nutraceutical have the potential to play a role in healthy eating and to contribute to the prevention and treatment of diseases so that how functional components in foods could expand the role of disease prevention and treatment. The Nutraceuticals are preferred due to

1. Since new molecule is difficult to discover and more expensive and risky than ever before, many pharmaceutical companies are now trying to Nutraceuticals so that there is undoubtedly a very huge and growing market.
2. The belief among consumers that these "food like substances" are either

harmless or least toxic as compared to conventional pharmaceuticals.

3. Increased healthcare costs with conventional pharmaceuticals, recent legislation and scientific discoveries.
4. Inappropriate dietary habits are seen as contributing to the leading cause of deaths of due to coronary heart disease, certain type of cancers etc., the role of Nutraceuticals in treating these conditions is thus speculated.
5. The emergence of diet-disease relations have lead to search of specific constituents of plants, animals and minerals having a beneficial role for our mental and physical health.
6. Nutraceuticals are gaining popularity as people are relying on them for safeguarding their health and avoiding side effects associated with drugs as well.
7. As public knowledge in this field has evolved, manufacturers have sought to fulfill their appetite for these products resulting in exploding market. Japan, USA, UK is the world leaders in the Nutraceuticals market. These are around 5000 established Nutraceuticals products, worldwide.
8. Long history of use and better patient tolerance as well as public acceptance.
9. Renewable source, Cultivation and processing environmental friendly and local availability.
10. Plants constitute to be a major source of new lead generation.

RISING HEALTH CONSCIOUSNESS: THE MAJOR GROWTH DRIVER

Consumer today are more aware when it come to health, which makes them go for nutritional supplements.

1. **Aging baby boomers:** Energy and preventive care early senior, health maintenance care late seniors, rising heart and bone problems among aged population.
2. **Rising health consciousness:** Concern on health during second half of life, concern on maintaining the healthy/youthfulness, paradigm shift towards preventive health care.
3. **Dissatisfaction with modern medicine:** Increased side effects, rising healthcare cost in modern treatment.
4. **Increase acceptance of alternative treatments:** Economical, less side effects, use in diseases which are untreated by modern medicine, increased standardization of products.

NUTRACEUTICALS – WHAT ARE THEY?

Nutraceuticals are natural bioactive, chemical compounds that have health promoting, disease preventing or medicinal properties. Nutraceuticals are found in a mosaic of products emerging from

(a) The food industry,
(b) The herbal and dietary supplement market,
(c) Pharmaceutical industry, and
(d) The newly merged pharmaceutical/agribusiness/nutrition conglomerates.

- It may range from isolated nutrients, herbal products, dietary supplements and diets to genetically engineered "designer" foods and processed products such as cereals, soups and beverages.
- It is often difficult to distinguish among nutrients, food additives and drugs independent of the matrix (food or pill) in

which it is taken a dietary supplement can sometimes be food like and other times drug like.

- One way to differentiate between food and drugs could be examining how people are exposed to them. Drugs can be found sometimes in foods, and can participate in the metabolism.
- However, these substances are not normally exposed in humans at the dose at which they exert their beneficial effect.
- Some dietary supplements are drug like when ingested in amount that could never be achieved in the diet, even though they are essential nutrients when ingested in smaller quantities. e.g., tryptophan is an essential amino acid required for metabolism and incorporation into proteins at low dose in humans. At high dose, it increases brain 5-hydroxytryptamine levels and thus acts as a drug to treat insomnia. Polyunsaturated fatty acid likes leptin and statins that increases bone formation.
- The Nutraceutical containing phytosterols are effective in lowering LDL cholesterol. Proteins and non-proteins of bovine milk fat globule membrane are potent Nutraceutical that effective as anticancer, anticholesterolemic, coronary heart disease.
- The Nutraceuticals of plant origin may evolve to be considered a vital aspect of dietary disease-preventive food components. Many years ago, the National Institute of health does not support researches that are focused on dietary means to solve health problems. Noteworthy is the recent establishment of Centers for study of alternative medicine around the world. Careful studies are being done on the various phytonutrients for their role in the prevention of chronic degenerative diseases.
- The sources of Nutraceuticals include ginseng, spirulina, gingko biloba, amino acids, glucosamine, chondroitin and *Aegle marmelos* that are to be formulated and consumed or administered internally under the supervision of a qualified medical practitioner and intended for the specific dietary management of a disease or condition for which distinctive nutritional requirements, based on recognized scientific principles, are established by medical evaluation.

CLASSIFICATION

The food products used as Nutraceutical contain the following except Probiotics; all the components are in fruits, vegetables and different type of herbal foods.

1. Antioxidant
2. Prebiotics
3. Probiotics
4. Omega 3 fatty acids
5. Dietary fibers

ANTIOXIDANTS

Antioxidants are substances, which retard or prevent deterioration, damage or destruction caused by oxidation. Fortunately, the body has an army of antioxidants for damage limitation. Antioxidant form an integral part of the Nutraceutical market. During the last few years' research has confirmed that many have the common disease and ailments of 21st century (CVS, diabetes, cataracts, high blood pressure, infertilities, respiratory infection, and rheumatoid arthritis) are associated with tissue deficiency and/or low dietary levels of compounds called antioxidants. The oxygen is consumed in the body during metabolism by process called oxidation. During oxidation free radicals are generated. These free radicals at a molecular level burn everything they touch. Antioxidants are power full electron donors and react with free radical damage the biomolecules. The formed antioxidant radical is stable and unreactive. Antioxidants are quite large in number and diverse in nature which oppose the process of oxidation largely by neutralizing free radicals at relatively small concentrations have the potential to inhibit to inhibit the oxidants chain reactions. Dietary antioxidants and some accessory molecules, such as zinc and certain vitamins are important in maintaining free radical scavenging systems, biosynthetic capacity, membranes, enzymes and DNA. Antioxidants are found in the vegetable oils. E.g. Soybean oil, canola oil, corn oil, oat oil, wheat germ oil, palm oil, evening prime rose oil.

FREE RADICALS

A free radical has defined as any species capable of independent existence that contain one more unpaired electron. Unpaired electron makes the molecule unstable and highly reactive. They are mainly derived from oxygen and nitrogen. Free radicals are short lived. Most of the free radicals are formed in the body from oxygen are super oxide, hydroxyl radical, nitric oxide, singlet oxygen, peroxyl radical, hydrogen peroxide and alkoxyl. The sources of free radicals are both endogenous and exogenous.

The free radicals disrupt the equilibrium of biological systems by damaging their major constituents' molecules (lipids, proteins, carbohydrates and DNA) that eventually lead to cell death.

ACTION OF ANTIOXIDANTS

Antioxidants are used to prevent the damage at the cellular level by using the following mechanisms:

- They may reduce the energy of the free radical
- Preventive (suppress radical formation)
- Repair repair damage and reconstitute membranes)

PROBIOTICS

Probiotics are live microbial food ingredients, which are beneficial to health. The prerequisite for probiotic action include survival in and adhesion to specific areas of the gastrointestinal tract and competitive exclusion of pathogens or harmful antigens. Probiotics are situated as health or functional foods whereby they are ingested for their purported positive advantages in the digested tract and/or systemic area like the liver, brain, vagina or blood stream. Colon is the most densely populated region of the gastrointestinal tract and harbors an estimated 500 different bacterial species.

PROBIOTIC BACTERIAL SPECIES

The various types of bacteria that are having the Probiotics characteristics are:

- Lactobacilli
- Lactobacillus rhamnosus
- Lactobacillus reuteri
- Lactobacillus case
- Bifidobacterium

- Bifidobacterium lactis
- Bifidobacterium longum
- Bifidobacterium breve
- Bifidobacterium infantis
- Streptococcus
- Lactococcus
- Lactococcus platinum
- Lactococcus reuteri

CHARACTERISTICS OF PROBIOTIC BACTERIA

Bacteria should have the following features:

1. GRAS (generally recognized as safe)
2. *In vitro* resistance to hydrochloric acid and pancreatic juice
3. Produce antimicrobial substances
4. Compete with bad bacteria to adhere on the gut wall.
5. Compete for the nutrients and stimulate immunity and
6. Alter the intestinal micro flora balance, inhibit growth of harmful bacteria, promote good digestion, boost immune function and increase resistance to infection.

PREBIOTICS

Prebiotics are the substances, which reach to colon in intact form i.e. without getting depleted by the gastric pH and digestive acids. These prebiotics also selectively promote the growth of colonel probiotic bacteria; hence they act as fertilizers for these bacteria. These are collective term for non-digestive but a fermentable dietary carbohydrate that may selectively stimulates growth of certain bacterial groups' resident in the colon, such as *Bifidobacteria, Lactobacilli* considered to be beneficial for the human host. e.g. –inulin, which is soluble dietary fibers and resistant to digestive enzyme and thus reaches to large intestine or colon essentially intact, where it is fermented by resistant bacteria, *Lactobacilli*. A range of oligosaccharides have been tested using various *in vitro* methods, animal models and human clinical trials are –

1. Fructo oligosaccharides
2. Inulins
3. Lactilol
4. Lactulose
5. Galacto-oligosaccharides
6. Soybean oligosaccharides
7. Lactosucrose
8. Isomalto-oligosaccharides

THE FOOD COMPONENTS OR INGREDIENTS (PREBIOTICS)

A prebiotic nature has been attributed to many food components that the food or food components

1. Resists host digestion, absorption and absorption processes.
2. Fermented by the microflora colonizing the gastrointestinal system.
3. Selectively stimulates the growth and/or the activity of one or a limited number of bacteria with the gastrointestinal system.

POLYUNSATURATED FATTY ACIDS

Essential fatty acids are needed for normal growth and development but cannot be synthesized by our body. Omega-3 fatty acids belong to this class. Long chain omega-3 fatty acids such as eicosapentaoic acid and docosagexanoic acids are built up in algae and plankton and the fish living on them. The natural vegetable oils and marine animal oils containing polyunsaturated fatty acid belong to Linoleic group (omega 6-type and omega 3-fatty acid) help to reduce cholesterol formation/deposition and prevent thromboxane formation. E.g. safflower oil, corn oil, soybean oil, mustard oil and marine fishes. Evening primrose oil, flax oil, hemp seed, borage seed.

The following are diseases for which polyunsaturated fatty acids are preferred.

- Heart disease and stroke
- Rheumatoid arthritis
- Inflammatory arthritis
- Inflammatory bowel disease
- Asthma
- Cancer
- Chronic lung failure
- Kidney transplant

DIETARY FIBRES

Dietary fibres are used in health food products for normalization of intestinal transit time. They have dual effect on intestinal transit. First effect is on the bulk faeces, which are often increased, in substantial proportion 127% after ingestion of 20g of wheat bran, this action with insoluble fibres. The other effect if dietary fibres are upon the duration of transit, which gets normalized around in 48 hours. Long transit time gets shortened and short transit get longer. Dietary fibres are categorized into two groups

WATER SOLUBLE FIBRES

Soluble fibres dissolve in water and form a gel that binds the stool and inhibit the non-propulsive colon contractions, helps in bulking of stool and their quick passage through digestive tract. Oats, dried beans, legumes, chicory.

WATER INSOLUBLE FIBRES

Insoluble fibres are present in brown rice, banana, vegetables and whole grains. Source of dietary fibres are –

- Fresh fruit: Apple, orange, apricot, plum, pineapple with fibres 18%-30%
- Vegetables: Cabbage, carrot, lettuce, onion, tomato with fibres 9%- 12 %

Table 99.1 lists the nutraceuticals available in market.

Table 99.1

Nutraceuticals available in market

Brand name	Components	Function
Z-trim	Wheat	Zero calorie fat replacer
Linumlife	Lignan extract flax	Prostate health
Fenulife	Fenugreek galactomannon	Control blood sugar
Teamax	Green tea extract	Potent antioxidant
Marinol	ω 3 FA, DHA, EPA	Heart health protection
Clarinol	CLA	Weight loss ingredient
Cholestaid	Saponin	Reduce cholesterol

METHOD TO ENHANCE ACTIVE COMPONENTS IN FOOD

- Manipulating the diet to get maximum level of active components
- Combination of food ingredients rich in nutraceuticals
- Fortifying food with active ingredients
- By fermentation of food products
- Changing food habits to natural type of diet

CONCLUSION

- Nutraceuticals are present in most of the food ingredients with varying concentration
- Concentration, time and duration of supply of nutraceuticals influence human health
- Manipulating the foods, the concentration of active ingredients can be increased
- Diet rich in Nutraceuticals along with regular exercise, stress reduction and maintenance of healthy body weight will maximize health and reduce disease risk

REFERENCES

1. Baichwal R.S. 'Developments in nutraceuticals' Pharma Times, 1999, pp.19-20.
2. Khan M.A., Khan N.A., Qasimi I.A., Ahmad G. and Zafar S. 'Study of antidiarrhoeal activity of a herbal test formulation in rats', Journal of Science and Pharmacy, 2004, Vol.5, No.2, pp.45-49.
3. Rishi R.K. 'Nutraceuticals: Borderline between food and drug?' The Pharma Rev., 2006, pp.51-53.
4. Dhami V.P.S. and Chopra K. 'The world of nutraceuticals', The Eastern pharmacist, 2000. pp.29-30.
5. Mani, T.T., Mukherjee, P.K., Manimaran. S. and Suresh, B. 'Indian herbal drug development- problems and prospects' Pharma Times, 2002, Vol. 34, pp.13-14.
6. Samanta M.K., Mukherjee P.K., Prasad M.K. and Suresh B. 'Development of natural products', The Eastern Pharmacist, 2000, pp.23-27.
7. Prasana R. 'Nutraceuticals to gain ground globally', The Pharma Rev., 2006, pp.55-56.
8. Dureja D., Kaushik D. and Kumar V. 'Developments in nutraceuticals', Indian journal of pharmacology, 2003, Vol.35, pp.363-372.
9. Hauselmann H.J. 'Nutripharmaceuticals for osteoarthritis', Best Practice and Research Clinical Rheumatology, 2001, Vol.15, No.4, pp.597-607.
10. Ojha S.K., Nandave M. and Arya D.S. 'Dietary nutraceuticals: A promising approach in management of cardiovascular diseases', Indian Drugs, 2006, Vol.43, No.3, pp.181-190.
11. Beliveau R. and Gingras D. 'Green tea: prevention and treatment of cancer by nutraceuticals' The Lancet, 2004, Vol.364, pp. 1021-1022.

CHAPTER 100

PHARMACOECONOMICS

DEFINITION

- Pharmacoeconomics has been defined as "The description and analysis of the costs of drug therapy to health care systems and society."
- Pharmacoeconomic research identifies, measures, and compares the costs (i.e., resources consumed) and consequences (i.e., clinical, economic, humanistic) of pharmaceutical products and services.

OBJECTIVES

- Objectives of Pharmacoeconomics and outcomes research must originate within three dimensions when considering results and value of healthcare (Fig. 100.1).

PHARMACOECONOMIC METHODOLOGIES (FIG. 100.2)

- Cost minimization
- Cost utility
- Cost-consequence Analysis
- Cost-of-illness Evaluation
- Cost benefit
- Cost effectiveness

COST-MINIMIZATION ANALYSIS

When two or more interventions are evaluated and demonstrated or assumed to be equivalent in terms of a given outcome or consequence, costs associated with each intervention may be evaluated and compared.

Example

Drug therapy may be the evaluation of two generically equivalent drugs in which the outcome has been proven to be equal, although the acquisition and administration costs may be significantly different

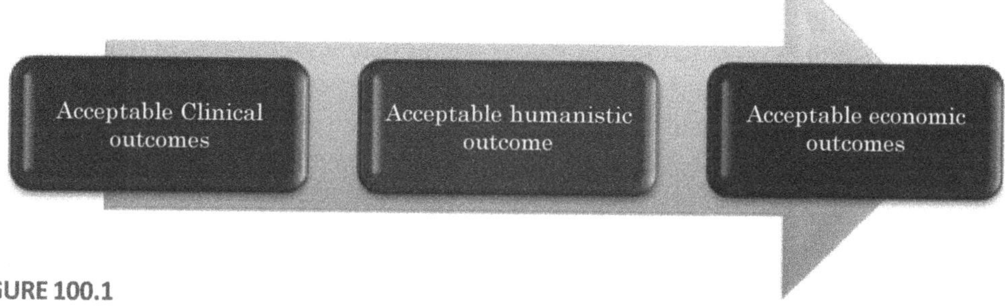

FIGURE 100.1

Objectives of pharmacoeconomics.

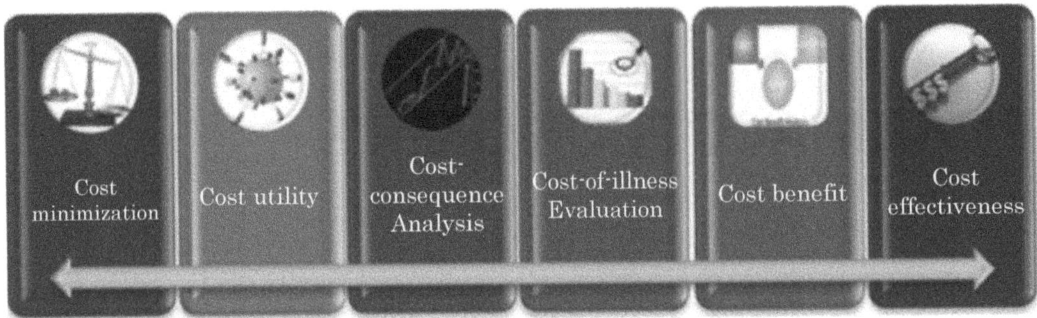

FIGURE 100.2

Pharmacoeconomic methodologies.

COST-BENEFIT ANALYSIS

- Cost-benefit analysis *is* a basic tool that can be used to improve the decision-making process in allocation of funds to healthcare programs. Cost-benefit analysis consists of identifying all of the benefits that accrue from the program or intervention and converting them into dollars in the year in which they will occur.
- This stream of benefit dollars is then discounted to its equivalent present value at the selected interest rate. Ideally, all benefits and costs resulting from the program should be included.
- Cost-benefit analysis often has been used when comparing the value of dissimilar programs where the outcomes are in different units (e.g., cost-benefit of having a neonatal care program versus a cardiac rehabilitation program)

COST-EFFECTIVENESS ANALYSIS

- It is defined as a series of analytical and mathematical procedures that aid in the selection of a course of action from various alternative approaches.
- Cost-effectiveness analysis has been applied to health matters where the program's inputs can be readily measured in dollars, but the program's outputs are more appropriately stated in terms of health improvement created (e.g., life-years extended, clinical cures).
- An important point to be considered in both cost-benefit and cost-effectiveness analysis is that a program/treatment providing a high benefit (effectiveness)-to-cost ratio in terms of value to society may not be valued in the same way by all members of society.
- For example, drug therapy that reduced the number of patient-days in an acute care institution may be positive from a third-party payer's point of view, but not necessarily from the view of the institution's administrator who operated under a fixed level of revenue and depended on a fixed number of patient-days to meet expenses. What is viewed as cost-beneficial for society as a whole may be viewed differently by plan sponsors, administrators, health providers, governmental agencies, or even individual patients.

COST-UTILITY ANALYSIS

- It is an economic tool in which the intervention consequence is measured in terms of quantity and quality of life. It is much the same as cost-effectiveness analysis, with the added dimension of a particular point of view, most often that of the patient. Quite often the results of cost-utility analysis are expressed in the intervention cost per quality-adjusted life-year
- Although cost-utility analysis has been used somewhat successfully to aid in decisions regarding healthcare programs (e.g., surgery vs. chemotherapy), instruments that are reliable and sensitive enough to detect changes with drug treatments (e.g., one antihypertensive agent vs. another) are still needed.

COST-OF-ILLNESS EVALUATION

- Cost-of-illness studies are important to pharmacoeconomic evaluations of new therapies.
- By evaluating the humanistic impact of disease and the resources used in treating a condition prior to discovery of a new intervention, the pharmacoeconomist can effectively establish a baseline for comparison.
- Although the value and methodologies of cost-of-illness studies have been debated, they remain prevalent in the Pharmacoeconomic literature.
- As with all pharmacoeconomic evaluation, when conducting or evaluating the cost-of-illness, it is important to carefully consider the design and intent of the study. There is value in having baseline information, but absolute conclusions regarding the value of an intervention versus an alternative can be made only after direct comparison.

COST-CONSEQUENCE ANALYSIS

- It is defined as one "in which costs and effects are calculated but not aggregated into quality adjusted life-years or cost-effectiveness ratios."
- Simply, this type of analysis comprises a listing of all relevant costs and outcomes of drug therapy or healthcare intervention including direct medical costs, direct nonmedical costs, indirect costs, clinical outcomes, utility impacts, and quality-of-life impacts. Cost-consequence analysis provides the most comprehensive presentation of information describing the value of an intervention and has the advantage of being more readily understandable and more likely to be applied by healthcare decision-makers.
- Another potential weakness of cost-consequence analysis is that all of the data are not always of comparable quality.
- Cost-consequence analyses in the literature often include a variety of data from clinical trials and other sources, since no single source is adequate to provide the breadth of information required.
- Imputation and extrapolation are often necessary. Despite these considerations, cost-consequence analysis remains a useful approach to presenting relevant information for a wide range of healthcare concerns.

OTHER ISSUES OF IMPORTANCE

Two further issues are crucial in understanding the approach utilised by health economics to evaluate drug use.

PERSPECTIVE

The 'cost-effectiveness' of any health service intervention in large part depends upon from whose point of view the study is conducted. A range of potential perspectives can be adopted from the most limited (impact of changes on a single drug budget) to the societal where all indirect costs are studied a well. Given that the aim of economic analysis is to make the best use of all of society's resources, the societal perspectives considered the most appropriate, but a health care manage with a limited budget might be tempted to place increased emphasis upon costs that are imposed upon his area. A study of migraine from the perspective of the health service alone would be likely to ûnd that the use of Sumatriptan in migraine (a very high cost drug in an area which previously cost the health service very little) was highly undesirable. In contrast a study taking a societal perspective that incorporates all of the additional costs imposed upon the migraine sufferer might come to the opposite conclusion.

TIMING OF COSTS AND BENEFITS

Frequently the investment of health service resources occurs over a different time scale to the period during which patients experience the health benefits. For example a surgical intervention to improve cardiovascular functioning represents an investment of resources. Now to achieve health beneûts over a number of years. In comparison pharmacological interventions, to achieve the same benefits, create continuous costs and benefits into the future. Therefore in order to compare two such interventions with different profiles of costs and benefits, it is necessary to 'discount' them to their Net Present Value. In general, costs incurred in the future are discounted at an annual rate set by the Treasury (currently 6%). The extent to which future health beneûts should also be discounted remains an area of controversy within health economics. While it is relatively easy to accept that £100 spent now is 'worth' more than £100 spent in 5 years time, the theoretical basis for comparing the value of a healthy year now with a healthy year in 5 years time is not as obvious. Given such controversy, the most sensible approach is to analyse the sensitivity of the results obtained from the economics analysis to the discounting of future health benefits by presenting future health benefits both in a discounted and an undiscounted form.

PHARMACOECONOMIC AND DRUG DISCOVERY

Clinical trials are used to evaluate the efficacy and safety of therapies. The relationships between pharmacoeconomic evaluations and clinical trials are threefold.

1. The pharmacoeconomic evaluation may be a secondary objective of a trial designed primarily to study safety and efficacy.
2. The pharmacoeconomic evaluation may be the principal purpose of a clinical trial.
3. A pharmacoeconomic evaluation may be done retrospectively using clinical data obtained in previous trials.

PHARMACOECONOMIC GUIDELINES

Researchers and evaluators continue to develop and refine guidelines for

Pharmacoeconomic analysis. The uses and subject of the proposed guidelines are as follows:

1. Methodological guidelines would guide researchers to appropriately design, conduct, analyze, and report economic and humanistic evaluations.
2. Reimbursement and pricing guidelines would outline the content, presentation, and evaluation of Pharmacoeconomic data to determine or justify the price or reimbursement of a pharmaceutical product.
3. Approval guidelines would set the standards acceptable to particular government to obtain approval to market a new product.
4. Promotional guidelines would set the criteria for the use of Pharmacoeconomic data in support of pharmaceutical promotion to prescribers and consumers.

PHARMACOECONOMIC CHALLENGES

- One of the biggest challenges for Pharmacoeconomic research lies in the education of those who are going to be evaluating the data derived from this research.
- Although the end users of Pharmacoeconomic research data would like to have simple, clear-cut answers to their questions regarding the allocation of resource and the healthcare benefits derived from them, in actuality, the answers are quite complex.
- Pharmacoeconomics remains an art as well as a science. Even though the science may be perfectly clear, applying that science must be done artfully using professional judgment.
- Just as it is impossible to develop an algorithm for the treatment of a disease that is appropriate for all patients, it would be impossible to develop one for making Pharmacoeconomic decisions.
- In the end, the user of Pharmacoeconomic research data must be able to evaluate the scientific appropriateness and robustness of the research and make a decision regarding its usefulness in a particular situation.
- To do this, evaluators will need to understand the basic principles of Pharmacoeconomic research.
- The challenges of Pharmacoeconomic research are inexhaustible; many are addressed within the chapters of this book.
- The real challenge, however, is not identifying the tools of Pharmacoeconomic research, but rather discovering how and when to use them.

CONCLUSION

- Applied PE has been the "missing link" in pharmacy.
- PE principles and methods can be successfully applied in the "real world" to enhance decision making.
- PE can be applied to any therapeutic area, using a variety of application strategies.
- Application of PE to the "real world" is a new dimension, challenge and opportunity for hospital pharmacy.

REFERENCES

1. Aberg-Wistedt A, Cressell T, Lidberg Y, Liljenberg B, Osby U. Two-year outcome of team-based intensive case management for patients with schizophrenia. Phychiatr Serv 1995;46:1263-6.
2. Lieu AT, Cochi SL, Black SB, Halloran ME, Shinefield HR, Holm,es SJ, etal. Cost-effectiveness of a routine varicella vaccnination program for US children. JAMA 1994; 271:375-81.
3. Drummond M. Cost –of-illness studies. Pharmacoeconomics 1992: 2:1-4.
4. Davey PJ, Leeder SR. The cost of migraine. More than just a headache? Pharmacoeconomics 1992;2:5-7.
5. Klarman H.Present status of cost-benefit analysis in the health field. Am J Public Health 1967;57: 1948-58.
6. Crystal R, Brewster A. Cost-benefit and cost-effectiveness analysis in the health field: an introduction. Inquiry 1966; 3:3-13.
7. Klarman H. Application of cost/benefit analysis to health services and the special case of technological innovation. Int J Health Serv Res 1974;4:325-52.
8. MacKeigan LD, Bootman JL. A review of cost-benefit and cost-effectiveness analyses of clinical pharmacy services. J Pharm Marketing manage 1988;2:63-84.
9. Russell LB, Gold MR, Siegel JE, Daniels N, Weinstein MC. The role of cost-effectiveness anlaysis in health and medicine. Panel on Cost-Effectiveness in Health and Medicine. JAMA 1996:276: 1172-7.

CHAPTER 101

Pharmacogenomics

INTRODUCTION TO PERSONALIZED MEDICINE

The goal of personalized medicine is to individualize health care by using knowledge of patients' health history, behaviors, environments, and, most importantly, genetic variation when making clinical decisions. Research on genetics has provided advances that can be used to more accurately predict the risk of developing certain diseases personalize screening and surveillance protocols and, in some cases, prevent the onset of disease. In certain cases, genetics can also be used to diagnose diseases and tailor therapies and disease management strategies. These advancements in personalized medicine rely on knowledge of how a patient's genotype (genetic makeup) influences his or her phenotype (observable traits or characteristics). Using the principles of personalized medicine, health care providers may be better equipped to move beyond the "one-size-fits-all" approach that defined much of patient care in the past, to care that is appropriate for unique patient subgroups.

PHARMACOGENOMICS

- Pharmacogenomics is the study of how an individual's genetic inheritance affects the body's response to drugs. The term comes from the words pharmacology and genomics and is thus the intersection of pharmaceuticals and genetics.
- Pharmacogenomics combines traditional pharmaceutical sciences such as biochemistry with annotated knowledge of genes, proteins, and single nucleotide polymorphisms.
- Combines many different fields: Genetics, genomics, molecular biology, pharmacology, pharmaceutics, toxicology, population biology, and statistics.
- Pharmacogenomics holds the promise that drugs might one day be tailor-made for individuals and adapted to each person's own genetic makeup. Environment, diet, age, lifestyle, and state of health all can influence a person's response to medicines, but understanding an individual's genetic makeup is thought to be the key to creating personalized drugs with greater efficacy and safety.

GENES COMMONLY INVOLVED IN PHARMACOGENOMIC DRUG METABOLISM AND RESPONSE

There are several genes responsible for differences in drug metabolism and response. Among the most common are the Cytochrome P450 (CYP) genes, encoding enzymes that control the metabolism of more than 70% of prescription drugs. People who carry variations in certain CYP genes often do not metabolize drugs at the same rate or extent as in most people, and this can influence response in many ways. Other genes known to affect drug response encode the receptors for regulatory molecules such as neurotransmitters, hormones, cytokines and growth factors, and cellular proteins such as enzymes, transporters, carriers, ion channels, structural proteins and transcription factors. Variations in these genes can lead to poor response and adverse drug reactions by disabling, inactivating, interfering with, or inaccurately inducing the signaling mechanisms or cellular machinery that must function for the body to respond properly to the drug; or by causing side effects that prevent continued use of the drug. Selected drugs whose safety and efficacy are affected by gene variations

METABOLIZER PHENOTYPE

The metabolizer phenotype describes the patient's ability to metabolize certain drugs and is based on the number and type of functional alleles of certain genes that a patient carries. These genes most commonly encode the CYP enzymes. The metabolizer phenotype can range from "poor," used to describe patients with little or no functional activity of a selected CYP enzyme, to "ultra-rapid," used to describe patients with substantially increased activity of a selected CYP enzyme. Depending on the type of CYP variation present, the patient's metabolizer phenotype and the type of drug (active pharmacologic agent or inactive prodrug precursor), therapeutic drug response is often suboptimal. The table 101-1 on the following page summarizes the effects of CYP variation on therapeutic efficacy.

For example, poor metabolizers are unable to metabolize certain drugs efficiently, resulting in a potentially toxic build-up of an active drug or the lack of conversion of a prodrug into an active metabolite. In contrast, in ultra-rapid metabolizers, an active drug is inactivated quickly, leading to a sub therapeutic response, while a prodrug is quickly metabolized, leading to rapid onset of therapeutic effect.

Table 101.1

Effects of CYP variants on therapeutic efficacy

Metabolizer phenotype	Active drug (inactivated by metabolism) Drug $\xrightarrow{\text{Enzyme}}$ Inactive Metabolite	Prodrug (needs metabolism to produce active metabolite) Prodrug $\xrightarrow{\text{Enzyme}}$ Active Metabolite
Poor	Increased efficacy; active metabolite may accumulate; usually require lower dose to avoid toxic accumulation	Decreased efficacy; prodrug may accumulate; may require lower dose to avoid toxic accumulation, or may require alternate drug
Ultra-rapid	Decreased efficacy; Active metabolite rapidly inactivated; usually require higher dose to offset inactivation	Increased efficacy; Rapid onset of effect; may require lower dose to prevent excessive accumulation of active metabolite

SOME DRUGS AND FOODS CAUSE ALTERED METABOLIZER PHENOTYPE

Certain drugs mimic the effect of genetic variations, effectively causing changes in metabolizer phenotype. For example, quinidine is an inhibitor of CYP2D6 activity. A patient taking quinidine is therefore a CYP2D6 poor metabolizer, similar to someone who carries a loss-of function variation in CYP2D6. In those patients, drugs that require the activity of CYP2D6, such as atomoxetine, will not be metabolized at the same rate as in most people. Certain foods can also mimic the effects of genetic variations. One of the most common examples is grapefruit juice, which is an inhibitor of CYP3A4. In people regularly drinking grapefruit juice, drugs that require the activity of CYP3A4, such as diazepam, will not be metabolized at the same rate as in most people.

WHAT MAKES PHARMACOGENOMICS POSSIBLE TODAY?

1. Sequencing of the human genome reveals 2.9 billion base pairs that are constant, narrowing down variability to about 3 million base pairs, of which 100,000 capture the full human variation and <10,000 may be pharmaceutically relevant.
2. Advances in genome sequencing technology make possible addressing those individual base pairs.
3. Automatization and miniaturization significantly drive down cost of DNA sequencing reaction.
4. Computer technology and computer networks facilitate handling of data.

CURRENT IMPACT

1. Pharmacogenomics broadly adopted in drug discovery and development phases in the pharmaceutical industry.
2. Pharmacogenomics research heavily invested upon by public and private companies
3. Pharmacogenomics seen as the future of medicine – so called personalized medicine.

CURRENT DEVELOPMENTS

1. Laboratory pharmacogenomic testing
2. Case-specific genetic testing
3. Race-based medications

FUTURE TRENDS

1. Point-of-care (Doctor's office/ Pharmacy) genetic testing.
2. Genetic profiling as part of a person's medical history.
3. Genetic-based medications.

PHARMACOGENOMICS IN THE CLINICAL SETTING

Awareness of the influence of gene variations on patient response to certain drugs can help physicians decide which type of drug therapy may be appropriate, and identify cases in which a patient isn't responding as anticipated to a drug. The examples that follow illustrate three categories for which pharmacogenomic knowledge can help inform therapeutic decisions: predicting and preventing adverse reactions, determining the efficacy of a drug for a particular patient, and predicting the optimal drug dose.

USING PHARMACOGENOMICS TO PREDICT AND PREVENT ADVERSE DRUG REACTIONS

Several drugs can cause severe or life-threatening reactions in patients with variations in genes that encode proteins that metabolize or are targets of the drugs. Knowing about patients' genetic variations can help physicians avoid drugs that may cause adverse reactions.

EXAMPLES OF DRUGS IN THIS CATEGORY

Abacavir (Ziagen®) is a nucleoside reverse transcriptase inhibitor used in combination with other antiretrovirals to treat HIV infection. An immunologically-mediated hypersensitivity reaction occurs in 5–8 %of patients taking abacavir, usually during the first six weeks after initiation of therapy. The hypersensitivity symptoms include a combination of fever, rash, gastrointestinal tract symptoms and respiratory symptoms that become more severe with continued dosing. Discontinuation of abacavir therapy results in reversal of symptoms. The abacavir hypersensitivity described above is associated with a variant allele of the major histocompatibility complex, HLA-B*5701. Patients who carry the HLA-B*5701 allele have an increased risk for developing a hypersensitivity reaction.HLA-B*5701 screening before abacavir treatment results in a significantly reduced number of hypersensitivity cases. The abacavir product labeling recommends genetic testing to detect the presence of HLA-B*5701.

CASE STUDY

JS is a 35 year-old man who has recently been diagnosed as HIV positive. Before initiating abacavir anti-retroviral therapy, his physician orders genetic testing to determine whether he carries the HLA-B*5701 allele, knowing that JS would develop fever, rash, nausea and fatigue if he carried the variant allele. The test confirmed that JS carries the HLA-B*5701 allele.

How did genetic testing help JS and his physician?

Knowing that JS carried the HLA-B*5701 variation indicated that he would likely experience a hypersensitivity reaction. JS's physician will probably not include abacavir in his antiretroviral regimen.

USING PHARMACOGENOMICS TO PREDICT EFFECTIVENESS

Several drugs are sub therapeutic or ineffective in patients with variations in genes that encode drug-metabolizing proteins or targets of the drugs. Knowing about patients' genetic variations can help physician's select drug therapies that will be most effective for individual patients. Below is an example of a drug in this category.

Clopidogrel (Plavix®) is a platelet inhibitor used in the treatment of a number of cardiovascular diseases. It is often prescribed for secondary prevention following acute coronary syndromes and for those undergoing percutaneous coronary intervention. However, despite clopidogrel treatments, up to one-quarter of patients experience a sub therapeutic antiplatelet response, resulting in a higher risk for ischemic events. Clopidogrel is a prodrug; its antiplatelet properties are exerted once it is converted to an active metabolite. A cytochrome P450 enzyme, CYP2C19, mediates the conversion of clopidogrel into the active metabolite. Patients who carry certain variations in CYP2C19 are considered poor metabolizers and show reduced ability to convert clopidogrel into its active metabolite, resulting in a diminished antiplatelet effect. Further, these patients are more likely to have an ischemic event following clopidogrel therapy. Approximately 2%–20 % of patients (depending on ethnicity) are likely to carry CYP2C19 variations.

CASE STUDY

JM is a 58 year-old man who recently had an acute myocardial infarction. To prevent subsequent ischemic events, JM's physician recommends antiplatelet therapy and prescribes clopidogrel. Six months later, JM suffered another acute MI, and his physician suspects that the patient has been non-adherent, or alternatively, that clopidogrel therapy may have been ineffective.

How would genetic testing help JM and his physician?

Determining JM's CYP2C19 genotype may reveal that he carries a variant that diminishes the antiplatelet effect of clopidogrel. If this were the case, alternative anti-platelet therapies may have been considered, reducing the chance that JM would suffer a second cardiac event. In patients taking both clopidogrel and the proton pump inhibitors omeprazole or esomeprazole, diminished antiplatelet activity and adverse cardiac outcomes have been observed. It is thought that omeprazole and esomeprazole inhibit the activity of CYP2C19, making patients who take these drugs de facto CYP2C19 poor metabolizers, similar to someone who carries a loss-of function variation in CYP2C19. In these patients, drugs that require the activity of CYPC19, such as clopidogrel, will not be metabolized at the same rate as in most people.

USING PHARMACOGENOMICS TO PREDICT OPTIMAL DOSE

Genetic variations can lead to an altered dosage regimen. Knowing whether a patient carries these genetic variations can assist physicians in determining optimal therapeutic dose. An example of a drug with an altered dosage regimen in patients with certain genetic variations is warfarin.

Warfarin (Coumadin®) is the most widely-prescribed anticoagulant used to treat and prevent thromboembolic diseases. It is metabolized by the CYP2C9 enzyme, and its anticoagulant effect is mediated by the enzyme VKORC1. Variation in the CYP2C9 gene causes some patients to have slow metabolism of warfarin and a longer half-life of the drug, resulting in higher than usual blood concentrations of warfarin and greater anticoagulant effect. Certain variations in the VKORC1 gene result in reduced activity of the enzyme and subsequently reduced synthesis of coagulation factors. The combination of slow warfarin metabolism caused by CYP2C9 gene variations and reduced coagulation caused by VKORC1 gene variations increases the risk of bleeding during warfarin therapy. Warfarin has a narrow therapeutic index; variations in CYP2C9 and VKORC1, in addition to several other patient characteristics, make it difficult to predict the effective dose. Those carrying certain CYP2C9 and VKORC1 variations are likely to require altered doses and may require prolonged time to reach a stable maintenance dose. The prevalence of these CYP2C9and VKORC1 variations is variable among racial and ethnic groups: up to 17 % of Caucasians, 4 % of African-Americans and less than 2% of Asians carry at least one variant of CYP2C9; while 37

%of Caucasians, 14 % of African-Americans, and 89 %of Asians carry at least one variant in VKORC1.

CASE STUDY

ML is a 65 year old woman who has recently been diagnosed with Atrial fibrillation. To reduce the risk of stroke and other thrombotic events, ML's physician recommends warfarin therapy. To estimate the initial dose, ML's clinical characteristics (age, sex, weight, diet) were considered. However, ML will need to return to the clinic every day for INR monitoring until a stable dose is determined, and then every few weeks thereafter for maintenance monitoring.

How would genetic testing help ML and her physician

Determination of ML's CYP2C9 and VKORC1 genotype would reveal whether she carries any Variations that alter her ability to metabolize and respond to warfarin. Knowing about any gene Variations before initiating therapy allows for more accurate initial dosing and faster INR Stabilization, and can reduce the risk for bleeding or clotting events.

PHARMACOGENOMICS AND GENETIC TESTING

Genetic tests that detect variations in the genes that control metabolism and response to certain drugs are commercially available. Costs and insurance coverage are variable, depending on the type of test ordered. Hospital and reference laboratories as well as clinical geneticists are valuable sources of information on the best test to order and interpretation of results.

ANTICIPATED BENEFITS OF PHARMACOGENOMICS

- **More powerful medicines:** Pharmaceutical companies will be able to create drugs based on the proteins, enzymes, and RNA molecules associated with genes and diseases. This will facilitate drug discovery
- **More accurate methods of determining appropriate drug dosages:** Current methods of basing dosages on weight and age will be replaced with dosages based on a person's genetics —how well the body processes the medicine and the time it takes to metabolize it. This will maximize the therapy's value and decrease the likelihood of overdose.
- **Better vaccines:** Vaccines made of genetic material, either DNA or RNA; promise all the benefits of existing vaccines without all the risks. They will activate the immune system but will be unable to cause infections. They will be inexpensive, stable, easy to store.
- **Better, safer drugs the first time:** Instead of the standard trial-and-error method of matching patients with the right drugs, doctors will be able to analyze a patient's genetic profile and prescribe the best available drug therapy from the beginning. Not only will this take the guess work out of finding the right drug, it will speed recovery time and increase safety as the likelihood of adverse reactions is eliminated.
- **Advanced screening for disease:** Knowing one's genetic code will allow a person to make adequate lifestyle and environmental changes at an early age

so as to avoid or lessen the severity of a genetic disease. Likewise, advance knowledge of particular disease susceptibility will allow careful monitoring, and treatments can be introduced at the most appropriate stage to maximize their therapy.

- **Improvements in the drug discovery and approval process:** Pharmaceutical companies will be able to discover potential therapies more easily using genome targets. Previously failed drug candidates may be revived as they are matched with the niche population they serve. The drug approval process should be facilitated as trials are targeted for specific genetic population groups providing greater degrees of success.
- **Decrease in the overall cost of health care:** Decrease in the numbcr of adverse drug reactions, the number of failed drug trials, the time it takes to get a drug approved, the length of time patients are on medication, the number of medications patients must take to find an effective therapy, the effects of a disease on the body (through early detection), and an increase in the range of possible drug targets will promote a net decrease in the cost of health care.

BARRIERS TO PHARMACOGENOMICS PROGRESS

- Complexity of finding gene variations that affect drug response
- Limited drug alternatives
- Disincentives for drug companies to make multiple pharmacogenomic products
- Educating healthcare providers

MORE BUSINESS

1. Pharmacogenomics may drive new business models based on developing preventive therapy for patients with genetic predispositions to disease.
2. Blockbuster drugs of today probably not possible if individual genetic variation becomes integrated with drug prescription, due to reduced market sizes.
3. Incorporation of genetic information into the diagnosis of disease and prescription of drugs will lead to new service industry.
4. Pharmacogenomics will foster safer, less toxic drugs

CONCLUSION

Pharmacogenomics represents the current state of cumulative human knowledge of how drugs work and why they work the way they are thought to work. Pharmacogenomics impacts all scientific fields of research studying how drugs work, and is based on the same assumptions on which those fields are based. Quite possibly, just as computer technology has had a great influence on pharmacy practice; Pharmacogenomics will help shape the practice of pharmacy in the future. It is important to note that the field of Pharmacogenomics is still developing, with new findings being rapidly reported. Clinical trials and other studies focusing on the benefits, risks and cost-effectiveness of using genetic information to inform drug therapy are underway. In the meantime, physicians and health care providers should be familiar with the concept that genetic variations can cause their patients to respond unexpectedly to drug therapy, and that in some cases, it may be appropriate to use genetic testing to guide therapeutic decisions.

REFERENCES

1. Collins FS. 2010. The Future of Personalized Medicine. NIH Medline Plus 5(1):2–3.
2. Lesko L. Regulatory Perspective on Warfarin Relabeling with Genetic Information. May 2007.
   Presentation at the 9th National Conference on Anti-Coagulation Therapy. www.fda.gov/downloads/Drugs/ScienceResearch/ResearchAreas/Pharmacogenetics/ucm085563.pdf. Accessed June 23, 2010.
3. Belle DJ, Singh H. (2008). Genetic Factors in Drug Metabolism. Am Fam Physician 77(11):1553–1560.
4. Indiana University Division of Clinical Pharmacology. P450 Drug interaction Table. 2010.
5. GlaxoSmithKline. Ziagen® (abacavir sulfate) product labeling. 2010.
6. Mallal S, Phillips E, Carosi G, Molina JM, Workman C, Tomazic J et al. (2008). HLA-B*5701 screening for hypersensitivity to abacavir. N Engl J Med 358(6):568–579.
7. Ellis KJ, Stouffer GA, McLeod HL, Lee CR. Clopidogrel pharmacogenomics and risk of inadequate platelet inhibition: U.S. FDA recommendations. (2009). Pharmacogenomics10(11):1799–1817.
8. Simon T, Verstuyft C, Mary-Krause M, Quteineh L, Drouet E, Meneveau N et al. (2009). Genetic determinants of response to clopidogrel and cardiovascular events. N Engl J Med 360(4):363–375.
9. Shuldiner AR, O'Connell JR, Bliden KP, Gandhi A, Ryan K, Horenstein RB et al. (2009) Association of cytochrome P450 2C19 genotype with the antiplatelet effect and clinical efficacy of clopidogrel therapy. JAMA 302(8):849–857.
10. Mega JL, Close SL, Wiviott SD, Shen L, Hockett RD, Brandt JT et al. Cytochrome p-450 polymorphisms and response to clopidogrel. N Engl J Med 2009; 360(4):354–362.
11. Bristol Meyers Squibb/Sanofi Pharmaceuticals Partnership. Plavix® (clopidogrel bisulfate) product labeling. 2011.
12. Ho PM, Maddox TM, Wang L, Fihn SD, Jesse RL, Peterson ED, Rumsfeld JS. (2009). Risk of Adverse Outcomes Associated With Concomitant Use of Clopidogrel and Proton Pump Inhibitors
13. Gage, BF. (2006). Pharmacogenetics-Based Coumarin Therapy. Hematology ASH Educ Prog Book. 467–473.
14. Reider MJ, Reiner AP, Gage BF, Nickerson DA, Eby CS, McLeod HL et al. (2005). Effect of VKORC1 Haplotypes on Transcriptional Regulation and Warfarin Dose. N Engl J Med 352(22):2285–2293.
15. Bristol Meyers Squibb Company. Coumadin®(warfarin sodium) product labeling. 2010.

PART - IV CASE STUDIES

102 Cardiovascular Case Studies

103 Respiratory Case Studies

104 Central Nervous System Case Studies

105 Gastro Intestinal Case Studies

106 Infection Case Studies

107 Endocrine Case Studies

108 Malignant Case Studies

109 Skin Case Studies

110 Liver Case Studies

111 Miscellaneous Case Studies

CHAPTER 102

Cardiovascular Case Studies

CASE STUDY – 1 – ANGINA

Mr. Robert a 58 years old taxi driver of Indian Origin attends community pharmacy with a prescription for glyceryltrinitate (GTN) spray 400 micro grams 1 or 2 puffs as required. He tells you that his doctor think he has angina and asked him to use the spray the next time he gets any minor chest pain or tightness.

Mr. Robert returns after few days complaining of headache after using the spray. He is reluctant to use the spray again. He asks pharmacist advise on managing his headache. He also smokes nearly 10 cigarettes a week and asks if he should now stop.

1. **What typical symptoms could a patient with angina present with?**
   (A) Chest tightness or heaviness which may be brought on by exertion or relieved by rest. It may radiate to one or both arms, the neck, jaw or teeth. Other associated symptoms include dyspnoea (shortness of breath) nausea, sweating and faintness.
2. **What are the risk factors for developing angina?**
   (A) Hyperlepidemia, smoking, hypertension, lack of exercise, poor diet, obesity, heavy alcohol consumption, contraceptive pills, stress and strain.
3. **What are the side effects of GTN spray?**
   (A) Postural hypotension, tachycardia, throbbing headache, dizziness, less commonly nausea, vomiting, heartburn, flushing.
4. **Mr. Robert's headache may be caused by the use of GTN spray. What can you recommend to him to help manage his headache?**
   (A) It is recommended that no more than 3 metered doses are taken at any 1 time and that there should be a minimum interval of 15 minutes between consecutive treatment. Mr.Robert may be advised to take paracetamol 500 mg tablets every 6-8 hrs to relieve his headache. If the headache persists or is sever he should arrange to see his doctor to discuss the treatment.
5. **What advice would you give Mr.Robert in relation to his smoking?**
   (A) Any one with angina should quit smoking. Smokers have a higher incidence of ischaemic heart disease and greater risk of dying. Nicotine

replacement therapy can be recommended as part of smoking cessation programme.

CASE STUDY – 2 – ATRIAL FIBRILLATION

Mr. Richard (62 Years) is admitted to emergency assessment unit at his local hospital complaining of palpitations, breathlessness and dizziness. He has 4-day history of some dizziness and palpitations. In the last 24 hrs he experienced additionally shortness of breath. He collapsed at home and was then admitted to hospital via emergency department. He experienced similar symptoms 2 months ago but did not seek medical advice and seemed to recover quickly.

Following information is obtained:

Previous Medical history:

Hypertension (diagnosed 3 years ago) no previous history of cardiovascular disease. The patient is a regular cigarette smoker (more than 20 per day) and drinks approximately 25 units of alcohol per week.

Drug history: No known allergies Mr. Richard has been prescribed Lisinopril tablets 10mg daily but was poorly compliant with treatment.

DIAGNOSIS : ATRIAL FIBRILLATION

Relevent test results : Full blood count, liver function tests, electrolytes and renal function were all normal at admission and throughout the admission up to discharge.

Mr. Richard is subsequently transferred to cardiology ward where his continuing atrial fibrillation is latest can fumed as persistent atrial fibrillation. As the ward clinical pharmacist you are responsible for daily renew of drugs chest and advice medical and nursing staff on drug treatment.

1. **What is atrial fibrillation?**

   (A) Atrial Fibrillation is an arrhythmia in which electrical activity in the atria is disorganized. The AV node receives more electrical impulses than it can conduct and most are blocked resulting in irregular ventricular rhythm.

2. **What are the most common signs and symptoms exhibited by patents with atrial fibrillation? Indicate which of these signs and symptoms the patients in exhibiting.**

   (A) Symptoms : Breathlessness/dyspnoea, palpitations, syncope or dizziness, chest discomfort or stroke/ ischaemic attack.

   Signs : - Irregular pulse, ventricular rate 120-180 beats per minute. ECG shows fine oscillations of the baseline with no clear P-waves. Rapid and irregular QRS rhythm.

3. **What are the two options in terms of treatment strategy that may be employed to manage atrial fibrillation. Indicate what would be the appropriate strategy that you could recommend to doctor managing the patient and why you think this could be the case.**

(A) The two options are rate control or rhythm control. Rate control is the most appropriate in this case as Mr. Richard is 624 Years old. Atrial fibrillation appears to be of long standing and may have been present 2 months ago. His lisinopril shall be stopped as his B.P will be controlled with beta blocker.

4. **Assuming a rate control strategy to be used what class of drug should be the first line treatment for the particular patient? If the first line drug was contraindicated what class of drug could be used as alternative treatment.**

   (A) A Beta-blocker in suitable first line treatment for rate control. A rate limiting calcium channel blocker could be used in those where beta-blocker is not suitable, such as asthmatics.

5. **Assuming the patient to be discharged on a beta-blocker and aspirin, what counseling does he require?**

   (A) Mr. Richard need to be advised to take his medication regularly. If he experiences any problems he should talk to his GP or pharmacist.

He should be advised to take aspirins in morning after food. The tablet may be dispersed in water or taken whole with water. The beta-blocker should be taken regularly. Mr.Richard should be told that if he experiences side effects with this medication, such as dizziness, he should not stop taking it suddenly but should speak with his GP or pharmacist.

CASE STUDY – 3 – MYOCARDIAL INFARCTION

Mr. William B a 70 year old retired bank employee complains of chest pain after climbing stairs at his daughter house. In the ambulance he is administered aspirin 300 mg on arrival at hospital and subsequent examination and review by the admitting doctor the following information is obtained.

Previous Medical History

Hypertension (10 years) type 2 diabetes mellitus (Recently diagnosed, currently diet controlled). The patient is a regular cigarette smoker (More than 20 per day) and drinks nearly 20 units of alcohol per week. He has osteoarthritis of the knee.

Family History

Father died following myocardial infarction at 60 Years of age. No material history of cardiovascular disease.

Drug History

Allergies

Trimethoprim Mr. William has been taking diclofenac tablet 75 mg (twice daily)and nifedipine 20 mg (twice daily). Bothe were stopped on admission.

Signs and symptoms – on examination:

Temperature	- Normal
BP	- 160/90 mmHg
Heart rate	- 75 beats per minute regular
Respiration rate	- 13 breaths per min

No basal crackles in lungs

An ECG taken immediately on arrival reveals ST elevation of 3 mm in inferior leads.

DIAGNOSIS: MYOCARDIAL INFARCTION.

Relevant test results : Full blood count, Liver function tests, electrolytes and renal function, total cholesterol , blood glucose were taken at admission.

1. **What further diagnostic and biochemical tests should be ordered to help confirm the diagnosis?**
   (A) Troponin: Troponin enzymes consist of tropinin T,C and I which are located within cardiac and skeletal muscle. Cardiac isoforms of tropinin T and I are exclusively expressed in cardiac myocytes. They act as sensitive and specific markers of cardiac damage. An initial rise in tropinin may be seen as early as 3 to 4 hrs after cardiac event and is usually measured on admission to hospital. However a rise in tropinin may be delayed therefore the initial measurement taken on admission is repeated by a further blood sample 12 hrs after the onset of chest pain. The troponin assay has prognostic information that can determine mortality risk in acute coronary syndrome and define which patients may benefit from aggressive medical therapy and early coronary revascularization.

Creatine kinase (CK) occurs in high concentration in the brain, cardiac and skeletal muscle and is elevated in the blood with muscle damage. A rise in CK in seen in acute myocardial infarction but also in other conditions. The more specific marker is creatine kinase MB (CK-MB) which is an isoenzyme of creatine – kinase that is more specific for cardiac muscle damage. CK or CK-MB will rise approximately 4 hours after on acute cardiac event and will reach peak after 24 hours and will remain raised for 3-4 days.

2. **What is myocardial infarction and what are the classic symptoms?**
   (A) Myocardial infarction occur when the blood supply to a part of heart is interrupted. This is most commonly due to occlusion (blockage) of coronary artery following rupture of an atherosclerotic plague in wall of artery. The resulting ischemia and acute shortage of oxygen supply can cause damage and or death of heart muscle (myocardium). Symptoms are severe cardiac pain, Chest tightness, sweating, breathlessness, nausea and dyspnoea.
3. **Explain the mechanism of action of thrombolytics such as reteplase in acute myocardial infarction.**
   (A) Fibrinolytic agents such as reteplase enhance their breakdown of occlusive thrombosis by the activation of plasminogen to form plasmin.
4. **Following the initial dose of heparin (5000 units) what dose of heparin should be administered by I.V infarction and for how long?**
   (A) Intraveneous infusion of heparin 1000 units per hour starting after the second reteplase bolus. Heparin should be administered for at least 24 hours preferably 48-72 hours arming to keep activated partial thromboplastin time (APTT) values 1.5-2 times normal.

5. **What classes of drugs should be initiated as secondary prevention treatment following acute myocardial infarction in the patient.**
   (A) Beta-blockers, statins, ACE inhibitors; antiplatelet therapy with aspirin.
6. **As this patient has type 2 diabetes mellitus**
   (a) Which drug/drug class mention above as standard secondary prevention may cause problems in this patient.
   (b) What problems may be experienced in the use of this drug/drug class in a patient with type 2 diabetes mellitus.
   (A) Beta-blockers may be a problem in this patient because they can mask the usual signs of hypoglycemia. An alternative would be a rate limiting calcium channel blocker such as diltiazem, nifedipine, Amlodipine.
7. **If this patient is initiated on statin as cholesterol lowering treatment when should the total cholesterol next be checked following drug initiation.**
   (A) After 8-12 weeks minimum interval of at least 6 weeks.
8. **What counseling should the patient receive regarding the side effects of statins?**
   (A) Simvastatin, like other inhibitors of HMG-COA reductase occasionally causes myopathy manifested as muscle pain, tenderness or weakness. Myopathy sometimes take the form of rhabdomyolysis with or without acute renal failure secondary to myoglobinuria and very rare fatalities have occurred.

   Concomitant prescribing of drugs that increase the plasma statin concentration (Fibrates) will increase the risk of muscle toxicity.
9. **Mr. William experiences a chest infection 4 days post admission and is prescribed amoxicillin 500 mg 3 times daily and erythromycin 500 mg 4 times daily. What problems may this cause with patients statin therapy.**

   Erythromycin may cause increase in serum levels of simvastatin. The committee on safety of medicine (CSM) has advised that this should not be co-prescribed with simvastatin. At this instance pharmacist should check local policies for management of hospital acquired chest infection/pneumonia to ascertain first and second line choices. If Erythromycin or any macrolide cannot be avoided then a practical way is to avoid taking any dose of simvastatin for the duration of the course of macrolide.

CASE STUDY – 4 – HEART FAILURE

Mr.Roy is a 70 years old man who was admitted in the emergency department complaining of increasing shortness of breath. He has woken in the middle of night, struggling for breath. On arrival at hospital and on subsequent examination and review by the duty doctor the following information is obtained.

History of presenting complain

Shortness of breath and tiredness increasing over the last two months and is able to walk approximately 20 kilometers

Past Medical History

Ischaemic heart disease over 12 years myocardial infarction 2 years ago Hypertension – 15 years.

Social History

The patient is a regular cigarette smoker (more than 30 per day) and drinks approximately 50 units of alcohol per week.

Drug history on admission : No Known allergies.

Signs and symptoms on examination :

Temperature	-	Normal
BP	-	120/80 mmHg
Heart rate	-	90 beats per minute, Irregular
Swelling of ankles		
Weight	-	95 Kg
ECG	-	Normal
CXR	-	Cardiomegaly

Biochemistry results on admission day:

Na^+	-	Normal
K^+	-	Normal
Urea	-	17 mmol/L (0-7.5 mmol/L)
Creatinine	-	170 micromol/L (35-125 micromaol/L)
TC	-	Normal
Blood Glucose	-	Normal
Bilirubin	-	Normal
ALT	-	Normal
Alk phos	-	Normal

Thyroid function tests were also performed and are within normal range. A full blood count parameters were normal and within range.

***Diagnosis*: Diagnosis of acute heart failure is male.**

1. **What signs and symptoms patient experiences that he has heart failure? Does he have right or left sided heart failure or both?**

   (A) Symptoms

   (a) Shortness of breath (lung contusion) left sided heart failure

   (b) Lethargy/ tiredness

   (c) Swelling of ankles and pitting to the knees

Signs

1. Increasing weight due to increased fluid retention
2. Cardiomegaly on CXR.
3. Increased fluid retention in the lungs due to left sided heart failure.

   The patient has both left and right sided heart failure as he is showing signs and symptoms like swelling of ankles and lung congestion.

2. **What systems is adopted to classify heart failure in well accepted classification based on severity of symptoms.**

   (A) The new York Heart Association (NYHA) classification is well accepted classification based on severity of symptoms.

Class 1 – No symptoms with normal physical activity

Class II – Slight limitation and shortness of breath on moderate to sever exertion.

Class III – Marked limitation of activity , less than ordinary activity causes shortness of breath

Class IV – Severe disability, dyspnea at rest, no physical activity possible without discomfort.

3. **What drug treatment should be inhibited for immediate relief of oedema associated with acute heart failure.**

   (A) Diuretic therapy such as furosemide would be appropriate. The aim of furosemide treatment is to relieve symptoms such as shortness of breath and to make patient more comfortable. A dose of furosemide 40 mg twice daily would be appropriate.

4. **What parameter should be monitored for treatment of oedema?**

   (A) Blood pressure : To ensure it as normal. BP should be maintained regularly throughout day.

   Heart Rate: To maintain normal around 70-80 beats per minute

   Patient Body weight : Patients weight to be monitored on daily basis to ensure that excess fluid is removed.

   Fluid balance: The total amount of fluid the patient consumes and excretes must be monitored.

   Urea and electrolytes – Sodium, potassium, urea and creatinine require close daily monitoring. The main aim is to normalize and to avoid in particular, drops in electrolysis such as sodium and potassium . other electrolytes such as magnesium and calcium need to be checked regularly.

5. **What are the main aims of drug treatment in acute heart failure?**

   (A) Ensure appropriate diuretic therapy.

   Relieve congestion and to monitor the patient for improvement in signs and symptoms such as shortness of breath, swelling of ankles etc.

   Monitoring of Weight Loss

   Maintaining BP and Heart rate

   Monitoring of urea and electrolysis

6. **What side effects can occur while initiating the therapy with ACE inhibitor and how can these side effects can be minimized?**

   Initially after first drug therapy hypertension may occur while ACE inhibitors are introduced. This effect may be partiality pronounced if the patient is taken high dose of loop diuretic. Temporary withdrawal of loop diuretic could be considered but not appropriate. In such case, it may cause rebound pulmonary oedema. ACE inhibitor at low dose (Ramipril 1.25 mg daily at night while the patient is lying down).

CHAPTER 103

Respiratory Case Studies

CASE STUDY – 1 – ASTHMA

Julie a 32 years old woman weighing 80 kg was admitted to casualty ward with history of increased breathlessness and wheezing, over last 4 days. She is known to have had asthma for 15 years and has smoked more than 10 cigarettes per day since the age of 18 years. Her last hospital admission was 2 months ago. She lives alone in 10th floor. On medical examination the following were found

- **Audible wheeze throughout the chest**
- **Not able to speak in sentences**
- **Tachycardia – pulse 130 beats per minute**
- **Tachypnoeic – respiratory rate 25 breaths per minute**

1. **Explain why this patient is tachycardic and tachypnoeic?**

   (A) Tachy cardia is an increase in heart rate over 100 beats per minutes. This is due to excessive use or side effects of beta agonist, it can be used by anxiety and Panic which a patient may experience during asthma attack. Tachypnoeic is an increase in respiratory rate due to airway narrowing and constriction.

2. **Describe what other tests would be of importance in this patient at the time of admission?**

   (A) Other tests would be helpful in this patient are FEV1,FVC and blood gases. The spirometry values provide data not only on the expiration of air but also on the time taken for forced expiration. (FEV1- Forced Expiratory Volume, FVC- Forced Vital Capacity). In normal patients it would be in the region of 75% and in patients with obstruction the ratio FEV/FVC will be reduced.

3. **Explain how the severity of acute asthma is estimated and what investigation should be done.**

   (A) Patients should be assessed by GP every 3 months. Pharmacist should routinely review the patents if medication alters and at least every 3 months. The following symptoms should be assessed

   (a) Episodic wheeze

   (b) Cough

   (c) Shortness of breath

   (d) Number of attacks

Investigation include

(a) Peak expiratory flow rate

(b) Lung function tests

(c) Skin prick tests to identify allergens

Clinical features of acute severe asthma include

(a) Inability to speak continuously

(b) Respiratory rate 725 breaths per Minute

(c) Tachycardia 110 beats per minute

Life threatening characteristics include

(a) Silent chest and cyanosis

(b) Exhaustion confusion and coma

(c) Bradycardia or hypotension

4. What are the aims of asthma treatment?

(A) The aims of asthma treatment are

- Effective control of asthma symptoms
- Positive quality of life
- Minimal acute hospital admissions.

5. Critically review the Non-Pharmacological therapies that are available for people with asthma.

(A) Non-Pharmacological therapies include

- Lifestyle (Exercise and stop smoking)
- Avoidance of precipitating factors (Pollutants, House dust mites, Pollens and fungal spores)
- Flu vaccination
- Avoidance of medicines like aspirin, NSAIDS etc.
- Occupational hazards (Veterinary medicines, Baking, Laundry).

6. Discuss the role of asthma management plan for this patient?

(A) Understand disease

(B) Can analyze the medicine why it is prescribed and how it should be monitored

(C) Appropriate health outcomes

(D) Effective chronic disease management will prevents exacer-bations and hospital admissions.

CASE STUDY – 2 – COPD

Mr. John 75 Years old man admitted to hospital very short breath. He used to work in docks as clerk and has smoked 50 cigarettes daily for 25 years and stopped 3 years ago. His previous medical history includes COPD, recurrent infective exacerbation, type 2 diabetes mellitus on insulin 20 units b.d for 15 years, retinopathy, Ischemic heart disease, coronary artery bypass graft, HT,MI, Atrial fibrillation, High cholesterol.

The patient was discharged from hospital 2 weeks ago with antibiotics. There was same improvement but still very short of breath at rest. 5 days ago with worsening shortness of breath over previous week, the patient took clarithromycin 500 mg bid. Four days ago he took prednisolone 30 mg daily but has now stopped with no improvement. He is using nebuliser 8 times daily (salbutamol + Ipratropium). Because he was no better his daughter called an amubulance.

On arrival he had shortness of breath on exertion, Cough, Chronic, Chronic wheeze, No chest pain, No palpitations, ankle swelling no worse than moral, both legs sollens to upper calf, orthopnoea. The patient sleeps up right and gets paroxysmal nocturnal dyspnoea if lying flat.

Systems Review : Bowels - OK; Genetourinary – poor stream, No haematuria, No dysuria, No allergies.

Medicines: Aspirin 300 mg O.D, Diltiazen 300 mg O.D, Bendroflumethazide 2.5 mg O.D, Losartan 50 O.D, Furosemide 80 mg O.D, Atorvastatin 10 mg O.D, Carbocisteine 500 mg q.D.S, insulatard 20 i.u b.d, Ferrous Sulfate 300 mg t.d.s, omeprazole 20 mg O.D, Salbutamol 2.5 mg Ipratropium 500 µg t.d.s nebulised.

Diagnosis: Infective exacerbation of COPD with heart failure.

1. **Discuss the role of smoking history and calculate the total pack years this patient has been smoking to.**

   (A) Cigarette smoking is the single most important risk factor for developing COPD. Smoker with impaired lung function are likely to die from a atherosclerotic vascular disease. Some smokers are very susceptible to impaired lung function. Total pack years in calculated in this manner

   $$\frac{50 \times 25}{20} = 62.5 \text{ pack year.}$$

2. **Critically review the Johns list of medicines.**

   (A) Aspirin

3. **Describe pharmaceutical care plan for continued treatment of the patient.**

   (A) See Table 103.1

Table 103.1

Case issues and plan

Case Issues	Care Plan
Patient understanding of medicines	Discuss with patient the need for each medicine
Use of Medicine devices	Monitor and assure the use of nebulizer
Blood Glucose	Check the hemoglobin (HBA1C) review the dose of insulin
Monitor for chest infection	Raised WCC with raised neutrophils will require antibiotics.
Monitor patients nutrition	Check the patients BMI and record dyspnoea score
Verify the use of vaccines	pneumococcal and flu vaccination are recommended
Action plans	Patient is encouraged to take prompt action, this may involve the use of antibiotics and oral steroids.
Patient organization	Discuss with patient the availability of patient support including british lung foundation

CHAPTER 104

Central Nervous System Case Studies

CASE STUDY – 1 – A CASE OF INSOMNIA

Mr. Antony 21 years old student came to the local pharmacy last week with a 5 days prescription for diazepam 10 mg tablets are to be taken at night. The drug was prescribed to him by his GP. Mr. Antony started suffering from insomnia. During the day he feels very tired, anxious and tearful. It is now 3 days since he taking the prescription but he claims he is still not able to sleep properly.

1. **How is insomnia defined?**
   (A) Insomnia is characterized by the inability to sleep and or to remain asleep for a reasonable period. The sleep disturbance is observed at least 3 times per week and at least one month.
2. **What are the risk factors for its development?**
   (A) The most common risk factors for development of insomnia are as follows
   - Depression
   - Excessive use of alcohol
   - Excessive use of caffeine
   - Stress, pain
   - Hypomanic/Manic Episodes
   - Circadian rhythm sleep disorders
   - Nocturnal polyuria, diabetes, kidney diseases hormonal imbalances
   - Sleep apnoea etc.
3. **What are the side effects of diazepam?**
   (A) The most common side effects of benzodiazepines are drowsiness, Muscle weakness, lightheadedness, dizziness, ataxia, blurring of vision, confusion and apathy.
4. **What alternative preparation could you recommend for Mr. Antony?**
   (A) Diazepam is better indicated if insomnia is associated with day time anxiety, other benzodiazepine prescribed include Nitrazepam, Flurazepam, Loprazolam and Temazepam.

The sedative anti psychotic promethazine hydrochloride is sometimes used to facilitate sleep with 25-50 mg recommended dose.

5. **What counseling could you give Mr. Antony?**

Relevent sleep hygiene, some traditional remedies for insomnia have included drinking warm milk before bed time, taking warmbath in evening, exercising vigorously for half an hour in afternoon having light evening meal, avoiding mentally stimulating activities, making sure to get up early in the morning and to go to bed at reasonable hour. Distraction in the bedroom, including excessive light and noise should be avoided.

CASE STUDY – 2 – A CASE OF DEMENTIA, ALZHEIMER'S TYPE

Wife of Mr. Peter who is 68 years old female seeking some advice from the pharmacist and she is concerned about behavioral changes in her husband from the last few months. His mood is very volatile, somewhat unpredictable, his memory and concentration seem to be very poor and at times he may be very impulsive. For the first time he is now using words and language that are rude and vulgar. Local psychiatrist assessed that Mr. Peter is mildly confused with both decreasing in BP and Sodium level. He was finally diagnosed with ALZHEIMER'S type dementia.

1. **What are Alzheimer's type dementia clinical signs and symptoms?**

   (A) Alzheimer's disease is a neuro-degenerative disease characterized by progressive cognitive deterioration accompanied by neurological, psychiatric and behavioral disorders. This is characterized by loss of short term memory (Amnesia) accompanied by relative integrity of older memories. As the disorder Progresses cognitive impairment extends to domains of language (Aphasia) skilled movements (Apraxia) recognition (Agnosia) decision making and planning.

2. **What are the suitable treatment option for Mr. Peter?**

   (A) Donepezil, Galantamine and Rivastigmine should be used as treatment for moderate stages of AD.

3. **Out line pharmaceutical care plan for Mr. Peter. What are the goals of therapy in Alzheimer's dementia?**

   (A) People with dementia may develop symptoms such as depression, restlessness, aggressive behavior and psychosis (Delusions and Hallucinations) possible medications to be prescribed include atypical antipsychotics. Sodium valproate and carbamazepine are sometimes advised to reduce aggression and agitation. Ant depression may be helpful not only in improving persistently low mood but also in controlling both irritability and rapid mood swings. Tricyclic anti-depressants such as amytryptylime, imipramine are likely to increase confusion and might also cause dry mouth, blurred vision, constipation, difficulty in urination and hypotension.

4. **Describe the prognosis and long term complications of Alzheimer's dementia.**

   (A) People with AD eventually loose the ability to carryout the daily activities such as dressing,undressing toileting, travelling, handling money. As a result they require high level of utmost care on them.

5. **What are the social pharmacy issues related to Mr. Peter case?**

   The patient should be helped to lead an active life with interesting and stimulating daily advertises. By minimizing distress and agitation and limiting the use of sedative drugs.

CASE STUDY – 3 – A CASE OF SCHIZOPHRENIA

Mr. Sam 28 years old research student comes to pharmacy in distresses state. His mood is volatile, smells of body odours and he has sensations of insects crawling under his skin. Last few days he has been sick and absolutely convinced that all this is because his neighbour some how puts some toxic gases in to this house. He bought some of his vomit to be analyzed so that he will be able to take appropriate action against his neighbour.

1. **What are the typical signs and symptoms of schizophenia?**

   (A) The disease in often described in terms of positive and negative symptoms. Positive symptoms include delusions, auditory hallucinations and thought disorders. Negative symptoms include flat, blunted or constricted affect and motion, poverty of speech and lack of motivation. The patient may show both disorganized speech and behavior.

2. **Is there any laboratory data in making diagnosis of schizophrenia?**

   (A) The diagnosis is based on self-reported experiences of the patient. There are no reliable biological markers for schizophrenia, though studies suggest that genetics and neurobiology are contributory factors.

3. **Describe pharmaceutical care plan in the case reported.**

   (A) The meaningful approach could take is to make sure that the patient is referred to GP for an immediate assessment by community mental health team. The patient need to be compulsorily admitted in psychiatric ward.

4. **Expand the prognosis and comorbidity issues relevant to the condition of schizophrenia.**

   (A) Women tend to show higher recovery rates than men. Acute and sudden onset of schizophrenia is associated with higher rates of recovery while gradual onset is associated with lower rates. Comorbidity is also high with both depression and anxiety disorders.

5. **Any alternative non-pharmacological therapies for the treatment of schizophrenia?**

   (A) Cognitive behavioral psychotherapeutic approach may be offered. This may focus on direct symptoms reduction, social functioning and insight.

CHAPTER 105

Gastro Intestinal Case Studies

CASE STUDY – 1 – DUODENAL ULCER

Mr.Bob is 57 years old man who was admitted after starting to pass black stools. He has 2 days history of severe stomach pain and has suffered with indigestion for some months. He is life long smoker with mild chronic cardiac failure for which he is taking enalapril maleate 5 mg twice daily for 2 years. He also started taking naproxen 500 mg twice daily for arthritis. His Hb was reported as 10.38%, platelets 162 × 10^9/L, he was mild tachycardic 90 beats per minute and has slightly low BP 160/75 mmHG. He return from endoscopy this morning and has been newly diagnosed as having bleeding duodenal ulcer.

1. **What risk factors does Mr. Bob have for bleeding peptic ulcer?**

   (A) The prevalence of peptic ulcer increases with age and *Helicobacter pylori* infection increases with age. Mr. Bob is 57 years old and peptic ulcer are more common in smokers and alcoholics. Further Mr. Bob is taking NSAID drug naproxen which is associated with ulceration.

2. **Has his treatment appropriate?**

   (A) Mr. Bob is not very old and is not shocked and active bleeding has not been reported. He had the fluid replacement as blood was not needed as he did not have any signs of hypovolemic shock and his Hb levels are above 10 gm.

3. **Should Mr. Bob be given proton pump inhibitor? If yes what would you recommend?**

   (A) Mr. Bob had recent bleed and in this situation he should be given an infusion of omeprazole which may prevent the bleeding by stabilizing the clotting process. There fore it would be advisable to start omeprazole 40 mg twice daily by oral route.

4. **What would be next stage of treatment for Mr. Bob?**

   (A) Mr. Bob needs full-dose PPI for 4 to 6 weeks to heal ulcer. He should be tested for H.Pylori if the test is positive he should have eradication treatment.

5. **What medication Mr. Bob should continue?**

   (A) Enalapril Maleate - 5 mg twice daily
   Furosemide - 40 mg daily
   Omeprazole - 20 mg twice daily

If possible NSAID should be permanently stopped and consideration to be given to manage pain relief. Paracetamol would be safer drug with an opoid such as codeine, however as he has rheumatoid arthritis. It is unlikely that this paracetamol will control his pain and in such case lowest dose of ibuprofen should be initiated. When his treatment for ulcer healing is completed he should take PPI (Omeprazole 20 mg) daily for gastroprotection.

1. **What counseling is required for Mr. Bob?**
   (A) Simple life style advice, avoiding fatty foods, reducing weight, giving up smoking.
2. **What follow should Mr. Bob have?**
   (A) He should be retested for H.Pyroli and if this test is positive further course of eradication treatment using different antibacterial combination is required. He should also be reviewed and given advice on life style and management of dyspeptic symptoms.

CASE STUDY – 2 – ULCERATIVE COLITIS

Mrs. Tina has been admitted with acute severe ulcerative colitis. This is her 3rd flar this year. This time she has 5 day history of bloody diarrhoea with severe abdominal pain. On average she is opening her bowels and 8 times a day. She is commonly taking mesalazine 800 mg 3 times daily as prednisolone 20 mg daily. She has fever and pulse rate of 95 beats per minute. She is due to have abdominal x-ray and stool culture.

1. **Why is she consuming mesalazine?**
   (A) This is useful in maintaining remission in patients with ulcerative colitis.
2. **What adverse effects should Mrs. Tina particularly aware of?**
   (A) The most important adverse effects (Stevens johnson syndrome, pancreatits, agranulocytosis) are rare all patients should be advised of symptoms such as bleeding, bruising, purpura, sore throat, fever or malaise.
3. **What signs and symptoms indicate that she need to be admitted**
   (A) Her symptoms (more than six motions a day) increased pulse rate recent temperature suggest systemic disease which requires urgent attention.
4. **Why is she having abdominal X-ray and stool cultures done?**
   (A) Stool cultures to rule out infective cause of the disease. Abdominal X-ray to exclude toxic dilation of colon are bowel perforation which require surgical attention.
5. **Why is surgery likely?**
   (A) In ulcerative colitis surgery (A colectomy) offers hope of cure by removing the diseased portion of GIT. This contrasts with crohn's disease while surgery is undertaken for symptomatic relief.
6. **What is the importance and use of cyclosporine?**
   (A) Cyclosporine is used to suppress the immune system and has rapid onset of action. The cyclosporine will be

given through a drip if it is successful in controlling the disease she will be given oral treatment

7. **What drugs would you expect Mrs.Tina to use?**
   (A) Cyclosporine – 6-8 mg/kg per day
   Prednisolone – 40-60 mg daily
   Co-trimoxazole – 300mg 3 times daily
   Mesalazone – 800 mg 3 times daily
8. **What future treatment she likely to receive?**
   (A) Cyclosporine will be tailed off as azathioprine (1.5 – 2.5 mg/kg per day) is slowly started. This will be continued for 3to6 months to allow azathioprine to start working. Co-trimoxazole will be discontinued when cyclosporine is stopped. Patient often remain on corticosteroids.

CASE STUDY –3 – GASTRO OESOPHAGEAL REFLUX

James is 4 months old baby born at 35 weeks gestation. He has been in hospital since birth with variety of problems. He is now feeding enterally via bottle he has been on feed thickners and ranitidine for last month for Gastro Oesophageal reflux but symptoms still persist.

1. **What is gastro Oesophageal reflux and what are the main symptoms?**
   (A) Spontaneous regurgitation of gastric contents in to the oesophagus is defined as gastro Oesophageal reflux. When reflux leads to recurrent regurgitation or vomiting problems start to rise, irritability and abnormal posturing may also become common.
2. **What alternative class of drugs may work in the same way as ranitidine but more effective?**
   (A) Proton pump inhibitors block the acid production more completely than ranitidine and may achieve greater acid control.
3. **Name 3 prokinetic agents which could be added to the regimen?**
   (A) Domperidone, Metoclopramide and Erythromycin.
4. **What is the rational use of these products?**
   (A) By increasing speed of transit of stomach contents through digestive track.
5. **Briefly mention the potential issues of domperidone, metoclopromide and erythromycin?**
   (A) Domperidone – widely used, unlikely to cause CNS side effects as it does not cross BBB.
   Metoclopromide – Very effective, main disadvantage is possibility of central side effects due to ability to cross BBB.
   Erythromycin – Known to increase peristalsis through the gut.
6. **What is the potential risk of using metronidazole along with ranitidine suspension?**
   (A) Ranitidine suspension is formulated with alcohol as an excipients. Metronidazole may react with the alcohol in the blood to cause disulfiram like reaction leading to flushing and tachycardia.

CHAPTER 106

Infection Case Studies

CASE STUDY – 1 – MENINGITIS

Mr.Raju a 19 years old student presents himself to the GP with severe headache, vomiting and photophobia since early morning. On examination the patient has fever and he is unable to touch his chin to his knees. He does not have rash and is alert. The doctor administered benzyl penicillin I.V 1.2 g and the patient was transferred urgently by ambulance to accident and emergency ward. Mr.Raju weighs 70 kg is a smoker and takes caffeine tablets. Prior to examination but otherwise takes no regular medication. He remembers receiving meningitis vaccine at school, on arrival to hospital his vital signs are recorded as follows. Heart rate – 125 beats per minute, Temp - 101^0 F, Respiratory rate – 28 breaths /minute , BP-100/70 mm Hg.

Planned investigation include

- Lumbar Puncture and CSF Analysis
- Blood Cultures
- Coagulation Screen
- Urea and electrolytes and full blood count
- Liver function tests

The patient is diagnosed with suspected meningitis and the treatment plan is as follows.

- Cefotaxime I.V 2 g q.d.s
- Dexamethasone 10 mg q.d.s

  Aedonv I.V 700 mg t.d.s

  Paracetamol 500 mg q.d.s

  Cyclizine I.V 50 mg t.d.s

  Enoxaparin S.C 40 mg O.D (Post Lumber Puncture)

1. What are the signs and symptoms of meningitis and meningococcal septicemia (Bloodstream Infection)?

(A) The clinical signs of meningitis are

(a) Fever

(b) Neck stiffness

(c) altered mental state

(d) Headache

Three other classical signs of meningitis are

(a) Dislike of bright lights (Photophobia)

(b) Vomiting

(c) Rash

Additional signs and symptoms that may indicate septicemia are

(a) Severe pain and aches in limbs and joints

(b) Very cold hands and feet

(c) Shivering

(d) Rapid breathing

(e) Red or Purple spots

(f) Diarrhea and Stomach Cramps

2. What are the important pathogens and appropriate treatment options for bacterial meningitis?

(A) The main organism causing bacterial meningitis are N. Meningitidis, diplococcus pneumoniae and streptococcus pneumoniae, H.influenzae also accounts. Due to the increasing resistance to penicillin in pneumococcal and H.influenzae the 3rd generation cephalosporins, cefotaxime and cefatrixone are currently recommended as first line agents for patients hospitalized with suspected bacterial meningitis. The drugs of choice is penicillins, cephalosporins allergic patients is chloramphenicol.Addition of ampicillin or amoxicillin is recommended in patients over 55 years of age to cover listeria. In several clinical trails dexamethasone demonstrated significant beneficial effect in pneumococcal and meningococcal meningitis.

3. Which antibiotic regimens achieve therapeutic concentration in CSF and which should be avoided?

(A) Ampicillin, Amoxicillin, cefotaxime and Ceftriaxone administered IV to achieve peak CSF levels and are effective against streptococcus pneumonia, Neisseria meningitis and H.influenzae. Benzylpenicillin achieves peak CIF levels and are reliable for treating strains of streptococcus pneumonia and N.meningitidis, but not H.influenzae and therefore cefotaxime or ceftriaxone are more reliable for H.influenzae meningitis.

4. What is the rational for prescribing acyclovir in cases of suspected meningitis?

(A) Acyclovir is prescribed to treat encephalitis (inflammation of brain parenchyma) caused by herpes herpes simplex virus. Symptoms of encephalitis include fever, headache, mental status (Lethargy, Irritability, behavioral and personality charges).

5. What are the goals of therapy in community acquired bacterial meningitis?

(A) The goals of therapy are to control the infection and minimise morbidity and mortality. Early recognition of septicaemia and timely intervention by administering high-flow of oxygen and providing volume resuscitation and identification of pathogen for treatment purpose and quick administration of antibiotics in activity ill-patients.

6. How therapy is monitored?

(A) Close observation and maintain of vital signs during treatment, serum c-reactive protein and white cell count should be monitored and repeated examination of CSF.

7. What are the potential long term complications of meningitis?

(A) Fatality rate of meningitis due to streptococcus pneumonia and N.Meningitidis are 35% and 15%, long term neurologic problems like hearing loss my occur.

8. What are social pharmacy issues including life style?

(A) Patients with meningococcal meningitis should be isolated after atleast 48 hrs of antibiotic therapy of prevent spread of infection to others. Spread of meningococcal infections between family member and close contacts and chemo-prophylaxis is recommended preferably within 24 hours. Rifampicin 600 mg twice for 2 days.

Smoking is a risk factor for carriage of meningococcal bacteria and the patient in advised to stop smoking. Health workers who has administered mouth to mouth resuscitation or had prolonged face to face contact with patient require prophylactic treatment.

CASE STUDY – 2 – DIABETIC FOOT INFECTION

Mr. Peter 59 years old person is admitted in accident and emergency ward by his daughter due to fatigue, weakness, confusion and drowsiness. Mr. Peter has 15 years history of type-2 diabetes mellitus and hyper-cholesterolemia, he also has history of IHD and underwent coronary artery bypass grafting1 year ago. He consumes half a bottle of red wine per day and smokes pipe. He is allergic to penicillin and his medications are

Metformin tablet 850 mg t.d.s, rosiglitazone tab 4 mg b.i.d , atorvastatin 40 mg O.D, ezetimibe 10 mg O.D, amoldipine 10 mg O.D, furosemide 40 mg O.D, Aspirin 75 mg O.D, perindopril 4 mg O.D, and gabapentin 600 mg t.d.s, ISMO 60 mg O.D, Glyceryl Trinitrate Spray 400-800 µg.

On examination he appears confused, disoriented and has an inflamed foot ulcer, on close inspection the wound is deep penetrating to ligaments and muscle but a probe–to-bone test for osteoporosis is negative. The area surrounding the ulcer appears cellulitic. The patient is diagnosed with hyper osmolar non-ketotic (HONK) Syndrome infection of a diabetic foot ulcer and treatment pain is sodium chloride 0.9% I.V 1L per hour.

Insulin (Actrapid) I.V 1 L unit

Piperacillin – tazobactam I.V 4.5 g t.d.s

co-codamol 500 mg tab q.d.s

cyclizine I.V 50 mg t.d.s

Enoxaparin S.C 40 mg O.D

1. **What are the signs and symptoms of foot infection in diabetic patients?**

   (A) Neuropathy of the sensory, motor and autonomic nerves, impaired neutrophil function all contribute for the development of foot ulcer in diabetic patients. Features associated include cellulitis, lymphangitis, sinus tract formation, osteomyelitis septic arthritis, abses formation, development of gangrene. Clinical diagnosis of infection is based on the presence of pus, warmth, erythema, swelling and pain.

2. **What are likely pathogens?**

   (A) *Staphylococcus aureus, streptococcus pyogenes, staphylococcus aureus, streptococcus epidermidis, streptococci, E.coli, Klebsiella proteus and seudomonas species.*

3. What are the goals of therapy in diabetic foot infection?

(A) To control the infection, stabilize the patient to minimize morbidity and mortality and reduce the risk of amputation.

4. What is the prognosis and long term complication of diabetic foot ulcer?

(A) Foot ulcer cause morbidity and impaired quality of life and is a risk factor for amputation of lower extremity. The Lifetime risk of foot ulcer is 15% for diabetic patients 25% of ulcers. result in surgical removal of bone.

5. What are the relevant life style issues?

(A) Pharmacist can educate public about self care and self monitoring of the feet. Patients are advised to check the feet daily wash in warm water, encouraged to wear well-fitted shoes. Good control of blood pleasure and removal of corns etc.

CHAPTER 107

Endocrine Case Studies

CASE STUDY –1– TYPE 2 DIABETES

Mr.Stephen is over weight despite being on the maximum dose of metformin and gliclazide. His HbAIC is 9% and on examination has neuropathy developing in his feet. He is taking ramipril 10 mg, simvastatin 40 mg, Aspirin 75 mg. Her BP was 130/80 mmHg and TC was 4.0 mmol/L. There is no microalbuminuria present.

1. **What are the clinical issues?**

   (A) The patients diabetes is not well controlled as he has neuropathy and high blood sugar levels. His weight must be controlled by diet and exercise otherwise he may develop insulin resistance and require injection.

2. **What are the macrovascular and microvascular complication of this conditions?**

   (A) Macrovascular complications – related to cardiovascular system His BP, cholesterol being controlled.

   Microvascular complication - Include neuropathy, nephropathy, retinopathy. Already the patient is having neuropathy which could lead to amputation if not controlled.

3. **What is HbAIC?**

   (A) RBC are components of haemoglobin. Glucose sticks to the hemoglobin to make glycosylated hemoglobin molecule (HbAIC). The more glucose present in the blood, the more HbAIC will be present.

4. **How insulin therapy be introduced?**

   (A) If fasting glucose > 6 mmol/<, add intermediate acting insulin 6-10 units at bed time. Increase dose by 1-2 units every 3 days until blood glucose levels reached.

   If fasting glucose is normal but day time glucose levels are above target level, add intermediate acting insulin 6-10 units at breakfast time increase by 1-2 units every 3 days until target is reached.

5. **What different type of insulin are available?**

   (A) Short acting – Soluble / Aspart/Lis pro
   Intermediate acting – Isophane/
   Biphasic Lispro / Biphasic Isophane
   Long acting – Protamine zinc/
   Glargine

6. **Describe pharmaceutical care plan and include goals of therapy?**

   (A) Life style – Smoking cessation, Weight loss, increase exercise levels

Blood glucose levels – to be controlled

Blood pressure – Less than 135/75 mm Hg

Lipids – Total cholesterol within limits

Antiplatelet treatment to be continued.

7. **What monitoring doses Mr. Stephen require?**

    (A) Twice daily checking blood glucose levels

    BP to be monitored as well Hb/AIC

    Lipid profile every 6 months to be checked

    Review with consultant

Malignant Case Studies

CASE STUDY – 1 – TREATMENT OF ADVANCED COLORECTAL CANCER

Mrs. Susan 52 Years old servant is admitted in a hospital as inpatient in oncology ward with symptoms from colon cancer. She was referred to hospital oncology team 2 weeks ago for colonoscopy and biopsy of a colonic man as well CT scan. Her oncology consultant has admitted her for FOLFOX systemic cytotoxic treatment. At the time of admission her lab results were as follows.

Hb-8.8g/dl; WBC-7.2×10⁹/L, platelets - 346×10⁹/L Na-139 mmol/L Na-139 mmol/L kᵗ-2.6 mmol/L urea – 10.7 mmol/L, creatinine – 126 mmol/l. Total bilirubin – 17 ì mol/L ALT – 30 units, ALP-101 ì/l, GGT – 42 units/L. Mrs. Susan consultant oncologist chemotherapy regimen is given below.

Oxaliplatin 85 mg I.V infusion over 2 hrs day 1
Folinic acid 200 mg I.V infusion over 2 hrs day 182
5- Fluorouracil 400 mg I.V bolus day 182
5- Fluorouracil 600 mg I.V infusion day 182
repeated every 14 days for 4 to 6 cycles.

The oncologist prescribes I.V hidration for first 24 hrs to correct Mrs. Susn's hypokalaemia

Sodium Chloride 0.9% 100 mL/I.V infusion potassium chloride 40 mmol over 12 hrs.

Sodium Chloride 0.9% 500 mL/I.V infusion potassium chloride 20 mmol over 12 hrs.

1. What arc thc signs and symptoms of bowel cancer that alert health care professional?

(A) Patients with colorectal cancer develop the follows 4 symptoms.

1. Abdominal pain and discomfort
2. Change in bowel habit.
3. Rectal bleeding – blood from rectus that is darker in colon mixed with stool is more likely.
4. Anemia
5. Anorexia and weight loss any combination of these symptoms should prompt patient to be referred to specialist for investigations.

2. Evaluate Mrs. Susan Lab results?

(A) Significant abnormalities can be seen

1. Hb levels are lower indicates anemia; it may have resulted from bleeding.

2. Potassium levels are low leads to hypokalaemia. The development of hypokalemia in patients may often occur due to diarrhoea or vomiting caused by abdominal pain and discomfort.
3. Urea and creatinine levels are high, this may occur as results of dehydration from excessive fluid loss. Renal impairment is due to compressing of the ureters.

3. What are the typical side effects of FOLFOX Regimen?

(A) Bone marrow suppression, nausea and vomiting, diarrhea, stomatitis, alopecia, neurological toxicity, peripheral neuropathy characterized by dysaesthesia and paraesthesia, sensation of dysphagia (Difficulty swallowing) laryngospasm and bronchospasm, abnormal tongue sensation and feeling of chest pressure. 5 fluorouracil may produce hand-foot syndrome (Palmoplantar Eryth-rodysaesthesia) results in dry reddend and painful area on extremeties of hands and feet.

4. How nausea and vomiting, stomatitis and hand foot syndrome side effects be managed?

(A) Nausea and Vomiting : - Prophylactic administation of anti emetics such as metoclopramide or domperidone and severe manifestations may be managed by delay or dose modifications of chemotherapy cycle.

(B) Stomatitis : - This can be relieved by the administration of mouth care products like antiseptics or local analgesic preparations.

(C) Hand – foot syndrome : - Pyridoxine tablets to manage this effect the dose of 5- fluorouracil component need to be modified.

5. What patient parameters to be followed to monitored treatment effectiveness?

(A)

1. Subjective measure of disease reduction in symptoms of cancer.
2. Tumor markers and these markers to be monitored by serum samples.
3. Objective measure of disease by CT scan etc.

6. What patient parameters to be followed to maintain treatment toxicity?

(A) Haematological parameters.
Neurologial Toxicity
Hepatic and renal function
Any other toxic or side effects.

7. What overall goal treatment for Mrs.Susan?

(A) To prolong her life by controlling tumor growth in primary and meta states.

(B) To improve her quality of life

(C) To minimize intolerable side effects or treatment.

(D) Dosage adjustments Advising medical and nursing staff

(E) Ensuring supportive medication and anti emetics.

CHAPTER 109

Skin Case Studies

CASE STUDY – 1 – SEVERE ACNE

Miss. Sujana 18 years old girl comes to pharmacy with her regular prescription for Microgynon 30. Two months ago she complained of problem with ACNE and the pharmacist recommended her to try an over the counter topical benzoyl peroxide formulation. Miss. Sujana did not show any improvement from the treatment and she taken an appointment with her GP. She presents a new prescription for oxytetracycline tablets 500 mg b.d.

1. **What is ACNE?**

   (A) This is an inflammatory diseases of sebaceous glands and hair follicles of the skin. It is characterized with eruption of pimples especially on the face.

2. **Explain the type of topical formulation of benzoyl peroxide available.**

   (A) Benzyl peroxide is available as brevoxyl cream, panoxyl aquagel/ cream, compound preparations with anti microbials and also available on benzamycin gel.

3. **Why aqueous gel be recommended instead of alcoholic gel?**

   (A) Alcoholic preparations are not recommended for patients with sensitive skin an aqueous gel would be more suitable.

4. **How to counsel the patient regarding the use of topical formulation of benzoyl peroxide.**

   (A) Apply once are twice daily preferably after washing with soap and water. Treatment should be started with lower strength formulations, adverse effects include skin irritation, Scaling and redness. If this occurs the patient need to reduced the frequency of application. Benzyl peroxide formulation can also cause bleaching of clothes.

5. **How could you counsel Miss. Sujana to take oxytetracycline tablets**

   (A) Oxytetracycline tablets to be taken 4 times a day, two times for the treatment of acne (250 mg twice a day). These tablets should be taken 1 or 2 hours before or after meals, followed by glass of water. Milk, Food and antacids should not be taken at the same time as they may interfere and affect the absorption and make medicament less effective.

6. **What are the common side effects of Oxytetracycline?**

(A) Vomiting, Nausea, Diarrhea, Dysphagia and Oesophageal irritation.

7. **What are the alternative treatment options for Acne instead of tetracycline's?**

When tetracycline's are not tolerated orcontraindicated, erythromycin is an alternative. If erythromycin has problems with resistance and GIT adverse effects than doxycycline may be prescribed, minocycline is second line treatment.

CASE STUDY – 2 – ACUTE CELLULITIS

Mrs. Rani mother of 12 Years old keerti came to the pharmacy with a prescription. The prescription requesting pencillin V oral solution 250 mg/5 ml four times a day and flucloxacillin 125 mg/5ml four times a day, 30 minutes before food. Mrs. Rani enquires information about her daughter condition, cellulitis from the patients medication record keerti was recently treated for athlete's foot.

Few days later Mrs. Rani came to pharmacy for advice mentioning her daughter has developed a red rash on her back.

1. **What is cellutitis?**

(A) Cellulitis is a skin infection of the dermis and subcutaneous tissue. It is characterized by redness, swelling, pain and inflammation. Common symptoms is fever. Cellulitis is caused by bacterial infection most commonly streptococcus and staphylococcus.

2. **What are the risk factors for developing cellulitis?**

(A) Risk factors include athlete's foot, swollen legs or obesity, poorly controlled diabetes.

3. **Does keerti have any of the risk factors for developing cellulitis.**

(A) Athletes foot is fungal skin infection that result in cracked skin between the toes, through these breaks bacteria will enter and multiply under the surface resulting in cellulitis.

4. **Why should penicillin V and flucloxacillin should be taken on empty stomach?**

(A) Both penicillin V and flucloxacillin should be taken is an empty stomach since they are not absorbed well in to the blood stream. Taking these medicines on an empty stomach helps to improve absorption profile.

5. **What are the side effects of penicillin?**

(A) Common side effects are GIT disturbances (Nausea, Diarrhea) Hypersenstivity (Rash, Urticaria) and super infection (Candida infection)

6. **Co–amoxiclav is an alternative treatment to penicillin V and flucloxacillin. What does this formation contain?**

(A) Co–amoxiclav consists of amoxicillin abroad spectrum penicillin and clavulanic acid is a beta-lactemase, inhibitor. It is available as tablets, oral suspension and as an injectable formulation.

7. **Penicillin should be used with caution in renal impairment why?**
   (A) Penicillins are mainly cleared by renal tubular secretion and therefore should be usual with caution in renal impairment as penicillin half life is increased.

8. **How common are allergic reactions to penicillin?**
   (A) Allergic reaction to penicillin occur 1-10%.

9. **What alternative treatment for penicillins?**
   (A) Alternative treatment for cellulitis is macrolide antibiotic erythromycin.

CASE STUDY – 3 – ATOPIC ECZEMA

Mr. Rakesh 38 years is taking asthma medication for 10 years and occasionally suffers from eczema. His regular prescription is salbutamol inhaler 100 µg /metered 1-2 puffs and clenil modulite 100 g/ dose 2 puffs twice daily. He presents to pharmacy with new prescription for betnovate scalp application.

Few days later Mr. Rakesh returns to pharmacy complaining of severe symptoms, with redness on area of scalp and the skin has crusted appearance. Mr. Rakesh is advised to see GP.

1. **What is atopic eczema?**
   (A) This is chronic inflammatory skin condition and it is characterized by itchy red rash associated with skin flexures and other diseases such as asthma and hay fever.

2. **What is the main cause of atopic eczema?**
   (A) Atopic eczema occurs in individuals who are genetically predisposed when exposed to environmental irritants (abrasives, soaps, detergents, temp/humidity and allergies (Dust mites, polen, moulds etc). It may be worsened by endogenous factors hormones and stress.

3. **What are the main therapies available for treating atopic eczema?**
   (A) Skin dryness if treated with emollients, topical corticosteroids are generally used, oral antibiotics may be indicated for moderate to severe infection. Other therapies include ichthammol paste (reduces itching) zinc oxide (exudating eczema) newer treatments options include tacro-limus.

4. **Explain the terms glucocorticoid and mineral corticoids activity.**
   (A) Glucocorticoid activity refer to anti-inflammatory, immunosuppressive activities (Diabetes). Dexamethasone shows significant gluco-corticoid activity. Mineral corticoids refer to effects on both fluid and salt balance (Sodium and water retention, Potassium loss). Fludrocortisones shows mineral corticoid activity.

5. **How should betnovate scalp applications be applied?**
   (A) Initially apply to affected area of scalp both morning and evening. The bottle should be gently squeezed until the affected area is covered with thin layer of the liquid

which may be rubbed in to the scalp, wash hands after use.

6. **Beclomethasone (as dipropionate) is pro-drug. Explain the pharmacodynamics involved.**

   (A) Beclomethasone is a pro drug with weak glucocorticoids receptor binding activity. It is hydrolysed via esterase enzymes to the active metabolite beclomethasone – 17 – mono-propionate (B-17 MP) which has high topical anti inflammatory activity.

7. **How is beclomethasone (as dipropionate) metabolized. State the metabolites involved?**

   (A) Beclomethasone under goes extensive first pass metabolism and is rapidly excreted from systemic circulation. The main active metabolite is beclomethasone -17 monopropionate and minor inactive metaboliteare beclomethasone – 21 monopropionate and beclomethasone.

8. **Discuss both systemic and local adverse effects of corticosteroids.**

   (A) Systemic side effects are GIT disturbance, Musculoskeletal effects, Neuro Psychiatric effects and ophthalmic effects. Local side effects include stretch marks, blood vessels dilation, bruising and discoloration.

9. **Mr. Rakesh worsening symptoms are probably due to bacterial infection. What is the most common cause of bacterial infected eczema?**

   (A) Staphylococcus aureus is the most common cause of bacterial infected eczema, 90% of atopic eczema patches are colonized by this organism.

10. **What is the first line treatment for bacterial eczema?**

    (A) Flucloxacillin is recommended as first line oral antibiotics. If the patient is allergic to penicillin then erythromycin is prescribed.

CHAPTER 110

Liver Case Studies

CASE STUDY – 1 – ALCOHOLIC CIRRHOSIS, MANAGEMENT OF BLEEDING AND HEPATIC ENCEPHALOPATHY

Mrs. Kanthi 56 years old was admitted to acute medical ward with malaise, distended abdomen, swollen ankles and jaundice. It was also noticed that she smelt of alcohol and was showing signs of alcohol with drawl. Mrs. Kanthi weight 64 kg with acute and her lab data is

Total proteins – 49 g /L; Albumin – 20g/L bilirubin – 114 μ mn/l.

ALP – 382 14/L ALT – 88 /l, GGT – 306 iu/L

Diagnosis of alcoholic cirrhosis of liver was made based on liver function tests abdominal with assumed, CT scan and liver biopsy.

1. **What is cirrhosis of liver?**
   (A) This is histological development of regenerative nodules surrounded by fibrous bands, it is an advanced stage of liver fibrosis.
2. **What are the possible causes of cirrhosis?**
   (A) Alcoholic liver disease and hepatitis C and B are most common causes of cirrhosis, genetic causes of cirrhosis include haemochromatosis and wilson's disease, epidemiological studies have Identified that regular alcohol consumption, obesity, insulin resistance or diabetes, hypertension and hyperlipidaemia are possible causes.
3. **What other clinical signs and symptoms may Mrs. Kanthi Show?**
   (A) Mrs. Kanthi has shown itching, jaundice, dark urine, pale stool, abdominal pain, nausea, fatigue, bleeding, hepatic encephalopathy, hapatomegaly ascites, distended abdominal veins, and she may also present with the signs like, irritability, anxiety, tachycardia, tremors, sweating, confusion and hallucinations.
4. **What treatment would you recommend to reduce the risk of bleeding?**
   (A) At increased risk of bleeding Vit K can be given as injection or orally konakion is Phytomenadione 10 mg/ml may be administered by slow I.V injection or by infusion in glucose 5%. Alternatively Phytomenadione tablets may be used.

5. What medication would you advice Mrs. Kanthi to avoid bleeding risk?

(A) Medications known to increase the risk of bleeding in cirrhotic patients include aspirin, clopidogrel, dipyridamole, corti-costeroids, NSAIDS, Heparin and Warfarin.

6. What treatment options are available to help Mrs. Kanthi abstain from alcohol?

(A) Disulfiram is an aversine therapy that works by inhibiting acetaldehyde dehydrogenase. Interaction between disulfiram and alchohol can result in severe reactions such as MI, Congestive heart failures, respiratory depression and death. Acamprosate is indicated for maintenance of abstinence in alcohol dependent adults. It appears to decrease brain hyper excitability during alcohol withdrawl which may reduce alcohol consumption. The recommended period of treatment with acomprosate is one year.

7. What is hepatic encephalopathy? What are the clinical signs and symptoms?

(A) Hepatic encephalopathy is a neuropsychiatric syndrome which may complicate all types of liver diseases. Mrs.Kanthi presented with signs of hepatic encephalopathy including flapping tremor of hands, intellectual deterioration, slurred speech, Confusion, drowsiness and irritability.

8. What factors may precipitate hepatic encephalopathy?

(A) The various factors that may precipitate hepatic encephalopathy are

(1) Hypokalemia
(2) Diarhoea and Vomiting
(3) Constipation
(4) Gastrointestinal hemorrhage
(5) Infection especially Peritonitis
(6) CNS depressant drugs such as opioids or benzodiazepines

9. Mention any two treatment options for the management of Mrs. Kanthi hepatic encephalopathy?

(A) Provision of supportive care, identification and removal of precipitating factors, reduction in nitrogenous load from the gut. The dose of lactulose should be two soft stools without diarrhea. Lactulose is metabolized in the colon to lactic acid and formic acid causing PH of the color to drop from 7 to 5.

Neomycin is a non-absorbable antibiotic which may be used to reduce the number of bacteria in the blood that normally breakdown proteins. Neomycin therapy is limited to 1 week but some absorptions may occur with risk of nephrotoxicity and ototoxicity.

CHAPTER 111

Miscellaneous Case Studies

CASE STUDY – 1 – PULMONARY TUBERCULOSIS

Mr. Raju is a 47 years old patient returned from Celyon with cough, malaise, weight loss and night sweats. Sputum culture showed acid fast bacilli, 3 days later mycobacterium tuberculi was isolated.

1. **What is TB what causes it and what is the most common source of infection?**
   (A) Tuberculosis is an infection with mycobacterium tuberculi, the most common source of infection is lungs. Infection spreads by inhalation of infected droplets.
2. **What drugs could be used to treat?**
   (A) Capreomycin, Cycloserine, Ethambutol, Isoniazid, Pyrazinamide, Rifampicin and Streptomycin.
3. **Are there any problems with drugs and how they can be managed?**
   (A) Isoniazid can cause convulsions and therefore should be prescribed with caution in patients with epilepsy. Isoniazid is an enzyme inhibitor and may increase carbamazepine levels.

   Rifampicin is an enzyme inducer and may decrease carbamazepine levels.
4. **Mr. Raju need 750 mg of streptomycin daily. Why was this reduced and how its should be maintained?**
   (A) The dose of 750 mg is given to patients over 40 years of age. Streptomycin is an aminoglycoside antibiotic it is associated with ototoxicity and nephrotoxicity. Rifampicin can cause renal failure, hyperbilurubinaemia or serve hepatotoxicity and other side effects. Streptomycin can cause renal and ototoxicity. The combination of refampicin and streptomycin increases risk of streptomycin induced renal failure.

   Rifampicin is an enzyme inducer and can increase the incidence and severity of isoniazid induced hapatitis. Carbamazepine is an enzyme induction agent and intereacts with isoniazid increasing its hepatotoxicity. Isoniazid is an enzyme inhibitor may increase carbamazepine levels so this must be checked in time.

PAEDIATRIC CASE STUDIES

CASE STUDY – 2 – CROUP

A middle aged woman comes to pharmacy with a young girl who is 6 months old, she complains that her daughter has a harsh cough which sounds like a bark and it is terrible at night and really struggles to get sleep. She is keen to have medicines that can be inhaled in steam but not to have anything other than this. The Pharmacist decide that the child must have croup.

1. **What is Croup?**

   (A) Croup is most commonly caused by para influenza virus and presents with night time symptoms of barking cough. Hoarseness, inspiratory stridor and respiratory depression may be present. Although both upper and lower airways may be affected it is primarily related to upper airway.

2. **Should steam therapy be recommended by community pharmacist?**

   (A) If the child is having Croup she should be referred to hospital immediately, many Croup patients may recover with no treatment however if they get worse quickly, the therapy is based on maintaining airways and hydration. Menthol and Eucalyptus may help ease congestion and thus assist breathing.

3. **What is the first line treatment to moderate croup?**

   (A) Glucocorticoids are the first line treatment for mild to moderate Croup. They are effective via many routes (inhaled, oral or parenteral) but Dexamethasone given orally as one single dose or in two divided doses.

4. **Are there side effects related to use of glucocorticoids?**

   (A) Side effects include bone demineralization, Immuno-suppression, Cushingoid symptoms etc.

5. **What other treatment has been shown to be effective in serve Croup?**

   (A) Nebulised adrenaline should be considered for infants with moderate to severe symptoms of Croup.

6. **How does this treatment work?**

   (A) Adrenaline works by stimulating alpha-adrenergic receptors resulting in constriction of arterioles, resorption of intestinal fluid and decrease of oedema in infraglottic region.

CASE STUDY – 3 – ASTHMA

A 4 year old boy comes to accident and emergency ward with severe asthma attack, this is the third in the last 3 months. He started on nebulised, salbutamol, intravenous aminophylline and oral prednisolone. The symptoms include tachycardia, rapid breathing, unable to talk due to breathlessness. 3 days later he is discharged on salbutamol, beclometosone inhalers plus leukotriene antagonist.

1. **What is asthma?**

   (A) Asthma is a chronic inflammatory disease affecting the airways. Inflammatory mediators like prostaglandins, histamines cause damage to bronchial epithelium and cause bronchial constriction.

2. How does early childhood asthma present?

(A) Coughing at night.

3. What are the common symptoms?

(A) Common symptoms include

(1) Shortness of breath

(2) Cough

(3) Wheezing

(4) Tightness at chest region

4. What route of administration Beta$_2$ agonist is usually used?

(A) Beta 2 agonists are usually inhaled so that medicines goes straight to lungs reducing the amount entering systemic circulation and reducing side effects.

5. What are the main side effects of this class of drugs?

(A) Tremors, Headache, Peripheral dilations, Palpitation, tachycardia.

6. What is the role of leukotrienes antagonist?

(A) This effect can be antagonized using Montelukast.

7. What preparation are available and be most suitable?

(A) Both Montelukast and zafirlukast are most suitable and they may be mixed with spoonful of food and taken immediately.

8. What are the other main devices used to administer medications in asthma?

(A) Metered dose inhalers, Dry powder devices, Breath actuated metered dose inhalers and nebulizers.

CASE STUDY – 4 – OSTEOPOROSIS

Mrs. Reshma 72 years lady with well-controlled asthma using high dose steroid inhalers and occasional oral courses, She came to show her wrist which is in plaster cast, her orthopedic consultant has sad that she got osteoporosis and wants to send her for special x-ray and start treatment.

1. How is osteoporosis characterized?

(A) Osteoporosis is characterized by micro-architectural determination of bone issue and low bone mass leading to bone fragility and risk fracture.

2. What are the risk factors for this condition and which are relevant to Mrs. Reshma?

(A) Mrs.Reshma has history of long term steroid use. Other risk factors include poor intake of dietary calcium, lack of weight, previous fracture, premature menopause, excessive alcohol intake, long episodes of amennorrhoea before menopause and hyperparathyroidism.

3. What is the special x-ray?

(A) Bone mineral density (BMD) is measured using dual energy x-ray absorptiometry (DEXA) usually at the neck of femur (on hip). Other methods of measuring bone density such as ultrasonography of the heel are available.

4. What are the main goals of therapy?

(A) To increase bone mineral density and reduce the fracture possibility.

5. What drug treatments are available?

(A) Bisphosphonates – must be taken on empty stomach as they chelate with metal ions in food. Increases bone mass when given with calcium and Vit D.

Calcitonin – Require dietary calcium intake.

Calcitriol – Need to monitor plasma calcium and creatinine.

Raloxifene – Does not reduce menopausal vasomotor symptoms.

Strontium ranelate – Must be taken on empty stomach as it chelates with metal ions in food.

Teriparatide – Only by injection.

6. What important measures would patients need to take?

(A) Life style measures, such as cessation of smoking, weight bearing exercise calcium and Vit D supplements.

Patient risk factors are:

1) Balance gait or mobility problem 2) Poly Pharmacy 3) Visual impairment 4) Postural Hypotension

Environmental risk factors include

a) Poor lighting b) Steep stairs c) Loose carpets d) Slippery floor e) Badly fitting foot wear f) Lack of safety equipment

Older people risk factors

(a) Previous fragility fractures
(b) Live in unsafe housing conditions
(c) Afraid of falling
(d) Frequent unexplained falls

PART - V PROBLEMS

112 Problems based on Paediatric Dose Calculations

113 Problems based on Clearance

114 Problems based on Absorption Half Life

115 Problems based on Elimination Half life

116 Problems based on Area Under Curve (AUC)

117 Problems based on Wagner Nelson Method

118 Problems based on One Compartment Oral Absorption

119 Problems based on Two Compartment Model IV Bolus

120 Problems based on Non Compartmental Analysis

CHAPTER 112

Problems based on Paediatric Dose Calculations

YOUNG'S FORMULA

Child Dose =

$$\times\left(\frac{\text{Age in years}}{\text{Age in years}+12}\right)\text{adult dose}$$

1. What will be the dose of a child of 5 years, if the adult dose of a drug is 400 mg

   Given data: Age in years = 5 years; adult dose = 400 mg

   Formula: Young's formula =

   $$\left(\frac{\text{Age in years}}{\text{Age in years}+12}\right)\text{adult dose}$$

   Substitution: $\frac{5}{5+12}\times 400 = 117.64$ mg

2. The antipsychotic drug haloperidol can be given in the dose of 5mg two or three times a day. What will be dose of a child of 5 years

   Given data: Age in years = 5 yrs; Adult dose = 5mg

   Formula: Young's formula =

   $$\left(\frac{\text{Age in years}}{\text{Age in years}+12}\right)\text{adult dose}$$

   Substitution: $\frac{5}{5+12}\times 5 = 1.4$ mg

3. If the adult dose of a drug is 60 mg. What is the dose for a child of

   (a) 6 years

   Given data: Age in years = 6 years; Adult dose = 60 mg

   Formula: Young's formula =

   $$\left(\frac{\text{Age in years}}{\text{Age in years}+12}\right)\text{adult dose}$$

   Substitution: $\frac{6}{6+12}\times 60$

   (b) 8 years

   Given data: Age in years = 8 years; Adult dose = 60 mg

   Formula: Young's formula =

   $$\left(\frac{\text{Age in years}}{\text{Age in years}+12}\right)\text{adult dose}$$

   Substitution: $\frac{8}{8+12}\times 60$

4. The adult dose of a drug is 5mg. What will be the dose for a 3 years old infant

   Given data: Age in years = 3 Years; Adult dose = 5 mg

   Formula: Young's formula =

   $$\left(\frac{\text{Age in years}}{\text{Age in years}+12}\right)\text{adult dose}$$

Substitution: $\frac{3}{3+12}\times 5 = 1\text{mg}$

5. What is the dose of 6 years old child .If the average adult dose is 1.5 mg

   Given data: Age In years = 6 years; Adult dose = 1.5 mg

   $$\times\left(\frac{\text{Age in years}}{\text{Age in years}+12}\right)\text{adult dose}$$

   Formula: Young's formula

   $$=\left(\frac{\text{Age in years}}{\text{Age in years}+12}\right)\text{adult dose}$$

   Substitution: $\frac{6}{6+12}\quad 1.5 = 0.5\text{mg}$

DILLING'S FORMULA

$$\text{Child Dose} = \frac{\text{Age in years}}{20}\times\text{adult dose}$$

1. The antipsychotic drug haloperidol can be given in the dose of 5 mg, two to 3 times a day. Calculate the dose of a child of 5 years

   Given data: Age in years: 5 years; Adult dose = 5 mg

   Formula: Dilling's formula =

   $$\frac{\text{Age in years}}{20}\times\text{adult dose}$$

   Substitution: $\frac{5}{20}\times 5 = 1.25\text{mg}$

2. If the adult dose of ampicillin is 250-500 mg can be given three to four times a day. What will be the dose of a child of age of 10 years?

   Given data: Age in years: 10 years; Adult dose = 250-500 mg

   Formula: Dilling's formula =

   $$\frac{\text{Age in years}}{20}\times\text{adult dose}$$

   (a) Substitution : $\frac{10}{20}\times 250 = 125\text{mg}$

   (b) Substitution : $\frac{10}{20}\times 500 = 250\text{mg}$

3. Calculate the dose for a boy of 16 years, when the adult dose is 100 mg.

   Given data: Age in years: 16 years; Adult dose = 100 mg

   Formula: Dilling's formula =

   $$\frac{\text{Age in years}}{20}\times\text{adult dose}$$

   Substitution: $\frac{16}{20}\times 100 = 80\text{mg}$

4. If the actual dose of allopurinol is 200 mg. What is the dose for,

   Child of 12 years

   Given data: Age in years: 12 years; Adult dose = 200 mg

   Formula: Dilling's formula =

   $$\frac{\text{Age in years}}{20}\times\text{adult dose}$$

   Substitution: $\frac{12}{20}\times 200 = 120\text{mg}$

   (a) Child of 16 years

   Given data: Age in years: 16 years; Adult dose = 200 mg

   Formula: Dilling's formula =

   $$\frac{\text{Age in years}}{20}\times\text{adult dose}$$

Substitution: $\frac{16}{20} \times 200 = 160\text{mg}$

COWLING'S FORMULA

Child Dose

$$= \frac{(\text{Age in years} + 1)}{24} \times \text{adult dose}$$

1. What will be the dose of a child of 10 years, If the adult dose is 500 mg

   Given data: Age in years: 10 years; Adult dose = 500 mg

   Formula: Cowling's formula =

   $$\frac{(\text{Age in years} + 1)}{24} \times \text{adult dose}$$

   Substitution: $\frac{(10+1)}{24} \times 500 = 229.16\text{mg}$

2. The maximum daily dose of a drug is 120 mg. How much of is should be Given for a child of

   (a) 11 years

   Given data: Age in years: 11 years; Adult dose = 120 mg

   Formula: Cowling's formula =

   $$\frac{(\text{Age in years} + 1)}{24} \times \text{adult dose}$$

   Substitution: $\frac{(11+1)}{24} \times 120 = 60\text{ mg}$

   (b) 15 years

   Given data: Age in years: 15 years; Adult dose = 120 mg

   Formula: Cowling's formula =

   $$\frac{(\text{Age in years} + 1)}{24} \times \text{adult dose}$$

   Substitution:

   $$\frac{(15 + 1)}{24} \times 120 = 80\text{ mg}$$

FRIED'S FORMULA

Child Dose =

$$\frac{\text{Age in months}}{150} \times \text{adult dose}$$

1. The antipsychotic drug haloperidol can be given in the dose of 5 mg. 2-3 times a day, what will be the dose for a 6 months old infant.

   Given data: Age in months = 6 months; Adult dose = 5 mg

   Formula: Fried's formula =

   $$\frac{\text{Age in months}}{150} \times \text{adult dose}$$

   Substitution: $\frac{6}{150} \times 5 = 0.2\text{ mg}$

2. The average adult dose of a drug is 250 mg. what is the dose for 8 months old infant.

   Given data: Age in months = 8 months: Adult dose = 250 mg

   Formula: Fried's formula =

   $$\frac{\text{Age in months}}{150} \times \text{adult dose}$$

   Substitution: $\frac{8}{150} \times 250 = 13.3\text{ mg}$

3. Calculate the dose for 9 months old infant. If the adult dose is 100 mg.

   Given data: Age in months = 9 months: Adult dose = 100 mg

   Formula: Fried's formula =

   $$\frac{\text{Age in months}}{150} \times \text{adult dose}$$

   Substitution: $\frac{9}{150} \times 100 = 6\text{ mg}$

4. If the adult dose is 60 mg, how much it can be given to a
   (a) 6 months old
   Given data: Age in months = 6 months: Adult dose = 60 mg
   Formula: Fried's formula =
   $$\frac{\text{Age in months}}{150} \times \text{adult dose}$$
   Substitution: $\frac{6}{150} \times 60 = 2.4\,\text{mg}$
   (b) 24 months old infant
   Given data: Age in months =24 months: Adult dose = 60mg
   Formula: Fried's formula =
   $$\frac{\text{Age in months}}{150} \times \text{adult dose}$$
   Substitution: $\frac{24}{150} \times 60 = 9.6\,\text{mg}$
5. What is the dose for 8 months old infant, If the average adult dose is 200 mg
   Given data: Age in months = 8 months: Adult dose = 200 mg
   Formula: Fried's formula =
   $$\frac{\text{Age in months}}{150} \times \text{adult dose}$$
   Substitution: $\frac{8}{150} \times 200 = 10.6\,\text{mg}$
6. What is the dose for 9 months old infant, If adult dose is 25 mg
   Given data: Age in months = 9 months: Adult dose = 25 mg
   Formula: Fried's formula =
   $$\frac{\text{Age in months}}{150} \times \text{adult dose}$$
   Substitution: $\frac{9}{150} \times 25 = 1.5\,\text{mg}$

BASTEOD'S FORMULA

Child dose =
$$\frac{\text{Age in years } + 3(\text{adult dose})}{30}$$

1. The adult dose of paracetamol is 500 mg. what will be the dose. For a child of 4 years.
   Given data: Age in years = 4 years: Adult dose = 500 mg
   Formula: Basteod's formula = Age in years + 3 (adult dose) /30
   Substitution: $\frac{4 + 3(500)}{30} = 50.1\text{mg}$
2. If the adult dose of a drug is 100 mg. How much of it can be given to a patient of,
   (a) 9 years
   Given data: Age in years = 9 years: Adult dose = 100 mg
   Formula: Basteod's formula = Age in years + 3 (adult dose) /30
   Substitution: $\frac{9 + 3(100)}{30} = 10.3\,\text{mg}$
   (b) 12 years
   Given data: Age in years =12 years: Adult dose = 100mg
   Formula: Basteod's formula = Age in years + 3 (adult dose) /30
   Substitution: $\frac{12 + 3(100)}{30} = 10.4\,\text{mg}$

GAUBIN'S FORMULA

Gaubin's formula age	Parts of adult dose
Under 1 year	1/12
1-2 yrs	1/8
2-3 yrs	1/6
3-4 yrs	1/4
4-7 yrs	1/3
7-14 yrs	1/2
14-20 yrs	2/3
21-60 yrs	full adult dose
60-70 yrs	4/5

1. If the adult dose of a Paracetamol is 500 mg. What will be the dose for a child of 5 years

   Given data: Adult dose = 500 mg; Age = 5 years

   Formula: Child dose = 1/3 × part of adult dose

   Substitution: 1/3 × 500 = 166.6 mg
2. Chlorpromazine as antipsychotic drug can be given to adult in a dose of 5 mg two (or) three times a day. What will be the dose for a person of 6 years?

   Given data: Adult dose = 5 mg; Age = 6 years

   Formula: Child dose = 1/2 × part of adult dose

   Substitution: 1/2 × 5 = 4 mg

CLARK'S FORMULA

Child dose

$$= \frac{\text{Weight in kg}}{60} \times \text{adult dose}$$

Child dose

$$= \frac{\text{Weight in lg}}{150} \times \text{adult dose}$$

PROBLEMS BASED ON BODY WEIGHT

CLARK'S FORMULA

1. If the adult dose is 100 mg what would be the dose for a child of 30 kg

   Given data: Adult dose = 100mg; Body weight = 30 kg

   Formula: Child dose =

   $$\frac{\text{Weight in kg}}{60} \times \text{adult dose}$$

   Substitution: $= \frac{30}{60} \times 100 = 50$ mg
2. Calculate the dose for a child of weight

   (a) 12 lb

   (b) 15 lb if adult dose is 100 mg

   Given data: Adult dose = 100 mg; weight = 12 lb, 15 lb

   Formula: Child dose =

   $$\frac{\text{Weight in lg}}{150} \times \text{adult dose}$$

   Substitution:

   (a) 12/150 × 100 = 8 mg

   (b) 15/150 × 100 = 10 mg
3. What will be the dose for a 40 lb child if the average adult dose of Medicament is 10mg.

   Given data: Adult dose = 10mg; Body weight = 40 lb

   Formula: Child dose =

   $$\frac{\text{Weight in lg}}{150} \times \text{adult dose}$$

   Substitution: $= \frac{40}{150} \times 10 = 2.66$ mg

4. Calculate the dose of a drug for a child who weighs 28 lb if average adult dose is 100 mg.

   Given data: Adult dose = 100mg; Body weight = 28Lb

   Formula: Child dose =

$$\frac{\text{Weight in lg}}{150} \times \text{adult dose}$$

Substitution: $= \frac{28}{150} \times 100 = 18.6\,\text{mg}$

PROBLEMS BASED ON BODY SURFACE AREA

Child dose =

$$\frac{\text{Body surface area of child}}{\text{Body surface area of adult}} \times \text{Adult dose}$$

1. Calculate a dose for a child that has a body surface area, of 0.57 m^2 when the adult dose is 50 mg and the adult body surface area is 1.73 m^2

   Given data:

   Child body surface area = 0.57 m^2

   Adult body surface area = 1.73 m^2

   Adult dose = 50 mg

   Formula: Child dose =

$$\frac{\text{Body surface area of child}}{\text{Body surface area of adult}} \times \text{Adult dose}$$

Substitution: = 0.57/1.73 × 50 = 16.47 mg

2. What is the dose for an individual who has 1.21 m^2 Body surface area when the adult dose is 4,00,000 units

   Given data: Adult body surface area = 1.73 m^2

   Body surface area of child = 1.21m^2

   Formula: Child dose =

$$\frac{\text{Body surface area of child}}{\text{Body surface area of adult}} \times \text{Adult dose}$$

$$\frac{1.21}{1.73} \times 400{,}000 = 279768.78 \text{ units}$$

3. If the average adult dose of a drug is 50 mg. What is the dose for a child who has body surface area of 1.21m^2

   Given data: Body surface area of child = 1.21m^2

   Adult body surface area = 1.73 m^2

   Child dose

Substitution $= \frac{1.21}{1.73} \times 50$

$= 21.67$ mg

Problems based on Clearance

1. Penicillin has total clearance of 15 mL/min. calculate the elimination rate for when the plasma drug concentration Cp is 2 μg/mL and 10 μg/mL

Solution:

(a) Clearance =

$$\frac{\text{Rate of elimination}}{\text{Plasma drug concentration}}$$

Given data: Clearance = 15mL/min;

Cp = 2 μg/mL

$$15 = \frac{\text{Rate of elimination}}{2}$$

Rate of elimination = 30 μg/min

(b) Cp = 10μg/mL; clearance = 15 mL/min

Rate of elimination = clearance × Cp

= 15 × 10 = 150 μg/min

2. Determine total body clearance for a drug in a 70 kg male patient. The drug follows kinetics in one compartment model and has elimination half life of 3 hrs with an apparent volume of distribution of 100 mL / kg

Solution:

Total clearance = 0.693 × V_d / $t_{½}$

V_d = 100 mL/kg = 100 × 70kg (body wt.) = 7000 mL

$t_{½}$ = 3 hrs

Total clearance = 0.693 × 7000/3 =1617 mL/hr

3. A new antibiotic is actively excreted by the kidney V_d is 35 L in normal adult the $t_{½}$ of the drug is 33.3 minutes .What is the clearance ?

Total clearance = 0.693 × $V_d/t_{1/2}$

V_d = 35 L; $t_{1/2}$ = 37.3 min

cl_t = 0.693 × 35000/37.3 = 650 mL/min

4. A single 250 mg oral dose of an antibiotic is given to an young man of age 33 yrs. Creatinine clearance levels are 122 mL/min and his weight is 78 kg. From the literature the drug is known to have an apparent volume of distribution equal to 21% of body weight and an Elimination half life of 2 hrs. The dose is normally 90% bioavailable. urinary excretion of the unchanged drug is equal to 70% of absorbed

(a) What is the total body clearance for this drug

(b) What is the renal clearance for this drug

Solution:

(a) Total body clearance = 0.693 × $V_d/t_{1/2}$

V_d = 21/100 × 78 = 16.38 L (or) 16380 mL

Total clearance = 0.693 × 16380/120 = 94.6mL/min

(b) Unchanged drug = 70%

K_E = 70% of Elimination constant

$$K_E = \frac{0.693}{t_1/2} \times 0.7 = 0.242\text{hr}^{-1}$$

Renal clearance = $V_d \times K_E$

= 0.242 × 16380 = 3963mL/hr

5. Theophylline is effective in the treatment of bronchitis at a blood level of 10-20µg/mL at therapeutic range. Theophylline follows first order kinetics, the average $t_{1/2}$ for 3 hrs and range = 1.8-6.8 hrs. The average V_d is 30 L.

   (a) What is the average, upper and lower clearance limits for Theophylline

   (b) The renal clearance of theophylline is 0.36 L/hr. What is Km, Ke assuming all non clearance is due to metabolism.

Solution:

(a) Total clearance = 0.693 × $V_d/t_{1/2}$

Average clearance = 0.693 × 30/3.4 = 6.114 L/hr

Lower clearance = 0.693 × 30/6.8 = 3.05 L/hr

Upper clearance = 0.693 × 30/1.8 = 11.55 L/hr

(b) Renal clearance = 0.36

Ke = renal clearance/V_d = 0.36/30 = 0.102 hr^{-1}

Total clearance = renal clearance – non renal clearance

= 6.11 – 0.36 = 5.75 L/hr

Non renal clearance = km × V_d

Km = non renal clearance/V_d

= 5.75/30

= 0.191 hr^{-1}

CHAPTER 114

Problems based on Absorption Half Life

When a drug is administered by extravascular route, absorption is a pre requisite for its therapeutic activity. A large number of plasma concentration time profiles can be described by a one compartment model with first order absorption and elimination.

- After extra vascular administration, the rate of change in the amount of drug be dx/dt is the difference between the rate of absorption i.e., dx_{ev}/dt and rate of elimination dx_E/dt.

dx/dt = Rate of Absorption – Rate of Elimination

$$dx/dt = dx_{ev}/dt - dx_E/dt$$

- For the drug that follows one compartment model, the plasma concentration time profile is characterized by absorption phases, post absorption phase and elimination phase.
- During absorption phase ; Rate of absorption > Rate of elimination i.e., $dx_{ev}/dt > dx_E/dt$.
- At peak plasma concentration, the rate of absorption is equal to rate of elimination

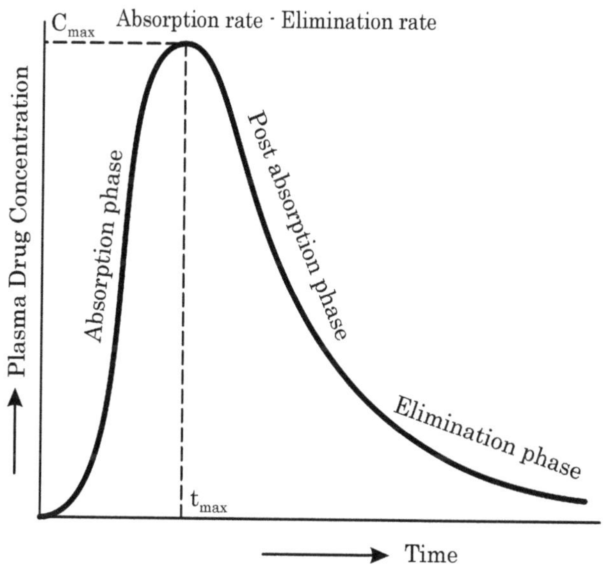

and the change in the amount of drug in the body is zero i.e.,

$dxev/dt = dx_E/dt$

During post absorption phase there is some drug at the extravascular site, still remaining to be absorbed and the rate of elimination at this stage is greater than absorption rate i.e.,

$dxev/dt < dx_E/dt$

- After the completion of drug absorption, its rate becomes zero & the plasma level-time curve is characterized only by the elimination phase.

Absorption rate constant: It can be calculated by the method of residual curves also known as feathering, peeling & stripping method.

- For a drug that follows one compartment kinetics and administered extra-vasucularly, the concentration of drug in plasma is expressed by a biexponential equation i.e.,

$$C = \frac{Ka\ Fxo}{V\bar{d}\ (Ka - KE)}\ [e^{-k_E t} - e^{-k_a t}]$$

where, $k_a Fxo/V_d\ (ka - k_E) = A$ = Hybrid content

$$C = A\ [e^{-k_E t} - e^{-k_a t}]$$

$$C = A\ [e^{-kEt} - Ae^{-kat}]$$

During elimination phase, $Ka >> K_E$

$e^{-k_a t} = 0$ $\quad e^{-kEt}$ = has some finite value

At this time the equation will reduce to $C = A.e^{-kEt}$

$\text{Log } C = \text{Log } A = k_E t/2.303$

Log C = extrapolated line

Log A = y intercept

$K_E t/2.303$ = Slope of linearity.

Subtraction of true plasma concentration values form extrapolated value gives residual concentration Values. (Cr)

$$(C - C) = C_r = A.e^{-ka.t}$$

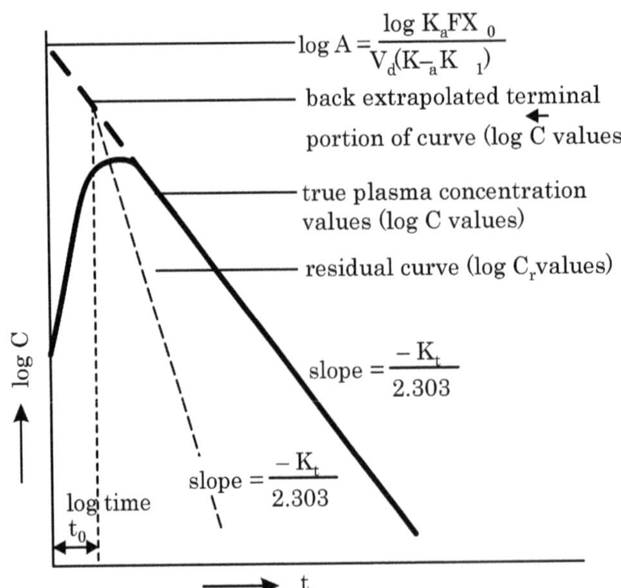

Applying log on both sides, we get

Log Cr = Log A – Kat/2.303

A plot of log Cr Vs t yields a straight line with aslope – ka/2.303,

Y intercept = log A.

Absorption half life can be computed from ka using the relation 0.693/ka

This technique works best when the difference between Ka and K_E is large.

1. The 59 kg male patient receives 2mg/kg of an antibiotic orally. The following plasma concentration versus time data is obtained. Assume that the drug follows one compartment model. Calculate absorption half life.

Time (hrs)	Conc. (μg/ml)
0.25	2.2
0.5	3.8
0.75	5
1	5.8
1.5	6.8
2	7.1
2.5	7.1
3	6.9
4	6.2
6	4.8
8	3.5
12	1.9
18	0.8
24	0.3

Solution:

Time (hrs)	Conc. (μg/mL)	Extrapolated values	Residual values
0.25	2.2	11.0	8.8
0.5	3.8	10.5	9.25
0.75	5	10.0	5
1	5.8	9.1	3.3
1.5	6.8	8.8	2
2	7.1	8.4	1.3
2.5	7.1	7.9	0.8
3	6.9	7.4	0.5
4	6.2		
6	4.8		
8	3.5		
12	1.9		
18	0.8		
24	0.3		

By, semi log plot of concentration Vs time

Slope = $\log Y_2 - Y_1/X_2 - X_1$ =0.38

Ka = 2.303 × 0.38

= 0.875 hr^{-1}

$t_{1/2}$ = 0.693/0.875 = 0.792 hrs

Report: By semi log plot of concentration Vs time, ka was found to be 0.792 hrs^{-1}.

2. The administration of 10 mg of new drug solution through oral route, plasma samples are withdrawn at different time intervals and corresponding data was found as,

Time (hrs)	Conc. (µg/mL)
0.25	2.85
0.5	5.43
0.75	7.75
1	9.84
2	16.7
4	22.15
6	23.01
10	19.09
14	13.9
20	7.97

Solution:

Time (hrs)	Conc. (µg/mL)	Extrapolated values	Residual values
0.25	2.85	48	45.15
0.5	5.43	47	41.57
0.75	7.75	46.5	38.75
1	9.84	43	33.16
2	16.7	40	23.3
4	22.15	34	11.85
6	23.01	29	5.99
10	19.09		
14	13.9		
20	7.97		

By, semi log plot of concentration Vs time

Slope = $\log Y_2 - Y_1/X_2 - X_1$ = 0.15

Ka = 2.303 × 0.15 = 0.34 hr^{-1}

$t_{½}$ = 0.693/ka

= 0.693/0.34 = 2.03 hrs

Report: By semi log plot of concentration Vs time, ka was found to be 2.03 hrs^{-1}

CHAPTER 115

Problems based on Elimination Half Life

When a drug that distributes rapidly in the body is given in the form of rapid IV injection and takes about 1-3 minutes for complete circulation. The general expression for rate of drug presentation to body is,

dx / dt = Rate in (availability) – Rate out (elimination)

Since rate of absorption is absent, the equation becomes

dx/dt – ratc out

If the rate out follows first order kinetic – then,

$$dx / dt = k_E x^- \quad ...(115.1)$$

Where,

K_E = first order elimination

X = amount of drug in the body at any time 't' remaining to be eliminated

Negative sign indicates = drug being eliminated

On integration of above equation (115.1)

$$\text{In } x = \text{In } x_0 - k_E t$$

$$x = x_0 - e^{-K_E t}$$

$$\text{Log } x = \log x_o - \frac{K_E t}{2.303}$$

Since it is difficult to determine directly the amount of drug in the body, advantage is taken of fact that a constant relationship exists between drug concentration in plasma and amount of drug C Thus,

$$x = V_d C$$

It is a pharmacokinetic parameter that permits the use of drug concentration in place of C.

$$\text{Log } C = \text{Log } Co - kt/2.303$$

Elimination half life: It is also called as biological half life. It is the time taken for amount of drug in body as well as plasma concentration to decline one half or 50% of its initial value so,

$$t_{½} = \frac{0.693 \times V_d}{\text{Clearance (Total)}}$$

Clearance: It is an important parameter in clinical drug application & is useful in evaluating mechanism by which a drug is eliminated by whose organism /particular organism.

$$\text{Clearance} = \frac{\text{Rate of elimination}}{\text{Plasm a drug conc.}}$$

$$Cl_t = dx /dt/c$$

Since, $dx/dt = – K_E x$ (from eq. (115.1))

$Cl_t = K_E\ x/c$ (since $x/c = V_d$)

$Cl_t = K_E \times V_d$

$Cl_t = 0.693 \times V_d / t_{1/2}$

(since $K_E = 0.693 / t_{1/2}$)

Problems:

1. Estimate K_E, $t_{½}$ for IV injection based on one compartment model

Time (hrs)	0.25	0.5	1	2	4	6
Du (mg)	160	140	200	250	188	46

Solution:

Time (hrs)	Du(mg)	Cumulative	$D_u^{\infty} - D_u$	Log ($D_u^{\infty} - D_u$)
0.25	160	160	824	2.91
0.5	140	300	684	2.83
1	200	500	484	2.68
2	250	750	234	2.36
4	188	938	46	1.66
6	46	984	0	-

From the graph plotted log ($D_u^{\infty} - D_u$) Vs time,

$K_E = 2.303 \times 0.33$ (slope = 0.33 form the graph)

$= 0.759\ \text{hrs}^{-1}$

$$t_{½} = \frac{0.693}{0.759} = 0.913\ \text{hrs}$$

2. A 50 kg women was given a single IV dose of an antibacterial dug at a dose level of 6 mg/kg. Blood samples were taken at different time intervals (C_p) was determined in the plasma fraction of each blood sample and The following data is obtained.

Time (hrs)	0.25	0.50	1.00	3.00	6.00	12.0	18.0
C_p (µg/mL)	8.21	7.87	7.23	5.15	3.09	1.11	0.40

Solution:

Time (hrs)	C_p (µg/ml)	LogC_p
0.25	8.21	0.91
0.50	7.87	0.89
1.00	7.23	0.85
3.00	5.15	0.71
6.00	3.09	0.48
12.0	1.11	0.45
18.0	0.40	-

(a) Estimate K. $t_{1/2}$, V_d.

$K = 2.303 \times 0.07$ (slope = 0.07 from the graph of log C_p versus time)

$t_{½} = 0.693 / K$

$$= \frac{0.693}{0.168} = 4.125\ \text{hrs}$$

V_d = dose / Cp°

$= 6 \times 50 / 8.21$

$= 36.5$ L

(b) This antibacterial drug is not effective at a plasma concentration of less than 2, µg/mL. What is the duration of activity of drug

$\text{Log } C_p = \text{Log } C_p^{\,0} - Kt / 2.303$

$0.168t / 2.303 = 0.91 - 0.30$

$0.168t = 0.61 \times 2.303$

$t = 0.61 \times 2.303 / 0.168$

$= 8.362$ hrs

(c) How long would is take for 99.9% of drug to be eliminated

99.9%

$t_{½}$	Amount of drug eliminated	Amt.remained
1	50%	50%
2	75%	25%
3	87.5%	12.25%
4	93.75%	6.25%
5	96.87%	3.125%
6	98.43%	1.562%
7	99.21%	0.195%
8	99.6%	0.197%
9	99.79%	0.048%

Report:

(a) $K = 0.168 hrs^{-1}$, $t_{½} = 4.125 hrs$,
$V_d = 36.5$ L

(b) t = 8.362 hrs

(c) It takes 10 $t_{½}$ for 99.9% of drug to be eliminated

3. A new drug was given in a single IV dose of 200 mg to an 80 kg adult male patient. After 6 hrs, the plasma drug concentration of drug was 1.5 mg for 100 mL of plasma assuming that V_d is 10% of body weight, compute the total amount of drug in the body after 6 hrs

Given data: $x_o = 200$ mg

V_d = 10% of body weight = 10/100 × 80
= 0.1 × 80 = 8000mL = 8L

Cp = 1.5 mg / 100mL

$V_d = x/c$

8000 = x/1.5/100

x = 12000/100 = 120mg

$\text{Log } x = \log x_0 - kt/2.303$

Log 120 = Log 200 – kx6 /2.303

$K = 0.088 \ hr^{-1}$

$t_{½} = 0.693/k$

= 0.693/0.088

= 7.8 hrs

4. A new antibiotic drug was given in a single IV bolus of 4mg/kg to 5 healthy male adults ranging in age from 23-30 yrs. Average rate of person is 75 kg. The pharmacokinetics of plasma drug con curve fits a one compartment model. The equation of the curve that best fits the data is.

$Cp = 78 \times t^{-0.46t}$

Determine the following

Assume unit of mg/mL for Cp and hours t

(a) What is $t_{½}$

(b) What is V_d

(c) What is plasma level of drug after 4 hrs

(d) How much of drug is left in the body

Solution:

(a) $t_{½} = 0.693$ /k
= 0.693 / 0.46 = 1.50 hrs

(b) $V_d = x / c$
= 390 / 78
= 3.84 L

(c) Plasma level,
$\text{Lop } Cp = \log Cp^0 - K_t / 2.303$
= Log 78 – 0.46 × 4 / 2.303
= 1.8 – 1.046 × 4/2.303
= anti log (1.092)
= 12.38 µg/mL

(d) Drug left
$x = C \times V_d$
= 12.38 × 3.84 = 47.42 mg

5. If the amount of drug in the body declines from 100% of dose to 25% of dose in 8 hrs. What is the elimination half left of this drug

$\log x = \log x_0 - k_E t / 2.303$

Log 25 = Log 100 – k × 8/2.303

1.39 = 2 – k × 8 / 2.303

$K = 1.73 \ hr^{-1}$

$t½ = 0.693/k$

$= 0.693/1.73 = 4$ hrs

6. The adult male patient (age = 35 years, weight = 72 kg) with urinary tract infection was given a single IV bolus of antibiotic (dose = 300mg) The patient was instructed to empty his bladder prior to being medicated. After dose administration the patient saved his urine specimens for analysis. The urine specimens were analyzed for drug content and sterility (lack of bactericide) the drug assays gave the following results.

Time in hrs	0	4	8
Amt of drug in urine (mg)	0	10	26

Assuming first order elimination, calculate elimination half life for the antibiotic in this patient

Solution:

Time (hrs)	d_u	$d_u / \Delta t$	t*	Log du/dt
0	0	–	–	–
4	100	25	4/2 = 2	1.39
8	26	6.5	84/2 = 6	0.81

From the graph, Log du/dt versus t*

Slope = 1.39 – 0.81 / 6 – 2

= 0.58/4 = 0.145

$K_E = 0.145 \times 2.303 = 0.33$

$t_{½} = 0.693/0.33$

= 2.1 hrs

7. Elimination half-life of a drug is 6 hrs and drug follows first order kinetics. If single IV dose of 200mg is given to an adult male patient (68kg) by IV bolus injection. What percent of dose is lost in 24 hrs?

Solution:

$t_{½}$	Amount eliminated	Percent drug remaining
6	50%	50%
12	50+25 = 75%	25%
18	75 + 125 = 87.5	12.5%
24	87.5 + 6.25 = 93.75	6.25%

$t_{½} = 6$hrs

1 day = 24 hrs as the drug has t½ of 6 hrs totally $6 \times 4 = 24$ hrs. As per this the drug lost in 24hrs is 93.75%.

∴ Percentage of drug lost in 24 hrs is 93.75%

8. A single IV bolus injection containing 500 mg of cephamandole naphthate is given to an adult female patient of 63 yrs, 55 kg for septicemia injection. The apparent V_d is 0.1L/kg and elimination half life is 0.75hrs. Assuming the drug is eliminated by first order kinetics. Calculate
   (a) Cp_o
   (b) Amount of drug in body 4 hrs after dose is given.

Solution:

$V_d = 0.1 \times 5.5$

= 5.5 L

$5.5 = \frac{x}{c}$

$= \frac{500}{c}$

C = 90.9 mg / L

$Cp = C_o.e^{-KEt}$

$\log x = \log x_0$

$X_o = 500$

log x = log 500

log x = 2.698 – 0.4012 × 4

log x = 1.098

x = 12.53 mg

The C_p of Cephamandole IV bolus injection is 90.9 mg/L. Amount of drug in body 4 hrs after dose is given is 12.53mg.

CHAPTER 116

Problems based on Area Under Curve (AUC)

Area under curve represents the total integrated area under the plasma level time profile and expresses the amount of drug that comes into systemic circulation after administration. It is expressed in µg.mL/hr. It is helpful in evaluating the bioavailability of a drug from its dosage form as it represents extent of absorption Area under curve is calculated by trapezoidal rule.

$$AUC_0^\infty = AUC_0^t + AUC_t^\infty$$

$$AUC_0^t = \Sigma_{t=0}^{[t=n]} (Cn_{-1} + C_n) /2 \times (t_n - t_{n-1})$$

$$AUC_t^\infty = C^* / K_E$$

PROBLEMS

1. A 59 kg male patient receive 2 mg/kg antibiotic orally. The following plasma level concentration vs time data was obtained assume that the drug follows one compartment open model and is completely absorbed calculate AUC

Time	0.25	0.5	0.75	1	1.5	2	2.5	3	4	6	8	12	18	24
C_p	2.2	3.8	5	5.8	6.8	7.1	7.1	6.9	6.2	4.8	3.5	1.9	0.8	0.3

Solution:

Time (hrs)	Cp (µg/mL)	Log C
0.25	2.2	0.34
0.5	3.8	0.57
0.75	5	0.69
1	5.8	0.76
1.5	6.8	0.83
2	7.1	0.85
2.5	7.1	0.85
3	6.9	0.83

Time (hrs)	Cp (µg/mL)	Log C
4	6.2	0.79
6	4.8	0.68
8	3.5	0.54
12	1.9	0.27
18	0.8	–0.09
24	0.3	–0.52

$AUC_0^t = ½ (C_1 + C_2) (t_2 - t_1)+.....$

$AUC_0^t = ½ [(0 + 2.2) (0.25 - 0) + (3.8 + 2.2) (0.5 - 0.25) + (5 + 3.8) (0.75 - 0.5) + (5.8 + 5) (1.0 - 0.75) + (6.8 + 5.8) (1.5 - 1.0) +$

(7.1 + 6.8) (2 – 1.5) + (7.1 + 7.1) (2.5 – 2) + (6.9 + 7.1) (3 – 2.5) + (6.2 + 6.9) (4 – 3) + (4.8 + 6.2) (6 – 4) + (3.5 + 4.8) (8 – 6) + (1.9 + 3.5) (12 – 8) + (0.8 + 1.9) (18 – 12) + (0.3 + 0.8) (24 – 18)]

= 1/2 (0.55 + 1.5 + 2.2 + 2.7 + 6.3 + 6.95 + 7.1 + 13 + 22 + 16.6 + 21.6 + 16.2 + 6.6)

= ½ × 130.5

AUC_0^t = 65.25

$AUC_t^{\infty} = C^*/K_E = 0.3/0.145$

= 2.068 μg hr/mL

[K_E is determined by plotting a graph bet log c and time and it is 0.145]

$AUC_0^{\infty} = AUC_0^t + AUC_t^{\infty}$

= 65.25 + 2.068

= 67.318 μg.hr/mL

Report: AUC was found to be 67.318 μg. hr/mL

2. A person administered 50 mg of drug orally. The following data was obtained.

 Calculate AUC.

Time	0	1	2	3	4	5	6
C_p	0	5.5	9.2	14.9	10.3	7.3	2.2

Solution:

Time (hrs)	Cp (μg/mL)	Log C
0	0	0
1	5.5	0.740
2	9.2	0.963
3	14.9	1.073
4	10.3	1.012
5	7.3	0.863
6	2.2	0.342

$AUC_0^t = ½ (C_1 + C_2) (t_2 - t_1) + \ldots$

= ½ [(5.5 + 0) (1 – 0) + (9.2 + 5.5) (2 – 1) + (14.9 + 9.2) (3 – 2) + (14.9 + 10.3) (4 – 3) + (10.3 + 7.3) (5 – 4) + (7.3 + 2.2) (5 – 6)]

= 1/2 (5.5 + 14.7 + 24 + 25.2 + 17.6 + 9.5)

= ½ × 96.6

= 48.3

$AUC_t^{\infty} = C^*/K_E = 2.2/0.34 = 6.47$ μg hr /mL

[K_E is determined by plotting a graph bet log c and time and it is 0.340]

$AUC_0^{\infty} = AUC_0^t + AUC_t^{\infty}$

= 6.47 + 48.3

= 54.77 μg hr/mL

Report: AUC was found to be 54.77 μg hr/mL

CHAPTER 117

Problems based on Wagner Nelson Method

It is used for calculating absorption constant. It involves determination of ka from percent unabsorbed –time plots.

Percent drug unabsorbed at any time is calculated by

$\% \text{ ARA} = [1 - X_A/X_A"] \times 100 =$

$[1 - C + K_E(AUC)_0^t/K_E(AUC)_0"] \times 100$

1. An 45 kg male received 10 mg/kg of an antibiotic orally. The following plasma concentration versus time data is obtained. Assume that the drug follows one compartment open model. Calculate k_a using Wagner nelson method.

Time (hr)	Cp (μg/mL)
0.25	2.2
0.5	3.8
0.75	5
1.0	5.8
1.5	6.8
2.0	7.1
2.5	7.1
3	6.9
4	6.2
6	4.8
8	3.5
12	1.9
18	0.8
24	0.3

Solution:

From The Plot of log Cp versus Time

$\text{Slope} = Y_2 - Y_1 / X_2 - X_1$

$= 0.07$

$K_E = 0.07 \times 2.303 = 0.161$

From The Plot of log $(1 - \frac{xA}{xA\infty}) \times 100$ versus Time

$\text{Slopc} = Y_2 - Y_1 / X_2 - X_1$

$= 0.32$

$K_a = 0.32 \times 2.303 = 0.73 \text{ hr}^{-1}$

2. A 55kg woman has administered with 10 mg/kg of an antibiotic. The following concentration versus time data was obtained. Calculate k_a using Wagner nelson method.

Time (hr)	Cp (μg/mL)
0.5	1.87
1	3.65
2	7.31
3	8.67
4	9.12
5	8.45
6	6.12
8	4.86
10	3.11
12	2.45
18	1.12
24	0.06

Time	Cp	Log cp	$(AUC)_0^t$	Cum. $(AUC)_0^t$	K_E $(AUC)_0^t$	Cp+ K_E $(AUC)_0^t$	x_A^{∞}	x_A / x_A^{∞}	$(1-\frac{xA}{xA^{\infty}})\times 100$	$\log(1-\frac{xA}{xA^{\infty}})\times 100$
0.25	2.2	0.34	0.28	0.28	0.04	2.24		0.20	80	1.90
0.5	3.8	0.57	0.75	1.03	0.16	3.96		0.36	64	1.80
0.75	5	0.69	1.1	2.13	0.34	5.34		0.49	51	1.70
1	5.8	0.76	1.35	3.48	0.56	6.36		0.58	42	1.62
1.5	6.8	0.83	3.15	6.63	1.06	7.86		0.72	28	1.44
2	7.1	0.85	3.47	10.11	1.62	8.72		0.80	20	1.30
2.5	7.1	0.85	3.55	13.66	2.19	9.29	10.79	0.86	14	1.14
3	6.9	0.83	3.50	17.16	2.76	9.66		0.87	11	1.04
4	6.2	0.79	6.55	23.71	3.81	10.01		0.92	8	0.90
6	4.8	0.68	11.00	34.71	5.58	10.38		0.96	4	0.60
8	3.5	0.54	8.30	43.01	6.92	10.42		0.96	4	0.60
12	1.9	0.27	10.80	53.81	8.66	10.56		0.97	3	0.47
18	0.8	-0.09	8.10	61.91	9.96	10.76		0.99	1	0
24	0.3	-0.52	3.3	65.21	10.49	10.79		1	0	-

Solution:

Time	C_p	Log cp	$(AUC)_0^t$	Cum. $(AUC)_0^t$	$K_E (AUC)_0^t$	Cp+ $K_E (AUC)_0^t$	x_A^{∞}	x_A / x_A^{∞}	$\left(1-\frac{xA}{xA^{\infty}}\right) \times 100$	$\log\left(1-\frac{xA}{xA^{\infty}}\right) \times 100$
0.5	1.87	0.271	0.467	0.467	0.084	1.954		0.136	86	1.934
1	3.65	0.562	1.380	1.847	0.333	3.980		0.278	72	1.857
2	7.31	0.863	5.480	7.370	1.326	8.640		0.605	39	1.591
3	8.67	0.938	7.99	15.317	2.757	11.430		0.800	20	1.301
4	9.12	0.959	8.895	24.200	4.356	13.480		0.943	6	0.778
5	8.45	0.926	8.785	32.980	5.936	14.390		1.007	0	-
6	6.12	0.786	7.28	40.260	7.246	13.370	14.28	0.936	6	0.778
8	4.86	0.686	10.98	51.240	9.223	14.080		0.985	1	0
10	3.11	0.492	7.97	59.210	10.657	13.770		0.964	3.6	0.556
12	2.45	0.389	5.56	64.770	11.658	14.110		0.988	1	0
18	1.12	0.049	10.71	75.480	13.586	14.710		1.030	-3	-
24	0.06	−1.200	3.54	79.020	14.223	14.280		1	0	-

From The Plot of log C_p versus Time

Slope = $Y_2 - Y_1 / X_2 - X_1$

= 0.08

$K_E = 0.08 \times 2.303 = 0.180\ hr^{-1}$

From The Plot of $\log (1 - \frac{xA}{xA^{\infty}}) \times 100$

versus Time

Slope = $Y_2 - Y_1 / X_2 - X_1$

= 0.26

$K_a = 0.26 \times 2.303 = 0.59\ hr^{-1}$

CHAPTER 118

Problems based on One Compartment Oral Absorption

FIRST ORDER ABSORPTION MODEL

This model assumes a first order input across gut wall and 1st order elimination from the body. This applies to oral absorption of drugs in solution (or) rapidly dissolving dosage forms such as tablets, capsules and suppositories.

In case of a drug given orally the dosage form first disintegration if it is given as a solid then the drug dissolves in to fluids of GIT. Only the drug is solution is absorbed in to the body. The rate of disappearance of drug from GIT is described by

$$\frac{dDG_1}{dt} = -k_a DG_1 F$$

Where K_a – 1st order absorption constant

F – Fraction absorbed

DG_1 – Amount of drug in solution in GIT at any time 't'

Integration of above equation gives

$$\frac{dDG_1}{dt} = D_{oe} - kat$$

Where, D_o – dose of drug

The rate of drug elimination is described by first order rate process for must of drug $= - KD_B$

The Rate of drug change in body is

$$\frac{d_{DB}}{dt} = \text{Rate in} -$$

Rate out

$$\frac{d_{DB}}{dt} = FK_a DG_1 - KD_B$$

Where F-Fraction of drug absorbed systemically since the drug in GIT follows 1st order decline the amount of drug in GIT at any time "t" = $D_{oe\,-\,kat}$

$$\frac{d_{DB}}{dt} = FK_a \left(D_{oe\,-\,kat}\right)^{-KDB}$$

The value of F may vary from one for fully absorbed drug to zero to that is completely unabsorbed this can be indicated general oral absorption equation for calculation of drug concentration (CP) in plasma at any time "t" is given below.

$$C_p = \frac{Fk_a D_o}{vd\left(k_{a-k}\right)}\left(e^{-K_E T} - e^{-kat}\right)$$

The maximum plasma concentration after oral dosing is C_{max} and the time needed to reach maximum concentration is t_{max}. independent of dose and dependent on rate constant on absorption and elimination k.

At sometimes peak concentration on the rate of drug absorbed = Rate of drug eliminated.

Therefore the net rate of concentration change can be obtained by differentiating the above equation.

$$C_p = \frac{Fk_a D_o}{vd(k_{a-k})}\left(K_{e^{-kt}} + Ka_{e^{-kat}}\right)$$

This can be simplified as

$$K_{e^{-kt}} = ka.e^{-kat}$$

$$t_{max} = \frac{In\left(\frac{ka}{k}\right)}{k_a - k}$$

$$t_{max} = \frac{2.303\log\left(\frac{ka}{k}\right)}{ka^{-k}}$$

1. A single oral dose of 100 mg was given, drug follows one compartment model and equation is C_p=45 ($e^{-0.17t} - e^{-0.15t}$) estimate

   (a) t_{max} (b) C_{max}

   (c) t1/2

   (A) Equation $C_p = (e^{-0.17t} - e^{-0.15t})$

$$t_{max} = \frac{2.303\log\left(\frac{ka}{k}\right)}{ka^{-k}}$$

$$= \frac{2.303\log(1.5/0.7)}{1.5-0.7}$$

$$= \frac{2.303\ \log 8.82}{1.33}$$

$$= \frac{2.17}{1.33}$$

$$= 1.63 \text{ hrs}$$

$$C_p = 45\ (e^{-0.17 \times 1.63} - e^{-1.5 \times 1.63})$$

$$= 45\ (e^{-0.27} - e^{-2.44})$$

$$= 45\ (0.76 - 0.08)$$

$$= 45\ (0.68)$$

$$= 30.6 \text{ mg/ml}$$

$$\frac{t}{2} = \frac{0.693}{0.17}$$

$$= 4.07 \text{ hrs}$$

Report

From the given data, t_{max}, C_{max} and t1/2 were found to be 1.63 hrs, 30.6 μ/ml , 4.07 hrs.

2. The equation that best fits the P^k of paracetamol after oral administration of 500 mg dose.

$$c = 1.18(e^{-0.24t} - e^{-1.6t})$$

Assuming one compartmental kinetics. Determine t_{max}, C_{max}, t1/2 and absorption half life.

$$t_{max} = \frac{2.30\ \log\ kd/k}{ka - k}$$

$$= \frac{2.30\ \log\left(\frac{1.6}{0.24}\right)}{1.6-0.24}$$

$$= \frac{2.30\ \log\ (6.66)}{1.36}$$

$$= \frac{2.303 \times 0.82}{1.36}$$

$$= \frac{1.89}{1.36}$$

$$= 1.38 \text{ hrs}$$

$c = 1.18\ (e^{-0.24 \times 1.38} - e^{-1.6 \times 1.38})$

$= 1.18\ (e^{-0.33} - e^{-2.20})$

$= 1.18\ (0.71 - 0.11)$

$= 1.18\ (0.6)$

$= 0.708$ mg/ml

$$\text{Elimination half life} = \frac{0.693}{KE}$$

$= 0.693/0.24$

$= 2.88$ hrs

$$\text{Absorption half life} = \frac{0.693}{Ka}$$

$= 0.693/1.6$

$= 0.43$ hrs

Report

Form the given data, t_{max}, C_{max}, elimination half life and absorption half life were found to be 1.38 hrs, 0.708 µg/ml, 2.88 hrs, 0.43 hrs.

3. Plasma samples were withdrawn after administration of 10 mg of new drug solution through oral route. Estimate KE & Ka values. Give the equation for plasma drug concentration using

Time	Cp
0.25	2.2
0.5	3.8
0.75	5
1.5	6.8
2	7.1
2.5	7.1
3	6.9
4	6.2
6	4.8
8	3.5
12	1.9
18	0.8
24	0.3

Time	Cp	Extrapolated Values	Residual Values
0.25	2.2	10.8	8.6
0.5	3.8	10.4	6.6
0.75	5	10	5
1	5.8	9.8	4
1.5	6.8	9	2.2
2	7.1	8.2	1.1
2.5	7.1		
3	6.9		
4	6.2		
6	4.8		
8	3.5		
12	1.9		
18	0.8		
24	0.3		

$$Cp = \frac{FK_aD_o}{vd(K_a - K)}\left(e^{-KEt} - e^{-Kat}\right)$$

$= 10.8\ (e^{-0.13t} - e^{-0.96 \times t})$

Report

From the given data, K_E was found to be 0.13 hrs^{-1} Ka was found to be 0.96 hrs^{-1}. The equation for plasma drug concentration was 10.8 ($e^{-0.13t} - e^{-0.96t}$).

CHAPTER 119

Problems based on Two Compartment Model IV Bolus

1 Central Compartmet ↓ K_E	K_{12} ⟶ ⟵ K_{12}	2 Peripheral Compartment

K_{12} & K_{21} be the first order distribution rate constants depieting drug transfer between the cental and peripheral compartments and let subscripts p & c defined central and peripheral compartment.

The rate of change in drug concentration in the central compartment is given by

$$\frac{dc_c}{dt} = K_{21}C_p - K_{12}C_c - K_E C_c$$

Extending the relationship x = vdc

$$\frac{dc_c}{dt} = \frac{K_{21}.X_p}{V_p} - \frac{K_{12}.X_c}{V_c} - \frac{K_E C_c}{V_c} \quad ...(1)$$

Where X_c & X_p are amounts of drug in the cental and peripheral compartments respectively.

V_c & V_p are the apparent volumes of cenral and peripheral compartment.

The rate of change in drug concentration in peripheral compartment is

$$\frac{dc_c}{dt} = K_{12}C_c - K_{12}C_p$$

$$\frac{K_{12}.X_c}{V_c} = \frac{K_{12}.X_p}{V_p} \quad .....(2)$$

Integration of equation 1 & 2 yields the concentration of the drug in the central and peripheral compartment at any given time 't'.

$$C_c = \frac{X_o}{V_c}\left[\left(\frac{K_{21} - \alpha t}{\beta - \alpha}\right)e^{-\alpha t} + \left(\frac{K_{21} - \beta}{\alpha - \beta}\right)e^{-\beta t}\right]$$

$$C_p = \frac{X_o}{V_p}\left[\left(\frac{K_{12}}{\beta - \alpha}\right)e^{-\alpha t} + \left(\frac{K_{21}}{\alpha - \beta}\right)e^{-\beta t}\right]$$

X_o - IV bolus dose, α & β are hybrid first order constants for the rapid distribution phase and slow elimination phase which depend upon first order rate constants such as K_{12}, K_{21}, K_E.

K_{12}, K_{21} → Micro constants

Relation between hybrid and micro constants

$\alpha + \beta = K_{12} + K_{21} + K_6$

$\alpha \ \beta = K_{21} \ K_E$

$C_c = Ae^{-at} + Be^{-bt}$

C_c = Distribution exponent + elimination exponent A & B are resolved by method of residuals

$$A = \frac{X_o}{V_c}\left(\frac{K_{21}-\alpha}{\beta-\alpha}\right) = C_o\left(\frac{K_{21}-\alpha}{\alpha-\beta}\right)$$

$$B = \frac{X_o}{V_c}\left(\frac{K_{21}-\beta}{\alpha\ \ \beta}\right) = C_o\left(\frac{K_{21}-\beta}{\alpha-\beta}\right)$$

C_o- Plasma drug concentration

$C_o = A + B$

$$K_E = \frac{\alpha\ \beta C_o}{A\beta + \beta\ \alpha}$$

$$K_{12} = \frac{AB(\beta-\alpha)^2}{C_o\,(A\beta+\beta\alpha)}$$

$$K_{12} = \frac{A\beta + B\alpha}{C_o}$$

1. The pharmacokinetics of amirinone after a single IV bolus injection of 75 mg was studied in 14 healthy adult male. The pharmacokinetics of this drug followed two compartment open model and fits the following equation.

   $C_p = A.e^{-at} + B.e^{-bt}$

   $A = 4.62 + 12.0\ \mu g/ml$

   $B = 0.64 + 0.17\ \mu g/ml$

   $a = 8.94 + 13\ hr^{-1}$

   $b = 0.19 + 0.06\ hr^{-1}$

   Estimate

   (a) Volume of central compartment

   (b) Transfer constant K_{12} & K_{21}

   (c) Volume of tissue compartment

   (d) Elimination half life amirinone after the drug has equilibrated with tissue compartment

Solution:

$C_p = A.e^{-at} + B.e^{-bt}$

$= 4.62\ e^{-8.94t} + 0.64\ .\ e^{-0.19 \times t}$ □

(a) Volume of central compartment =

$$\frac{D_o}{A+B}$$

$$vd = \frac{x}{c}$$

$$75\ mg \rightarrow \frac{75\times1000}{4.62+0.64}$$

$$= \frac{75{,}000}{5.26}$$

$= 14{,}258$ ml

$$(b)\ K_{12} = \frac{AB(\beta-\alpha)^2}{C_o\,(A\beta+B\alpha)}$$

$$= \frac{4.62\times0.64(0.19-8.94)^2}{5.26\left[(4.62\times0.19)+(0.64\times8.94)\right]}$$

$$= \frac{2.96(76.56)}{5.26(0.877+5.72)}$$

$$= \frac{226.31}{34.70}$$

$= 6.52\ hrs^{-1}$

$$K_{21} = \frac{A\beta + B\alpha}{C_o}$$

$$= \frac{(4.62\times0.19)+(0.64\times8.94)}{4.62+0.64}$$

$$= \frac{0.877+5.72}{5.26}$$

$= 1.25\ \text{hrs}^{-1}$

(c) $V_p K_{12} = V_t K_{21}$

$$V_t = \frac{14.258 \times 6.52}{1.25}$$

$$V_t = \frac{92962}{1.25}$$

$= 74,369$ ml

$$\text{(d) Elimination half life} = \frac{0.693}{\beta}$$

$= 0.693/0.19$

$= 3.64$ hrs

Time	C_p µg/ml
0	70
0.25	53.8
0.5	43.3
0.75	35
1.0	29.1
1.50	21.2
2.0	17.0
2.5	14.3
3.0	12.6
4.0	10.5
5.0	9.0
6	8
7	7

Report

From the given data:

(a) Volume of central compartment was found to be 14,258 ml

(b) Transfer constants & were found to be 6.52 hrs^{-1} and 1.25 hrs^{-1}.

(c) Volume of tissue compartment was found to be 74,369 ml

(d) Elimination half life was found to e 3.64 hrs.

2. A drug was admixture by rapid IV injection into 70 kg adult male and blood samples were withdrawn over a 7 hr period and assayed for intact drug. The results were tabulated below. Using the method of residuals. Calculate the values for intercepts A & B, Slopes α, β, K_{12} & K_{21}

B → 17 (Extrapolated)

A 53 (Residual)

$$K_E = \frac{\alpha\beta(A+B)}{A\beta + B\alpha}$$

Time	C_p	Extrapolated Values	Residual
0	70	17	53
0.25	53.8	16.5	37.3
0.5	43.3	16	27.3
0.75	26	15.5	19.5
1.0	29.1	15	14.1
2	17	13	4
2.5	14.3	12.5	1.8
3	12.6		
4	10.5		
5	9		
6	8		
7	7		

$$= \frac{(1.28 \times 0.11)(53+17)}{(53 \times 0.11)(17 \times 1.28)}$$

$$= \frac{0.14 \times 70}{5.83 + 21.17}$$

$$= \frac{9.8}{27.59}$$

$= 0.35$

$$K_{12} = \frac{AB(\beta-\alpha)^2}{C_o(A\beta+B\alpha)}$$

$$= \frac{53\times17(0.11-1.28)^2}{70(53\times0.11+17\times1.28)}$$

$$= \frac{901(1.36)}{70(5.83+21.76)}$$

$$= \frac{1225.36}{1931.3}$$

$$= 0.63 \text{ hrs}^{-1}$$

$$K_{21} = \frac{A\beta+B\alpha}{A+B}$$

$$= \frac{5.83+21.76}{70}$$

$$= \frac{27.59}{70}$$

$$= 0.39 \text{ hrs}^{-1}$$

Report

From the given data

(a) A, B was found to be 53,17

(b) a, b were found to be 1.28 hrs^{-1}, 0.11 hrs^{-1}

(c) K_{12}, K_{21} were found to be 0.63 hrs^{-1}, 0.39 hrs^{-1} .

CHAPTER 120

Problems based on Non Compartmental Analysis

Non-Compartment analysis is also called as model independent method and doesn't require the assumption of specific compartment model. It is based on assumption that the drugs or metabolites follow linear kinetics.

It is based on statistical moments theory that involves collection of experimental data following a single dose of the drug.

If one considers the time course of drug concentration in plasma as a statistical distribution curve MRT is equal to $\frac{AUMC}{AUC}$.

MRT Mean Residential time ie average amount of time spent by the drug in the body before being eliminated

AUMC = Area Under First Moment Curve

$$AUMC = \int_0^\infty . ct\ dt$$

AUC = Area Under Zero Moment Curve

$$AUC = \int_0^\infty . cdt$$

MRT is useful in calculating the steady state volume of distribution. It is the ratio of amount of the drug in the body at steady state to clearance state.

$$MRT = \frac{Vd^{ss}}{clt}$$

$$CLT = \frac{dose}{(AUC)_0^\infty}$$

1. After an IV dose 500mg of an antibiotic. The plasma concentration time data were collected and the area under curve was completed to be 20 mg/lit. hr. The $(AUMC)_0^\infty$ area was found to be 100 mg / lit.hr². Calculate MRI, vdss°, Clt.

Solution:

$$MRT = \frac{AUMC}{AUC}$$

$$= \frac{100}{20} = 5 \text{ hrs}$$

$$ClT = \frac{dose}{(AUC)_0^\infty}$$

$$= \frac{500}{20} = 25 \text{ lit. hrs}^2$$

Report

From the given data, MRT,Clt, Vd^{ss} were found to be 5hrs, 25 lit.hr, 125 Lit.hrs^2 .

APPENDIX-I

General Medical Abbreviations

A

AA - Alcoholics anonymous
AA - African american
AA - Amino acid
AAA - Abdominal aortic aneurysm
AAL - Anterior axillary line
A>B - Air conduction greater than bone conduction
ABBI - Advanced breast biopsy instrument
ABC - Aneurysmal bone cyst
ABD - Abdomen
ABG - Arterial blood gas
ABI - Ankle to brachial index
ABP - Androgen binding protein
Abx - Antibiotics
ac - Ante cibum (before meals)
AC - Abdominal cicumference
AC - Adriamycin, cyclophosphamide
ACA - Anterior cerebral artery
ACBE - Air contrast barium enema
ACE - Angiotensin-converting enzyme
ACLS - Advanced cardiac life support
ACS - American cancer society
ACT - Activated clotting time
ACTH - Adrenocorticotropic hormone
ADA - American diabetes association
ADA - American dental association
ADA - American dietetic association
ADCC - Antibody dependent cell-mediated cytotoxicity
ADH - Antidiuretic hormone
ADHD - Attention deficit hyperactivity disorder
ADI - Acceptable daily intake
ADL - Activities of daily living
ADR - Adverse drug reaction
AED - Automated external defibrillators
AES - Adult emergency service
AF - Afebrile
AF - Acid-fast
AF - Anterior fontanel-aortofemoral
AF - Atrial fibrillation
AFB - Acid-fast bacillus
AFI - Amniotic fluid index
AFP - Alpha fetoprotein
AH - Auditory hallucination
AHA - American heart association
AHG - Antihemophilic globulin
AI - Aortic insufficiency
AIDS - Acquired immune deficiency syndrome
AIHA - Autoimmune hemolytic anaemia
AIS - Abbreviated injury scale
AKA - Above the knee amputation

AKA - Also known as al - left ear
ALA - Aminolevulinic acid
ALL - Acute lymphoblastic leukemia
ALOC - Alternate level of care
ALS - Amyotrophic lateral sclerosis
ALS - Advanced life support
ALT - Alanine transaminase
AMA - Anti-mitochondrial antibodies
AMA - Against medical advice
AMA - American medical association
AMA - Advanced maternal age
AMI - Acute myocardial infarction
AMI - Anterior myocardial infarction
AML - Acute myeloblastic leukemia
AMN - Adrenomyeloneuropathy
AMP - Ampicillin
AMS - Altered mental status
ANA - Anti-nuclear antibodies
ANC - Absolute neutrophil count
ANCA - Antineutrophil cytoplasmic antibody
ANP - Atrial natriuretic peptide
A&O - Alert and oriented
AOB - Alcohol on breath
AOM - Acute Otitis media
AP - Anteroposterior
AP - Angina pectoris
AP - Acid phosphatase
APA - Antiphospholipid antibody
APC - Atrial premature contraction
APD - Afferent pupillary defect
APR - Abdominal perineal resection
APR - Anterior posterior repair
APTT - Activated partial thromboplastin time
APUD - Amine precursor uptake and decarboxylation
ARDS - Adult respiratory distress syndrome
ARF - Acute renal failure
ARF - Acute rheumatic fever
AROM - Artificial rupture of membrane
ART - Anti-retroviral therapy
ART - Assisted reproductive technology
AS - Aortic stenosis
ASA - Acetylsalicylic acid (aspirin)
ASAP - As soon as possible
ASCAD - Atherosclerotic coronary artery disease
ASCAD - Atherosclerotic cerebral artery disease
ASCUS - Atypical squamous cells of unknown significance
ASD - Atrial septal defect
ASHD - Atherosclerotic heart disease
ASPD - Antisocial personality disorder
ASO - Anti-streptolysin O
ASP - Antisocial personality
AST - Aspartate aminotransferase
AT - Atraumatic
AT - Ataxia-telangiectasia
ATLS - Advanced trauma life support
ATN - Acute tubular necrosis
ATP - Adenosine triphosphate
au - Both ears
AV - Atrioventricular
AV - Arteriovenous
AV - Aortic valve
AVP - Arginine vasopressin
AVM - Arteriovenous malformation
AVN - Atrioventricular node
AVR - Aortic valve replacement
AVRT - Atrioventricular re-entrant tachycardia

A&W - Alive and well
AXR - Abdominal x-ray
AZT - Zidovudine

B

B1 - Billroth 1 gastroduodenostomy
B2 - Billroth 2 gastrojejunostomy
BAD - Bipolar affective disorder
BAL - Blood alcohol level
BB - Bundle branch
BBB - Blood brain barrier
BBB - Bundle branch block
BBT - Basal body temperature
BC - Blood culture
BC - Birth control
BCG - Bacille Calmette-Gurein (tuberculosis vaccine)
BCx - Blood culture
BE - Barium enema
BE - Bacterial endocarditis
BFP - Biological false positive
BIB - Brought in by
BIBA - Brought in by ambulance
bid - bis in dies (twice a day)
BKA - Below the knee amputation
BLS - Basic life support
BM - Bowel movement
BM - Black male
BMD - Bone mass density
BMI - Body mass index
BMR - Basic metabolic rate
BMT - Bone marrow transplant
BP - Blood pressure
BPD - Biparietal diameter
BPP - Biophysical profile
BPH - Benign prostatic hypertrophy
BRB - Bright red blood
BRBPR - Bright red blood per rectum
BS - bowel sounds
BS - Breath sounds
BSA - Body surface area
BSO - Bilateral salpingo-oophrectomy
BTL - Bilateral tubal ligation
BUFA - Baby up for adoption
BUN - Blood urea nitrogen
BW - Black woman
BW - Birth weight
Bx - Biopsy

C

c - Cum (with)
Ca - Calcium
CA - Cancer
CAB - Carotid artery bruit
CABG - Coronary artery bypass graft
CAD - Coronary artery disease
CAE - Carotid endartectomy?
CAGE - Cut down, annoyed, guilty, eye-opener
CAH - Chronic active hepatitis
CAH - Congenital adrenal hyperplasia
CAH - Command auditory hallucination
CAO - Chronic airway obstruction
CAP - Community acquired pneumonia
CAP - Chest, abdomen, pelvis
CAT - Computed axial tomography
CBC - Complete blood count
CBD - Common bile duct
CBF - Cerebral blood flow
CC - Chief complaint
CCB - Calcium channel blocker
CCE - Clubbing, cyanosis, edema

CC - Chief complaint
CDC - Centers for Disease Control and Prevention
CEA - Carcinoembryonic antigen
CF - Caucasian female
CF - Cystic fibrosis
C/F - Chills, fever
CF - Citrovorum factor (leucovorin)
CFT - Complement fixation testing
CFTR - Cystic fibrosis transmem-brane conductance regulator
CGD - Chronic granulomatous disease
CHD - Congenital heart disease
CHF - Congestive heart failure
CIN - Cervical intraepithelial neoplasia
CJD - Creutzfeldt-Jacob disease
CK - Creatine kinase
CLL - Chronic lymphocytic leukemia
CM - Case manager
CMF - Cyclophosphamide, methotrexate, fluorouracil
CML - Chronic myeloid leukemia
CMT - Cervical motion tenderness
CMV - Cytomegalovirus
CN - Cranial nerve
CNS - Central nervous system
CO - Cardiac output
COLD - Chronic obstructive lung disease
COMT - Catechol-O-methyl-transferase
COPD - Chronic obstructive pulmonary disease
CP - Chest pain
CP - Cerebral palsy
CPAP - Continuous positive airway pressure
CPC - Clinicopathologic conference
CPCR - Cardiopulmonary-cerebral resuscitation
CPD - Cephalopelvic disproportion
CPI - Chronic uteralplacental insufficiency
CPK - Creatine phosphokinase
CPP - Cerebral perfusion pressure
CPR - Cardiopulmonary resuscitation
CRF - Chronic renal failure
CRH - Corticotropin releasing hormone
CRI - Chronic renal insufficiency
CRL - Crown rump length
CRH - Corticotropin-releasing hormone
C/S - Cesarean section
C&S - Culture and sensitivity
CSF - Cerebrospinal fluid
CSF - Colony stimulating factor
CST - Contraction stress test
CSW - Case social worker
CT - Computed tomography
CTA - Clear to auscultation
CTZ - Chemoreceptor trigger zone
CUPS - Cancer of unknown primary site
CV - Cardiovascular
CVA - Cerebral vascular accident
CVA - Costovertebral angle
CVOD - Corporal veno-occlusive dysfunction
CVS - Chorionic villus sampling
c/w - Consistent with
CW - Caucasian woman
CVP - Central venous pressure
CVS - Chorionic villous sampling
CXR - Chest x-ray
CYA - Cover your ass
CYE - Charcoal yeast extract

D

D5W - 5% dextrose in water
D5WNS - 5% dextrose in normal saline
D50W - 50% dextrose in water
DA - Developmental age
DA - Dopamine
DAG - Diacyl glycerol
DAP - Draw-a-Person Test
DAP - Diaminopimelic acid
DAT - Dementia of the Alzheimer type
DAW - Dispense as written
D/C - Discontinue
DC - Discharge
D&C - Dilation and curettage
DCIS - Ductal carcinoma in situ
DDAVP - Diamino-8-D-arginine vasopressin
DDC - Dideoxycytidine
DDI - Deoxyadenosine
Ddx - Differential diagnosis
D&E - Dilation and evacuation
DEB - Diepoxybutane
DES - Diethylstilbestrol
DEXA - Dual emission x-ray aborption
DFS - Disease free survival
DH - Dermatits herpetiformis
DHEA - Dehydroepiandrosterone
DHEAS - Dehydroepiandrosterone sulfate
DHT - Dihydrotestosterone
DI - Diabetes insipidus
DIC - Disseminated intravascular coagulation
DICC - Dynamic infusion caverno-sometry and cavernosography
DIT - Diiodotyrosine
DKA - Diabetic ketoacidosis
DM - Diabetes mellitus
DMD - Duchenne's muscular dystrophy
DMPA - Depo-provera
DMSA - Dimercaptosuccinic acid
DNA - Deoxyribose nucleic acid
DNKA - Did not keep appointment
DNR - Do not resuscitate
DO - Disorder
DOA - Dead on arrival
DOA - Date of admission
DOB - Date of birth
DOE - Dyspnoea on exertion
DOT - Directly observed therapy
DP - Dorsalis pedalis
DPI - Dry powder inhaler
DPL - Diagnostic peritoneal lavage
DPT - Diptheria, pertussis, tetanus
DSA - Digital subtraction angiography
DSD - Detrusor-external sphincter dyssynergia
DSM - Diagnostic and Statistical Manual on Mental Disorders
DST - Dexamethasone suppression test
DT - Delirium tremens
DTaP - Diptheria, tetanus, acellular pertussis
DTP - Diptheria, tetanus, pertussis (vaccine)
DTR - Deep tendon reflex
DUB - Dysfunctional uterine bleeding
DV - Domestic violence
DVT - Deep venous thrombosis
Dx - Diagnosis

E

EBI - Exercise induced bronchospasm
EBL - Estimated blood loss
EBV - Epstein-Barr virus
EC - Eye contact
ECASA - Enteric coated acetylsalicylic acid
ECC - Emergency cardiac care
ECF - Extracellular fluid
ECG - Electrocardiogram
ECMO - Extracorporeal membrane oxygenation
ECR - Endocavitary radiation
ECT - Electroconvulsive therapy
ECV - External cephalic version
ED50 - Effective dose in 50% population
EDC - Estimated date of confinement
EDD - Estimated delivery date
EDP - Emotionally disturbed person
EDTA - Ethylenediaminetetraacetic acid
EEG - Electroencephalogram
EF - Ejection fraction
EFW - Estimated fetal weight
EGA - Estimated gestational age
EGC - Early gastric cancer
EGD - Esophagogastroduodenoscopy
EGF - Epidermal growth factor
EHBA - Extrahepatic biliary atresia
EHEC - Enterohemorrhagic e. coli
EIEC - Enteroinvasive e. coli
EKG - Electrocardiogram
ELISA - Enzyme-linked immunosorbent assay
EMD - Electromechanical dissociation
EMG - Electromyogram
EMS - Emergency medical services
EOMI - Extraocular muscles intact
EPEC - Enteropathogenic e. coli
EPP - End plate potential
EPS - Extrapyramidal syndrome
EPS - Expressed prostatic secretions
EPS - Exophthalmos-producing substance
ERCP - Endoscopic retrograde cholangiopancreatography
ERP - Effective refractory period
ERV - Expiratory reserve volume
ESL - English as second language
ESR - Erythrocyte sedimentation rate
ESS - Empty sella syndrome
EST - Exercise stress test
ESRD - End stage renal disease
ESWT - Extracorporeal shock wave therapy
ETC - Electron transport chain
ETEC - Enterotoxic e. coli
EtOH - Ethanol (alcohol)
EVS - Endovaginal sonography
EW - Emergency ward

F

F - Father
F - Female
FAP - familial adenomatous polyposis
FAS - Fetal alcohol syndrome
FB - Foreign body
F/C - Fever, chills
FDA - Food and Drug Administration
FEF - Forced expiratory flow
FEN - Fluids, electrolytes, nutrition
FEV - Forced expiratory volume

FFP - Fresh frozen plasma
FH - Family history
FH - Fundal height
FHR - Fetal heart rate
FL - Femur length
FM - Fetal movement
FNA - Fine needle aspiration
FNF - Finger to nose
FNH - Follicular nodular hyperplasia
FOB - Father of baby
FOBT - Fecal occult blood testing
FRC - Functional residual capacity
FROM - Free range of motion
FS - Finger stick
FSE - Fetal scalp electrode
FSH - Follicle stimulating hormone
FT - Full term
FTP - Failure to progress
FTT - Failure to thrive
F/U - Follow up
FU - Fluorouracil
FUO - Fever of unknown origin
FVC - Forced vital capacity

G

G6PD - Glucose-6-phosphate dehydrogenase
GA - Gestational age
GABA - Gamma-amino butyric acid
GAD - Generalized anxiety disorder
GAF - Global assessment of function
GBM - Glioblastoma multiforme
GBS - Guillain-Barré syndrome
GC - Gonococcal
GCS - Glasgow Coma scale
GDM - Gestational diabetes mellitus
GERD - Gastroesophageal reflux disease
GETA - General endotracheal anesthesia
GIFT - Gamete intrafallopian transfer
GFR - Glomerular filtration rate
GGT - Gamma-glutamyl transferase
GMC - Generalized medical condition
GnRH - Gonadotropine releasing hormone
GH - Growth hormone
GHRH - Growth hormone releasing hormone
GI - Gastrointestinal
GIST - Gastrointestinal stromal tumor
GLT - Glucose loading test
GSW - Gunshot wound
GTD - Gestational trophoblastic disease
GTP - Guanosine triphosphate
GTT - Glucose tolerance test
GU - Genitourinary

H

HA - Headache
HA - Hemolytic anaemia
HAV - Hepatitis A virus
HBV - Hepatitis B virus
Hb - Haemoglobin
HC - Head circumference
hCG - Human chorionic gonadotropin
hCS - Human chorionic somatom-ammootropin
hct - Hematocrit
HCTZ - Hydrochlorothiazide
HCV - Hepatitis C virus
HDL - High density lipoprotein
HDV - Hepatitis D virus
HEENT - Head, eyes, ears, nose, throat

HEPA - High efficiency particulate air
HEV - Hepatitis E virus
HIAA - 5-hydroxyindoleacetic acid
HIB - Hemophilus influenzae type B
HIDA - Hepatobiliary iminodiacetic acid
HIV - Human immunodeficiency virus
HKS - Heel knee shin
HLA - Human leukocyte antigen
hMG - Human menopausal gonadotropin
HMO - Health maintenance organization
HNPCC - Hereditary nonpolyposis colon cancer
HP - Hospital police
HPA - Hypothalamic suppression test
HPI - History of present illness
hPL - Human placental lactogen
HPV - Human papillomavirus
HR - Heart rate
HRCT - High resolution computed tomography
HRT - Hormone replacement therapy
HSG - Hysterosalpingogram
HSV - Herpes simplex virus
HTLV - Human T-cell leukemia virus
HTN - Hypertension
HUS - Hemolytic uremic syndrome
HVA - Homovanillic acid

I

IA - Intraarterial
IBD - Inflammatory bowel disease
IBS - Inflammatory bowel syndrome
IBW - Ideal body weight
IC - Inspiratory capacity
IC - Immunocompromised
ICA - Internal carotid artery
ICD-9 - International Classification of Diseases, 9th Revision
ICH - Intracerebral hemorrhage
ICM - Intensive case manager
ICP - Intracranial pressure
ICU - Intensive care unit
I&D - Incision and drainage
ID - Infectious diseases
IDDM - Insulin dependent diabetes mellitus
IFN - Interferon
IGF - Insulin-like growth factor
IHSS - Idiopathic hypertrophic subacute stenosis
IL - Interleukin
IM - Intramuscular
IMA - Internal mammary artery
IMA - Inferior mesenteric artery
IMV - Inferior mesenteric vein
IMV - Intermittent mandatory ventilation
INH - Isoniazid
INO - Internuclear opthalmoplegia
INR - International normalized ratio
I&O - Ins and outs
IOC - Intraoperative cholangiogram
ION - Ischemic optic neuropathy
IOR - Ideas of reference
IP - Inpatient
IPF - Idiopathic pulmonary fibrosis
IPPB - Intermittent positive pressure breathing
IPV - Inactivated polio vaccine
IQ - Intelligence quotient
IRV - Inspiratory reserve volume
ISS - Insulin sliding scale

ISS - Injury severity score
ITP - Idiopathic thrombocytopenic purpura
IUD - Intrauterine device
IUFD - Intrauterine fetal death
IUGR - Intrauterine growth restriction
IUI - Intrauterine insemination
IUP - Intrauterine pregnancy
IUPC - Intrauterine pressure catheter
IV - Intravenous
IVC - Inferior vena cava
IVCD - Intraventricular conduction delay
IVDSA - Intravenous digital subtraction angiography
IVDU - Intravenous drug use
IVF - Intravenuous fluids
IVF - *In vitro* fertilization
IVH - Intraventricular hemorrhagc
IVIG - Intravenous immune globulin
IVP - Intravenous pyelogram
IVP - Intravenous push

J

JCV - JC virus
JGA - Juxtaglumerular apparatus
JP - Jackson-Pratt (tube)
JRA - Juvenile rheumatoid arthritis
JVD - Jugular venous distension

K

KS - Kaposi sarcoma
KUB - Kidney, ureter, bladder (x-ray)

L

LA - Left atrium
LAAM - L-a-acetylmethadol
LAHB - Left anterior hemiblock
LAD - Lymphadenopathy
LAD - Left anterior descending
LAD - Leukocyte adhesion deficiency
LAP - Leukocyte alkaline phosphatase
LAFB - Left anterior fascicular block
LAR - Low anterior resection
LBBB - Left bundle branch block
LBP - Lower back pain
LBW - Low birth weight
LCIS - Lobular carcinoma in situ
LCME - Liaison Committee on Medical Education
LD50 - Lethal dose in 50% population
LDH - Lactase dehydrogenase
LDL - Low density lipoprotein
LDR - Labor and delivery room
LE - Lower extremity
LE - Leukocyte esterase
LES - Lower oesophageal sphincter
LEV - Levamisole
LFD - Low fat diet
LFT - Liver function test
LGA - Large for gestational age
LGV - Lymphogranuloma venereum
LH - Luteinizing hormone
LIH - Left inguinal hernia
LLL - Left lower lobe
LLQ - Left lower quadrant
LMP - Last menstural period
LOA - Left occiput anterior
LOC - Loss of conciousness
LOC - Level of conciousness
LOF - Loss of fluid
LOP - Left occiput posterior
LOS - Length of stay
LOT - Left occiput transverse

LP - Lumbar puncture
LPFB - Left posterior fascicular block
LPHB - Left posterior hemiblock
LR - Lactated Ringer's
LSB - Left sternal border
LSD - Lysergic acid diethylamide
LSO - Left salpingo-oophrectomy
LTX - Leukotrienes
LUL - Left upper lobe
LUQ - Left upper quadrant
LV - Left ventricle
LVH - Left ventricular hypertrophy

M

M - Mother
M - Male
MABP - Mean arterial blood pressure
MAC - Mycobacterium avium intracellulare complex
MAC - Minimum alveolar concentration
MAI - Mycobacterium avium intracellulare
MAOI - Monoamine oxidase inhibitor
MAP - Mean arterial pressure
MAS - Meconium aspiration syndrome
MAT - Multifocal atrial tachycardia
MBC - Minimal bacteriocidal concentration
MCA - Middle cerebral artery
MCH - Mean corpuscular haemoglobin
MCHC - Mean corpuscular haemoglobin concentration
MCL - Mid clavicular line
MCO - Managed care organization
MCTD - Mixed connective tissue disease
MCV - Mean corpuscular volume
MD - Muscular dystrophy
MDD - Maximum daily dose
MDD - Major depressive disorder
MDE - Major depressive episode
MDI - Metered dose inhaler
MEA - Multiple endocrine adenomatosis
MEC - Mininum effective concentration
MEFR - Maximal expiratory flow rate
MEN - Multiple endocrine neoplasia
MHC - Major histocompatibility complex
MHPG - 3-methoxy 4-hydroxy-phenylglycol
MI - Myocardial infarction
MIC - Minimal inhibitory concentration
MIF - Müllerian inhibiting factor
MIT - Monoiodotyrosine
MLD - Metachromatic leukodystrophy
M&M - Morbidity and mortality
MMEFR - Maximal mid-expiratory flow rate
MMFR - Maximal mid-expiratory flow rate
MMM - Moist mucous membrane
MMPI - Minnesota Multiphasic Personality Inventory
MMR - Measles, mumps, rubella (vaccine)
MOPD - Mechlorethamine, vincristine (Oncovin), procarbazine, prednisone
MR - Mental retardation
MRA - Magnetic resonance angiography

MRCP - Magnetic resonance cholangiopancreatography
MRDD - Maximum recommended daily dose
MRG - Murmurs, rubs, and gallops
MRI - Magnetic resonance imaging
MRM - Modified radical mastectomy
MRPN - Medical resident progress note
MRSA - Methicillin-resistant Staphylococcus aureus
MRT - Medical review team
MRT - Magnetic resonance tomography
MS - Multiple sclerosis
MS - Mental status
MS - Mitral stenosis
MS - Morphine sulfate
MSAFP - Maternal serum alpha-fetoprotein
MSD - Mean sac diameter
MSE - Mental status examination
MSG - Monosodium glutamate
MSH - Melanocyte stimulating hormone
MSO4 - Morphine sulfate
MV - Mitral valve
MVA - Motor vehicle accident
MVI - Multivitamin
MVP - Mitral valve prolapse
MVR - Mitral valve replacement
MVV - Max voluntary ventilation

N

NAD - No acute distress
NAD - Nicotinamide adenine dinucleotide
NBT - Nitroblue tetrazolium reduction test
NC - Normo-cephalic
NC - No change
NC - Nasal canula
NCI - National Cancer Institute
ND - Non-distended
NDI - Nephrogenic diabetes insipidus
NE - Norepinephrine
NEC - Necroting enterocolitis
NGT - Nasogastric tube
NHL - Non-Hodgkin's lymphoma
NIDDM - Non-insulin dependent diabetes mellitus
NIF - Negative inspiratory force
NIH - National Institutes of Health
NKDA - No known drug allergies
NM - Neuromuscular
NMS - Neuroleptic malignant syndrome
NOS - Not otherwise specified
NPH - Neutral protamine Hagedorn (regular insulin)
NPO - Nil per os (nothing by mouth)
NPV - Negative predictive value
NS - Normal saline
NSAID - Nonsteroidal anti-inflammatory drug
NSR - Normal sinus rhythm
NST - Nonstress test
NSVD - Normal spontaneous vaginal delivery
NT - Non-tender
NTD - Neural tube defect
NTD - Nothing to do
NTG - Nitroglycerine
N/V - Nausea, vomiting
NVD - Normal vaginal delivery

O

OA - Occiput anterior
OAA - Oxaloacetic acid
OCD - Obsessive compulsive disorder
OCG - Oral cholecystography
OCP - Oral contraceptive pills
OCT - Oxytocin challenge test
ODD - Oppositional defiant disorder
OGTT - Oral glucose tolerance test
ON - Optic neuritis
OOB - Out of bed
OP - Occiput posterior
OPD - Outpatient department
OPV - Oral polio vaccine
ORIF - Open reduction & internal fixation
OS - Overall survival
OSA - Obstructive sleep apnea
OTC - Over the counter

P

PA - Posteroanterior
PA - Physician's assistant
PA - Pulmonary artery
PA - Patient
PAC - Premature atrial contraction
PAH - P-aminohippuric acid
PAP - Pulmonary artery pressure
PAT - Pulseless atrial tachycardia
PBC - Primary biliary cirrhosis
PBP - Penicillin binding protein
PCA - Patient controlled anesthesia
PCA - Posterior cerebral artery
PCB - Polychlorinated biphenyls
PCN - Penicillin
PCO - Polycystic ovaries
PCOS - Polycystic ovarian syndrome
PCP - Pneumocystis carinii pneumonia
PCP - Phencyclidine
PCP - Primary care physician
PCR - Polymerase chain reaction
PCTA - Percutaneous transluminal angioplasty
PCWP - Pulmonary capillary wedge pressure
PD - Peritoneal dialysis
PD - Parkinson's Disease
PDA - Patent ductus arteriosus
PDGF - Platelet derived growth factor
PE - Pulmonary embolism
PE - Physical exam
PEA - Pulseless electrical activity
PEF - Peak expiratory flow
PEEP - Positive end expiratory pressure
PEG - Percutaneous endoscopic gastrostomy
PEG - polyethylene glycol
PERRLA- Pupils equal in size, round and reactive to light and accommodation
PES - Paediatric emergency service
PET - Positron emission tomography
PFT - Pulmunary function test
PG - Prostaglandin
PICC - Peripherally inserted central catheter
PID - Pelvic inflammatory disease
PICU - Paediatric ICU
PIF - Prolactin inhibiting factor
PIH - Pregnancy induced hypertension
PKD - Polycystic kidney disease
PKU - Phenylketonuria

Plt - Platelet
PMA - Psychomotor agitation
PMD - Primary medical doctor
PMH - Past medical history
PMI - Point of maximal impulse
PML - Progressive multifocal leukoencephalopathy
PMP - Post menopausal
PMR - Psychomotor retardation
PMR - Proportionate mortality rate
PMS - Premenstrual syndrome
PND - Paroxysmal nocturnal dyspnoea
PNET - Primitive neuroectodermal tumor
PNS - Peripheral nervous system
PNV - Pre-natal vitamins
PO - Per os (by mouth)
PO - Parole officer
POC - Products of conception
POD - Post operative day
POEM - patient oriented evidence that matters
PPD - Purified protein derivative (tuberculosis test)
PPD - Pack per day
PPN - Peripheral parenteral nutrition
PPROM - Preterm premature rupture of membrane
PPV - Positive pressure ventilation
PPV - Positive predictive value
PR - Per rectum
PRBC - Packed red blood cells
PRN - As necessary
PROM - Prolonged rupture of membrane
PSA - Prostate serum antigen
PSA - Polysubstance abuse
PSE - Present State Examination
PSH - Past surgical history
PSS - Progressive systemic sclerosis
PSTT - Placental site trophoblastic tumor
PSUD - Polysubstance use disorder
PSVT - Paroxysmal supraventricular tachycardia
PT - Prothrombin time
PT - Physical therapy
PT - Patient
PT - Posterier tibialis
PTA - Prior to admission
PTA - Percutaneous transluminal angioplasty
PTC - Percutaneous transhepatic cholangiogram
PTCA - Percutaneous transluminal coronary angioplasty
PTFE - Polytetrafluoroethylene
PTH - Parathyroid hormone
PTL - Preterm labor
PTSD - Post-traumatic stress disorder
PTT - Partial prothrombin time
PTU - Propylthiouracil
PTX - Pneumothorax
PUBS - Percutaneous umbilical blood sampling
PUD - Peptic ulcer disease
PVC - Premature ventral contraction
PVR - Pulmonary vascular resistance
PVR - Pulse volume recording
PVS - Persistent vegetative state
PVT - Pulseless ventricular tachycardia

Q

qd - Once a day
qh - Once every hour

qhs - Once every day at night
qid - Four times a day
QNS - Quantity not sufficient
qod - Every other day

R

RA - Right atrium
RA - Rheumatoid arthritis
RA - Room air
RAD - Reactive airway disease
RAIU - Radioactive iodine uptake
RAM - Rapid alternating movements
RBBB - Right bundle branch block
RBC - Red blood cell
RCA - Right coronary artery
RDI - Recommended daily intake
RDS - Respiratory distress syndrome
RDW - Red blood cell distribution of width
REE - Resting energy expenditure
REM - Rapid eye movements
RF - Risk factor
r/g/m - Rubs, gallops, murmurs
RHD - Rheumatic heart disease
RID - Radial immunodiffusion
RIH - Right inguinal hernia
RIMA - Reversible inhibitors of monoamine oxidase A
RISS - Regular insulin sliding scale
RLL - Right lower lobe
RLQ - Right lower quadrant
RN - Registered nurse
ROA - Right occiput anterior
ROM - Rupture of membrane
ROP - Right occiput posterior
ROS - Review of symptoms
ROT - Right occiput transverse
RPF - Renal plasma flow
RR - Respiratory rate
RRP - Relative refractory period
RRR - Regular rate and rhythm
RSB - Right sternal border
RSO - Right salpingo-oophrectomy
RSV - Respiratory syncytial virus
RTA - Renal tubular acidosis
RTC - Return to clinic
RTF - Residential treatment facility
RTS - Revised trauma score
RUL - Right upper lobe
RUQ - Right upper quadrant
RV - Right ventricle
RV - Residual volume
RVH - Right ventricular hypertrophy
Rx - Treatment
RXN - Reaction

S

SA - Sinoatrial
SA - Suicide attempt
SAB - Spontaneous abortion
SAD - Schizoaffective disorder
SAD - Seasonal affective disorder
SAH - Subarachnoid hemorrhage
SAM - S-adenosylhomocysteine
SBE - Subacute bacterial endocarditis
SBO - Small bowel obstruction
SBP - Spontaneous bacterial peritonitis
SBS - Shaken baby syndrome
SC - Subcutaneous
SCID - Severe combined immuno-deficiency disease
SCT - Sentence Completion Test
SD - Standard deviation

SDA - Same day admission
SEM - Systolic ejection murmur
SES - Socio-economic status
SFNA - Stereotactic fine needle aspiration
SGA - Small for gestational age
SGOT - Serum glutamic oxaloacetic transaminase
SI - Suicidal ideations
SIADH - Syndrome of inappropriate antidiuretic hormone
SICU - Surgical ICU
SIDS - Sudden infant death syndrome
SIL - Squamous intraepithelial lesions
SL - Sublingual
SLNTG - Sublingual nitroglycerin
SLE - Systemic lupus erythematosus
SMA6 - Sequential multiple analyzer series 6 (electrolyte panel)
SMA - Superior mesenteric artery
SMA - Spinal muscle atrophy
SMR - Sexual maturity rating
SMV - Superior mesenteric vein
SMX - Sulfamethoxazole
SNF - Skilled nursing facility
SOB - Shortness of breath
SP - Suprapubic
S/P - Status post
SPA - Sperm penetration assay
SPECT - Single photon emission computed tomography
SPEP - Serum protein electrophoresis
SQ - Subcutaneous
SR - Sustained release
SROM - Spontaneous rupture of membrane
SS - Social security
SSE - Sterile speculum examination
SSE - Subacute spongiform encephalopathy
SSLF - Sacral spinous ligament fixation
SSPE - Subacute sclerosing panencephalitis
SSS - Sick sinus syndrome
SSS - Scalded skin syndrome
SST - Somatostatin
STD - Sexually transmitted disease
STSG - Split thickness skin graft
SV - Stroke volume
SVC - Superior vena cava
SVE - Sterile vaginal examination
SVR - Systemic vascular resistance
SVT - Supraventricular tachycardia
SW - Social work
SWL - Shock wave lithotripsy
Sx - symptom

T

TAH - Total abdominal hysterectomy
TAHBSO- Total abdominal hysterectomy, bilateral salpingo-oophrectomy
TAPVR - Total anomalous pulmonary venous return
TAS - Transabdominal sonography
TAT - Thematic Aperception Test
TB - Tuberculosis
TBI - Traumatic brain injury
TBG - Thyroid binding globulin
TBW - Total body water
T&C - Type and cross (blood)
TC - Thought content
TC - Therapeutic community
TCA - Tricyclic antidepressant
TCBS - thiosulfate citrate bile salts sucrose

TCH - Tetrahydrocannabinol
TCP - Transcutaneous pacing
TD - Tardive dyskinesia
TD50 - Toxic dose in 50% population
TDF - Testes-determining factor
TEE - Transesophageal echocardiogram
TEM - Transanal endoscopic microsurgery
TFT - Thyroid function test
TGA - Transient global amnesia
TGA - Transposition of the great arteries
TGV - Transposition of the great vessels
THC - Transhepatic cholangiogram
THC - Tetrahydrocannabinol
TI - Therapeutic index
TIA - Transient ischemic attack
TIBC - Transferrin iron-binding capacity
tid - Three times a day
TIG - Tetanus immunoglobulin
TIPS - Transjugular intrahepatic portosystemic shunt
tiw - Three times a week
TLC - Total lung capacity
Tm - Maximal temperature
TM - Tympanic membrane
TME - Total mesorectal excision
TMP - Trimethoprim
TNF - Tumor necrosis factor
TNM - Tumor, node, metastasis
TOA - Tubo-ovarian abcess
TOC - Tubo-ovarian complex
TOL - Trial of labor
TOS - Thoracic outlet syndrome
TP - Thought process
tPA - Tissue plasminogen activator
TPN - Total parenteral nutrition
TPR - Total peripheral resistance
T&R - Treated & released
TRAM - Transverse rectus abdominis myocutaneous (flap)
TRH - Thyrotropin releasing hormone
T&S - Type and screen (blood)
TSH - Thyroid stimulating hormone
TSS - Toxic shock syndrome
TSST - Toxic shock syndrome toxin
TT - Thrombin time
TTE - Transthoracic echocardiogram
TTN - Transient tachypnea of the newborn
TTP - Thrombotic thrombocytopenic purpura
TURP - Transurethral resection of the prostate
TURBT - Transurethral resection of bladder tumor
TV - Tidal volume
TXA2 - Thromboxane A2

U

UA - Urinalysis
UC - Ulcerative colitis
UE - Upper extremity
UO - Urine output
UPJ - Ureteral pelvic junction
URI - Upper respiratory infection
US - Ultrasound
USOH - Usual state of health
UTI - Urinary tract infection
UTO - Unable to obtain

V

VA - Ventriculoatrial
VATS - Video-assisted thoracoscopy
VB - Vaginal bleeding
VBAC - Vaginal birth after caesarean section
VC - Vital capacity
VCUG - Voiding cystourethrogram
VDRL - Venereal Disease Research Laboratory (syphilis test)
VF - Ventricular fibrillation
VH - Vaginal hysterectomy
VH - Hallucination
VIN - Vulvar intraepithelial neoplasia
VIP - Vasoactive intestional peptide
VIP - Voluntary interruption of pregnancy
VLDL - Very low density lipoproteins
VMA - Vanillylmandelic acid
VNS - Visiting nurse service
VPC - Ventricular premature contraction
VRS - Volume reduction surgery
VS - Vital signs
VSD - Ventricular septal defect
VSS - Vital signs stable
VT - Ventricular tachycardia
VZV - Varicella zoster virus

W

WAIS-R - Wechsler Adult Intelligence Scale, Revised
WAGR - Wilm's tumor, aniridia, genitourinary malformation, mental retardation
WAS - Wiskott-Aldrich syndrome
WB - Whole blood
WBC - White blood cell
WCST - Wisconsin Card Sort Test
WD - Well developed
W/D - Withdrawal
WF - White female
WIC - Walk in clinic
WISC-R - Wechsler Intelligence Scale for Children, Revised
WM - White male
WN - Well nourished
WNL - Within normal limits
WPPSI - Wechsler Preschool and Primary Scale of Intelligence
WPW - Wolf-Parkinson-White
w/r/r - Wheezing, ronchi, rales

X

XRT - External radiation therapy
XST - Extra strength Tylenol

Z

ZE - Zollinger-Ellison syndrome

APPENDIX-II

Glossary of Medical Terms

ABC: The 'ABC' of resuscitation or life support means to check Airways, Breathing and Circulation.

ACHALASIA: *Achalasia* is a serious condition that affects the esophagus.

ACROMEGALY: *Acromegaly* is a hormonal disorder that develops when your pituitary gland produces too much growth hormone during adulthood.

ACUTE: When applied to a medical condition, this term means 'of severe, sudden, but short duration'.

ACUTE MYOCARDIAL INFARCTION: Onset of sudden damage to part of the heart muscle, usually due to blockage of the heart's (coronary) arteries. Synonymous with a heart attack.

ADDICTION: In the context of this handbook, the habitual taking of drugs or alcohol due to a physical and/or psychological dependency.

AFEBRILE: Without fever.

AIDS: Autoimmune dificiency Syndrome.

ALCOHOLISM: Where any physical, mental or social problem caused by alcohol is present.

ALLERGY: Sensitivity to a foreign substance, resulting in a physical reaction such as rash or hay fever.

AMBULANT: Able to walk.

AMYOTROPHIC LATERAL SCLEROSIS: *Amyotrophic lateral sclerosis* (*ALS*), also known as Lou Gehrig's disease and motor neurone disease (MND), is a specific disease that causes the death of neurons which control voluntary muscles.

ANAEMIA: A decrease in the concentration of red blood cells or of HAEMOGLOBIN in the blood. May cause pallor (paleness) of the skin.

ANGINA: Cardiac pain due to poor blood supply to the heart.

ANOREXIA: Loss of appetite.

ANOXIA: Without oxygen.

ANTEROGRADE AMNESIA: Anterograde amnesia is a loss of the ability to create new memories after the event that caused the **amnesia**, leading to a partial or complete inability to recall the recent past, while long-term memories from before the event remain intact.

ANTI-ANXIETY (medication): Prescribed drugs used to treat anxiety disorders.

ANTIBIOTIC: A drug that destroys bacteria.

ANTIBODY: A substance produced by the immune system to fight invading organisms such as viruses.

ANTIDEPRESSANT (medication): Prescribed drugs used to treat depression.

ANTIPSYCHOTIC (medication): Prescribed drugs used to treat psychosis.

ANXIETY: A state of tension affecting the mind and the body. Anxiety can range from acute (short term) to chronic (long term).

APERIENT: A laxative (to move the bowels).

APHTHOUS STOMATITIS: *Aphthous stomatitis* is a common condition characterized by the repeated formation of benign and non-contagious mouth *ulcers* (aphthae) in otherwise healthy individuals.

APPENDICITIS: Inflammation of the appendix, a hollow finger-like projection of the colon.

ARREST: Used in a medical sense, this means a cessation of bodily activity (for example, cardiac arrest means that the heart has stopped beating and respiratory arrest means cessation of breathing).

ARTHRITIS: Inflammation of a joint.

ASTHMA: A lung disease characterised by difficulty in breathing and by coughing and wheezing.

ATAXIA: A jerky unsteadiness of the limbs and body due to disease in a particular part of the brain.

AURA: A visual disturbance occurring prior to an epileptic fit.

AUTOIMMUNE DEFICIENCY SYNDROME: Commonly referred to as AIDS, it implies loss of immune system function. Due to late stage HIV infection.

BACTERIA: Microscopic organisms that cause infection and which can reproduce themselves.

BARRETT'S ESOPHAGUS : *Barrett's esophagus* refers to an abnormal change (metaplasia) in the cells of the lower portion of the esophagus.

BASELINE BLOOD TEST: Basic tests done in initial stages of a medical investigation.

BCG: The 'Bacille Calmett-Guerin' (tuberculosis or TB) vaccination.

BRONCHIAL: Of the larger airways of the lungs.

BRONCHIECTASIS: *Bronchiectasis* is a disease in which there is permanent enlargement of parts of the airways of the lung.

BRONCHITIS: Infection of the larger airways of the lungs.

BRONCHOGENIC CARCINOMA: **Bronchogenic carcinoma** is a malignant neoplasm of the lung arising from the epithelium of the bronchus or bronchiole.

BUDD-CHIARI SYNDROME: *Budd-Chiari syndrome* is an uncommon condition induced by thrombotic or nonthrombotic obstruction of the hepatic venous outflow and is characterized by hepatomegaly, ascites, and abdominal pain.

CARNEY'S TRIAD: Carney triad (CT) is characterized by the coexistence of three types of neoplasms, mainly in young women,including gastric gastrointestinal stromal tumor, pulmonary chondroma, and extra-adrenal paraganglioma.

CAROTID: The large artery beside the larynx which is ideal for emergency checking of the pulse.

CAROTID ENDARTERECTOMY: **Carotid endarterectomy** (CEA) is a surgical procedure used to reduce the risk of stroke by correcting stenosis (narrowing) in the common **carotid** artery or internal **carotid** artery.

CEREBELLAR HEMANGIOBLASTOMA: *Hemangioblastomas* are rare tumors that occur in blood vessels of the brain and spinal.

CEREBRAL PALSY: Cerebral palsy refers to a group of neurological disorders that appear in infancy or early childhood and permanently affect body movement and muscle coordination Cerebral palsy (CP) is caused by damage to or abnormalities inside the developing brain that disrupt the brain's ability to control movement and maintain posture and balance.

CHEYNE-STOKES RESPIRATION: *Cheyne–Stokes respiration*/ÈtƒejnÈstoŠks/ is an abnormal pattern of breathing characterized by progressively deeper and sometimes faster breathing.

CHRONIC: Long term.

CHRONIC THROMBOEMBOLIC PULMONARY HYPERTENSION: Chronic thromboembolic pulmonary hypertension (CTEPH) is a distinct pulmonary vascular disease caused by chronic obstruction of major pulmonary arteries that is amenable to cure by pulmonary endarterectomy (PEA).

CIRRHOSIS: Condition of the liver where it becomes shrunken, hardened and fails to function normally.

COGNITION: The area of more sophisticated mental functioning (intelligence, judgment, insight, memory and so on).

COMA: A persistent state of unconsciousness.

CONCUSSION: Loss of consciousness due to severe head injury.

CONJUNCTIVITIS: Pinkeye (also called *conjunctivitis*) is redness and swelling of the conjunctiva, the mucous membrane that lines the eyelid and eye surface.

CORONER: A magistrate appointed to investigate the cause of death in certain situations, for instance a sudden unexpected death.

CPR: Cardio-Pulmonary-Resuscitation (active combined resuscitation of the heart and lungs).

CRICOPHARYNGEAL DYSFUNCTION: **Cricopharyngeal dysfunction** is a narrowing at the level of the upper oesophageal sphincter caused by failed or incomplete sphincter opening as a result of lack of pharyngoesophageal coordination or reduction in the muscular compliance of the upper oesophageal sphincter.

CRISIS ASSESSMENT TEAM (CAT): A community based emergency psychiatric service.

CROHN'S DISEASE: *Crohn's disease* is an inflammatory bowel *disease* (IBD). It causes inflammation of the lining of the digestive tract, which can lead to abdominal pain, severe diarrhea, fatigue, weight loss and malnutrition.

CUTANEOUS FISTULAS: A fistula is an abnormal communication between two epithelialized surfaces; an enterocutaneous fistula (ECF), as the name indicates, is an abnormal communication between the small or large bowel and the skin.

DELIRIUM TREMENS (the DTs): A serious state of delirium due to alcohol withdrawal. Due to overactivity of the nervous system.

DERMATOMYOSITIS: *Dermatomyositis* is an idiopathic inflammatory myopathy with characteristic cutaneous findings that occur in children and adults.

DELUSION: A false idea or belief held by a person that cannot be corrected by reasoning.

DEMENTIA: Partial or total loss of personality and other significant mental functions, due to mental deterioration, but without psychosis.

DEPENDENCY: Describes an ongoing need for a substance to prevent unpleasant symptoms. May be psychological or physical.

DEPERSONALISATION: A subjective experience where there is a feeling of being disconnected from the body or from the immediate environment.

DEPRESSION: An unpleasant, unhappy state of mind and body with significant impairment of memory, concentration and other mental processes. Physical activity is also slowed.

DERMATITIS: Inflammation of the skin.

DETOXIFICATION: Removal over time of toxic (drugs/alcohol etc.) substances from the body.

DIABETES: A disease with abnormally high blood sugar. Due to lack of insulin.

DIABETIC: A patient with diabetes.

DIAGNOSIS: Determination of the cause and severity of a disease.

DIAPHORESIS: *Diaphoresis* is the medical term used to describe excessive, abnormal sweating in relation to your environment and activity level.

DIFFUSE ESOPHAGEAL SPASMS: **Diffuse esophageal spasm** (DES) is a condition characterized by uncoordinated contractions of the **esophagus**, which may cause difficulty swallowing (dysphagia) or regurgitation.

DISORIENTATION: Inability to recognise time or surroundings or identify oneself or another person.

DOWN SYNDROME: *Down syndrome* (DS or DNS), also known as trisomy 21, is a genetic disorder caused by the presence of all or part of a third copy of chromosome 21.

DRUG WITHDRAWAL: The process where a toxic substance (drug) is naturally removed from the body. Subjectively unpleasant.

DUCTAL ADENOCARCINOMA: Pancreatic ductal adenocarcinoma is a type of exocrine pancreatic cancer. It develops from cells lining small tubes in the pancreas called ducts (duct cells in the diagram above). These carry the digestive juices, which contain enzymes, into the main pancreatic duct and then on into the duodenum (first part of the small intestine).

DUPEYTRON'S CONTRACTURE: Deformity of the hand, with the fingers in a claw-like position.

DYSBETALIPOPROTEINEMIA: **Familial dysbetalipoproteinemia** or type III hyperlipoproteinemia (also known as "remnant hyperlipidemia", "remnant hyperlipoproteinaemia", "broad beta disease" and "remnant removal disease") is a condition characterized by increased total cholesterol and triglyceride levels, and decreased HDL levels.

DYSPHAGIA: Dysphagia is the medical term for the symptom of difficulty in swallowing.

DYSPNOEA: Difficulty in breathing.

ECG: Electrocardiogram. An electrical recording of activity of the heart. May indicate either angina or a heartbeat rhythm problem.

ECT: Electroconvulsive Therapy. Used in the treatment of severe depression.

EEG: Electro-encephalogram. An electrical recording of brain activity.

ELECTROENCEPHALOGRAPHY: *Electroencephalography* (EEG) is an electrophysiological monitoring method to record electrical activity of the brain.

ELECTROMYOGRAM: An **electromyogram** (EMG) measures the electrical activity of muscles when they're at rest and when they're being used.

ELECTROOCULOGRAPHY (EOG/ E.O.G.): It is a technique for measuring the corneo-retinal standing potential that exists between the front and the back of the human eye. The resulting signal is called the *electrooculogram*.

EMPHYSEMA: Emphysema is a long-term, progressive disease of the lungs that primarily causes shortness of breath due to over-inflation of the alveoli (air sacs in the lung).

EMPHYSEMA: A lung disease with loss of lung tissue. Occurs in cigarette smokers.

ENDOMETRIAL CARCINOMA: *Endometrial cancer* is a *cancer* that arises from the *endometrium* (the lining of the uterus or womb). It is the result of the abnormal growth of cells that have the ability to invade or spread to other parts of the body.

EPIDIDYMAL CYSTADENOMA: Papillary *cystadenomas* of the *epididymis* are the benign tumours of the *epididymis* .

EPILEPSY: The occurrence of convulsions (involuntary bodily movements) due to abnormal electrical discharges in the brain.

EPISCLERITIS: It is a benign, self-limiting inflammatory disease affecting part of the eye called the episclera. The episclera is a thin layer of tissue that lies between the conjunctiva and the connective tissue layer that forms the white of the eye (sclera).

EPISTAXIS: Bleeding of the nose.

ERUPTIVE CUTANEOUS XANTHOMATOSIS: The sudden *eruption* on the skin of crops of pink papules (firm pea-sized bumps) with a creamy center.

ERYTHEMA NODOSUM: *Erythema nodosum* (EN) is an acute, nodular, erythematous eruption that usually is limited to the extensor aspects of the lower legs.

ESOPHAGEAL ADENOCARCINOMA: *Esophageal cancer* is a disease in which malignant (*cancer*) cells form in the tissues of the *esophagus*. The *esophagus* is a muscular tube that moves food and liquids from the throat to the stomach. The most common types of *esophageal cancer* are squamous cell *carcinoma* and *adenocarcinoma*.

ESOPHAGECTOMY: *Esophagectomy* (US English) or Oesophagectomy (British English) is the surgical removal of all or part of the esophagus.

FEBRILE: The presence of fever.

FEVER: A temperature above the normal level of 37 degrees Celsius.

FISTULA: A site where one bodily organ has formed an abnormal opening into another.

FITS: 1. The occurrence of epilepsy. 2. The street name for hypodermic syringes.

FRACTURE: A broken bone.

GALLSTONES: A common disease where firm 'stones' accumulate in the gall bladder.

GASTRITIS: Inflammation of the lining of the stomach, with pain and/or vomiting.

GASTRO-ENTERITIS: Inflammation of the stomach and intestine, with vomiting and/ or diarrhoea.

GASTROENTEROPATHY: *Gastro-enteropathy* manifesting in upper gastrointestinal symptoms, delayed gastric emptying, constipation, diarrhea and fecal incontinence occurs frequently in patients with diabetes mellitus and represents a significant health care burden.

GENERIC: When used in regard to health care, implies nonspecialised, or not specifically related to, a particular group, service, company etc.

GILBERT'S SYNDROME: *Gilbert's syndrome* (GS) is a mild liver disorder in which the liver does not properly process bilirubin.

GOODPASTURE'S SYNDROME: *Goodpasture syndrome* is a rare but serious autoimmune disease that attacks the lungs and kidneys. The disease occurs when the body's immune system mistakenly produces antibodies against collagen in the lungs and kidneys.

GUILLAIN-BARRÉ SYNDROME: *Guillain–Barré syndrome* (*GBS*) is a rapid-onset muscle weakness caused by the immune system damaging the peripheral nervous system.

GUILLAIN-BARRÉ SYNDROME: *Guillain–Barré syndrome* (*GBS*) is a rapid-onset muscle weakness caused by the immune system damaging the peripheral nervous system.

HAEMATEMESIS: Vomiting of pure blood or blood mixed with stomach contents.

HAEMATOMA: Medical name for a well demarcated 'bruise'.

HAEMATURIA: Blood in the urine.

HAEMOGLOBIN: A complicated iron-containing protein and found in red blood cells. It carries oxygen to the tissues.

HAEMOPTYSIS: Coughing up of blood.

HAEMORRHAGE: Loss of blood from the body, either internally or externally.

HALLUCINATION: A false sensory perception of one or more of the senses (vision, hearing, taste, smell, touch).

HASHIMOTO'S DISEASE: Hashimoto's disease is a condition in which your immune system attacks your thyroid, a small gland at the base of your neck below your Adam's apple.

HEART ATTACK: A general term referring to an acute affliction of the heart. Usually refers to ACUTE MYOCARDIAL INFARCTION, but may be used to describe acute onset of a disturbance to heartbeat rhythm.

HEART DISEASE: Any disease affecting the heart.

HEART FAILURE: Where the heart fails to perform its job of pumping blood to the lungs and to the remainder of the body.

HEMATOSPERMIA: Hematospermia is defined as blood in the semen. While often perceived as a symptom of little significance, blood in the ejaculate can cause great concern to the men who experience it.

HENOCH–SCHÖNLEIN PURPURA: *Henoch-Schonlein purpura* (*HSP*) is a disease involving inflammation of small blood vessels.

HEPATITIS: Inflammation of the liver; usually due to toxic substances such as alcohol or to viral infections such as the Hepatitis C virus.

HEPATOJUGULAR REFLUX: The *hepatojugular reflex* is a distension of the jugular veins that occurs when the abdomen is compressed for 10 to 30 seconds.

HEPATOSPLENOMEGALY: Hepatosplenomegaly (commonly abbreviated HSM) is the simultaneous enlargement of both the liver (*hepatomegaly*) and the spleen (*splenomegaly*).

HEPATOSPLENOMEGALY: It is a disorder where both the liver and spleen swell beyond their normal size, usually due to an infection such mononucleosis or viral hepatitis. It may also be a sign of another more serious illness such as a lysosomal storage disorder.

HERNIA: The abnormal protrusion of the contents of one part of the body into another.

HERNIA: A *hernia* occurs when an organ pushes through an opening in the muscle or tissue that holds it in place.

HOSPICE: A small hospital for the terminally ill.

HUMAN IMMUNODEFICIENCY VIRUS: A virus which infects the human immune system, impeding its operation.

HUNTINGTON DISEASE: *Huntington disease* is a progressive brain disorder that causes uncontrolled movements, emotional problems, and loss of thinking ability (cognition).

HYPERCAPNIA: *Hypercapnia*, also known as hypercarbia and CO2 retention, is a condition of abnormally elevated carbon dioxide (CO2) levels in the blood.

HYPERGLYCAEMIA: A blood sugar level above normal, which is indicative of diabetes.

HYPERREFLEXIA: *Hyperreflexia* (or hyper-reflexia) is defined as overactive or overresponsive reflexes.

HYPERTENSION: Blood pressure above normal; sometimes inaccurately used to describe stress.

HYPERTROPHIC OSTEOARTHROPATHY: *Hypertrophic osteoarthropathy* (HOA) is a syndrome of clubbing of the digits, periostitis of the long (tubular) bones, and arthritis.

HYPERVENTILATION: Breathing at a rate above normal, and often due to anxiety.

HYPOGLYCAEMIA: A low blood sugar level. Usually due to an excessive insulin dose.

HYPOTENSION: Low blood pressure.

HYPOTHERMIA: A low body temperature, which may be life threatening.

INCONTINENCE: Loss of control of the bladder and/or bowel.

INFECTION: Invasion of the body by harmful organisms that cause disease.

INFLAMMATION: The body's reaction to injury. Signs of inflammation are redness, heat, swelling and tenderness.

INSOMNIA: Inability to sleep.

INSULIN: A substance produced by the pancreas; needed to convert sugar to energy. Lacking in diabetics.

INTRAVENOUS: Within the vein, as with injections into a vein.

IRITIS : *Iritis* (i-RYE-tis) is inflammation that affects the colored ring around your eye's pupil (iris). The iris is a part of the middle layer of the eye (uvea), so *iritis* is a type of uveitis, also known as anterior uveitis.

ISCHAEMIA: Lack of blood supply to an area of the body. For example, cardiac ischaemia, which may cause angina. If severe, cardiac ischaemia may cause a heart attack.

JAUNDICE: Yellow discolouration of the skin and eyes due to liver disease.

KAPOSI'S SARCOMA: Kaposi sarcoma is a cancer that causes lesions (abnormal tissue) to grow in the skin; the mucous membranes lining the mouth, nose, and throat; lymph nodes; or other organs.

KORSAKOFF'S SYNDROME: Sufferers show amnesia and confabulation (filling in gaps in memory by guessing); due to the end stage of alcoholism. Connected with the Alcohol Related Brain Injury Syndrome.

LARYNGECTOMY: Laryngectomy is the removal of the larynx and separation of the airway from the mouth, nose and esophagus. In a total **laryngectomy** the entire larynx is removed; in a partial **laryngectomy** only a portion is taken out.

LEPTOSPRIOSIS: Leptospirosis is an infection caused by corkscrew-shaped bacteria called *Leptospira*. Signs and symptoms can range from none to mild such as headaches, muscle pains, and fevers; to severe with bleeding from the lungs or meningitis. If the infection causes the person to turn yellow, have kidney failure and bleeding, it is then known as **Weil's disease**. If it causes a lot of bleeding into the lungs then it is known as **severe pulmonary hemorrhage syndrome**

LIPOMATOUS HYPERTROPHY: *Lipomatous hypertrophy* of the interatrial septum (LHIS) is a relatively uncommon disorder of the heart characterised by benign fatty infiltration of the interatrial septum.

LYME DISEASE: *Lyme disease* is caused by a bacteria, Borrelia burgdorferi, that's transmitted to humans through a bite from an infected black-legged or deer tick.

LYMPHOGRANULOMA VENEREUM: Lymphogranuloma venereum (LGV) is a chronic (long-term) infection of the lymphatic system. It is caused by any of three different types (serovars) of the bacterium Chlamydia trachomatis. The bacteria spread by sexual contact. The infection is not caused by the same bacteria that cause genital chlamydia.

LYMPHOGRANULOMA VENEREUM: Lymphogranuloma venereum (LGV) is a chronic (long-term) infection of the lymphatic system. It is caused by any of three different types (serovars) of the bacterium Chlamydia trachomatis. The bacteria spread by sexual contact. The infection is not caused by the same bacteria that cause genital chlamydia.

MANIA: An elated, overactive state of mind and body, with restless-ness and euphoria.

MANIPULATION (medical): Manual movement of a body part to more acceptable position.

MANTOUX TEST: A skin test given to assist in the diagnosis of tuberculosis.

MENINGITIS: Inflammation of the meninges, a collection of three protective membranes surrounding the brain.

MENINGOENCEPHALITIS: *Meningoencephalitis* is inflammation of the meninges (the tissue which covers the brain and spinal cord) and brain tissue.

MIGRAINE: A headache with specific characteristics and due to disturbances to the blood vessels in the head.

MORBIDITY: 1. Description of the outcomes of disease. 2. The relative incidence of a particular disease in a specific locality.

MUNCHAUSEN SYNDROME: An aberrant condition involving fabrication of an illness to attract medical attention. Sufferers seek numerous medical consultations with different doctors.

MYCETOMA: Mycetoma is a chronic infection of skin and subcutaneous tissue.

NAUSEA: An unpleasant sick feeling in the stomach area.

NEBULISER: A device powered by an air pump which converts a liquid to a fine spray for inhalation. Often used by asthma sufferers.

NEURITIS: Inflammation of neural tissue.

NEUROSIS: A mental condition with many variations, but most commonly with anxiety due to various causes such as stress or previous difficult life experiences. The personality is usually not severely affected.

NIGHT SWEATS: Excessive night-time sweating May indicate serious disease, for example TB.

ODYNOPHAGIA: *Odynophagia* is pain when swallowing. The pain may be felt in the mouth or throat and can occur with or without difficulty swallowing.

OEDEMA: Fluid in the tissues.

OESOPHAGUS: The part of the digestive tract between mouth and stomach. Synonymous with the gullet.

ORGANOMEGALY: Organomegaly is the abnormal enlargement of organs. For example, clitoromegaly is the enlargement of the clitoris, and cardiomegaly is enlargement of the heart. Visceromegaly is the enlargement of abdominal organs.

ORIENTATION: The ability of a person to reliably establish their position regarding time, place and persons.

OVERDOSE: Administration of an excessive amount of a drug or substance into the body.

ORTHOPNEA: *Orthopnea* or orthopnoea is shortness of breath (dyspnea) that occurs when lying flat, causing the person to have to sleep propped up in bed or sitting in a chair.

PALLIATIVE CARE: Care aimed at minimising pain and suffering without aiming to effect a cure.

PALPITATIONS: Awareness of the heartbeat; not necessarily due to heart disease.

PANCREAS: A gland that lies behind the stomach. It produces insulin.

PANCREATITIS: Inflammation of the pancreas organ.

PARALYSIS: Loss of movement of any part of the body due to nerve damage.

PARANOIA: A form of schizophrenia involving delusions, hallucinations, fears of persecution, and undue suspicion of others.

PAROXYSMAL NOCTURNAL DYSPNEA: **Paroxysmal nocturnal dyspnea** or **paroxysmal nocturnal dyspnoea** (PND) refers to attacks of severe shortness of breath and coughing that generally occur at night.

PAROXYSMAL SUPRAVENTRICULAR TACHYCARDIA: *Paroxysmal supraventricular tachycardia* (PSVT) is episodes of rapid heart rate that start in a part of the heart above the ventricles.

PATHOLOGICAL: Related to an abnormality or disease.

PEDICULOSIS: Infestation of the skin by the pediculosis louse. Also known as scabies.

PEPTIC: Related to stomach acid, as in 'peptic ulcer'.

PERICARDITIS : Pericarditis is inflammation of the pericardium (the fibrous sac surrounding the heart).

PERITONEAL CARCINOMATOSIS: **Peritoneal carcinomatosis** is a rare type of **cancer** that occurs in the **peritoneum**, the thin layer of tissue that covers **abdominal** organs and surrounds the **abdominal** cavity. The disease develops when cancers of the appendix, colon, ovaries or other organs spread to the **peritoneum** and cause tumors to grow.

PELVIC INFLAMMATORY DISEASE: An infection of all or part of the female reproductive tract.

PERSONALITY DISORDER: A behavioural disorder that is not due to anxiety, mood disturbance or psychosis.

PHARYNGECTOMY: A *pharyngectomy* is the total or partial surgical removal of the pharynx, the cavity at the back of the mouth that opens into the esophagus at its lower end.

PHLEBITIS: Inflammation of a vein.

PHOBIA: An irrational fear of a situation, person or object.

PLUMMER-VINSON OR PATERSON-KELLY SYNDROMES: Plummer–Vinson syndrome (PVS), also called Paterson–Brown–Kelly syndrome or sideropenic dysphagia, is a rare disease characterized by difficulty in swallowing, iron deficiency anemia, glossitis, cheilosis and esophageal webs.

PNEUMONIA: Infection of the lung tissue.

PNEUMOTHORAX: Condition with increase in air pressure in the chest cavity resulting in collapse of the lung.

PNEUMOTHORAX : A *pneumothorax* is an abnormal collection of air in the pleural space that causes an uncoupling of the lung from the chest wall.

POLIOMYELITIS: *Poliomyelitis*, often called polio or infantile paralysis, is an infectious disease caused by the poliovirus.

POLYARTICULAR ARTHRITIS: This is a kind of rheumatoid arthritis that causes swelling and pain in numerous joints.

POLYMYOSITIS: Polymyositis (PM) is a type of chronic inflammation of the muscles (inflammatory myopathy) related to dermatomyositis and inclusion body myositis.

PRESBYESOPHAGUS: Presbyoesophagus is term that has been traditionally used to describe the manifestations of degenerating motor function in the aging oesophagus.

PROCTITIS OR COLITIS : *Proctitis* is an inflammation of the lining of the rectum. The rectum is a muscular tube that's connected to the end of your colon.

PROGNOSIS: The likely final medical outcome of an illness, in terms of time and condition.

PSYCHOSIS: An extreme derangement of the mind, due to mental illness, with total loss of judgment, memory and insight. It may be a temporary, intermittent or permanent condition.

PSYCHOSOMATIC: Bodily symptoms associated with a nervous complaint or psychological disorder.

PSYCHOTHERAPY: Counselling treatment for mental illness.

PULMONARY: Of the lungs or bronchial system.

PULMONARY CHONDROMA: *Pulmonary chondromas* are rare, benign cartilaginous tumours of the lungs, and form part of the Carney triad although they can also arise sporadically.

PULMONARY EMBOLUS: Lodgment of an embolus (mobile blood clot) in the lung tissue.

PULSE: The rhythmic expansion of an artery which can be felt.

PYODERMA GANGRENOSUM: *Pyoderma gangrenosum* is a condition that causes tissue to become necrotic, causing deep ulcers that usually occur on the legs.

RAPPORT: The situation whereby a facilitative and empathic understanding develops between the health care worker and his/her client/patient.

RECKLINGHAUSEN'S NEUROFIBROMATOSIS: Von **Recklinghausen's** disease (VRD) is a genetic disorder characterized by the growth of tumors on the nerves. The disease can also affect the skin and cause bone deformities. ... **neurofibromatosis** type 2 (NF2) schwannomatosis, which is a variant of NF2.

RENAL PAPILLARY NECROSIS: Renal papillary necrosis is a disorder of the kidneys in which all or part of the renal papillae die.

RETINAL HEMANGIOMATOSIS: *Retinal* capillary *hemangioma* is a benign *retinal* hamartoma that may be associated with von Hippel-Lindau (VHL) disease.

RHINORRHEA: **Rhinorrhea** or rhinorrhoea is a condition where the nasal cavity is filled with a significant amount of mucus fluid. The condition, commonly known as a runny nose, occurs relatively frequently. **Rhinorrhea** is a common symptom of allergies (hay fever) or certain diseases, such as the common cold.

SARCOIDOSIS: *Sarcoidosis* is an inflammatory disease that affects multiple organs in the body, but mostly the lungs and lymph glands.

SCABIES: An inflammatory skin condition due to the pediculosis louse.

SCHATZKI RINGS: A **Schatzki ring** or **Schatzki**–Gary **ring** is a narrowing of the lower esophagus that can cause difficulty swallowing (dysphagia). The narrowing is caused by a **ring** of mucosal tissue (which lines the esophagus) or muscular tissue.

SCHIZOPHRENIA: A nervous disorder characterised by disturbances to normal thought processes.

SEPSIS: Infection.

SHOCK:
1. A state of dangerously low blood pressure.
2. A state of mental distress.

SIGN (of illness): An observable indication of illness.

SINUS:
1. Facial sinus: A cavity in the skull bones.
2. An abnormal opening in a body organ, e.g. skin sinus (an opening in the skin that is discharging).

SPIDER ANGIOMATA: A **spider angioma** (also known as a **nevus araneus**, **spider nevus**, **vascular spider**, and **spider telangiectasia**) is a type of telangiectasis (swollen blood vessels) found slightly beneath the skin surface, often containing a central red spot and reddish extensions which radiate outwards like a spider's web.

SPLEEN: A richly perfused organ in the upper left abdominal area which is unfortunately prone to trauma. It is part of the immune system.

SPUTUM: Phlegm (secretions coughed up from the lungs).

STEATOHEPATITIS: *Steatohepatitis* is a type of fatty liver disease, characterized by inflammation of the liver with concurrent fat accumulation in liver.

STEATORRHEA: Steatorrhea (or steatorrhoea) is the presence of excess fat in feces. Stools may be bulky and difficult to flush, have a pale and oily appearance and can be especially foul-smelling. An oily anal leakage or some level of fecal incontinence may occur.

STERNUM: The middle chest bone where ribs from each side of the body meet.

STEROID: A group of chemical substances produced by the adrenal glands. May have anabolic (body building), or anti-inflammatory, or other properties.

STOMACH ULCER: An ulcer within the lining of the stomach. Synonymous with peptic ulcer.

STROKE: The result of damage to part of the brain; usually associated with weakness, numbness or paralysis.

STURGE-WEBER SYNDROME: Sturge-Weber syndrome (SWS) is a **neurological** disorder marked by a distinctive **port-wine stain** on the forehead, scalp, or around the eye. This stain is a birthmark caused by an overabundance of capillaries near the surface of the skin. Blood vessels on the same side of the brain as the stain may also be affected.

SYDENHAM CHOREA: Sydenham chorea (SD) is a neurological disorder of childhood resulting from infection via Group A beta-hemolytic streptococcus (GABHS), the bacterium that causes rheumatic fever.

SYMPTOM: A specific feeling or physical manifestation due to an illness.

SYSTEMIC LUPUS ERYTHEMATOSUS (SLE): It is also known simply as **lupus**, is an autoimmune disease in which the body's immune system mistakenly attacks healthy tissue in many parts of the body.

SYNDROME: A group of symptoms due to a particular disease.

TETANUS: A serious bacterial infection beginning in unclean wounds, and at risk of causing paralysis.

THIAMINE: Vitamin B1. An important vitamin needed for the heart and brain; often low in alcoholics.

THYROTOXICOSIS: *Thyrotoxicosis* is the condition that occurs due to excessive thyroid hormone of any cause and therefore includes hyperthyroidism.

TINNITUS: *Tinnitus* (TIN-ih-tus) is the perception of noise or ringing in the ears.

TOLERANCE: A process where the body adapts to administration of a foreign substance, resulting in the need for more of the drug to achieve the same effect.

TOURETTE'S SYNDROME: *Tourette syndrome* is a complex disorder characterized by repetitive, sudden, and involuntary movements or noises called tics.

TRANSFERENCE: The unconscious tendency to transfer to another person significant feelings and attitudes that are your own and which are excessive.

TRANSHEPATIC CHOLANGIOGRAPHY : Percutaneous *transhepatic cholangiography* (PTC) is a radiographic technique employed in visualisation of the biliary tract, and can be used as the first step in a number of percutaneous biliary interventions (e.g. percutaneous *transhepatic* biliary stent placement)

TRANSNASAL ESOPHAGOSCOPY : Transnasal esophagoscopy (TNE) is a safe and inexpensive way to examine the esophagus in patients at risk for esophageal cancer and other disorders. TNE doesn't require sedation, unlike other techniques widely used to look into the esophagus.

TUBERCULOSIS: A serious bacterial infection of the lungs or (sometimes) of the kidneys. Also referred to as 'TB'.

TUBEROERUPTIVE XANTHOMAS: Tuberoeruptive xanthomas are dermal papules with an inflammatory component, while tuberous xanthomas are larger, non-inflammatory lesions that can extend beyond the dermis to the subcutaneous tissues.

TUBEROUS SCLEROSIS: Tuberous sclerosis complex (TSC) is a rare multisystem genetic disease that causes benign tumors to grow in the brain and on other vital organs such as the kidneys, heart, liver, eyes, lungs, and skin.

ULCER: Loss of the surface tissue layer of an organ (e.g. skin, stomach lining and cornea) is known as *ulceration*.

URGENCY (of symptoms): Sudden involuntary urges to pass urine, etc.

UROLOGICAL: Of the bladder, kidneys or urinary system.

VENTRICULAR HYPERTROPHY: Ventricular hypertrophy (LVH) is a condition in which the muscle wall of heart's pumping chamber (**ventricle**) becomes thickened (**hypertrophy**).

VIRUS: An infective particle much smaller than bacteria. Requires 'host' cells (for example human cells) to reproduce. Not destroyed by antibiotics.

VON HIPPEL-LINDAU DISEASE: Von Hippel-Lindau syndrome (VHL) is a hereditary condition associated with tumors arising in multiple organs. The tumors in VHL include **hemangioblastomas**, which are blood vessel tumors of the brain, spinal cord, and eye. The **eye tumors** are also called retinal angiomas.

WEGENER'S GRANULOMATOSIS: Granulomatosis with polyangiitis (GPA), formerly known as Wegener granulomatosis, is a rare multisystem autoimmune disease of unknown etiology. Its hallmark features include necrotizing granulomatous inflammation and pauci-immune vasculitis in small- and medium-sized blood vessels.

WHEEZE: Breathing characterised by a whistling noise. Usually due to asthma.

WHIPPLE'S DISEASE: *Whipple disease* is a rare bacterial infection that primarily affects the small intestine caused by a gram-positive bacterium, Tropheryma whippelii.

WILSON'S DISEASE: Wilson's disease, also known as hepatolenticular degeneration and progressive lenticular degeneration, is a rare genetic **disorder** that causes copper poisoning in the body.

WOLFF-PARKINSON-WHITE [WPW] SYNDROME: *Wolff–Parkinson–White syndrome* (*WPW*) is a *disorder* due to a specific type of problem with the electrical system of the heart which has resulted in symptoms.

ZOLLINGER-ELLISON SYNDROME: Zollinger-Ellison syndrome is a rare condition in which one or more tumors form in your pancreas or the upper part of your small intestine (duodenum). These tumors, called **gastrinomas**, secrete large amounts of the hormone **gastrin**, which causes your stomach to produce too much acid.

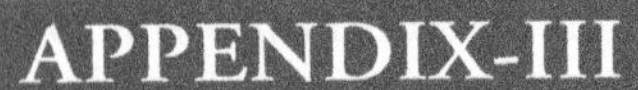

APPENDIX-III

Drug Induced Disorders

Table AIII-1

Drug induced renal disorders

Glomerular Injury		
Mechanism	**Disease**	**Drug**
Alterations to the rennin-angiotensin system/ prostaglandin synthesis	Functional / hemodynamic effect	NSAIDS/CNIs
Podocyte injury, possibly immune (T-cell) mediated	MCD	NSAIDS
Podocyte injury, with phenotypic alterations	FSGS	Pamidronate
Inhibitions of lysosomal enzyme	Phospholipidosis	Chloroquine
Immune complex deposition	MGN/ Lupus-like glomerulonephritis	Gold/Penicillamine/ Hydralazine
ANCA	Crescentic/necrotising glomerulonephritis	Infliximab / Propylthiouracil
Endothelial damage	TMA	CNIs/ Bevacizumab
ANCA: antineutrophil cytoplasmic antibody; CNIs: calcineurin inhibitors; FSGS: food and segmental glomerulosclerosis: MCD: minimal change disease; MGN: membranous glomerulonephritis; NSAIDS: non-steroidal anti-inflammatory drugs; TMA: thrombotic microangiopathy		
Vascular Injury		
Mechanism	**Disease**	**Drug**
Endothelial/myocyte damage	TMA	CNIs
Cell antibody mediated	Inflammatory vasculitis	Various antibiotics
Capillary/ischemic damage	Analgesic nephropathy	Combination analgesics
CNIS: calcineurin inhibitors, TMA: thrombotic microangiopathy.		

Table AIII-1 *contd...*

Tubulointerstitial Injury		
Mechanism	**Disease**	**Drug**
Direct cellular toxicity	ATN/Nephrogenic diabetes insipidus	Cisplatin / Lithium
Changes in osmotic gradient across cell membrane	Osmotic nephrosis	Plasma volume expanders / IVIG
Cast formation obstructing tubules	Tubulointerstitial nephritis/ATN	Various drugs / Sirolimus
Crystal deposition/Calcification	Tubulointerstitial nephritis/ATN/ Nephrocalcinosis	Diethylene glycol/ Indinavir/Oral sodium phosphate purgative.
ATN: acute tubular necrosis; IVIG: intravenous immune globulin		

Table AIII-2

Drug induced haematological disorders

Syndrome	Examples of Associated Drugs
Immunohemolytic anaemia	Pencillins, cephalosporins, alpha-methyl-DOPA, oxaliplatin, Fludarabine, anti - Rh D antiglobulin
Nonimmune hemolytic anaemia	Ribavirin, phenazopyridine, chloroquine,
Methhemoglobinemia	Phenazopyridine, dapsone, benzocaine, prilocaine
Megaloblastic anaemia	Trimethoprim, pyrimethamine, diphenyhydantoin
Sideroblastic anaemia	Isoniazid, chloramphenicol, linezolide
Aplastic anaemia	Chloramphenicol, gold NSAIDs, Diphenylhydantoin
Pure red cell aplasia	Azathioprine, chlorpropamide, Isoniazid, erythropoietin
Immune thrombocytopenia	Quinine, quinidine, heparin, vancomycin, sulfas, pencillins, glycoprotein II b - III a inhibitors
Thrombotic microangiopathy	Quinine, quinidine, clopidogrel, ticlopidine, cylosporine A, Mitomycin-C, cisplatin
Platelet dysfunction	Pencillins, beta-Lactam antibiotics, aspirin, NSAIDS Estrogens, tamoxifen, asparaginase, heparin
Hypercoagulability	Bevacizumab, thalidomide/lenalidomide, COX-2 inhibitors, erythropoietin
Circulating anticoagulants	Isoniazid, Hydralazine, procainamide
Hypoprothrombinemia	Cephalosporins, pencillins, sulfas, Antithyroid drugs, procainamide, sulfas ,captopril, phenothiazines
Neutropenia	Diphenylhydantoin, Rituximab
Neutrophilia	Glucocorticoids, lithium, G-and GM-CSF
Eosinophilia	Pencillins, sulfas, allopurinol, diphenyhydantoin
Polycythemia	Erythropoietin, anabolic steroids, diuretics
Acute leukemia/myelodyplasia	Alkylating agents, topoisomerase II inhibitors

Table AIII-3

Drug induced liver disorders

Drugs that may cause Acute Dose-Independent Liver Damage (Resembling Acute Viral Hepatitis)			
• Acebutolol • Indomethacin • Phenylbutazone	• Labetalol • Probenecid • Cimetidine	• Quinine • Diltiazem • Naproxen	• Ethionamide • Phenelzine • Tricyclic Antidepressants
• Allopurinol • Isoniazid • Phenytoin	• Maprotiline • Pyrazinamide • Dantrolene	• Ranitidine • Enflurane • Para-Aminosalicylic Acid	• Halothane • Phenindione • Valproic Acid
• Atenolol • Ketoconazole • Piroxicam • Carbamazepine	• Metoprolol • Quinidine • Diclofenac • Mianserin	• Sulfonamides • Ethambutol • Penicillin's • Sulindac	• Ibuprofen • Phenobarbital • Verapamil
Drugs that may Cause Acute Fatty Infiltration of the Liver			
• Adrenocortical Steroids	• Tetracyclines		
• Phenothiazines • Sulfonamides • Antithyroid Drugs • Phenytoin	• Isoniazid • Salicylates • Valproic Acid • Methotrexate		
Drugs that may cause Cholestatic Jaundice			
• Chlorpropamide • Erythromycin • Amoxicillin/ Clavulanate	• Danazol • Glyburide • Carbimazole	• Haloperidol • Ketoconazole • Norethandrolone	• Penicillamine • Tolbutamide • Nitrofurantoin
• Cloxacillin Flecainide	• Diazepam	• Sulfonamides	• Phenothiazines
• Azathioprine • Cyclophos-phamide	• Gold • Cephalosporins	• Mercaptopurine • Oral Contraceptives	•Tricyclic Antidepressants • Nonsteroidal
• Flurazepam	• Disopyramide	• Tamoxifen	• Phenytoin Troleandomycin
• Captopril	• Griseofulvin	• Methyl testosterone	• Anti-Inflammatory Drugs
• Cyclosporine • Flutamide	• Chlordiazepoxide • Enalapril	• Oxacillin • Thiabendazole	• Propoxyphene • Verapamil

Table AIII-3 *contd...*

Drugs that may cause Liver Granulomas (Chronic Inflammatory Nodules)
• Gold
• Phenytoin
• Aspirin
• Hydralazine
• Procainamide
• Carbamazepine
• Isoniazid
• Quinidine
• Chlorpromazine
Drugs that may cause active chronic hepatitis
• Acetaminophen (Chronic Use, Large Doses)
• Dantrolene
• Methyldopa
• Isoniazid
• Nitrofurantoin

Table AIII-4

Drug induced pulmonary disorders

Drugs causing common clinical presentations of pulmonary toxicity		
Asthma	**Interstitial pneumonia or fibrosis**	**Pleural effusion**
Aspirin Beta-blockers Cocaine	Amphotericin B Bleomycin Busulfan	Amiodarone Anticoagulants Belomycin
Dipyridamole Hydrocortisone Interleukin-2	Carbamazepine Chlorambucil Cocaine	Bromocriptine Busulfan Granulocyte-macrophage colony stimuli-ting factor (GM-CSF)
Methylphenidate Nitrofurantoin	Cyclophosphamide Diphenylhydantoin	Interleukin-2
Protamine Sulfasalazine Timolol	Flecainide Heroin Melphalan	Methotrexate Methysergide Mitomycin-C
Vinca alkaloids (with Mitomycin)	Methysergide	**Pulmonary infiltrate with Eosinophilia**
Bronchiolitis obliterans organizing Pneumonia	Nitrosoureas	Amiodarone
Amiodarone	Procarbazine Silicone	Amphotericin B Diphenylhydantoin
Bleomycin	Tocainide	Ethambutol
Cocaine	Vinca alkaloids (with Mitomycin)	Etoposide

Table AIII-4 *contd...*

Drugs causing common clinical presentations of pulmonary toxicity		
Asthma	**Interstitial pneumonia or fibrosis**	**Pleural effusion**
Cyclophosphamide	**Noncardiac Pulmonary edema**	GM-CSF
Methotrexate	Cocaine	Isoniazid
		Methotrexate
Mitomycin-C	Cytarabine	Minocycline
Penicillamine	Gemcitabine	Mitomycin -C
Radiation	Heroin	Nitrofurantoin
Sulfasalazine	Hydrochlorothiazide	Para-aminosalicylic acid
		Procarbazine
Tetracycline, Minocycline	Methadone	Radiation
		Sulfasalazine
Drug-induced systemic lupus erythematosus	Mitomycin-C	
	Phenothiazines	
Diltiazem	Sulfasalazine	
Diphenylhydantoin		
Hydralazine	Anticoagulants Azathioprine	Sulfonamides
Penicillamine	plus 6-mercaptopurine	Tetracycline
Para-aminosalicylic acid	Cocaine	Trazodone
Minocycline	Mineral oil	**Pulmonary vascular disease**
Isoniazid	Nitrofurantoin	Appetite suppressants
Hydrochlorothiazide	Radiation	(dexfenfluramine, fenfluramine,
Streptomycin		phentermine)
Sulfonamides		Cocaine
		Heroin
		Methadone
Hypersensitivity infiltrate		Methylphenidate
Azathioprine plus		Nitrosoureas
6-mercaptopurine		Radiation
Methotrexate		Busulfan
Methylphenidate Fluoxetine		
Radiation		

Colour Plates

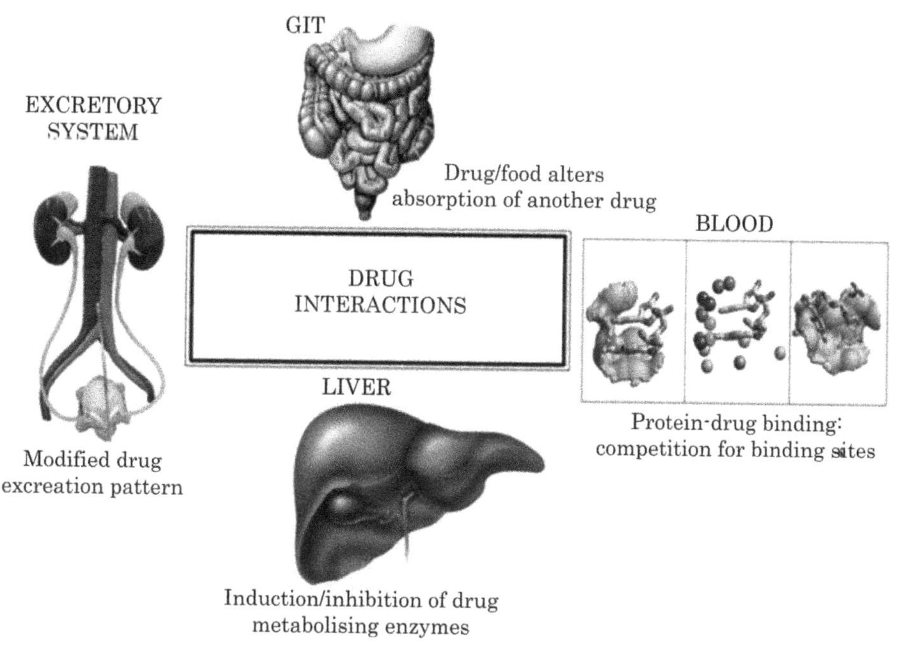

FIGURE 8.1

Pharmacokinetic interactions.

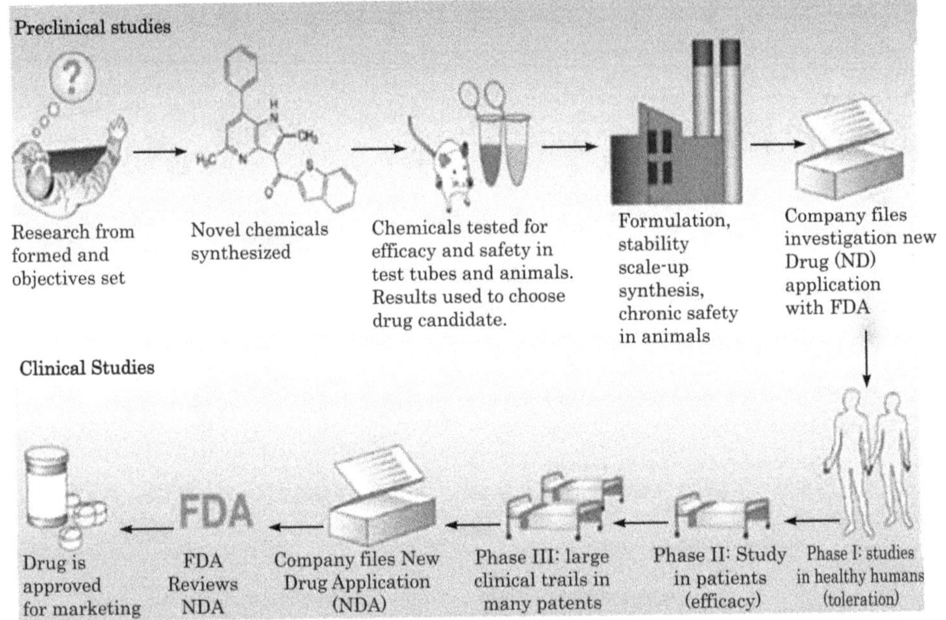

FIGURE 14.2

Preclinical and clinical studies.

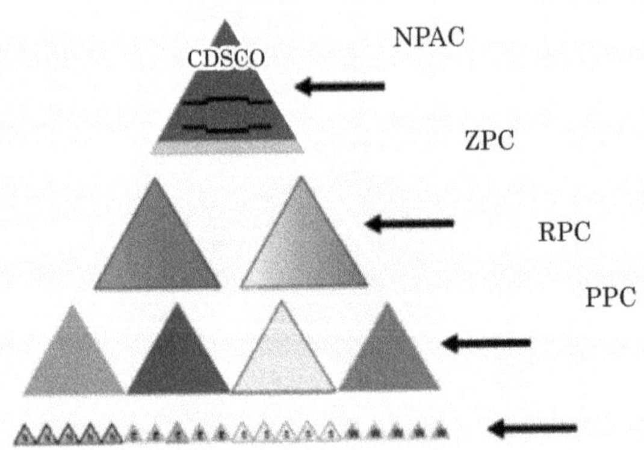

FIGURE 14.3

National pharmacovigilance programme.

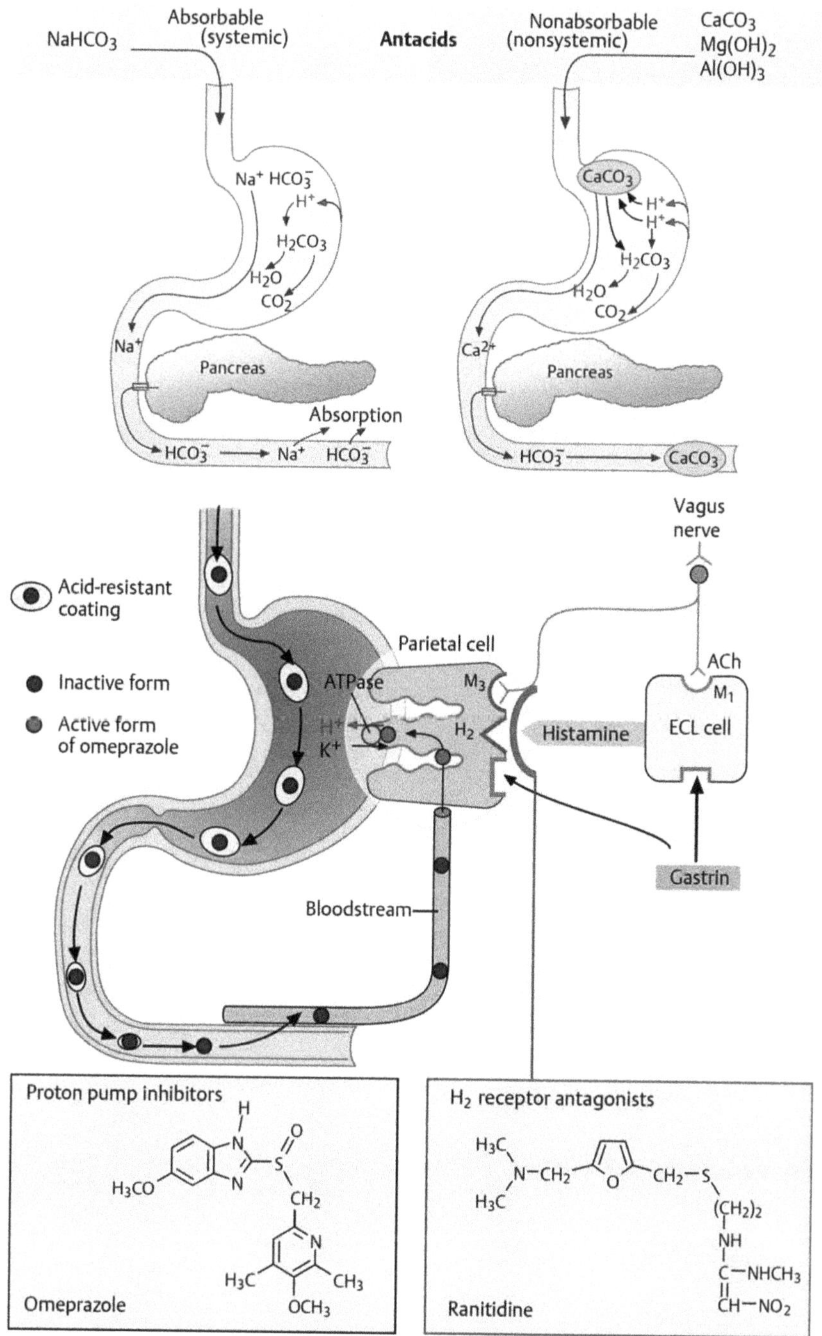

FIGURE 22.3

Drugs used to lower and neutralize gastric acid.

(Source : Colour Atlas of Pharmacology, 3rd edition, Page no.171)

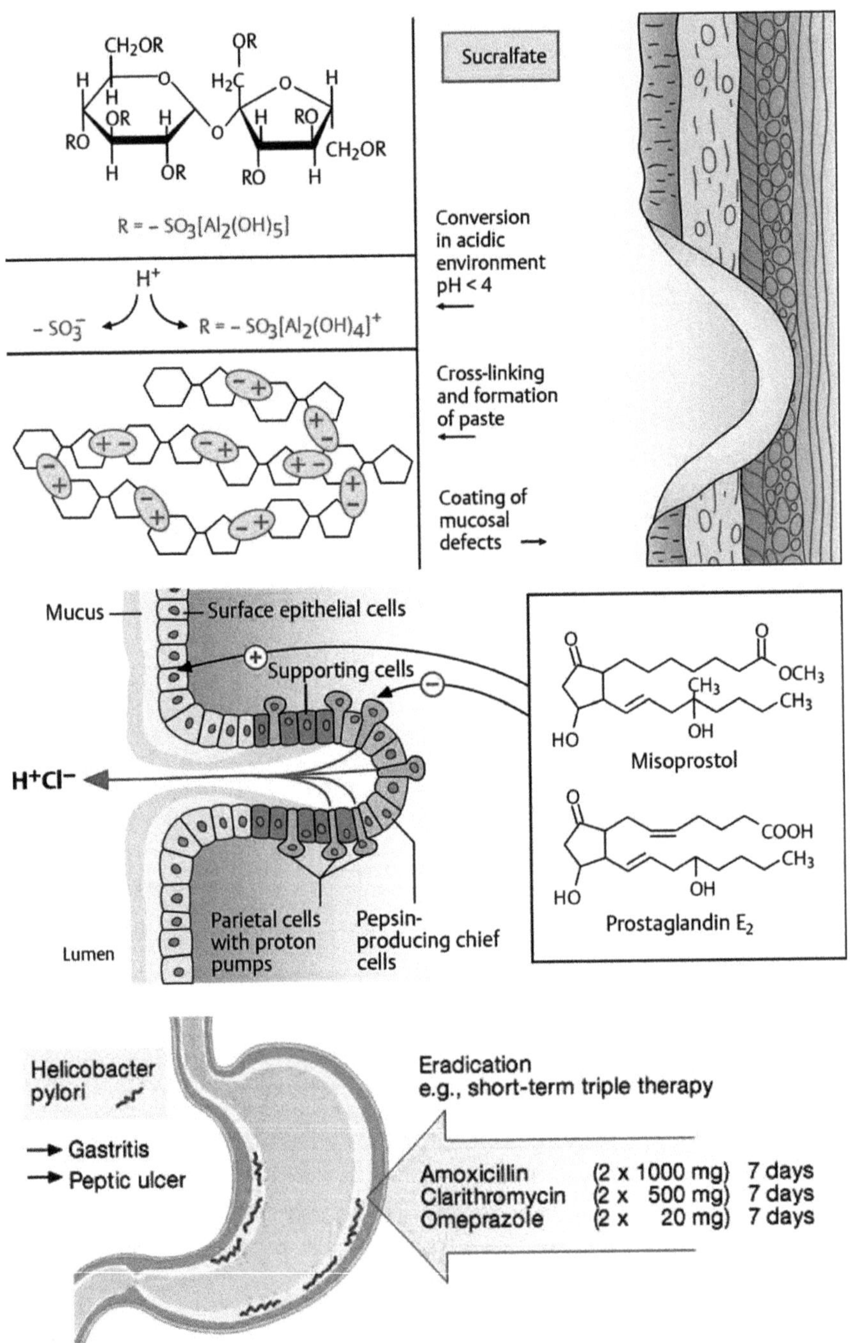

FIGURE 22.4

Protective effects of sucralfate, misoprostol and helicobacter eradication.

(Source : Colour Atlas of Pharmacology, 3rd edition, Page no.173)

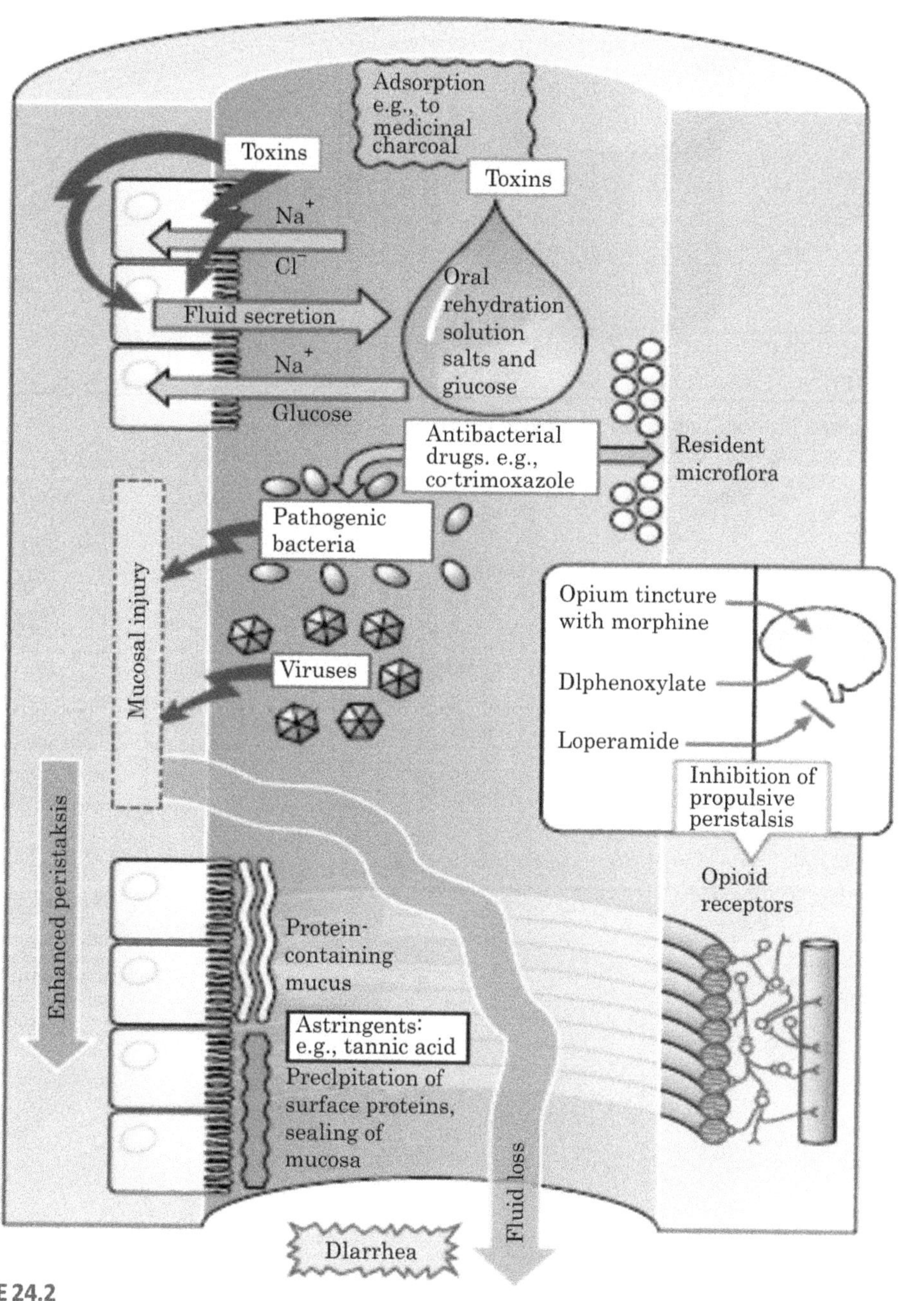

FIGURE 24.2

Anti diarrheals and their site of action.

(Source : http://intranet.tdmu.edu.ua/data/kafedra/internal/pharmakologia/classes_stud/en/pharm/prov_pharm/ptn/Pharmacology/3%20year/14%20Gastrointestinal%20agenrs%20-1..htm)

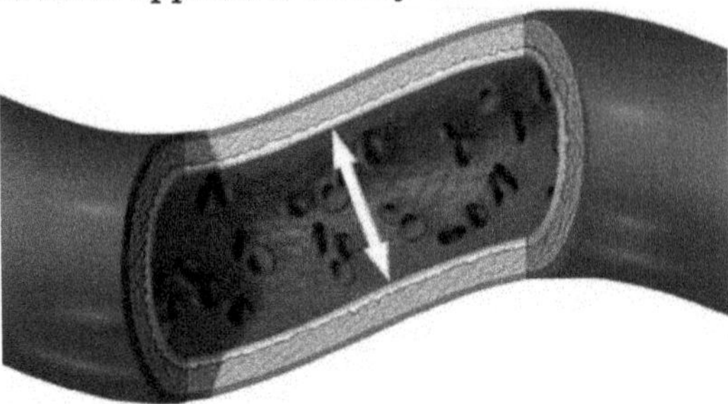

FIGURE 40.1

Blood pressure in blood vessels.

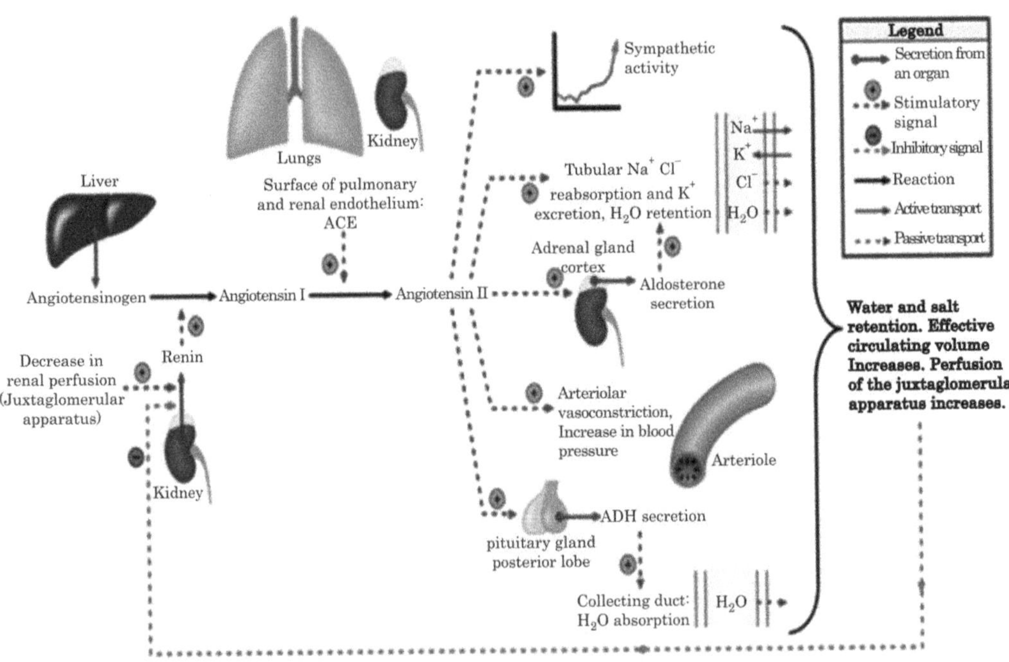

FIGURE 40.2

Rennin - angiotensin - aldosterone system.

(source: https://en.wikipedia.org/wiki/Renin%E2%80%93angiotensin_system)

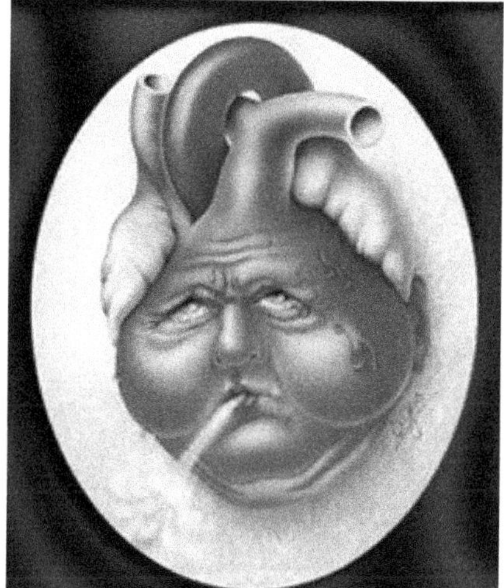

FIGURE 41.1

Heart failure.

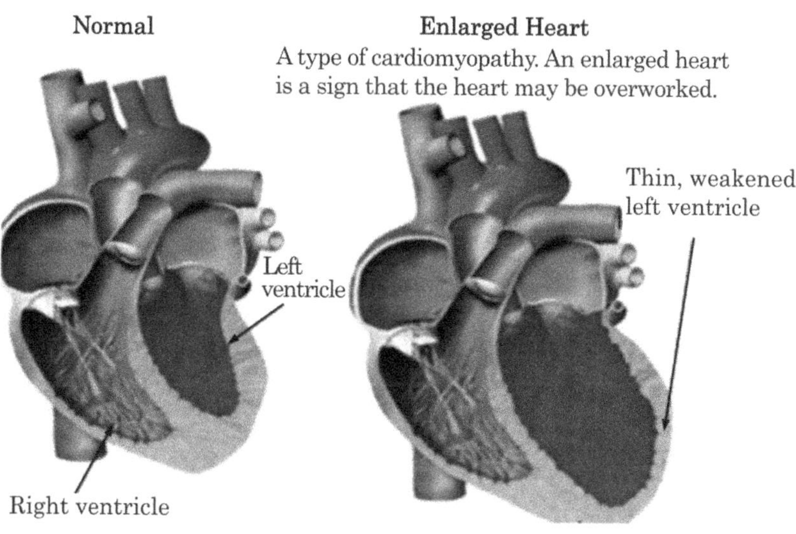

FIGURE 41.2

Normal and enlarged heart.

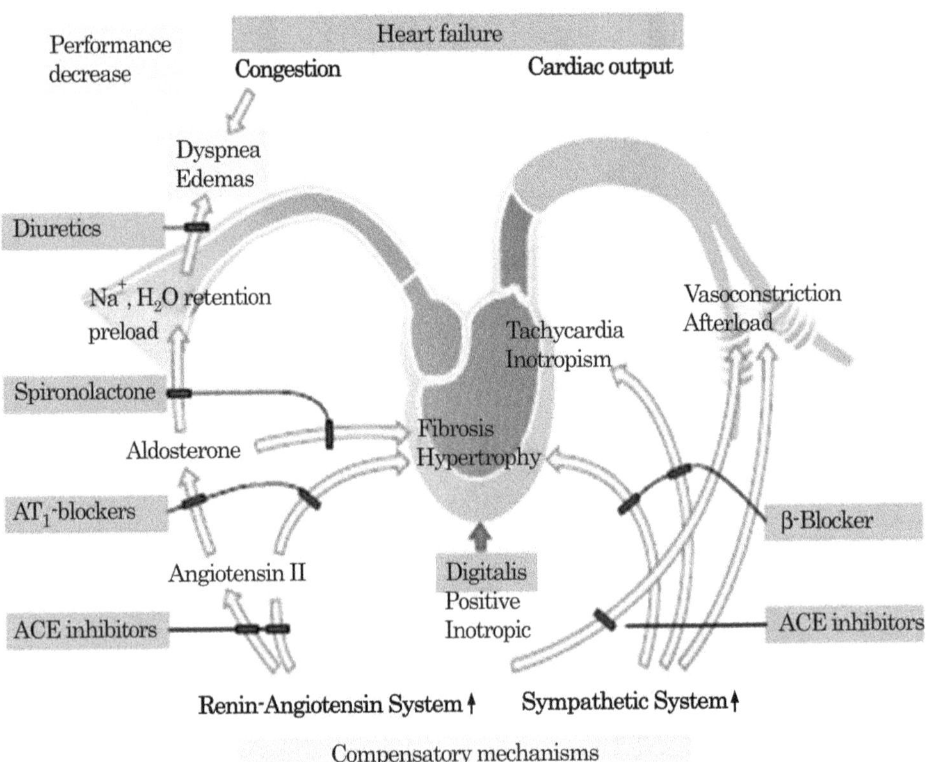

FIGURE 41.3

Congestive heart failure and its drug treatment.

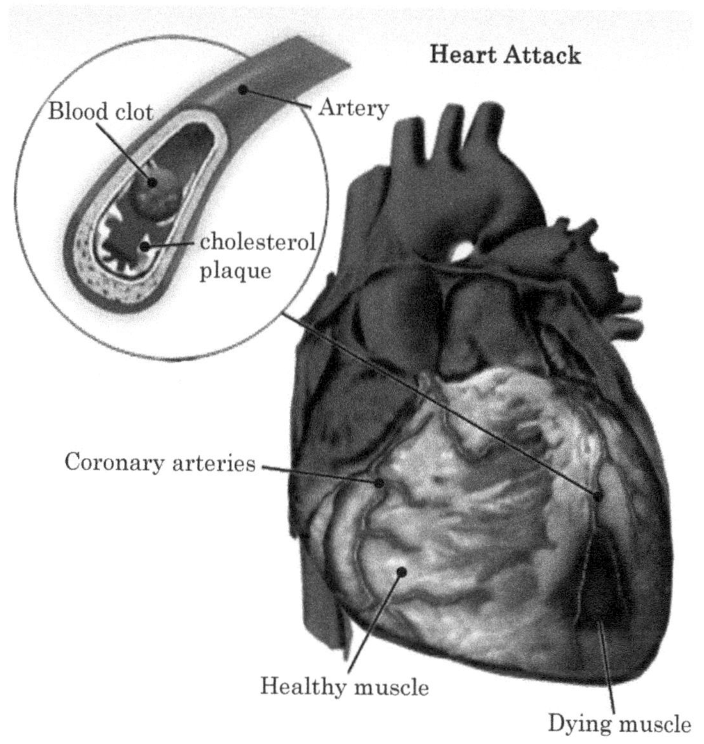

FIGURE 44.1

Heart attack.

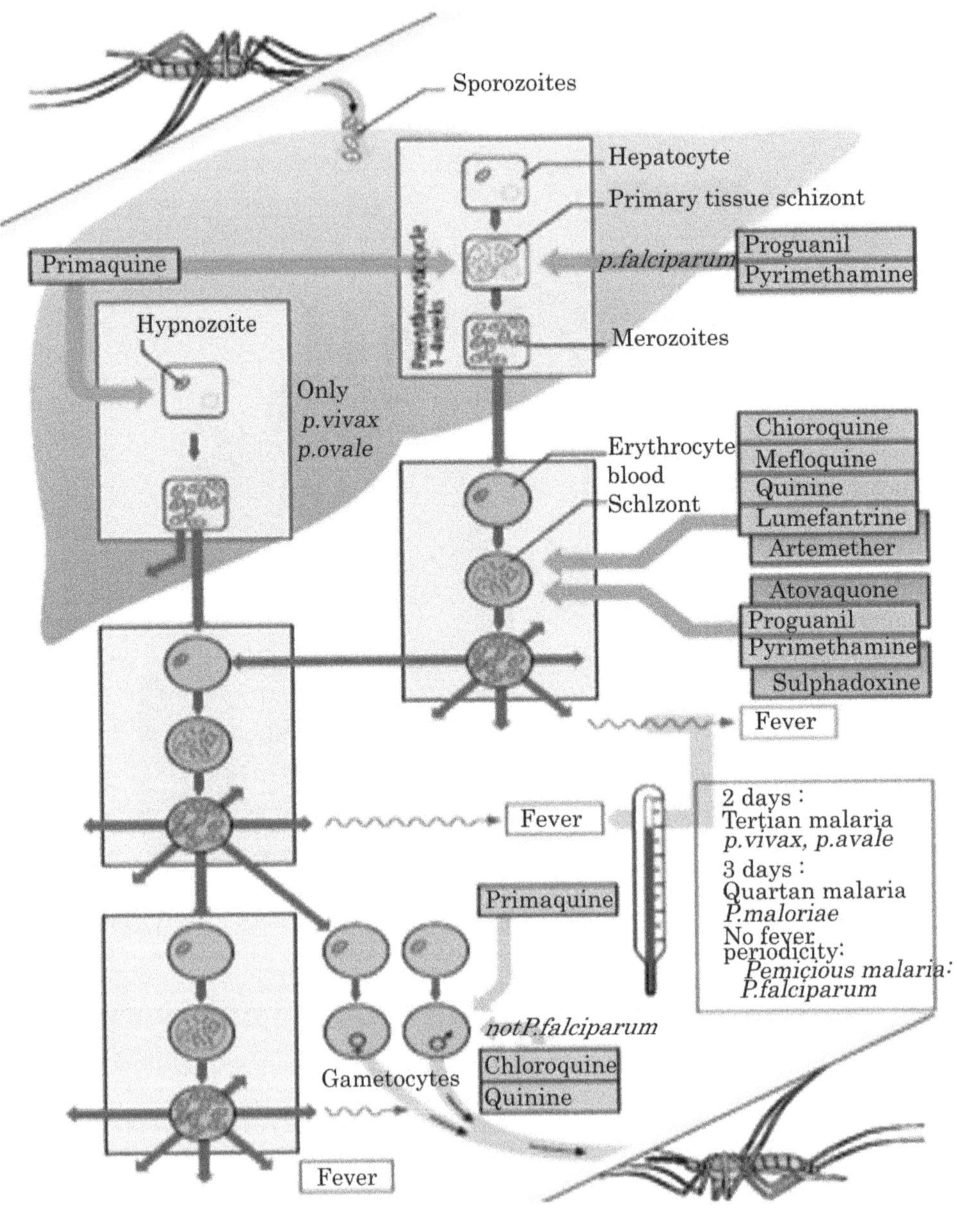

FIGURE 72.1

Life cycle plasmodium falciparum.

Source : Colour Atlas Of Pharmacology ,3rd edition ,Page no.295)

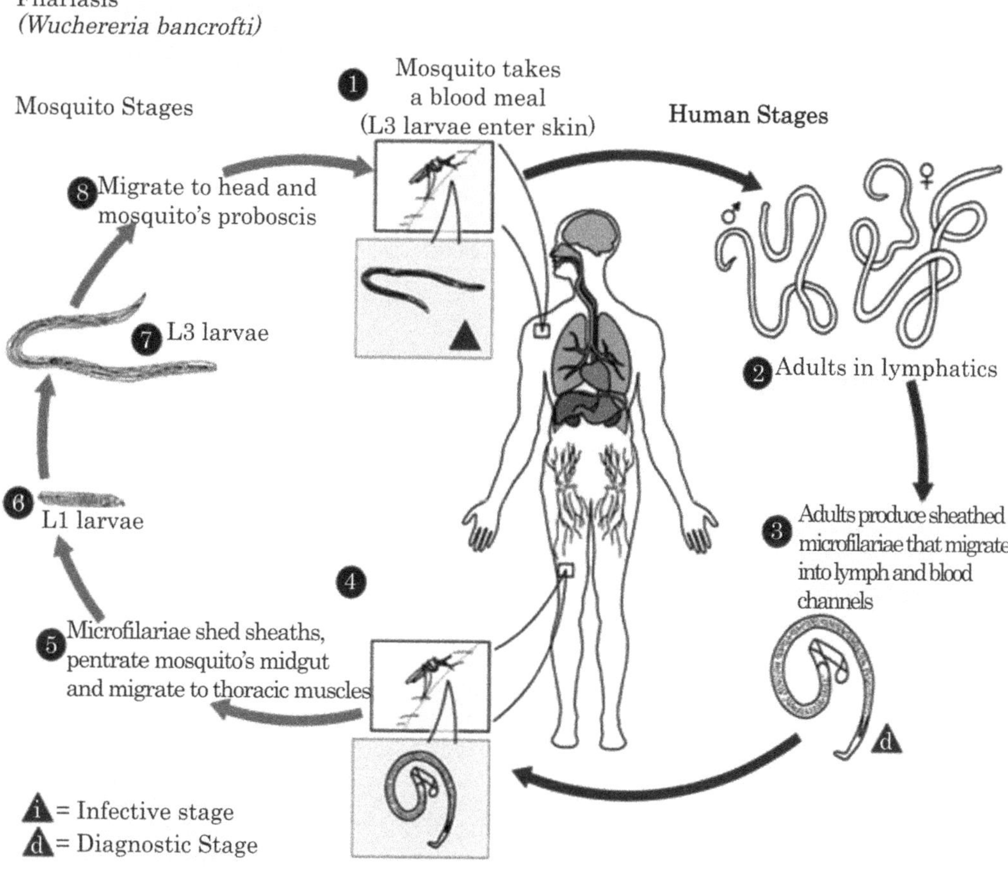

FIGURE 73.1

Wuchereria bancrofti life cycle.

(Source : http://www.parasitesinhumans.org/wuchereria-bancrofti-lymphatic-filariasis.html)

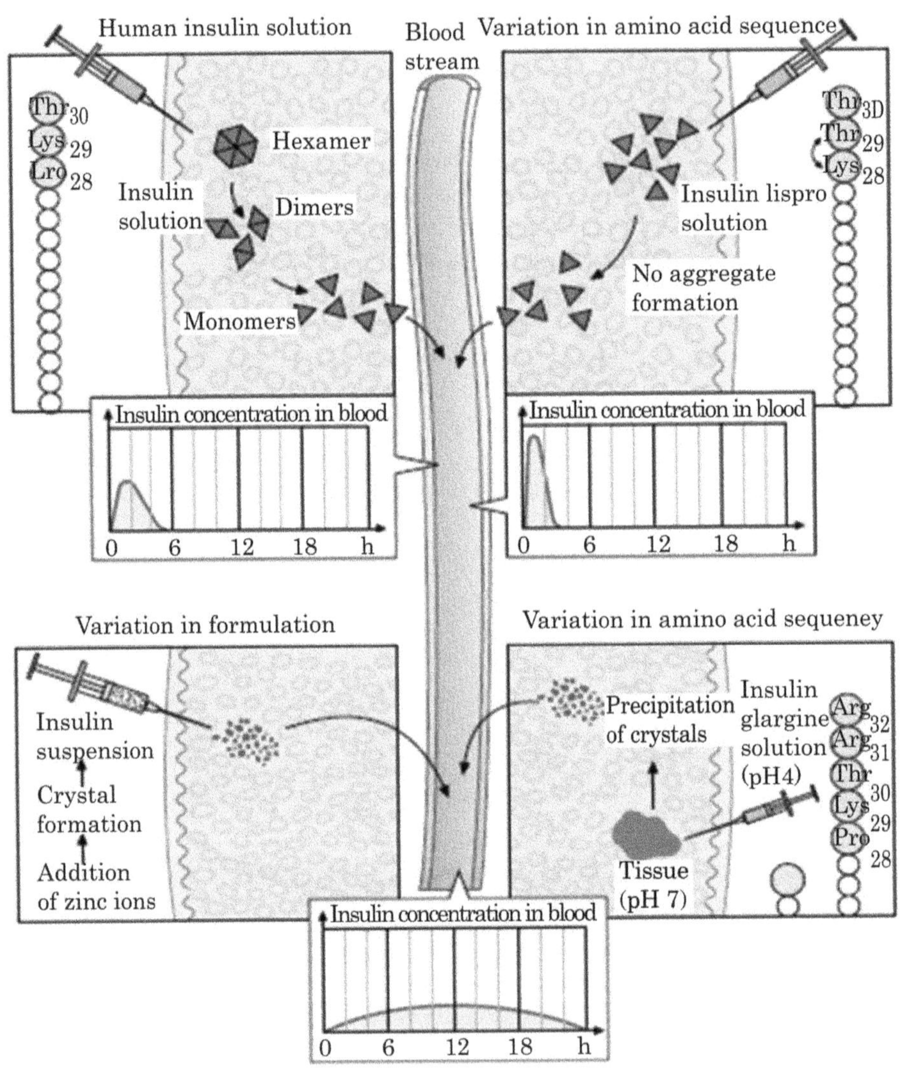

FIGURE 76.2

Human insulin release from injection site.

(Source : Colour Atlas Of Pharmacology ,3rd edition ,Page no.259)

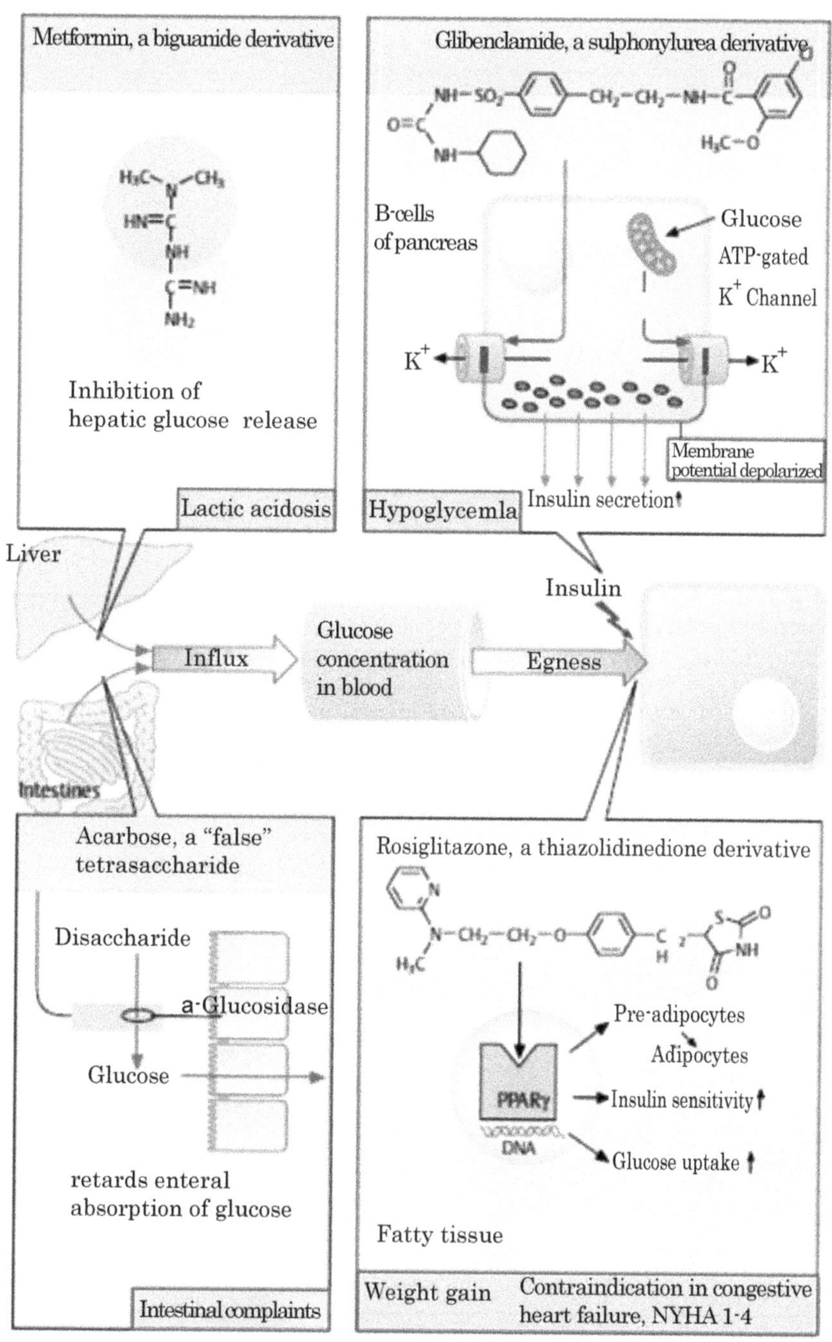

FIGURE 76.3

Oral antidiabetics.

(Source : Colour Atlas Of Pharmacology, 3rd edition, Page no.265)

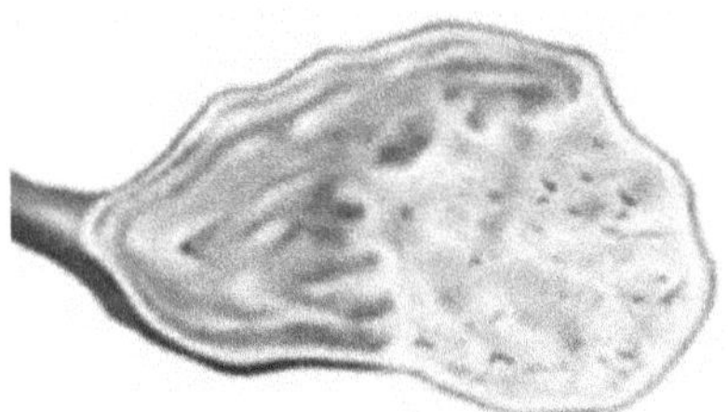

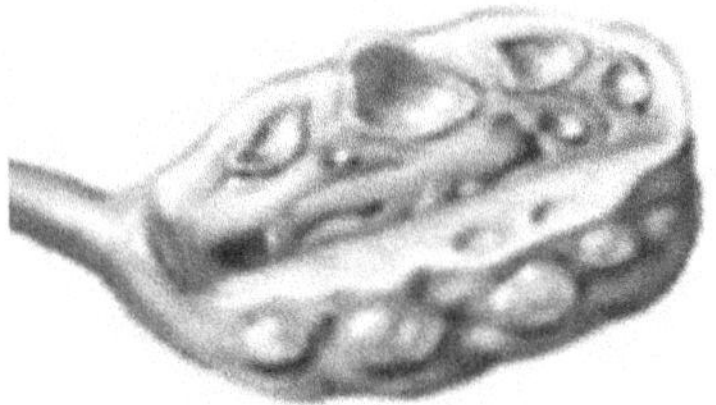

FIGURE 80.3

Ovarian tumor and polycystic ovary.

(Source : https://hubpages.com/health/PCOS-and-tips-on-dealing-with-it)

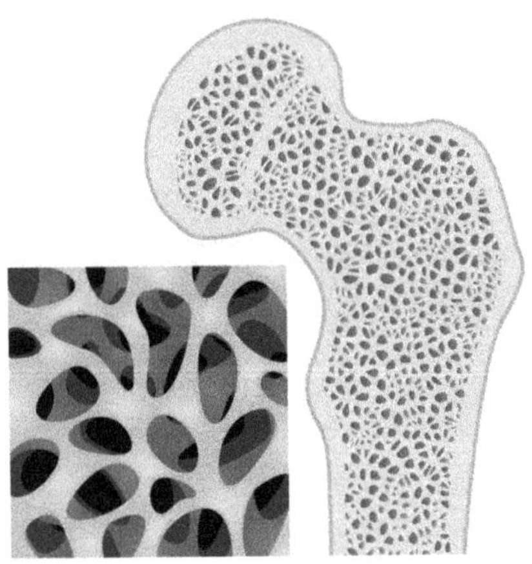

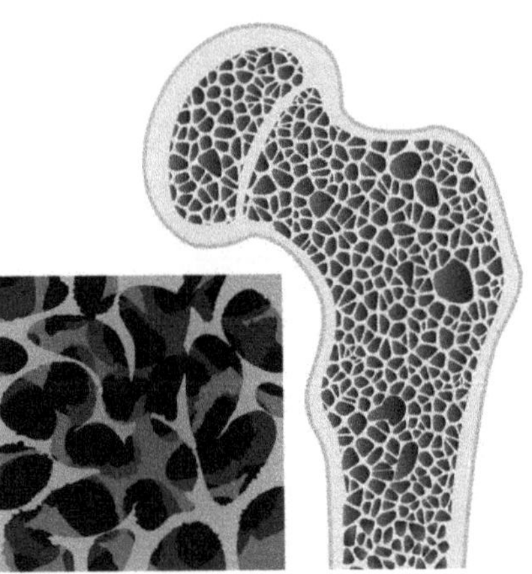

FIGURE 80.4

Bone osteoporosis.

(source : http://rehabilitaciontacna.com/osteoporosis-y-osteopenia/)

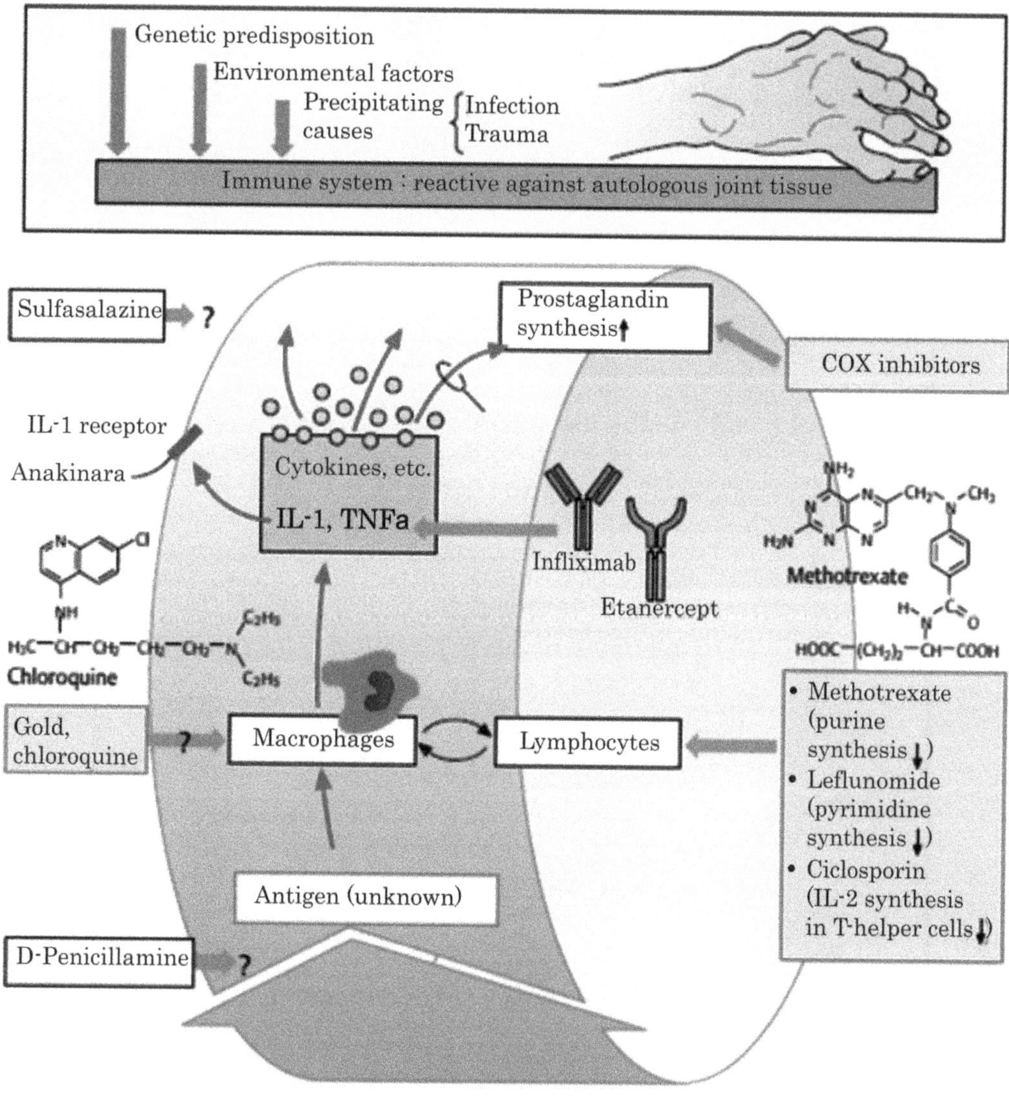

FIGURE 89.1

Anti rheumatoid drugs.

(Source : Colour Atlas of Pharmacology , 3rd edition ,Page no.333)

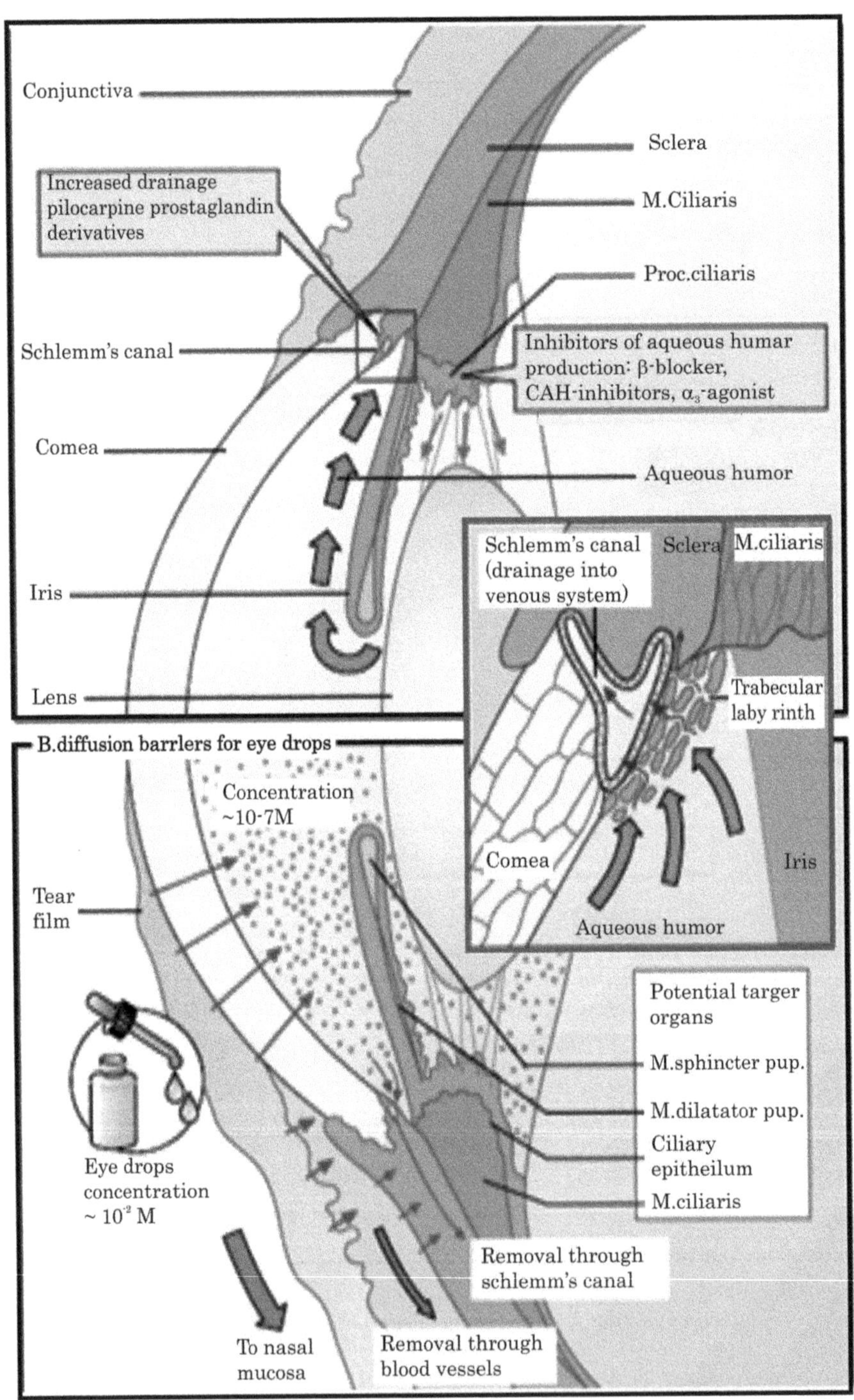

FIGURE 92.1

Local pharmacotherapy of glaucoma.

INDEX

[131I]meta-iodobenzyl guanidine scan 785
5-HT model 536
5-HT/NE link hypothesis 551
5α-reductase inhibitors (dutasteride and finasteride) 368
α-adrenergic antagonists 367
α-Aminobutyric acid (GABA) receptor model 536
α-Lipotropin 767
β-amyloid protein aggregation 528

A

A definitive diagnosis of AP 350
A medication history 27
Abdominoperineal excision of rectum 875
Abiraterone acetate 859
Abstinence 673
ACE inhibitors 320
Acetaminophen 343
Achalasia, alachrymia syndrome 761
Acne vulgaris 949
Acne vulgaris (ACNE) 949
Acromegaly 778
ACTH 766
Acupuncture 583
Acute ethanol intoxication and hangover 970
Acute migraine therapiesa 576
Acute pancreatitis (AP) 348
Acute paroxysms 779
Acute viral gastroenteritis 659
Additional iatrogenic causes of dysphagia 290
Adenine dinucleotide 302
Adjuvant biologic therapy 848
Adjuvant radiotherapy for rectal cancer 880
Adrenal carcinoma 740
Adrenal crisis 771
Adrenal hemorrhage 752
Adrenomyeloneuropathy and adrenoleukodystrophy 760
Advanced glycation end products (AGES) 380
Aetiology of colon and rectal cancer 862
Aetiopathogenetic theories 581
Age 919
Alcoholic hepatitis 302
Alcoholism 970
Aldehyde dehydrogenase 302
Aldosterone antagonists 285
Alkylating agents 882
Allopurinol 386

Alpha-methyldopa 320
Alpharadin 860
Alteplase 591
Alteration in bowel habit 868
Alzheimer's disease (AD) 528
Ambrisentan, randomized, double-blinded, multicenter, efficacy study (ARIES I & II) 470
Ambulatory ph monitoring 274
Aminoglutethimide 850
Aminoketon 558
Amiodarone 319
Amoxapine 557
Amylase 284
Anabolic steroids 308
Anabolic steroids 977
Anal cancer 878
Anastrozole, letrozole, and exemestane 850
Angiotensin II receptor blockers 591
Anorectal examination 869
Antagonists 574
Anthracyclines 850
Antibiotic stewardship 128
Antibiotics 345, 953
Anticoagulants 346
Anticoagulation 134, 752
Antidepressants 344, 533, 542, 545, 575
Anti-endotoxin therapy in sepsis 679
Antiepileptics 341
Antihypertensive agents 320
Antihypertensive treatment 377
Antimetabolites 882
Antipsychotics 533
Anti-serotoninergic drugs 574
Antituberculosis agents 341
Anxiety disorders 536
Arylpropionic acids 571
Ascites 281
Aspiration devices and distal embolic protection 434
Aspirin 591
Assertiveness 16
Assess the actual problem using soap format data 73
Associations of addison's disease 756
Associations of pheochromocytoma 776
Asthma 132, 141
At the early phase of sepsis 680
At the late phase of sepsis 681
Atrial flutter 436
Atrophic adenocarcinoma 853
Atypical features 738
Autoimmune adrenal failure 748

B

Bacillary dysentery (shigellosis) 656
Background diabetic retinopathy 921
Bacteremia (fungemia) 675
Bacterial infections 653
Balloon-like hepatocytes 303
Barium radiography 274
Basal steroid measurement 762
Beneficial actions of corticosteroids in sepsis 679
Benign prostatic hyperplasia (BPH) 356
Benzodiazepine anti anxiety agents 542
Benzodiazepines 546
Benzoyl peroxide 952
Beraprost 472

Beta blockers 320
Beta-lactam antibiotics (penicillins/cephalosporins) 345
Bevacizumab 851
Bilateral adrenalectomy 743
Biochemical diagnosis 781
Biogenic amine hypothesis 551
Blastomycosis 751
Body language 145
Bone and joint involvement 477
Bone-targeting agents in advanced prostate cancer 860
Bosentan trial of endothelin antagonist therapy (BREATHE-1) 469
Brachytherapy 880
Breast cancer 842
Bright light therapy 554
Bronchopulmonary 757
Building rapport 17
Bupropion 566
Buspirone therapy 544

C

Cabazitaxel 861
Cabozantinib 861
Calcium channel blockers 320, 467, 573
Caliciviruses 660
Campylobacteriosis 658
Cancer 482
Capecitabine, vinorelbine, or gemcitabine 850
Carbamazepine 534
Cardiac ascites 282
Cardiac causes 436
Cardiomyopathy 443
Cardiovascular 756
Cardiovascular disease 132
Care of drugs and drugs cabinets in wards 88
Carotid doppler studies 589
Case presentation 137
Catecholamine metabolites 781
Categorize quality of evidence 48
Causes of adrenal hemorrhage 753
Causes of ascites 281
Causes of atrial flutter 436
Causes of haemoptysis 483
Cerebellar hemangioblastoma 775
Chemotherapy 881
Chest radiograph 872
Chlorpromazine/phenothiazines 344
Cholelithiasis 778
Cholesterol 284
Chronic atrial flutter 437
Chronic daily headache (CDH) 584
Chronic pancreatitis 351
Chronic pancreatitis (CP) 348
Client education 29
Clinical assessment of degree of dehydration in children based on percentage of body weight loss 652
Clinical pharmacology of the cholinesterase inhibitors 532
Clinical presentation 352
Clinical presentation of acute hepatitis A 311
Clinical presentation of alzheimer's disease 529
Clonidine suppression test 784
Closing 16

Coagulation/fibrinolysis pathway 681
Collection of information 74
Colon cancer: surgical procedures 873
Colonography/virtual colonoscopy 871
Common medical conditions, substance use disorders, and medications associated with depressive symptoms 553
Common medical illnesses associated with anxiety symptoms 540
Communication 83
Communication with other healthcare professionals 159
Community pharmacists as gateway practitioners 129
Compensatory anti-inflammatory response syndrome 675
Complement blockade 681
Complications (Acute addisonian crisis) 767
Complications of pheochromocytoma 781
Computed tomography 871
Computerized tomography 785
Computerized tomography of the adrenals 764
Concept of microalbuminuria 372
Condition 675
Condoms 673
Consequences of the pharmacist as a skilled communicator 15
Consequences of the pharmacist as an unskilled communicator 16
Consistency between sites 130
Constitutional 755
Control of hyperlipidemia 377
Coronary plaque fissuring or rupture 430
Coronary stenting 434
Corticosteroids 308
Cotton wool spots 923
CR 547
CR, controlled 548
Creating the search strategy 38
Critique of drug therapy 138
Cushing's syndrome 733
Cyproterone acetate 754
Cystic fibrosis 475
Cysts 842
Cytokines 305
Cytotoxic antibiotics 882

D

Deep retinal haemorrhages 923
Define the clinical question 34
Definitions of terms related to sepsis 675
Degrees of severity of acne 951
Dermatological 756
Designer drugs 976
Detrimental actions of corticosteroids in sepsis 679
Develop a conclusion and recommendation 53
Development of therapeutic goals 73
Diabetes 141
Diabetes mellitus 135
Diabetic maculopathy 922
Diabetic retinopathy 918
Diabetic retinopathy risk factors 918
Diagnosis of alcoholic hepatitis 305
Diagnosis of BPH 366
Diagnostic criteria for obsessive compulsive disorder 597

Diagnostic tests for ascites 282
Dialysis in the treatment of diabetic patients with end-stage renal disease (ESRD) 380
Dietary recommendations in renal stone disease 387
Disclosing personal information 16
Disease 758
Disease management 126
Diuretics (pulmonary & systemic oedema) 467
DNA methylation 864
DNA-repair genes 862
Document in the client's chart 29
Donepezil 531
Donepezil, rivastigmine, and galantamine 531
Dosage of endothelin receptor antagonists used in pulmonary arterial hypertension 470
Double-contrast barium enema 870
Drug abuse 961
Drug addiction 961
Drug choices for anxiety disorders 541
Drug dependence 961
Drug dependence and drug abuse 961
Drug related problems 73
Drug therapy and follow-up of syphilis 665
Drug therapy of the patient 142
Drug-induced adrenocortical insufficiency 753
Drug-induced liver disease 318
Drugs associated with anxiety symptoms 540
Drugs used in the treatment of generalized social anxiety disorder 548
Drugs used in the treatment of panic disorder 547
Ductal adenocarcinoma 852
Duloxetine 558
Dyslipidaemia and DN 374
Dysphagia 289
Dysphagia treatment 291

E

Early manifestations 738
Ectopic ACTH syndrome 740
Education 129
Effects on other evidence-based 36
Elderly patients at increased risk 82
Electroconvulsive therapy (ECT) 553
Elevated blood pressure 590
Emergency surgery 874
Emotional health 13
Endoanal ultrasonography 871
Endocrine disorders 290
Endocrine factors 842
Endocrine neoplasia (Men) 774
Endocrine therapies used for metastatic breast cancer 849
Endocrine therapy 849
Endometrial carcinoma 852
Endoscopy 274
Endothelin receptor antagonists 468
Enterotoxigenic (choleralike) diarrhea 654
Enzalutamide 860
Epididymal cystadenoma 775
Epoprostenol (Flolan) 471
Ergotamine 572
Error types 85
Erythromycin (0.5%) or tetracycline 666
Escherichia coli 655

Esophageal manometry 274
Esophagitis 291
Ethanol 967
Etiological diagnosis of addison's disease 764
Etiological diagnosis of cushing's syndrome 739
Etiology of addison's disease 748
Etomidate 754
Evaluate literature 39
Evaluating the outcomes 76
Evaluation of patients with suspected drug-induced hepatotoxicity 318
Evaluation of pituitary hormones 766
Evaluation of therapeutic outcomes 351
Evidence-based medicine 33
Exclusion of other causes of liver damage 319
Expanding the role of pharmacy technicians 131
Explaining 16
Explaining and educating patients to improve concordance 157
Extent and pattern of abuse 963
Extent and pattern of abuse 965
External beam radiotherapy 880
Extraadrenal endocrine dysfunction in addison's disease 766
Exudates 922

F

Facial expression 147
Factors influencing alcoholinduced liver injury 304
Factors influencing pharmacist involvement in disease management 129
Faecal occult blood test 870
Fatigue 885
Feedback 156
Fibrinolysis versus direct PCI 432
Filtration of mediators 680
Fine needle aspiration cytology 843
Flexible sigmoidoscopy 870
Fluorescein angiographic evaluation 925
Fluorescein angiography 930
Follicular hyperkeratosis 949
Format of case presentation 137
Fulvestrant 850
Functional assessment of pulmonary arterial hypertension 468
Fungal diseases 750
Further treatment: chemotherapy and radiotherapy 879
Future strategies for the treatment of diabetic nephropathy 380

G

Galantamine 531
Gallstones and alcohol abuse 348
Gastroesophageal reflux disease (GERD) 272
Gaze or eye contact 147
General therapeutic principles 545
Generalized anxiety disorder 537, 540
Genetic factors 919
Genetics 304
Genital herpes 667
Genitourinary involvement 477
GI infections 651
Glomerulopathy 371
Glucagon provocative test 785

Glucocorticoid therapy 769
Glucose 284
Glycaemic control and DN 372
Goals and objectives of ward round 71
Gonadal 757
Gonorrhea 663
Goserelin, leuprolide, or triptorelin 850

H

H+/K+-atpase (acid proton pump) inhibitors 276
H_2-receptor antagonists 275
Haemoptysis in children 483
Haemorrhages 921
Hallucinogens 973
Hartmann's procedure 875
Hemodynamic support 683
Hemoptysis 482
Hemorrhagic stroke 588
Hepatic involvement 477
Hepatitis A 310
Hepatitis B 311
Hepatitis B immune globulin 315
Hepatitis C 315
Hepatitis C virus 305
Hepatotoxic drugs requiring chronic monitoring 340
Herbs that balance hormone levels 955
Herbs to combat infection and inflammation 956
Heteroarylacetic acids 571
High mobility group-l (HMG-l) 682
High-intensity focused ultrasound for prostate cancer 857
Histoplasmosis 750
History of pharmacists' involvement in patient care 127
History taking by clinical pharmacist 70
HMG-COA reductase inhibitors 344
Hormones 953
However 132
Hyperglycaemia 918
Hyperlipidemia 133
Hypertension 132, 918
Hypertrophic cardiomyopathy 443

I

Identifying problems 74
Idiopathic hemoptysis 483
Iloprost 472
Immediate management and stabilization 431
Impact of the pharmacist in managing specific diseases 131
Inattentiveness to patients 15
Incidence of alcoholic hepatitis 30 304
Incidence of diabetic retinopathy 918
Incorrect administration technique 86
Indole and indene acetic acids 571
Infection 478, 782, 675
Information sources 28
Inhaled bronchodilators 480
Inhibitors of inducible nitric oxide synthase (INOS) 680
Inotrope and vasoactive drug support 683
Interleukin-l receptor antagonists 679
Intermediate-lobe pathology 735
International headache society (IHS) 567
Interpersonal communication 144
Interviewing the person 28

Intestinal involvement 476
Intraoperative ultrasonography 872
Intraretinal microvascular abnormalities (IRMA) 923
Invasive (dysentery-like) diarrhea 656
Ipilimumab 860
Irinotecan 883
Iron deficiency anaemia 868
Ischaemic heart disease 430
Ischemic stroke 588
Isotretinoin 953
Isotretinoin and birth defects 955
Isotretinoin and psychiatric problems 954
Isotretinoin and serious health problems 954
Ivacaftor 480
Ixabepilone 851

K

Ketoconazole 753
Kidney cysts or tumors 775

L

Labelling and dispensing in patient prescriptions 87
Labelling and dispensing out patient prescriptions 87
Labelling and medication: general 86
Lactate dehydrogenase 284
Laparoscopic surgery 876
Lapatinib 851
Large volume paracentesis 287
Laryngoscopic examination 274
Left hemicolectomy 874
Legislative efforts 131
Levels of evidence—specific study design characteristics 49
Lipid-lowering agents 344
Liquid radioactive sources 880
Listening 16
Liver transplantation 309
Local excision 876
Locally advanced breast cancer (Stage III) 848
Logical reasoning 33
Loop diuretics 286
Lossa 652
Low doses of glucocorticoids 681
Lower esophageal sphincter (LES) pressure 279
Low-protein diet 377
Lung transplantation 480
Lymphoepithelioma-like carcinoma 853

M

Macrolides 345
Macronodular hyperplasia 739
Macrophage migration inhibitory factor (MIF) 681
Macroscopic appearance 775
Magnetic resonance imaging 843
Magnetic resonance imaging 871
Major depressive disease 551
Malignant ascites 282
Mammography 843
Management of the patient with advanced renal involvement 379
Management of the patient with mild to moderate renal involvement 378
Maprotiline 557
Maprotiline and amoxapine 556
Marijuana 971

Massive hemoptysis 485
Measurement of adrenal antibodies 765
Medication counseling tips 160
Medication errors and their prevention 85
Medication history taking tips 29
Medication related problems 140
Medication-related problems & proposed interventions 140
Medications used in the treatment of dysphagia 292
Medicine activities 36
Memantine 532
Mental health 13
Metastatic breast cancer (Stage IV) 849
Metastatic disease 751
Microaneurysms 921
Microbiological culture and gram stain 283
Microsatellite instability and dna-repair genes 863
Migraine 567
Migraine in children 568
Migraine variants 568
Mineralocorticoid replacement 770
Mirtazapine and progestins 747
Miscellaneous agents 882
Mitotic spindle inhibitors 882
Mixed serotonin-norepinephrine effects 558
Mobile/tethered/operable tumours 880
Monoamine oxidase inhibitors 558
Motility disorders 291
MRP's and PI's 140
Mucosal biopsy and cytology 274
Multiple 774
Multiple item checklists 40
Multiple questions 150
Multiple-organ dysfunction syndrome 675
Muscular disorders 290
Musculoskeletal 757

N

Neisseria gonorrhoeae 663
Nephropathy 919
Neurofibrillary tangles 528
Neuropathic disorders 290
Neuropharmacotherapy 744
New therapies in hormone relapsed disease 859
Newer treatments for hypertension 381
Next-generation antiandrogens 860
Nicotinamide 302, 347
Nicotine 966
Nicotinic acid 344
Nitrofurantoin 345
Nocturnal acid reflux 279
Non pharmacological treatment 553
Nonbenzodiazepine antianxiety agents for generalized anxiety disorder 541
Nonmassive hemoptysis 485
Non-pharmacological approaches 83
Nonspecific routine tests 761
Nonsteroidal anti-inflammatory drugs (NSAIDS) 342, 532, 569
Non-verbal communication 16, 145
Noradrenergic model 536
Nutritional factors 304

O

Obsessive–compulsive disorder (OCD) 596

Obsessive-compulsive symptom groups: clinical examples 599

Ocular factors 920

Omission error 85

Oncocytic adenocarcinoma 853

Oncogenes 862, 863

Opening 16

Opioids 963

Oral 651

Organizing the pertinent information 53

Organ-specific antibodies in polyglandular autoimmune syndrome 760

Oropharyngeal stage 289

Other 'potassium- sparing' diuretics 286

Other adverse effects of chronic abuse 966

Other ascitic fluid tests 284

Other medical therapies 309

Other questions to determine the effectiveness/compliance 29

Other therapies 571

Outcomes & endpoints 142

Outpatient assessment 869

Oxazepam and other benzodiazepines 534

Oxygen free radical scavengers 681

P

Palliation in colonic cancer 874

Palliative radiotherapy for advanced colorectal cancer 881

Pancreatic cysts & tumors 775

Pancreatic involvement 476

Panic disorder 537, 545

Panproctocolectomy 878

Pathogenesis of alcoholic hepatitis 303

Pathological assessment 843

Pathology 303

Pathophysiology 351

Pathophysiology of GERD 272

Patient access 129

Patient care planning 68

Patient counseling 144

Patient satisfaction and concordance are related 15

Patients who should always be counseled 161

Patients who should be counseled at certain intervals 161

Patients with BPH can present with a variety of signs and symptoms 366

Pegylated interferon comparison 317

Perineal prostatectomy 856

Periodic hormonogenesis 740

Persuading 16

Pharmaceutical care plan 68

Pharmacist interventions 141

Pharmacokinetic characteristics of triptans 578

Pharmacokinetics of benzodiazepine anti anxiety agents 543

Pharmacological actions on central nervous system 972

Pharmacological causes 290

Pharmacological management 444

Pharmacological therapy of hemorrhagic stroke 593

Pharmacological therapy of ischemic stroke 590
Pharmacological treatment of atrial flutter 439
Pharmacotherapy of cognitive symptoms 531
Pharmacotherapy of noncognitive symptoms 533
Phenelzine, tranylcypromine 556
Phenoxybenzamine 786
Pheochromocytoma 774
Phosphodiesterase-5 inhibitors 471
Photocoagulation 926
Physical health 13
Phytotherapy 368
Pico approach defined 35
Pituitary ablation 930
Pituitary radiation 743
Pituitary-dependent cushing's disease 739
Pituitary-dependent hypercortisolism 733
Plaened 1002
Plan development 74
Plasma catecholamines 783
Plasma lipids 919
Platelet glycoprotein llb/IIIa inhibitors (GP llb/IIIa) 433
Polyglandular deficiency syndromes 758
Polypharmacy 82
Polypharmacy and medication errors 82
Positron emission tomography 872
Possible treatment plans in cushing's syndrome based on etiology 745
Post traumatic stress disorder 538, 546
Postoperative radiotherapy 881
Postsynaptic changes in receptor sensitivity 551
Posture 147
Potassium citrate 386
Practitioner-patient interaction 14
Pravastatin and lovastatin 533
Precipitating factors for a paroxysm 778
Pregnancy 920
Pregnancy in the patient with diabetic nephropathy 381
Preoperative radiotherapy 880
Preproliferative diabetic retinopathy 922
Prescriptive role of clinical pharmacist 138
Presentation of genital herpes infections 668
Presentation of trichomonas infections 670
Prevention 82
Prevention of medication error 86
Prevention of STDS 673
Primary adrenal insufficiency 747
Primary hypothalamic etiology 734
Primary PAH 466
Primary pituitary disorder 735
Principles of surgery 873
Probing questions 149
Problem 33
Problem assessment 74
Problems based on non compartmental analysis 1066
Problems based on one compartment oral absorption 1059
Problems based on two compartment model iv bolus 1062
Procainamide 320
Prognostic features in alcoholic

hepatitis 306
Prolactin 767
Proliferative diabetic retinopathy 923
Promotility agents 276
Prompting questions 149
Prophylactic migraine therapies 578
Prophylactic treatment of migraine 572
Prophylaxis of HBV 313
Propionibacterium acnes 949
Prostanoids 471
Prostate cryoablation 858
Prostate-specific antigen 854
Protein kinase C (PKC) 381
Proximity and orientation 147
Pseudomembranous colitis (clostridium difficile) 655
Psychiatric 757
Psychiatric agents 344
Psychogenic dysphagia 290
Puberty 919
Pulmonary arterial hypertension - types & causes 466
Pulmonary arterial pressure 466
Pulmonary hypertension 466
Pulmonary involvement 477
Pulmonary venous hypertension 483
Putative syndrome pediatric autoimmune neuropsychiatric disorders associated with Streptococcal infection 598
Pygeum africanum 368

Q

Questioning 16
Questioning mnemonics 152
Questions to ask 28
Quinidine 320, 438

R

Radioimmunodetection 872
Radiology 870
Radiotherapy 879
Radiotherapy for locally advanced rectal cancer 881
Rarer causes of primary adrenal failure 754
Rationale for pharmacologic treatment 467
Reasonable outcomes 139
Reassurance strategies 17
Recklinghausen's neurofibromatosis 774
Recommendations for antibiotic therapy 653
Recommended hepatitis C virus treatment dosing 3174
Reconciliation and documentation 29
Rectal bleeding 868
Rectal cancer: first-line adjuvant treatment 876
Rectal cancer: surgical procedures 875
Reference to tradition 33
Regular medication review 82
Rehydration therapy 651
Rehydration therapy (ORT) 651
Relaxation training 583
Renal 757
Reperfusion therapy 432
Retinal hemangiomatosis 775
Retinopathy 381
Retrieve pertinent information 37
Rewarding effect 961

Rifampin 754
Right hemicolectomy 873
Risk factors for stone formation 383
Risk factors for stroke 588
Risks and side effects of acne treatments 954
Rivastigmine 531
Rotaviruses 659

S

Salicylates 342
Salicylic acid 952
Salmonellosis 657
Scientific method 33
Screening for polyglandular failure syndrome 766
Secondary adrenal insufficiency 747
Secondary PAH 466
Sedative–hypnotics 966
Selected syndromes associated with common sexually transmitted pathogens 662
Selective serotonin reuptake inhibitors 558
Sepsis 675
Septic shock 675
Serenoa repens 368
Serotonin 567
Serum ascites albumin gradient 283
Setting up of a data-base of the patient 73
Severe sepsis 675
Sexually transmitted diseases 661
Sigmoid colectomy 874
Sigmoidoscopy 869
Signs and symptoms of pharyngeal dysphagia 289
Simplify 83
Single contrast barium enema 870
Sinus involvement 475
Sipuleucel-T 860
Sitaxsentan to relieve impaired exercise trials (stride 1 and 2) 470
Soap analysis – pwdt 138
Social anxiety disorder 538, 546
Social health 13
Societal health 13
Soluble guanylate cyclase stimulator riociguat 473
Some common causes of ascites 282
Specific 443
Specific commonly used drugs that have hepatotoxicity 319
Specific search terms 36
Spiritual health 13
St. john's wort 556
Stages of alzheimer's disease 529
Stages of DN 372
Staphylococcus aureus and staphylococcus epidermidis 949
Stenting 874
Steps for managing polypharmacy 82
Stimulants 964
Stoma formation 878
Stone composition 383
Stroke 588
Sturge-weber syndrome, and carney's triad 774
Subarachnoid hemorrhage 590

Subtotal colectomy 877
Suggesting/advising 16
Summarized hospital course 138
Surgical causes 290
Surgical intervention 368
Sustained hypertension 780
Sweat glands 475
Symptom of gastroesophageal reflux and esophagitis 273
Synchronous tumours: surgical management 877
Synthetic hormones 345
Syphilis 663
Systemic causes 437
Systemic inflammatory response syndrome 675

T

Tacrine 531
Tamoxifen 850
Tamoxifen and raloxifene 851
Targeting androgen receptor signaling 859
Taxanes 850
Taxoids/taxanes 882
Tension-type headache 579
Tests for infectious disease 765
Tetracycline 345
The “classic” presentation 736
The 5-step evidence-based medicine 33
The acne scale 950
The APC gene 865
The DCC gene 866
The MCC gene 866
The metyrapone test 763
The multistep model for colorectal carcinogenesis 865
The need for good communication 13
The p53 gene 866
The pharmacist’s role 128
The pharmacist’s role in preventing antibiotic resistance 128
The rapid ACTH stimulation test 763
The RAS oncogene 867
The relationship of blood pressure to DN 373
The role of DA 551
The role of pharmacists in disease management 127
The role of the pharmacist in disease management 126
The selective serotonin reuptake inhibitors (SSRIS) 556
The therapeutic approach to the patient with diabetic nephropathy 374
The use of transplantation in the treatment of diabetic patients ESRD 380
The well-defined clinical question 35
Therapeutic endpoints 139
Thiazide diuretics 386
Three types of alternative treatments for acne 955
Thyrotropin-releasing hormone (TRH) 734
Time to treatment is paramount 432
Tips for defining the clinical question 37
TNM staging 844
Tolerance 961
Toll-like receptors 680
Topoisomerase I inhibitors 882
Toremifene 850

Total colectomy 877
Total mesorectal 875
Traditional colorectal surgery 877
trans rectal ultrasound (TRUS) 854
Transrectal ultrasoundguided biopsy 855
Transsphenoidal pituitary microsurgery 742
Trastuzumab 851
Trauma 752
Treatment 386, 437, 467
Treatment for acute intoxication 970
Treatment for alcoholism 971
Treatment of acid-base and electrolyte disorders 378
Treatment of acne scars 954
Treatment of cardiac complications 378
Treatment of comorbid conditions associated with diabetes mellitus and kidney involvement 381
Treatment of genital herpes 669
Treatment of opioid dependence 964
Treatment of tension-type headache 583
Treatment of trichomoniasis 671
Treatment of underlying cause 771
Treatment regimens for miscellaneous sexually transmitted diseases 672
Treatment to fit the type and severity of ACNE 950
Treprostinil 472
Trial and error 33
Triazolopyridines 558
Tricyclic antidepressants 556
Triptans 572
Tuberculosis 749
Tuberculous peritonitis 282
Tumor markers 284
Tumour suppressor genes 862, 863
Type I polyglandular autoimmune syndrome 759
Type II polyglandular autoimmune syndrome 759
Types of ACNE 950
Types of ward rounds 71

U

Ultrasonography 872
Ultrasonography and electroretinography 926
Ultrasound 843
Unauthorized drug error 85
Untreated pheochromocytoma 775
Unusual manifestations 780
Unusual manifestations of pheochromocytomas 781
Urinary catecholamines 782
Urinary stone disease 383
Urolithiasis 383
Urtica dioica 368
Using the internet as a resource 39

V

Vaccination 129
Vardenafil (Levitra) 471
Various steps in pharmaceutical care plan 73
Venlafaxine 557
Venous abnormalities 923
Ventricular rate 437
Verbal communication 145
Viral hepatitis 310

Vitamins and minerals 956
Vitrectomy and vitreolysis 929
VMA (vanillylmandelic acid) 782
Von hippel-lindau disease 774, 777
Von recklinghausen's disease 776
Von recklinghausen's neurofibromatosis 774

W

Ward rounds 70
Waterhouse-friderichsen syndrome 747, 752
Withdrawal (syn. abstinence) syndrome 961
Written communication 159
Wrong dose error 85
Wrong preparation of a dose 86
Wrong rate error 85, 86
Wrong route error 85
Wrong-time error 86

Y

Yersiniosis 659

www.ingramcontent.com/pod-product-compliance
Ingram Content Group UK Ltd.
Pitfield, Milton Keynes, MK11 3LW, UK
UKHW060019200726
13845UKWH00046B/89

9 789386 819635